COMMUNITY HEALTH NURSING

COMMUNITY HEALTH NURSING
Caring in Action

Janice E. Hitchcock, RN, DNSc

Professor and Associate Director
Department of Nursing
Sonoma State University
Rohnert Park, California

Phyllis E. Schubert, RN, DNSc, MA

Nurse Educator (Retired)
California State University System
Fresno and Rohnert Park, California
Nurse Therapist, Private Practice
Carmichael, California

Sue A. Thomas, RN, EdD

Professor
Department of Nursing
Sonoma State University
Rohnert Park, California

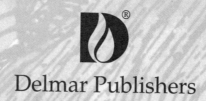

Delmar Publishers

an International Thomson Publishing company

Albany • Bonn • Boston • Cincinnati • Detroit • London • Madrid
Melbourne • Mexico City • New York • Pacific Grove • Paris • San Francisco
Singapore • Tokyo • Toronto • Washington

Cover Design: Scott Keidong
Cover Illustration: Sergio Sericolo

Delmar Staff:

Publisher: William Brottmiller
Acquisitions Editor: Cathy L. Esperti
Developmental Editor: Marah Bellegarde

Project Editor: Christopher Leonard
Production Coordinator: Sandra Woods
Art and Design Coordinator: Jay Purcell
Editorial Assistant: Darcy M. Scelsi

COPYRIGHT © 1999
Delmar is a division of Thomson Learning. The Thomson Learning logo is a registered trademark used herein under license.

Printed in the United States of America
2 3 4 5 6 7 8 9 10 XXX 04 03 02 01 00 99

For more information, contact Delmar, 3 Columbia Circle, PO Box 15015, Albany, NY 12212-0515; or find us on the World Wide Web at http://www.delmar.com

International Division List

Japan:
Thomson Learning
Palaceside Building 5F
1-1-1 Hitotsubashi, Chiyoda-ku
Tokyo 100 0003 Japan
Tel: 813 5218 6544
Fax: 813 5218 6551

Australia/New Zealand
Nelson/Thomson Learning
102 Dodds Street
South Melbourne, Victoria 3205
Australia
Tel: 61 39 685 4111
Fax: 61 39 685 4199

UK/Europe/Middle East:
Thomson Learning
Berkshire House
168-173 High Holborn
London
WC1V 7AA United Kingdom
Tel: 44 171 497 1422
Fax: 44 171 497 1426

Latin America:
Thomson Learning
Seneca, 53
Colonia Polanco
11560 Mexico D.F. Mexico
Tel: 525-281-2906
Fax: 525-281-2656

Canada:
Nelson/Thomson Learning
1120 Birchmount Road
Scarborough, Ontario
Canada M1K 5G4
Tel: 416-752-9100
Fax: 416-752-8102

Asia:
Thomson Learning
60 Albert Street, #15-01
Albert Complex
Singapore 189969
Tel: 65 336 6411
Fax: 65 336 7411

Library of Congress Cataloging-in-Publication Data

Hitchcock, Janice E.
    Community health nursing : caring in action / Janice E. Hitchcock, Phyllis E. Schubert, Sue A. Thomas.
        p. cm.
    Includes bibliographical references and index.
    ISBN 0-8273-6485-7
    1. Community health nursing. 2. Public health nursing. I. Schubert, Phyllis E. II. Thomas, Sue A. III. Title
    [DNLM: 1. Community Health Nursing. 2. Public Health Nursing.
    WY 106 H674c 1999]
    RT98.H58 1999
    610.73'43—dc21
    DNLM/DLC
    for Library of Congress   98-46716
                                                                CIP

DEDICATION

To the memory of my husband and to my family of origin. I continue to feel their sustenance and caring. To my friends, to whom my gratitude is beyond words for their unfailing support and love.

J. E. H.

To my family and friends with my love and appreciation for their encouragement and support.

P. E. S.

To my friends and colleagues, both in Australia and in the USA, whose continued support and encouragement throughout this project is highly appreciated.

To the memory of my parents and other family members who were committed to community development and participation as highly respected leaders in their communities—they truly cared.

S. A. T.

To nursing students past, present, and future. They continue to teach us and, we hope, in some measure, this book will repay them for all that they have given us.

CONTENTS

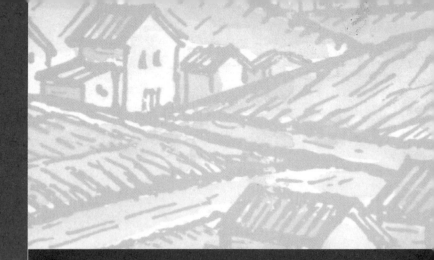

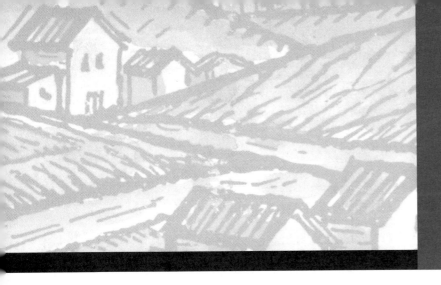

CONTRIBUTORS

David Becker, MSRN, CS, CNAA
Associate Professor
Massachusetts Bay Community College
Wellesley Hills, Massachusetts
   Chapter 23: Mental Health and Illness

Anne L. Biggins, RN, RM, Psych, BN, MPHC
Lecturer
School of Nursing
Faculty of Health Science
The Flinders University
Adelaide, South Australia, Australia
   Chapter 10: Population-Focused Practice

Patricia Biteman, RN, MSN
Lecturer
Humboldt State University
Arcata, California
   Chapter 28: Rural Health

Claire Budgen, RN, BSN, MSN, PhD
Professor
Okanagan University College
Kelowna, BC, Canada
Adjunct Professor
University of British Columbia
Vancouver, British Columbia, Canada
   *Chapter 13: Program Planning, Implementation,
   and Evaluation*

Peter I. Buerhaus, PhD, RN, FAAN
Director, Harvard Nursing Research Institute
Assistant Professor, Department of Health Policy and
Management
Harvard School of Public Health
Cambridge, Massachusetts
   Chapter 4: Health Care Economics

Doris Callaghan, RN, BScN, MSc
Professor
Okanagan University College
Kelowna, British Columbia, Canada
   Chapter 21: Chronic Illness

Gail Cameron, RN, BSN, MN
Professor
Okanagan University College
Kelowna, British Columbia, Canada
   *Chapter 13: Program Planning, Implementation, and
   Evaluation*

Nancy Kiernan Case, RN, PhD
Associate Dean
School for Health Care Professions
Director, Department of Nursing
Regis University
Denver, Colorado
   Chapter 5: Philosophical and Ethical Perspectives

Suzanne Chubinski, RN, BSN, MA
Case Manager Critical Care
Parkview Hospital
Fort Wayne, Indiana
   Chapter 26: Nutrition

Gregory L. Crow, RN, EdD
Professor of Nursing
Sonoma State University
Rohnert Park, California
   Chapter 4: Health Care Economics

Rebekah Jo Damazo, RN, MSN
Associate Professor
California State University—Chico
Chico, California
   Chapter 20: Communicable Diseases

**Jenny E. Donovan, RN, RM, MCHN, DipApp/Sci, BN,
MSc**
Lecturer in Nursing
The Flinders University
Adelaide, South Australia, Australia
   Chapter 10: Population-Focused Practice

Linda G. Dumas, RN, PhD
Associate Professor
College of Nursing
University of Massachusetts
Boston, Massachusetts
Chapter 25: Substance Abuse

Laurel Freed, RN, MN, PNP
Professor of Nursing
Sonoma State University
Rohnert Park, California
Chapter 31: Power, Politics, and Public Policy

Susan S. Gardner, RN, ANP, MS
Assistant Professor of Nursing
Department of Nursing, Baccalaureate Nursing Outreach
Program
Weber State University
Ogden, Utah
Chapter 14: The Varied Roles of Community Health Nursing

Nancy Gilien, MPH, RN, BSN
Nursing Consultant, Private Practice
Napa, California
Chapter 22: Developmental Disabilities

Barouk Golden, MS, RN
Public Health Nurse Case Manager
Department of Public Health, California Children's
Service
San Francisco, California
Clinical Faculty
Mental Health, Community and Administrative Nursing
University of California—San Francisco
San Francisco, California
Chapter 23: Mental Health and Illness

Mary Beatrice Hennessey, RN, MSN
Instructor
College of Nursing
University of Massachusetts
Boston, Massachusetts
Chapter 25: Substance Abuse
Chapter 27: Homelessness

Joan Heron, RN, PhD
Professor of Nursing (Retired)
California State University, Fresno
Fresno, California
Chapter 9: Health-Promotion and Disease-Prevention Perspectives
Chapter 18: Frameworks for Assessing Families

Gail P. Howe, MA
Marriage, Family, Child Counselor
Kelseyville, California
Chapter 26: Nutrition

Margaret H. Kearney, PhD, RN-C
Associate Professor
Boston College
School of Nursing
Chestnut Hill, Massachusetts
Chapter 20: Communicable Disease

Harriett J. Lionberger, DNSc, RN
Nursing Consultant
Napa, California
Chapter 6: Cultural and Spiritual Perspectives
Chapter 7: Environmental Perspectives
Chapter 8: Caring Communication and Teaching/Learning

Carol A. Lockhart, PhD, RN, FAAN
President
C. Lockhart Associates
Tempe, Arizona
Chapter 3: Health Care Delivery in the United States

Judy J. Miller, BSN, MSN
Nursing Consultant in Gerontology/Long Term Care
San Luis Obispo, California
Chapter 17: Care of Young, Middle, and Older Adults

Lindsey K. Phillips, RN, MS
Quality Assurance/Utilization Review Systems Consultant
Huckleberry Youth Programs
San Francisco, California
Chapter 11: Epidemiology

Michelle Porter, RN, MSN, FNP
Family Nurse Practitioner
Sutter Medical Group of The Redwoods
Santa Rosa, California
Chapter 24: Family and Community Violence

Relda J. Robertson-Beckley, PhD
Assistant Professor
San Francisco State University
San Francisco, California
Executive Director
Nurses in Action
Oakland, California
Chapter 16: Care of Infants, Children, and Adolescents

Ruth Roth, MS, RD
Clinical Dietician
Parkview Hospital
Fort Wayne, Indiana
Chapter 26: Nutrition

Mary Jo Starsiak, MSN, RN
Contra Costa Community College District
Martinez, California
Chapter 9: Health-Promotion and Disease-Prevention Perspectives

Andrea Wass, RN, BA, Mhlth Sc, DRM, MRCNA
Lecturer, School of Health
University of New England
Armidale, New South Wales, Australia
Chapter 12: Assessing the Community

Susanne F. Wilkey, RN, MS
Former Assistant Professor of Nursing
Department of Nursing, Baccalaureate Nursing Outreach Program
Weber State University
Ogden, Utah
Chapter 14: The Varied Roles of Community Health Nursing

Eileen M. Willis, RN, BEd, MEd
Senior Lecturer
School of Nursing
Faculty of Health Science
The Flinders University
Adelaide, South Australia, Australia
Chapter 10: Population-Focused Practice

Marshelle Thobaben, RN-C, MS, APNP, FNP, PHN
Professor of Nursing
Humboldt State University
Arcata, California
Chapter 28: Rural Health

Janice A. Young, RN, MS
Tuberculosis Nurse Consultant
California Department of Health Services
TB Control Branch
Berkeley, California
Chapter 11: Epidemiology

REVIEWERS

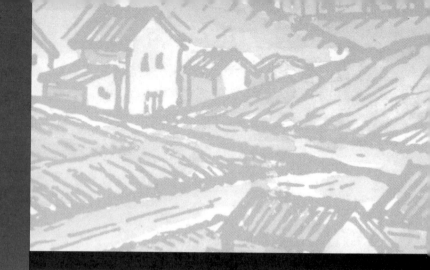

Marie H. Ahrens, RN
University of Tulsa
Tulsa, Oklahoma

Dodi Alexander, MN, ARNP
University of Florida
Gainesville, Florida

Margaret M. Anderson, EdD, RN-C, CNAA
Northern Kentucky University
Highland Heights, Kentucky

Linda C. Baumann, PhD
University of Wisconsin—Madison
Madison, Wisconsin

Henrietta Bernal, PhD
University of Connecticut
Storrs, Connecticut

Judy Hayes Bernhardt, RN, MPH, PhD
East Carolina University
Greenville, North Carolina

Rose Marie Bolton, BS, MS
Redlands Community College
El Reno, Oklahoma

Emily O. Bond, PhD
Southeastern Louisiana University
Hammond, Louisiana

Sharon Burt, MSN
San Diego State University
San Diego, California

Susan E. Closson, MSN, RNCS
Valdosta State University
Valdosta, Georgia

Catherine Cover, MS
University of South Carolina
Columbia, South Carolina

Julie Dewitt
Andrews University
Barren Springs, Michigan

Elizabeth O. Dietz, EdD, RN, CS
San Jose State University
Sunnyvale, California

Lois Ellis, CRNA, EdD
Retired
Indiana Wesleyan University
Marion, Indiana

Carmel A. Esposito, BSN, MSN, PhD
Trinity Health System School of Nursing
Steubenville, Ohio

Dorcas C. Fitzgerald, MSN, RN
Youngstown State University
Youngstown, Ohio

Susan Gaskins, BSN, MPH, DSN
University of Alabama
Tuscaloosa, Alabama

June Helburg, EdD, RN
The University of Rochester
Rochester, New York

Patricia M. Huber, MSN
University of Kansas Medical Center
Kansas City, Kansas

Ruth Knollmueller, PhD
University of Kentucky
Lexington, Kentucky

Piper J. Larson
Wisconsin Indianhead Technical College
Superior, Wisconsin

Nancy Rudner, DrPh, RN
University of North Carolina—Charlotte
Charlotte, North Carolina

PREFACE

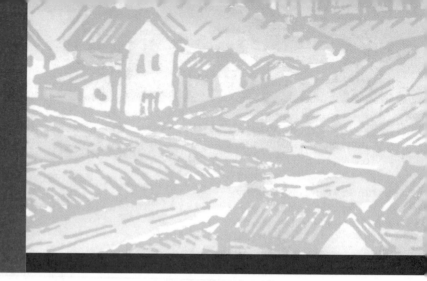

Community Health Nursing: Caring in Action is a comprehensive text designed for nursing students and practicing nurses to provide a foundation in community health nursing practice. This exciting new text prepares nurses to take advantage of the opportunities and challenges present when working in the community and the everchanging health care system.

Throughout history, community health nurses have been an integral part of health promotion and disease prevention activities as well as health care reform. With the evolving health care system and challenges that clients face in the community, the importance and necessity of community health nurses continues. There is growing awareness of the importance of strategies to promote health and prevent disease at global and national levels. More and more, there is an increasing need for nurses to care for clients in the community and provide them with services designed to promote, protect, and preserve their health. The importance of addressing aggregate needs through program planning in partnership with the community has emerged as a major strategy to improve the health of the community. With the increased complexity of health care, client advocacy is imperative.

With these issues and countless others encountered in today's world, the goals of this text are to provide a broad-based perspective of the many dimensions of community health and community health nursing.

CONCEPTUAL FRAMEWORKS

Community Health Nursing: Caring in Action was written and designed with the reader in mind. The text builds on knowledge and skills common to all nurses, including nursing process, nursing theory, communication process, human development, and nursing care of individuals. It provides opportunities for the reader to critically apply the knowledge presented and to learn how to seek answers to questions that arise. The conceptual approach to this text is based on the following:

- *International perspectives* are interwoven as nursing is challenged to meet the health care needs of people, both nationally and internationally. It is no longer possible in today's world to look only at regional health concerns. A sense of global connectedness is necessary. The text includes contributors from Canada and Australia, countries with well recognized public and community health systems, to enhance an international perspective.
- *Caring frameworks* are used as a basis for practice. We believe that nursing and nursing education must focus on building caring environments to promote health and healing. Caring requires a partnership between students and faculty and with clients as well as other health care professionals. It requires respect for the student's ability to think and practice and respect for the client's right to make health decisions coupled with their capacity to make appropriate decisions when given adequate health related information.
- *Community and family concepts* are stressed throughout to prepare the student to work in the community with the family as a unit, not just with individuals within the family. Population-focused practice as well as multidimensional family dynamics and family aspects are emphasized throughout the text.
- *Alternative/complementary health practices* including healing modalities, energetic healing, visualization, and imagery are incorporated. The concept of mutual connectedness provides a framework for examining the nature of healing processes and outcomes.
- *Healthy People 2000 objectives* are discussed throughout the text.

ORGANIZATION

Unit I introduces the student to the practice of community health nursing as a population-focused specialty, with a presentation of caring as central to practice and an overview of caring models. The historical perspective is discussed with an emphasis on health and healing.

Unit II highlights the many dimensions of the current

health care system including transformations and economic issues related to the health care system.

Unit III provides the foundations of community health nursing. Philosophical, ethical, cultural, spiritual, and environmental perspectives are explored as well as the many dimensions of caring communication, defined as teaching/learning and counseling/communication. Issues in health promotion and disease prevention are explored.

Unit IV focuses on caring for populations with an emphasis on the application of the nursing process at the community level. Aggregate populations are examined along with an exploration of population-focused practice and epidemiology as a public health science. Community assessment, program planning, implementation, and evaluation are discussed in detail. The roles of the community health nurse take many forms and these roles are examined and explained as well.

Unit V emphasizes caring for individuals and families in the community. Community health nurses work with families in their homes, schools, and other settings. The many aspects of the home visit are delineated and discussed. The growth and development of individuals from infancy through old age are examined. Because nurses work with individuals in all phases of the life cycle, they are expected to understand what is considered normal and recognize deviations from this pattern. Risk factors at each stage of development are emphasized. The multidimensional nature of families is explored through a discussion of frameworks for assessing families and family environments and an exploration of family functioning. The relationship of these matters to the health of the family is explored.

Unit VI deals with issues regarding the care of vulnerable populations, that is, those populations that are at high risk for health problems. Problems such as communicable disease, chronic illness, developmental disabilities, mental health problems, family and community violence, substance abuse, nutritional problems, homelessness, and rural health issues are discussed. These are all major health problems that the community health nurse deals with on a regular basis. Communicable disease, chronic disease and illness, and developmental disabilities have long been the focus of community health nursing. Mental health, substance abuse, family violence, and homelessness are community health problems that the community health nurse must also address because of the magnitude in the community. Nutrition is a core element in health, yet nutritional problems have often been inadequately identified by nurses who can be overwhelmed by the client's more acute health concerns. Rural health needs continue to challenge the resources of community health nurses.

Unit VII addresses issues of health care delivery worldwide. National and international health perspectives are discussed. Global health care delivery issues are explored.

Also addressed in this unit are public policy issues and the related concerns of power and politics in health care and health care delivery systems. It is imperative in today's and tomorrow's world of health care that all nurses understand and participate at these levels.

The final chapter, Chapter 32, provides a vision for community health nursing practice to consider. We have addressed the present needs of community health nursing and at the same time, envisioned the future of community health and the nurse's role within it.

SPECIAL FEATURES

There are numerous special features in *Community Health Nursing: Caring in Action* designed to stimulate critical thinking and self-exploration, and to encourage readers to synthesize and apply critical knowledge presented in the text:

Reflective Thinking boxes encourage readers to examine their own personal views on given topics in order to identify their own thoughts and feelings, and to understand the varying viewpoints they may encounter in clients and coworkers. These boxes are designed to encourage reflection on an issue from a personal context, to raise awareness, and to stimulate critical thinking and active problem solving.

Decision Making boxes encourage the reader to develop sensitivity to ethical and moral issues and guide the reader to think critically in community health nursing practice and be active in problem solving.

Research Focus features outline findings from current research and offer discussions of their impact on nursing practice.

Perspectives offer community health insights from the perspective of nursing students, faculty, practicing nurses, and clients. This true-life feature allows the reader to see the types of issues, experiences, and people encountered while practicing in the community.

Community Nursing View features real-world scenarios to help the reader make the connection between theory and practice more easily. This feature offers critical thinking questions that allow the reader to assess and act within the nursing environment while reinforcing knowledge of the nursing process in assessing, diagnosing, identifying outcomes, planning care, performing interventions, and evaluating the outcomes of the care.

EXTENSIVE TEACHING AND LEARNING PACKAGE

Classroom Manager

This comprehensive, resource-packed CD-ROM includes:

Conversion Grids

- **Conversion Grids** are provided for the major published community health texts to make your transition to Hitchcock, Schubert, Thomas/*Community Health Nursing: Caring in Action* smooth.

Instructor's Manual

- **Key terms and definitions** are listed by chapter to create a comprehensive glossary.
- **Instructional strategies** center on the competencies presented in each chapter and include 3 to 5 questions for the instructors to pose to students to pique their interest. These strategies also include possible answers.
- **Case Study/Theory Application** feature includes community health scenarios that allow the student to apply theory and offer the instructors helpful hints to stimulate discussion, individual exercises, group exercises, and Internet activities to reinforce the theory application.
- **Suggested answers** to the decision-making type questions presented in the Community Nursing View feature of the text.

Computerized Testbank

- Electronic testbank in IBM format includes 800 NCLEX-style questions.
- Electronic gradebook automatically calculates grades, tracks student performance, prints student progress reports, organizes assignments, and more to simplify administrative tasks.
- On-line testing feature of the computerized test bank allows exams to be administered on-line via a school network or stand-alone PC.

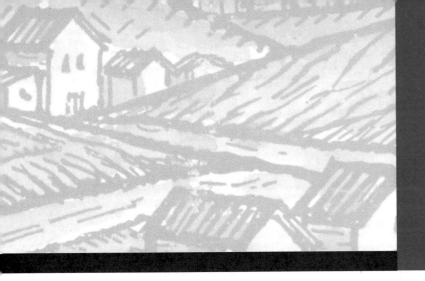

ACKNOWLEDGMENTS

The authors wish to acknowledge the many people who have been a part of the creation of this textbook. Those who have contributed chapters have worked unstintingly to share their expert knowledge in exceptionally well written manuscripts. Their endeavors reflect a vision of the future of nursing and an enthusiasm and pride in the profession.

Students and colleagues have greatly enriched the book through generous contributions of their own clinical and personal experiences. These offerings have significantly helped to make the chapters come alive and give life to the theories and concepts presented in the text. The nursing faculty at Sonoma State University have been very understanding of our sometimes harassed states and enthusiasm about our project. They have always been available to help whenever we have needed it.

Many thanks and deep appreciation to Dr. Harriett Lionberger, who edited several chapters that needed significant revisions, illuminating the essential meaning of the chapters. We want to thank Gini Longhitano who, out of friendship, answered a multitude of phone calls and conveyed many messages, often unintelligible to her, when we were not available. We would also like to thank Dr. Barbara Place from Melbourne, Australia, Fellow of the Royal College of Nursing, Australia, for her ongoing support of our efforts to increase the international focus in this text. She was consistently available to share her valuable ideas in a variety of ways.

The staff at Delmar have been consistently encouraging and supportive when, at many points, we were not sure we could complete the daunting tasks of developing a textbook. They always came through with ideas and resources when they were needed. We would like to particularly thank Holly Skodal Wilson who introduced us to the idea of sharing our thoughts about community health nursing with a larger audience. Beth Williams, editor, helped launch us on our way. Beth's direction was consistently helpful.

Cathy Esperti, editor, and Marah Bellegarde, developmental editor, have taken us to the completion of this project, and have dealt with the many issues and concerns that arise as work comes to a close with graciousness and patience. Darcy Scelsi, Sandy Woods, Jay Purcell, Christopher Leonard, and Gail Farrar have been invaluable. They were always happy to answer our many questions and were quick to return phone calls and e-mails, something that we valued highly.

We especially want to thank all our reviewers, whose comments were invariably helpful and who often enlightened us with different perspectives which added considerably to the final outcome of the text.

Finally, we apologize if we have missed anyone. It was not intentional. We have valued everyone who has contributed to this project in any way. Without you, we would never have made it.

ABOUT THE AUTHORS

Janice E. Hitchcock received her diploma in nursing from New England Deaconess Hospital, Boston, Massachusetts. She obtained her Baccalaureate degree from Simmons College, Boston, Massachusetts, her Master's degree in psychiatric-mental health nursing/community health nursing, and her Doctorate in Nursing Science from the University of California, San Francisco. Dr. Hitchcock is a licensed Marriage, Family and Child Counselor (MFCC) and, while continuing to teach, she also maintained a private practice in individual, couple, and family therapy for 15 years. She is currently a Professor and Associate Director in the Department of Nursing at Sonoma State University, Rohnert Park, California.

Dr. Hitchcock has worked in and taught psychiatric-mental health nursing and community health nursing for nearly four decades. She also teaches communication theory, human sexuality, and family theory. She was a founding faculty member of the Second Step nursing program at Sonoma State University in 1972. This program was the first of its kind to be accredited by the National League for Nursing. More recently, she helped to initiate a basic Baccalaureate program at the same University.

Since the early 1980s she has taught a general education course in human sexuality that is well received by students from all disciplines. She has a special interest in gay health care and has worked with Master's degree students in the nursing department and throughout the country who have replicated her doctoral research in which she developed a basic social process called "Personal Risking." This process evolved from a grounded theory analysis of interviews with lesbians in the San Francisco Bay Area regarding their decision-making process of self-disclosure of their sexual orientation to health providers.

Dr. Hitchcock has a number of publications to her credit and is a member of several professional organizations, including the American Nurses Association, American Public Health Association, American Association of Sex Educators, Counselors, and Therapists, American Association of Marriage and Family Therapists, and the Society for the Scientific Study of Sex.

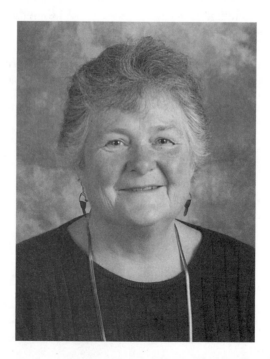

Phyllis E. Schubert received her basic nursing education in a diploma program at Los Angeles County General Hospital in California. She earned a Baccalaureate degree in nursing, a Master's degree in community health nursing with a school nursing focus, and a second Master's degree in counseling from California State University, Fresno. She earned a Doctor of Nursing Science degree in community health nursing with a focus in holistic nursing practice from the University of California, San Francisco.

Dr. Schubert's career in nursing has spanned the field of nursing and has included medical-surgical nursing, long-term care, school nursing in elementary and secondary schools in programs for migrant and learning disabled children, and in-patient psychiatric evaluation and care of children. She has served on nursing faculties while teaching community health nursing, nursing theory, communication skills, and holistic nursing approaches at California State University, Fresno, and Sonoma State University in Rohnert Park, California. Since retiring from the California State University System, she co-founded Nursing Therapeutics Institute in Cotati, California, an organization dedicated to the practice, education, and research of holistic nursing therapies and approaches; she has also provided health promotion and healing therapies for clients in private holistic nursing practice settings.

She has been practicing and teaching Therapeutic Touch (TT) for over 20 years, and is recognized as a qualified teacher of TT by the Nurse Healers—Professional Associates, Inc. and is thus a member of the Therapeutic Touch Teachers Cooperative. She is certified by Jin Shin Jyutsu, Inc. of Scottsdale, AZ to practice Jin Shin Jyutsu® (JSJ) and to teach JSJ self-help classes; and is certified by the Academy for Guided Imagery of Mill Valley, CA to practice Interactive Guided Imagery. She currently holds membership in the American Nurses Association/California, the Society for Rogerian Scholars, Nurse Healers—Professional Associates, Inc., the International Association of Interactive Imagery[SM], and the National Health Ministries Association. She is especially interested in the area of spiritual health, the role of the parish nurse, and developments within the field of parish nursing.

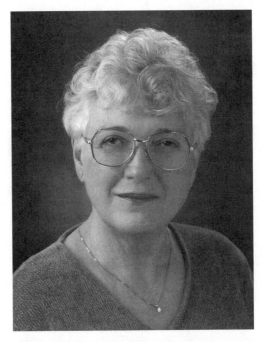

Sue A. Thomas received her Baccalaureate degree in nursing at University of California, San Francisco, attending both University of California, Berkeley and University of California, San Francisco. Her Master's degree in community health nursing, with a focus on administration and supervision, was obtained from Boston University School of Nursing. A Doctor of Education in Organization and Leadership was received from the University of San Francisco.

Dr. Thomas' professional career in nursing has included a variety of experiences both in the USA and in Australia. Her clinical practice in San Francisco included a variety of areas: medical-surgical nursing, public health nursing in San Francisco's multicultural communities, school nursing within the context of public health nursing, and supervision of staff in public health nursing. She is a professor of nursing who has been responsible for coordinating the community health nursing program at Sonoma State University in California, teaching both community health nursing theory and clinical courses. She has also taught graduate courses in leadership and management as well as graduate and undergraduate research, and has recently served as Graduate Coordinator. Prior to teaching at Sonoma State University, Dr. Thomas taught community health nursing theory and practice at San Francisco State University.

One of Dr. Thomas' major interests is international health and international nursing. She has also taught in Australia, primarily in the Melbourne area, at La Trobe University School of Nursing. She was a Visiting Fellow at the Royal Melbourne Institute of Technology School of Nursing (formerly Phillip Institute of Technology) in Melbourne. In addition, she served as nursing consultant in a variety of capacities, one of which was Curriculum Consultant at Deakin University (formerly Victoria College). In addition to teaching and consulting in Australia, Dr. Thomas was the International Coordinator of the 1992 International Caring Conference held in Melbourne, Australia—co-sponsored by the International Association for Human Caring and the Royal College of Nursing Australia, with nurses from 14 countries represented. She was one of the charter members of the International Association for Human Caring, having served for a number of years in the 1990s on the Board and as a Board Officer. Dr. Thomas is currently a member of the Editorial Review Board for the *International Journal for Human Caring*.

In addition, Dr. Thomas has participated as a co-investigator in a collaborative research team since the early 1990s, most recently having completed a cross-national study focused on care delivery patterns. Three earlier studies were published in refereed journals. The cross national study was presented at the Sigma Theta Tau, Int. International Research Congress in Utrecht Netherlands, July 1998.

Dr. Thomas is also especially interested in the delivery of care to vulnerable populations, the emerging field of parish nursing, and the study of caring worldwide. She currently serves on the Advisory Council for a Nursing Center designed to meet the needs of the homeless and near homeless in an Interfaith Council Agency in the NorthBay region in California. Dr. Thomas is currently a member of the American Public Health Association, Sigma Theta Tau, Int., the International Association for Human Caring, and the American Nurses Association/California.

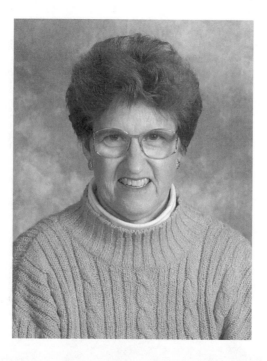

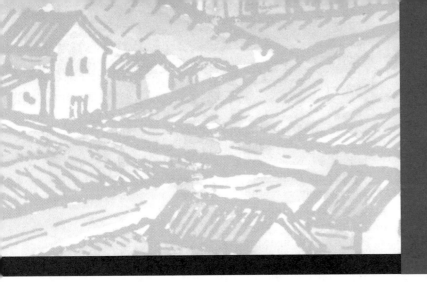

BOXED FEATURES

Decision Making

Research Focus

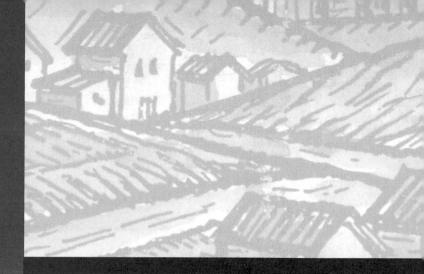

LIST OF SELECTED FIGURES

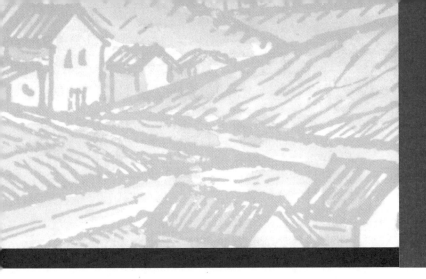

LIST OF SELECTED TABLES

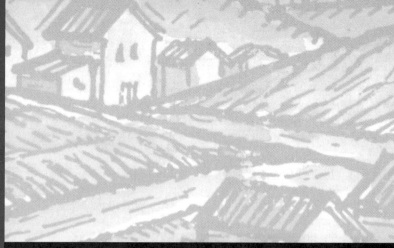

HOW TO USE THIS TEXT

▲ COMMUNITY NURSING VIEW

Featuring real-world scenarios, the Community Nursing View will help you make the connection between theory and practice more easily. Decision making type questions allow you to assess and act within the nursing environment while reinforcing your knowledge of the nursing process of assessing, diagnosing, identifying outcomes, planning care, performing interventions, and evaluating the success of your care. Read the background story and answer the questions. Share your answers with your classmates and discuss the responses.

◄ DECISION MAKING

This feature allows you to assess and act within the community nursing environment by offering the opportunity for you to think critically and problem solve as well as allowing you to develop sensitivity to ethical and moral issues. You may choose to read through each one and explore the situation before reading the chapter. Then as you read through the chapter, readdress each Decision Making and reevaluate your original thoughts. If you choose to read them as you go through the chapter, perhaps write your thoughts down, then go back and look at them at a later date.

RESEARCH 🔍 FOCUS

Factors Influencing Exposure of Children to Major Hazards on Family Farms

STUDY PROBLEM/PURPOSE

The purpose of this descriptive study was to understand factors that influence parents' decisions to expose children to major hazards on family farms.

METHODS

The study involved a two-phase descriptive study that was based on planned change and using mail survey research methods. A representative sample of 1,255 Wisconsin dairy farmers was drawn from a stratified random sample of 6,000 dairy farmers. Eighty-nine percent of these farmers agreed to participate in the study. They provided data about factors that influence their decision to expose children younger than 14 years to driving a tractor with more than 20 horsepower; being a second rider on a tractor without a cab that is driven by the father; and being within 5 feet of the hind legs of a dairy cow. Fathers' behavioral intentions to expose their children to these major farm hazards and factors influencing those intentions were measured.

FINDINGS

Multivariate analyses revealed that attitudes, subjective norms, and perceived control accounted for up to three-fourths of the variance in fathers' behavioral intentions. On a seven-point scale from very likely to very unlikely, they were quite likely to allow children 10 to 14 years old to drive a tractor and less likely to allow a child to be near a dairy cow or to be an extra rider on a tractor without a cab. For all three high-risk behaviors, multivariate analyses revealed that it was the father's attitude toward the behavior that accounted for his allowing a child to engage in it. The child's grandparents and mothers exerted a little influence, and health care providers exerted only modest influences on fathers' feelings of social pressure.

IMPLICATIONS

A comprehensive approach to childhood agricultural injury prevention is needed. Strategies that may influence farmers in allowing their children to be exposed to major hazards on farms include individual counseling, educational resources, group activities, and community-based initiatives.

SOURCE

From "Factors Influencing Exposure of Children to Major Hazards on Family Farms" by B. C. Lee, L. S. Jenkins, J. D. Westaby, 1997, Journal of Rural Health, 13(3), pp. 206–215.

◀ **RESEARCH FOCUS**

The Research Focus emphasizes the importance of research in nursing by linking theory to practice. A useful learning tool, these boxes focus attention on current issues and trends in nursing.

🌀 REFLECTIVE THINKING 🌀

Perception of Mental Retardation

The parents and siblings of a child being provided dietary treatment for a metabolic disorder underwent psychological testing as part of the evaluation of treatment outcomes. The mother's IQ scores placed her in the moderate to mild range of mental retardation.

The young woman was beautiful, wore stylish and expensive clothes, and was well groomed. Her manner was sweetly dignified. She asked questions that encouraged the other person to talk at length while she listened attentively.

Her husband, a prominent professional man, explained that his wife's family had accepted her condition and had provided every advantage. She went to private school with no suggestion of "special" classes. She took art classes at the local community college so she could be perceived as having gone to college. Her family carefully trained her in social skills and household care.

She was unable to plan and shop for an elaborate meal or manage her child's special diet, but she had a housekeeper to assist her. She could not chair a committee meeting, but she presided well at their dinner parties.

Her husband esteemed her for what she was: a loving wife, mother, and graceful companion. Their common interests were their children, extended families, social life, and travel. Her husband helped her to avoid situations she could not handle.

• Should this woman be considered mentally retarded? Consider her ability to meet social and cultural expectations. Consider her support system.

• How might your perception of her be influenced by applying to her the system of definition and classification of the American Psychiatric Association? Of the American Association on Mental Retardation?

▲ **REFLECTIVE THINKING**

These boxes deal with self-reflection and opinions on various ethical and social issues. It may be useful to keep a journal in which you write down your immediate response to each box on a chapter to chapter basis. At the end of each chapter, review your journal entries and ask yourself how your values will affect your nursing care

Perspectives...

Insights of a Public Health Nurse

I work as a public health nurse for a large county health department serving poor children and their families. One of the most important things I do is serve as an advocate. Advocacy has become even more important recently because families do not know how or are not able to navigate the health care system and need someone who can help with the managed care process. Because there are so many problems in the changing system, families often need an advocate to help them get needed services. Agents of vendoring services often do not tell clients about available services, and the nurse has to seek out the information for families.

Being an advocate for my clients is so very important. A non-English-speaking family was referred to me because the physician wanted to remove an 8-year-old daughter from the family home. The girl had cystic fibrosis, and failure to thrive had been an issue. The physician was accusing the parents of not giving the child her nighttime feedings containing medication and nutrition. The social worker from Child Protective Services and I made a home visit and found everything in place for the feedings. The mother showed me her equipment and supplies, demonstrated how she gave the feedings, and showed me the records. There was no problem, and the child seemed to be doing very well.

I made an appointment with the mother and child and went with them to see the physician. Everything checked out fine, and the child had gained weight. A resident physician who spoke Spanish saw the child and was very kind to the mother. But the primary physician came into the room after the resident physician had left and continued to insist that the child was not being fed and must be removed from the home. The mother cried all the way home, and I could not comfort her very well because I do not speak Spanish.

I checked out the medical records and talked with people to put the story together. A note posted to the medical record by a physician indicated that the child needed night feeds but that the physician assumed the vendoring agency would not approve because of the cost. As a result, the night feeds had not even been requested! The child had eventually been hospitalized due to weight loss but gained back the weight while in the hospital. Because the child had gained weight during the hospital stay, the physician assumed the child was not getting the night feeds because of negligence on the part of the mother. After the confusion had been cleared up, the physician decided against removing the child from her home, and she is doing well. I am really glad we were there for her and for her family. The language barrier makes things even harder.

I see a lot of children in foster homes who are really suffering. These children *really* need advocates. Because the licensing agencies are not allowed to make unannounced visits to these homes, I have to be their ears and eyes when I make home visits. Probably about half of the foster parents care about the children and are doing a good job. But the other half do not care at all and are just doing foster care for the money: The kids are a commodity. They were probably better off with their biological parents. We need an organization of health care workers just to be advocates for the foster kids in this county.

—*Paula, RN, PHN*

◀ **PERSPECTIVES**

These boxes provide real-life, sensitive stories about community health nursing through the eyes of the student, faculty, nurse, and client. They are here to help you get a more personalized look at nursing in the community and help you to develop a sensitivity to the needs, fears, and issues you will face in community health practice. It may be helpful for you to keep a running journal of your own experiences in the field—did a certain family affect you in some way, did you work with an experienced community health nurse who was a wonderful mentor, or did you help research a community health issue and what was that experience like?

Nursing and Caring in the Community

This unit introduces the student to the practice and history of community health nursing and the importance of the concepts of caring, collaboration and partnership as they pertain to nursing, specifically community health nursing.

UNIT I

Caring in Community Health Nursing

Sue A. Thomas, RN, EdD

Caring is the foundation stone of respect for human dignity and worth upon which everything else should be built . . . . When all else fails, as it eventually must in the lives of all of us, a society that gives a priority to caring . . . is worthy of praise.

—Callahan, 1990, p. 149

COMPETENCIES

Upon completion of this chapter, the reader should be able to:

- Identify the major goal of community health nursing practice.
- Discuss the definitions of community health and public health nursing.
- Describe the focus of community health nursing practice.
- Discuss caring as the context for nursing practice.
- Describe the concept of caring in specific relation to community health nursing.
- Discuss the meaning of caring in nursing.
- Consider the importance of establishing caring partnerships with individuals, families, and groups.
- Define *health, health promotion, health protection, healing,* and *disease prevention.*
- Define public health and its focus.

Community health nurses have a rich tradition of providing care to individuals, families, and communities. They are committed to social justice, health promotion, health protection, disease prevention, and the facilitation of healing. The major goal of community health nursing is the preservation and improvement of the health of populations and communities worldwide. In order to accomplish this goal, community health nurses practice in the neighborhoods and homes of individuals and families in the United States as well as in other nations. Community health nurses are keenly aware of the special application of human caring to their practice.

Community health nurses are leaders in improving the quality of health care for individuals, families, and communities. They have the knowledge and skills to work in geographically and culturally diverse settings, from large cities to isolated rural areas. Community health nurses work with many families and groups within their communities and in a variety of community health agencies, from state and national health departments to community-based neighborhood groups. The services they provide range from examining infants in a clinic setting to providing case-management services to frail elders in the home. Community health nurses also carry out epidemiologic investigations and participate in health-policy analysis and decision making. They are in a position to contribute to the development of community-based systems that address the current and projected health needs of populations.

This book focuses on the unique contributions that community health nurses make to improving the health of our communities and on the nature of the knowledge that these nurses must have in order to practice in the community. An emphasis on caring in this book demonstrates the authors' belief that caring is a vital force for human growth, fulfillment, promotion of health, and survival. In this opening chapter, which serves as an introduction to subsequent chapters, community health nursing is viewed within the context of caring for the health of individuals, families, and populations. This approach requires a discussion of the concept of caring and its significance to community health nursing. To illustrate the caring mission of community health nursing practice, this chapter also explores the concepts of health, public health, social justice, health promotion, health protection, disease prevention, and healing.

DEFINITION AND FOCUS OF COMMUNITY HEALTH/PUBLIC HEALTH NURSING

The focus of community health nursing is the health of populations. **Health** is defined as a state of well-being resulting from harmonious interaction of body, mind, spirit, and the environment. **Community health** is achieved by meeting the collective needs of the community and society by identifying problems and supporting community participation in the process. Community health nursing's scope of concern and commitment is to the entire population as distinguished from a designated individual or family focus. Community health nurses work with individuals and families within the context of the larger community. The goals of care are health promotion, health protection, the prevention of illness, and healing. Health-promotion activities and prevention efforts may be directed at the total population or at individuals and families within that population **aggregate**, or subgroup. Because the focus is the community, nurses must be prepared to promote the health of the community through health-promotion activities and prevention efforts that address the health problems of populations.

DECISION MAKING

Community Awareness

• What existing health problems are you aware of in your community?

• If you were a community health nurse, what activities might you propose to decrease the health problems in your community?

• What activities are currently taking place in your community to address identified health problems?

Considerable discussion and debate have centered on the definition and focus of public health nursing and community health nursing practice. Public health nursing has certain characteristics and is viewed as a specialized field of practice within the broad arena of community health nursing (Williams, 1996). This view is consistent with those recommendations developed at a Consensus Conference on the Essentials of Public Health Nursing Practice and Education, sponsored by the Division of Nursing in 1984.

Freeman (1963) provides a classic definition of **public health nursing**:

Public health nursing may be defined as a field of professional practice in nursing and in public health in which technical nursing, interpersonal, analytical, and organizational skills are applied to problems of health as they affect the community. These skills are applied in concert with those of other persons engaged in health care and through comprehensive nursing care of families and other groups and through measures for evaluation or control of threats to health, for health education of the public, and for mobilization of the public for health action (p. 34).

The American Public Health Association (APHA) Ad Hoc Committee on Public Health Nursing (1981) put forth the following definition of public health nursing in the delivery of health care:

Public health nursing synthesizes the body of knowledge from the public health sciences and professional nursing theories for the purpose of improving the health of the entire community. This goal lies at the heart of primary prevention and health promotion and is the foundation for public health nursing practice. . . . Identifying subgroups (aggregates) within the population which are at high risk of illness, disability, or premature death, and directing resources toward these groups, is the most effective approach for accomplishing the goal of [public health nursing] (p. 10).

Williams (1996) proposes one of the major factors that should distinguish public health nursing from other areas of specialization in nursing is practice that is community based and population focused, noting that a population focus is historically consistent with public health philosophy.

In 1980, the American Nurses Association (ANA) defined **community health nursing** as follows:

Community health nursing is a synthesis of nursing practice and public health practice applied to promoting and preserving the health of populations. The practice is general and comprehensive. It is not limited to a particular age group or diagnosis and is continuing, not episodic. The dominant responsibility is to the population as a whole; nursing directed to individuals, families, or groups contributes to the health of the total population. Health promotion, health maintenance, health education and management, as well as coordination and continuity of care are utilized in a holistic approach to the management of the health care of individuals, families, and groups in a community (p. 2).

The Task Force on Community Health Nursing Education, Association of Community Health Nursing Educators (ACHNE) (1990), described the terms *community health nursing* and *public health nursing* as synonymous, stating that

Community health nursing is the synthesis of nursing theory and public health theory applied to promoting and preserving the health of populations. The focus of community health nursing practice is the community as a whole, with nursing care of individuals, families, and groups being provided within the context of promoting and preserving the health of the community (p. 1).

Common to each of these various definitions is the provision of nursing service to the population as a whole. The ANA definition is important in that it addresses the care provided at individual, family, and group levels in relation to improving the health of the community. The APHA and ACHNE definitions focus on care to the community as a whole and consider the individual or family only when viewed as members of groups at risk (Muecke, 1984). Each of the definitions is important in addressing the health of populations.

The most current update of the definition of public health nursing was proposed in 1996 by the American Public Health Association, Public Health Nursing Section:

Public health nursing is the practice of promoting and protecting the health of populations using knowledge from nursing, social, and public health sciences. . . . The primary focus of public health nursing is to promote health and prevent disease for entire population groups. Public health nurses work with other providers of care to plan, develop, and support systems and programs in the community to prevent problems and provide access to care (pp. 1, 2).

Early public health nursing pioneers demonstrated the distinction between the definitions. In the late 1800s, Lillian Wald, at Henry Street Settlement House, New York City, and Mary Brewster, New York City Visiting Nurse Service, not only focused on the importance of working with individuals and families in the community but also recognized the need to become social activists. They worked toward the improvement of health education and health standards in their communities. Both Wald and Brewster recognized the need to bring nursing services into the homes of those who were experiencing poor health and who were living under unhealthy conditions in the community. Their vision extended beyond caring for families during illness to include a reform agenda aimed at effecting pub-

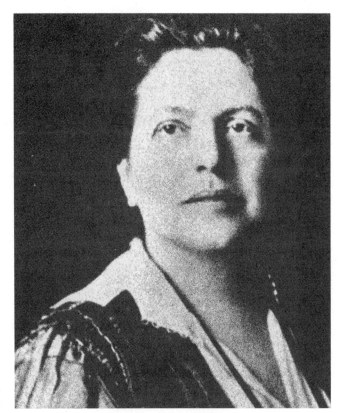

Lillian Wald. *Photo courtesy of American Nurses Association.*

lic policy to improve the unhealthy conditions in their city. Early public health nurses led many of the policy revolutions that helped bring family planning, workplace safety, and maternal child health services to populations in need (Salmon, 1993).

Wald (1971) and her colleagues utilized direct clinical nursing practice in the home combined with collective political activities as their two major approaches to improve the health of the **community**, a group of people sharing common interests, needs, resources, and environment. Although these early public health nurses worked closely with individuals and families within communities, they realized that the social and environmental **determinants of health** (factors that influence the risk for health outcomes, such as pollution, poverty, and child labor) required collective action aimed at improving the social and environmental conditions. The need to affirm direct clinical practice and social activism as the two approaches applied in community health nursing practice is just as pertinent today. Interesting parallels exist between our late–20th-century dilemmas and those confronted by Wald and her public health nurse associates over 100 years ago (Buhler-Wilkerson, 1993). Now, as then, frightening diseases, alienation of the poor, a problematic economic climate, and unmet health care needs of populations at great risk constitute serious health care issues. This is clearly a moment in time when nurses can provide assistance in meeting societal needs for community-based health care.

ꙮꙮ REFLECTIVE THINKING ꙮꙮ

Social Mission of Nursing

* What does social activism mean to you?

* What feelings arise for you when you consider the level of poverty in your community? What does poverty mean to you?

* What do you think are the unmet needs in your neighborhood?

INTRODUCTION TO CARING IN COMMUNITY HEALTH NURSING

Caring is defined as those assistive, enabling, supportive, or facilitative behaviors toward or for another individual or group to promote health, prevent disease, and facilitate healing. Historically, community health nurses have worked to establish caring **partnerships** with families and communities. As such, they focus on developing relationships with those they serve, basing their services on the **empowerment** (enabling others to acquire the knowledge and skills needed for informed decision making and affording others the authority to make decisions that affect them) of others and on fostering mutual respect and cooperation. The nurse's facilitation of a humane and healing environment is central to community nursing practice.

Community health nurses manifest their caring perspective through their work with individuals, families, and groups as well as through their participation in formulating public policy. Many community health nurses work with marginalized populations—the poor or disenfranchised. Consistent with the definition of caring, they work to develop trusting relationships with the families and communities in order to promote health, prevent disease, and facilitate healing. Community health nurses are thus essential instruments of caring and can assist in transforming the present and future health care system by demonstrating actions that are courageous, competent, compassionate, and creative at local, state, national, and international levels. As Roach (1991) suggests,

> The nursing profession, by its very nature and mandate, has the great privilege of standing in the health care world with a tradition of . . . caring. Its power for moving the world toward a more humane resolution of the crises it now experiences is both formidable and reassuring (p. 8).

Nurses offer important means of assessing the health of populations and the impact of environmental hazards on that health, establishing open lines of communication within the community and conveying information about health hazards and **risks**. As trusted health professionals,

nurses are frequently able to enter and move within communities in ways not possible for others. The community health nurse knows ways to reach out to people, facilitate growth in the direction of wholeness and health, and encourage the development of trust.

Population-Focused Practice

It is important to understand that population-focused practice is central to community health nursing; this perspective is different from that of nursing practice focused primarily on providing services to individuals and families. Population-focused practice is discussed in greater detail in Chapter 10, but an introduction is in order here.

Population-focused practice, as differentiated from individual practice, is based on the notion that an understanding of the population's health is critical. A population's problems and strengths (assets) are defined (diagnoses) and solutions (interventions) are proposed in contrast to diagnoses and interventions at the individual client level. The population focus is consistent with public health philosophy and is a fundamental principle that distinguishes community health nursing from the other nursing specialties.

A population focus requires thinking upstream, looking beyond the individual. McKinlay (1979) challenged health professionals to focus more on **upstream thinking**, "where real problems lie" (p. 9). Upstream strategies focus on identifying and modifying economic, political, and environmental variables that are contributing factors to poor health worldwide. For example, a population focus would require consideration of those who may need particular services but who either have not entered the health care system or do not have access to an acceptable, compassionate service system (e.g., homeless or near homeless elderly persons with untreated hypertension, diabetes, or foot infections; nonimmunized children). **Downstream thinking** refers to a microscopic focus characterized primarily by short-term, individual-based interventions. Figure 1-1 tells the story of a successful population-focused practice.

The Meaning of Caring for Community Health Nurses

The concept of caring is central to community health nursing practice. It is a constructive concept: that is, one that affirms those qualities that foster health and facilitate healing. Caring provides both the context and energy for nurses to work in diverse communities ranging from isolated rural areas to the crowded cities.

Caring is a dynamic state of consciousness (Gaut, 1993a) where nurses' thoughts, feelings, and actions determine how deeply they care about the communities they serve, the nature of their work with individuals, families, and groups as well as their participation in public policy making and change. The power of caring enables community health nurses to awaken those energies that

Figure 1-1 Population-Focused Practice: Caring in Action

In 1991, a committee was formed by a group of professional women committed to eliminating elder homelessness in Boston. The committee, called the Committee to End Elder Homelessness (CEEH), continues to exist to this day. The original and continuing Board President is Anna Bissonnette, RN, MS, a community health nurse and faculty member at Boston University School of Medicine. Bissonnette was also a founder of CEEH. Her vision, leadership, and activism in advocating for the rights of elders helped increase public awareness of the problem of elder homelessness. She has worked to reach out to elders at risk and to create housing and health-service options for homeless individuals. The CEEH has conducted a comprehensive survey to determine the extent of elder homelessness, worked to create a shared-living home for formerly homeless women in Jamaica Plain, sponsored apartments for homeless men and women, and developed an extensive outreach program to assist the homeless. In 1996, CEEH launched its most recent project: the renovation of a former warehouse into 40 apartments for homeless elderly men and women who are coping with mental and/or physical health problems. The project was completed in 1997. Health services are provided within this South-Boston facility, creating a model assisted-living program. Because of the ingenuity, compassion, and commitment with which Anna Bissonnette and her committee have worked to meet the health care needs of people in their community, Bissonnette received the Robert Wood Johnson Leadership Award in 1994 and, more recently, the Massachusetts Gerontology Louis Lowy Award in addition to being recognized by the mayor of Boston for her advocacy for justice for the elderly homeless.

illuminate and enable their participation in social transformation. As community health nurses become engaged in creating new possibilities for the health care system worldwide, social transformation becomes a reality.

To meet the health needs of the population, the community health nurse brings a sensitivity to the many individuals and groups in the community, with respect for their cultural lifeways and patterns, spiritual needs, values, health beliefs, and methods of managing their unique problems. The practice of community nursing is diverse and adaptable to different age and socioeconomic groups as well as cultural and ethnic groups in a variety of settings. Within the context of this diverse nursing practice, the nurse has the opportunity and responsibility to foster health by providing a caring presence in the company of human vulnerability and suffering. At the population level, the community health nurse would demonstrate caring by, for example, examining the prevalence of hypertension among different age, racial, gender, and socioeconomic groups, identifying those subpopulations with the highest rates of untreated hypertension, and

determining those programs that could reduce the prevalence of untreated hypertension.

An increasing number of nurses worldwide are recognizing the power of caring in relation to their work with individuals, families, and communities. Caring enables nurses to identify problems, recognize possible solutions, and implement those solutions (Benner & Wrubel, 1989) within the context of a healing environment. **Holism** is the belief that living beings are interacting wholes who are more than the mere sum of their parts. A caring, holistic practice perspective "enlarges the notion of the human from a duality of mind and body, to one that respects the simultaneous and continuous interaction of person, environment and health" (Gaut, 1993a, p. 167). As such, human beings are viewed in the context of the **ecological system** (the interrelationship between living things and their environment)—as part and parcel of a whole. Health and healing, together with the concept of wholeness, are integrated in family and community life.

Believing that caring is central to nursing practice, nurse scholars have studied dimensions of caring in different contexts. An increasing number of nurses from countries around the world are interested in studying care and caring from philosophical, **epistemologic** (pertaining to the nature and foundation of knowledge), economic, administrative, educational, and practice perspectives. Human caring is viewed as one of the most essential characteristics that assist people to maintain health, recover from illness, and die with dignity. As Roach (1991) succinctly states, "Caring is the expression of our humanity, and it is essential to our development and fulfillment as human beings" (p. 8).

The earliest studies of caring in nursing trace back to the early 1960s and the Gadsups of New Guinea, when Leininger (1977) identified various perceptions of caring, such as protection, nurturance, and surveillance. On the basis of her early work, Leininger (1977) went on to describe the phenomena of care and caring as an essential human need, necessary for health, well-being, human development, and survival. In subsequent work, Leininger

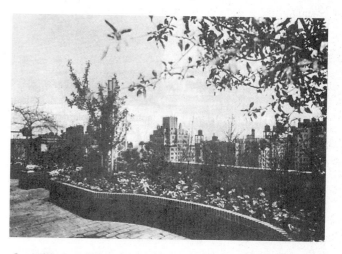

Community health nurses provide care to people in a variety of settings.

further explored the concept of caring from a combined anthropological and nursing perspective, with the cultural meaning of human caring being the focus of concern. Leininger's important discoveries related to the concept of caring laid the foundation for other researchers to follow.

The concept of caring continues to receive increased attention and emphasis in health care and nursing. In addition, caring has been recognized as an important concept to many other disciplines, as reflected in the various meanings of human caring described by those in the sociobehavioral sciences, anthropology, fine arts, psychoneuroimmunology, philosophy and ethics, and theology (Lakomy, 1993). Lakomy points out that "the meanings of caring have suggested both diversity and a universal theme" (1993, p. 181). An understanding of caring in a variety of contexts is therefore imperative for community nursing. The systematic study of caring; the development of theoretical models of caring; the significance of caring in relation to individual, family, and community outcomes; and the examination of caring from health-policy perspectives and in comparative contexts are of major importance.

The implications of caring for community health nurses are clear. A caring perspective requires the community health nurse to approach individuals, families, and groups from a holistic viewpoint, where principles of wholeness, harmony, and healing speak strongly to the nature of health.

Definitions of Caring

Caring has been defined in a number of different ways. A review of the various definitions suggests a diversity in the conceptualization of caring. Each of the definitions is important for community health nurses to examine because each has implications for practice. Leininger (1991) defines caring as "those actions and activities directed toward assisting, supporting, or enabling another individual or group with evident or anticipated needs to ameliorate or improve a human condition or lifeway" (p. 4) or to face death. Larson (1986) defines caring as the intentional attitudes and actions that convey emotional concern and physical care and that promote a sense of safeness and security in another.

Other definitions of caring emphasize that caring is a motivation to protect the welfare of another person or to assist that person to grow and actualize the self (Mayeroff, 1971; Gaylin, 1976).

Fry (1993) states that human caring "is a moral concept when caring is directed toward human needs and is perceived as a duty to respond to need" (p. 176). Watson (1985) characterizes caring as the moral ideal of nursing; a commitment, an intention. Caring has also been conceptualized as the human mode of being (Roach, 1991). As the human mode of being, caring is not unique to nursing but, rather, is unique in nursing as the concept

which subsumes all the attributes descriptive of nursing as a human, helping discipline. Nursing is no

Figure 1-2 Dimensions of Caring

Compassion

Competence

Confidence

Conscience

Commitment

Roach (1991) proposed that caring involves five different expressions.

more or no less than the professionalization of the human capacity to care through the acquisition and application of the knowledge, attitudes, and skills appropriate to nursing's prescribed roles (p. 9).

Roach proposes a helpful categorization of the concept of caring, stating that caring involves a number of different expressions. She identified these expressions as the five Cs: compassion, competence, confidence, conscience, and commitment (see Figure 1-2). These dimensions of caring have significance for community health nurses as these nurses develop partnerships with individuals, families, and communities.

Caring provides the central focus for community nursing practice. Community health nurses work with vulnerable populations—the wounded and those who are suffering. Because the community health nurse enters into the lives of people in their homes, in schools, in clinics, and in other settings, it is essential that nurses develop a philosophical and ethical framework to guide and evaluate their nursing practice. Understanding the meaning of caring is central to developing effective relationships and to promoting health and **wellness** (a group's progression to a higher level of functioning) within the context of community nursing practice.

REFLECTIVE THINKING

The Meaning of Caring

• What does caring mean to you?

• What are some examples of a nurse who demonstrates caring behaviors with families and populations?

• How might you feel if you thought a nurse was uncaring?

RESEARCH FOCUS

The Interdisciplinary Means of Caring

STUDY PROBLEM/PURPOSE

The concept of caring has received increased attention and study in nursing and nursing research. Caring has also been addressed by other disciplines. The purpose of this study was to examine the nature and meaning of caring from an interdisciplinary perspective.

METHODS

Hermeneutics, the understanding and interpretation or explanation of texts, was the methodology used for the study. Sixteen experts were interviewed regarding the specific discipline's knowledge base related to human caring. A nonstructured, tape-recorded interview was conducted, with the interview focused on the expert's meanings of caring and the discipline's exemplary literature and knowledge base in human caring. Computerized literature searches were also conducted. The Ethnograph software program was used to assist with data manipulation.

Nine disciplines were selected to participate in the discovery and identification of human caring literature. Those disciplines were psychoneuroimmunology, fine arts, sociobehavioral sciences, anthropology, humanities, philosophy, ethics, theology, and nursing. Exemplary literature included a classical foundation as well as representative works on human caring.

FINDINGS

The study revealed that the meanings of human caring were not discipline specific; rather, the meanings were shared by many disciplines. Seven major themes for human caring emerged from the interdisciplinary analysis. The meanings of caring were related to the essence of person/being; genuine relationships/encounters; decisions/choices; genuine dialogue; experiential process; healing modalities; and human/economic resource exchanges.

All nine disciplines selected to participate in the study shared meanings of human caring related to the themes of essence of person/being; genuine relationships/encounters; and healing modalities. The meaning of caring from a decision-making/choices perspective was conveyed in the literature from ethics and nursing. Caring as genuine dialogue was portrayed in fine arts, humanities, philosophy, theology, and nursing. The literature for fine arts, humanities, ethics, theology, and nursing described caring as an experiential process—a catalyst for human growth and development. Caring in relation to human/economic resource exchanges was found to be pertinent in anthropology, ethics, and nursing.

IMPLICATIONS

The findings from the interdisciplinary analysis of the meanings of human caring provide an opportunity to access, retrieve, and integrate the caring literature for use in practice education and research. In examining and creating the meanings of human caring, it is imperative that the meanings of caring, from an interdisciplinary perspective, not be stifled by applying a constricting definition to the concept.

SOURCE

From The Interdisciplinary Meanings of Caring by J. M. Lakomy (1993). In D. A. Gaut (Ed.), A Global Agenda for Caring (pp. 181–189), New York: National League for Nursing. Copyright 1993 by National League for Nursing Press.

Caring Themes and Models

Just as no consensus exists regarding the definition of caring, the concept itself can be viewed through different lenses. As Brown (1986) explains in her study of clients' perceptions of caring, caring is always understood in a context. In other words, various behaviors may be experienced as caring, depending on the needs and values of the individual, family, or group.

Whether caring is viewed as a human trait, a moral imperative or ideal, an affect, an interpersonal relationship, or a therapeutic intervention (Morse, Solberg, & Neander, 1990), community health nurses must learn to identify the meanings that the various conceptual categories have for them. Nurses must also learn to identify the meaning of caring from the perspectives of the individuals, families, and communities they serve.

Fry (1991, 1993) developed a helpful description of the models of human caring that emphasizes the various attributes of the concept. A **model** provides a frame of reference for members of a discipline to guide their thinking about observations and interpretations (Fawcett, 1989). A conceptual model refers to ideas about individuals, groups, situations, and events of interest. Models are based on the concepts considered to be relevant. The first, and most widely used, model of caring is the cultural model developed from anthropological and sociological studies of caring behaviors in various cultural groups. The cultural model relates caring to cultural beliefs, practices, and human survival (Leininger, 1984). It is discussed in greater detail in Chapter 6.

A feminist model of caring relates human caring to the perspective of feminine moral development (Gilligan, 1977) and identifies caring as an attitude that can be learned and nurtured through education (Noddings, 1984). Noddings describes caring as an attitude that expresses our earliest memories of being "cared for." The feminist model has received a great deal of attention in nursing.

Another model, described as a humanistic model of caring, relates human caring to a **moral obligation** or duty (Pellegrino, 1985). Pellegrino believes that caring as a professional duty is an obligation to promote the good of someone—to promote the welfare and well-being of the client.

Humanistic models of caring have been developed by a number of nurse scholars (Gadow, 1980, 1985; Gaut, 1981, 1984; Ray, 1981, 1987; Watson, 1985; Roach, 1989). These authors characterize caring as an intention, a will, a commitment, and an ideal. Caring is viewed as a way of being that is supported by a philosophy of moral commitment directed toward preserving humanity and protecting human dignity.

Fry (1991) proposes an obligation model of caring, which emphasizes compassion, doing good for others, and competence. The purpose of caring is directed toward the good of the individual. Fry (1993) also proposes a covenant-oriented model of caring, which emphasizes the presence of fidelity in relationships. Fidelity between persons flows from the covenant made between persons when they exist in particular relationships with each other: teacher and student, nurse and client, mother and child. Nurse caring, as proposed in this model, embodies **compassion**: doing for others, respect for persons, and the protection of human dignity.

Thus different conceptual approaches have been developed in the attempt to understand the phenomenon of human caring. Each of the models of caring is important because it indicates that caring encompasses different dimensions in a variety of contexts. In community health nursing, caring is more than an ideal, a commitment, or a sentiment; it is a science, an art, an action, and definitely not an exercise in passivity. Caring is a moral obligation that requires nurses to manifest those acts and processes directed toward meeting expressed or anticipated human needs in ways that are perceived as competent, compassionate, supportive, and growth enhancing.

THE CONTEXT FOR COMMUNITY HEALTH NURSING

The major goal of community health nursing is the preservation of the health of individuals, families, groups, and communities through a focus on health promotion, health protection, and health maintenance. In order to accomplish this goal, the community health nurse is oriented toward health and the identification of populations at risk. For the purpose of illustrating the caring mission of community health nursing as a population-focused practice, the concepts of health, public health, social justice, health promotion, health protection, disease prevention, and healing are explored.

Health

The term *health* has been defined in a number of different ways and is an evolving concept. The World Health Organization (WHO) (1974) formulated a classic definition of health as "a state of complete physical, mental, and social well-being and not merely the absence of disease or infirmity" (p. 1). This definition of health introduced the area of social well-being, thereby linking health and social life, health and social policy. The WHO definition thus called attention to the multidimensional nature of health. The WHO views health within the social context. Health is not only a personal responsibility but is influenced by the physical and social environments.

Pickett and Hanlon (1990) describe health as being on a continuum and emphasize the absence of disability. They state that "a disease or injury is any phenomenon that may lead to impairment" (p. 5). Kickbusch (1989) suggests that we need to reexamine our understanding of health itself in view of both the changing lifestyles of our societies and the new, more inner-directed values emerging in industrialized countries. Value orientations today view human beings in the context of the ecological system, with the individual a part of a whole. In this context, the health of an individual is related not only to the physical self but also to the mind and spirit. Kickbusch (1989) states, "Health is integrated in family and community life, is dependent on the physical as much as on the socioeconomic environment. It is constituted through the interaction of human biology and personal behavior and is created within a totality of culture and biosphere" (p. 48).

Health, as Pender (1996) points out, is increasingly recognized as a concept that is not only multidimensional but applicable to individuals and population aggregates as well. Health is a dynamic process inherent in the life experience of families and communities.

Over the course of time, views on health and illness have diverged significantly and in various systems of sociocultural values. Differences can be noticed among subcultures, smaller communities, and individuals. Thus, health is a complex phenomenon that is given form and meaning according to how it is perceived (Nijuis, 1989). It is, therefore, imperative that the community health nurse examine the ways individuals, families, and communities define health.

Public Health

Many attempts have been made to define the term *public health*, and, clearly, the definitions have changed over time. Early definitions focused on the sanitary measures utilized against nuisances and health hazards (Pickett & Hanlon, 1990). With the bacteriologic and immunologic discoveries of the late 19th and early 20th centuries and the development of techniques for the application of these discoveries, the concept of disease prevention was added. Public health then came to be viewed as an integration of sanitation and medical sciences. Today, public health is also regarded as a social science.

One of the best known and most widely accepted definitions of public health is the one formulated by Winslow in 1920 (Hanlon & Pickett, 1984):

Public Health is the science and art of (1) preventing disease, (2) prolonging life, and (3) promoting health and efficiency through organized community effort for

a. the sanitation of the environment
b. the control of communicable infections
c. the education of the individual in personal hygiene
d. the organization of medical and nursing services for the early diagnosis and preventive treatment of disease
e. the development of social machinery to ensure everyone a standard of living adequate for the maintenance of health, so organizing these benefits enables every citizen to realize his birthright of health and longevity (p. 4)

A more recent definition of public health was published in the 1988 Institute of Medicine (IOM) Report, which addressed the future of public health. In that report, **public health** was defined as "organized community efforts aimed at the prevention of disease and promotion of health" (Institute of Medicine [IOM], 1988, p. 41). Public health was also described as "what we, as a society, do collectively to assure the conditions in which people can be healthy" (IOM, 1988, p. 41).

In its 1988 report, the Institute of Medicine indicated that the mission of public health could be addressed by both private and public groups as well as by individuals but that the government had a specific function: ensuring that the vital elements are in place and that the mission is adequately addressed (IOM, 1988). In order to clarify the government's role, the report refers to the core functions of public health at all levels of government: (1) assessment of the population and monitoring of the population's health status and disseminating that information; (2) policy development, which refers to developing policies that use scientific knowledge in decision making for the purpose of promoting the health of the population; and (3) assurance, which refers to the role of public health in making sure that basic, communitywide health services are available and accessible as well as ensuring that a competent public health staff is available.

Organized public health efforts a century ago were developed in the political arena of social reform. Many of the public health pioneers were social-policy reformers. They were pioneers in relation to promoting an under-

standing of the relationship between health, work, labor, housing, and sanitation, from the perspectives of various disciplines and political alignments (Kickbusch, 1989). Various sectors of the community worked together to bring about the major changes in the health of populations at the turn of the century. Much of this early innovation was introduced by local authorities at the city level. The early public health efforts were linked to social policy, environmental health, and housing policy. These efforts were viewed as an expression of societal progress.

Over the past 100 years, the focus of public health has changed. Kickbusch (1989) contends that public health has become medicalized, with a primary focus on large-scale, disease-based interventions. These interventions have focused primarily on the organization of medical services rather than on systems that promote health and prevent illness. The link to social policy has become less obvious. Measures such as health promotion, prevention, environmental protection, and social interventions have become less important in a system focused on disease and disease intervention.

Since the late 1980s, however, the WHO (1989) has recognized the need to reaffirm the basic tenets of the "old public health," to create a renaissance of public health thinking and action. Public health is once again based on a "social and ecological understanding of health" (WHO, 1989, p. 44) with public health in a stage "where it aims to move from planning for sick factors to truly planning for health. That implies setting goals for policy action and not just goals to alter individual and family behavior" (pp. 46–47). The WHO (1989) articulated the goal that, by the year 2000, all people in all countries should have a level of health that enables them to work productively and to participate actively in the social life of the community in which they live.

In 1989, Kickbusch, from the WHO, pointed out that the link between political action, social reform, and public health efforts—characteristic of the earlier public health approach—had to be reestablished. Public health efforts also had to be linked to societal planning and to a notion of social change (Kickbusch, 1989). Since 1989, action has taken place at local, state, national, and international levels to improve the health of cities and communities. In Chapter 2, these actions are discussed in greater detail.

∞ REFLECTIVE THINKING ∞

The Meaning of Health

• What does the term *health* mean to you?

• How would you describe the health of your community?

• What health-promotion activities that might transform the health of your community would you support?

Community health nurses have a very significant role to play in terms of planning for the transformative process that must occur.

Social Justice

Social justice is the mission of public health. With its focus on the protection and preservation of the health of the population, public health has an egalitarian tradition. **Social justice** is that form of justice that entitles all persons to basic provisions such as adequate income and health protection. In the event that persons are not able to provide for their basic necessities, collective action is taken to make such necessities available. In public health, therefore, collective action addresses a health ethic that focuses on health and the identification of populations at risk in order to promote and preserve health. Thus, public health policy addresses not only lifestyle changes but also social and environmental factors that impinge on health. It should be pointed out here that, in the United States, the predominant model of justice is the *market justice* model, a model that assigns entitlement based on that which has been gained through primarily individual efforts.

Health Promotion and Health Protection

I believe promotion of health is far more important than the care of the sick. I believe there is more to be gained by helping every man learn how to be healthy than by preparing the most skilled therapists for service to those in crises (Henderson, 1993, p. 40).

The concepts of health promotion, health protection, and disease prevention are crucial ones in relation to understanding the mission of public health and, thus, community health nursing. Breslow (1990) points out that current ideas of health promotion are evolving "in a milieu that reflects recent life extension and health improvement and recognizes that factors other than medical service largely determine health" (p. 11).

Health promotion can be defined as those activities related to individual lifestyle and choices and designed to improve or maintain health. Noack (1987) emphasizes that health promotion comprises those efforts directed toward the protection, maintenance, and improvement of **health potential** (the ability to cope with environmental changes) and, hence, **health balance** (the state of well-being resulting from the harmonious interaction of body, mind, spirit, and the environment). Thus, there is an individual as well as a community component to health promotion. The individual component seeks to improve health potential through immunizations, adequate nutrition, education, counseling, exercise, and social support. The community component aims to improve the health of the community through multisectoral, holistic, political,

legislative, and administrative efforts. The community's health is sustained through the maintenance or establishment of health services, healthy working environments, information networks, and self-help programs.

Probably the most widely cited definition of health promotion (Breslow, 1990) can be found in the Ottawa Charter for Health Promotion (1987):

Health promotion is the process of enabling people to increase control over, and to improve, their health. To reach a state of complete physical, mental, and social well-being, an individual or group must be able to identify and to realize aspirations, to satisfy needs, and to change or cope with the environment. Health is, therefore, seen as a resource for everyday life, not the objective of living. Health is a positive concept emphasizing social and personal resources, as well as physical capabilities. Therefore, health promotion is not just the responsibility of the health sector, but goes beyond healthy lifestyles to well-being (p. iii).

This Ottawa definition of health promotion reflects an integration of community and personal efforts by a focus on enabling individuals or groups, through social action, to improve their health. The WHO (1989), European Region, considers health promotion as the process of enabling individuals and communities to increase their control over the determinants of health and thus improve their health. Health promotion is viewed as a unifying concept for those who recognize the need for change in the ways and conditions of living in order to promote health. As noted by the WHO, European Region (1984):

Health promotion best enhances health through integrated action at different levels on factors influencing health—economic, environmental, social, and personal. Given these basic principles, an almost unlimited list of issues for health promotion could be generated: food policy, housing, smoking, coping skills, social networks (p. 3).

As consensus on the meaning of health promotion evolves, social action to strengthen members of society

DECISION MAKING

Health Promotion

• What activities or programs in your community emphasize health promotion?

• How might you find out about such activities?

• Do any of the "health programs" in your community benefit you or your family? If so, how? If not, how might you assist in developing a program of benefit to you? To others in your community?

will surface as a central tenet. Health promotion can act as a mediating strategy between people and their environments, combining personal choice with social responsibility. As a principle, health promotion involves the whole population in the context of their everyday life. Thus, health promotion involves close cooperation between all sectors of the community—including government—to ensure that the total environment is conducive to health.

Health promotion therefore includes strategies (U.S. Department of Health and Human Services [USDHHS], 1991) related to individual and family lifestyles coupled with personal choices made in a social context that significantly influence overall health. Examples include increased physical activity, improved nutrition, decreased tobacco use, decreased use of alcohol and other drugs, family planning with the goal of fewer teen pregnancies and unwanted pregnancies, reduced family violence, improved mental health, and the development of educational and community-based programs in schools and workplaces.

Two important public health tenets clearly underlie the concept of health promotion: a multisectoral approach and community involvement. If health promotion best enhances health through integrated action, and if health emerges from the influence of a variety of factors, then close cooperation among different sectors of the community is needed. With health promotion becoming more prominent on the health agenda, care must be taken to reach out to those populations most in need. In the United States, those who have historically been neglected in relation to health matters are the poor, racial and ethnic minority groups, and elders. Health promotion activities in the workplace and in schools and other neighborhood sites are ways to reach out to all people.

Health protection refers to activities designed to actively prevent illness, detect illness early, thwart disease processes, or maintain functioning within the constraints of illness (Pender, 1996). Health protection includes environmental or regulatory strategies that confer protection on large population groups specific to occupational health and safety, environmental health, food and drug safety, oral health, and unintentional injuries (USDHHS, 1991).

Disease Prevention

Disease prevention is another major concept central to public health and the caring mission of community health nursing. **Disease prevention** refers to those activities designed to protect persons from disease and its consequences. In order to understand the concept of prevention, Leavell and Clark (1958) proposed the classic definition delineating three levels of prevention. These levels are defined and examples are provided in Figure 1-3.

Primary prevention—activities designed to prevent a problem or disease before it occurs

Secondary prevention—activities related to early diagnosis and treatment, including screening for diseases

Tertiary prevention—activities designed to treat a disease state and to prevent it from further progressing

Disease prevention is not synonymous with health promotion. The relationship between health promotion and disease prevention, as Breslow (1990) suggests, may be viewed more accurately as a continuum ranging from "extreme infirmity to bounding health" (p. 13). A person's degree of health may be found somewhere on the con-

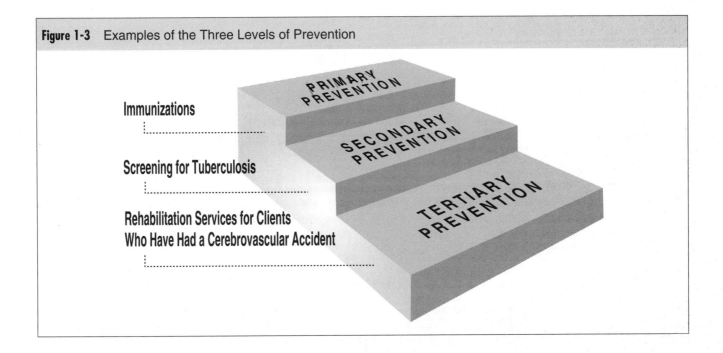

Figure 1-3 Examples of the Three Levels of Prevention

tinuum. Health promotion focuses on facilitating the maintenance of a person's current position on the continuum relative to age, with movement toward the positive end. Disease prevention, however, focuses on preventing specific diseases that carry one to the negative end of the health spectrum.

Many industrialized nations have reached a point at which health, rather than merely the control of disease, is on the agenda of health care priorities. Although diseases must continue to be confronted, coupled with ways to minimize them, a focus on health is also needed. Community health nurses as well as other health professionals have a special role in health promotion, health protection, and disease prevention: to delineate the prospects for preserving life and extending health for most persons, to determine the barriers to achieving health potential, and to advocate the social and personal actions necessary to meet these ends.

Healing

Healing has emerged as an important concept to nursing and public health. Healing enhances, promotes, and preserves the individual, family, or group. The term *healing* is derived from the word *hale*, meaning "whole." Thus, the literal meaning of healing is "becoming whole."

Healing refers to wholeness and balance. Implicit in this concept is a recognition of the unity of life and an

REFLECTIVE THINKING

Community Involvement

• Do you know of nurses in your community who demonstrate an interest in the health of the populations who live there? If so, how are those nurses involved in health care?

• How would you assess your own involvement in your community? What role do you think you could play in the future?

emphasis on the harmony between persons and their environment. **Healing** is therefore defined as the restoration of health, harmony, and well-being to the body, mind, spirit, and environment.

Human caring transactions with persons and communities requiring health care services have the capacity to promote healing processes, to ease suffering. When community health nurses work with families and groups within the context of a caring environment, the potential for self-healing arises. The recognition of the healing power within individuals, families, and communities, and the use of that power to promote health and well-being, is a central mission of community health nursing.

Perspectives...

Insights of a Community Health Nurse

Reflections

We ponder and reflect
listening
to the sounds of our own voices.
Coming together
to reach out to others,
Aspiring to care
in ways that are our own.

We open ourselves
learning about others
Learning about living, loving,
dying.

We are enriched, touched,
by those
who have taught us
so much.

We learn once again
to share our own light
experience our own energy.
Soaring
like a bird in flight
Seeking
new ways of being
and becoming.

—*Sue A. Thomas, November 1990*

CARING FOR POPULATIONS: POPULATION-FOCUSED PRACTICE

As was the case over 100 years ago, nurses today are in a position to participate in transforming our health care systems. Community health nurses can participate by contributing to the development of a unifying structure for the delivery of comprehensive, quality health care—a system focused not only on disease control and prevention but on health promotion as well. The Pew Health Professions Commission commented on the failure of health services to manage a person's safe passage through the health care system so that health is enhanced, illness prevention is incorporated, and death is dignified (Shugars, O'Neil, & Bader, 1991). Broad-based case management and coordination of care are services needed to facilitate "safe passage."

With a focus on providing care to populations, community health nurses are able to participate in coordinating health care services. Further, they possess a practice knowledge indispensable in a quality health care system: practice in providing case management as well as health education services to vulnerable populations; skill in coordinating care and developing trusting relationships through the establishment of caring partnerships with members of the community; and knowledge of the personal, environmental, political, social, spiritual, and cultural dimensions of health.

Community health nurses work in a variety of settings in the community, including homes, clinics, schools, workplaces, and organizations. They are also involved as members of health-planning agencies and councils, and they serve their communities as elected political officials. Community health nurses are concerned about the needs of those who do not receive health care services as well as the enhancement of health for those who do have access to the health care system. They are skilled in providing services to populations at high risk for illness, aging populations, homeless persons, children and adults with chronic illnesses and disabilities, persons struggling with alcohol and chemical dependencies, families trying to cope with violence in their homes and neighborhoods,

COMMUNITY NURSING VIEW

Heather Voss was an RN–BSN student at Sonoma State University who recognized the need for a nursing center in Marin County, California—a center designed to provide free nursing health care services to the homeless and near-homeless population. This center would become a program in an interfaith council agency serving the homeless and near-homeless population. Heather believed that in order to enhance health promotion, disease prevention, and healing in a very vulnerable population, nursing services should be based on the philosophy of caring practice—respect, compassion, competence, and dignity. Her vision became a reality in 1995 with the opening of a nursing center staffed by nurses and nurse practitioners. The center provides basic health services, health screening and referral, and case management. It continues today as a well-recognized community service, one that provides professional, compassionate health services.

Nursing Considerations

ASSESSMENT
• What did Heather observe that may have precipitated her action to create a nursing center?

This center is a part of an agency that serves the homeless, near-homeless population primarily.

DIAGNOSIS
• Lack of adequate housing is an obvious issue for the homeless population.
• Identify other possible problems faced by the homeless and formulate a nursing diagnosis for each.

OUTCOME IDENTIFICATION
• What outcomes would be expected for the populations served?

PLANNING/INTERVENTIONS
• Provide a plan for reaching the vulnerable population to be served by the center.
• How would the services offered be publicized?
• What interventions would be offered?

EVALUATION
• What would indicate that the center succeeded in its initial goal to enhance health promotion, disease prevention, and healing?
• How might client satisfaction be determined?

and persons confronting the return of acute or chronic communicable diseases (Zerwekh, 1993).

As Williams (1996) indicates, community health nurses must use a population-focused approach to practice. Although individuals and organizations may be responsible for subpopulations in the community (e.g., a health department responsible for a teen-parent program), population-focused practice addresses the larger community. Inherent in such an approach is examination of the health needs of the population and of the nature of the health care resources designed to meet those needs. The community is viewed as a whole, and questions are raised about its overall health and those factors contributing to that health. A population focus in community health nursing uses a scientific approach based on assessment of the community or population. This assessment is used for planning, intervention, and evaluation purposes at individual, family, aggregate, and population levels.

In planning and providing care to populations, community health nurses are interested in the phenomena of human care, caring, and healing. The perspective of the nurse is a holistic vision of the community's health. In order to promote individual, family, and community health, a holistic approach requires partnerships among many different sectors in the community. Partnerships based on the principles of empowerment, cooperation, and negotiation facilitate the creation of an environment where transformation can occur.

An increasing number of nurses are awakening to the possibilities of caring—caring about families, organizations, communities, nations, and the biosphere. As these nurses reaffirm caring as a concept with central importance in the study and practice of nursing, the possibilities of transformation become a reality where community health nurses fulfill their obligations in human caring through effective nursing practice.

Key Concepts

- The focus of community health nursing is caring for the health of individuals, families, and communities.

- The preservation and improvement of health of populations give direction to community health nursing practice.

- The ANA, APHA, and ACHNE definitions of community health nursing emphasize the synthesis of nursing and public health knowledge as a foundation for the scope of practice.

- The concept of caring is of central importance in community health nursing.

- A caring perspective requires the community nurse to approach individuals, families, and groups from a holistic view.

- The creation of caring partnerships with individuals, families, and communities is basic to community health nursing practice.

- The concepts of social justice, health, health promotion, health protection, disease prevention, and facilitation of healing are central to community health nursing.

- Principles of wholeness, harmony, and healing are important in understanding the nature of health.

- Community health nurses work in a variety of community settings, as well as serve as members of agency boards, planning teams, and councils.

Historical Development of Community Health Nursing

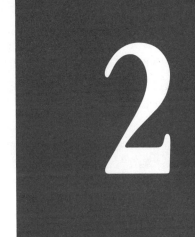

Sue A. Thomas, RN, EdD

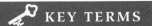 **KEY TERMS**

epidemic
incidence
pandemic
prevalence
primary health care
vital statistics

No occupation can be intelligently followed or correctly understood unless it is, at least to some extent, illumined by the light of history interpreted from the human standpoint.

—Dock & Stewart, 1938, p. 3

COMPETENCIES

Upon completion of this chapter, the reader should be able to:

- Discuss the significance of examining community health nursing from a historical perspective.
- Describe the development of major public health events in Europe and the United States.
- Examine the central elements of two major international initiatives for community health.
- Describe the contributions of the early public health nursing leaders who played a central role in the development of nursing practice in the community.
- Identify the major contributions of early public health leaders.
- Discuss the evolution of major organizations relative to public health and community health nursing.
- Describe the ways whereby World War I and World War II influenced the development of community health nursing.
- Discuss the impact on community health nursing of the health model that grew out of the Healthy Cities projects.

To understand the nature of community health nursing and the factors influencing its development, one must examine the historical context. This chapter describes early practices that formed a foundation for the organizations and methods we now term *public health* and *community health nursing*.

Community health nursing, as discussed in Chapter 1, was introduced as a term in 1980 by the American Nurses Association to broadly identify those nurses whose focus of practice is the community. *Public health nursing*, a term introduced earlier in the history of nursing, is often called community health nursing today. Public health nursing, however, is viewed as a specialty area in community health nursing, as are school nursing, hospice and home health nursing, occupational health nursing, and an emerging area of practice called parish nursing. In this view, public health nursing takes place within a public agency funded by governmental sources to protect the public health, such as in a county or state health department. The terms *community health nursing* and *public health nursing* are used interchangeably in this chapter.

This chapter further traces the evolution of modern practices. Donahue (1991) succinctly summarizes the meaning of historical knowledge to nursing when she states that history enables one to speculate and reflect, throwing light on the origins of persistent

Table 2-1 Pre-Christian Era Events Related to Public Regulation of Health Practices

ERA	EVENT
ca. 3000 B.C.	Sewage disposal system developed in Egypt (Hanlon, 1964).
ca. 2000 B.C.	Code of Hammurabi specifies health practices and regulates physician conduct in ancient Babylonia (Anderson, Morton, & Greene, 1978).
ca. 1500 B.C.	Hebrews' Mosaic law specifies personal and community responsibilities for maternal and child health, communicable disease control, sewage disposal, etc. (Anderson, Morton, & Greene, 1978).
498 B.C.	In Rome, office created to supervise health concerns such as garbage removal and sewage systems (Winslow, 1923).

problems and issues and thus providing a basis for analysis. This analysis may provide insight into possible resolutions. As Keeling and Ramos (1995) also emphasize, in order to fully understand their heritage, nurses must study nursing history.

A review of nursing history also expands the knowledge base of nurses and promotes understanding of the social and intellectual origins of the profession (Booth, 1989; Friedman, 1990; Donahue, 1991). Community health nursing has developed from social pressures that exist in new as well as familiar forms. As Keeling and Ramos (1995) point out, current practice and health care dilemmas "are not easily understood nor challenges addressed in the absence of such insight" (p. 31).

HISTORICAL BACKGROUND OF PUBLIC HEALTH EFFORTS

This section provides a broad overview of the historical and political influences on public health activities, thereby laying the foundation for the sections on public health nursing and community health nursing. Although this information is discussed separately with regard to European and American history, the accompanying tables interlace events of all geographic areas in order to show their temporal relationships.

International Background

Early historical evidence suggests that personal as well as community hygiene and health care were practiced during the pre–Christian era. Many primitive tribes developed practices such as the removal of the dead and the burial of excreta, along with rules against fouling tribal quarters (Hanlon, 1964). Whether these practices were based more on superstition than on concerns surrounding sanitation is unknown. What can be surmised is that many primitive people recognized the existence of disease and engaged

in various activities to drive away the evil spirits of disease (Hanlon & Pickett, 1984).

Table 2-1 lists some early activities that reflect an interest in public health. Early Greek civilization, for example, emphasized personal cleanliness, exercise, and nutrition—health-promotion activities still encouraged today (Hanlon, 1964). Around 1500 B.C., the Hebrews were practicing public health measures, such as protection of food and water supplies as well as specific disease control (Anderson, Morton, & Green, 1978).

The Middle Ages

When the Christian era began, a change in philosophy toward community health and personal health began to emerge. The early Christian Church, representing the thinking of the time, believed that Roman and Grecian life patterns, as discussed previously and in Table 2-1, focused on the body rather than the soul. The resulting philosophical shift to emphasizing neglect of the body for the purposes of enhancing the spiritual self led to a number of health problems (Kelly, 1981).

Because of the decline in community and personal prevention efforts during the Middle Ages, **epidemics** (disease rates beyond the usual frequency) of terrifying **pandemic** (worldwide epidemic) proportions occurred. Bubonic plague, for example, appeared in China, Egypt, India, Armenia, Europe, and other locations. The total mortality from bubonic plague is estimated to have been more than 60 million. In France, only one-tenth of the population is said to have survived. Over time, other diseases such as syphilis, diphtheria, streptococcal infections, dysenteries, and typhoid also took their toll (Pickett & Hanlon, 1990).

Early Christianity did, however, emphasize personal responsibility for the care of others and organized care of the sick to help meet the needs of society (Brainard, 1985). The sick, poor, and needy were cared for in hospitals, asylums, and almshouses.

The Renaissance

In Europe, after a depressing period associated with a focus on disease as punishment for sin, the concept of human dignity began to resurface. Intellectual inquiry and the search for scientific truth emerged. The Renaissance (A.D. 1500–1700) also led to awareness of society's responsibility for the health and welfare of its citizens. Of particular interest to community health nursing was the growing interest in care of the ill and aged in their homes. Founding of the Sisters of Charity in France set the stage for the emergence of visiting nurse services. (The work of these sisters and of St. Vincent de Paul is discussed further in the section on establishment of community and public health nursing practice.) See Table 2-2 for a list of events and actions that occurred during the Renaissance (including Colonial American events, to be discussed later).

The Industrial Revolution

The Industrial Revolution of the 1700s had a major influence on the health of the community. Industrialization and rapid urbanization throughout Europe resulted in higher infant mortality, poor working conditions, occupational diseases, overcrowding in poor urban areas, and populations vulnerable to epidemic infectious diseases (Ashton, 1992). The emphasis on industry and production overshadowed many of the gains made during the Renaissance. Similar conditions were taking place in the late 1700s in the United States.

The 18th and 19th Centuries in Europe

During the 18th and 19th centuries, the growth of populations in Europe led to greater emphasis on sanitation and **vital statistics** (the systematic use of data from registration of life events such as birth, deaths, and marriages to track health and social needs). There was a high **incidence** (frequency of new cases in a specified population) and **prevalence** (number of existing cases) of infectious diseases such as smallpox, cholera, and tuberculosis. The poor were living in "appalling, unsanitary conditions, crowded into slums" (Ashton, 1992, p. 1), where they were vulnerable to epidemic infectious disease.

In response to growing public awareness of existing sanitary and social problems, Great Britain enacted the first sanitation legislation in 1837. During this period, death rates were high in cities such as Liverpool, where more than half of the children of working-class families died before age five. The average age at death was 22 years for tradespeople, 36 years for gentry, and 16 years for laborers (Pickett & Hanlon, 1990).

In the 1840s public health, as it is known today, began with Edwin Chadwick in Great Britain. In 1842 Chadwick became known for his significant "Report on an Inquiry into the Sanitary Conditions of the Labouring Population of Great Britain." One result of this report was the establishment in 1848 of a General Board of Health in England (Hanlon & Pickett, 1984). Improvements soon followed with the enactment of legislation concerning factory management, child welfare, care of the aged and the mentally ill, education, and other social reform measures. Chadwick's answers to the appalling conditions of the poor— sewers, housing improvements, and water supply—had more to do with urban planning than with health services as we know them today.

Historical Development in America

On the North American continent, public health problems were recognized quite early by the colonists, who set the stage for later development. Table 2-2 lists some 17th-century European and Colonial American health-related events.

Colonial America

As early as 1639, a mandate by the Massachusetts Bay Colony required official reporting of vital statistics. Similar laws were enacted by the Plymouth Colony (Chadwick, 1937). Very little further progress of a public health nature occurred prior to the American Revolution, although temporary boards of health were established in response to particular epidemic health problems such as yellow fever, smallpox, typhoid fever, and typhus. The first permanent board of health was established in 1780.

With the development of the Marine Hospital in 1798 came the provision of health care to sick and disabled merchant seamen. The hospital concept was of particular significance because it was the beginning of what later came to be known as the U.S. Public Health Service (Hanlon, 1964). A public health committee formed in New

Table 2-2 Health-Related Events of the 17th Century	
YEAR(S)	**EVENT**
1601	Elizabethan Poor Law enacted in England addresses care for the aged and disabled.
1600s	St. Vincent de Paul founds order of Sisters of Charity in France to care for the sick and poor at home.
1639	Massachusetts and Plymouth colonies mandate reporting of births and deaths (Chadwick, 1937).
1647	Massachusetts passes legislation prohibiting pollution of Boston Harbor.
1669	First visiting nurses sponsored by St. Vincent de Paul in France.

York City at about the same time focused on sanitation and other health-related measures. The term *public health* has since been used to refer to government-run health services, which now constitute only one segment of the broader concept of community health.

The 18th and 19th Centuries in America

As can be inferred from Table 2-3, few major health-related events occurred in the 18th century. Although the United States expanded considerably during the first half

Table 2-3	Events of the 18th and 19th Centuries That Influenced Community Health Nursing
YEAR(S)	**EVENT**
1701	Massachusetts enacts laws regarding isolation of smallpox victims and ship quarantine.
1780	First permanent local board of health organized in Petersbury, Virginia (Public Health Service [PHS], 1958).
1789–1799	Boards of health established in Philadelphia, New York, Baltimore, and Boston (PHS, 1958).
1798	U.S. Congress creates Marine Hospital.
1812	Irish Sisters of Charity founded in London, initiating home visiting by nuns.
1837	Great Britain enacts first sanitation legislation.
1839	American Statistical Society founded by Shattuck.
1842	Chadwick's Inquiry into the Sanitary Conditions of the Labouring Population of Great Britain published (Pickett & Hanlon, 1990).
1844	Healthy Towns associations formed in London in response to threats posed by urbanization and industrialization and to enact legislation to improve public health (Finer, 1952).
1848	Public Health Act passed in Parliament in London, unifying the organization of public health efforts.
	General Board of Health for England established to deal with child welfare, care of mentally ill and disabled, and other social actions.
1850	Shattuck's Report of the Sanitary Commission of Massachusetts published.
1854	Nightingale begins her involvement in the Crimean War, addressing environmental and health care issues.
1859	Rathbone promotes establishment of district nursing in Liverpool, England.
1869	First state board of health established in Massachusetts.
1870	Second state board of health established in California.
1872	American Public Health Association founded.
1875	Ward-Richardson shares vision of "Hygeia: A City of Health in England" to encourage passage of Public Health Act in Great Britain, which included prevention measures and occupational health and safety (Cassedy, 1962).
1876	Pasteur and Koch usher in the mechanistic biomedical paradigm, with its emphasis on identification and treatment of germ-related causes of disease (Duhl & Hancock, 1988).
1877	First home visiting nurses employed by a volunteer agency in the United States.
1879	Ethical and Cultural Society of New York employs four nurses in dispensaries.
1882	American Red Cross founded by Clara Barton to supply nurses for service during World War I.
1885–1886	Visiting Nurse associations established in Buffalo and Philadelphia.
1892	School nursing established in London.
1893	Henry Street Settlement founded by Lillian Wald.
	Dock, Robb, and Nutting organize the American Society of Superintendents of Training Schools for Nurses in the United States and Canada.
1895	Vermont Marble Company employs first occupational health nurse.
1896	First rural nursing service in United States started by Ellen M. Wood in Westchester County, New York.
1898	Los Angeles becomes the first city to hire a nurse in an official health department.

of the 19th century, public health activities did not advance. Epidemics of smallpox, yellow fever, and other infectious diseases crossed the land. In Massachusetts, the tuberculosis death rate exceeded 300 per 100,000 population in 1850; during the same time period, infant mortality was estimated at approximately 200 per 1,000 live births (Hanlon, 1964). As the United States grew, the number of cities increased, and the poor, as in Europe, crowded into substandard housing with unsanitary conditions, thereby creating the environment for illnesses to flourish (Rosen, 1958).

In response to the problems that emerged during the late 1700s and that continued into the 1800s, some larger cities, such as New York and Philadelphia, established city health departments. These city departments—along with the first state Board of Health, established in 1869—set the stage for the four levels of official public health action, now including national and international agencies.

Lemuel Shattuck, public health pioneer, issued a Census of Boston, which revealed startling statistics about the high infant- and maternal-death rates. Shattuck's 1850 report of the Sanitary Commission of Massachusetts has been viewed as one of the most remarkable reports in U.S. history, and one well ahead of its time (Hanlon, 1964). The report included a discussion of present and future public health needs of Massachusetts as well as of the nation. The report provided information related to environmental, food, drug, and infectious-disease patterns and recommended keeping vital statistics records. Although Shattuck's visionary report called for these and many other reforms that seem modern even today, it "remained almost unnoticed by the community or by the profession for many years, and its recommendations were ignored" (Hanlon, 1964, p. 50).

Not until 1869, 19 years later, was the first state board of health established in Massachusetts, as earlier recommended by Shattuck. This state health department, under Dr. Henry Bowditch's leadership, focused on public and professional education related to hygiene, housing, communicable diseases, and living conditions of the poor, among other issues. By the end of the 19th century, 18 other states had established state health departments; in the early part of the 20th century, the remaining states followed suit.

With the increased focus on the public's health toward the end of the 19th century, people became more concerned about the plight of the poor, and, as a result, greater emphasis was placed on the abolition of child labor, improved housing, and maternal and child health. Many voluntary organizations were founded, including the Red Cross, the American Society for the Control of Cancer, and the National Tuberculosis Association. The American Public Health Association (APHA), founded in 1872, became the formal organization for public health professionals (Fee, 1991). Formation of the APHA represented a significant advance in public health expansion. Its early meetings focused on aspects of sanitation, transmission and control of diseases, longevity, hygiene, and other subjects (Hanlon & Pickett, 1984). The APHA today

remains a major organization in the United States, serving its members and the public with information and advocacy for improvement of health in communities throughout the nation.

The 20th Century

Soon after the turn of the century, the U.S. Public Health Service (USPHS) was created. This federal service actually began in 1902, with the Public Health and Marine Hospital Service. Renamed the U.S. Public Health Service in 1912, it grew rapidly as U.S. society became increasingly complex and experienced several wars and economic depressions (Hanlon & Pickett, 1984).

The chief officer of the USPHS became the Surgeon General, with the passage of federal legislation mandating federal involvement in health promotion. In the early years of the 20th century, health needs of special population groups began to be recognized, leading to development of federal programs related to maternal and child health, sexually transmitted diseases, mental illness, and other health concerns. Today, the USPHS is the most important federal health agency. Table 2-4 lists 20th-century events that influenced community health nursing.

INTERNATIONAL INITIATIVES IN PUBLIC HEALTH

The study of international initiatives in public health during the 20th century provides the background necessary to understand public health projections for the next century. Particularly from the 1930s through the early 1970s, public policy on health in Great Britain and many other countries, including the United States, was dominated by a treatment orientation, with the implicit assumption that "magic bullets could be provided by the pharmaceutical industry for all conditions" (Ashton, 1992, p. 3).

By the early 1970s, however, the therapeutic approach was being challenged. Most countries, including developing countries, were experiencing a crisis in health care costs. Many had adopted the Western pattern of building large hospitals that incorporated highly trained professionals. Such facilities took up the bulk of the health care

Table 2-4	Events of the 20th Century That Influenced Community Health Nursing
YEAR(S)	**EVENT**
1902	Lina Rogers, on loan from Henry Street Settlement House, starts school of nursing in New York.
1904	Los Angeles becomes the first city in the United States to hire school nurses.
1909	Metropolitan Life Insurance Company offers visiting nurse services to policyholders in New York (first national system of insurance coverage for home-based care).
	First White House Conference for Children held.
1910	Mary Adelaide Nutting starts first postgraduate course in public health nursing at Teacher's College, Columbia University, New York.
1911	Metropolitan Life Insurance Company initiates visiting nurse services throughout the United States.
1912	U.S. Children's Bureau and U.S. Public Health Service created.
	American Red Cross Town and Country Nursing Service established.
	National Organization for Public Health Nursing (NOPHN) formed, with Lillian Wald as first president.
1920	U.S. legislation giving women the right to vote passes.
1921	Shepherd-Towner Act passes, authorizing grants to states to provide care to at-risk maternal aggregates.
1922	Harlem Committee of New York Tuberculosis and Health Association established, based on Mabel Staupers' community assessment.
1923	Goldmark Report published, recommending that nursing education be offered in institutions of higher learning.
1925	Frontier Nursing Service started by Mary Breckinridge in Kentucky.
1930	National Institutes of Health created in the United States.
1934	Mabel Staupers appointed as first nurse executive of National Association of Colored Graduate Nurses.
	Pearl McIver becomes the first public health nurse hired by the U.S. Public Health Service.
1935	Social Security Act passes in U.S. Congress, establishing Old Age, Survivors, and Disability Insurance (OASDI) program.
1952	NOHPN absorbed into the National League for Nursing (NLN).
1953	U.S. Department of Health, Education, and Welfare created.
1963	NLN requires baccalaureate nursing programs to include public health nursing content and practice in the curriculum, as recommended in 1951.
1964	Economic Opportunity Act passes, providing funds for neighborhood health centers, Head Start, and other community programs.
1966	Comprehensive Health Planning and Public Health Services Act passes.
	Social Security Act amended to include Medicare program.
	Development of Healthy Cities Projects begins throughout the world, continues through 1993.
1967	U.S. Congress passes Medicaid provision of Social Security Act to provide care for the poor.
1974	LaLonde Report ("A New Perspective on the Health of Canadians") published in Canada.
	National Health Planning and Resources Development Act passes in United States as an attempt to create systematic health care planning.
1976	McKeown's statistical analysis of infectious disease mortality in England and Wales published.
1978	International Conference on Primary Health held, resulting in the World Health Organization (WHO) initiative known as the Alma Ata declaration on Primary Health Care.
1981	Global Strategy for Health for All by the Year 2000 agreement adopted by member nations of WHO.
1983	Prospective payment system (DRGs) instituted under Medicare.
1985 and 1991	WHO Regional Office for Europe publishes Targets for Health for All reports.

Continued

Table 2-4	Events of the 20th Century That Influenced Community Health Nursing *(Continued)*
YEAR(S)	**EVENT**
1986	Ottawa Charter for Health Promotion developed at the First International Conference on Health Promotion, held in Canada.
	1990 Health Objectives for the Nation published.
	Healthy Cities Project created, WHO European Office.
1988	Health for All Australians report developed in response to WHO's Health for All initiative.
1989	New Zealand Health Goals and Targets for the Year 2000 report published.
1990s	Health care systems in Western and developing nations undergo restructuring.
1990	U.S. Healthy People 2000 Objectives published.
1986–1993	Healthy Cities Projects developed throughout the world.
1993	First International Healthy Cities and Communities Conference held in San Francisco.
1996	U.S. Healthy People 2000, Midcourse Review and 1995 Revisions published.
2000	Projected publication of U.S. Healthy People 2010.

budget, leaving little funding for rural areas or for primary care. From the problems associated with this development, the two concepts of primary health care and emphasis on community development began to surface (Ashton, 1992).

In Great Britain, McKeown's (1976) statistical analysis demonstrated that most of the decline in infectious disease mortality in England and Wales between 1840 and 1970 occurred before medical therapeutic intervention. This analysis resulted in a revived interest in public health and prevention efforts. McKeown concluded that a number of factors contributed to improved health outcomes in Great Britain. These were:

- Limitation of family size,
- Increase in food supplies,
- A healthier physical environment, and
- Specific preventive and therapeutic measures.

A review of international literature specific to public health refers to McKeown's work as a benchmark for what has become known as the New Public Health. This approach seeks a synthesis of the environmental and personal preventive and the therapeutic eras in public health history. It focuses on public policy as well as personal behavior and lifestyle (Ashton, 1992).

The LaLonde Report, "A New Perspective on the Health of Canadians," published in Canada in 1974 and discussed in Chapter 30, has been viewed as a restatement of earlier public health reports on sanitary conditions among laboring populations. The LaLonde Report has been applied at different levels in various nations (Ashton, 1992).

Declaration of Alma Ata

Since the LaLonde Report, the World Health Organization (WHO) has generated several initiatives. At the Interna-

tional Conference on Primary Health Care, held in 1978 at Alma Ata, participants from 143 countries identified primary health care as the best possible way to attain health for all by the year 2000. The Alma Ata Declaration, referred to as Health for All by the Year 2000, resulted in countries throughout the world taking action to create national initiatives focused on implementing primary care measures to improve the health of their people. Health itself was described as a basic human right and worldwide social goal (Basch, 1990).

Primary health care emphasizes the preventive rather than the curative end of the health care continuum. This approach to care focuses on equity, community participation, accessibility of services, and the importance of the environment in relation to the health of individuals and communities (Lamont & Lees, 1994). The Alma Ata primary health care focus, by its very nature, requires a coordinated, intersectoral approach. It is transdisciplinary, broad in nature, and a more integrated approach to the health and social well-being of the community.

The central elements of both WHO initiatives, the Alma Ata Declaration and the Healthy Cities Project (discussed below), are a focus on the poor and disenfranchised; the need to reorient the focus of medical and health systems away from hospital care and toward primary health care; the importance of a consumer focus in health care; and the creation of partnerships between public, private, and voluntary sectors. The concept of health promotion embedded in these initiatives reaffirms the importance of public policy and environmental action as well as personal lifestyle.

Health for All by the Year 2000

The WHO policy of Health for All by the Year 2000 resulted in the setting of goals and targets to improve the public's health worldwide. Two years after Health for All was adopted by WHO in 1981, the U.S. Surgeon General's Report on Health Promotion and Disease Prevention was developed, subsequently resulting in the publication of the Healthy People 2000 Objectives in 1990 (USDHHS, 1990). The WHO's European Regional Office published the first set of Targets for Health for All in 1985 (WHO, 1985). This report was updated in 1991 on the basis of broad representation from the various European member states (WHO, 1991). In 1988, Australia published its first national goals and targets for population health for the year 2000 and beyond (Health Targets and Implementation Committee, 1988). In 1989, the New Zealand Health Charter was developed, making area health boards accountable to the New Zealand government for achieving objectives in order to justify their budgets. With the change in government in 1990, however, New Zealand abandoned these goals and targets (Green, 1996).

The Australian and U.S. approaches, in contrast to the New Zealand model, provided opportunities for states and communities to decide whether to adopt or adapt the national health objectives in their own policies and plans. These approaches have been effective ones. In the United States, for example, the process and objectives have survived several changes of government. Four presidents and six secretaries of Health and Human Services (as of 1996) have assisted the U.S. health-promotion and disease-prevention objectives through the various transitions in government without changing the general direction of the Healthy People 2000 Objectives (Green, 1996). As Lee (1996) notes, an interstate network is in place in 41 states and 2 territories to translate the national objectives to meet state needs and priorities. This interstate network has resulted in consensus-building efforts, effective consultation procedures, coalition building activities, and a willingness to revise and improve the objectives (Green, 1996). In 1996, 70% of the local health departments in the United States were using Healthy People 2000 as a framework for health promotion and disease prevention.

As can be seen, the WHO initiative Health for All by the Year 2000 has resulted in the creation of a momentum among nations that embodies the spirit of partnership, collaboration, and consensus building. It is anticipated that through the process of working together, we can build healthier cities and communities worldwide.

Healthy Cities and Communities

The Healthy Cities initiative was started in 1986 by the European office of the WHO. A proposal that included four to six cities was developed. This project was thought by many world cities and towns to be a useful vehicle for translating the WHO Health for All by the Year 2000 strategy and the 30 European Targets for Health for All into local programs.

In 1993, the first International Healthy Cities and Communities Conference was held in San Francisco, California. Participants from around the world gathered to discuss various activities related to the creation of the Healthy Cities Project and actions to improve the health of those in their communities. The conference was very successful, providing the opportunity for participants to share their experiences with each other—participants from countries such as Australia and countries in Asia, South America, Europe, and North America.

The WHO initiatives indicate recognition of the need to reduce fragmentation of services—to work toward creating seamless, integrated health care systems that focus on consumer needs. The challenge today, as we move toward the 21st century, is whether the global initiatives of the 1990s can be as effective as the national initiatives established in Britain in the 1840s. As Ashton (1992) points out, "It is imperative that broad-based professional, public, and political coalitions be built to tackle the problems which confront us" (pp. 10–11).

Duhl (1992), one of the primary leaders of the WHO Healthy Cities Project, suggests that if living areas contain diverse groups, cultures, values, and goals, as they do in cities throughout the world, then "a new means must emerge for dealing with health" (p. 17). The values built into the Health Promotion, Healthy Public Policy, and Healthy Cities initiatives are such a response. The Healthy Cities model, known in Canada as Healthy Communities, respects diversity, encourages participation, and calls for equity, asking that providers and consumers sit together, explore perceptions of health needs, investigate various visions, and create responsive systems. Duhl goes on to say, "For those of us who believe that

DECISION MAKING

Creating Community Partnerships

Building partnerships among organizations in the community reflects an effort to improve the nature of health care delivery and, ultimately, the health of the community. Through collaboration, health care problems and issues can be and are being addressed in a more comprehensive way. Creating partnerships between providers and consumers is another endeavor to enhance care delivery.

• What types of activities have occurred in your community in relation to creating partnerships for health care delivery?

• What do you think about the idea of creating partnerships among organizations to enhance health care delivery? What about partnerships between providers and consumers? What does consumer-focused care mean to you?

• How might you participate in the process?

health, holism, holy, healing, and whole are similar, Healthy Cities offers a chance to bring all our separate parts together as we help our own cities" (p. 20).

EVOLUTION OF COMMUNITY HEALTH NURSING—CARING AND HEALING PRACTICE

Caring and Healing in Community Health Nursing

Over the past century, community health nurses have demonstrated courage and commitment in providing care to people in their communities. In the United States as well other countries, community health nursing, also known as public health nursing, can trace its origins to those first nurses who provided care to poor people in their homes, neighborhoods, workplaces, schools, and clinics. In Great Britain, Australia, Canada, the United States, and other nations, these nurses were frequently the only providers of care to underprivileged individuals and families. They also visited families in outlying areas, traveling by many different modes of transportation. Among early community health nurses, caring for the people included raising needed funds for services and political support. In this way, community health nurses fulfilled social as well as professional roles.

In San Francisco in November 1993, the American Public Health Association recognized the outstanding contributions of public health nurses to improving the health of their communities. That year, public health nurses in the United States celebrated a century of caring—caring for communities, aggregates, and families. Across the nation, nurses came together to honor their founders—leaders such as Lillian Wald, Mary Brewster, Margaret Sanger, and Lavinia Dock. Public health nursing in the United States began with those nurses, who provided nursing services to needy families in their homes.

The first public health nurses were caring women with compassion for the communities they served. They recognized the overwhelming health problems in the late 1800s and committed themselves to providing care to families in homes, their workplaces, schools, neighborhoods, and clinics, reaching out to care for those in their communities (American Public Health Association, 1993).

Public health nurses have served people of all ages and have practiced in a variety of settings, focusing on health promotion, disease prevention, treatment, and rehabilitation in their efforts to address health needs (Freeman, 1964). The early public health nurses were able to mobilize community resources in creating enlightened models for care—models that are still relevant today. Many of the early nursing leaders were involved in the social issues of their time, including women's suffrage, public health, and child labor laws (Donahue, 1991), as discussed in subsequent sections.

The Legacy of Florence Nightingale—The Evolution of Modern Nursing

Nursing is an art; . . . it requires as exclusive a devotion, as hard a preparation as any painter's or sculptor's work; for what is having to do with dead canvas or cold marble, compared with having to do with the living body; the temple of God's spirit? (Nightingale, 1867, in Styles & Moccia, 1993, p. 149).

Florence Nightingale, the woman credited with establishing modern nursing, was born in 1820 to an established English family. She was well educated and concerned about hygiene and health (Goodnow, 1933). In her youth, Nightingale longed to be a nurse; however, nursing was not yet a recognized field of study. Further, being a nurse was viewed as less than socially desirable; therefore "respectable" people did not do the work.

Not until she was 31 years of age did Nightingale enter nurse's training under the direction of Pastor Fliedner at Kaiserwerth Hospital on the Rhine in Germany. Nightingale also studied the organization of the Sisters of Charity in Paris as well as nursing systems in Austria, France, Germany, and Italy (Dock & Stewart, 1925).

In 1854, Nightingale responded to the Crimean War at Scutari in Turkey, where she became a pioneer in improving conditions for wounded soldiers. When Nightingale arrived at Scutari, she found that the hospital, built for 1,700 patients, actually held 3,000 to 4,000 wounded men. The men were lying naked, and there were no beds, no blankets, no laundry, and no eating areas (Goodnow, 1933).

Nightingale not only made major reforms in hospital operations within a few months; she also recognized the importance of keeping statistical information about the death rates of soldiers in the Crimean hospital, comparing these rates with the death rates in hospitals in Manchester and in or near London.

ҩ҂ REFLECTIVE THINKING ҩ҂

The Legacy of Florence Nightingale

- What do you think were Florence Nightingale's most important contributions?

- What were some of her contributions that have relevance for today?

Because of Nightingale's meticulous attention to maintaining statistical records, she was able to clearly demonstrate that, by the end of the Crimean War, her reforms had resulted in lower death rates of soldiers. Nightingale also established community services and activities for soldiers, such as rest-and-recreation facilities. In addition, care for families was organized (Dock & Stewart, 1925).

Florence Nightingale demonstrated, in an exemplary way, that public health principles are central to health care services. One of her greatest contributions was in relation to sanitation reform. As noted by Cohen (1984) and Grier and Grier (1978), Nightingale was concerned about the environmental determinants associated with health and disease. She also demonstrated the value of utilizing statistics to describe population factors, statistics that could be used for political advocacy on behalf of the population aggregate. The development and application of statistical procedures continued after her return to London, at the close of the Crimean War in 1856.

Florence Nightingale was a visionary, and she left a rich legacy to those of us in the latter part of the 20th century and beyond. Styles (1992), in her commentary for a commemorative edition of Florence Nightingale's *Notes on Nursing*, describes Nightingale as

> our enduring symbol. . . . She represents many of the values we continue to hold dear. The origins of many of today's nursing movements can be traced to the Nightingale legacy. She was preaching vehemently about the environment, the community (or district), sanitation, hygiene, healthy living, and preserving the vitality of patients more than a century before primary health care was elevated to the rank of worldwide gospel at Alma Ata (pp. 72–75).

Nightingale was influential in the reformation of hospitals and in promoting public health policies for the British Sanitary System (Kalisch & Kalisch, 1982). She was the first nurse to exert political pressure on government, taking social action at a time when nursing was not a recognized or highly valued endeavor.

Establishment of Community Health Nursing and Public Health Practice

Community health nursing began in 1669 with the first visiting nurses, who were sponsored by St. Vincent de Paul in Paris. St. Vincent de Paul organized the Sisterhood of the Dames de Charité, introducing the principles of visiting nursing and social welfare. He focused on helping people to help themselves. The work of the sisterhood emphasized the belief that home visiting required not just kindness and intuition but also sound knowledge of scientific principles (Maynard, 1939). The voluntary association of friendly visitors established by St. Francis de Sales to care for the sick poor in their homes represents another early form of visiting nursing (Dolan, 1978).

Other early forerunners of community health nursing were the first two nursing orders in Great Britain. Mary Aikenhead (Sister Mary Augustine), who started the Irish Sisters of Charity in Dublin in 1812, developed a nursing model whereby the nuns visited the sick in their homes. The community health nursing movement owes its further development to William Rathbone of Liverpool, England, a Quaker who in 1859 became impressed by the skilled care his wife received during a fatal illness. As Gardner (1919) states, "It is to Mr. Rathbone that we owe the first definitely formulated district nursing association" (p. 14). A philanthropist, Rathbone promoted the establishment of district nursing, or visiting nursing service, for the sick poor of Liverpool. Rathbone believed that if nursing care could help his wife, who had the money to purchase services, those who were sick and poor might benefit from the needed services even more.

Rathbone employed Mrs. Mary Robinson, the first nurse to visit the sick poor in their homes. She was not only to provide therapeutic nursing care for the sick but also was to instruct the patients and their families in the care of the sick, the maintenance of hygienic practices in the home, and those things that contributed to healthful living. The service provided was so effective that Rathbone decided to establish a permanent district nursing service in Liverpool (McNeil, 1967). Liverpool was organized into 18 districts, each of which would have a nurse and a social worker to meet the needs of its communities.

In order to obtain qualified nurses who would be able to do this difficult work, Rathbone asked for assistance from Florence Nightingale, who helped him establish a training school for visiting nurses in affiliation with the Roy Infirmary of Liverpool. From the beginning, Nightingale referred to the graduates of the visiting nursing program as "health visitors." The model was very successful and eventually expanded to the national level under voluntary agencies (Rosen, 1958).

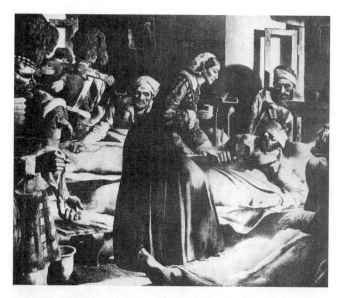

Florence Nightingale in the Crimea. *Photo courtesy of Parke, Davis, a division of Warner-Lambert Company.*

Community Health Nursing in the United States

In the United States, as in Great Britain, community health nursing developed from district and home visiting, with the first nurses employed in 1877 by the Women's Branch of the New York City Mission, a voluntary agency (Waters, 1912). Frances Root, a graduate nurse, was the first salaried U.S. nurse to provide nursing care to the sick poor in their homes. In 1878, the Ethical Culture Society of New York employed four nurses in dispensaries to serve in an ambulatory care role in the community. These nurses worked under the supervision of a physician, incorporating health teaching as well as illness care in their practice (Brainard, 1985).

Within the next few years, the idea spread, with nursing associations, later called visiting nursing associations, established initially in Buffalo and Boston in 1885 and in Philadelphia in 1886. These associations relied on support from lay contributions and on small service charges. The Boston Instructive Visiting Nurse Association emphasized the community health nursing education role as well as care of the sick, ushering in the beginning of the health-promotion focus that now characterizes community health nursing. By 1890, visiting nurse services were organized in 21 U.S. cities (Novak, 1988).

Visiting nursing in the United States, as in Great Britain, was begun by people who were concerned about the conditions in which the poor lived. Then, as now, many of the most serious public health problems were in poverty-stricken communities, with hunger, family violence, homelessness, crime, youth alienation, deterioration of the physical environment, and unemployment clearly evident.

Contributions of Lillian Wald and Others

In 1893, Lillian Wald and Mary Brewster cofounded the first organized public health nursing agency, or settlement house, in New York City. They rented an apartment in lower Manhattan, beginning what came to be known as the Henry Street Settlement, eventually the New York Visiting Nurse Association. Mary Brewster and Lillian Wald were able to obtain funds from philanthropists in order to offer care to needy persons. It was Wald, a nurse, who coined the title *public health nurse*. Wald used the word *public* so that all people would know that this type of service was available to them (Haupt, 1953). Wald claimed that she selected the title *public health nurse* to emphasize the community value of the nurse, whose service attitudes were built on an understanding of the social and economic problems associated with illness and disease.

Wald and Brewster developed a model based on the premise that nurses should be available to anyone who needed them, without the intervention of a doctor, thereby highlighting nursing as an independent profes-

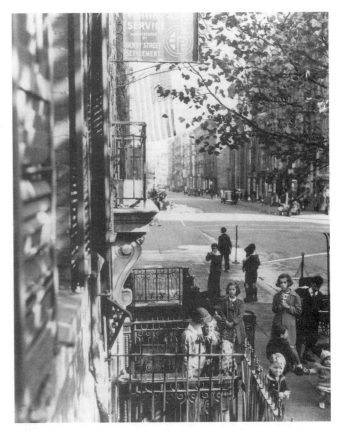

Nurses at the Henry Street Settlement in New York City.
Photo courtesy of the Visiting Nurse Service of New York.

sion. Wald's settlement house was different from the other visiting nursing services of that time, the latter of which were associated with sectarian organizations or dispensaries. Wald believed that the nursing agency should not be associated with a religious institution or with one physician. Further, she believed that nurses should live in the neighborhood where they provided services in order to more fully understand the needs of the families they served. Both Wald and Brewster lived in the area of the Henry Street Settlement.

Like Nightingale, Lillian Wald and Mary Brewster were wealthy young women and trained nurses who traveled a different path than did many other women in their social class. They were very concerned about the care of the poor, who faced overwhelming physical, social, emotional, and economic problems. Henry Street Settlement went beyond the individual efforts of community health nurses of earlier times. Lillian Wald had a vision that public health nurses would be available to those in need in homes, in workplaces, in schools, on street corners, in clinics—anywhere that people in need lived, worked, played, and died.

As director of the Henry Street Settlement House, Wald is legendary not only for her nursing accomplishments but also for her dedication to social reform. Wald and Brewster's collective vision focused not only on direct care and cure activities with families but also on education and the alleviation of the social causes of disease.

Perspectives...

Excerpt from *The House on Henry Street*

From the schoolroom where I had been giving a lesson in bedmaking, a little girl led me one drizzling March morning. She had told me of her sick mother, and gathering from her incoherent account that a child had been born, I caught up the paraphernalia of the bedmaking lesson and carried it with me.

The child led me over broken roadways—there was not asphalt, although its use was well established in other parts of the city—over dirty mattresses and heaps of refuse—it was before Colonel Waring had shown the possibility of clean streets even in that quarter—between tall, reeking houses whose laden fire-escapes, useless for their appointed purpose, bulged with household goods of every description. The rain added to the dismal appearance of the streets and to the discomfort of the crowds which thronged them, intensifying the odors which assailed me from every side. Through Hester and Division streets we went to the end of Ludlow; past odorous fishstands, for the streets were a market-place, unregulated, unsupervised, unclean; past evil-smelling, uncovered garbage-cans; and—perhaps worst of all, where so many little children played—past the trucks brought down from more fastidious quarters and stalled on these already overcrowded streets, lending themselves inevitably to many forms of indecency. The child led me on through a tenement hallway, across a court where open and unscreened closets were promiscuously used by men and women, up into a rear tenement, by slimy steps whose accumulated dirt was augmented that day by the mud of the streets, and finally into the sickroom.

All the maladjustments of our social and economic relations seemed epitomised in this brief journey and what was found at the end of it. The family to which the child led me was neither criminal nor vicious. Although the husband was a cripple, one of those who stand on street corners exhibiting deformities to enlist compassion, and masking the begging of alms by a pretense at selling; although the family of seven shared their two rooms with boarders—who were literally boarders, since a piece of timber was placed over the floor for them to sleep on—and although the sick woman lay on a wretched unclean bed, soiled with a hemorrhage two days old, they were not degraded human beings, judged by any measure of moral values.

In fact, it was very plain that they were sensitive to their condition, and when, at the end of my ministrations, they kissed my hands (those who have undergone similar experiences will, I am sure, understand), it would have been some solace if by any conviction of the moral unworthiness of the family I could have defended myself as a part of a society which permitted such conditions to exist. Indeed, my subsequent acquaintance with them revealed the fact that miserable as their state was, they were not without ideals for the family life, for society, of which they were so unloved and unlovely a part.

That morning's experience was a baptism of fire. Deserted were the laboratory and the academic of the college. I never returned to them. On my way to my comfortable student quarters my mind was intent on my own responsibility. To my inexperience it seemed certain that conditions such as these were allowed because people did not know, and for me there was a challenge to know and to tell. When early morning found me still awake, my naive conviction remained that, if people knew things—and "things" meant everything implied in the condition of this family—such horrors would cease to exist, and I rejoiced that I had had a training in the care of the sick that itself would give me an organic relationship to the neighborhood in which this awakening had come.

To the first sympathetic friend to whom I poured forth my story, I found myself presenting a plan which had been developing almost without conscious mental direction on my part.

—Lillian Wald

From The House on Henry Street *(pp. 4–9) by L. Wald, 1971, New York: Dover Publications. (Original work published 1915, New York: Henry Holt.) Copyright 1971 by Dover. Used with permission.*

Wald and Brewster both recognized that their activities influenced the making of health policy.

The work of Lillian Wald and the other nurses at Henry Street Settlement ultimately led to the first White House Conference for Children, held in 1909. Wald's political ingenuity and social activism contributed to the creation of the Children's Bureau, established by Congress in 1912 to oversee child labor laws that focused on the well-being of children (Kelly, 1981). Wald was also recognized for her contribution to improving housing conditions in tenement districts; establishing city recreation centers; instituting classes for handicapped children; and improving services to immigrants.

Wald supported the teaching of public health nursing courses at Teacher's College, Columbia University, and was the founder of the National Organization for Public Health Nursing, serving as its first president (Kaufman, Hawkins, Higgins, & Friedman, 1988). Wald's two-pronged approach helped shape nursing practice—practice that went beyond simply caring for families during illness episodes to the practice of social activism, encompassing an agenda for reform in the health industry, in recreation, in education, and in housing.

Wald's friend Lavinia Dock, a nurse who practiced at Henry Street Settlement, was also a social activist and an early feminist. Although she was vocal regarding many social issues, Dock saw the disenfranchisement of women as central to the issues in nursing and society in the early years of the 20th century. As such, she was committed to women's suffrage and participated actively in protests and demonstrations until the 1920 passage of the 19th amendment to the U.S. Constitution, which gave women the right to vote. Dock's vocal active role regarding suffrage served to alienate other nursing leaders of the time.

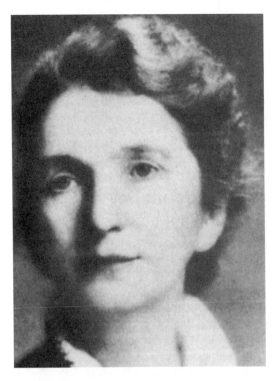

Margaret Sanger. *Photo courtesy of American Nurses Association.*

The expanding concept of public health coupled with the valuable contributions of nurses at Henry Street Settlement as well as of visiting nurses in district nursing organizations led to the direct employment of nurses by official health departments in the United States. The service provided, however, was visiting nursing care for the sick poor rather than educational or health-promotion activities such as those that Wald had incorporated in New York City. The first official public health nurse, paid for by tax funds and responsible to the health officer, was assigned to the Los Angeles Settlement Association in 1898. By 1913, as more nurses were employed, the health department added a bureau of municipal nursing. The first state to legally approve public health nurse employment by local boards of health was Alabama in 1907 (Hanlon, 1964).

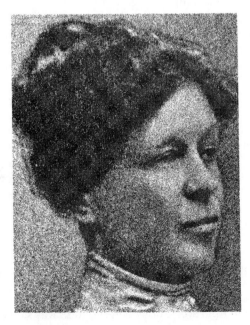

Lavina Lloyd Dock. *Photo courtesy of American Nurses Association.*

☙❧ REFLECTIVE THINKING ☙❧

Visions of Nursing Leaders

It is important to examine the visions of early nursing leaders and to consider how these visions might be relevant today.

- What relevance do the visions of the early community health nursing leaders hold for today?

- How do you think our public health problems today compare with those of Lillian Wald's period?

- What problems do you see in your own community? How should they be handled? By whom?

Margaret Sanger, another public health nurse who also played a politically important role in New York, was concerned about the health problems of factory workers. She was primarily concerned with those working poor women who had unwanted pregnancies. Sanger was instrumental in promoting public birth control education and access. A social and political activist, Sanger opened the first birth control clinic in the United States, in Brooklyn, New York (Kelly, 1971).

Expanding Community Health Services

In 1909, the effectiveness of health visits by nurses in preventing disease and death among the poor was recognized. Lillian Wald and Lee Frankel, founder of the Metropolitan Life Insurance Company, Welfare Division, proposed to the Metropolitan Life Insurance Company board of directors that providing nursing services to its policyholders could be a cost-effective investment because doing so could reduce mortality and would limit the benefits paid by the company. Wald and Frankel recommended that Metropolitan Life hire visiting nurses to care for policyholders during illness. The two principles underlying the insurance coverage for nursing services were that the company would utilize existing public health nursing services rather than employing their own, if at all possible, and that services would be available to anyone, with payment based on the ability to pay. Both of these principles continue today in health agencies in the United States.

Metropolitan Life Insurance Company began providing nursing services on an experimental, three-month basis in June 1909. Nurses from the Henry Street Settlement visited sick Metropolitan Life policyholders referred by agents in one section of the city. Results were compared with those for similar policyholders in another section of the city who did not receive nurse visits. The three-month experiment was such a success that the Metropolitan Life directors authorized an extension of the program to cover policyholders throughout the city (Hamilton, 1989), resulting in the first national system of insurance coverage for home-based care.

By 1911, Metropolitan Life started offering nursing services throughout the United States. Wherever possible, Metropolitan Life contracted with visiting nurse associations to provide care; when this was not possible, the insurance company employed its own nurses to provide care. By 1916, the services of a visiting nurse were available to 90% of the insurance company's 10.5 million policyholders in 2,000 Canadian and U.S. cities. By 1925, Metropolitan Life reported that 240,000 lives had been saved, translating to an estimated savings of $43 million for the company (Hamilton, 1989).

For many years, Metropolitan Life Insurance Company financed approximately one third of the budgets of most visiting nurse associations. After 44 successful years, the Metropolitan project ended in 1953. The shift from volun-

tary responsibility for health care to professional community organizations was one of the major reasons for the change. The Metropolitan project, however, demonstrated how nursing and a business endeavor could work together to accomplish their goals; contributed to the establishment of a cost-accounting system for visiting nurse associations that is still in use today; demonstrated that nursing services could reduce deaths from infectious diseases; and educated nurses in relation to marketing services and recruitment (Haupt, 1953).

School Nursing

The health of mothers and children was yet another concern of Lillian Wald and other social activists of her time. The nurses from Henry Street Settlement and other service programs identified children who had been excluded from school because of illness. (The preceding perspective box, which contains an excerpt from Lillian Wald's notes, highlights the conditions in which some children were living.)

By 1902, the health conditions of school children in New York City, for example, were of major concern. Many students had diseases such as pediculosis, trachoma, ringworm, scabies, and impetigo. Fifteen to 20 children in each school were being sent home daily. This high level of school absence due to the childhood illnesses convinced Wald to contact Dr. Lederle, Commissioner of Health in New York City, whom she convinced to try a school nursing experiment (Buhler-Wilkerson, 1985).

Lina Rogers, a public health nurse from Henry Street Settlement, was loaned to the New York City Health Department to work in a school (Dock & Stewart, 1925). Subsequently, other nurses from Henry Street Settlement were assigned to three other New York City schools in a pilot project. This project was so successful that school nurses were hired on a widespread basis. These nurses provided health teaching to students and their families, treated minor infections, and performed physical assessments.

The concept of school nursing soon spread to other parts of the United States. Los Angeles became the first city to hire nurses in schools (Gardner, 1952). School nursing began with an emphasis on preventing the spread of communicable diseases and treating other problems associated with school-age children. By the 1930s, however, school nursing also incorporated a focus on health-promotion activities such as casefinding, integrating healthy lifestyle concepts in the curriculum, and maintaining a safe and healthy physical school environment (Igoe, 1980).

Rural Nursing

In cities and towns, public health nursing was developing rapidly; in rural areas, however, progress was slower. The first rural nursing service was established by Ellen Morris Wood in Westchester County, New York, in 1896. In 1906, a nursing service for both the well-to-do and the poor was started in Salisbury, Connecticut.

In addition to her work in the city, Lillian Wald was also concerned about providing health services to those in rural areas. In 1912, she asked her wealthy friend Jacob Shiff to donate money to the American Red Cross so that it could establish a rural nursing service. She was successful in her actions, convincing the American Red Cross to direct its attention to creating a new department, the Town and Country Nursing Service. The service extended community health nursing services to rural areas (Brainard, 1985). The purpose of the service was to provide rural areas and small towns with public health nurses and to supervise the work of these nurses. The Town and Country Nursing Service later became known as the Bureau of Public Health Nursing.

Another important development in the expansion of rural nursing and community health outreach programs was the work of a nurse named Mary Breckinridge. Breckinridge played a vital role in community health by founding the Frontier Nursing Service (FNS) of Kentucky. She was committed to promoting the health care of disadvantaged women and children and used part of the money left to her by her grandmother to start the FNS (Browne, 1966).

The first health center organized by Breckinridge was established in a five-room cabin in Kentucky in 1925. By 1930, six outpost nursing centers had been built. Through fund-raising efforts, Breckinridge was able to provide leadership in establishing medical, surgical, and dental clinics and 24-hour nursing and midwifery services, serving nearly 10,000 people over 700 square miles. The FNS continues today, playing a vital role in the delivery of community health nursing services.

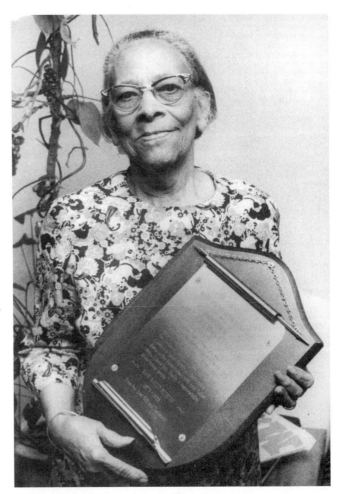

Mabel K. Staupers. *Photo courtesy of Foundation of the New York State Nurses Association, Guilderland, NY.*

Occupational Health Nursing

Occupational health nursing is another area of focus in community health nursing. Margaret Sanger, PHN, was instrumental in addressing the health problems of factory workers (women, in particular) in the lower East Side of Manhattan. In addition, Vermont's Governor Proctor hired nurses to address the health needs among those who lived in the villages associated with the Vermont Marble Company (Novak, 1988). By 1897 the Employees Benefit Association of John Wanamaker's department store in New York City had hired nurses to provide services to employees in their homes. These nurses soon expanded their role to include disease and injury prevention and first aid in the workplace. From 1910 to 1919, the number of firms employing nurses grew from 66 to 871 (Brainard, 1985).

Equality in Nursing and Services to Special-Population Groups

In the early 1900s, injustices in the U.S. health care system were apparent, particularly in relation to community health services for African Americans and the poor. Mabel K. Staupers recognized these injustices and devoted her life to improving community health services for African Americans in Philadelphia and Harlem (Mosley, 1995). She is recognized as a renowned nursing leader who clearly demonstrated caring in practice.

When Staupers was 13, her family moved to Harlem from the British West Indies. After completing her high-school education, she decided to become a nurse. In 1914, segregation in schools of nursing limited African American women's choices to Chicago, New York, and Washington, D.C. Mabel attended and graduated in 1917 from the Training School for Nurses at Freedman's Hospital in Washington, D.C. (Mosley, 1995).

Like many African American nurses at that time, Staupers, after receiving her nursing diploma, was employed primarily to care for patients of her own race in hospitals and in private duty nursing. Staupers worked as a nurse in the District of Columbia area until 1920, when she returned to New York City and noted the living and health conditions in the African American community. In Harlem alone, many African American women were dying from childbirth complications. The mortality rate from tuberculosis among African Americans of all ages was three to four times that of the general population of New York

City. In fact, tuberculosis was Harlem's major killer (Harding, 1926).

Health services in the Harlem community were very limited (Mosley, 1995). Staupers joined two physicians, Louis T. Wright and James L. Wilson, in opening the Booker T. Washington Sanitorium, the first African American–owned and African American–managed hospital in Harlem. She served as director of nurses there, helping to relieve the suffering among the people in the community.

Staupers later left the sanatorium. After working for a time in Philadelphia as a director of nurses, Staupers returned to New York, where she was hired to work with the New York Tuberculosis and Health Association. She conducted a survey of Harlem's community health needs, and, as a result, the Harlem Committee of the New York Tuberculosis and Health Association was established in 1922 (Osofsky, 1966).

According to Osofsky (1966), the major efforts of the Harlem Committee focused on eradicating tuberculosis. The committee, however, did not view its role as being limited to this cause and subsequently organized health clinics to provide services ranging from social hygiene and nutrition to prenatal care. Serving as the executive secretary of the committee for 12 years, Staupers attracted public attention and was commended for her work. She organized health-education activities provided in churches, schools, and other organizations. She also helped organize free prenatal dental care for expectant mothers who were registered with the Visiting Nurse Association; free dental service for children in schools; neighborhood health-education programs in Harlem; a health-examination service; nutrition classes for children; a free diagnostic clinic for those unable to pay; and a health-information program (Kiernan, 1952). Eventually, the various services developed by Staupers became a part of the Central Harlem Health Center.

In addition to her outstanding leadership in community health characterized by her efforts to establish community-based outreach health care services in Harlem, Staupers was also an activist in the struggle for equality in the professionalization of African American nurses, who sought the opportunity to work in a variety of agencies. In 1934, Staupers was appointed the first nurse executive of the National Association of Colored Graduate Nurses

(NACGN); in 1949, she was elected president. Staupers was a very active executive director and president, significantly influencing the professional process for African American nurses in relation to job placement, promotion, educational opportunities, and curriculum improvements in African American schools of nursing. Among the American Nurses Association, the National League for Nursing Education, and the National Organization for Public Health Nursing, Staupers also made significant inroads in increasing awareness of the problems encountered by African American nurses (Mosley, 1995).

NURSING ORGANIZATIONS AND NURSING EDUCATION

Beginning in the late 19th century in the United States and Canada, the value of organized efforts among nurses was recognized. In 1893, Isabel Hampton Robb led the effort to create the American Society of Superintendents of Training Schools of Nursing in the United States and Canada. This society, which later became known as the National League for Nursing (NLN) (Goldwater & Zusy, 1990; Kelly, 1991), established training standards and promoted collaborative relationships among nurses. In 1895, the Nurses Association Alumnae of the United States and Canada was formed, later becoming the American Nurses Association (ANA). The purposes of this organization were to strengthen nursing organizations, promote ethical standards, and improve nursing education (Lancaster, 1996).

By 1911, efforts were being made to standardize nursing services outside the hospital. A joint committee was organized with representatives from the ANA and the American Society of Superintendents of Training Schools. Lillian Wald served as chairperson. The committee recommended the formation of a new organization to meet the needs of community health nurses. After considerable discussion with representatives of such organizations as city and state boards of health and education, visiting nurse associations, tuberculosis leagues, hospitals, dispensaries, day nurseries, settlements, and churches and other charitable organizations, the National Organization of Public Health Nursing (NOPHN) was formed. This was the first national nursing organization to have a paid staff and a designated headquarters (Fagin, 1978).

Following the development of the NOPHN, public health nursing expanded to meet societal needs. Allen (1991) points out the ways whereby the development of district nursing, and later public health nursing, fostered the concepts inherent in holistic nursing. To public health nursing, nursing meant caring for the whole person, family, friends, neighbors, and the community in relation to health and illness needs. As Allen comments:

The ideas of wholeness implicit in the public health nursing movement were important in providing its direction, significant in the notion that it was a type of nursing set apart and above other specialties, and

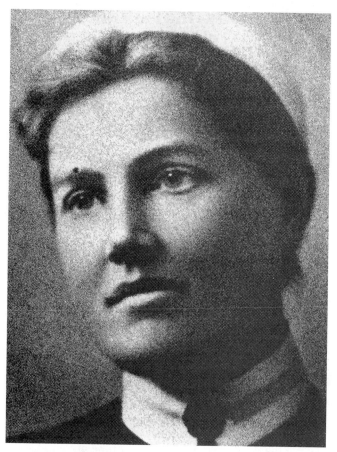

Isabel Hampton Robb. *Photo courtesy of American Nurses Association.*

crucial to the movement of nursing education into the universities and nursing's recognition as a profession (p. 75).

It became apparent that public health nursing called for special educational preparation. Traditionally, all nurses were prepared in apprentice-type programs in hospitals. The curriculum was determined by hospital needs and under the direction of physicians. The focus of study was individual-illness–oriented and did not adequately prepare the nurse to provide services in a community setting. Public health nurses in the community functioned more independently, performed casefinding and health teaching, made referrals, and viewed their domain as the community—serving individuals, families, and population aggregates from a holistic perspective.

With the recognition that community health nurses needed additional preparation beyond the hospital-based curriculum, nursing leaders in the United States, after considerable debate, decided that all nurses needed some community health training. Basic undergraduate courses began to include community health in the curriculum, with Boston offering the first undergraduate community health nursing course (Lancaster, 1996).

As community health nursing grew, and the broad scope of community health nursing became more apparent, the need for postgraduate work in community nursing also became apparent. In 1910, Mary Adelaide Nutting

started the first postgraduate community health nursing course at Teacher's College in conjunction with the Henry Street Settlement (Deloughery, 1977). Because of community health nursing's concerns with social and educational problems, many of the early university-based public health nursing programs were offered through teacher's colleges or university departments of social work in sociology. By 1921, 15 colleges and universities in the United States offered courses in public health nursing, meeting the standards set forth by the NOPHN (Jensen, 1959).

In 1923, a landmark study called the Report of the Committee for Study of Nursing Education was published. This study, which began in 1919, came to be known as the Goldmark Report. Under the auspices of the Rockefeller Foundation, the Committee for the Study of Public Health Nursing Education began with a focus on public health nursing education. The following year, however, the focus expanded to nursing education in general. The report findings affected not only public health nursing but all of nursing as well. The report recommended that nursing education take place in institutions of higher learning. Subsequently, Yale University School of Nursing and the Frances Payne Bolton School of Nursing at Case Western Reserve University opened in 1923. Community health nursing content was included in both programs (Tinkham & Voorhies, 1977).

In addition to the offering of community health nursing content at institutions of higher learning, a change in the employment of public health nurses occurred in the 1920s. Prior to this time, most public health nursing services were provided by voluntary agencies such as the American Red Cross and other organizations. During the 1920s, however, official governmental agencies such as local and state health departments began to incorporate public health nursing services (Tinkham & Voorhies, 1977).

Schools of nursing expanded throughout the United States during the 1920s. Collegiate programs in nursing increasingly included content in public health, with the first basic collegiate program in nursing accredited in 1944. That program included adequate preparation in community health so that graduates did not have to take additional courses to practice public health nursing (National Organization of Public Health Nursing, 1944). Beginning in 1963, the NLN required baccalaureate nursing programs to include public health nursing content and practice in order to be considered for accreditation.

THE INFLUENCE OF THE WAR YEARS ON COMMUNITY HEALTH NURSING

Both World War I and World War II affected the development of public health programs and of community health nursing. This section illustrates the particular ways that many aspects of community health nursing and life in general changed because of these wars.

World War I and After

By the time World War I began in 1917, the role of the community health nurse was well established. The onset of World War I, however, required thousands of nurses to work for the war effort, leaving very few to provide services in the public health setting. The American Red Cross helped maintain community health nursing by establishing a roster of nurses who could be asked to supply health care services. These services focused on educational programs for the community as well as the control of communicable diseases (Roberts, 1954).

During World War I, a nurse was loaned to the U.S. Public Health Service from the NOPHN to establish a community health nursing program for military outposts. This program resulted in the first community health service to become a part of the federal government (Gardner, 1919).

After World War I, many changes occurred that affected community health nursing, such as economic prosperity and the use of the automobile. The automobile enabled nurses to reach rural areas and to provide services to those in areas that were less accessible. Public health services expanded throughout the nation. Many federally funded relief projects utilized nurses, resulting in the recognition that federally employed nurses were needed to provide consultation to the states. Public health, as noted by Smillie (1952), became a subject of nationwide interest and importance. By 1920, 28 states had statewide public health nursing programs; 5 of these states included divisions of public health nursing within their state health departments (Roberts, 1954).

One of the major events that also occurred after World War I was the Great Depression. By the early 1930s, the effects of the Depression were clearly evident. Salaries decreased, unemployment was rising, and public health nursing services had to be reduced. Because public health nursing had formulated its objectives, however, and had developed a sound basis for organization, it was able to withstand the Depression. The need for services increased, and public health nursing was able to respond (Tinkham & Voorhies, 1977). The results of the Depression required that the federal government assume more responsibility for the general welfare of the people, largely because there was a growing realization that the good of the people was central to the government's mission (Tinkham & Voorhies, 1977).

In 1934, Pearl McIver, a well-qualified public health nurse, became the first nurse employed by the U.S. Public Health Service to provide consultant services to the states for nurses working in federal relief projects. Prior to 1936, as noted by Lancaster (1996), "only a few states had budgeted community health nursing positions" (p. 13). By 1936, however, all states were allocating budget funds for some type of public health nursing consultant position.

In 1930, the National Institutes of Health (NIH) was created, providing federal support for health care research in the United States. After the Great Depression of the 1930s, the federal government expanded health and social welfare programs. The first of these initiatives was the Social Security Act in 1935, which addressed the financial needs of elders through the Old Age, Survivors, and Disability Insurance (OASDI) program. In 1966, the Social Security Act was amended to create the Medicare program, which provides health care insurance for older Americans. In 1967, Medicaid was passed to provide health insurance for low-income Americans.

World War II and After

After World War II began in 1941, many nurses joined the army and navy nurse corps. In response to the increased need for nurses, the National Nursing Council, comprising six national nursing organizations, assisted by the U.S. Department of Education, asked for and received $1 million to increase nursing-education facilities. The U.S. Public Health Service administered these nursing-education funds.

World War II, like World War I and the Great Depression, had a major effect on community health nursing. Specifically, the war resulted in an expansion of community health nursing practice and health care delivery. The prosperous postwar economy affected community health nursing practice. Furthermore, even greater numbers of community health nurses found it possible to see far more people thanks to the increased use of the automobile.

A particularly important effect of World War II on community health nursing had to do with returning veterans. During the war, approximately 15 million U.S. servicemen were exposed to quality health care, some of them for the first time. Further, wartime service called attention to the poor health of many young and middle-aged males. The high-quality, broader scope of care received by veterans during the war led them to expect the same on the home front. Local health departments thus soon found themselves besieged not only by a burgeoning group of clients who expected high-quality services but also by a sudden increase in accidents, emotional problems, alcoholism, and other health problems not previously considered to be a part of their responsibility (Roberts & Heinrich, 1985).

When the war was over in 1945, President Harry Truman presented to Congress the following proposals for a health care system (Kalisch & Kalisch, 1982):

1. Prepayment of medical costs with compulsory insurance and general revenues
2. Protection from loss of wages as a result of sickness
3. Expansion of services related to the public's health, including maternal and child health services
4. Governmental aid to medical schools for research
5. Increased construction of hospitals, clinics, and medical institutions (p. 21)

National health insurance was proposed; however, charges of socialism from the American Medical Association ended the debate about national coverage in 1949 and 1950 (Kalisch & Kalisch, 1995). But increased demand for services led to an increase in funding for specific health problems such as venereal disease, cancer, tuberculosis, and mental illness. Increased demand also led to new arrangements for financing health care and a subsequent expansion of the health insurance industry (Ginzberg, 1985).

Local health departments also increased significantly in the United States. By 1955, 72% of all counties in the continental United States had full-time local public health services, with public health nurses composing a large proportion of the staffing. During the 1950s, interest increased in nurse midwifery, equality and advancement of African American nurses in public health, cost analysis studies, and improved coordination of organized nursing (Roberts & Heinrich, 1985).

The 1960s brought a revolution in health care in the United States that affected public health and public health nursing. The Economic Opportunity Act provided funds for neighborhood health centers, Head Start, and many other community programs designed to improve the health of the community. Programs for maternal and child health, mental health, mental retardation, and public health training also saw increases in funding. New programs funded care for elders and the poor. As Lancaster (1992) notes, however, the revised act did not include coverage for preventive health care, and home health care was reimbursed only when ordered by a physician. Funding for home health services, however, resulted in the rapid expansion of home health agencies, including for-profit agencies. At the same time, however, there was a decline in many health-promotion and disease-prevention activities because of limited funding. Today, home health care is one of the major growth areas in the health care industry.

In 1965, the nurse practitioner movement began at the University of Colorado, with the development of the first pediatric nurse practitioner program. This program prepared nurses to provide comprehensive well-child care in ambulatory settings (Ford & Silver, 1967). This development set the stage for nursing's role expansion into providing primary health care to select populations. The early public health movement was the forerunner of today's primary care movement (Fagin, 1978). Public health nurses were the first nurse practitioners, and although many remained in public health, others left to work in a variety of clinical arenas. In public health agencies, nurse practitioners have continued to play an important role in providing primary health care to individuals and families in inner cities, rural areas, and other underserved areas.

In the 1970s, community health nurses played important roles in the hospice movement, the birthing center initiative, drug and substance abuse programs, day care for elders and those with disabilities, and rehabilitation services in long-term care (Roberts & Heinrich, 1985). Prevention once again was viewed as critical at the federal level, and cost effectiveness emerged as a new concern for health care. Because nurses were viewed as cost-effective providers of primary care, the way was cleared for community nursing to expand into new areas.

REFLECTIVE THINKING

Community Health Nursing Contributions

• What characteristics do you think community health nurses must have in order to be effective in the health care arena?

• How do you think nurses might participate in improving the health of their communities?

In this new economic climate, nurses in other specialty areas of nursing, including medical-surgical, maternal and child health, and psychiatric, began to work with individuals and families outside the hospital setting (Ruth & Partridge, 1978). Public health nurses had been the first to promote the idea that nursing could best meet the total health needs of people, and their focus continued to include aggregates as well as individuals and families in the community.

THE INFLUENCES OF THE 1980s AND 1990s

The 1980s ushered in a period of change throughout the world. The Healthy Cities concept linked the Health Care for All initiative to an implementation model that is being utilized today as a model for change and development in community health.

In the United States, cost effectiveness of health care became a major concern. Health-promotion and disease-prevention programs were assigned lower priority as funding was shifted to meet increased costs of hospital care and technological medical procedures. In 1983, a prospective payment system for hospital care based on diagnosis related groups (DRGs) was instituted under Medicare. Ambulatory services and home health care grew rapidly. People were more often expected to assume caregiving roles for family members and for themselves. Health education, a major role of public health nursing since Lillian Wald's time, became more important. Self-care became more of a focus in health care approaches. With decreased funding came fewer nurses in official public health agencies. The number of nurses in home health care, however, increased. Other community outreach centers were developed, such as community nursing centers and linkages with schools.

The 1990s brought restructuring of the health care systems in the United States and other Western nations, a process that continues today. Increasingly, nursing care is being delivered in community settings, with greater emphasis being placed on primary health care, case management, long-term care management, and the care of the acutely ill in their homes and in other ambulatory settings.

It is projected that consumers in the future will play an even more important role as informed participants in making decisions about their own care. In addition,

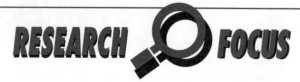

The Caring Connection in Nursing: A Concept Analysis

STUDY PROBLEM/PURPOSE

The concept of connection has been used in the nursing literature in the context of a caring relationship in nursing; however, the concept needs further description. Because caring is viewed as the essence of nursing, it is important to examine the concept of connection within the caring context. The purpose of this study was to conduct a concept analysis in order to explicate the concept of "connection" in relation to the caring literature in nursing.

METHODS

The process of concept analysis was used, incorporating the methods of Walker and Avant (1995) and Rodgers (1989). Publications for the proceedings of the Caring Conferences for the International Association for Human Caring over the past two decades were the primary sources of information and CINAHL was used to search the nursing literature for the key word *connection* under the subject of caring.

FINDINGS

The concept analysis of connection was identified as a dynamic concept that has different meanings depending on whether the term is used as a verb or a noun. Connection was viewed as an outcome, a consequence of the process of connecting. Establishing a meaningful connection with the client was one of five conceptualizations found in the nursing literature.

Critical attributes, the process attributes (those related to connecting) included (1) effective communication skills (being present, empowering, attending, listening) and (2) intentionality (involves choice or the decision by the nurse to engage in the nurse–client relationship; includes co-presence, depth in the relationship, and transcendence).

As an outcome, connections included synchrony, rhythm, harmony, and unity. Connection enables healing.

IMPLICATIONS

The concept of connection is one that can be most important in nursing education and practice, a concept that is central to the caring mission of nursing. The moments of connection make a difference in the lives of individuals and families, moments that can be ones of healing and transcendence. The concept of connection in nursing is embedded in the caring literature. The special moments shared with clients can be ones of harmony, healing, and diminishing of vulnerability, thereby fostering opportunities to enhance healing. Establishing connections with clients should be modeled by experienced nurses and nourished in beginning nurses. The caring connection in nursing is needed.

SOURCE

From "The Caring Connection in Nursing: A Concept Analysis" by M. H. Wilde, 1997, International Journal for Human Caring 1(1), pp. 18–24.

---

ambulatory, primary health care systems are expected to assume an increasingly significant place in health care. These projections apply not only in the United States but also in Australia, Canada, Great Britain, and other Western nations. One of the major reasons for the reconfiguration of health care delivery systems is cost containment. Community health nurses, as well as other nurses, are in a prime position to assist in the paradigm shift. Nurses must, however, take leadership roles in emphasizing the need for humanistic care and practice, rather than focusing primarily on the principles of economic rationalism. Community health nurses will have to cooperate with other health professionals and consumers in order to develop comprehensive advocacy programs that will promote and protect the health of people.

At the National and International Case Management Conference in Melbourne, Australia, in July 1995, participants from Australia, Great Britain, and the United States talked about practice issues, ideas, and concerns related to health care practice and the need for case management. Various case-management models were discussed, whether the setting was long-term care, ambulatory care, acute care, or home care. A focus on consumer needs and on a more community-responsive system that encourages consumer decision making was stressed. Nursing was identified as central to the process of working together with other disciplines in ensuring that consumers receive comprehensive care in a seamless system. Health providers and consumers alike recognize that the health care system is difficult to negotiate and that consumers clearly need

COMMUNITY NURSING VIEW

A public health nurse is working in a neighborhood of ethnically diverse, low-income people. The nurse makes home visits to various clients, including 75-year-old Emanuel, who receives assistance from an in-home support service program. Emanuel lives alone in an apartment and has a history of alcohol abuse, which has been successfully treated. He attends Alcoholics Anonymous. He has a variety of medical problems that require long-term care-management services. The nurse has been visiting Emanuel in his home for the past month.

During the nurse's most recent home visit, Joan, a neighbor from next door, makes a visit to Emanuel's home. Before the nurse leaves, Joan asks the nurse to take her blood pressure. Joan complains that she has been having headaches and blurred vision for the past two days, is worried about her blood pressure, and will soon be evicted from her apartment with nowhere to go. Joan states that she lives alone, has a car, and may be forced to stay in a storage room. Joan says that she understands that public health nurses help people in need of services. When asked about access to health care, Joan states that she receives medical care from a nonprofit health maintenance organization (HMO) in the same town but that she has neither seen nor called her doctor yet. "I have been so busy and so stressed. I know I should have gone or at least called. I thought that you could help me when Emanuel told me you would be visiting today." This is the first time that the nurse has met Joan.

Nursing Considerations
ASSESSMENT
- What additional data are needed to assess Joan's situation?
- How would a knowledge of community health nursing history affect assessment in this situation?

DIAGNOSIS
- On the basis of the information given, what diagnosis would be made?

OUTCOME IDENTIFICATION
- What outcome would be expected for Joan?

PLANNING/INTERVENTIONS
- How might the issue of impending homelessness be addressed?
- How might the public health nurse respond to this situation?
- What actions might be taken?

EVALUATION
- What would indicate that the plan and intervention were successful?

assistance in moving through the system. Community health nurses have played and continue to play an important role in this process.

A basic principle of community health nursing, then, is to understand the concerns of the people they serve. The community health nurse sees where people work, play, worship, live, study, and die. Community health nurses work with groups, families, and individual clients as well as function in multidisciplinary teams and programs. They participate in identifying the strengths of the communities they serve as well as in defining and addressing health problems. They have worked and continue to work with people in their own environments.

Community health nurses have fostered the caring, healing, and health model of nursing, a model that must once again come to the forefront. In the early days, community health nurses worked to create community models of caring. Today, community health nurses must partici-pate with other disciplines and with consumers in creating healthier communities, with health viewed in its broadest sense, from a holistic perspective.

Key Concepts

- To understand the nature of community health nursing and future developments, one must examine the historical context of early public health and community health nursing efforts.
- A number of factors influenced the development of community health nursing: early Christianity, the Industrial Revolution, heightened public awareness of community problems, two major wars, a major economic depression, and social action on the part of community health nursing leaders.

- The Health for All and Healthy Cities initiatives are rooted in a spirit of partnership, collaboration, and consensus building.

- The mission of public health nursing has historically been twofold: personal advocacy and social activism.

- Since their inception, the roles of community health nurses have been multifaceted, complex, and challenging.

- Public health and community health nursing organizations matured as a result of both the vision of the nurses themselves and evolving community needs.

- The years during and after the two world wars brought expansion of health care concepts as well as new roles for community health nurses.

- An intersectoral approach to planning and implementing health care for all is basic to public health philosophy.

Health Care in the United States

This unit highlights the many dimensions of the United States health care system including the current health care delivery system, the steps being taken to change it, and the economic aspects that affect health care delivery.

UNIT II

Health Care Delivery in the United States

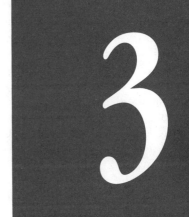

Carol A. Lockhart, PhD, RN, FAAN

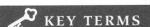
Many Americans are critical about our health care system. But not nearly as many are knowledgeable about it. Maybe I should call it our health scare system, or our health care non-system. Unfortunately, there is no system in the way Americans scramble for health care.

—*Koop, 1991, p. 302*

COMPETENCIES

Upon completion of this chapter, the reader should be able to:

- Describe how health services are planned and organized in the United States.
- Discuss the influence of the U.S. political culture on the health care system.
- Identify the role of health insurance and public health in providing access to health care services.
- Examine the definitions and incentives relating to managed care.
- Identify the types of health service organizations that deliver care.
- Describe the responsibilities of public health organizations at national, state, and local levels.
- Discuss the focus of community nursing organizations and centers and their potential role in health-service delivery.
- Discuss the influences on the consumer's choice of health services.
- Describe the paradigm shift that is beginning in health care.
- Describe the focus of community health nursing under the new paradigm.

Public health organizations and the community health nurses working within them are committed to caring for the populations, families, and individuals that make up a community. Most nations, particularly the industrialized nations, have an organized national health system whose goal is to deliver the full range of available care to its citizens. Through such a system, the government defines and sets national health goals that are supported by modifying the national system. Although the goals are not always achieved, there exists a national direction and plan for the health care offered to the citizens of the given country.

This, however, is not true of the United States. Whereas we do deliver sophisticated and technologically advanced health care services and, in many senses, the best individualized care in the world, we do not have a national system for delivering that care or for ensuring our population's health and well-being. A system presumes ". . . a coordinated body of methods or a scheme or plan of procedures" (Random House Webster's College Dictionary, 1992, p. 1356). In the United States, health care is treated as a private business rather than a publicly produced good or service that should be available in some coordinated way to all citizens as part of citizenship. A wide range of services are offered through individual private practitioners, organizations, and programs. Although services are sometimes coordinated between the various providers, this is usually not the case, and there exists no specific responsibility for doing so.

The federal government in the United States usually takes the lead in defining the health-related goals for the nation, as was done in the case of *Healthy People 2000: National Health Promotion and Disease Prevention Objectives* (U.S. Department of Health and Human Services [USDHH], 1990). Multiple private groups, associations, and like bodies, such as the National Academy of Science's Institute of Medicine, also provide overall public policy direction through publication of reports such as *The Future of Public Health* (Institute of Medicine, 1988). This report defines goals and a direction for public health into the next century. Accomplishing the suggested goals, however, is difficult because no nationally organized delivery system or responsible party is charged with achieving them, and there is no way to require private providers to work toward them.

This seemingly impossible and improbable situation constitutes the subject of this chapter. Community health nurses deal with whole communities, not just with single individuals, practitioners, or institutions. To be able to understand and assist a community to achieve or maintain a certain health status, community health nurses must know how health care is financed, organized, and delivered in the United States, including the strengths U.S. health care offers and the gaps or failures that limit it. This chapter, then, explores the ways that health care services are organized and delivered and the impact that this has on populations and on community health nursing practice.

HEALTH CARE IN THE UNITED STATES

Health care in the United States is provided by a wide range of people and encompasses both the organized health care services and the informal health care (attention and protection) offered by individuals, families, and friends. Self-care and the care offered to children, loved ones, and friends on a daily basis actually constitute the bulk of the health care provided in this country.

Organized health care services, including public health, are the organized delivery components of health care wherein services are offered by individual practitioners, organizations, and institutions to the client or consumer of the services (Rakich, Longest, & Darr, 1992). Increasingly, the dominant, Western **allopathic** (practices derived from scientific models and technology) medical model of health care is being challenged to acknowledge and incorporate alternative modes of care such as **osteopathy** (a system of medical practice based on the theory that diseases are due chiefly to a loss of structural integrity), **homeopathy**, [a system of medical practice that treats certain diseases by the administration of small doses of a

remedy (drugs) that would, in healthy persons, produce symptoms of the disease being treated] and **complementary** health care services such as those offered by Eastern medicine, traditional healers, and folk medicine. Complementary health care services are those not used in general medical practice and have not been tested by scientific study in the United States. These services are used by clients in addition to their mainstream medical care. In acknowledgment of this trend, the National Institutes of Health, the health research arm of the federal government, created an Office for Alternative Medicine in 1991. Further discussion of alternative/complementary care practices is included in Chapter 6.

Regardless of the health care model, payment to the provider of services may come wholly or in part from the individual, the employer, government tax revenue, or voluntary organizations that choose to support specific services as part of a charitable mission. These four types of payors finance the delivery of health care services in the United States (see Figure 3-1). Although the bulk of the money spent in the system goes to allopathic health care services, it is estimated that many billions of dollars are spent on alternative medicine, with the vast majority of this money coming from the individual's own pocket (Eisenberg, 1993). (See Chapter 4 for a more in-depth discussion of health economics.)

The Political Foundation of Health Care

No look at U.S. health care can be undertaken without first understanding the political context within which the delivery system developed. Elazar (1966) describes the political culture of this country as being one of: (1) individualism; (2) civil liberties; (3) equality (of process, not outcomes); (4) popular sovereignty and representative democracy; (5) belief in private property, capitalism, and the free market; (6) rationality, which is reflected in self-interest and competition; (7) a Protestant work ethic; and (8) separation of church and state. Our country is a federation of states whose citizens have chosen to decentralize power throughout federal, state, county, and local governments. Nowhere in our nation do we look to a central authority or body to dictate the lives of our citizens. Centralized control is against every belief and structure we have created as a nation.

Not surprisingly, then, the United States has consistently supported a health delivery approach that allows as much individual and state/local government control as possible. We have supported health care as a private business not only because we are a capitalist nation but also because this approach fits with the beliefs we hold about ourselves as individuals and about the role of government.

In the United States, government's role in our lives is generally expected to be limited rather than enhanced by public-policy decisions. Even when government's role is expanded, new programs are designed to fit with and build on existing law and on our independent and busi-

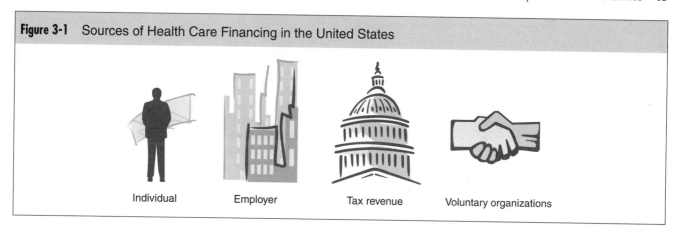

Figure 3-1   Sources of Health Care Financing in the United States

Individual   Employer   Tax revenue   Voluntary organizations

ness-centered market approach to health care. Incremental or gradual change rather than wholesale modification characterizes our political process. Proposals that seek to enlarge government—even generally positive federal and public health programs—are often criticized by legislators and individuals as being too intrusive and contrary to the political philosophy of the country. In the political environment of the 1980s and 1990s, federal programs have been changed to reduce the requirements that states must meet to qualify for program funding. Block grants (lump sums of money) or other approaches are allowing states to set their own rules and regulations to a significant degree. Welfare reform and Medicaid (health care for the poor) reforms that allow use of managed care are two examples of this reform trend.

Payors have financed the creation of a health system rich in resources. We have used those resources to develop medical research and technology that place us at the forefront of medical care and quality worldwide but that do not necessarily ensure optimal health-status outcomes for our people. We use billions of dollars each year to provide wonderful physical structures, machines and instruments, new pharmaceuticals, and well-prepared health professionals. We expect our science and technology to fix most things, including poor health and disease. But whether a person has access to all these riches and enjoys their benefits depends in great part on whether that person has insurance and where that person lives.

TYPES OF HEALTH INSURANCE AND THE UNINSURED

Nearly all health services in the United States are financed through private insurance purchased by an employer or through public insurance paid for with tax revenues from local, state, or federal taxes. A much more limited number of services are offered to the public as part of general public health programs or by charitable organizations.

Private insurance is offered by employers, usually with the employee paying some share of the premium cost. Employer-provided insurance covered 64% of the U.S. population under 65 in 1996, whereas individually purchased private insurance accounted for only 7.0% of the people insured during this same time period (Employee Benefit Research Institute, 1997). The Civilian Health and Medical Program of the Uniformed Services (CHAMPUS) functions like a private insurance plan but is actually a publicly funded insurance program for the U.S. military and their dependents. This program allows military personnel to obtain care in the private health care market. Approximately 2.9% (1997) of the insured population is covered by CHAMPUS, which like private insurance plans, has a specified list of benefits, payments, and requirements that may change slightly each year in response to financing and program modifications.

The federal Medicare and Medicaid programs, created in 1965, represent the bulk of publicly financed insurance. Medicare, Title XVIII of the Social Security Act of 1965, is the public insurance program for those over age 65 and others who have certain health conditions such as end-stage renal disease (ESRD). It is funded by federal taxes and by a premium for physician-related care (Medicare Part B) and hospital (Medicare Part A) deductibles paid by either the covered individual or, possibly, another governmental program such as Medicaid. Pharmaceuticals are not covered unless the insuree has agreed to participate in a managed care plan. Part A provides payment for hospital services, home health services, and extended care facilities. Part B provides coverage for physician services and for services other than hospitalization. It covered an estimated 37.5 million people in federal fiscal year 1996 (U.S. House of Representatives Committee on Ways and Means, 1996).

Medicaid (Title XIX of the Social Security Act of 1965) is the other major public insurance program, serving 12.1% of the populace under 65 (Employee Benefit Research Institute, 1997). Those eligible are deemed "the poor," but the definition of this designation is determined by and varies among the states. Medicaid, unlike Medicare, is a jointly funded federal and state program, with the federal government setting minimum requirements and the states setting the criteria for eligibility and service payment levels. The share each pays varies according to the services covered and the wealth of the state.

Federal health programs serve as a significant source of revenue for providers. All but a few people over age 65 and many disabled persons are on Medicare. Under Medicaid, once a person is determined eligible by virtue of income (means), the program will meet whatever health care costs are incurred. Both programs have seen increased costs and increased numbers as the elderly population grows and as new categories of eligible individuals are added to meet the continuing need for care by so many.

The Uninsured and the Underinsured

In a given year, somewhere between 80% and 85% of the population has access to insurance in one form or another. Some people, however, may lose their insurance for short or long periods for a variety of reasons, including (1) being unable to pay the premium; (2) having a **pre-existing condition** (health problem that was diagnosed or treated or that existed prior to issuance of an insurance policy) that an insurer either refuses to cover (thereby making the person uninsurable) or delays covering for fear that the insuree will need care and cost money; (3) becoming ineligible for Medicaid or some other government-related program; (4) changing jobs or going to work for a company that does not offer insurance, such as is often the case in farming, housekeeping, and other job situations where people are employed in low-wage jobs; or (5) going to work for an employer who passes most of the cost of insurance on to the employee, an expense that the employee cannot afford. In other words, an uninsured person may be almost anyone, and in 1996, the uninsured accounted for 17.7% of the population (Employee Benefit Research Institute, 1997).

Those who are unemployed, self-employed, or who work in small businesses often have difficulty buying health insurance because they lack the purchasing and bargaining power of large organizations. Many uninsured persons either have made too much money in the previous year to qualify for a public program or do not make enough money to feel that they can afford to purchase insurance on their own; and many of those who do purchase insurance are financially limited to buying policies that offer little in the way of services, in effect rendering insurees underinsured.

Yet another segment of the uninsured are employed by employers who do contribute to the cost of insurance, but these individuals are healthy and do not believe they will need care. They therefore choose not to use any of their income to buy health insurance. Young adults often fall into this category of the uninsured.

A number of health-reform efforts at both federal and state levels have repeatedly attempted to extend coverage to the uninsured and uninsurable. In the absence of some mandatory national or state programs, millions will at some time in their lives find themselves without health insurance coverage and therefore limited in the health care they can hope to receive.

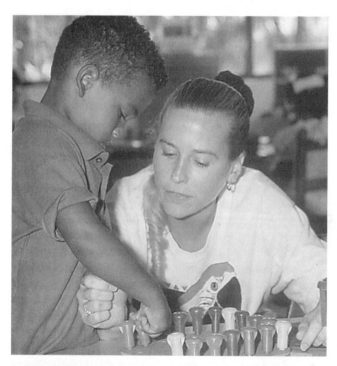

In order for this day care worker to have health care insurance, she must pay the entire cost herself. Unfortunately, her wage is not adequate to cover this expense along with her other living expenses. Consequently, she does without insurance.

Those persons without insurance, those denied insurance because of their health status, and those with inadequate insurance or with public or private insurance that purposely restricts access to certain care, to timely care, or to quantities of care are faced with rationing of the health services. Rationing is not new in the United States. For years the uninsured have been denied health services or have received limited services only. Although rationing in one form or another has always existed in the U.S. health system, not until the last 15 to 20 years has it been purposely used to help control ever-increasing health care costs. At one time, the ability to charge some payors higher prices left room for providers to offer services for free or at reduced cost to select clients. This practice of shifting the cost of care from one payor to another is becoming increasingly limited under current payment and delivery schemes such as managed care.

For the majority of employed insured individuals and families, the impact of rationing efforts is minimal or, at least, acceptable. These insurees pay a small portion of their health care costs—a portion that is within their financial means—and the insurance pays for most, if not all, of the costs associated with the services they require. For the uninsured and underinsured and for many persons covered by Medicare and Medicaid, sharing in the cost of care may be a much greater burden depending on the size of their share. Those who find the financial burden too great may forgo necessary care because of associated costs.

The proportion of the nation's income and expenditures that goes toward buying health care has steadily climbed over the years. At the same time, other things such as housing, food, and education continue to demand our dollars. Resources available to fund the health care system, thus, are not unlimited. This dictates judicious use of resources and services on the part of community health nurses and others who seek to ensure that the national population has access to needed services to ensure an acceptable health status.

HEALTH INSURANCE AND MANAGED CARE

Health insurance began in the 1930s as a plan to pay hospitals fees for services provided to clients. That plan (the third party) became Blue Cross. A short time later, a Blue Shield plan was developed to pay physicians fees (Williams & Torrens, 1999). Other insurance approaches grew out of these initial efforts.

Indemnity insurance plans (which pay a cash benefit to the insured) have largely used **fee-for-service (FFS)** payment approaches, wherein fees are paid for a single episode of care, mostly, acute episodes of care. As a payment system, insurance is not responsible for the health care delivery system that provides the care and coordinates its various components to ensure a person either stays well or is returned to maximum attainable health status. By adopting a fee-for-service payment approach,

providers of care had the opportunity to increase the number of single services they delivered in order to increase the number of fees received (income or profit). The more fees paid, the greater the revenue generated for the provider (physician, hospital, etc.) and the greater the cost to the insurance company and the private or public payor (individual, company, or government) purchasing the insurance. Utilization of health service increased under these conditions, as did the dollars spent to provide the services. This is the genesis of much of the concern regarding rising health service costs in the last quarter of this century, because the federal insurance schemes (Medicare, Medicaid, and CHAMPUS) and employer insurance traditionally used fee-for-service as their primary payment approach.

The rising cost of health care and the fragmentation and inefficiency of the existing health care delivery structure have prompted the largest payors for health care services (both employers and government) to question whether the current system deserves their support. Increasingly, they are turning to managed care in the hope that it will provide the quality and quantity of care needed to ensure people's health and well-being.

Managed care refers to a variety of organizational arrangements, some of which are even now evolving. Managed care, however, seeks to provide, coordinate, and manage the services offered to the client, all within one financing and delivery system. In other words, the financing, payment, and delivery components are all linked within the managed care plan and thus should be able to decrease episodes of fragmented care and unnecessary utilization while improving care cost efficiency and effectiveness.

By moving to managed care, payors change the financial and operating incentives facing providers. With managed care, a set price is established and prepaid (paid in advance) to the health corporation for the care being delivered. It may be paid per person or per head (**capitation**) on a monthly basis, per illness, per day, or per any defined group of services. Capitation refers to a health insurance mechanism wherein a fixed amount is paid per person to cover services. If the insuree does not need the care or uses only a little, the managed care plan still keeps the money paid to it. If the insuree uses more care than the total of the prepayment, the managed care organization must provide the necessary services and absorb the added cost. This is considered the risk managed care faces for doing business. Table 3-1 compares the potential consequences of the incentives that characterize the fee-for-service and managed care capitation approaches.

In addition to increased use of managed care, payors are using their purchasing power by banding together in business coalitions, alliances, and various affiliated groups to purchase care directly from networks of providers instead of insurance companies and managed care plans. Rather than having to take the price offered by an insurance company or plan, these large groups negotiate premium rates on their own. In some cases, these groups control the health care purchasing for so many people that they can, to a significant degree, set the price they are willing to pay. As networks, the managed care plans and insurance companies compete with each other to enroll employer, Medicaid, and Medicare clients. The effort by purchasers to introduce competition into a health care market that is seen as having little real competition is termed **managed competition**. The hope is that such competition will force insurers and providers to lower their prices in order to capture more business and gain access to more people able to pay for health care coverage.

The impact of these changes is that caregivers and institutions must shift from seeking to provide as many services as possible under a fee-for-service payment approach to keeping the client well and providing fewer services so as to protect their best interests in an atmosphere of prepayment and negotiated contracts. In a fee-for-service system, the concern is that a client might receive too many or unnecessary services; in a prepaid system, the concern is that too few services might be given in order to save the provider and the managed care plan money.

Managed Care

Prepaid health plans have existed in the United States since the mid-1800s. They were initially most active on the West Coast and became firmly entrenched there when Kaiser Industries created the Kaiser Permanente Health Plan in 1938 to care for its shipbuilding employees (Davis, Collins, & Morris, 1994). Not until the early 1970s, however, did the term **health maintenance organization** (HMO) begin to be used to describe the concepts related to the comprehensive financing and management of health services (Luft & Trauner, 1981).

Until the late 1980s, HMOs were owned primarily by private not-for-profit organizations and hospitals. By the late 1980s, much of the ownership had moved to private for-profit insurance companies and investors (Davis et al., 1994). Along with that change came a blurring of the HMO structure and definition and increasing use of the term *managed care organization*.

Originally, HMOs were defined as either group or staff model organizations. **Medical group model HMOs** have their own facilities and equipment but contract with a medical group practice for the physician services they need. **Staff model HMOs** employ full-time salaried physicians to provide care in HMO-owned facilities. Care is closely monitored in both models, with clients and physicians able to see only those people participating in a given HMO. Clients who seek care outside the HMO list of participating physicians/providers must have referrals to do so or must pay for the services out of their own pockets. Many people are reluctant to pay for care on their own and, even when they have questions or believe they need further attention, often hesitate to challenge the HMO or fail to seek outside care, even if it may mean their lives. For this reason, knowing the ways to challenge a decision and to file a grievance in any insurance plan or HMO is important for both client and nurse.

Table 3-1 Possible Outcomes of Fee-for-Service and Managed Care Capitation Payment Approaches	
FEE-FOR-SERVICE	**MANAGED CARE USING CAPITATION**
Increased services	Decreased services
Single service	Continuum of services
Episodic care	Prevention/wellness care
Emphasis on specialty care	Emphasis on primary care/case management
Shift of costs to other payors	Cost management within premium
Independent providers	Integrated providers
Limited peer review	Extensive peer review
Little or no financial risk	Managed care plan and providers placed at financial risk

Note: It is important to remember that these are potential consequences of the different payment approaches; the likelihood and severity of these consequences (harm to the patient) depend on the philosophy and perspective of the individual and groups providing the care.

Independent practice association (IPA) HMOs are a variation on the original HMO models and began as a competing model that allowed physicians to remain entrepreneurs in their own private practices and offices. IPAs contract with single physicians or single-specialty group practices (such as a group of obstetrician/gynecologists) to see IPA/HMO clients in their private offices. The physicians maintain their own practices and, unlike in group or staff model HMOs, see clients from several plans and those with other types of insurance.

Network model HMOs are another variation on a theme. Rather than contracting with single physicians, these HMOs contract with one or more large, multispecialty physician group practices that serve clients from a number of sources. Both IPAs and networks are growing faster than group and staff model HMOs because their structures allow some continuing independence not afforded by the closed group and staff models (Davis et al., 1994). Again, clients are restricted to the IPA and network providers, who are generally less closely controlled by the managed care plan than are the physicians participating in group or staff model HMOs. Another version of networks now offers the services of physicians and hospitals contracting directly with the payor (such as a large employer group) rather than with a managed care plan.

Payments to the physicians in any of these HMO models may be made through capitation, fee-for-service, and/or bonus arrangements that are based on whether the number of services utilized falls within a predicted or specified range. Physicians practicing under capitation and bonus arrangements share in the financial risk to the plan; if they order too much care, their share of profit from the payments will fall. The financial risk faced by the physician is something that both clients and community health nurses should be aware of because the care made available may be influenced by whether a physician or physician group will lose money if additional tests or services are provided.

Demand for some of the elements of managed care without all the limitations prompted the creation of preferred provider organizations (PPOs) and point-of-service plans. **Preferred provider organizations** contract with providers, typically on a discounted fee-for-service basis, and offer clients financial incentives to use the services of the discounted providers. If clients use a PPO provider, the costs are less to them than if they use a provider who does not contract with the PPO. When clients use a nonparticipating provider, they pay a greater percentage, or even all, of the costs associated with care. In a **point-of-service plan**, clients need not specify whether they will use services in a fee-for-service, HMO, or PPO approach until they seek care. They pay more for the freedom afforded by such a plan and pay different prices depending on the approach they use.

The clear differences that once existed between types of managed care organizations and insurance companies are blurring. Managed care concepts are being incorporated into traditional insurance plans. Since the early 1980s, payors (employers and government) have de-

manded that providers accept increasing review and direction regarding the use of health services. Such **utilization review (UR)** is now part of nearly all health insurance and health maintenance organizations. Prehospital admission screening, requirements for second surgical opinions, ambulatory laboratory services, and a host of other approaches are designed to monitor and control the utilization of health care services. Only 5% of insurance-supported services have no utilization review (Sullivan & Rice, 1991). Thus, 95% of the insured population, whether they are in managed care plans or not, are having managed care principles applied to the services they receive.

It is unclear whether managed care will deliver all it seems to promise. Providing care in a more consistent manner and with defined goals for client outcomes and improved health, however, would seem an improvement on the existing splintered system within which payment dictates practice and clients often lose their way, even when they have insurance and money for care.

Because managed care, at its best, does support the general philosophy and approach of public health and well-being, community health nurses are particularly interested in these developments. Many of the managed care efforts to date, however, have been so focused on managing costs and acute medical services that they still have much to do in the way of supporting primary prevention and care. Public health services and prevention approaches have been, and continue to be, poorly integrated into insurance and managed care practices. Efforts to link approaches to care that can improve the health status for whole populations are and will remain a focus of public health agencies and community health nurses well into the next century. A summary of types of managed case plans is found in Table 3-2.

COORDINATION AND INTEGRATION OF HEALTH CARE SERVICES

The organizations and individuals who offer health services are usually independent providers. Physicians, hospitals, nursing homes, rehabilitation programs, and others provide care within the scope of their services and often leave clients to find and manage the other services they might need.

The local delivery system the client must turn to has also been left to its own devices in determining, planning, and designing the services that are to be made available within a community. "Hospitals can open or close according to community resources, preference, and the dictates of an open market for hospital services. Also, physicians are free to establish their practice where they choose" (De Law, Greenberg, & Kinchen, 1992, p. 151). To the extent planning is done in this country, it is done largely in response to budgetary decisions and is based on the amount of funds available in private businesses or public coffers.

Table 3-2 Types of Managed Care Plans

HEALTH MAINTENANCE ORGANIZATION (HMO)	PREFERRED PROVIDER ORGANIZATION (PPO)	POINT-OF-SERVICE PLAN (PSO)
Organization designed to provide health benefits to an enrolled population for a fixed periodic amount to be paid by purchaser.	Contracts with providers typically on a discounted fee-for-service basis and offers client incentives to use the services of the discounted providers.	Clients do not need to specify whether they will use services in fee-for-service, HMO, or PPO approach until they go for care. Clients pay more for this freedom of choice.

Group Model

Has own facilities but contracts with a medical group practice to provide physician services. May own hospital or may contract with other hospitals.

Staff Model

Has salaried physicians who provide care. May own hospital or may contract with other hospitals.

Independent Practice Association (IPA) Model

Contracts with single physician or single specialty group practice. Physicians maintain own practice in own office and see clients from different insurance plans.

Network Model

Multispecialty physician group practices that serve clients from a number of sources.

Community health planning, which sought to direct the location and size of facilities and equipment, was popular during the 1970s and early 1980s. In the years since popularity diminished, largely because the political climate at national and state levels shifted away from a regulatory approach and toward deregulation under Presidents Reagan and Bush. It has continued to do so under a Republican-controlled Congress and a national conservative trend. There are no health planning requirements at the federal level, and states require health planning to varying degrees (De Law et al., 1992). Construction of hospitals and nursing homes as well as purchase of some large-capital investments such as magnetic resonance imaging machines may be reviewed in some states. Even so, most buildings and equipment are eventually purchased and developed as an organization or individual wishes, as long as that organization or individual has the required funds.

Governmental and charitable programs are frequently left to fill the gaps created when private providers do not, or will not, offer a service in a particular locale. In many cases, the areas left unserved are inner cities or small rural communities, where income levels may mean that residents do not have the insurance or resources to buy health care. To fill this gap in available care, the government develops or encourages development of a geographically well positioned range of services to afford individuals access to acceptable and desirable care. In many such programs, community health nurses are key providers, such as in community health and mental health centers. Uncertain and often dwindling funding makes the future of such programs precarious, however.

Until recently, almost all health care was controlled by locally owned organizations or hospitals that had little or no relationship with each other. Now, health services may actually be part of larger, private health plans, alliances, and corporations with national, state, and local offices, facilities, or programs. Where facilities are located (or purchased) is increasingly dictated by the ways that the national organizations plan to compete for clients. Many smaller and locally owned organizations cannot compete or survive in this kind of environment and are being bought by or are merging with larger systems. For the community health nurse, a work setting that was once a locally owned and run visiting nursing service or home health agency may thus now be part of a larger statewide or national organization.

OWNERSHIP OF HEALTH DELIVERY ORGANIZATIONS

Health services are delivered to the insured and uninsured alike by private and public entities. Private ownership can be divided into two categories: (1) not-for-profit, voluntary, or charitable entities and (2) for-profit, investor-owned entities. Public or governmental ownership rests with government bodies at the federal, state, and local levels, where tax dollars are used directly to purchase care or deliver services. (The structure of government-owned public health organizations is discussed in greater detail later in this chapter.)

Private physicians' offices and those of nurse practitioners and other health professionals, hospitals of all

Figure 3-2 Types of Private Ownership in the Health Care Service Delivery System

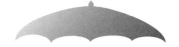

NOT-FOR-PROFIT (Voluntary/Charitable)

Sectarian or religiously affiliated

Community-based groups

Fraternal organizations (e.g., Shriners, Kiwanis)

Business and industry (e.g., Kaiser-Permanente Plan)

Unions

Disease-specific groups (e.g., Cancer Society)

Foundations (e.g., Pew, Robert Wood Johnson)

Professional associations

Some insurance companies (e.g., some Blue Cross/Blue Shields)

FOR-PROFIT (Investor Owned)

Individually owned

Partnerships

Limited liability companies

Corporations

types, nursing homes, managed care organizations, clinics, freestanding surgical centers, psychiatric facilities, and any and all other entities or groups that provide services may fall within the definition of private for-profit or not-for-profit ownership.

Historically, private not-for-profit voluntary health care institutions were developed by religious and charitable organizations that received tax-free status in return for the good they provided the community. The behavior and charitable mission of these groups dictated their services, and any profit was returned to the institution or group to enhance or expand services. In the case of private for-profit organizations, by contrast, profit is a stated goal, and taxes are paid by the organizations. The designation of an organization as for-profit or not-for-profit indicates nothing about the quality of the care and services provided.

Today, the difference between private not-for-profit and for-profit entities is becoming blurred. Both types of organizations are struggling to deliver services within a health care setting where costs are outpacing the ability of these organizations to absorb them. Cost consciousness is prompting many to limit whom they serve, downsize their organizations, merge with other organizations to achieve economies of scale, sell, or close. When not-for-profit groups are sold to for-profit groups, government and the courts are supporting the position that the money accrued under tax-free status should not go to the for-profit entity making the purchase. Instead, the "profits" are to be used to create foundations that will continue to have a community/charitable goal. Such foundations may represent a significant source of money for local health programs in coming years.

In order to understand the incentives, issues, and disputes that arise surrounding both defining the services to be delivered and paying for those services, it is important to know who owns a health care business. Figure 3-2 displays the types of private health care institutions and organizations from which individuals receive their care. The

private health services delivery sector and the businesses that support it—such as pharmaceutical companies and medical equipment and supply companies—constitute what many refer to as the "health care industry." The word *industry* has been applied to health care in recent years because it describes the nature of the business attitude and processes that now dominate health care.

HEALTH SERVICE ORGANIZATIONS

Health service organizations (HSOs) are formed to deliver care, with the number and variety of organizations created and influenced by both the ways we choose to finance and pay for that care and the technology available. Payors are further influencing those choices by asking that the dollars spent result in more than just a tally of the number of services provided. They are asking that the services actually produce outcomes of value to the client and that plans and providers be able to report on outcomes for the populations to which they provide care—a positive step toward improved health status.

‍‍ REFLECTIVE THINKING ‍‍

Impact of Different Types of Health Care Systems

• What are the strengths and weaknesses of a privately owned, business-oriented health care system?

• What impact does a private system of care have on health and wellness?

• What role do you think government should play in the health care system?

Following is a brief discussion of some of the most common types of health service organizations, including public health organizations. The inclusion of public health in this discussion is intentional, because as simply one component of the U.S. organized health care system, public health must be examined within the context of that system. It should be further noted that the following discussion can by no means be considered exhaustive, because new health service organizations and groupings of services are constantly being created.

The Public Health System

Ellencweig and Yoshpe (1984) suggest that public health services are intended to protect the community against the hazards of group living. This is a simple statement, but it encompasses the goal that community health nurses work toward and that public health has always sought to do for populations.

During the latter half of the 19th century, communicable diseases were spurred by unsafe drinking water and food and by poor sanitation. People died of acute gastrointestinal and respiratory tract infections such as pneumonia. Tuberculosis was one of the few diseases with which people lived long enough to have the disease be considered chronic. Public health efforts designed to improve sanitation and food handling reduced the number of people affected by communicable diseases or eliminated many such diseases (Rakich et al., 1992).

By the early 1900s, attention had shifted from general public health issues affecting whole communities to single acute episodes of illness experienced by individuals. Developing technologies, medications, and health insurance helped encourage this shift in focus from public health to acute illness.

At the public level, services and programs respond to broad community needs that are not usually addressed by privately owned and more narrowly defined service providers. While privately owned entities do indeed provide research and education, these efforts do not always coincide with all the perceived needs of the public. Consequently, government (primarily at the federal level) funds extensive research and education believed to be in the interest of national goals for health and safety. Public health and welfare are further protected by the public (governmental) sector through regulation, licensing, and monitoring of select health services, health professionals, and health programs (primarily at the state and local levels). When the private sector is involved, it is most often as a contractor to government or as a grant recipient implementing programs planned by government or by private foundations.

The Institute of Medicine's report *The Future of Public Health* defines the mission of public health "as fulfilling society's interest in assuring conditions in which people can be healthy" (1988, p. 7). To do this, public health agencies at different levels of government provide the epidemiologic and community assessment necessary to

define health need; develop and modify the policies, laws, and programs required to respond to that need; and work to ensure that the programs are implemented in a manner so as to have the desired effect. This process is not simple, because actions are carried out largely within the political arena and in a setting where government budgets dictate much of that which can or cannot be done. Furthermore, elected officials most often think in terms of immediately fulfilling campaign promises, rather than in planting the seeds of positive impact 10 or 15 years hence when a preventive public health program they earlier supported might finally demonstrate success.

Federal, state, and local levels of government may provide any or all of the following: direct services, research, education, development/planning, and regulation of health care services. Table 3-3 indicates the range of health-related services offered by state and local governmental bodies. The majority of public health–related services provided are under state or local direction because the Constitution grants the states the power and responsibility to protect the public health. Core public health

Table 3-3 Examples of State and Local Public Programs and Services

Direct/Contracted Services

Public health and primary care services

Mental health hospitals and services

City/county/university hospitals and medical schools

Nursing home care

Hospital districts or authorities

Animal control

Policy Development/Planning

Monitoring, data collection, analysis–epidemiologic assessment

Development/implementation of health laws and regulation

Regulation

Licensing of health care facilities (hospitals, nursing homes, etc.)

Licensing of health care agencies (home health, hospice, ambulances, etc.)

Licensing of health care professionals

Licensing of restaurants and food handlers

Regulation of environment (water, sewer, sanitation, air)

Education/Research

Health education, promotion, and disease prevention

Training/educational programs

Research (often as part of data gathering)

functions carried out by state and local governments, as suggested by the Association of State and Territorial Health Officials (1994), are related to the following: (1) monitoring the health of the population and developing policies to promote healthy behavior and health; (2) mobilizing and training specialists to investigate, prevent, and control epidemics, disease, and disasters; (3) organizing communities for action; and (4) protecting the public by monitoring and regulating medical services, the environment, the workplace, housing, food, and water.

Funds may be appropriated by any level of government for use in any of the activities carried out by a public health agency. Most often, however, we hear about the distribution of federal monies to the states, which may use the monies themselves or may in turn distribute the monies to local governments. The grants or allocations may be in lump sums (block grants, which have broad guidelines and allow the receiving group wide latitude in defining how grant money is used) or tied to an activity or service for which requirements are specified in detail.

Figure 3-3 lists the specific departments and agencies of the federal Department of Health and Human Services (USDHHS). While the USDHHS encompasses most of the agencies responsible for health at the federal level, other departments do have a health role, such as: (1) the direct services offered by the Department of Defense (Army, Navy, and Air Force), Veterans Affairs, and the Department of Justice (federal prisons); and (2) the regulatory roles filled by the Departments of Labor (Occupational Safety and Health Administration) and Agriculture (farm worker health and control of disease in animals), the Environmental Protection Agency, and the Department of the Treasury (alcohol, drug and firearms control).

Because the information presented in this section is not exhaustive, and organizational structures change with nearly every election, it is important for community health nurses to learn about their communities and how those communities relate to changing national, state, and local health priorities and programs. Today, the easiest way to stay current with regard to the organizational structure and function of a government entity is via the Internet.

As the 21st century approaches, continuing advancements in technology and care are fostering a demographic transition. Individuals who might once have died now live long lives, even with ongoing illnesses or conditions. Today, acute episodes of illness may in fact be exacerbations of existing chronic conditions. Rather than treatment of single episodes of illness, the management of chronic conditions over time for people of all ages, and particularly for the elderly, is taking center stage in health care. Demand is growing for health services to positively influence the health of the population served and to manage health conditions with which people live on an ongoing basis. The direction of change is back toward concern for the health status of populations and the public's health, a direction that was missing in the U.S. health care delivery system in the latter half of the 20th century. Of all the funds spent on health care in 1993, for instance, less than 1% was invested in population-based public health activities (U.S. Department of Health and Human Services [USDHHS], 1994). Public health is and will continue to be in competition for its share of available health care funding. Its often unseen importance to the community and the individual makes it difficult to gain support for increasing public health–related services and dollars. As more of these services are presumed to be part of the scope of services offered in managed care settings, cooperation between public health agencies and private bodies will be increasingly necessary to ensure that the needs of the population are addressed.

Figure 3-3 Organization of the Federal Department of Health and Human Services

Office of the Secretary (OS)—Director of HHS

Administration for Children and Families (ACF)

Administration on Aging (AOA)

Agency for Health Care Policy and Research (AHCPR)

Agency for Toxic Substances and Disease Registry (ATSDR)

Centers for Disease Control and Prevention (CDC)

Food and Drug Administration (FDA)

Health Care Financing Administration (HCFA)—Medicaid and Medicare Administration

Health Resources and Services Administration (HRSA)

Indian Health Services (IHS)

National Institutes of Health (NIH)

Program Support Center (PSC)

Substance Abuse and Mental Health Services Administration (SAMHSA)

Primary Health Care Systems

Primary health care as an organizational movement officially began at the 30th World Health Organization (WHO) Assembly in 1977 with the adoption of a resolution identifying the goal of health attainment that would enable citizens of the world to live socially and economically productive lives. As a WHO member nation, the United States endorsed primary health care as a way to achieve the goal of Health for All by the Year 2000.

Primary health care has been defined as essential care made universally accessible and available to individuals and families within a community, with an emphasis on disease prevention, health promotion, community involvement, multisectoral cooperation, and a cost that the community and country can afford (World Health Organization, 1978). The primary health care system includes a comprehensive range of services such as public health, prevention, diagnostic, therapeutic, and rehabilitative services. Primary health care services are community focused with an emphasis on health promotion and preventive services. Primary health care services include health education, nutrition, maternal–child health care, family planning, immunization, prevention and control of locally endemic diseases, treatment of commonly occurring diseases and injuries, provision of essential medications, and safe water and basic sanitation. Primary health care is part of public health, acute, long-term health and mental health care settings.

Hospitals

Today's hospitals primarily offer secondary and tertiary care or the acute care required for both simple and complex problems (specialty care) requiring 30 or fewer days of medical, surgical, and nursing care or emergency services. Hospitals have been a part of society for thousands of years as houses for the ill, poor, and dying. Not until the latter half of the 19th century, however, did improvements in technology allow for the beginnings of safe and effective organization and delivery of services. Discoveries and advances in antisepsis, asepsis, inhalation procedures, and anesthesia made it possible for invasive surgery to be planned and effective as opposed to being the last of a number of poor options for saving a life. Developments in radiography, blood typing, and clinical laboratories plus increased understanding of clinical care and client responses allowed hospitals to offer improved medical and surgical interventions (Rakich et al., 1992).

The work of Florence Nightingale in British hospitals also brought improvements and understanding in the areas of sanitation and the organization and operation of hospitals (Kopf, 1991). Nightingale's use of fundamental public health and epidemiologic principals provided direction for the development of all health services, and her efforts at training nurses to work in the hospital helped increase the use of organized hospital services and laid the basis for today's hospital nursing practice.

Most hospitals were created as private, not-for-profit corporations responding to community need and the needs of the poor. Every community wants a hospital of its own. In recent years, however, hospitals (particularly small hospitals) have begun to close as falling occupancy rates, controls on length of hospital stays, movement of care to the community, and mergers reduce the need and competition for hospital beds. If clients do not require intensive medical or nursing care, they are discharged to recover at home. Even with such changes, however, hospitals received nearly 44% of all monies spent for health care in the United States in 1991 (Letsch, 1993).

Psychiatric hospitals differ from acute care hospitals, both in the type of care they provide and in ownership. Most were created as public facilities where the mentally ill were warehoused and often committed involuntarily. Not until after World War II, when technological advances prompted by the war led to the development of psychoactive drugs, were the mentally ill given new hope for control over and recovery from their conditions. In response to the changes facilitated by medication and treatment advances, the 1963 Community Mental Health Center Act sought to foster the movement of mental health clients from psychiatric hospitals to community-based centers where they could be treated outside an institutional setting. This shift, combined with further advances in the development of medications and treatments, fostered the expectation that clients could and should be treated more appropriately in the community. The resources necessary to adequately implement such an approach, however, have never been forthcoming, leaving many mental health clients with inadequate treatment and community supports such as housing.

Insurance coverage for mental health services has been limited. Private insurance pays more readily for physical care than for mental health care and, typically, provides only limited coverage for psychiatric problems. Thus, public funding may be the only recourse for a mental health client, but, often, this funding is also limited. Insurance parity, or equality of treatment and payment for physical and mental health services, has been enacted into law in some states, but it is still a goal to be achieved nationally in the 21st century.

Ambulatory Surgery

Technology has helped reduce the amount of time clients must remain in the hospital. For years, select surgeries have been performed with the client being admitted and discharged from the hospital on the same day. Only since the early 1970s, however, have large numbers of surgeries been performed on an outpatient (rather than as a hospital inpatient) basis (Morgan, 1986). Hospitals, freestanding surgical centers, and physicians' offices today offer surgery to the ambulatory patient.

By not admitting clients for overnight care, the use of costly hospital facilities, 24-hour nursing care, and ancillary services such as food and laundry is avoided. Clients spend the day and return to their homes to heal.

The interest in reducing both hospital costs and the cost of health care in general has contributed to the rise in same-day surgery. Short-acting anesthetics, new surgical procedures, and technology that allows for very small incisions that heal quickly have all contributed to the growth of outpatient surgical procedures. In some cases, insurance will pay for certain surgeries only if they are performed on an outpatient basis.

Long-Term Care Facilities and Home- and Community-Based Care

Long-term care refers to the range of services that people with functional impairments require to be maintained "in safety and dignity, and to pursue the most meaningful lives that their disabilities permit" (Fogel, Brock, Goldscheider, & Royall, 1994, p. 1). The need for long-term care arises when individuals can no longer maintain them-

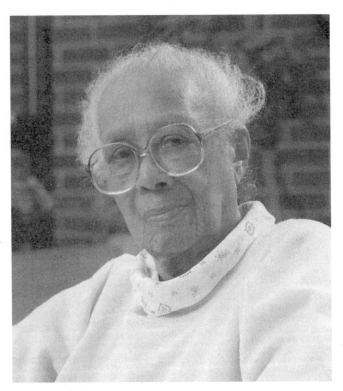

The growing number of elders with chronic health conditions increases the need for home and community-based services and quality long-term care facilities.

selves without assistance or supervision because of mental, physical, or social impairment and because the environments within which they live cannot or will not offer them the support they need.

The United States and other industrialized nations are facing growing populations of elderly individuals. Health care and technology have allowed individuals to live longer lives with chronic conditions that may impair their health or functioning without causing death. Growing numbers of elders require assistance and care to maintain themselves in: (1) their homes, with family members, nurses, and others providing intermittent care and support; (2) residential housing, where they can live in some variation of congregate housing and receive limited amounts of support from people employed to assist those living there; (3) community day care settings, where families can leave elders during work hours and then return to take their elderly family members home in the evening; and (4) nursing homes, where various levels of care are offered according to the clients' needs.

Nursing Homes

Nursing homes are probably the best known long-term care facilities. They grew out of the community almshouses, or poorhouses, and, later, the privately owned "boarding houses" sponsored by churches and those caring for the wealthy aged. Social Security legislation passed in 1935 included an Old Age Assistance (OAA) program, which paid for residents of private facilities meeting min-

imal requirements set by the federal government, thereby encouraging small, private, for-profit boarding houses to increase in number in response to the private-market financial incentive (Rakich et al., 1992). The law specified coverage for private facilities only, primarily because the private sector had the most effective lobbying efforts.

By 1950, nursing homes were licensed in every state (American Nursing Home Association, 1993). Whereas Medicare provides limited funding for skilled nursing care services, Medicaid pays for many of the nursing home beds in use in this country. The federal Medicare program specifies the requirements that must be met by nursing home facilities, but the states perform the compliance reviews and provide state licensing. Stryker (1988) notes that the model for nursing home care is based on a hospital medical disease model rather than on a model focusing on quality of life. This focus limits the social supports available to nursing home clients. In some cases, clients who need only social supports could more appropriately remain at home. Some funding exists for such support services but, where offered, the services are bound by regulation and constraints that limit the total availability of services.

Costs for nursing home care accounted for 9.1% of the spending for personal health care in 1991. Nursing home costs constitute the fourth largest expense behind those for hospitals, physician services, and pharmaceuticals. Nursing home care will have significant budget implications as the number of elderly persons increases into the next century (Letsch, 1993). Alternatives to nursing homes will become more important to elected leaders as the number of elders requiring assistance increases—and as those same elders use the power of their votes to have their demands met.

Home Health Care

Home care services are provided by home health agencies, visiting nursing services, some public health agencies, and private companies. Lillian Wald is credited with establishing the first continuing program in the United States, with the creation of the Visiting Nursing Service of New York City in 1893 (Mudinger, 1983). Wald's vision significantly shaped the character and content of community health nursing.

Home health care is usually thought of in terms of the definition used by the Medicare program, which covers physician care, skilled nursing services, physical therapy, occupational and speech therapy, social work services, and home health aide services. Skilled nursing care is defined as intermittent, part-time services delivered by a nurse in the residence of a homebound client.

In 1960, home health care was so rarely used that it was not included in the calculations of national health care expenditures. By 1980, however, home health care accounted for $1.3 billion and by 1991 $9.8 billion of the total expenditures for national health care (Letsch, 1993). It is expected that expenditures for home health care and other long-term care services will increase as the number

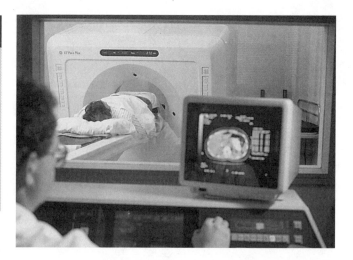

MRI and CAT scan services are examples of the many diagnostic and surgical services offered by ambulatory programs. Photo courtesy of Ed Eckstein/Corbis.

of elders continues to surge with the aging of the post–World War II baby boomers.

Hospice

The modern version of hospice was developed in the 1960s in England by Cicely Saunders, MD (Manning, 1984). It spread to the United States, where independent, community-based programs using volunteers trained to deal with death and dying provided care to clients and their families.

Hospice programs focus on palliative care and comfort for the client who is expected to die within the near future. Support is offered to the client and family during and after the death of the ill family member. Today, volunteers and an interdisciplinary team of health professionals and chaplains work to provide a wide range of physical and emotional supports to clients and families.

Ambulatory Care

Ambulatory care is care delivered in an office or other setting at the time and place of the client's choosing. Once the care is provided, the client returns to home or work. Ambulatory care constitutes much of the primary care offered in this country and, often, the first point of contact for the client with the health care system.

Physicians' offices, emergency rooms, and outpatient clinics of acute care hospitals, urgent care centers, and freestanding clinics and centers offer ambulatory/primary care. Walk-in diagnostic imaging centers and mobile mammography examinations are examples of the growing variety in types of ambulatory settings and services.

As is the case with ambulatory surgery, ambulatory care settings offer increasingly sophisticated and complex treatments to clients who simply stop in for care and then go on their way. Emergency rooms are frequently used to provide ambulatory care. The cost of the care, however, is far more expensive than if it was delivered in a physician's office or clinic. In order to shift clients whose cases are not true emergencies to the less expensive clinic setting, some hospitals are establishing ambulatory clinics in conjunction with their emergency rooms. Insurance companies discourage the use of the emergency room as an ambulatory care site. Most, in fact, reduce the amount they will contribute and require a greater out-of-pocket payment by the client than if the client had been seen in another ambulatory care site.

Community Nursing Organizations/Community Nursing Centers

Community nursing organizations (CNOs) or centers (CNCs) also offer ambulatory/primary care services. A CNO can be a single setting where clients visit, but, more often, encompasses a wide range of services offered by nurses in a variety of practice arrangements and settings in the community. Both CNOs and CNCs offer nurse-managed services to clients across the continuum of care in the home, community, hospital, or nursing home setting (Aydellotte et al., 1987; Riesch, 1990; Sharp, 1992). They usually offer both illness-management services (comparable to a medical acute care model) and nursing care and coordination. Advanced practice nurses offer the acute care to clients and bill insurance companies if possible (Safriet, 1992). Community health and other nurses offer nursing care, coordination, and education. The majority of the care provided by advanced practice, community health, and other nurses is not reimbursable under insurance; thus, other payment sources such as grants and direct contracts with employers, city and state governments, and others must replace the unavailable insurance revenue (Lockhart, 1994).

Although the CNO has a difficult time as an independent financial entity, the model for care is being adopted by groups of providers who want to use the approach to market coordinated care to the public. Advanced practice, community health, and other nurses are serving as the first contacts and managers of care for

RESEARCH 🔍 FOCUS

The Use of Health-Risk Appraisal in a Nursing Center: Costs and Benefits

STUDY PROBLEM/PURPOSE

Health promotion and disease prevention are important components of the services offered in nursing centers and are being used increasingly in the work setting. Health-risk appraisals are widely used to provide a baseline of information about the education and services a client might need. Whether the appraisals and subsequent interventions lead to long-term behavior change has not been adequately documented, nor have the costs and benefits derived by the client and the employer. This study sought to answer these questions by examining one cohort of university employees seen at a nurse practitioner–managed employee health clinic.

METHODS

The population sample was drawn from new hires at the University of Texas, Houston. Data were collected during the period between September 1992 to August 1993. Of the 847 new employees, 418 (52%) voluntarily participated in the health-risk appraisal offered during a health-screening examination given to all new hires. The tool used was the Life Survey by Wellsource. Data provided by the university were tabulated and the risk analysis completed by Wellsource. Results and suggestions for education and other activities were provided to the client by the clinic.

An analysis was done of the relationships among selected health indices as well as of the characteristics of the employees who voluntarily participated in the program. Cost, extent of long-term behavioral change, and client and organizational perceived benefit were examined.

FINDINGS

The health-risk appraisals were based on self-reported data. Efforts were made to ensure confidentiality, but as new hires, clients may have been hesitant to admit to poor health habits while working

in a large university and medical center. Insurance rebates for positive health behaviors may also have led to bias in reporting. Reports of positive attitudes and behavior did not match the poor fitness, heart health, health practices, and stress/coping found on physical examination and interview, all of which suggest the findings cannot be generalized but do offer direction for further research.

The cost of the health-risk appraisal used was $37.50 per employee. This particular appraisal approach was deemed to be expensive and time consuming but did provide useful information that helped a number of clients change risky behaviors, particularly those behaviors related to exercise and nutrition. In the long run, these changes should result in improved health status. Use of a shorter, less costly version of the tool is being considered as are efforts at using it with a more narrowly defined and targeted population, both of which should reduce costs and improve outcomes.

IMPLICATIONS

The study adds to the body of literature on efforts at health promotion and prevention within the work setting and, particularly, those provided by a nurse-run clinic. It identified a number of variables that could skew the findings in studies of this type. Such information is important to know in order to design other more rigorous studies that can more clearly define clinical, professional, and organizational influences on the care provided and outcomes achieved. The study was too short to shed much light on the long-term effects on clients or on employer health care costs over time. Studies of this type are still needed if research is to assist in showing the clinical and cost benefits of health promotion and disease prevention for populations.

SOURCE

From "The Use of Health-Risk Appraisal in a Nursing Center: Costs and Benefits by T. Mackey and J. Adams, B. Murphy (Ed.), (1994). In Nursing Centers: The Time Is Now *(pp. 254–265), New York: National League for Nursing Press. Copyright 1994 by National League for Nursing Press.*

various institutions, employers, and insurance companies. They are expected to do so in increasing numbers as payors demand coordinated care for insured individuals. Although CNCs began to expand in the early 1960s, the American Nurses Association (Aydellotte et al., 1987) and Glass (1989) suggest their origins lie in the public health nursing centers, nurse settlements, and rural nursing services of 100 years ago.

INFLUENCES ON HEALTH SERVICES DELIVERY

As has already been discussed, multiple influences affect the health care system and the ways it operates. Figure 3-4 presents one model (Lockhart, 1992) for analyzing those influences as they affect the choices and purchases made by consumers and their providers. This model highlights the structures that shape a consumer's choice of services within the health care delivery system. It also can be used to analyze the influences on local, state, or national approaches to care and can help community health nurses identify areas where they or others can seek to intervene as advocates for clients.

The outer circle of the figure identifies the overall influences of socio/cultural, political, economic, demographic, and environmental events. The cultural diversity of our nation, increases or decreases in the population, and/or the ages of population members all change the type and number of services needed and wanted. In 1997 women represented 46% of the work force and will reach parity with men in the next century. They will require specific services, particularly those relating to children (Judy & D'Amico, 1997). Social issues such as drug use, homicide, and other crimes also influence the types and number of services required to respond to the population's needs and demands.

Whereas at one point in time we could chart our country's economic future by how well the economy and production were managed, today our economic future is linked to the global economy and thus surges or declines along with the economies of other countries throughout the world. Turns in the economy affect the wealth of individuals and the nation and, thereby, the money both are willing to commit to health services.

Politically, our nation changes its focus as leaders change and espouse what are called conservative or liberal agendas. It is increasingly difficult to define exactly what those terms mean; however, it is true that whoever holds political power sets the agenda for establishing laws and regulations and determining the availability of education and services for such things as birth control, abortion, and acquired immunodeficiency syndrome (AIDS).

The environment in which all this transpires is more healthy or less healthy depending on the attitudes and beliefs of the politicians and society within which we live and, thereby, the efforts undertaken to ensure clean air, safe drinking water, soils free of contaminants, and other factors that create not only a safe but a pleasant environment. The ways that those safeguards affect the viability of industry and business influence whether certain rules and regulations are enacted. The ultimate cost to the health of the population is often weighed against the cost of the loss of jobs.

The laws, regulations, technology, and financing depicted in the second outermost circle in Figure 3-4 are all affected by the influences in the outermost circle, just discussed. Although the political influences on laws and regulations may be the most obvious, the choices and trade-offs made in response to the political, economic, social, demographic, and environmental factors in the outermost circle affect all the variables in the second outermost circle. The results shape our country's financial well-being and, therefore, the number of dollars believed available to provide health care to our population.

Financing for health care insurance is done primarily through the employment setting for the working popula-

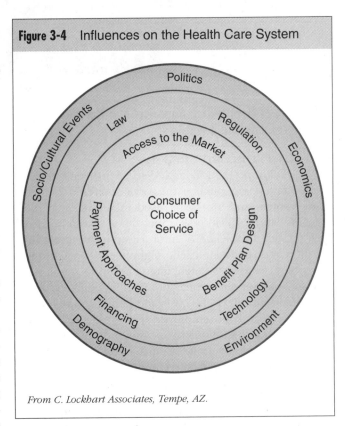

Figure 3-4   Influences on the Health Care System

From C. Lockhart Associates, Tempe, AZ.

tion and through government for the elderly and specific populations. Those who provide the financing and the amounts available ultimately define which health and public health services are offered and the ways they are offered, particularly with regard to health technology. The passage or failure of laws, regulations, and policies that (1) make it easy or difficult to bring new technology to market and (2) allow for or restrict payment for that technology dictates the technology that will be developed and used.

In Figure 3-4, the third and last set of influences on consumer choice—payment approaches, benefit plan design, and access to the market—are all specific to the ability to offer and purchase a service in the health care market.

Who has access to the market in order to provide services is dictated by both who is licensed to care for clients and who is eligible to be reimbursed for the care provided. Nurse access to the market is limited sometimes by law but most often by a program, plan, or insurance policy that excludes nurses from the definition of a provider, limits the services for which nurses will be paid, or pays an amount different from (usually less than) that paid to other providers offering the same service. In addition, the design of the benefit plan determines the type of services eligible for payment under the plan. If a service or provider, including a public health provider, is not listed as one of those eligible for payment or coverage, the client and provider must decide whether to pursue the service at the client's own expense.

All the items listed in the circles of influence act on each other and on the consumer. Finally, the consumer's personal choices, listed in the center of the circle of influ-

Figure 3-5 Technological Methods

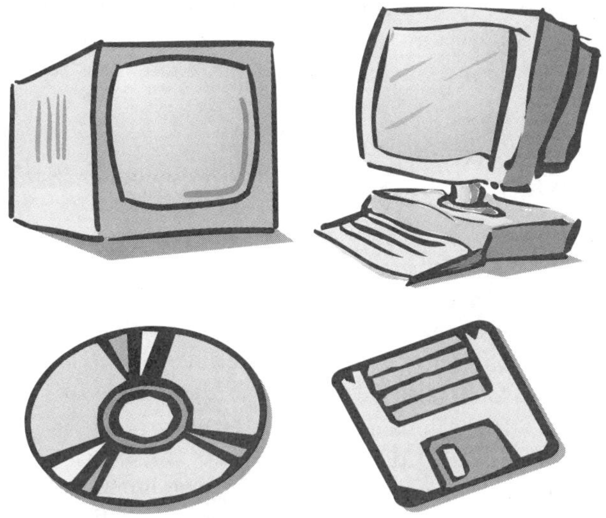

What are your thoughts regarding the delivery of care through these technological methods? What about the quality of care? What sort of care could be offered through these methods?

threat of government-imposed change with actions the industry believes address perceived failures in the system. Individual practices and institutions are becoming part of larger systems through outright purchase or contracts. Large organizations with national systems of care are evolving, organizations that will seek to offer outcome-specific, cost-effective, and efficient care to employers and government purchasers for use by employees and Medicaid and Medicare enrollees across the country.

As this consolidation and reorganization of the health care delivery system continues, it is expected that a relatively few large and privately owned organized systems of care will control the delivery of health services in the United States. Employer-based coverage will continue to be the primary method of financing health services. Nearly all delivery options offered to privately or publicly funded individuals will be within some version of a managed care system. Fee-for-service health insurance will constitute only a small portion of the private insurance offered throughout the country. In other words, health care of the 21st century is expected to look different from that of the 20th century.

ences in Figure 3-4, are shaped by considerations such as the following:

• What is the quality of the service?
• How much of it will I need (quantity)?
• How much does it cost (price)? Can I afford to share in the cost or to pay for it completely on my own?
• Where is it offered (location)? Is it convenient to my home? Can I get there from where I live?
• Can I afford the time? Does it require time away from work? Loss of pay?
• What are my preferences for care? Do I simply like a certain physician or nurse?

When buying health care, the strength of these last influences may vary because individuals may not have enough information to make a choice or may have so little responsibility for the cost of the service that they simply go where their physician or plan suggests. This is in part the reason that health care really does not resemble a normal market for goods and services. Even so, consumer choices are influenced by these factors, and as health care continues to change, one of the changes will be demand for greater involvement of clients in the choices and uses of the services offered them.

REFORMING HEALTH CARE IN THE UNITED STATES

National and state health care reform efforts during the 1990s spurred the health care industry to respond to the

A Paradigm Shift

The model, or **paradigm**, under which health care is currently delivered is undergoing a shift. The various changes previously discussed as being under way do not constitute a true paradigm shift, however. In a paradigm shift, as described first by Thomas Kuhn (1986), the underlying beliefs about a thing are shaken and changed forever.

To date, the primary change in health care has been a movement of the payment system away from fee-for-service and toward some level of managed care and prepayment. Prepayment refers to a system that provides health care services to clients for a basic fee, one fee covering all services. New on the horizon is the expectation that a price paid for services should deliver an expected outcome of defined quality. What that quality should be in regard to the design of the delivery system is not yet clear. Discussion regarding the definition of quality will likely continue well into the 21st century.

But even these changes do not really represent a paradigm shift, because the model of care that underlies the delivery of services is the same model we have used throughout the 20th century. The focus is on acute episodes of care provided to individuals by single practitioners. Thus, although practitioners may be operating in a newly linked or larger system, to a great extent, the care and the delivery are much the same as they have always been. The paradigm shift, then, is largely rhetorical at this point. Health for the client is often a stated but poorly defined goal of the insurance and managed care systems being created. Cost controls, new quality demands, and compliance with payment requirements have made the system different than it was a few years ago; but these things have not yet changed the underlying beliefs, expectations, and practices of those operating in the system. A true shift will require time and the education of both providers and consumers.

Health care reform, a paradigm shift, is a goal nursing has consistently embraced and endorsed. In 1993, to add to a growing national momentum for change, 62 nursing organizations put forward *Nursing's Agenda for Health Care Reform* (American Nurses Association, 1993). This document supports efforts to ensure access to a core of essential health care services for all at an affordable cost. Health care would be restructured to focus on consumers and to work toward wellness and care rather than illness and cure.

This agenda and others like it have been put forward by groups and individuals who want to see a true paradigm shift within the health care system. That shift is about changing the purpose for which the system is created and then designing the delivery system, services, payment, and financing to ensure that health and well-being are attainable for the population served. This is a far greater change than simply modifying payment or even restructuring the delivery system; it requires that we ask anew which services are needed (whether or not they are currently covered by insurance) and how best to deliver them to ensure healthy populations.

Answering questions about those things needed to keep people healthy requires consideration of more than just acute medical care. It requires examining the human ecosystem with regard to the ways it influences health and determining that which must be done to support or change those influences in a given individual, family, or community. It also requires consideration of the ways that consumer choices are, or might conceivably be, influenced to support health. Instead of reacting, a reformed health care system should consider how to proactively influence positive health and lifestyle choices through the design of the system and the services offered.

Designing a proactive, positive health system requires leadership by people who understand clients and the full range of care and services they might need. Nurses, and particularly community health nurses, understand the human ecosystem and the holistic nature of health care and services. In addition, community health nurses understand how to meet the needs of populations. Community health nurses should thus play a primary role in defining the new paradigm in health care. Membership on local, state, and national governmental and private health planning boards and committees can afford community health nurses the opportunity to speak to the character of the care and services needed in a responsive health care system operating under a new paradigm. Three key concepts in that new paradigm are discussed next.

Consumer Sovereignty and Responsibility

Consumer sovereignty is a major paradigm shift from traditional values that view professional autonomy above other consumer values. Consumer sovereignty, as used here, suggests that clients have the power, authority, and responsibility to be involved in their health care and services. Personal health care involves the daily choices and actions taken to ensure ongoing health. Health care services are used to prevent disease, promote health, and treat illness. Consumers' choices may be limited by some rationing method, but within the scope of the choices available, the consumer should have a say about what is or is not done.

The Center for Biomedical Ethics of the University of Minnesota conducted an interdisciplinary research project that examined the values framework of the U.S. health care system (Priester, 1992). An assessment of the current values of professionals and the public alike placed professional autonomy above all other values including client autonomy, consumer sovereignty, client advocacy, access to care, and quality of care.

The concept of consumer sovereignty is contradictory to the way our current health care system operates but is consistent with our political and cultural philosophy. Consumers have surrendered control of their health to health professionals. In no other areas of their lives do Americans do this. A true paradigm shift demands that consumers exercise control over their health status.

Women will be significant players within any redefined system, because they are the primary purchasers and managers of health care for their families and themselves. Community health nurses must therefore help educate women to be informed and assertive consumers empowered to make choices and able to manage the health status of themselves and their families.

Population projections suggest that the United States will become even more culturally diverse in the next century. Community health nurses must be comfortable with and part of the cultures and races represented throughout the nation. Diversity will be a reality, and community health nurses themselves must both reflect that diversity and allow it to shape the type and manner of services they provide to clients.

Wellness and Care

This text proposes wellness and care (as opposed to illness and cure) as the preferred model for health services. This still-evolving paradigm is one that nursing can support and advance.

Perspectives...

Insights of a Community Health Nurse

The United States health care system is undergoing major change—rapid and dramatic. In the United States, economics, access, and quality are major issues that are being addressed in a number of different ways. One of the major changes, the shift from acute to community-based care, has resulted in the expansion of nursing services in the community. A greater emphasis is placed on developing community partnerships and population-focused practice. Rather than seeing clients apart from their environment, clients are viewed within the context of community in order to ensure that all aspects of health are considered. In addition to the previously mentioned changes, there is also a focus on multidisciplinary care that emphasizes care from a variety of different professionals working in a coordinated system around client needs.

The various changes in the U.S. health care system are having a significant impact on community health nursing and the role of faculty in teaching students to prepare for practice. In the early development of nursing, people were cared for in their homes. Hospitals were developed to assist in the care of the homeless and poor. Today, and in the future, a vast majority of health care services will continue to be provided in the home once again, in schools, in community-based centers, in faith communities, and in other settings. As the population ages, there will be an even greater need for long-term care management services for clients in

their homes, as well as home health services following hospital discharge. There will also be a need for improved coordination of care services for young families—child bearing and child-rearing. Vulnerable population groups such as the homeless and near homeless will require creative, innovative partnerships in communities to address their health care needs. As community health nursing faculty, we have a major role to play in preparing students for these changes.

I think that community health nurses have a vital role to play in building caring communities—communities where partnerships are fostered, where multidisciplinary and community members work together to identify client health care needs and services to meet those needs provided at a cost that the community can afford. In my work with students, I focus on the imperative for delivering caring, compassionate services to families in the midst of change. I also stress the importance of functioning as a member of the multidisciplinary health team and provide opportunities for students to experience the process. We explore the meaning of caring within the context of community and discuss the need for working to develop a seamless health care system where partnerships among institutions and agencies will ultimately enhance health and healing. As community health nursing faculty, we must provide opportunities for students to participate in such efforts.

—*Sue A. Thomas, RN, EdD*

Biotechnology developments and genetic research currently under way will ultimately provide the information necessary to predict who will become ill and develop certain diseases and conditions. Such predictions will be able to be made long before we learn how to change the genes that cause the related problems, however. Research by physicians, nurses, and others will help define ways that clients can maintain wellness. It will also identify the personal care and health services needed by individuals in order to prevent crossing from wellness into illness states requiring cure. This paradigm, again, is different from the one that currently exists. This paradigm presumes people can be taught and assisted in their efforts to remain well

and that this approach will work to a significant degree. Rather than meaning that people will not have chronic and other health problems, this paradigm presumes that enough support and education will be provided to clients to help them make the choices and take the actions necessary to limit any health risks. This, then, is a proactive approach to keeping people well, rather than a retrospective effort at curing that which has already gone wrong. Again, community health nurses must be at the forefront of change.

The advances made will also raise significant ethical issues. Individuals will need to learn to manage the courses of their own health and plan their lives in light of the knowledge that they carry genes that may negatively affect their health. Because the outcomes will dictate the approaches to well-being for the client populations they serve, community health nurses must be in the forefront of the ethical debates that will arise.

The education and care community health nurses offer will increasingly be provided with the help of electronic media, computers, video, and other technology, facilitating provision of care across communities and into rural and isolated areas. Clinical practice guidelines and general care guidelines being developed by the Agency for Health Care Policy and Research, professional associations, insurance companies, and managed care plans will seek to identify the most likely range of services, education, and actions needed to achieve a positive health outcome. Guidelines and outcomes definition will of necessity require the input of professionals and consumers alike. Community health nurses should seek to participate in guidelines development at all levels to ensure that public health and care concerns are addressed.

Care in the Community

As previously stated, care is moving from institutions to the community. Hospitals and institutional settings are increasingly used for only limited periods of time when clients are acutely ill, with clients being discharged home for most of their recovery. In response, some nurses are moving to the community to serve the clients. Still others are working to provide care to a defined population across the continuum of settings serving the clients. Community health nurses must take on leadership and management roles in such programs and must help define how community nursing organizations and other nurse-managed services can provide significant components of

COMMUNITY NURSING VIEW

A public health nurse is working in a county with a significant number of homeless and near homeless persons. In the county, an Interfaith Council agency serves this population and is known for its compassion and outreach to them. The agency provides counseling, clothing, assistance with job placement, and a day service center where the homeless can take showers, use phones, etc. The nurse has visited the program site and identified the need for developing a nursing center there, a nursing center that would provide basic health screening and follow-up, treatment of minor conditions, case management, and client advocacy. Many of the clients who use the agency programs have indicated that they would definitely like to have a nursing center available to them. Many of them have indicated that they feel "safe," "respected," and "treated with dignity" at the Interfaith agency.

Nursing Considerations

ASSESSMENT
• What information would you need from the agency director and staff to assist in deciding whether to initiate the development of a nursing center?

• What questions would you ask to obtain the information?

DIAGNOSIS
• Identify several nursing diagnoses that may pertain to the health needs of the homeless population.
• Which of the listed diagnoses could be addressed by having a nursing center in the community?

OUTCOME IDENTIFICATION
• What outcomes would indicate that the nursing center had achieved its objectives?

PLANNING/INTERVENTIONS
• Who would need to be involved in the planning process?
• What services could be offered?
• Would outside financing be needed? If so, when could it be obtained?

EVALUATION
• What process could be used to determine the type of outcome measurements that would provide the evaluation data needed?

the prevention, primary care, community-based services and client-centered care required in the new paradigm. The community health nurse will need to work with government and managed care plans to monitor and assess both the health status of the populations served and the impact of the service provided on the entire community within which the community health nurse works. We are on the threshold of a new health care paradigm and a new millennium. What we do as practitioners will influence the ultimate shape of both.

≋ Key Concepts

- Health services in the United States are, to a great extent, privately planned and organized, with little local, state, or national governmental input.

- The U.S. political culture fosters individualism and entrepreneurial efforts in the economy and in all sectors of society, including health care.

- Privately or publicly provided health insurance is the primary vehicle through which people gain access to health services. In the absence of insurance, individuals must pay out of their own pockets or face going without services except in emergencies.

- Within one financing and delivery system, managed care seeks to provide, coordinate, and manage the services offered to clients in an effort to improve quality while controlling costs and utilization.

- A wide range of health-service organizations exist, with new configurations being created in response to changes in financing and delivery demands.

- Community nursing organizations/centers offer ambulatory care and community nursing services focusing on primary care and prevention.

- The consumer's choice of health services is affected by political, economic, social/cultural, demographic, and environmental factors and a wide range of approaches and practices that derive from these factors.

- A true shift in the underlying beliefs about health care would require that the health of the client be defined as the goal for the delivery of health services.

- Wellness and care, consumer sovereignty, and community-based care are concepts that would characterize a health care system operating under a new paradigm.

Health Care Economics

Gregory L. Crow, RN, EdD

We live in a universe of creative emergence.

—*Wilber, 1996, p. 25*

COMPETENCIES

Upon completion of this chapter, the reader should be able to:

- Describe the U.S. health care system, including the way whereby it functions.
- Define general and health care economic terms.
- Discuss the federal, state, and local governmental roles in health care.
- Identify the mechanisms by which health care costs are controlled.
- Compare and contrast the European health care financing model with that of the United States.
- Describe the ways that emerging health care financing trends shape health care in the United States.
- Apply the concept of caring to health care economics.

The American health care system is in the midst of unparalleled change. The paradigm, or model, under which the U.S. health care system operates changed dramatically after 1983, when the federal government introduced diagnosis related groups as a means of controlling health care costs. While economics is playing a significant role in the paradigm shift, numerous other factors must be understood in order to put these changes in context such as consumer demand for the most up-to-date therapies, an aging population, and living longer with chronic illness. Change begins with understanding. Community health nurses must understand the U.S. health care system in order to influence it in ways that clearly demonstrate nursing's commitment to protecting the public's health.

Policymakers, employers, health care providers, insurance companies, and consumers are searching for ways to enhance, provide, and control allocations of finite health care resources. Figure 4-1 illustrates the sources and the targets of the U.S. health care dollar in 1996 (Health Care Finance Administration [HCFA], 1997a). As can be seen, governmental programs (Medicare, Medicaid, and other) accounted for $0.47 of every dollar spent; private health insurance, out-of-pocket payments, and other private sources accounted for the remainder. The targets of this spending demonstrate that most health care dollars continue to be spent on acute hospital care. Figure 4-2 demonstrates that from 1960 to 1996, national health care expenditures rose from $26.9 to $1,035.1 billion. At the same time, out-of-pocket nonreimbursable expenses rose from $13.1 billion nationally to $622 billion (HCFA, 1998b).

The HCFA (1997a) predicts that if the United States is unable to check health care cost increases, the total dollar amount for U.S. health care expenditures will reach $1.7 trillion by the year 2000 and will reach $16.0 trillion by the year 2030. The United States can ill afford such a future. Measures must therefore be put in place now to prevent

Figure 4-1   The Nation's Health Dollar Expressed in Cents per Dollar: 1996

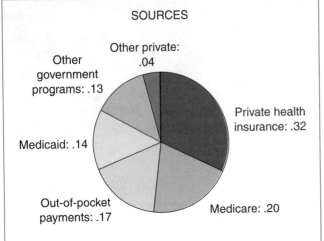

SOURCES

Other private: .04
Other government programs: .13
Private health insurance: .32
Medicaid: .14
Out-of-pocket payments: .17
Medicare: .20

TARGETS

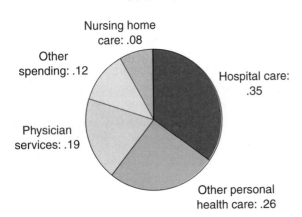

Nursing home care: .08
Other spending: .12
Hospital care: .35
Physician services: .19
Other personal health care: .26

From Health Care Finance Administration, "Medicare Bulletin," March 1998.

Figure 4-2   National Health Care Expenditures: 1960–1996

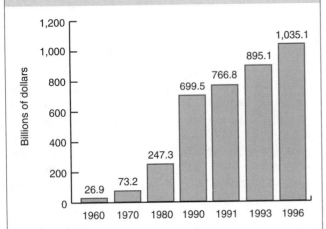

Billions of dollars

Year	Amount
1960	26.9
1970	73.2
1980	247.3
1990	699.5
1991	766.8
1993	895.1
1996	1,035.1

From Health Care Finance Administration, Data extracted from Health Care Finance Administration home page. Available: http://www.HCFA.gov. May 1997.

the potentially catastrophic consequences of rising costs and lack of reform, and economics will play an ever-expanding role in health care reform, evaluation, and system maintenance.

Richard Lamm (1994), former governor of Colorado, cites the driving forces in the rise of health care costs as being:

1. The dramatic increase in the elderly population
2. Technological advances
3. Consumer demands and expectations
4. Lack of consumer price sensitivity
5. Medical malpractice premiums
6. A collective inability to recognize resources as being finite

This chapter seeks to provide an overview of general and health care economics and their influencing factors. A discussion of those factors contributing to rising health care costs and of the cost-control measures that have been or could be put in place to curb this trend is also included in this chapter. Because of the nature of the content, some pertinent material that was discussed in Chapter 3 is reinforced in this chapter.

ECONOMICS

The first step in wisdom is "getting things by their right names" (Wilson, 1998, p. 13). Because economics plays such a vital role in health care, community health nurses must increase their knowledge and awareness of those forces that shape health care financing in the United States. Specifically, the nurse must understand a number of terms in order to understand the economics of health care.

Economics is the science concerned with the ways that society allocates scarce resources commonly known as goods and services (Duffy, 1993). Economics addresses the supply and demand on the part of an environment for a product or service. Examples of economic health care environments are individual consumers, insurance companies, employers, and state and federal governments. Resources include inputs such as labor, capital, and technology. Resources are considered scarce when society demands more resources and goods than are generally available. Economics viewed from a market perspective is divided into macroeconomics and microeconomics.

Macroeconomics

Macroeconomics is one of two major economic theories. The prefix *macro* means "large," indicating that **macroeconomics** is the study of the market system on a large scale. Macroeconomics focuses on the aggregate performance of all markets in a market system and on the choices made by that large system in an economy (Duffy, 1993). In health care, one macroeconomic market is the entire U.S. health care system, including the way that it performs in terms of profit, loss, and efficiency.

Microeconomics

Microeconomics is the second major economic theory. The prefix *micro* means "small," indicating that **microeconomics** is the study of the market system on a small scale. Microeconomics focuses on the individual markets that make up the market system and on the choices made by small economic units such as individual consumers and individual firms (Duffy, 1993). One example of a microeconomic system is the individual consumer or small-business owner and the ways that these markets interact and influence each other in the provision of health services. Macroeconomics and microeconomics are both influenced by economic policy formulated at federal, state, and local levels.

The state microeconomic system can influence the federal macroeconomic system because the number of state enrollees in health care plans, partially funded by federal programs, can rise or fall depending on state law or policy. As the number of state enrollees rises or falls, the amount of funds transferred from federal macroeconomic programs to state microeconomic programs will fluctuate. Vice versa, the federal macroeconomic system can influence the state microeconomic system by limiting the total amount of dollars available for funding or by establishing federal laws that influence how states spend health care dollars.

Economic Policy

Economic policy is a course of action intended to influence or control the behavior of an economy. Economic policy is typically implemented and administered by the government (Wessels, 1993). The U.S. federal, state, and local governments are attempting to develop economic policies to control health care costs. It should be noted, however, that the U.S. health care system, or market, has not reacted to health care economic policy in the manner that other markets have typically responded to governmental policy decisions. Typically, as a commodity becomes scarce, the price increases, and, conversely, as the market becomes flooded with a commodity, the price goes down. Regardless of health care policy, supply, or demand, however, the United States has experienced a consistent increase in costs associated with health care.

Federal, state, and local governments have traditionally attempted to control health care costs via economic policy, financing, and reimbursement. **Financing** is the amount of dollars that flow from payors to an insurance plan, either private or governmental. **Reimbursement** is the flow of dollars from the insurance companies to providers or hospitals. The flow of dollars within health care is focused on a market, whether that market be local, state, or federal.

Market System

A **market system** is a mechanism by which society allocates scarce resources (Duffy, 1993; Wessels, 1993). In the United States, several types of market systems allocate scarce health care resources. The federal government allocates resources via programs such as Medicare, Medicaid, and the U.S. Public Health Service. At the state level, public health service and community district hospitals represent the primary sources in the market system. On the private side of the health care market system are profit and not-for-profit health maintenance organizations, private hospitals, insurance companies, and group or individual medical practices (Mechanic, 1994). The way that a market system operates in terms of efficiency or waste affects the gross domestic product of the country in question.

Gross Domestic Product

The **gross domestic product (GDP)** is all the goods and services produced for domestic use by a nation in one year and represents a microeconomic theoretical base. It also constitutes a way of comparing one nation with another in terms of economic function. In comparative studies, the collective health care expenditures of each of a number of nations are often each expressed as a percentage of the GDP (Duffy, 1993). One factor that influences the GDP is the theory of supply and demand for a product or service. The GDP does not take into account any products produced by another nation and transported to the United States for consumption. Therefore the GDP is concerned only with goods and services produced and consumed within the borders of the United States in a one-year period.

Supply and Demand

Supply and demand is a microeconomic theory. In every market system, there are both buyers and sellers. The buyer's willingness to purchase a particular product or service is referred to as **demand.** The seller's willingness to supply a particular product or service at a cost is referred to as **supply**. Obviously, there are costs associated with supply and demand. In market systems other than health care, as the supply increases, the demand and the associated cost of purchasing a product decrease. The opposite is true when supply decreases: As the demand goes up and the amount of product declines or remains stable, the price increases because the product is scarcer. Changes in demand usually are related to changes in:

1. Prices of related goods
2. Incomes of the buyers
3. Preferences
4. Expectations

Changes in supply usually are related to changes in:

1. Prices of other goods
2. Prices of inputs
3. Technology (Duffy, 1993; Enthoven, 1993; Wessels, 1993)

The price of gasoline illustrates the concept of supply and demand. In the summer months, vacations result in increased demand for gasoline. If the supply of gasoline remains constant or declines as the demand increases, the price increases. The gasoline producers are able to increase the price of gasoline because the demand has increased and the public is willing to pay more for the product.

This relationship between supply and demand has not generally held true in health care, however, where costs continue to rise regardless of supply and demand. A major goal of health care reform is to force the health care market to react in a predictable fashion to the theory of supply and demand by creating market systems based on the competitive model of microeconomics used in other market systems such as retail (Enthoven, 1993). The supply and demand ratio often affects the cost of goods and services. This effect can result in inflation within a market system. Historically, the health care industry has not responded in the fashion typical of the supply and demand cycle. Whether health care is abundant or scarce, price increases. This phenomenon has baffled and frustrated health care economists for decades. With the understanding that competition usually drives down cost, the federal government introduced the competitive model to health care in the hopes of stabilizing prices.

Inflation

Inflation, a rise in the general level of prices, is a term generally associated with macroeconomic theory (Duffy, 1993; Wessels, 1993). Inflation is closely related to the concepts of supply and demand discussed earlier. A frustrating aspect of inflation and its relation to health care in the United States is that our costs appear to inflate whether or not there is ample supply or decreased demand. In fact, as the supply of health care during the Kennedy and Johnson administrations increased, the cost increased as well. Currently, the federal government is attempting to control the cost of health care by decreasing the supply and controlling how health care dollars are spent. While inflation has not proceeded at the rate it did in the 1970s and 1980s it nonetheless is still increasing. Federal and state governments and consumers are turning to managed care and managed competition as a means to control the inflationary tendencies of health care costs.

HEALTH CARE ECONOMIC TERMS

The following discussion highlights health care economic terms with which the nurse should become familiar.

Capitation

Capitation is a dollar amount established to cover the cost of health care services delivered to a person for a specific length of time, usually one year. The term usually refers to a negotiated, per capita (per person) rate to be paid periodically by a managed care organization to a health care provider. The provider is then responsible for delivering or arranging for the delivery of all health services required by the covered person under the conditions of the provider contract. Capitation may also refer to the amount paid to a managed care organization by the HCFA on behalf of Medicare or Medicaid recipients or by a state (HCFA, 1998a).

Case Management

Case management is the process whereby all health-related matters of a case are managed by a physician or nurse. Nurse and physician case managers coordinate designated components of health care, such as appropriate referral to consultants, specialists, hospitals, and services. Case management is intended to ensure continuity of services and accessibility and to negate the provision of fragmented services and redundant care and the misutilization of facilities and resources. It also attempts to match the appropriate intensity of services with the client's needs over time (HCFA, 1998b).

Co-payment

Co-payment is a cost-sharing arrangement whereby the person who is insured pays a specified charge (e.g., $10.00 for an office visit). The person is usually responsible for payment at the time that the service is rendered (HCFA, 1998a).

Diagnosis Related Groups (DRGs)

Diagnosis related groups is a prospective cost reimbursement classification system for inpatient services based on diagnosis, age, sex, and presence of complications. It is used as a means of both identifying costs for providing services associated with given diagnoses and reimbursing hospitals and select other providers for services rendered. The amount of payment is predetermined (HCFA, 1998b).

Fee for Service

Fee for service is a payment system whereby nurses, physicians, hospitals, and other providers are paid a specific amount for each service performed as it is rendered and identified by a claim for payment. Because costs of providing care vary depending on geographic location, fees also vary depending on region of the United States (HCFA, 1998b). For instance, the cost to build and operate a hospital in downtown San Francisco is more expensive than in rural California. In general, the costs of property, labor, and supplies are higher in cities as opposed to rural settings.

Managed Care

Reinhardt (1994) defines **managed care** as the external monitoring and comanaging of an ongoing provider–client relationship to ensure that the provider delivers *only* appropriate care. Staines (1993) notes that if all acute health care services were delivered through managed care systems, national health care expenditures might be decreased by as much as 10%. Managed care is seen as a means to control cost while also maintaining quality and access to appropriate care. Managed care is also a mechanism for introducing competition into the health care market and, thereby, for making the health care market respond in the expected fashion to the supply and demand cycle.

Managed Care Organization

A **managed care organization** is an entity that integrates financing and management and the delivery of health care services to an enrolled population. Managed care organizations provide, offer, or arrange for coverage of designated health services needed by members for a fixed, prepaid amount (HCFA, 1998a).

Managed Competition

Enthoven (1993) defines **managed competition** as "a purchasing strategy to obtain maximum value for employers and consumers" (p. 28). The theoretical foundation of managed competition is microeconomics, which rewards those suppliers who do the most efficient job of providing health care services that improve quality, cut costs, and satisfy consumers. The goal of managed care and managed competition is to limit expensive care that is unnecessary without interfering with appropriate treatment (Mechanic, 1994). Both managed care and managed competition are seen as potential strategies for third-party payors to control both the financial and reimbursement costs of the health care market.

Out-of-Pocket Expenses

Out-of-pocket expenses are expenses not covered by a health care plan and, thus, borne by the individual (HCFA, 1998a).

Preferred Provider Organization

A **preferred provider organization (PPO)** is a health care delivery system that contracts with providers of medical care to provide services at discounted fees to members. Members may seek care from nonparticipating providers but are generally penalized financially for doing so, via loss of discounts and higher co-pays and deductibles (HCFA, 1998b).

Prospective Cost Reimbursement

Prospective cost reimbursement is a method of paying all health care providers in which rates are established in advance. Providers are paid these rates regardless of the costs they actually incur. The best-known example of a prospective payment is the diagnosis related groups (DRGs) implemented by the Medicare program in 1983. DRG payments for each hospital are adjusted for differences in area wages, teaching activity, care to the poor, and other factors. DRGs, however, until recently applied only to hospitals, but did not apply to other facilities that provided services to Medicare beneficiaries. However, with the passage of the Balanced Budget Act of 1997 (BBA) (P.L. 105-33), the federal government implemented prospective payment systems for skilled nursing facilities in July 1998, and will do so for hospital outpatient departments in January 1999, long-term care hospitals and home health agencies in October 1999, and rehabilitation facilities in October 2000. The extension of prospective payments to these providers is expected to simplify payments and lower the growth of payments made by the Medicare program. Community health nurses can anticipate that as prospective payment systems cover the services that they have traditionally provided to Medicare beneficiaries, payment rates will become tighter and the financial health of many community agencies is likely to deteriorate.

Cost-Plus and Retrospective Reimbursement

Cost-plus reimbursement is reimbursement based on what a service costs, plus the addition of some percentage of profit. The cost of the service and the profit are predetermined and agreed upon by the provider and purchaser. **Retrospective cost reimbursement** is a type of reimbursement system that has no pre-established reimbursement rates and is commonly referred to as the fee-for-service system. In this system the provider would tally the cost of the service and send the bill to a third party, either the federal or state government programs such as Medicare or Medicaid, or to an insurance company. The third party would then reimburse the provider for services rendered. The fee-for-service system did have one minimal control mechanism. Providers were reimbursed on the basis of reasonable and customary charges. Reasonable and customary charges differed by region of the United States and by type of provider. For instance, a general practitioner would generally be reimbursed at a lower rate than a specialist. And the general practitioner in New York City would be reimbursed at a higher rate than a general practitioner in Kansas City because the cost of doing business in New York City is higher.

Third-Party Payor

Third-party payors for health care services vary and are determined by one's health care coverage. *Third party* refers to an entity other than the provider or the consumer that is responsible for total or partial payment of health care costs (Levit, Olin, & Letsch, 1992). Whether the third party pays all or a portion depends on the type of coverage. If the consumer is required to make partial payment, that payment is commonly referred to as a co-pay. For elderly persons, the third-party payor is Medicare; for the poor, it is Medicaid; and for the insured, it is the insurance company. The prevalence of third-party payors decreases the role that price plays in determining the supply and demand of health care services. Because the bill is sent directly from the provider to the payor, effectively bypassing the consumer, the consumer is unaware of the cost. Remember, the cost of a product is determined by the price that the consumer is willing to pay for that product. If consumers are not aware of the costs of their care, there is little incentive for providers to control those costs.

Medicare

Medicare Part A, or the Hospital Insurance (HI) program, helps pay for hospital, home health, skilled nursing facility, and hospice care for the aged and disabled. Part A is financed primarily by payroll taxes paid by workers and employers. The taxes paid each year are used mainly to pay benefits for current beneficiaries. Income not currently needed to pay benefits and related expenses is held in the HI trust fund and invested in U.S. Treasury securities. At age 65, people are automatically enrolled in Part A regardless of whether they are retired. A person and his or her spouse who have paid into the Social Security system via employment for 40 quarters or more are eligible for Social Security. People who have paid into the Social Security system for fewer than 40 quarters can enroll in Part A by paying a monthly premium. People who are totally and permanently disabled and are under age 65 may enroll in Part A after having received Social Security disability benefits for 24 months. People with chronic renal disease requiring dialysis or a transplant are also eligible for Part A after a 24-month waiting period.

A qualified hospital stay is one that meets the following criteria: (1) A doctor prescribes inpatient hospital care for an illness or injury. (2) The illness or injury requires care that can be provided only in a hospital. (3) The hospital participates in the Medicare program. (4) The hospital's utilization review committee agrees with the need for hospitalization.

A qualified nursing facility care stay must meet the following five criteria to be reimbursed by Medicare Part A: (1) The enrollee requires skilled nursing or rehabilitation services that can be provided only in a skilled nursing facility. (2) The enrollee was in a hospital for 3 days in a row, not counting the day of discharge, before entering the skilled nursing facility. (3) The enrollee is admitted to a facility within a short period of time (generally 30 days)

after leaving the hospital. (4) The condition for which the enrollee is receiving skilled nursing facility care was treated in the hospital, or arose while the person was receiving care in the hospital. (5) A medical professional certifies that daily skilled nursing or rehabilitation care is necessary.

Medicare Part A qualified home health care must meet the following four criteria: (1) The enrollee requires intermittent skilled nursing care, physical therapy, or speech-language therapy. (2) The enrollee is confined to home. (3) A physician determines that the enrollee needs home health care and sets up a plan for the person to receive care at home. (4) The home health agency providing the care participates in Medicare.

Medicare Part A also covers hospice care if the enrollee meets the following criteria: (1) The enrollee's physician and the hospice's physician certify that the enrollee is terminally ill. (2) The enrollee chooses to receive hospice care instead of the standard Medicare benefits for the illness. (3) The care is provided by a Medicare participating hospice program. See Table 4-1 for a summary of Medicare Part A benefits.

Medicare Part B, or the Supplementary Medical Insurance (SMI) program, pays for physician, outpatient hospital, and other services for the aged and disabled. Part B is financed primarily by transfers from the general fund (tax revenues) of the U.S. Treasury (approximately 75%) and by monthly premiums paid by beneficiaries. Income not currently needed to pay benefits and related expenses is held in the SMI trust fund and invested in U.S. Treasury securities (HCFA, 1997a).

Part B must be applied for at age 65 when enrolling in Medicare Part A. The monthly Part B premium is automatically deducted from the person's Social Security check (HCFA, 1998b).

Medicare Part B pays for a wide range of medical services and supplies. Medically necessary services of a physician are covered no matter where the enrollee receives them, whether at home, in the physician's office, in a clinic, nursing home, or hospital. Part B benefits have special requirements, and some are more strictly limited than others. The Medicare Part B premium covers physician services, hospital out-patient care, and durable medical equipment.

Ambulance services is one of the benefits that is strictly limited. Medicare Part B will pay for an ambulance when the ambulance, equipment, and personnel meet Medicare requirements, and if the transportation in any other vehicle could endanger the enrollee's health. Coverage is generally restricted to transportation between the enrollee's home and the hospital or the enrollee's home and a skilled nursing facility.

The enrollee is responsible for paying 20% of whatever the hospital charges, not 20% of a Medicare-approved amount. For some outpatient mental health services, the enrollees share can be as much as 50% of the Medicare approved amount. See Table 4-1 for a summary of Medicare Part B benefits. A further discussion of Medicare can be found later in this chapter.

Table 4-1   Medicare A and B Summary of Benefits

MEDICARE PART A

Who Is Eligible

A person is eligible for Medicare Part A if the person or his or her spouse worked for at least 10 years in Medicare-covered employment and the person is 65 years of age and a citizen or permanent resident of the United States.

Benefits

Inpatient hospitalization	Days 1–60 Medicare Part A pays except for the $760 deductible.	Days 61–90 Medicare Part A pays except for $190/day.	Days 91–150 Medicare Part A pays except for $380/day. (Note: beyond 150 with lifetime reserve days used, Medicare Part A pays nothing.)
Skilled nursing facility	Days 1–20 Medicare Part A pays the full cost of services.	Days 21–100 Medicare Part A pays all but $95/day.	After 100 days Medicare Part A does not pay for services.
Home health care	All services covered if enrollee meets the Medicare Part A criteria for home health care.	Medicare Part A pays the full cost of some medical supplies if billed through the home health agency.	Medicare Part A pays 80% of approved durable medical equipment such as wheel-chairs, hospital beds, oxygen supplies, and walkers.
Hospice care	Patient must elect to take the Medicare Part A hospice care instead of the standard Medi-care inpatient hospital benefits. The patient's physician must certify that the person suffers from a terminal illness.	Medicare pays the entire bill for hospice services.	There is a co-pay of $5 for each drug prescription.

MEDICARE PART B

Who Is Eligible

All Medicare Part A enrollees who elect to pay the monthly Part B premium of $43.80 are eligible.

Benefits

Medical expenses	Medicare Part B pays a portion of the bill for all medically necessary services.	Medically necessary services are physician care, physical and occupational therapy, medical equipment, diagnostic tests, and speech therapy.	Medicare pays 80% of approved amount after the enrollee pays the $100 annual deductible.
Preventive care	Medicare Part B will pay for services no matter where the enrollee receives them (inpatient or outpatient).	Medicare Part B pays for screening pap smears, breast prostheses following mastectomy, screening mammograms, artificial limbs, and eyes.	
Outpatient medications	Medicare Part B does not cover medications.		

From Health Care Finance Administration. Data extracted from Health Care Finance Administration home page. Available: http//www.HCFA.gov. Sept. 22, 1998.

Medicaid

Medicaid is a program funded by federal and state taxes and administered by the states. Medicaid pays for the health care of low-income persons. Services and eligibility differ from state to state; however, all states must provide certain federally mandated services in order to qualify for federal matching funds. Medicaid does not cover all peo-ple below the federal poverty line. Those mandated for coverage by the federal government are the following:

1. Recipients of Aid to Families with Dependent Children (AFDC)

2. Those people who are over age 65, blind, or totally disabled and who receive income from Supplemen-tal Security Income (SSI)

3. Pregnant women with incomes up to 133% of the federal poverty line

4. Children born after 1983 to families with incomes at or below the federal poverty line

A more detailed discussion of Medicaid can be found later in this chapter. Both Medicare and Medicaid rely on DRGs to finance and reimburse services they cover (HCFA, 1998a).

Health Maintenance Organization

Health maintenance organizations (HMOs) are a type of insurance. An HMO contracts with and enrolls individuals and groups to provide comprehensive health care services on a prepaid basis. These agencies can be profit or nonprofit. Health maintenance organizations emphasize preventive health services, and most provide inpatient and outpatient services (HCFA, 1998a). For a further discussion of HMOs, see Chapter 3.

FACTORS CAUSING UPWARD CLIMB OF HEALTH CARE COSTS

Issues related to health care costs underlie all aspects of the U.S. health care system and greatly influence all policy questions. Lee and Estes (1994) cite three basic reasons for the tremendous expenditure on health care in the United States:

1. Rising cost per volume of service
2. Per capita increase in volume of services
3. Growth in specific population groups such as elderly persons

A number of experts would additionally cite the introduction of advanced technology, rising administrative costs, client complexity, excess capacity, uncompensated care, and health care fraud as driving forces in the rapid and sustained increase in health care costs in the United States (Lamm, 1994). A brief discussion of these factors follows.

Cost per Volume of Service (CPVS)

Cost per volume of service (CPVS) is the cost associated with a particular volume of service. For example a community health agency knows the cost of doing a certain number of home visits for a particular type of client, such as a postoperative hip replacement. The costs associated with the care of the hip replacement client are supplies (dressings and drugs), equipment (bedside commode, trapeze, wheel chair), and staff salaries. The agency can

calculate the cost of care for a particular volume of clients and then staff the agency accordingly. The staffing procedure is directly linked to the amount of reimbursement an agency will receive for a particular diagnosis. The cost of that volume minus the rate of reimbursement is considered profit for the agency.

Per Capita Increase in Volume of Services (PCIVS)

Per capita increase in volume (PCIVS) is the increase in client days in the hospital, client visits in the ambulatory clinic, or home visits in the community health agency calculated over a one-year period. It is important to know exactly which services are increasing or decreasing so resources can be properly allocated to that service.

Growth in Specific Population Groups

Growth in specific population groups is a vital piece of information for any health care agency. Federal, state, local, and private agencies need to know the types of individuals they are serving to better plan service delivery. Population-based programs for specific groups such as the elderly or pregnant teenagers have very specific needs, and programs must be planned and financed with these needs in mind.

Advanced Technology

The introduction of advanced technology may or may not decrease the cost of care. In one example, Bodenheimer and Grunback (1998) note that the introduction of the laparoscopic cholecystectomy increased both the cost per volume of service and the number of procedures. They point out that laparoscopic technology shortened the operation time, decreased postoperative pain, and decreased length of hospital stay and recuperation. At first review this seems like a win-win situation for the client, the health care organization, and the physician. However, on closer examination the actual cost of the surgery increased. This technology greatly decreased the dangers of conventional surgery and drove up the per capita volume of cholecystectomies, and the total cost of this increased volume actually increased the cost of the cholecystectomy 11%.

Rising Administrative Costs

Administrative costs associated with the management of health care are expressed as a percentage. Rising administrative costs have been a concern because every dollar spent on administrative costs is a dollar not available for direct patient care. Bodenheimer and Grunback (1998) note that administrative costs have typically risen at a higher percentage than the cost of providing the care itself.

Client Complexity

Client complexity also adds to the cost of care. The more complex the client's needs, the more costly the care. For instance, a middle-aged man who has had a myocardial infarction and is also a brittle diabetic is likely to consume more health care resources than that same man without diabetes. Clients with complex needs are particularly suited for case management.

Excess Capacity

Excess capacity is a term usually associated with other service industries. The airline industry is said to have excess capacity if on the average airlines fly their planes with empty seats. Because an airline seat does not have anyone on it paying for the service, the cost of doing business for that airline goes up. As the number of empty seats increases, the cost of doing business also increases. This same concept can be applied to health care. With the introduction of advanced technology, we can reduce the length of stay in the hospital and home care. As clients take less and less time to recover, the total patient days will go down and the number of empty beds will increase—that is considered excess capacity.

Uncompensated Care

Uncompensated care refers to the personal health care rendered by hospitals or other providers without payment from the client or a government-sponsored or private insurance program. It includes both charity care, which is provided without the expectation of payment, and bad debts, for which the provider has made an unsuccessful effort to collect payment due from the client (Prospective Payment Assessment Commission, 1997).

Over the past two decades, whenever hospitals have complained that Medicare payments for services provided to beneficiaries are too low, administrators have asserted that they will be unable to continue providing charity care at the same level. The threat of further limited access to care for certain vulnerable populations has resulted in Congress's creating certain additional payments to hospitals that serve a relatively large volume of low-income clients (called the disproportionate share adjustment) (Prospective Payment Assessment Commission, 1997). Uncompensated care has also been raised by critics of for-profit hospitals who have argued that these hospitals have lower uncompensated care levels and hence provide less care to low-income people and those without health insurance. However, the evidence on this issue is mixed and far from conclusive. Nonetheless, in the years ahead, community health nurses can anticipate that as payments to hospitals become tighter, and

prospective payment systems are applied to non-hospital providers, the level of uncompensated care provided by community and other non-hospital providers will probably rise and threaten the financial stability of these organizations. As this occurs, the issue of uncompensated care will gain increasing attention by policymakers and community health agencies.

Health Care Fraud

The Medicare program defines fraud as the intentional deception or misrepresentation that an individual knows to be false or does not believe to be true and makes, knowing that the deception could result in some unauthorized benefit to himself or herself or some other person. The most frequent kind of fraud arises from a false statement or misrepresentation concerning payment under the Medicare program. Violators include physicians and other practitioners, hospitals and other institutional providers, clinical laboratories and medical devise suppliers, employees of providers and billing services, and beneficiaries or people in a position to file a claim for Medicare benefits. Examples of the most common forms of fraud include: billing for services not furnished; misrepresenting the diagnosis to justify payment; soliciting, offering, or receiving a kickback; unbundling or "exploding" charges; falsifying certificates of medical necessity, plans of treatment, and medical records to justify payment. Because each year the Medicare program makes several billion dollars in fraudulent payments, Congress and the Clinton administration have passed legislation aimed at identifying and severely penalizing those who commit fraud. In the years ahead, community health nurses can expect their employers to be increasingly cautious to avoid engaging in any fraudulent activities or risk the appearance of fraud.

GOVERNMENT IN HEALTH CARE

The question of the proper role of government in general as well as the relative distribution of power among federal, state, and local governments has been the subject of heated philosophical debates in health care reform circles. The rising costs of health care have overwhelmed third-party payors, leading them to decrease the total number of covered citizens. This has left a staggering 15.6% of the U.S. population—or an estimated 41.7 million people—without insurance (U.S. Bureau of the Census, 1997). The underinsured constitute an estimated additional 15 million people (U.S. Bureau of the Census, 1997). The uninsured and underinsured often seek health care through the most expensive and least effective avenue of the U.S. health care system: hospital emergency departments. Episodic care coupled with a lack of follow-up services may exacerbate both the person's illness and the financial woes of the health care system. An additional contributing factor to the numbers of uninsured and underinsured people is the inability of small and medium businesses to offer health insurance. As the price of providing health care insurance has increased, so has the inability of small to medium business owners to afford the cost of providing employee health insurance (Levit et al., 1992).

Himmelstein, Woolhandler, and Wolf (1992) note that lack of insurance affects ethnic groups differently. In 1992, for example, Hispanics accounted for the largest percentage of the uninsured, followed by African Americans, and then non–Hispanic Whites.

Race and ethnicity continue to be associated with lack of health insurance. In 1996, minority workers, especially Hispanic workers, were far more likely than Caucasians or African Americans to be uninsured. As illustrated in Figure 4-3, 38% of Hispanic workers and 25.7% of African-American workers were uninsured in 1996, compared with 14.7% of Caucasian workers (HCFA, 1997b).

Concomitantly, federal and state governments have also reduced health benefits covered by Medicare and Medicaid and state-sponsored programs, via reform of laws governing hospitals and physician-reimbursement policies. Additionally, employers have attempted to control the skyrocketing costs of health care by developing strategies that reduce cost, such as offering incentives for employees to reduce their use of health care services or charging a co-payment for services consumed. Walsey (1992) notes an alarming and growing trend among many employers, especially those in the service sector, of simply not providing access to health insurance coverage. (Service-sector jobs are those generally associated with low or minimal wage, such as retail store clerk and fast-food service worker.)

In terms of health and welfare, generally the U.S. system of government provides for the government to do

only that which private institutions either cannot or will not do. The role of the government has therefore historically been to intervene only when a remedy was needed for a failure of the private sector to provide a service. This rule of exception rather than of primary intervention on the part of government has led to the current uncoordinated, piecemeal health care system that while currently consuming 14% of the U.S. GNP (Levit et al., 1992; HCFA, 1998), does not provide comprehensive care for at least 41.7 million citizens who have no insurance (U.S. Bureau of the Census, 1997).

Over the past 200 years, the role of the U.S. government in the policy, organization, financing, and destiny of health care has evolved from that of a highly constricted provider of services and protector of public health to that of a major financial underwriter of an essentially private enterprise. Government policies and procedures have increasingly encroached on the autonomy of providers as a means to control costs (Levit et al., 1992; Walsey, 1992). As costs began to spiral upward and out of control, the government increasingly became the agency of cost control, access, and quality via programs such as Medicare and Medicaid.

Litman (1994) cites several distinct characteristics of government's role in the U.S. health care system:

1. Paying vendors to ensure availability of care
2. Policing the system to ensure standards
3. Providing direct funding to upgrade systems and educate the health care practitioner

THE CHANGING CLIMATE IN HEALTH CARE

Between 1961 and 1969, the federal government's role and responsibility began to change in relation to health care. During the Kennedy and Johnson presidencies, federal health care aid moneys were channeled through the state systems. The federal government began to direct federal support for local governments, nonprofit organizations, and private businesses and corporations to provide health care, health education, social services, and community development programs focused on the health of its citizens. Davis (1994) notes that with the passage of the Great Society legislation, and specifically Medicare and Medicaid, the federal government ushered in a new era of commitment to improving the health and well-being of the poor and elders, including increasing their access to health care services. In 1967, 19.5 million people were enrolled in Medicare; in 1996, the number was 35.3 million, an increase of 15.8 million. In 1997, 41.7 million people were without health insurance (HCFA, 1998a). Between 1960 and 1987, the time between the Great Society of presidents Kennedy and Johnson and the Reagan presidency, dramatic gains were made in the health and well-being of those covered by Medicare and Medicaid (Enthoven, 1994).

Figure 4-3 Percent of Uninsured Persons within Racial and Ethnic Groups: 1996

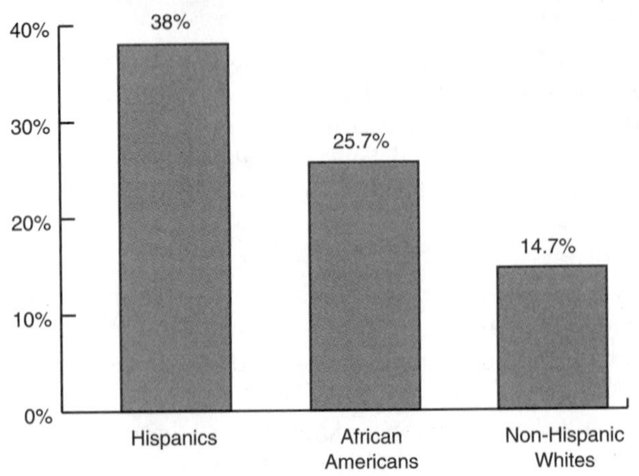

From Health Care Finance Administration, "Expenditure Panel Survey," March 1996.

In 1960, life expectancy at age 65 was 69.7 years for all races. In 1996, the figure was 80.4 years, an increase of more than 10 years. Data for the same year indicate that females of all races have the longest life expectancy at 84.2 years, compared with 78.2 years for males of all races (U.S. Bureau of the Census, 1997).

During the 1970s, President Nixon began his program of New Federalism and, with that, the move to a system that transferred revenues for state and local use with as few strings and regulations as possible. This system became known as block grants. Under President Nixon, block grants were given so that states and communities could use the monies for broad purposes that met their specific needs. President Nixon additionally believed that the federal government should play a significant role in providing health care and, thus, sought the direct support of both private and public institutions and systems that provided care (Litman, 1994).

The administrations of presidents Reagan and Bush accelerated the degree of change in health care policy that began with Nixon. The Reagan–Bush agenda had several specific aims, specifically to:

1. Reduce federal funding for domestic social welfare programs

2. Decentralize programs to states using block grants

3. Emphasize greater market forces to shape the health care system

4. Implement the DRG prospective payment system

Reagan and Bush attempted a variety of cost-control strategies at the federal, state, and local levels of government. Despite their efforts, however, health care costs continued to escalate (Enthoven, 1994; Litman, 1994).

During his first presidential campaign, President Clinton proposed that employers pay for much of the cost of health care and that federal subsidies be used for the purchase of insurance for low-income citizens. Clinton also wanted the federal government to provide subsidies to small-business owners for whom the universal mandate would be overly burdensome (Kronick, 1993; Enthoven, 1994). Without governmental subsidies, neither low-income people nor small-business owners would have been able to afford the Clinton mandate for employer-based health care coverage.

The Clinton administration advocated universal coverage through managed care, health alliances, and employer health care mandates. The Clinton plan included a guaranteed comprehensive health care package encompassing hospital and physician services, prescription drugs, and laboratory services. The plan also called for long-term care and expanded in-home services as well as prevention services for prenatal care, immunizations, and annual examinations (Enthoven, 1994; Enthoven & Kronick, 1994; Lundberg, 1994).

Although the Clinton plan failed as a total package, certain features of the plan were adopted in 1996 by the 104th Congress. Senators Kennedy and Kasselbaum drafted and the Congress passed a health care bill that prevents persons who change jobs from losing their health care benefits. The major disadvantages of the Kennedy–Kasselbaum bill were that mental health benefits were not covered and that no limitation was placed on the percentage of premium increase when a person transfers from one carrier to another.

As major payors, providers, and regulators of health care, the states are playing an ever-increasing role in the health care system. At no time in the history of the United States has this been truer than in the current throes of health care reform. Despite the fact that health care reform failed in 1994 in the 103rd Congress, several states have implemented their own health care reform measures. Moreover, states have come to regard fundamental changes in both the financing and delivery of health care as necessary to control costs and ensure access (Berrand & Schroeder, 1994). Stabilizing the Medicare Trust Fund constitutes the major focus of the 105th Congress. Potential health care reform measures include increasing the number of Medicare enrollees in managed care insurance plans, increasing the amount of co-pay for services and medications, and, perhaps, introducing means testing for level of coverage within the Medicare system. Means testing is a mechanism for determining the amount of money an enrollee might pay for services on the basis of his or her annual income (White House Fact Sheet, 1998).

President Clinton's 1998 budget contained proposals to continue to provide Medicare and Medicaid enrollees with both managed care and fee-for-service plans. Clinton also proposed to extend the Kennedy–Kasselbaum health portability plan to people in Medicare and Medicaid programs and, further, to improve access to medigap coverage (private health insurance that pays certain costs not covered by fee-for-service Medicare, such as Medicare co-payments and deductibles). President Clinton also proposed a series of new efforts to enroll uninsured children in health insurance programs. Of the 10 million uninsured children in 1997, nearly 90% had parents who worked but who did not have access to or could not afford health insurance. In response, President Clinton proposed an investment of $900 million over 5 years in children's health outreach programs (White House Fact Sheet, 1998).

Medicaid has constituted the fastest growing component in state budgets (Congressional Budget Office, 1995). The number of Medicaid recipients increased from approximately 10 million in 1967 to 37.5 million in 1996, an increase of 275%. The number of enrolled dependent children rose from 9.8 million in 1985 to 18.2 million in 1996, an increase of 80% (HCFA, 1996). If national health care reform does not pass soon, it may fall to the states to reform the U.S. health care system. Arguments can be made both for and against experimentation with health care reform at the state level, and these arguments often mimic those made at the national level. The main argument against state experimentation is that the states lack the financial resources and capacity necessary for health care reform. Furthermore, the business community sees health care insurance mandates and taxes as detrimental to small business (Berrand & Schroeder, 1994). Small-business owners often see additional programs mandated by the federal and state governments as increasing their cost of doing business. A small-business owner usually cannot absorb additional taxes and must therefore pass the additional cost of the tax on to the customer. As customers recognize that the cost of the service increases they must decide whether the service is now worth the cost. Organizations that are much larger can spread such a cost over many more customers and locations, thereby not noticeably increasing the cost of the service. One argument in favor of state experimentation is that the states offer arenas for both testing different forms of health care reform and gauging that which the general public as well as the business community is willing to support. It is further argued that the states are better positioned to develop specific systems targeted at specific state needs (Berrand & Schroeder, 1994).

For nearly three decades, health care spending has far outpaced economic growth in the United States. Between 1980 and 1991, in fact, national health expenditures increased twice as fast as did the GDP. As a result, the share of GDP devoted to health care grew from 8.9% in 1980 to 13.6% in 1995 and to 14.4% in 1997 (see Figure 4-4) (HCFA, 1998a).

For this reason, the cost of health care continues to attract the attention of the public, employers, insurance companies, federal and state governments, and policymakers. In 1960, the United States spent $124 per capita (per person) for health care; in 1990, the figure was $2,364, and in 1996 it was $3,295. By the year 2000, the per capita figure for health care is expected to rise to $5,712 (see Figure 4-5) (HCFA, 1997b). Of the 1996 amount, 88% was allotted for the purchase of medical care services or products, with the remainder dedicated to administrative costs.

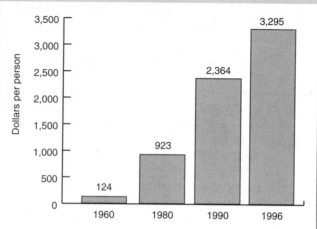

Figure 4-5   Per Capita Health Spending in the United States: 1960–1996

From Health Care Finance Administration. Data extracted from Health Care Finance Administration home page. Available: http// www. HCFA.gov. "Medicare Bulletin" January 1997b.

A recent study (Woolhandler & Himmelstein, 1997) estimates that administrative costs accounted for an average of 26% of total hospital costs in fiscal year 1994, up 1.2 percentage points from 1990. In 1991, the federal government spent $40.9 billion on health program administration, and in 1996, the amount had risen to $60.9 billion. In 1997, the federal government spent $0.26 of every dollar on costs to administer government-sponsored health care programs (HCFA, 1998b). Figure 4-6 displays the per capita out-of-pocket expenditures for given years from 1960 to 1996. As this figure illustrates, a dramatic decrease of over 50% occurred between 1960 and 1980. The enact-

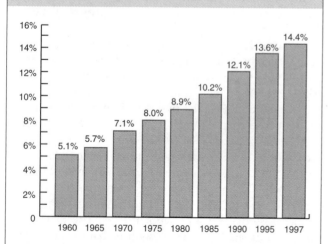

Figure 4-4   Health Care Expenditures As Percentage of GDP: 1960–1997

From Health Care Finance Administration, "Medicare Bulletin," January 1998.

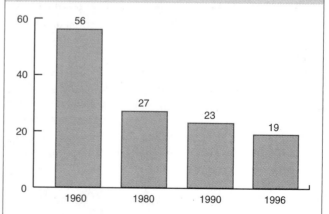

Figure 4-6   Per Capita Out-of-Pocket Spending As Percentage of Total Health Care Personal Expenditures: 1960–1996

From Health Care Finance Administration. Data extracted from Health Care Finance Administration home page. Available: http// www. HCFA.gov. "Medicare Bulletin" January 1997b.

ment of Medicare in the mid-1960s accounts in large part for this decrease (HCFA, 1997b).

COST CONTROLS

A myriad of initiatives designed to curb increases in health care expenditures have met with generally limited success (Kronick, 1993). Some such initiatives—such as prospective payment systems (DRGs), increased governmental regulation, audits, and controls on access to care—are meant to drive down costs. Other initiatives include managed care and the publishing of comparative pricing information to assist individuals and employers in selecting health care providers.

Cost controls are of two primary types: finance controls and reimbursement controls. **Finance controls** attempt to limit the flow of funds into public or private health care insurance plans. The intention is to force the plans to reduce the outflow of reimbursement. Finance controls can be further subdivided into two types: regulation and competition (Enthoven, 1993; Kronick, 1993).

Regulatory finance controls for public systems rely primarily on restricting the amount of state or federal tax revenues deposited into programs that fund health care programs such as Medicare or Medicaid. Another finance substrategy is to introduce competition into the market system. This strategy is used primarily in employment-based systems and takes advantage of market forces to constrain costs. Market forces rely on microeconomic principles to drive down costs. Competition forces providers and insurance plans to hold down costs in order to attract enrollees to their services (Enthoven, 1993; Kronick, 1993).

Reimbursement controls take several forms: price controls, utilization controls, and client cost sharing. The state and federal governments as well as insurance plans have enacted price-control mechanisms such as usual and customary reimbursement. In **usual and customary reimbursement**, the provider agrees to provide a service for a predetermined level of reimbursement (Enthoven, 1993). In **client cost sharing**, or co-pay, the client is required to pay for a portion of his or her health care. The intention is to make the consumer aware of the cost of care in the hope of driving down cost (Kronick, 1993).

Utilization controls are primarily geared toward controlling the supply side of the health care market. The primary strategy is to monitor the clinical activities of providers for the purpose of controlling costs (Enthoven, 1996). The provider is evaluated against other providers who offer similar services to determine the cost of care in relation to quality and outcomes. Providers who fall outside the pre-established norm are often sanctioned by the insurance plan. Sanctions can take many forms. Decreased referrals is one form of sanction, reimbursement made at the predetermined level regardless of the cost to the provider is another.

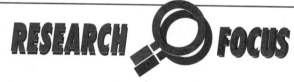

RESEARCH FOCUS

A Randomized Trial of Early Hospital Discharge and Home Follow-up of Women Who Have Unplanned Cesarean Section

STUDY PROBLEM/PURPOSE

To determine whether early discharge after unplanned cesarean section is safe and cost effective.

METHODS

Participants included 122 women randomly assigned to either early discharge with home follow-up care by a nurse specialist or to usual discharge time frame of 2 to 3 days.

FINDINGS

Women in the early discharge group went home 30.3 hours earlier than did those in the other group. Women discharged early expressed greater satisfaction with their care, and the charges for their home care were 29% lower than the charges for women discharged within the usual time frame.

IMPLICATIONS

Women who have had unplanned cesarean sections can be discharged early without compromising, and, in some cases, increasing satisfaction while at the same time controlling the cost of care. Reducing the cost of care and maintaining a quality service as judged by the client is thus a reachable goal. Maintaining quality while reducing the cost of care requires planning and client postdischarge support and education. Nurses have a responsibility to control costs whenever possible, and this study clearly indicates that this can be accomplished. To do so, nurses and other members of the health care team must continually undertake critical examination of the care process.

SOURCE

From "A Randomized Trial of Early Hospital Discharge and Home Follow-up of Women Who Have Unplanned Cesarean Section" by D. Brooten, 1994, Obstetrics and Gynecology, 84, pp. 832–834.

DECISION MAKING

The Nurse's Role in Controlling Health Insurance Costs

Employer-subsidized health insurance costs are increasing, which may result in increasingly fewer employers being able to offer health insurance to their employees.

• How can nurses help employers control insurance costs while enhancing the health of employees?

• What role can nurses take in an organization, and what programs might they design, to help create a healthier work environment with the concomitant benefit of curbing the rising costs of employer-based health insurance?

Actions to Control Costs

Although the introduction of the 1983 Medicare prospective payment system, known as DRGs, provided some respite from double-digit health care cost inflation, the majority of savings resulted from the decrease in the rates of hospital admissions under the DRG system. With the DRG system, Medicare established a fixed schedule of regionally appropriate fees paid for the treatment of each of the 475 DRGs. If the actual cost to the provider is lower than the DRG fee, the provider keeps the difference. If the cost of providing care is higher than the DRG fee, however, the provider absorbs the loss. The purpose of the prospective payment system was to encourage price sensitivity and, thereby, galvanize providers to control costs. The consumer and physician, however, did not feel price sensitivity, because the majority of savings were realized in decreased admission rates rather than in more efficient, appropriate, and cost-effective care. By the end of the third year of DRG (1986), the yearly increase in health care spending had risen to 10.7% of the GDP (Mechanic, 1994). In 1997, national health care expenditures as a percentage of GDP had risen to 14.4% (HCFA, 1998a).

An example of cost controls that take into account most of the variables mentioned earlier in this chapter is to control the types, rather than the numbers, of providers. Enthoven (1996) notes that increasing the proportion of general physicians may lead to savings for two reasons. First, generalists earn lower incomes than do specialists. Second, and of greater significance to overall cost savings, generalists appear to practice less resource-intensive care and, therefore, to generate lower overall health care expenditures. Furthermore, studies indicate that nurse practitioners can effectively perform many tasks of the primary care physician at a lower cost and an equal level of quality (Enthoven, 1996). Thus, the combination of increasing the numbers of generalists and using nurse practitioners as primary care providers may drive down costs while maintaining access and quality.

ACCESS TO HEALTH CARE INSURANCE

No single nationwide system of health insurance guarantees access to health care in the United States. The United States relies primarily on employers to voluntarily provide health insurance coverage to their employees and dependents. Although the popularity of employment-based insurance plans can be explained, in part, by their cost advantage over individual plans, the major reason for their dominance is that such plans are subsidized via federal and state taxes (Levit et al., 1992). In 1960, per capita personal health care expenditures were $124, with $69 (56%) being out-of-pocket expenses. In 1996, per capita health care expenditures had increased to $3,295, with $622 (18%) being out-of-pocket expenses. The dramatic decrease in out-of-pocket expenses from 56% in 1960 to 18% in 1996 (HCFA, 1997b) can be traced to the federal government and private and employer-based insurance programs taking an increasingly larger role in the financing of health care.

At first glance, the employment-based system seems to provide employees and dependents with insurance at very low costs, because employers generally pay most of the premium. Careful analysis, however, demonstrates that the employer's cost is largely shifted back to the employee in the form of lower wages and reduced benefits (Levit et al., 1992; Congressional Budget Report, 1993).

One of the most troubling developments in recent years is the increase in the number of employees and their dependents who do not have health insurance even though they are employed full time (Figure 4-7). This lack of coverage constitutes a particularly acute problem among certain groups of employees, such as those who work for small businesses or those who work for low wages, especially in the growing service sector of the U.S. economy. This expanding pattern is not accidental; rather, it reflects inherent weaknesses in the current system of employment-based insurance. As health care costs continue to grow unchecked, the disparity between those traditionally enjoying employment-based coverage and those uninsured in the small-business and service sectors will continue to grow. According to the U.S. Bureau of the Census statistics for 1997, of the 266.8 million total U.S. population, 225.1 million were with insurance, and 41.7 million were without insurance. One-fourth of the uninsured, or 10.6 million, were children. The majority of the insured, 187.4 million, were covered by private health

℗℘ REFLECTIVE THINKING ℗℘

Our Nation's Values in Health Care

If each nation's health care system is a reflection of its values, what values are being reflected in the U.S. health care system?

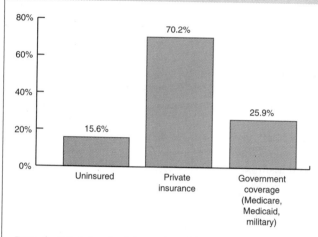

Figure 4-7 Insured/Uninsured As Percentage of U.S. Population: 1996

From the U.S. Labor Statistics and Health Care Finance Administration, Data extracted from the U.S. Labor Statistics and Health Care Finance Administration home pages. Available : http//www. govstarts.gov and http/www.HCPA.gov. March 1996.

Note: *Types of coverage are not mutually exclusive: i.e., persons may be covered by more than one type of health plan during the year.*

insurance, 163.2 million were covered by employment-based insurance, and Medicare and Medicaid insured 66.7 million (U.S. Bureau of the Census, 1997).

According to the Agency for Health Care Policy and Research (1996), three primary factors influence the growing number of uninsured and underinsured citizens. First, employment-based insurance is voluntary. Second, insurance companies practice risk sorting and restrictive underwriting. Under these practices, employers are assessed premiums on the basis of the health experience of their employees. Employers with high-risk employees, such as smokers or employees with pre-existing health conditions, pay higher premiums than do employers with low-risk employees. Third, some people rely on subsidized health care provided in the emergency rooms of public hospitals. The growing numbers of people who fall into this category are those who work 40 hours per week and do not have access to health care insurance, those who have been laid off, and the increasing numbers of homeless.

Health insurance obtained through the workplace is the primary source of private coverage for most Americans. Data from the 1997 Medical Expenditure Panel Survey (MEPS) (HCFA, 1997c) indicate that during the first half of 1996, on average, nearly two-thirds of nonelderly Americans (64.1%, or 148.5 million persons) obtained employment-related health insurance. The MEPS data also indicate that nearly one-fifth of nonelderly workers ages 16 to 64 (18.4%, or approximately 23 million persons) were without health insurance.

The importance of the workplace as a source of private health insurance, the incentives for inefficient health plan choice associated with the employment-based insurance system, and the size and composition of the employed

uninsured population have constituted ongoing public policy concerns. Specific issues receiving attention have included availability disparities, out-of-pocket costs, and tax treatment of employment-based coverage for workers in different employment circumstances. The inability of some workers or their dependents with health problems to obtain such coverage and the gaps in the continuity of work-related health insurance during employment transitions will constitute major areas of focus of Congress over the next five years (White House Fact Sheet, 1998).

HEALTH CARE PROGRAMS

Health insurance mandated and subsidized by the federal and state governments and offered via employers is receiving increased attention from the federal and state governments as a means of access to health care providers. For several decades, the United States has been faced with the problems of increasing numbers of uninsured and underinsured persons and rising health care costs. Finding options for insuring the growing numbers of uninsured and underinsured has become an increasingly important issue to policymakers, employers, and individuals as health care costs have skyrocketed over the last decade. Health spending's share of the economy grew from 9% to more than 12% between 1980 and 1990, and by another 1.5 percentage points between 1990 and 1993. From 1993 through 1997, health spending stabilized at roughly 13.5% of GDP, the longest period in which the health care sector has grown no faster than the rest of the economy in at least 30 years. However, the Congressional Budget Office (January 1998) projects that the growth in health spending will soon accelerate, and that national health expenditures will reach 15.5% of GDP by 2008 (or $2.055 trillion).

For the uninsured and underinsured, the rise in health care costs may mean a continued lack of health insurance. The resulting barrier to health care may, in turn, exacerbate or create health care problems that are potentially more costly and certainly detrimental to health and well-

✺✺ REFLECTIVE THINKING ✺✺

Consumers' Understanding of Our Health Care System

• What do you think is the proper role of the federal government in meeting the health care needs of its citizens?

• How would you educate the public regarding what to expect from a health care system operated via managed care?

• How can nursing help the public understand that the resources available to provide health care to U.S. citizens are finite?

being. For the insured, the continued rise in health care costs may make insurance unaffordable at some point, thereby forcing them into the ranks of the uninsured.

The vast majority of the U.S. population is covered by private health insurance. The U.S. Bureau of the Census (1997) estimated that 70.1% of the U.S. population under the age of 65 is covered by private insurance. Those under 65 years of age and their dependents obtain private insurance either through their employers or by purchasing such coverage directly from a nongroup health insurance plan. Between 1988 and 1993, the proportion of the nonelderly population covered by employer-based insurance dropped from 73.3% to 66.7%. The reasons for this decline include the increasing cost of insurance, competitive pressures on firms that forced the elderly to search for additional ways to cut costs, and changing industry and firm size trends (Prospective Payment Assessment Commission, 1997).

More than 1,000 private health insurance companies offer health insurance with various levels of coverage (DeLaw, Greenberg, & Kinchen, 1992). The federal government does not regulate insurance companies; this task is performed by state insurance commissioners. This lack of national regulation has led to a loosely structured delivery system organized at the local level and lacking a federal or intrastate influence on planning and coordination. Thus, little coordination exists between private and public programs.

Employment-Based Programs

Employment-based health insurance is basically a substitute for cash wages, a fact poorly understood. This employer subsidy has increased in recent years, rising from 6.9% of total compensation in 1991 to 8.3% in 1997 (U.S. Department of Labor, 1997). When employers pay wages in the form of health care benefits, the associated monies are not subject to personal or Social Security tax (Congressional Budget Office Report, 1992). This lack of tax revenue is one factor contributing to the underfunding of the Social Security Trust Fund and, therefore, to the potential bankrupting of Medicare and Medicaid as demand outstrips funding.

The majority of those with private health care insurance are covered for inpatient hospital services and physician services. Coverage for home health, outpatient services, and hospice vary greatly depending on the plan. Traditionally, industries with strong unions have the broadest health care benefit packages.

In 1996, only 5.4% of working union members were uninsured, compared with 20.1% of workers who were not union members. Over 90% of union workers held employment-based health insurance in 1996 (HCFA, 1997b).

Although nearly three-quarters (73.6%) of workers ages 16 to 64 obtained health insurance from their own or another employer (e.g., a spouse's), almost one-fifth (18.4%) of all nonelderly workers were uninsured

(Agency for Health Care Policy and Research, 1997). Whereas, certain types of workers were likely to obtain employment-related coverage, others were at risk of being uninsured. Employees of small businesses may face high premiums because their employers may not be able to take advantage of the risk pool (as the pool, or numbers of people insured, goes up, the risk and, therefore, the expense of providing insurance goes down) that larger companies enjoy. Low-wage workers who either are unable to afford health insurance when offered coverage or lack access to the kinds of jobs that provide health coverage often go uninsured. Working women were more likely than men to be covered by employment-related health insurance and were less likely to be uninsured. On the other hand, they were less likely to have employment-related health insurance in their own names, with 58.9% of male workers being policyholders compared with 50.5% of female workers. Minority workers, especially Hispanic workers, were far more likely than Caucasian workers to be uninsured (see Figure 4-3). Hispanic male workers were far less likely than all other workers to obtain employment-related health insurance and were more likely to be uninsured. In 1996, approximately one-half (49.7%) of Hispanic male workers obtained health coverage from an employer, and 43.5% were uninsured. Among African American workers, women were less likely to be uninsured. Although minority women workers were less likely to be uninsured than minority male workers, they still were much more likely to be uninsured than were employed Caucasian women. Among female workers, 29.9% of Hispanics and 22.2% of African Americans were uninsured, compared with 12.6% of Caucasians (HCFA, 1997c).

There were three primary reasons for the shift in who would be covered by health insurance. First, because the costs of providing health coverage rose at such alarming rates, the total number of employers who could offer this benefit decreased. Second, as co-payments were introduced as a means of controlling and sharing health insurance coverage, the number of employees who could afford coverage decreased. Third, the distribution of work shifted from manufacturing to the service sector, the latter of which traditionally has not provided health insurance

@@ REFLECTIVE THINKING @@

Health Care Access and the Unemployed

Perhaps you have known persons who have lost a job and, therefore, health insurance coverage for themselves and/or dependents. Describe the ways that these individuals or families were able to meet health care needs.

• Did the provision of health care become a central focus?

• Did the individuals or families outwardly express concern over the possibility of someone's getting ill?

coverage even for full-time work (U.S. Bureau of the Census, 1997).

Governmental Programs

Two governmental health care programs provide coverage for the aged, disabled, or poor: Medicare Parts A and B and Medicaid.

Medicare

Medicare is a national health insurance program for elderly and some disabled persons. It is the largest health insurer in the United States. As of January 1996, Medicare covered 13% of the population, or 35.2 million people, including virtually all elderly (over age 65 persons), and certain persons with disabilities. The program is financed by a combination of payroll taxes, general federal revenues, and premiums (HCFA, 1997b).

The 1997b Medicare program bulletin indicates that Medicare Part A pays for inpatient hospital services including room, meals, nursing care, operating room services, blood transfusions, special care units, drugs and medical supplies, laboratory tests, therapeutic rehabilitation services, and medical social services. Medicare also covers skilled nursing facility care for continued treatment and/or rehabilitation following hospitalization. Home health care services prescribed by a physician for treatment and/or rehabilitation of homebound patients, including part-time or intermittent nursing services, are also covered.

Medicare does *not* pay for long-term or custodial care. Also, personal convenience services (such as televisions and telephones), private-duty nurses, and the extra cost of a private room when not medically necessary are not covered.

In calendar year 1998, Medicare reimbursed for the first 60 days of inpatient hospital care minus a $760 deductible, for which the beneficiary was responsible. For days 61 through 90, Medicare paid for all covered services excepting a $190 per day co-insurance payment for which the beneficiary was responsible. From days 91 through 150, the beneficiary co-insurance rate was $380 per day, but coverage beyond 90 days in any benefit period was limited to the number of lifetime reserve days (the number of Medicare days not used in the current year available to the beneficiary and, thus, rolled over to the next year) (HCFA, 1998c).

In 1997, each beneficiary had 60 lifetime reserve days that could be used only once. If a beneficiary had been out of a hospital or skilled nursing facility for 60 consecutive days but was then readmitted to a hospital, a new benefit period began, and the beneficiary was again responsible for the $760 deductible for the first 60 days of inpatient care and for co-insurance for days 60 to 90 (HCFA, 1998c). If the services of a skilled nursing facility were needed for continued care of a beneficiary after at least three consecutive days of hospital inpatient care (not including the day of discharge), Medicare paid for all covered services for the first 20 days. From days 21 through 100, the beneficiary was responsible for paying $95 a day. Medicare did not pay for skilled nursing facility care beyond 100 days in each benefit period (HCFA, 1998c).

If a person is homebound and requires skilled care, Medicare will pay for medically necessary home health care including part-time or intermittent nursing care, physical and/or speech therapy, medical social services, and medical supplies. Equipment is reimbursed at 80%. For terminally ill patients, Medicare will pay for care from a Medicare-certified hospice, where the specialized care includes pain control, symptom management, and supportive services as opposed to curative services.

Medicare Part B, or the medical insurance supplementary coverage, pays 80% of approved charges and covered services in excess of the annual deductible of Medicare Part A. Part B is a voluntarily purchased program obtained through payment of a monthly premium. The Part B premium for 1998 is $43.80 per month, which is unchanged from the 1997 amount.

Medicare Part B generally does not cover routine physical examination, most dental care, routine foot care, hearing aids, preventive care, services not related to treatment of illness or injury, and outpatient prescription drugs to be self-administered. Screening pap smear and mammography examination are exceptions to the rule. Medicare Part B covers screening mammography examinations every two years for women ages 65 and over, annually for women ages 50 to 65, annually for women ages 40 to 50 at high risk of developing breast cancer, every two years for women ages 40 to 50 who are not at high risk, and one time for women ages 35 to 40 (HCFA, 1998c).

Medicare expenses are increasing faster than revenues, which, if expenditure controls are not enacted, could bankrupt the program early in the next century (Congressional Budget Office, 1995). Although there are numerous reasons for this path to bankruptcy, the primary factor is that fewer workers will be contributing to the program as the U.S. population continues to age. In 1960, there were five workers for each beneficiary; currently, there are three (White House Fact Sheet, 1998). Figure 4-8 demonstrates the rapid growth in Medicare payments from 1970 to 1996. In 1970, Medicare paid $7.3 billion; in 1996, the figure had increased to $197.8 billion, or a $192.5 billion increase (HCFA, 1997a). Table 4-1 summarizes Medicare benefits and limitations.

Medicaid

The HCFA *Medicaid Bulletin* (1997a) indicates that Medicaid is a health insurance program for certain categories of the poor and is administered by the states using federal matching funds. States administer the program on the basis of broad federal policies governing the scope of services, the level of payments, and group eligibility. Federal Medicaid law (Title XIX of the Social Security Act) authorizes federal matching funds to assist the states in providing health care for certain low-income persons. The states have considerable flexibility in structuring their programs.

Figure 4-8   Medicare National Health Care
Expenditures: 1970–1996

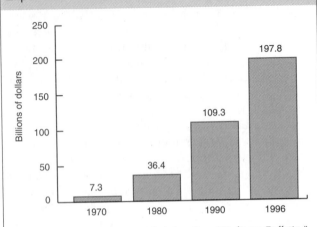

*From Health Care Finance Administration, "Medicare Bulletin,"
January 1998.*

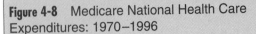

REFLECTIVE THINKING

Medicare and Medicaid

Do you know persons on Medicaid or Medicare?

• Are their health care needs being met?

• Do they fear hospitalization in terms of their financial viability? If so, what are they doing about it?

services can range from 50% to 80%; the lower the state's
per capita income, the higher the federal matching percentage. For the fiscal year 1996, the federal share of Medicaid expenditures was $87.0 billion, and the states' share
was $65.9 billion. From 1987 to 1996, Medicaid total pay-
ments (federal and state combined) increased dramatically. In 1987, total state and federal combined payments
were $47.7 billion for 23.1 million recipients. In 1990,
there were an additional 2.2 million Medicaid recipients
(25.3 million total) and a total combined payment of $68.7
billion. By 1996, there were 36.1 million recipients and a
combined payment of $152.9 billion, an increase of $105.2
billion dollars in eight years (see Figure 4-9) (HCFA,
1997b).

Eligibility for Medicaid is met when a person is both
poor and aged, disabled, pregnant, or the parent of a
dependent child. Medicaid recipients increased from
approximately 10 million in 1967 to 37.5 million in 1996,
an increase of 275%. The number of dependent children
enrolled rose from 9.8 million in 1985 to 18.2 million in
1996, an increase of 86%. Medicaid insures a larger percentage of children than it does persons in all other age
groups (HCFA, 1997a).

Enacted in 1965, the original Medicaid program covered four categories of care:

1. Inpatient and outpatient care
2. Laboratory and x-ray services
3. Physician services
4. Skilled nursing services

In 1972, amendments extended coverage to family planning. Because Medicaid is the only public program that
finances long-term care, significant and growing numbers
of middle-class elderly persons have become eligible for
Medicaid (DeLaw et al., 1992). Federal law and regulations specify a list of basic services that must be included
in any state Medicaid program. Services mandated to be
covered by state programs are: inpatient and outpatient;
services; physician services; laboratory and x-ray services,
nursing facility services for individuals 21 years of age and
over; home health care for persons eligible for nursing
facility services; family planning; rural health clinic services; nurse–midwife services; prenatal care; early and
periodic screening and diagnostic services for children
under age 21, as well as treatment for conditions identified in such screening.

On average, federal funds account for approximately
57% of the cost of the Medicaid program. The federal government's share of a state's expenditures for health care

Figure 4-9   Medicaid Enrollees and Total Federal
and State Program Payments: 1996

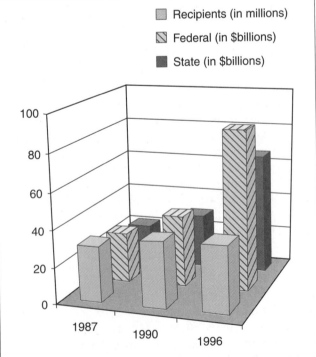

*From Health Care Finance Administration. Data extracted from
the Health Care Finance Administration home page. Available at
http://www.HCPA.gov. "Medicare Bulletin," January 1997.*

EMERGING TRENDS

The trends in health care economics, those either enacted or under consideration, are put forth in great part to improve access, control costs, control the rapid implementation of technology so that costs and benefits can be assessed, and to improve quality. Most would agree, however, that controlling costs is the paramount reason that employers, employees, third-party payors, and the federal and state governments are examining new mechanisms to provide health care.

Managed Care

Managed care has been a limited feature of the U.S. health care system for decades. The history of managed care shows the approach to have produced demonstrable savings over the better known fee-for-service system. Managed care systems integrate the delivery of services and the financing of those services (Enthoven, 1993; Enthoven & Kronick 1994). Inglehart (1994) notes that managed care is characterized by several factors:

1. Contracts with selected physicians and hospitals that furnish comprehensive health services exclusively to their members

2. Care delivered for a predetermined premium

3. Predetermined control over utilization

4. Member's receiving financial incentives for receiving care from a single provider

5. Some associated financial risk on behalf of the contracting physicians

Examples of such programs are HMOs and the Medicare prospective payment program known as DRG. Among HMOs, Group Health of Puget Sound (1945) and Kaiser Permanente Medical Program (1940) have been very successful for over 50 years at providing prospectively financed health care with outcomes matching those of other health care delivery systems. These early HMOs met with such success in part because they were pre-paid systems (managed care), they experienced very little competition given that the majority of health plans were fee for service, and they focused primarily on wellness (Enthoven & Kronick, 1994).

Managed Care in Medicare and Medicaid

Since 1993, the number of Medicare and Medicaid beneficiaries enrolled in managed care plans has grown considerably. As a result, the HCFA, which administers these two programs, is the largest purchaser of managed care in the country, representing 15.5 million Americans (HCFA, 1996).

As of February 1, 1996, almost 4 million Medicare beneficiaries—more than 10% of the total Medicare population—were enrolled in managed care plans. This represents a 67% increase in managed care enrollment since 1993. In 1995, an average of 68,000 Medicare beneficiaries voluntarily enrolled in HMOs each month. Medicare beneficiaries can enroll or disenroll in a managed care plan at any time and for any reason with 30 days notice (HCFA, 1996). By 1996, of the 35.2 million recipients of Medicare, over 60% were enrolled in managed care (HCFA, 1997a).

Medicaid managed care enrollment has grown even more. Since January 1, 1993, enrollment in Medicaid managed care plans increased 140%, including a 51% increase in 1995. As of June 30, 1995, 11.6 million Medicaid beneficiaries were enrolled in managed care plans, representing 32% of all Medicaid beneficiaries (HCFA, 1996). In 1996, a total of 31.5 million Medicaid recipients, or 70%, were enrolled in managed care plans (HCFA, 1997a). Currently, 49 states offer some form of managed care. Since 1993, states have utilized Medicaid waivers to increase enrollment in managed care and to develop other innovative changes to their Medicaid programs. Several states have used the savings resulting from managed care enrollment to expand both the number of individuals covered by Medicaid and the number of services covered under the program.

The federal government grants two types of Medicaid waivers: Section 1915(b) "free choice" waivers and Section 1115 demonstrations. Freedom of choice waivers permit states to require beneficiaries to enroll in managed care plans. To receive such a waiver, states must prove that these plans have the capacity to serve Medicaid beneficiaries who will be in the plan. States often use freedom of choice waivers to establish primary care programs and other forms of managed care. In 1995, HCFA approved five freedom of choice waivers (HCFA, 1997b).

Section 1115 demonstrations allow states to test new approaches to benefits, service eligibility, program payments, and service delivery, often on a statewide basis. The approaches are frequently aimed at saving money so as to allow states to extend Medicaid coverage to additional low-income and uninsured people. Since January 1, 1993, comprehensive care reform demonstration waivers have been approved for 12 states, and 8 such waivers have been implemented. When all 12 have been implemented, 2.2 million previously uninsured individuals are expected to receive health coverage (HCFA, 1997b).

Managed Competition

Enthoven (1993) notes that the precursor of the managed competition scheme is the pre-paid group practice association such as Kaiser Permanente Medical Care Program and other HMOs. Enthoven defines managed competition as "a strategy whereby consumers and employers reap maximal value for each dollar spent" (p. 27).

Managed competition, based on microeconomic principles, focuses on providing the best care while also restraining costs, improving quality, and satisfying consumers and their employers. President Clinton's national health care reform movement relied heavily on the concept of managed competition. He envisioned organizing the competition around health insurance purchasing cooperatives (HIPCs) that would compete with each other to attract consumers and employers on the basis of value, outcomes, and satisfaction. Value, outcomes, and satisfaction would be accomplished via the HIPCs' providing a standardized health care package at a fixed, per capita rate.

Global Budgets

Altman and Cohen (1993) propose that a national global health care budget would surpass all other health care cost strategies, because the target of a global budget is controlling total health care spending by controlling the product of price and value. **Global budgeting** practices are generally enacted to provide states with the maximal control over how monies are spent in the provision of health care at the state level, such as for Medicaid. A pre-established amount of money is shifted to the states from the federal government along with broad criteria for the ways that the money is to be spent and those outcomes

that should be reached. With global budgeting, the federal government's lump-sum payment to states would not be specifically targeted for a particular program within the state's health care system. The state would determine how much money each program would receive as well as which programs to offer.

Past efforts at controlling costs have focused primarily on constraining prices and service use. These approaches are, for the most part, piecemeal and are less likely than global budgeting to affect national expenditures (Altman & Cohen, 1993; Ashby & Greene, 1993). Global budgeting, which covers the entire population, has been implemented in Canada and several European countries. In his original health care reform package, President Clinton proposed global budgeting for all Medicare and Medicaid recipients beginning in 1996.

Although global budgeting may take several different forms, all forms of this approach set an overall spending limit that covers a defined set of services and specific groups. Ultimate accountability for administering a national global budget would fall to the federal government. As Ashby and Greene (1993) state, however, premium limits could be enforced via managed competition systems and rate setting. The obvious drawbacks are that global budgeting could negatively affect competition by encouraging providers to spend to the limit rather than seek savings.

Rationing

In one form or another, the U.S. health care system has used rationing to control access and cost. In general, **rationing** takes two forms. Implicit rationing, which limits the capacity of a system, and places specific dollar targets to that system so that the system may not exceed that amount. This usually requires the rationed system to prioritize services to be offered. A system would predetermine the services to be provided and the rate of reimbursement. This type of rationing is similar to the ethical concept of utilitarianism. Finite health care resources should be deployed so that they can do the greatest good for the greatest number of people. Explicit rationing, or the ability-to-pay scenario, is the most obvious strategy in the United States. The United States generally looks at health care as any other commodity or service to be purchased, which has made explicit rationing the dominant form of rationing in the United States. In an economic democracy, like the United States, as opposed to a social democracy, like Canada, a citizen's ability to obtain a service is determined by personal ability to pay for that service or by ability to obtain some sort of assistance (Medicaid) to obtain the service. Rationing of health care services and dollars is a very contentious topic in the United States. As the federal and state governments, insurance companies, HMOs, employers, and consumers attempt to control health care costs, the mechanism by which resources are allocated must change; however, some form of rationing will be necessary.

✪✪ REFLECTIVE THINKING ✪✪

Your Health Care Coverage

• How would managed care affect your access to health care?

• Would belonging to an HMO change your perspective of quality, cost, and access with regard to care?

• How has rationing of health care services affected your own state of health and well-being? Someone else's?

Figure 4-10   Comparison of National per Capita Health Care Spending in the United States and Selected European Countries: 1996

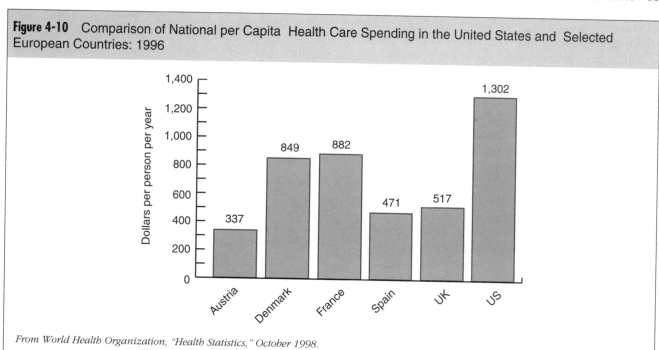

From World Health Organization, "Health Statistics," October 1998.

EUROPEAN HEALTH CARE FINANCING

Containing the cost of health care has become a goal of virtually all countries. Abel-Smith (1992) studied the ways that European nations control the cost of health care and concluded that it is technically possible to control health care cost via governmental policies that regulate supply rather than demand. According to World Health Organization (WHO) statistics, in 1996, (WHO, 1997) the United States outspent all European countries in per capita health care expenditures (see Figure 4-10). In terms of GDP, the United States outspends all other Western nations on health care (see Figure 4-11).

In providing social services such as health care, the U.S. government historically has become involved only when no remedy from the private sector could be found.

Figure 4-11   Comparison of National Percentage of GDP Spent on Health Care in the United States and Selected European Countries: 1996

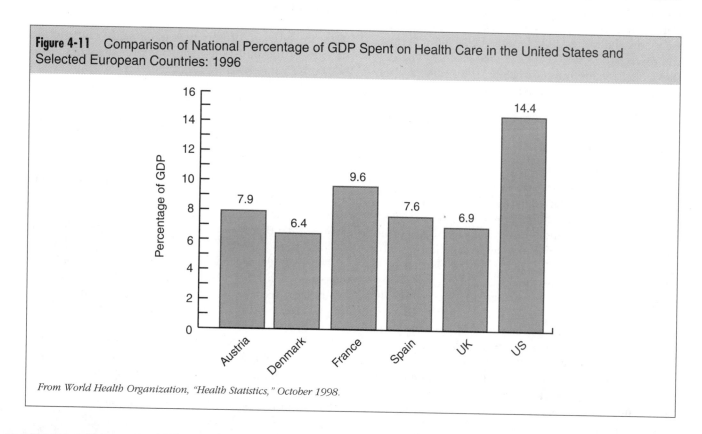

From World Health Organization, "Health Statistics," October 1998.

In Europe, conversely, governments establish a level of health care for all citizens ("Patients or Profits," 1998a).

In Europe, governments use finance controls as a means of controlling health care costs. Finance controls limit the flow of funds into health care, effectively placing a ceiling on spending with each fiscal year budget. European governments are also beginning to experiment with co-payments as a means to increase consumers' awareness of the cost of their care (Enthoven, 1994). Moreover, utilization controls are used in Europe to control the supply of health care services (WHO, 1998).

The methods used by various countries to control costs differ according to the ways those countries organize and finance health care. Control is more easily attained when the government owns health care facilities and pays health care professionals on a salaried basis. Controlling cost is made more difficult when health care providers are under contract with the government and bill for services they provide. Many European countries use rationing as a means of controlling health care expenditures. Implicit rationing limits the capacity of the health care system, and the Europeans clearly use implicit rationing at every level of their health care systems (Reinhardt, 1993; Enthoven, 1994; "Patients or Profits," 1998).

As compared with the U.S. government, European governments take a much more active role in the provision and financing of health care. The primary reason for this is that most European democracies are social democracies, in sharp contrast to the economic democracy of the United States. Social democracies typically provide some level of cradle-to-grave health care subsidized by a heavy personal tax base.

Many Americans view the level of taxes paid by people in western European countries as oppressive. In many European countries, such as Sweden, France, England, Germany, and Norway, the federal tax liabilities of citizens can reach 50% to 57% of total annual income, whereas in the United States our tax liability generally does not exceed 38% ("America's Bubble Economy," 1998b).

Supply and Demand

European nations impose cost containment primarily via consumer supply or demand or both. Abel-Smith (1992) notes that all European countries have used modest cost sharing as a means to reduce demand. Cost savings has not been a primary focus and is increasingly not used as a strategy. According to the *Economist* ("American's Bubble Economy," 1998) most Europeans have a form of private health insurance that pays the co-pay; they therefore do not share in the cost and do not experience price sensitivity.

Overall budgets for health care in many European countries are normally not increased if prices rise more than the government has projected (Abel-Smith, 1992; WHO, 1998). Because cost sharing (demand) has not proved overly effective in controlling costs in Europe, the main burden for economy in service has fallen on the hospitals (supply). Hospitals have been pressured to ration

supply by either closing smaller institutions or converting them to facilities that serve the chronically ill or the aged. Another approach to economizing is decreasing admissions. These two strategies have generally been effective in restraining expenditures.

Additionally, most European countries limit costly medical equipment in the public hospitals (Schieber & Poullier, 1991). Denmark, for example, has a central governmental body specifically responsible for assessing the costs and benefits of technology before implementation.

In many European countries, there has been a clear transfer of finance from hospitals to primary care as a means to control cost and access and to treat illness before it has reached the costly stage of tertiary care (Abel-Smith, 1992). Primary care is the predominant model of care in Europe. According to WHO statistics (1998), most European countries have a significantly higher percentage of primary care physicians than does the United States. Schieber and Poullier (1991) note that this trend seems to stem from the tough controls on hospital expenditures. These controls have proved to be more politically acceptable than have restraints on physicians and that which they authorize for care. National global budgets are also gaining in popularity among European countries as they, like the United States, search for mechanisms to control cost and access while increasing the health of their citizens.

HEALTH CARE ECONOMICS AND EXPRESSION OF CARING

With the advent of the national health care reform debates of the mid-1990s, the United States appears to be on the verge of associating the economics of health care with what some have called a moral imperative to provide basic health care services to *all* citizens of this country. As pointed out in Chapter 1, Fry (1994) defines caring as a moral concept, whereby efforts of caring are directed toward meeting human need, and caring is perceived as a *duty* to respond to that need. As indicated in the current chapter, European countries have long ago established that they have a moral obligation to provide basic health care service to their citizens, health care service that ensures access and quality while controlling costs.

Nurses in the United States are in a unique position to help ensure that the economics of health care in this country reflects the ways that neighborhoods, communities, cities, states, and the federal government *care* for themselves and for their most vulnerable citizens. For nurses, this represents a nationally focused expression of caring. Nursing organizations such as the American Nurses Association (ANA) have called for federally defined minimum standards for essential health care services. The central premises of ANA's health plan are as follows:

1. All citizens must have equitable access to essential health care services.

2. Primary care should play a more prominent role in health care in the United States.

3. Consumers must assume more accountability for their care.

4. A better balance must be created between the traditional illness and cure model and a wellness and care model.

5. Consumers must be protected from the costs of catastrophic illness (ANA, 1995).

As discussed in Chapter 6, Leininger (1981) posits that a culture guides decisions and actions. For nurses to be effective in changing the U.S. health care system so that it provides services to vulnerable populations, they must first understand the historical reasons for the establishment of that system. Knowing the traditional roles of the state and federal governments gives the nurse the historical perspective needed to take action without returning to past federal policies that no longer meet the health care needs of millions of U.S. citizens. The U.S. health care system has rarely changed quickly in relation to need; rather, it has changed incrementally. Enthoven (1994) notes that legislated change, while being necessary, fundamental, and far reaching, cannot be sudden and bear no resemblance to the past. Change that is so radical as to totally negate the past is much more difficult to accept than change that is balanced with some of the old and the new.

Nurses make up the single largest group of professional health care providers in the United States. United and coordinated efforts on the part of professional nursing organizations could bring about the needed change within our health care system via the paradigm of caring. However, it is necessary to first fully understand the source and evolution of the current "you're on your own" paradigm and the ways that the paradigm of caring (the moral duty to meet human needs) can be initiated to bring about desired changes. Specifically, all nurses must have a clear understanding of the economics of care. Without understanding the ways that our economic democracy operates, nurses stand little chance of influencing it. Nurses must also learn ways to be political at every level

DECISION MAKING

Your Curriculum and Health Care Economics

• How could your school of nursing better prepare you to manage the health care resources in community health nursing?

• Make a formal recommendation to your faculty on how they could incorporate contemporary health care financing trends into the curriculum at your school.

of health care—institutional, local, state, and federal. Politics has been described as the art of the possible. Without active and informed participation, however, nothing is possible.

A paradigm is a model or a way of thinking (Barker, 1992) and is amenable to change if certain conditions exist. New paradigms appear and are considered for implementation when old ways no longer serve the intended purpose. In other words, less effective paradigms take increasingly more time, money, and effort to solve increasingly fewer problems. This accurately describes the present condition of the U.S. health care system. How can nurses effect the paradigm shift from economics of overspending and serving increasingly fewer people to economics as an expression of caring for *all* citizens?

First, nurses must understand the theories of macroeconomics and microeconomics as applied to health care. Economics should be a part of undergraduate education to facilitate a broad understanding of the U.S. health care system and its spending habits. At the undergraduate level, students should study the economic as well as the social bases of health care. They should prepare budgets and analyze budget reports for positive and negative variances and the causes of those variances. No student should graduate from an undergraduate program if he or she cannot prepare and analyze a budget and understand and document the cost of the care that health professionals provide. Furthermore, nursing undergraduates should have gained a clear understanding of the macro- and microeconomic pressures that influence the allocation and spending of health care dollars at the institutional and local levels.

At the graduate level, particularly in nursing leadership and management programs, economics should be required for a minimum of one semester and, ideally, two semesters. These courses should focus on macro- and microeconomics as applied to managed care, managed competition, and global budgets. The usefulness of economic theory as a means of better understanding the ways that the U.S. health care system is financed should also be emphasized. At the graduate level, nursing students must be able to prepare and defend a workable business plan for any health care service or institution. Graduate students must have a better understanding of economics in general. In order for advanced practice nurses to fully participate in the economic health of their organizations, they must be able to actively and intelligently participate with other financial professionals. Nurses must learn that they can advocate simultaneously for the wellness of the client and the wellness of the organization.

A second means of effecting the paradigm shift is for nursing organizations and places of employment to further their efforts at getting nurses involved in the political aspects of the economics of the U.S. health care system. All economic policies are the result of a political process, a process that generally eludes most nurses. It is therefore imperative that nurses become familiar with and involved in the political process of health care policy formation, implementation, and evaluation (see Chapter 31).

Third, nurses must make their concerns known to can-

෮ REFLECTIVE THINKING ෮

Is the Government Responsible for Providing Health Care?

• Does the U.S. government have a moral obligation to provide health care for its citizens?

• Given that limited amounts of money are available to spend on health care, to whom would you give care first? Last? State the rationale for each of your answers.

• How does your community express its desire to care for its vulnerable citizens?

didates, office holders, and lobbyists who shape the national and, therefore, state and local health care systems. Such involvement on the part of nurses is central to bringing about a health care system that operationalizes caring in a financially responsible manner.

Economics will play an ever-increasing role in professional nursing. Because health care policy and economics are linked, nurses must increase their knowledge regarding economic principles and the ways that those principles affect the health of the nation. Community health nurses have long been committed to maintaining and improving the health of U.S. citizens. In order to fulfill this commitment, nurses must become health care economists who insist on full participation in the policies that shape the systems in which they work.

Perspectives...

Insights of a Clinical Nurse Educator and a Director of a Nurse Practitioner Program

"Your Money or Your Life," "Patients or Profits," and "Where Has the 'Caring' in Health Care Gone?"—all headlines from U.S. publications and all referring to managed care. About 10 years ago, a few hospitals and health systems in California tried to curb costs by rationing health care. The momentum grew, and currently, 160 million U.S. citizens are insured by a managed care insurance policy. The managed care industry has become one of the newest, largest, least understood, and perhaps most reviled aspects of the U.S. health care system.

As managed care companies continue to squeeze out traditional health insurance, clients are often caught unaware of newly placed restrictions on access and treatments, and nurses and physicians are concerned about both the state of health care for their clients and the health of their practices. Meanwhile, politicians are scrambling to introduce changes in managed care that please everyone—especially the voting public.

In one year, federal and state governments introduced more than 1,000 bills seeking to ban alleged abuses by medical profiteers; most such bills were tabled. In 1998, President Bill Clinton introduced his "Patient's Bill of Rights." If passed by Congress, this bill of rights will make it more difficult, if not

illegal in some cases, for insurers to deny payment for procedures. This legislation is very popular with a wide range of consumer groups and will more than likely be passed by Congress because HMOs in the United States are very unpopular. Survey after survey shows that the American people think HMOs care more about money than about patients ("How HMOs Decide," 1998).

It is hard to dispute that managed care companies are very unpopular. The news is not all bad, however. Before managed care came to the United States, health care costs were rising at an alarming rate. The United States spends more money per capita on health care than does any other Western nation, yet it does not rank number one in numerous outcome measures. Under managed care, the rate of inflation with regard to health care costs slowed somewhat, a feat achieved without a measurable drop in the quality of care. The best HMOs—and, yes, there are good HMOs—have devised techniques to allocate resources and measure outcomes, techniques that the rest of the world might replicate.

There is little doubt that terrible mistakes have been made under managed care; however, a question that must be asked is whether such mistakes also

Continued

Continued

happened under other forms of insurance and care. Because the emphasis in managed care appears to be strictly cost instead of cost *and* quality, many Americans believe that cheaper health care equates with poor-quality health care. The evidence suggests, however, that the HMO movement has saved money while maintaining previous standards of care.

Standards of care are much harder to measure than is money. For instance, it is impossible to demonstrate a link between health care delivery and life expectancy. Lifestyle choices such as diet, exercise, stress reactions, smoking, and substance abuse are not under the control of the HMO; yet poor choices in these areas greatly contribute to morbidity and mortality in the United States. Diet, level of stress, and whether to exercise, smoke, or abuse substances constitute individual choices—choices about which far too many Americans still seem to make poor decisions. If we are ever to change the way Americans view their part in maintaining their health and in promoting wellness, HMOs may be a route to doing so because they emphasize not only treatment of episodic illness but, more importantly, prevention.

The inability of the traditional fee-for-service systems to provide effective preventive care may contribute to the fact that the average American is no fitter than citizens in countries where far less is spent per capita on health care. Diabetes is a good basis on which to compare the health of Americans with that of citizens of other nations. In 1990, Americans with diabetes were twice as likely as their British counterparts to go blind or to have a limb amputated. Why? The British Health Service, which operates on a limited budget per citizen, appears to be more effective in ensuring that clients take their insulin, have regular eye exams, and generally manage diet and insulin more effectively.

Our government may play a very large role in what appears to be variation in health care quality across the nation. For Medicare alone, the federal government imposes over 22,000 pages of rules and regulations. Via overwhelming numbers of regulations that are at times more confusing than helpful, the government is attempting to micromanage health care. Many of these micromanagement regulations mandate specific treatments for specific conditions. This essentially forces the practitioner, whether nurse practitioner or physician, into a boiler plate or cookie cutter approach to health care. Many nurse practitioners and physicians feel these regulations interfere with the client–provider interaction.

Instead of the government (local, state, or federal) being seemingly always at battle with HMOs, providers, and the employers who purchase health care plans for their employees, we desperately need to develop a national health care policy that takes into account the nature of our economic system. We believe that Oregon and Hawaii are on the right track. These two states have decided that there is indeed enough money to cover the health care costs of their citizens and have engaged their citizens, insurers, governmental agencies, and employers in dialogue regarding meeting the health care needs of their citizens. The jury is still out on whether their efforts will be effective in the long run, but Oregon and Hawaii have instituted important changes that we should watch with an open mind.

The American health care system must continue to change. The types of change and the effectiveness of the changes should be guided by all of us—insurers, providers, citizens, and governments. Rather than holding on to a health care system that has served to maintain a lifestyle for a select number of providers at the expense of far too many citizens of this great country, our priority should be engaging in open, collaborative dialogue that focuses on system and individual accountabilities to ensure quality health care for all.

—Robert Geibert, RN, EdD
Wendy Smith, RN, DNS

COMMUNITY NURSING VIEW

Mrs. Yu has been referred to you for home care. She lives alone and has just left the hospital after two weeks, including three days in intensive care. She had been on a drinking binge for a week before her admission and was admitted to the hospital for severe esophageal and rectal bleeding. She was diagnosed with esophageal varices and rectal cancer. As soon as her esophageal bleeding was controlled, the rectal cancer was removed and she was given a colostomy. She was sent home with instructions for colostomy care and a warning that continued drinking would lead to further esophageal bleeding. You are making your first visit to her to supervise her colostomy care. The first question she asks is, "How much is all this going to cost me? I have no health care coverage and I'm afraid the cost will clean me out!" You know that her finances are good and she is expecting to pay for her hospital and home care. You realize that she speaks little English and will not understand her hospital bill, nor will she be able to easily contact the hospital and home care agency to get her questions answered. You want to help Mrs. Yu. Find answers to her questions.

Nursing Considerations

ASSESSMENT
- What information do you need to help Mrs. Yu understand the costs of her care?
- What agencies can you contact that can give you the information you need—not just for Mrs. Yu but for clients who use other agencies?
- If you can't get the data from the agencies, who else can you ask?
- What other information do you need to know about costs?

DIAGNOSIS
- Is there a diagnosis that would apply in this situation?

OUTCOME IDENTIFICATION
- What is the outcome you expect to achieve?

PLANNING/INTERVENTIONS
- How will you calculate the health care finance information you will need?

EVALUATION
- How would you evaluate your results?

≋ Key Concepts

- Nurses must thoroughly understand how the United States health care system functions in order to affect it in ways that promote wellness.
- Reasons for the rise in health care costs include rising cost per volume of service, per capita increase in volume of services, growth in specific population groups, advanced technology, rising administrative costs, client complexity, excess capacity, uncompensated care, and health care fraud.
- The major financial trends in the U.S. health care system are primarily focused at controlling increases in health care expenditures at the local, state, and federal levels.
- Government has become the agency of cost control, access, and quality through programs such as Medicare and Medicaid.
- Cost control mechanisms include DRGs, managed care, managed competition, global budgeting, and rationing.
- These cost controls primarily use three strategies: finance controls, reimbursement controls, and utilization controls.

- There is no nationwide system of health insurance that guarantees access to health care in the United States. Thus, many people do not have any health insurance or are underinsured.
- Three primary factors influence the growing number of uninsured and underinsured: Employment-based insurance is voluntary; insurance companies practice risk sorting and restrictive underwriting; and some people go without insurance because they are relying upon subsidized health care provided in the emergency rooms of public hospitals.
- Our health care system is divided into private and government sectors.
- Most European governments establish a level of health care for all citizens. They use financial and utilization controls to control spiraling health care costs. Their citizens bear the burden of high taxes to finance the health care system.
- Caring and economics are not antithetical concepts.
- Nurses must be aware of and active in politics and policy formulation, and they must understand how our health care systems are funded in order to change them.

Foundations of Community Health Nursing

The foundational knowledge required for application of caring in all community settings in which nurses serve aggregates is discussed in Unit III. The knowledge includes the study of philosophical and ethical, cultural and spiritual, and environmental perspectives, communication, teaching and learning, and health promotion and disease prevention.

5 Philosophical and Ethical Perspectives

6 Cultural and Spiritual Perspectives

7 Environmental Perspectives

8 Caring Communication and Teaching/Learning

9 Health Promotion and Disease Prevention Perspectives

Philosophical and Ethical Perspectives

Nancy Kiernan Case, RN, PhD

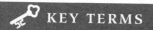
The ethically preferred world is one in which creatures are caring and cared for. Its institutions support and sustain caring while simultaneously reducing the need for care by eliminating the poverty, despair, and indifference that create a need for care.

—*Manning, 1992, p. 29*

COMPETENCIES

Upon completion of this chapter, the reader should be able to:

- Cite major ethical theories and principles that apply to community health nursing practice.
- Discuss the effect of a caring perspective on ethics in community health.
- Describe the essential components in an ethical decision-making model.
- Demonstrate the application of an ethical decision-making model in a dilemma that may occur in community health nursing.

Chapter 1 clearly presented caring as an essential feature of community health nursing practice. Caring is also an essential feature of evolving models of health care ethics (Leininger, 1990; Manning, 1992; Sherwin, 1992). Such models of health care ethics incorporate traditional theories and principles in the search for guidelines to live morally good lives. **Ethics** is the study of the nature and justification of principles that guide human behaviors and are applied when moral problems arise. The role of the professional community health nurse demands practice that bears moral responsibility for individuals, families, and communities as they grow toward full health potential.

This chapter discusses clients' rights and professional responsibility in community health, summarizes applicable classical ethical theories and principles, sets the ethical framework within caring, provides guidelines for ethical decision making, and examines some of the ethical issues unique to community health nursing practice.

CLIENT RIGHTS AND PROFESSIONAL RESPONSIBILITIES IN COMMUNITY HEALTH

The recognition of a client's rights concerning health care is considered one of the extensions of basic human rights (Annas, 1978). The right to health care is one of the basic human rights of clients recognized by the health care delivery system, in particular the public health system. Of course there are other client rights that are important, such as the rights to informed consent, to privacy, and to refusal of treatment; however, the major focus of this discussion will be on the right to health care.

The right to health care is a right to goods and services to improve and maintain the health that exists. It refers to a client's claim against the state or its agencies to provide certain types of health care services (Daniels, 1979). The right to health care has stimulated a considerable amount of discussion and debate in the United States such as what the government should provide, how access can be assured, and what services should be provided and by whom. Even with these debates the issues have not been resolved.

As the next century approaches, these discussions will continue with more focus on the roles of the government and of the private sector in providing health services. The societal obligations to citizens regarding basic health services and the responsibilities of health care providers in response to the client's right to health care must be explored. Equitable access to health care will continue to be a challenge for both the public and private health care sectors.

In response to client rights, community health nurses have responsibilities or duties that they are obligated to perform. In addition to caring, advocacy, and veracity, one of the major responsibilities is accountability. Moral accountability is addressed in the American Nurses Association Code for Nurses (1985). Moral accountability in nursing practice means that nurses are answerable for how they promote and protect health, as well as prevent disease and injury, while respecting client rights to self-determination in health care.

In community health nursing, whose primary emphasis is on aggregates rather than individual clients, moral accountability means that the nurses are accountable for how the health of population aggregates is promoted, protected, and met. In community health nursing, nursing actions are not only guided by the professional ethic of nursing but by the public health ethic, which places emphasis on the provision of accessible and available health services to maximize the health of the community. Thus, the need to explore ethical issues related to the right to health care is not new but has gained importance recently, particularly since the U.S. health care system is undergoing a major transformation due in part to factors associated with the high cost of health care, technology, increased awareness by an informed population, and a large aging population.

CLASSICAL ETHICAL THEORIES AND PRINCIPLES

In the past two decades, rapid advances in science and health care technology have precipitated a dramatic rise in the ethical dilemmas confronting health care professionals and the people to whom they provide care. Ethical dilemmas occur whenever ethical principles conflict. In such dilemmas, more than one resolution may be justifiable, but no one resolution satisfies all of the perspectives involved. Regardless of the setting, every nurse must

REFLECTIVE THINKING

What Is Your Code of Ethics?

• Do you believe that some actions are absolutely wrong in all circumstances? Give examples.

• Do you believe that you have an innate knowledge of right and wrong?

• How did you learn right and wrong? What was the influence of your parents? Society? Other forces?

• What are your thoughts about the ways that beliefs concerning right and wrong originate? To what degree do you believe that rules about right and wrong originate from a universal source? From within oneself?

Adapted from Ethics and Issues in Contemporary Nursing, *by M. A. Burkhardt & A. K. Nathaniel, 1998. Albany, NY: Delmar Publishers. Copyright 1998 by Delmar Publishers.*

anticipate ethical dilemmas in professional practice. Each nurse must be prepared to address the dilemmas by acquiring a thorough understanding of the theories, principles, decision-making models, and mechanisms to facilitate sound ethical decisions. Community health nurses face ethical dilemmas specific to their area of practice. Basic theories and principles provide universal guidelines for an underlying approach to ethical issues regardless of the setting for health care.

Basic Ethical Theories

Understanding ethical theories and principles is helpful to nurses in approaching ethical issues and decisions. It is important to remember that ethical theories are guides that are useful only in providing meaning for moral experience. Ethical decisions in health care are guided primarily by two classical ethical theories: deontology and teleology or, more specifically, one form of teleology called utilitarianism.

Deontology

Deontology is the classical ethical theory based on moral obligation or duty. **Moral obligation** refers to the duty to act in certain ways in response to moral norms. This theory suggests that the moral rightness or wrongness of human actions is determined by the principle or the motivation on which the action is based. From the deontological perspective, the consequences of an action neither drive ethical decisions nor serve as guides for ethical justification (Mappes & Zembaty, 1991; Ellis & Hartley, 1992; Munson, 1996; Beauchamp & Childress, 1994). Beauchamp and Childress (1994) indicate that the determination of rightness or wrongness of human actions may be based on religious traditions, an appeal to divine revelations, or intuition and common sense.

Utilitarianism

Utilitarianism is one form of teleology. **Teleology** is the ethical theory that determines rightness or wrongness solely on the basis of an estimate of the probable outcome. Unlike deontology, **utilitarianism** is based on usefulness or utility rather than moral obligation or duty. The utility of an action is determined primarily by an examination of its consequences. According to utilitarianism the rightness or wrongness of human actions is determined by an assessment of outcomes. The utility of an action is decided on the basis of whether that action would bring about the greatest number of good consequences as opposed to the least number of evil consequences and, by extension, greater good than evil in the world as a whole (Beauchamp & Childress, 1994).

To assist in distinguishing between the two theoretical positions, consider the issue of lying or withholding the entire truth concerning an issue. A deontologist's perspective suggests that lying, under any circumstances, is wrong because it violates the moral duty of veracity (truth telling). According to deontology, humans have a moral obligation to tell the truth regardless of the consequences. On the other hand, the utilitarian might argue that there are known circumstances in which lying would bring greater good and fewer evil consequences. Consider the circumstance of lying to an evildoer, one who would do unwarranted harm to an individual. If one lied to conceal the whereabouts of the individual, the utilitarian would evaluate the action as moral because of the greater good consequences. The utilitarian would argue that a world of such decisions would promote greater good than evil, despite the violation of the moral duty to tell the truth. The deontologist, however, would focus on the violation of the duty of veracity, declaring the act of lying ethically unjustifiable.

Another example to illuminate the differences between deontology and utilitarianism is the issue of abortion. Abortion, even to save the life of the mother, remains unjustifiable to the deontologist, because the action violates the moral duty to preserve life and to avoid killing. To the utilitarian, however, preserving the life of the mother may be justified by the greater number of positive (good) consequences. Preventing the death of the mother by aborting the fetus may allow the woman to return to her family, spouse, and other children or to contribute to society in general. The abortion of the fetus, while tragic to the utilitarian, represents fewer bad consequences than allowing the mother to die.

Although many health care professionals consider themselves utilitarians, an understanding of deontology is particularly helpful when ethical principles conflict. The ability to establish priorities among ethical principles or to establish the moral weight of ethical principles is fundamental to deontology. When confronted with ethical dilemmas, most health care professionals operate from a perspective carefully derived from aspects of both major classical theoretical positions.

Basic Ethical Principles

Several ethical principles that evolve from ethical theory apply in conflicts that occur in health care ethics. Beneficence, nonmaleficence, justice, and autonomy are among the ethical principles that influence decisions in health care ethics. Ethical rules represent another level of ethical perspective beyond theories and principles. Fidelity; veracity, and accountability are three ethical rules that exert a strong influence.

Beneficence

Beneficence is the principle of promoting the legitimate and important aims and interests of others, principally by preventing or removing possible harms (Mappes & Zembaty, 1991; Munson, 1996; Beauchamp & Childress, 1994). Because promoting the welfare of clients is explicit in the role of the professional nurse, beneficence becomes a complicated issue when benefit to one client conflicts with other ethical requirements such as benefit to another client and agency goals and other ethical principles such as client autonomy or the fair distribution of resources. Nurses must also consider whether client benefit should reflect overall benefit or be limited to health benefit.

As an example, a nurse's insistence on a low-sodium diet for an elderly client provides the greater health benefit for that client yet denies the client control over dietary choices and, thus, may deny the client pleasure, a sense of life quality, and autonomy (the experience of control over one's destiny). Underlying these considerations are significant questions regarding the meaning of benefit and who should define benefit in real-world treatment decisions. Is it the responsibility of the care provider, the client, or the client's family to decide the importance of dietary restrictions? In community health, the partnership between client and provider in decision making is essential.

Nonmaleficence

Nonmaleficence is the ethical principle that requires the care provider to do no harm. From an ethical perspective, nonmaleficence carries greater moral weight than does beneficence. A nurse must first be assured of doing no harm (nonmaleficence) before being ethically justified in trying to help or promote the legitimate interests of the client (beneficence). In illustration, consider a community health nurse who wishes to respect the right of a client to confidentiality regarding information about a disease state such as HIV status: That nurse must first be assured that keeping such information confidential for one client will not put other clients or the community at risk.

The avoidance of harm also seems inherent in the provision of professional nursing care. In practice, however, the nurse must constantly reflect on the multiple definitions and meanings of harm as well as on who is defining the term, remembering that the care provider's definition of harm may not coincide with that of the care recipient or the community.

Recent changes in the health care environment mean that nurses may be confronted with increased client loads in the face of reductions in time and resources. In such instances, the nurse must first be convinced that the reduction of resources has not also reduced the quality of care in a manner that exposes the client to increased risk. When safety and quality of care are affected, the nurse is morally justified in providing care (beneficence) only after being assured that no harm (nonmaleficence) will come as a result of the reduction in resources.

A less complex example of the moral weight of nonmaleficence over beneficence is the common ethical struggle of the nurse who becomes mildly ill and debates the benefits and burdens of seeing clients and, therefore, exposing them to the ailment or staying home to prevent such exposure but thereby denying care for those clients on that day.

Justice

Justice is the principle of fairness that is served when an individual is given that which is due, owed, or deserved. The principle of justice or fairness may be examined from two different perspectives. That which individuals feel is their due or is owed them, such as the political right to vote or the economic right to a fair wage, is evaluated or perceived as a benefit (entitlement theory). Responsibility owed by individuals to society, such as military conscription or taxes, may be evaluated or perceived as a burden. Both benefits and burdens are thus incorporated within the principle of justice.

In the current atmosphere of health care reform and increased recognition of the limitations of health care resources, the principle of justice, especially the more focused principle of distributive justice, takes on great importance. Distributive justice refers to the fair distribution and allocation of resources within the population. The importance of the principles of justice must be evaluated in light of benefits and burdens to individuals, groups in the community, and society in general.

The principle of justice, especially when applied to the allocation of scarce resources, is extremely complex. Although justice fundamentally suggests that equals should

be treated equally (egalitarian theory), there are examples in which unequal treatment is more just. In such an instance, an individual or group with a greater need receives a greater share of the resource under consideration. Competing interests are thus treated unequally but, perhaps, more fairly. An example of unequal but fair treatment occurs when a child with a chronic disease, such as cystic fibrosis, receives more of the available health care resources, such as home visits or access to necessary medications, than does a child with no chronic disease.

In a situation where the equal distribution of agency resources, such as personnel or time, results in care for all agency clients that is below a minimal standard of care, justice may be better served by the unequal distribution of the agency's resources. In other words, if the even distribution of a nurse's time leaves insufficient time at each visit for appropriate wound care for all clients, justice and client care may be better served by dividing the nurse's time on the basis of clinical criteria such as acuity of the wound or availability of other resources for each client rather than on simple division of the nurse's time. The requirement to prioritize resources according to need may be judged as unfair by those whose access to those resources is limited as a result. Careful allocation of an agency's resources within established guidelines may ultimately provide the greatest benefit to the most clients. Policy decisions regarding environmental needs within a community constitute other examples of allocation decisions made under the principle of justice.

The determination of that which is owed may be based on individual effort, merit, need, societal contribution, rights, or simple equal division (Beauchamp & Childress, 1994). Justice is a particularly important consideration in community health, an environment increasingly characterized by care limitations imposed by third-party payors. Limitations such as an arbitrary number of days of care for a given diagnostic category often do not coincide with individual disease trajectories or healing patterns and may not take into account the plans or policies within a specific community. In such instances, the community health nurse must discover a mechanism to perpetuate needed care for each client without jeopardizing the care available to all clients.

Autonomy

Autonomy, the principle of respect for persons, refers to an individual's right to self-determination. This principle of self-rule honors the right of competent individuals to make free, uncoerced, informed decisions while respecting the rights of others. Under the principle of autonomy, humans are recognized as unconditionally worthy, regardless of any special circumstances or that which they bring to others. Beauchamp and Walters (1994) emphasize the importance of the principle of autonomy:

> To respect the autonomy of self-determining agents is to recognize them as entitled to determine their own destiny, with due regard to their considered

evaluations and view of the world, *even if it is strongly believed that their evaluation or outlook is wrong and even potentially harmful to them* [italics added] (p. 29).

Although in recent years the principle of autonomy has been influential in health care ethics, its influence is beginning to wane somewhat. Autonomy will likely remain a pivotal principle in community health ethics, however, primarily because of the shift in power that occurs when care is provided in the client's home or immediate environment rather than on the "turf" of the provider. Community health practice has lead the way in developing partnerships between care providers and care recipients, especially for the purpose of making care decisions. Autonomy is thus a pivotal ethical principle in community health nursing.

Issues surrounding the harms that come from unhealthy lifestyles highlight ethical conflicts regarding autonomy. Clients who continue to smoke, eat poorly, refuse to exercise, or demonstrate inconsistency relative to medication or treatment routines may challenge the community health nurse's commitment to honoring the right of each client to make decisions (autonomy).

Informed consent, fidelity (promise keeping), and veracity (truth telling) all rely on the acceptance and exercise of autonomy. Informed consent requires that clients be given "the opportunity to choose what shall or shall not happen to them" (National Commission for the Protection of Human Subjects of Biomedical and Behavioral Research, 1978, p. 10). This means that clients must be provided with the necessary information to make decisions about their health care. The information provided to them must be at a level that they understand, and the consent must be voluntary and free of coercion (Beauchamp & Childress, 1994). The rules of *confidentiality*, so important in community health, also receive moral weight from the principle of autonomy. Clients maintain the right to full, accurate information and to protection of intimate and private information necessarily shared in the health care setting. All information regarding a client belongs only to that client, and only that client may grant permission for that information to be released publicly. Respect for each person dictates meticulous attention to the handling of client and family information.

Fidelity and Veracity

Fidelity, or promise keeping, is a rule of ethics that is fundamental to nursing practice in community health. Caring practice is based in large part on the development of a trusting relationship between care provider and care recipient. The expectations inherent in such trusting relationships are based on fidelity. **Veracity**, or truth telling, may be considered a type of promise keeping and is also essential to a trusting relationship. When care is delivered in the community, balance within the relationship may shift to the care recipient, but fidelity and veracity remain the moral responsibility of the care professional. This is true

DECISION MAKING

Outcomes of Client Empowerment

Upholding the view that clients know what they need opens nurses to the probability that some clients will make decisions that are inconsistent with what the nurse or other health team members think is best. Such decisions may have a relatively minor impact on a client's or family's health and well-being or may be judged to have potentially serious outcomes for the client or family.

- What factors must be considered when making decisions involving differing values between clients and nurses?

- Give examples of situations in which client empowerment might potentiate an ethical dilemma for you.

- If you thought that a client was making an unwise decision, how would you respond?

- Discuss your view regarding any limits or constraints on client empowerment.

Adapted from Ethics and Issues in Contemporary Nursing, *by M. A. Burkhardt & A. K. Nathaniel 1998, Albany, NY: Delmar Publishers. Copyright 1998 by Delmar Publishers.*

despite the fact that the care recipient may have greater control than in an agency setting simply because care is provided in the recipient's home or immediate environment. It is helpful for the community nurse to foster, acknowledge, and honor this shift in the balance of power between professional care provider and care recipient.

Accountability

According to the American Nurses Association (1985), "Accountability refers to being answerable to someone for something one has done. [It is] grounded in the moral principles of fidelity and respect for the dignity, worth, and self-determination of clients" (p. 8). Safe, autonomous practice is ensured through various processes of nursing accountability. Accountability is related to both responsibility and answerability (Leddy & Pepper, 1998). Because of the trust accorded nurses by society (gained through recognition of nurses' expertise) and the right given the profession to regulate practice (autonomy), individual practitioners and the profession must be both responsible and accountable.

Related to the concepts of autonomy and authority, accountability is an inherent part of everyday nursing practice. Each nurse is responsible for all individual actions and omissions. The ANA *Code for Nurses with Interpretive Statements* makes it clear that each nurse has the responsibility to maintain ethical and competent practice regardless of circumstances, stating that "neither

DECISION MAKING

Ethics and Confidentiality

• What would you do with confidential information regarding substance abuse or potential domestic violence on the part of a family member who is not your client and is not under your care?

• What is the professional and *ethical* response of the community health nurse?

physicians' orders nor the employing agency's policies relieve the nurse of accountability for actions taken and judgments made" (1985, p. 9). . . . The courts have tended to support this claim.

Many situations in community health care magnify the dilemmas that occur when the rights of some individuals conflict with the rights of other individuals, an agency, the community, or society or when ethical principles conflict with each other. Consider a situation in which a nurse providing care believes that as long as sufficient money is unavailable for full immunization programs, no money should be spent on organ transplantation programs, even to benefit a client. Further suppose that one of the clients to whom this nurse provides care is trying to raise public money for lung transplantation. The nurse's beliefs may interfere with his or her ability to provide adequate care to this client if those beliefs are not acknowledged and addressed.

Another situation often encountered in the community

is that of disagreement among family members regarding the intensity of intervention in long-term care. If the client desires continued high-level intervention but the family feels unable to sustain such care, the nurse provider may feel caught in the conflict.

Finally, the community health nurse may become involved in a case in which another agency is unable or unwilling to honor client decisions. A terminally ill teenager, for example, may have negotiated end-of-life decisions such as do-not-resuscitate (DNR) with family members and local emergency services but may find that school personnel are unwilling or unable to honor such an order while the teen is in school (Kuehl, Shapiro, & Sivasubramanian, 1992; Scofield, 1992; Strike, 1992; Younger, 1992).

Throughout health care, ethical principles sometimes conflict. A client's right to decide for self (autonomy) may conflict with the care provider's interpretation of that which is best for the client (beneficence). The allocation of scarce and precious resources on the basis of fairness (justice) may harm individuals or groups with lesser claims to those resources (nonmaleficence) yet provide the greatest good to the greatest number (utilitarianism).

Consideration of risks, benefits, and burdens must be an integral part of discussions surrounding these conflicts. Another challenge in the consideration of ethical rules, principles, and theories revolves around the question of whose rights prevail. Do the rights of a group or community automatically supersede the rights of an individual? The complexity of ethical issues demands a thorough, organized approach to adequately utilize ethical theories and principles in a context of care to facilitate appropriate resolution of conflicts. Table 5-1 summarizes some of the ethical principles influencing health care decisions.

Table 5-1   Ethical Principles Influencing Health Care Decisions

ETHICAL PRINCIPLE	DEFINITION	EXAMPLE
Beneficence	The principle of doing or promoting good that requires abstention from injuring others and promotion of the legitimate interests of others primarily by preventing or removing possible harms.	Teaching an elderly client about safety features in the home.
Nonmaleficence	The principle of doing no harm	Not leaving a client in acute distress.
Justice	The principle of fairness that is served when an individual is given that which he or she is due, owed, deserves, or can legitimately claim.	Providing nursing services regardless of ability to pay.
Autonomy	The principle of respect for persons that is based on recognition of humans as unconditionally worthy agents, regardless of any special characteristics, conditions, or circumstances.	Allowing a client to refuse a home visit.
Fidelity	The principle of promise keeping. The duty to keep one's promise or word.	Making a home visit at the agreed-upon time.
Veracity	The principle of truth telling. The duty to tell the truth.	Being honest; being authentic.

Perspectives...

Insights of a Community Health Nursing Professor

The value of caring in nursing is recognized as fundamental to the nursing role. It is a moral obligation that is practiced in response to the health needs and concerns of people who live in their various communities. This is the story of a client and a student community health nurse who provided nursing services to the client. The name and age of the client have been changed to protect her privacy. As the faculty member who worked with this student, I think it is important to share this story because it clearly exemplifies caring in practice.

Mrs. K., a 55-year-old widow who was a former teacher, lived alone in her apartment. She had few friends and one son who lived nearby; however, she did not see him very often. Mrs. K was a quadriplegic because of a car accident. She had a low income and received care provider assistance from the state; however, the provider coverage did not fund coverage for 24 hours a day or for nighttime hours. Mrs. K. was therefore alone at night. She was bedbound and could not move any body part, except to turn her head to the right. She was able to use a specially designed phone access system that allowed her to speak into a piece of equipment near her head. Thus, in the event of an emergency, she could call the emergency system in the county.

Mrs. K. was determined to stay at home as long as possible. She did not want and refused to go to an extended care facility.

The student community health nurse who visited Mrs. K. recognized the need to respect Mrs. K. and her request to remain at home as well as her need to maintain as much control as she could given the nature of her life situation. She identified Mrs. K. as an intelligent and courageous person who was very clear about what she wanted and didn't want. The student worked closely with the multidisciplinary team and identified that one of her most important roles was to serve as an active listener with Mrs. K., to take the time to hear the client's story, to assess and monitor the client's health condition, and to intervene as necessary. The student recognized that

Mrs. K. had a right to stay at home as long as possible and supported the social worker's actions when the police and fire departments were notified regarding the client's condition, in the event an emergency response was needed. The student worked closely with the care providers to ensure that they understood the need to report any changes in the client's condition to the social worker or public health nurse, changes that would prevent Mrs. K. from calling for emergency assistance at night, such as difficulty talking or difficulty in turning her head. By the time the semester ended, with the assistance of the social worker, Mrs. K. was able to find a family who needed housing to stay with her at night.

At the conclusion of the semester, Mrs. K. said to the public health nurse coordinator: "The student was simply wonderful—she took the time to hear my concerns. She was very helpful in assisting the providers to learn more about my condition. I wish she could stay longer—I really enjoyed talking with her. She respected me—she cared about me. She did not come in here and tell me what to do. She involved me in the decisions."

Coupled with the nursing care services at the client level, the student also took action in the broader political arena. In the state legislature, a bill had been introduced specific to expanding the number of allocated hours for care provider assistance for low-income severely disabled persons. The student recognized the opportunity to make her voice heard and wrote a letter to the legislator stating her support for the bill.

Caring is central to community health nursing practice. The student who manifested caring behaviors with Mrs.. K. made a difference. I believe that sharing our story provides a rich experience for others—we learn what connects us all. Stories help give us a sense of connection and community. We need to share our stories. This story is one about courage, hope, listening, sharing, compassion, trust, and political action.

—Sue A. Thomas, RN, EdD

PERSPECTIVES IN ETHICAL DECISIONS

Historically, ethical decisions in health care (bioethics and medical ethics) have relied almost exclusively on the formal application of ethical principles to resolve dilemmas. This system of theory and practice in ethics is known as principlism. In the past, **principlism** provided nurses, physicians, and the public with a simple and direct language and a structure within which to discuss the conflicts arising out of the rapid advances in health care technology that have spread to every aspect of the health care environment (DuBose, Hamel, & O'Connell, 1994).

Currently, health care ethics in the United States is moving toward the incorporation of broader perspectives in ethical dilemmas and decisions. Feminist, cross-cultural, and caring perspectives are among those moving health care ethics beyond principlism. There is great hope that the integration of these perspectives—especially the caring perspective—with principlism will promote greater understanding and acceptance of the meaning of the web of relationships that each individual brings to situations of ethical conflict. The diversity and complexity of the individuals, groups, and situations in the changing health care environment further highlight the need for broader perspectives. In an integrated ethical system, the principlist emphasis on autonomy and individual rights may become muted by the incorporation of community and societal values as well as by the interdependent relationships of the individual.

The caring perspective may help neutralize one criticism frequently directed toward principlism, that it "does not make space for emotion or take sufficient account of the notion of care in relationships" (DuBose et al., 1994, p. 3). Caring maintains the focus on the support, development, and importance of relationship. Therefore, the ethics of caring incorporates attention to specific, contextual relationship rather than to the abstract principles on which the principlist approach to ethical conflict and decision making is founded. In a feminist analysis of the limits of principlism, Gudorf (1994) points out that "more social principles—mutuality, community, solidarity, empathy, nurturance, wholeness or integrity, and relationality itself—are not lifted up, despite our knowledge of their importance for individual as well as community growth, health, and healing" (p. 167). New approaches to health care ethics seek to incorporate perspectives from caring and feminism in a manner that modifies "both the body of relevant principles and their interpretation," recognizing the "need to connect the use of principles with an examination of the concrete situation of those most at risk" (Gudorf, 1994, p. 168) in the ethical debate.

THE DECISION-MAKING PROCESS

Ethical dilemmas occur when principles conflict with one another or when the duties, rights, beliefs, and values of an individual conflict with those of another individual, of an agency, or of the greater society (Mitchell, 1990). Understanding ethical theories, principles, and rules is only a first step in reaching ethically defensible resolution to conflict situations arising in community health. Conflicts regarding community health care revolve around issues such as the actual or potential abuse of clients or care providers; the continuation of care when reimbursement for that care is no longer available; obvious differences in lifestyle values such as diet or substance abuse; and demonstration by the client of values different from those of the professional care provider, particularly in relation to levels of intervention or to the determination of futility of care.

Application of ethical theories and principles must be made in a manner that facilitates the creation of moral space, or an environment in which the formation, discussion, and application of moral standards can occur (Walker, 1993). An environment that provides moral space and that respects the values of all of the participants is essential. It is vital to acknowledge the effects of the multiple allegiances that nurses hold, the types of decisions being made, and the perspectives driving the decisions.

A decision-making process should be established for every setting where there exists potential for ethical conflict. A large number of ethical decision-making models are available in the literature (Silva, 1990; Husted & Husted, 1995; Benjamin & Curtis, 1992; Ellis & Hartley, 1992; Aiken & Catalano, 1994). Regardless of the model, however, six components are essential for adequately addressing ethical dilemmas (see Figure 5-1).

Essential Components of Decision-Making Models

Six essential components contribute to the adequacy of ethical decision-making models. Prior to encountering an actual dilemma requiring urgent resolution, every nurse should select and practice the application of an ethical

---

Figure 5-1 Decision Model Components

Each model should have a means of determining:

- Those who are involved in the issue, the decision, and the outcome
- All relevant information—medical, physical, social, spiritual, psychological, economic, emotional, and relational
- Options for potential resolution of the issue
- A process for reaching resolution
- A plan for action on the resolution
- A method of evaluating the process, the decision, and the outcome

decision-making model to gain facility in using a decision-making process.

Determining Involvement

Any decision-making model should provide a means of determining those who are involved in the decision making *and* in the outcome of the decision.

Gathering Data

Decision-making models must also provide means of gathering all relevant information. Information gathered should be factual and should encompass medical, psychological, spiritual, social, economic, resource, and emotional data. Information should be obtained beyond the obvious diagnosis, prognosis, and treatment options.

The development of an adequate database is essential to making "good"—that is, ethically justifiable—ethical decisions. Data collection provides an opportunity for the nurse to identify, define, and refine issues and to determine ownership of the problem, of the consequences, of the information, and of the decision itself. The nurse must be instrumental in the determination of all of these facets of data gathering.

Outlining Options and Consequences

Outlining options to reach potential resolution of the dilemma is the third component of any adequate decision-making model. Inherent in this component is an examination of the likely consequences of each option under consideration. In order to remain open to all practical options, especially to options that represent opposing viewpoints, a mechanism to identify and temporarily set aside values is helpful. The importance of considering divergent views cannot be overemphasized in the context of caring. Divergent views may encompass differing values regarding such things as life quality, standards of cleanliness in the home, aggressiveness of care, alternative therapies, the meaning of spirituality, or lifestyle in general.

The ability to recognize values as components in the decision-making process is critical when a nurse is engaged in ethical decision making. Although values initially must be set aside to accommodate consideration of all potential options, values return to the discussion before a choice is made. Without a discussion of the values of all persons involved, the resolution sought may be ethically justified but remain acontextual.

Process for Resolving Conflict

The fourth component of an adequate decision-making model is an identified process for resolving conflict. A number of practical issues must be addressed within the scope of this component. In order for conflict resolution to occur, issues such as ultimate responsibility and accountability for decisions, ways to reach consensus, ways to communicate the consensus, and steps to take if

agreement is impossible must be considered and agreed upon. A review of driving and restraining forces as well as the benefits, risks, and burdens of each option is also part of this process. The likelihood of a successful outcome also must be considered for each option. Selecting an option that cannot be acted upon within the confines of the law, for instance, would be counterproductive.

Planning for Action/Implementation

The fifth component of an adequate decision-making model is a plan for enacting the resolution. How is the decision to be carried out and by whom? Outlining options and consequences, resolving conflict, and enacting the resolution constitute the decision making itself.

Evaluation

The sixth and final essential component of an adequate decision-making model is a method of evaluation. This component encompasses evaluation not only of the decision but also of the consequences of the decision and of the decision-making process itself.

Together, then, these six components contribute to the adequacy of any decision-making model or framework, guiding whether the model is likely to foster ethically justifiable decisions. It should be clear that the process that occurs in ethical decision making parallels the nursing process utilized in clinical practice: gathering data—assessment; synthesizing data—analysis and diagnosis; outlining and selecting the options—planning; acting on the options—implementation; and evaluating the process and the decision—evaluation. On the basis of their experience in clinical decision making, nurses should thus feel confident in their ability to engage in ethical decision making. Figure 5-2 portrays the ethical decision-making model.

External Factors That Affect Decision Making

A number of factors affect the nurse's ability to make ethical decisions, even with an adequate decision-making

DECISION MAKING

Ethical Decision Making

• What would you do if a client did not tell the truth or withheld some information regarding care issues?

• Would your response be the same if the lack of truthfulness affected another family member? Another care provider? The client, but not in a manner related to the care you provide?

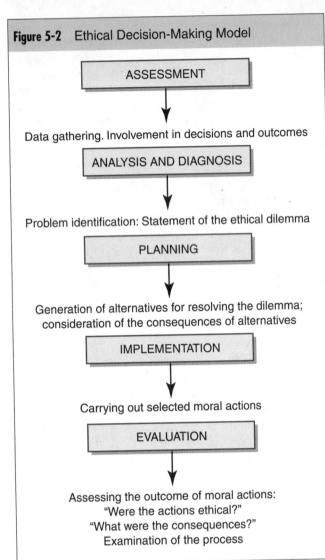

Figure 5-2   Ethical Decision-Making Model

ASSESSMENT

Data gathering. Involvement in decisions and outcomes

ANALYSIS AND DIAGNOSIS

Problem identification: Statement of the ethical dilemma

PLANNING

Generation of alternatives for resolving the dilemma; consideration of the consequences of alternatives

IMPLEMENTATION

Carrying out selected moral actions

EVALUATION

Assessing the outcome of moral actions:
"Were the actions ethical?"
"What were the consequences?"
Examination of the process

model and experience in clinical decisions in place. Among these factors are the multiple allegiances that encumber the nurse in practice; the type of decision being made—medical, legal, or ethical; environmental factors, or the atmosphere of the work setting; resources for decision making, such as the presence of and access to a formal decision-making system or process; and personal and professional values. All of these factors reflect the medical, legal, economic, and societal schema within which health care ethical decisions are made.

Multiple Allegiances

Nurses in all clinical settings are subject to the complexities of multiple allegiances. Multiple allegiances affect the interpretation of ethical conflicts as well as the decision-making process itself. As care managers, most professional nurses consider their role as client advocate to be fundamental. As members of interdisciplinary care teams, nurses practice in various levels of collegial relationships with a diverse group of other care providers. In some community situations, particularly in home health or hos-

pice, nurses depend on physicians' orders for part of the care they deliver. Many nurses in community health also provide independent care, engaging the client as an active participant in the care decision-making process. As clients and families become more active participants on the health care team, additional role definitions and allegiances evolve for the nurse in clinical practice. The caring relationship based on trust, integrity, and genuine presence on the part of the nurse is fundamental to the partnership between nurse and client.

The nurse is usually an employee of an agency or institution. Nurses therefore owe additional allegiance to their employers. In the community or in independent practice, the professional nurse may owe yet another type of allegiance, that to third-party payors. Personal, professional, community, and societal allegiances also place demands on the nurse in practice. It is therefore critical that each nurse maintain clarity regarding the effects of each allegiance on ethical issues, inherent values, and decision making. Figure 5-3 illustrates the multiple allegiances of the nurse that may affect decision making.

Decision Types

In the face of ethical conflicts, clarity regarding the nurse's allegiance should accompany a similar clarity regarding the type of decision being made. Health care (or medical), legal, and ethical aspects of conflicts are inextricably intertwined. A "good" or justifiable decision according to the standards of one discipline may not be justifiable according to the standards of the other disciplines. As an example, consider the Hmong family, whose newborn son is

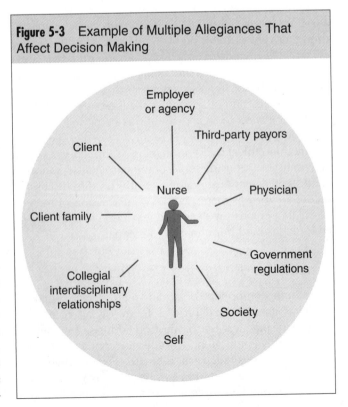

Figure 5-3   Example of Multiple Allegiances That Affect Decision Making

Employer or agency

Third-party payors

Client

Nurse

Physician

Client family

Government regulations

Collegial interdisciplinary relationships

Society

Self

DECISION MAKING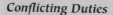

diagnosed at birth with Down syndrome (trisomy 21). The infant has a surgically correctable cardiac defect commonly found in clients with trisomy 21. Without surgical intervention, the infant is not expected to live into early childhood. According to the Hmong's religious, spiritual, and cultural beliefs, surgery is forbidden; intentional cutting of the human body is understood to kill the spirit or soul of the individual. From a medical perspective, denying a simple successful surgical repair of a cardiac defect represents a poor, unjustifiable decision.

From a legal perspective, Baby Doe rules and regulations should be considered. These regulations provide for the protection of handicapped infants against non-treatment decisions based on their actual or potential handicap. (For a complete review, interesting discussion, history, and summary of the Baby Doe rules and regulations see Pence, 1990). Babies with Down syndrome may face both mental and physical handicaps as a result of their genetic aberra-

tion and are therefore given protective consideration under the Baby Doe regulations. Although not legally binding, the regulations provide strong legal direction for health care decisions regarding infants with potential handicaps. From the legal perspective, decisions regarding care must not be made based on actual or potential handicaps. In the case of the Hmong infant, careful investigation must be undertaken to determine the motivation for refusing the surgery. From a legal perspective the decision is unclear, at best.

From an ethical perspective, sound decisions incorporate the significant values of everyone involved in the decision, particularly those who bear the greatest burden of the decision. Allowing the Hmong family to refuse surgery for their son because of their spiritual and cultural values represents an ethically justifiable decision that is medically unsound and legally in need of clarification. Supporting the genuine decision to love and care for their son within the confines of their own culture as an intact family committed to the natural consequences of refusing surgical intervention represents a contextual, caring, ethically justifiable decision. To suggest that the more desirable health care outcome resulting from surgery would be worth the ostracism and spiritual death of the Hmong family is to deny their moral experience and, furthermore, is based on values to which they do not ascribe.

Another example of the need to clarify the decision type involves the discipline of law. Numerous examples of legally sanctioned continued life support are questionable from the medical perspective and ethically unjustifiable or, at the very least, unsound. Without question, quality of life issues remain among the most poignant and complex ethical questions for care providers and recipients alike. Whenever confronted with an ethical dilemma, the community health nurse would be wise to obtain clarity regarding the type of decision being made. It is inappropriate to claim ethical justification for a decision derived solely from the standards or values of another discipline—most often the discipline of law. Nursing practice requires adherence to the law, but actions dictated by law should not automatically be assumed to be justifiable ethically.

As conflicts arise—as they are bound to in our pluralistic, culturally diverse world—it is critical that participants in the conflict and the decision-making process openly acknowledge the various perspectives that drive decisions. Each individual's perspective must be respected because it affects the understanding and use of ethical theories, principles, and rules and the decision-making process.

Environmental Factors

Agency and institutional constraints continue to be imposed on nursing practice, affecting the nurse's ability to participate in ethical decision making. Although early discussions of such constraints implicated acute care institutions, community care agencies have been shown to impose similar constraints. Since the late 1970s, nursing authors have identified some of the classic constraints on nurses. Sadly, many of these constraints still exist in the acute care setting and have extended to other practice settings such as community health.

These constraints include the roles and social positions of the nurse, physician, and care administrator, particularly as they exist within bureaucratic settings; the role and power of nursing leadership within the health care system; sexism; paternalism; and any limitations imposed on nursing practice that prevent moral agency in the nurse. **Moral agency** is the ability of the nurse to act according to professional moral standards. Each of these factors may be found to varying degrees within the community health practice setting.

Because of the more independent nature of practice in the community, the community health nurse may be less constrained by bureaucracy than is the nurse in the acute care setting, but agency administrators or governmental regulations may still inhibit the community health nurse in practice. Rules, regulations, policies, or procedures may assist in the smooth operation of an agency yet present barriers to appropriate care for an individual client or be poorly suited to the needs of the community itself.

In community health, the role relationship within the bureaucracy may be focused on nonphysician care providers, family members, or third-party payors as well as on physicians. Support from nursing colleagues, leaders, or supervisors may not be available to the nurse in community practice, particularly as community practice models continue to grow and restructuring of the delivery system moves forward. As awareness has increased regarding the potential harm of sexism and the inappropriateness of paternalism in health care, the signs and symptoms of both have become ever more subtle. Addressing ethical dilemmas in community health demands a keen awareness of even subtle environmental factors that may affect the nurse's ability to create, maintain, and enhance caring within that environment.

The development of collegial interdisciplinary relationships must continue in order to meet the needs of all clients in community health. Again, the multiple allegiances that encumber nurses are reflected among the interdisciplinary relationships that influence the caring environment and decisions within that environment. Conditions may exist within the care environment that affect professional relationships and, therefore, the nurse's ability to care. Administrative regulations, organizational constraints, and power structures within the environment are among those conditions and should be of primary concern to the nurse. It is important for the nurse to acknowledge, understand, and, in some cases, change those environmental factors that adversely affect the nurse's ability to maintain and enhance caring.

Resources for Decision Making

Closely related to environmental factors are the resources available to the community health nurse to facilitate ethical decision making. The presence of and access to a formal decision-making process has much to do with the nurse's ability to make and implement effective ethical decisions. Whereas most large acute care institutions have formal ethics committees in place, community agencies have only recently begun to develop formalized approaches to ethical decision making.

Bioethics committees in the United States were initially established to review policies and procedures; provide ethics education to committee members, the respective institution or agency, and the community at large; and supply active and retrospective case review and consultation when ethical conflict occurred (President's Commission, 1983; Smith & Veatch, 1987). The 1991 Joint Commission on Accreditation's (JCAHO) manual for hospital standards directed agencies seeking accreditation to demonstrate access to a formal ethical decision-making process and to have nurses represented in that process (Joint Commission, 1990).

Recent guidelines (Joint Commission, 1994; Joint Commission, 1996) directed agency ethics committees to become more responsible for the ethical environment. These regulations call on institutional ethics committees and, by implication, community agency ethics committees to set the ethical tone of the agency, to establish and implement a code of ethical behavior for members of the agency, and to integrate ethics into the daily life of the agency. Under these guidelines, the ethics committee is responsible for the ethical environment of the agency itself. The institutional bioethics committee is being asked "to support an environment of ethical practice" (American Health Consultants, 1995, p. 2). Community-based bioethics committees are being developed in response to the need for formal decision-making processes to respond to ethical challenges outside the acute care setting. Although most community health care agencies do not come under JCAHO review, it may be prudent for community-based ethics committees to be appropriately sensitive to these important JCAHO guidelines.

Community-based bioethics committees have been termed "third generation" ethics committees (Mason, 1995). First generation committees evolved as care review committees, abortion review committees, institutional review boards, prognosis committees, and dialysis patient–selection committees. Second generation committees are familiar to many as those that developed in the 1980s in acute care settings. Community health care agencies often have found it impossible to develop from within the resources needed for a formal ethics committee on the order of the second generation hospital-based ethics committees that blossomed in the 1980s (Ross, Glaser, Rasinski-Gregory, Gibson, McIver, & Bayley, 1993). The need for ethics education, policy review, and case consultation exists within community health agencies just as it does in the acute care setting. To address this need, third generation community-based ethics committees that combine and share resources across agencies have been initiated. Such committees, when available, may provide community health nurses with a formal process to address ethical conflicts encountered within the practice setting.

One example of a community-based ethics committee is the Denver Community Bioethics Committee. This committee is a model for community-based ethical review of health care decisions, primarily in long-term care facilities. As a noninstitutional volunteer committee, the members meet monthly and as needed for emergency consultation, to address issues and dilemmas involving long-term care clients or residents who lack decisional capacity. The committee was established through the Denver Department of Social Services with assistance from the Guardianship Alliance of Colorado to help agencies, facilities, and family members in the Denver metropolitan area negotiate difficult ethical issues related to the care of Social Service Department wards and long-term care clients or residents. Membership consists of 25 individuals including physicians, nurses, attorneys, social workers, clergy, adult protection administrators, nursing home ombudsmen, health care administrators, and an ethicist. All members have received ethics education. The committee focuses on issues related to the care of individuals who lack decisional capacity, including questions about life support and treatment termination. Access to the committee is by request through committee members. Anyone facing difficult health care decisions may access the committee (Mason, 1995).

A similar committee, the Montgomery County Department of Social Services' Ethics Committee in Rockville, Maryland, assists with difficult issues for clients with public guardians. On some occasions, the county committee has met jointly with a hospital ethics committee to resolve issues. The county committee has 17 members including nurses, physicians, clergy, social workers, and members of the community. This committee makes recommendations to the director of the Department of Social Services, who, in turn, makes recommendations to the court. Members of this committee also receive training in ethics and ethical decision processes. "Training encompasses ethical, religious, moral, and value implications of providing services to children and vulnerable adults" (American Health Consultants, 1994, p. 115).

In the absence of a community-based ethics committee, the nursing leadership within each agency as well as the individual nurse practicing in the agency bear the responsibility to investigate the possibility of developing such a committee. At the very least, access to other formalized assistance with ethical decision making should be sought. Individual community health nurses should understand those mechanisms that are available and the process to access those mechanisms.

Values

Personal and professional values significantly influence the community health nurse's ability to make and effect ethical decisions. The values that the individual nurse brings to the care setting as well as the values of everyone involved in an ethical conflict must be addressed. The nurse's values must remain clear in order to avoid confusing the nurse's personal or professional values with those of other care providers, the client, and the family. Unless each nurse maintains clarity regarding values, the very real danger exists that one set of values will inadvertently supersede another set of values in the conflict.

Respecting the values of all participants in a conflict situation is critical to reaching ethically justifiable resolution to ethical conflict. Understanding one's own values may facilitate remaining open to the values of others. Caring, as a core value in professional nursing, may enhance the ability of the practicing nurse to remain open and genuine in the face of differing and conflicting values. Health promotion and disease prevention, core values in community health, may not be shared by all those seeking care. Budget limitations, a client's or agency's orientation to the present rather than the future, or an interest in curing disease instead of taking measures to prevent the onset of disease represent the kind of value conflict encountered in community health.

Ethical Codes

Several nursing organizations have developed codes as guidelines for ethical conduct. The American Nurses Association (ANA) delineates the nurse's obligations to clients: "A code of ethics indicates a profession's acceptance of

REFLECTIVE THINKING

How Have Your Values Developed?

Think of three ideals or beliefs that you prize in your personal life. Try to trace each belief or ideal back to the earliest time in your life when you were aware of its importance or presence.

• When and how did you learn to view each belief or ideal as important?

• How have your beliefs and ideals changed or evolved over time?

• Where do you find your support for them?

• How prevalent do you think these beliefs or ideals are among other people?

• What do you think of people who hold different beliefs or ideals?

• Think of a time in your life when one of these beliefs or ideals has been challenged. How did you feel? How did you react?

Adapted from Ethics and Issues in Contemporary Nursing, *by M. A. Burkhardt & A. K. Nathaniel, 1998, Albany, NY: Delmar Publishers. Copyright 1998 by Delmar Publishers.*

Figure 5-4 American Nurses Association Code for Nurses

1. The nurse provides services with respect for human dignity and the uniqueness of the client, unrestricted by considerations of social or economic status, personal attributes, or the nature of health problems.

2. The nurse safeguards the client's right to privacy by judiciously protecting information of a confidential nature.

3. The nurse acts to safeguard the client and the public when health care and safety are affected by the incompetent, unethical, or illegal practice of any person.

4. The nurse assumes responsibility and accountability for individual nursing judgments and actions.

5. The nurse maintains competence in nursing.

6. The nurse exercises informed judgment and uses individual competence and qualifications as criteria in seeking consultation, accepting responsibilities, and delegating nursing activities to others.

7. The nurse participates in activities that contribute to the ongoing development of the profession's body of knowledge.

8. The nurse participates in the profession's efforts to implement and improve standards of nursing.

9. The nurse participates in the profession's efforts to establish and maintain conditions of employment conducive to high-quality nursing care.

10. The nurse participates in the profession's effort to protect the public from misinformation and misrepresentation and to maintain the integrity of nursing.

11. The nurse collaborates with members of the health professions and other citizens in promoting community and national efforts to meet the health needs of the public.

Reprinted with permission from Code for Nurses, with Interpretive Statements, *1985, © American Nurses Association, Washington, D.C.*

Figure 5-5 Canadian Nurses Association Code of Ethics for Nursing*

Health and Well-Being

Nurses value health and well-being and assist persons to achieve their optimum level of health in situations of normal health, illness, injury, or in the process of dying.

Choice

Nurses respect and promote the autonomy of clients and help them to express their health needs and values, and to obtain appropriate information and services.

Dignity

Nurses value and advocate the dignity and self-respect of human beings.

Confidentiality

Nurses safeguard the trust of clients that information learned in the context of a professional relationship is shared outside the health care team only with the client's permission or as legally required.

Fairness

Nurses apply and promote principles of equity and fairness to assist clients in receiving unbiased treatment and a share of health services and resources proportionate to their needs.

Accountability

Nurses act in a manner consistent with their professional responsibilities and standards of practice.

Practice Environments Conducive to Safe, Competent, and Ethical Care

Nurses advocate practice environments that have the organizational and human support systems, and the resource allocations necessary for safe, competent, and ethical nursing care.

This represents only one element of the code of values. For each value noted, the CNA Code of Ethics for Nursing provides obligations that provide more specific direction for conduct.

Reproduced with permission from the Canadian Nurses Association. Code of Ethics for Nursing, *1997, Ottawa: Author.*

the responsibility and trust with which it has been invested by society" (ANA, 1985). The ANA code of ethics can be found in Figure 5-4. The Canadian Nurses Association and the International Council of Nurses have also developed codes of ethics. These codes are presented in Figures 5-5 and 5-6, respectively.

ETHICAL DILEMMAS IN COMMUNITY HEALTH

Ethical dilemmas are universal in health care. The uniqueness of each health care setting, however, makes it appropriate to examine ethical dilemmas from the perspective of respective health care settings. Ethical issues in community health cover a spectrum as diverse as the agencies, client populations, and care providers in the community itself (Kane, Penrod, & Kivnick, 1993). Issues of client abandonment through care limitations, decisional capacity and competence, potential and actual client or provider abuse, lifestyle diversity, and compliance or cooperation with treatment regimes are addressed next.

Client Abandonment

The increasingly limited health care resources characteristic of the changing health care environment create issues of client abandonment, common in community health nursing centers. Although some have expressed concern regarding characterizing limitations imposed on care as "abandonment" (Reckling, 1989), community health nurses understand the terminology well. Restrictions and limitations on client care services have undeniably grown in response to the ever-increasing number, type, and complexity of payment systems and the significant limitations on health care resources.

Increasingly, coverage ends before the need for care ends. Nurses may be faced with critical decisions regarding the reporting of client care needs in order to place the client in the most advantageous light for continued receipt of coverage for needed care services. The nurse may also face conflict regarding the provision of care for which payment will not be forthcoming, thus potentially jeopardizing the economic stability of the employing agency or the level of care available to other clients.

> It often happens that when Medicare coverage expires, clients need ongoing care but are unable (or unwilling) to pay out of pocket for additional services. Rather than discharge such clients from care (and be liable to regulatory rebuke and legal challenge, not to mention moral quandary), an agency may continue care without reimbursement—at its own fiscal peril. . . . Agencies often have to choose between insufficient care and no care. When an agency assesses a client at a level of care for which funding is denied, the agency can offer a lower (but reimbursed) level of care or it can refuse to initiate or continue care. But refusing clients—or, worse, discharging them—can negate the whole purpose and mission of the agency. . . . Moral commitments bind the agency to the client in ways that wreak havoc with the autonomy of the agency and its commitment to the client's autonomy and well-being (Collopy, Dubler, & Zuckerman, 1990, p. 5).

REFLECTIVE THINKING

Conflicting Beliefs and Values

Consider a diabetic client who has progressed in the knowledge of self-care but who still requires further teaching, supervision, and practice in self-care skills.

- How will you manage personal beliefs and professional values that conflict with corporate practice or agency policy?
- How will you feel about having to cease care provision to this client when funding runs out?
- What will you do?

Figure 5-6 International Council of Nurses Code for Nurses

The fundamental responsibility of the nurse is fourfold: to promote health, to prevent illness, to restore health, and to alleviate suffering.

The need for nursing is universal. Inherent in nursing is respect for life, dignity, and rights of man. It is unrestricted by considerations of nationality, race, creed, color, age, sex, politics, or social status.

Nurses render health services to the individual, the family, and the community and coordinate their services with those of related groups.

Nurses and People

The nurse's primary responsibility is to those people who require nursing care.

The nurse, in providing care, promotes an environment in which the values, customs, and spiritual beliefs of the individual are respected.

The nurse holds in confidence personal information and uses judgment in sharing this information.

Nurses and Practice

The nurse carries personal responsibility for nursing practice and for maintaining competence by continual learning. The nurse maintains the highest standards of nursing care possible within the reality of a specific situation.

The nurse uses judgment in relation to individual competence when accepting and delegating responsibilities.

The nurse, when acting in a professional capacity, should at all times maintain standards of personal conduct that reflect credit upon the profession.

Nurses and Society

The nurse shares with other citizens the responsibility for initiating and supporting action to meet the health and social needs of the public.

Nurses and Coworkers

The nurse sustains cooperative relationships with coworkers in nursing and other fields. The nurse takes appropriate action to safeguard the individual when his care is endangered by a coworker or any other person.

Nurses and the Profession

The nurse plays the major role in determining and implementing desirable standards of nursing practice and nursing education.

The nurse is active in developing a core of professional knowledge.

The nurse, acting through the professional organization, participates in establishing and maintaining equitable social and economic working conditions in nursing.

Reproduced with permission from the International Council of Nurses. ICN Code for Nurses: Ethical Concepts Applied to Nursing, 1973, Geneva, Switzerland: Imprimeries Populaires.

RESEARCH FOCUS

Ethics and Case Management: Preliminary Results of an Empirical Study

STUDY PROBLEM/PURPOSE

Increased attention is being focused on case management in health care. This descriptive study of the ethical issues that emerge in case management as an approach to planning and allocating long-term care for elderly individuals is applicable to care-management issues in the community. The purpose of this study was to describe perceived ethical challenges from the perspective of a representative sample of case managers working in publicly subsidized case-management programs in 10 states.

METHODS

A sample of 251 case managers in the 10 states was selected to represent geographic and programmatic differences in case-management programs for long-term care. Telephone interviews of randomly selected case managers in each program were conducted by trained interviewers. Demographic data included age, gender, ethnicity, religion, education, income, and length of experience as a case manager. Type and range of case-management tasks performed were determined using a checklist. Attitudes toward aging, dependency, family responsibility, public assistance, and appropriate roles for case managers were collected from respondents using 5-point Likert scales.

Open-ended questions about ethical issues encountered by case managers on the job constituted the primary focus of each interview. Case managers were asked to identify ethical issues encountered in their jobs and discuss in detail the most difficult ethical issue faced as a case manager. Respondents were also asked about ethical issues that might occur in seven categories: "divergence between clients' interests or wishes and those of family members; divergence between clients' wishes and case managers' views of clients' needs; divergence between safety concerns and other values; client confidentiality and disclosure; interprofessional or interagency disagreements; agency policies giving rise to ethical issues; and public policies giving rise to ethical issues" (p. 8). Finally, respondents were asked a set of questions regarding how or whether case managers assessed the values and preferences of their clients; whether they observed any patterns in those values or preferences; and how or whether the values and preferences made a difference in the conduct of the case. Responses to the open-ended questions were coded to provide descriptions of ethical issues in case management. Responses were also tabulated by state, gender, age, religion, and length of time as a case manager.

FINDINGS

The findings revealed a wide range of specific issues including: admission to another care facility, client safety, confidentiality, agency policies, appropriateness of care, eligibility for care, decisions made about or for incompetent clients, rights of family members, and issues of coercion, especially those revolving around maximizing client autonomy. Responses in each of the seven categories were tabulated to demonstrate the specific issues in each of the categories. Conflicts between the client and family occurred most often when the family had different views from those of the client and/or the case manager regarding the decision to place the client in a care facility such as a nursing home. In this category, there were also conflicts of interest about money and the rights and responsibilities of the family, as well as disagreements among family members about the client.

Disparity between client needs and wants most often centered on a lack of safety or an unhealthy lifestyle. Disparities were demonstrated both when the client wanted more services than the case manager felt necessary or when the case manager felt more services were needed than the client desired or for which the client was willing to pay. A safe environment or healthy lifestyle was often at variance with other care goals. Privacy and confidentiality as they were related to disclosure of information to family members or agency providers were issues. The case managers, most of whom were not nurses, also encountered ethical issues with other professionals. Case managers encountered conflict with adult protection services, hospital personnel, social services, nursing home personnel, paraprofessional home care personnel, physicians, nurses, and mental health personnel. Interprofessional conflicts most frequently took the form of disagreements about care plans or the policies and practices of other agencies or providers. Confidentiality was an interprofessional issue of conflict as well.

Agency and public policies that were fraudulent, that constrained eligibility for services, that produced excess bureaucracy or excess paperwork, or that compromised confidentiality were major issues for case managers. Understaffing and underfunding and the availability of services were also sources of conflict.

Continued

Continued

IMPLICATIONS

The findings of this study indicate that case management is "indeed an ethical mine field" (p. 24). With clear implications for nursing in the community, the researchers summarized their findings in the words of one case manager: "She was expected to be all things to all people—to serve clients, family members, provider agencies, and the general community—and doing it right was difficult" (p. 25). The definition of competency and dealing with marginal

competency were particularly difficult for case managers. Eligibility policies and service limits added to the ethical conflicts. "The difficulty for case managers is exacerbated because they have the constant sense of dealing with important life-and-death matters in an imperfect world" (p. 25).

SOURCE

From Ethics and Case Management: Preliminary Results of an Empirical Study, by R. A. Kane, J. D. Penrod, & H. Q. Kivnick, 1993. In R. A. Kane & A. L. Caplan (Eds.), Ethical Conflicts in the Management of Home Care (pp. 7–25), New York: Springer. Copyright 1993 by Springer.

Nurses in the community most often choose to compromise regarding the care provided rather than abandon the client. The challenges are enormous for the nurse trying to provide optimal care within an atmosphere of cost containment, limited time, and restricted resources.

Decisional Capacity

Given the focus on the care provider–care recipient partnership in making care decisions in community health settings, community health nurses must assess the client's ability to make informed, uncoerced, competent decisions. In community health, the client is most often encountered at home or in the immediate community. Resources and collegial support that are available in an acute care setting are less accessible to the community health nurse who needs assistance in determining the client's capacity and competence to make appropriate health care decisions. The terms *competence* and *capacity* are often used interchangeably, although, in the past decisional competence was determined formally through the court system and capacity was usually determined more informally by the professional care providers in the health care system. Here, the term *capacity* is used to refer to the client's ability to make health care decisions. Capacity for making health care decisions assumes the ability to understand the nature, consequences, and alternatives of such decisions. In U.S. society, adults are presumed to have decisional capacity. Decisional capacity may be limited, however, according to the gravity of the decision and the weight of the consequences. Physicians are most often charged with the determination of health care decisional capacity. When a client has been judged incapable of making his or her own decisions, two models of surrogate decision making can be used: substituted judgment and best interest judgment.

Substituted judgment refers to a decision made on behalf of another who is unable due to age, developmental status, or medical condition to make the decision on her or his own behalf. Substituted judgment is made

"as if" the individual were making the decision. Such a surrogate decision is based on knowledge of the history, lifestyle, desires, prior decisions, and values of the individual for whom the decision is being made.

Best interest judgment is a less personal surrogate decision based on what a reasonable person in similar circumstances would decide. Best interest decisions differ from substituted judgment in that the standard for the decision is an unknown other rather than the known history and past decisions of the individual for whom the decision is being made (substituted judgment). A best interest judgment may very well not represent what the individual would decide were he or she able to do so.

The distinction between these two models is a particularly salient reminder to the nurse to acknowledge whose values are driving a surrogate decision—those of the client for whom the decision is being made (as in substituted judgment) or those of the individual making the decision (e.g., a family member or professional who is trying to determine what is in the best interest of the client). Caution must also be exercised in determining the need for a surrogate decision maker in the first place. To exercise such caution, one must understand individual state statutes regarding the process of assigning surrogates, the legal rights of surrogates, and any formal review of surrogates.

In examining a client's decisional competence or capacity, there is always the danger of the client's being judged incompetent purely on the basis of the client's making decisions different from those that would be made by the health care provider. It is unjust for health care professionals to award decisional capacity only to those with whom they agree. The right to make decisions for oneself (autonomy) is highly valued in our society. It is difficult to honor that right, however, when the client lacks the knowledge or skill to make decisions. In complicated medical situations, such as when religious or cultural beliefs conflict with prevailing medical opinion (as may be the case with Jehovah's Witnesses or Christian Scientists, whose religious beliefs forbid the use of specified medical treatments) or when family members disagree with each other, it is especially difficult to adequately evaluate the appropriateness of autonomous decisions.

Decisions regarding quality of life issues, made for another who is suffering from increased pain or progressive dementia, may be blurred by the values of the person making the decision. The blurring of values has the potential to affect the response of the care provider, who may have values different from the client or family. To the care provider who values life at all costs, the decision of a client or family to stop aggressive treatment may be viewed as incompetent. A care provider who holds quality of life in high esteem, however, may not question the competence of the client or family who makes such a decision.

Client/Provider Abuse

The awesome burdens of providing care to a relative in the home may lead to frustration that develops into some form of abuse. Providing intense care "represents a major commitment of time and energy to tasks that are mundane, unglamorous, repetitive, and labor intensive" (Collopy, Dubler, & Zuckerman, 1990, p. 4). Neglect and abuse may be inherent consequences of such care. Families in which violence or abuse have occurred in the past are unlikely to change because of the presence of the community nurse in the home. The community nurse is thus challenged to positively influence care provided in the home and seek additional resources to provide family members with appropriate respite. The safety of the nurse, the client, and the family members must always be considered.

Legal guidelines in cases of potential or actual client, family, or provider abuse are beyond the purview of this chapter. The professional responsibility of every nurse requires full knowledge and understanding of the law as it affects nursing practice. Beyond the law, however, the community health nurse should reflect on ethical responsibility in cases of actual or suspected abuse. It is important to consider the risks and benefits to client, provider, and family. Abuse may be physical, psychological, or financial. Providing care to clients in their daily surroundings renders the nurse vulnerable to physical or verbal

abuse from clients or family members. Resolution of situations involving abuse is difficult and complicated. Abuse by a family member of the client or the nurse threatens the safety of both client and nurse. It is often impossible to bring another provider into the situation, and abandonment of the client not only puts the client at greater risk for potential abuse but also exposes the client to a lack of care. Transfer of care to another provider or agency may be considered but must be done in conjunction with full disclosure of the risk to the safety of others. It is appropriate to question any agency policy requirement that places the nurse, the client, or a family member at risk.

Unreasonable risk to the safety of oneself or others should never be acceptable in community practice. No benefit will accrue if the care recipient or the care provider is harmed.

Lifestyle Diversity and Compliance

As discussed earlier in this chapter, the community health nurse may become intimately engaged in conflicts with clients regarding differing lifestyle beliefs. Clients who demand care but who are unable or unwilling to make lifestyle modifications to enhance and facilitate positive outcomes from care truly challenge health care providers. Clients who do not cooperate with medication and treatment regimes may likewise frustrate care providers. The nurse may begin to question the appropriateness of providing care to clients who do not accept responsibility for their own behaviors in the plan of care. Frustration may be magnified in situations where resources are limited and decisions about those who are to receive available care must be made.

Similarly, clients or families who demand care that is deemed unnecessary by the nurse highlight differing values among family members, clients, and care providers. Trying to understand the motivation for and desired outcome from the demanded care may help the nurse educate the client and family about more appropriate levels of care. The nurse must be assured, however, that such education is neither coercive nor directed toward changing the client's request merely because the client does not

COMMUNITY NURSING VIEW

The following excerpt is fictional, although the elements of the case are extracted from actual practice. Any resemblance to real individuals is purely coincidental.

Ms. Y. is a 47-year-old African American woman who for two years has received home health services under the auspices of the Public Health Visiting Nurse Agency. As a result of progressive symptoms of multiple sclerosis, she requires maximum assistance with activities of daily living (ADL) including personal care and hygiene, dressing, feeding, toileting, transfers, and exercise. On "good" days, she is able to ambulate with a walker. Home health aids provide most of her care during daily visits. On weekly visits, the RN provides medication assistance as well as ongoing assessment of nutritional status, skin integrity, ability to maintain care regimens, overall health status, and a monthly catheter change. Physical therapy visits are also provided through the agency. Most of her medical care is provided through a regional Multiple Sclerosis Center located in the next town. Despite the progression of her disease, Ms. Y. has remained communicative, with a bright personality and warm, smiling responses to her caregivers. Her home is located in a high-risk neighborhood where multiple assaults, murders, thefts, and acts of vandalism have occurred. Her husband, the only family care provider, is described as loud, belligerent, and verbally abusive. He also has documented alcohol and drug problems that appear to magnify his emotional responses. He has verbally and physically intimidated young female caregivers, has refused to allow male caregivers into the home, and has threatened staff with a gun on two occasions. Concerns have been expressed regarding actual or potential abuse of Ms. Y. She is considered to be competent to make decisions regarding her own care. Arrangements have been made for two-week respite periods during which Ms. Y. would be cared for out of her home. Mr. Y. receives money for providing care to her at home and is anxious to keep that source of financial support for them. Ms. Y. has been unwilling to leave her home or her husband.

Nursing Considerations

ASSESSMENT
- What are the nurse's responsibilities to the client? The agency? Mr. Y.? The community? Self and family?
- Does safety of the client or of the care provider come first? How might the safety of both be balanced in the situation described?
- What should be included in the assessment of the situation?

DIAGNOSIS
- State the ethical dilemma faced by the nurse.

OUTCOME IDENTIFICATION
- What outcomes would you anticipate that would help you determine if you had made an ethically justified decision?

PLANNING/INTERVENTIONS
- What alternatives are possible in this situation?
- Is it fair to assign staff to provide care to a client who has demonstrated need but whose care may compromise the safety of the staff?
- Is transfer to another agency ethical? If yes, under what circumstances?
- Discuss the relationship between client abandonment and the principles of nonmaleficence and beneficence?

EVALUATION
- How did you decide which alternatives were possible?
- Did you have the information you needed to make an ethically justifiable decision?
- What principles did you use to arrive at your decisions?

agree with the nurse or family. If this kind of disagreement is not resolved or if it is a true source of conflict, the nurse must involve others in a review of the conflict.

Review by an ethics committee may provide the nurse, the client, and the family with the knowledge and confidence that care options are offered in an unbiased manner, that the voices of all of the participants are respectfully heard, and that all options are carefully considered. Such committee review should be obtained to facilitate discussion of conflicts in an open, safe environment where all participants have equal power and voice in the discussion. Ideally, the ethics committee functions as facilitator of good decisions rather than as arbitrator of intractable conflicts.

Community health nurses face unique ethical challenges with far fewer resources and sometimes diminished collegial support as they seek to provide optimal care to clients and families throughout the community. Nurses must seek and seize opportunities for building multidisciplinary approaches both to providing care and to resolving the ethical conflicts that inevitably arise in the course of providing care. The role of nursing in influencing community values and health care policies must continue to expand to facilitate access to appropriate levels of care for all clients.

Key Concepts

- A caring perspective enhances the nurse's ability to resolve ethical conflict in a contextual way.

- Ethical theories, principles, rules, and values are important in the resolution of ethical conflicts in community health nursing.

- Analysis of any ethical issue must incorporate components of a decision-making process that allow for resolution of the acknowledged conflict.

- Six components are essential in any ethical decision-making model used to guide the resolution of ethical dilemmas: (1) a means of determining those who are involved in the decision; (2) a means of gathering all relevant information; (3) a process for outlining potential options for resolving the dilemma; (4) a process for resolving any conflict that arises; (5) a plan for implementing the selected resolution to the dilemma; and (6) a means of evaluating the decision, the process, and the resolution.

- Despite the development of the best possible database, complete data may not be available, and disagreements regarding the facts may occur.

- Both the direct and the indirect consequences of ethical decisions to all participants should receive attention before a resolution is selected.

- There are important distinctions among medical, legal, and ethical decisions.

- A multidisciplinary approach to ethical conflicts lends broad support and diverse perspectives to attempts at conflict resolution.

- Limited resources affect ethical decisions as well as the nurse's ability to provide optimal care.

Cultural and Spiritual Perspectives

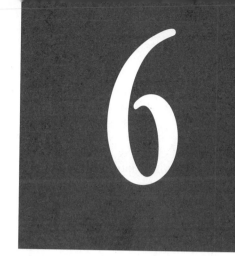

Phyllis E. Schubert, DNSc, RN, MA
Harriett J. Lionberger, DNSc, RN

KEY TERMS

- acculturation
- alternative health care
- caring
- centering
- chakras
- complementary health care
- cultural assessment
- cultural diversity
- cultural values
- culture
- culture-bound
- enculturation
- ethnicity
- ethnocentrism
- ethnomedicine
- folk health system
- healing practices
- holistic healing therapies
- holistic health
- holistic medicine
- homogeneity
- locus-of-control
- minority
- paradigm
- pattern appraisal
- race
- religion
- spiritual assessment
- spirituality
- transcultural nursing theory

Imagine how it [would feel] to always belong—belong in a diversified community, for it is the diversity in nature that gives the web of life its strength and cohesion. . . . Imagine being able to relax into our connectedness—into a web of mutually supportive relations with each other and with nature. . . . Imagine a world where what is valued most is not power but nurturance, where the aim has changed from being in control to caring and being cared for, where the expression of love is commonplace. . . . The very fact that you can imagine these things makes them real, makes them possible.

—Adair, 1984, p. 284

COMPETENCIES

Upon completion of this chapter, the reader should be able to:

- Discuss the importance of cultural understanding to community health nursing.
- Explore linkages among spirituality, culture, health beliefs, and health practices.
- Explore the effects of ethnocentrism and related concepts in nursing practice.
- Examine issues related to cultural differences between the nurse and the client.
- Discuss the emergence of alternative and complementary therapies in the Western world.
- Identify elements of spiritual assessment used in clinical practice.
- Explore the human search for purpose and meaning in life.
- Discuss the meaning of culturally appropriate health care.
- Examine transcultural nursing theory as an interpretation of caring.

Culture and spirituality are aspects of life that bring beauty and joy to human beings when differences among people are appreciated but that lead to conflict and misery when differences are met with intolerance. The community health nurse must have not only knowledge about spiritual and cultural beliefs and practices but also, and more important, understanding and wisdom in the implementation of that knowledge. Cultural issues continue to challenge the nurse, and continuous learning throughout one's professional life is essential because the beliefs that originate from cultural and spiritual life determine lifestyle, health, and **healing practices.** Healing practices are those intended to facilitate integration of one's whole self and relationships.

Leininger (1991) defines **culture** as the values, beliefs, norms, and practices of a particular group that are learned and shared and that guide thinking, decisions, and actions in a patterned way. **Cultural values** are those desirable or preferred ways of acting or knowing something that over time are reinforced and sustained by the culture and ultimately govern one's actions or decisions.

According to Moberg, **spirituality** was defined by the 1971 White House Conference on Aging as "the human belief system pertaining to humankind's innermost concerns and values, ultimately affecting behavior, relationship to the world, and relationship to God" (cited in Stuart, Deckro, & Mandle, 1989, p. 37). Wolf (1996) discusses spirituality as dealing with "the *recognition of unpredictable processes*" involving consciousness (p. 310; italics in original). Although spirituality is sometimes viewed as being in the domain of religion, some scholars such as Wolf relate this nonmaterial aspect of persons to processes perhaps of quantum physics.

Religion provides structure and tools for spiritual life and is considered not only an element of culture but also a link to the search for the spiritual meaning of life, a major determinant of health (Frankl, 1959). Other phenomena addressed in this chapter are the emerging **alternative** and **complementary health care** therapies in the United States, which reflect a blending of healing practices from various cultures with modern health science. These therapies are called alternative when they are used in place of standard medical practices, complementary when they are used in addition. For simplicity, the term alternative will be used in this chapter.

The aims of the chapter are to (1) promote understanding and respect for the vast diversity of meanings represented in the health beliefs and practices of clients and nurses; (2) introduce some useful tools for cultural and spiritual assessment; and (3) provide an introduction to alternative therapies used by clients of various belief systems, community health nurses in some settings, and other health care professionals. Transcultural nursing theory is presented as the framework for application of the previously mentioned concepts because this model is built on the practice of caring (discussed in Chapter 1). Caring is to cultivate, to nurture, and to support growth and is a major thread running through most cultures.

The chapter begins with a discussion of culture. Although religious practices are one aspect of culture, religion and the search for life meaning and purpose are considered separately as spiritual perspectives. We have elected to separate culture and spirituality, emphasizing that culture reflects our diversity whereas spirituality reflects that which unites us. A discussion of frameworks for understanding culture and spirituality in turn provides the framework for nursing assessment and intervention.

IMPORTANCE OF CULTURAL UNDERSTANDING TO COMMUNITY HEALTH NURSING

People of various cultural backgrounds create a rainbow of color and cultural diversity worldwide. The advancement of technology has led to increased contact among people of various cultures through travel and sophisti-

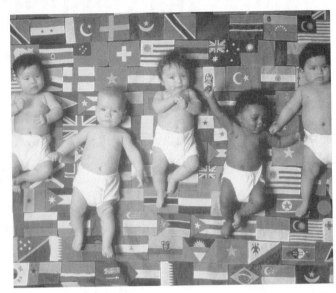

The United States is a melting pot of religions and cultures from all over the world. Photo courtesy of Jeffry W. Myers/Corbis.

cated communication systems. The United States has historically been considered a melting pot for those of many cultures. Native Americans and Mexicans, indigenous to this land, have been joined by people of cultures from around the globe. Statistics reported by the Bureau of the Census indicate that between 1980 and 1990, the U.S. Hispanic population rose by 53%, the Native American population by 39%, and the Asian population by 108%. Eight percent of Americans (or 19.8 million people) were born in other countries, and 32 million people spoke languages other than English at home.

Cultural diversity, the great variety of cultural values, beliefs, and behaviors, is expanding rapidly, requiring nurses to view health, illness, and nursing care from different perspectives (Grossman, 1994). Cultural diversity is recognized and accepted in theory, but in reality, intolerance for and prejudice against those with differing beliefs, values, and lifestyle practices often exist. Respect for such differences can help to create a healthier environment for humankind.

The community health nurse is confronted daily with clients and colleagues whose values differ from those of the nurse. The nurse who supports clients and colleagues within their own belief and value systems will be more likely to experience cooperation in the nurse–client or nurse–community relationship. In contrast, the nurse who insists on imposing her values on clients or colleagues will meet with resistance, conflict, and little or no progress toward resolution of the problems at hand. The work of health promotion and disease prevention in culturally diverse settings requires the nurse to be knowledgeable about various cultures, be respectful of all persons, and have insight regarding personal cultural beliefs. The following paragraphs provide some foundation for understanding the concept of culture and some related issues.

CONCEPTUAL FOUNDATIONS FOR TRANSCULTURAL ASSESSMENT

Culture, the full product of human concerns, helps us define who we are and what we believe, value, think, and feel. Culture dictates the way we address certain life events, including birth, death, puberty, childbearing, child-rearing, illness, and disease, and it influences our language, dietary habits, dress, relationships, and health behaviors. Culture shapes our personalities, families, and social organizations. It is a dominant force in the determination of health–illness caring patterns and behaviors. Because life transitions and health behavior are major focuses of nursing, it is imperative that cultural differences be a central issue in nursing practice. Culturally diverse nursing care employs appropriate variability to meet the needs of more than one aggregate (Giger & Davidhizar, 1995).

Understanding health and illness behavior is crucial to nursing care because behavior both affects and is affected by health status and healing processes. The nurse acknowledges that behavior is meaningful and that meaning is communicated through behavior. When behavior is examined from a cultural perspective, it becomes obvious that the client makes choices on the basis of his life-meaning and his view of his illness.

A transcultural nursing assessment is necessary to determine those cultural factors, ranging from religious views to folk cures, that may influence the client's health or illness behavior. An important part of this assessment is to determine the client's basic beliefs about the nature of health and disease (Grossman, 1994). For example, in some cultures, health is considered a gift from God and illness a punishment for sin. In other cultures, illness is thought to result from exposure to the elements, to witchcraft, or to evil spirits. In yet other cultures, health is understood as the balance of feminine (yin) and masculine (yang) energies, and a disharmony in this balance is thought to disturb body functioning. Members of other cultures believe that hot and cold forces are thrown out of balance during illness; these people will eat in a manner and exhibit behavior that they believe will balance these forces. Figure 6-1 lists some questions suggested by Kleinman (1980) that can be used to elicit information about health and illness beliefs.

Cultural assessment is an essential aspect of the nursing process because understanding of culture gives context to behaviors that might otherwise be judged negatively. If cultural behaviors are not recognized as such, their significance may be misunderstood by the nurse.

Two models for cultural assessment are presented here. The Leininger (1991) model is broad in scope and provides a systems approach to cultural understanding. Giger and Davidhizar (1995) propose a model that provides a basis for understanding culturally determined behavior.

Figure 6-1 Questions to Ask about Health and Illness Beliefs

- What caused this illness?
- Why did this illness start when it did?
- What does this illness do to you?
- How severe is this illness?
- What chief problems has this illness caused you?
- What do you fear most about this illness?
- What kind of treatment do you think would help?
- How do you hope to benefit from treatment?

These questions may be modified to fit the situation, depending on whether the client is an individual, a family, a group, or a population and whether the client is trying to achieve health maintenance, health restoration, or a higher state of wellness.

Adapted from Patients and Healers in the Context of Culture by A. Kleinman, 1980, Berkeley: University of California. Copyright 1980 by University of California.

The Leininger Sunrise Model

A culture is made up of educational, economic, political, legal, kinship, religious, philosophical, and technologic systems (see Figure 6-2). Each of these identified systems affects health.

Health needs are biological, psychosocial, and cultural and are met within a combination of two subsystems: a folk health system (primarily related to religious beliefs and practices) and the professional health system. Leininger (1991) points out that the greater the differences between folk and professional care practices, the greater the need for nursing care accommodations.

The **folk health system** refers to traditional or indigenous health care beliefs and practices. These are performed by local practitioners, are well known to the culture, and have special meanings and uses to heal or assist people to regain well-being or health or to face unfavorable circumstances (Leininger, 1991). *Professional health system* refers to those cognitively learned and practiced modes of assisting others that are obtained through formal professional schools of learning.

Folk medicine systems vary, but they often explain illness in terms of balances between the individual and the physical, social, and spiritual worlds and focus on personal relationships, perhaps involving many persons. Folk medicine classifies illness and disease as natural or unnatural. Natural illnesses are based on logical cause-and-effect relationships. Unnatural events are believed to occur when the harmony of nature is upset. They are unpredictable and may be considered a result of evil forces. Unnatural illness may be attributed to punishment for an evil act of some kind, for example.

Figure 6-2 Leininger's Sunrise Model to Depict Theory of Cultural Care Diversity and Universality

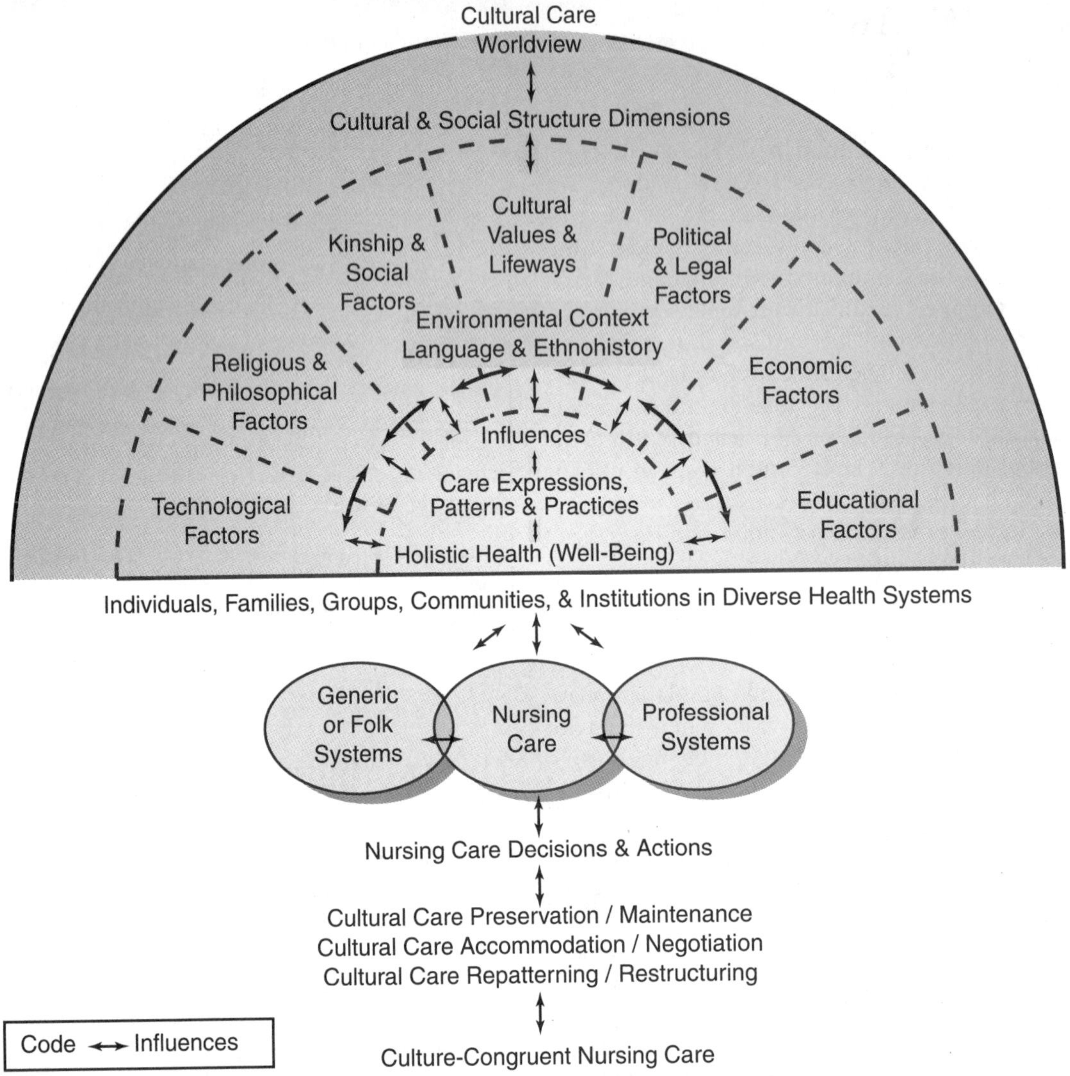

From Culture Care Diversity and Universality: A Theory of Nursing (p. 43) by M. Leininger, 1991, New York: National League for Nursing Press. Copyright 1991 by M. Leininger and NLN. Reprinted with permission from M. Leininger and NLN.

Although the cultural systems identified by Leininger represent all cultures within and outside the United States, discussion in this text addresses cultures only as they exist within the United States. This textbook is written from the perspective of the dominant culture looking at other cultures. Philosophical and religious systems and their impacts on values, beliefs, and health practices in general are discussed in the section on spirituality. Philosophy involves the search for theoretical and analytical knowledge of the nature of the universe, and religion the intuitive knowledge obtained through religious and spiritual practices.

The Giger and Davidhizar Model

The Giger and Davidhizar (1995) model proposes that culturally diverse nursing care take into account six cul-

tural phenomena that vary with regard to application and use yet are in evidence among all cultural groups: communication, space, time, environmental control, biological variations, and social organization. These phenomena vary not only across cultures but also with regard to caregiver response, recipient response, context of care, and goals of care. The six phenomena are discussed next.

Communication

Communication implies the entire realm of human interaction and behavior and is the means by which culture is transmitted. It provides the way we connect with each other, share information, and send messages and signals related to ideas and feelings. We affect each other by communicating with written or spoken language, gestures, facial expressions, body language, personal space, and

Language Barriers

Imagine that you are in another country where few people speak your language. You are well educated and speak the language of the land well but with a heavy accent. You realize people are pretending to understand you rather than asking you to repeat what you say. How do you feel? What might you do to deal with this situation?

symbols. Approximately 100 languages are spoken in the United States (Grossman, 1994), and interpreters are often necessary in community health nursing practice.

Communication may present barriers to the client–nurse relationship when the participants are from different cultural backgrounds. These barriers exist when the languages spoken and/or the communication styles, patterns, and understandings are different, leading to feelings of helplessness and alienation for one or more participants. These issues and suggestions for minimizing such barriers are further discussed in Chapter 8.

Space

An individual's comfort level is related to personal space—the area that surrounds a person's body and the objects in that area. Discomfort is experienced when this area is invaded. Personal space is an individual matter and varies not only with the situation but also across cultures. According to Giger and Davidhizar (1995), although some individual variations do exist, persons in the same cultural group tend to exhibit similar spatial behavior.

Because individuals are usually unaware of their own personal space needs, they often have difficulty understanding those of people from different cultures. What one person experiences as a physical expression of friendship, thus, may be interpreted as a threatening invasion of personal space by another. Individuals who step back from the nurse, do not directly face the nurse, or pull their chairs back from the nurse are nonverbally requesting more personal space. Because subtle variations in nonverbal signals can lead to misunderstanding, knowledge of cultural variations in nonverbal behavior is helpful to the community nurse.

Time

Giger and Davidhizar (1995) differentiate social time (duration, time passing) and clock time (points in time). Social time refers to patterns and orientations that are related to social processes and to the conceptualization and ordering of social life. Cultural patterns acknowledge social time such as dinner time, time for bed, prayer time, and gathering time. Whereas most cultures acknowledge social time, attention to clock time varies greatly across cultures.

In some cultures, clock time dictates most aspects of life, whereas in others, clock time is ignored or even scorned.

The temporal orientation of a group refers to a focus on either past, present, or future. Cultures or individuals who have a past orientation are generally resistant to change, whereas those with a future orientation tend to change more easily, as long as the existing order is not seriously threatened. Present-oriented persons or cultures tend not to adhere to strict, time-structured schedules. Those who are living in crisis and those who face homelessness, poverty, lack of transportation, and health problems tend to have a present temporal orientation, focusing on moment-to-moment survival. Such people often have difficulty keeping appointments in the health care system. Future orientation is requisite to disease-prevention efforts such as immunizations, use of condoms, and efforts toward earthquake safety. A future orientation, thus, dictates activities of the present, and knowledge of past efforts and their consequences provides information for planning the future.

Clock time is of paramount importance in the U.S. culture. Accordingly, time management is important to the economics, effectiveness, and efficiency of health care delivery in the United States. The varying temporal orientations of those served by the U.S. health care system may conflict with the prevailing clock-time orientation. Clients may interpret provider behaviors stemming from such conflicts as lack of caring.

Environmental Control

Beliefs about humankind's relationship with nature are important to health care. Cultural beliefs and values regarding the nature of the human–environment relationship vary on a continuum, from humans must dominate, to humans must live in harmony with, to humans are subjugated to nature. For example, a fatalistic attitude of "if I'm going to get cancer, I'll get it no matter what" will deter preventive care. Such beliefs determine one's perceived **locus-of-control** as being either internal or external, depending on whether one feels one's health is controlled by one's own behaviors and choices or by factors outside one's self. Specific examples of how these beliefs affect family health behavior are discussed later in this chapter.

Biological Variations

Biological variations are differences among people that are attributed to heredity, including body structure, skin color, and other visible physical characteristics; enzymatic and genetic variations; electrocardiographic patterns; susceptibility to disease; nutritional preferences and deficiencies; and psychological characteristics. People of different races tend to vary in height, body size, skin color, and other physical characteristics such as mongolian spots on the skin of African American, Asian, Native American, or Mexican newborns. Enzymatic variations make some health conditions more likely among people of certain races. For example, lactose intolerance is a problem for many Japanese, and inverted T waves in the precordial leads of an electrocardiogram is a common finding among African Americans but is considered abnormal among Caucasian Americans.

Susceptibility to disease is considered to have genetic or environmental origins, or a combination of the two. Sickle cell anemia is found predominantly in the African American population. Systemic lupus erythematosus is fairly common among women in general but is considered extremely rare among Asians, including Asian women.

Nutritional patterns also affect biological variation. Cultural differences in nutritional intake are addressed in Chapter 9. Nutritional patterns most likely affect body structure, susceptibility to disease, and many of the biological variations found among races and cultural groups.

Psychological characteristics also vary among racial groups. Feelings of insecurity may be related to cultural background. For example, psychological adjustment may be difficult for a Native American who has lived on a reservation but goes to a college where there are few, if any, other Native Americans. Mental health may be defined as a balance in a person's internal life and the person's adaptation to the outer reality. Normal behavior, then, is culturally determined, and psychological characteristics are based on enculturation processes. Other variables affecting mental health are family relationships, child-rearing practices, language, attitudes toward illness, social status, and economic status. Racism may be a major factor in the mental and physical health of minority groups.

Social Organization

The social organization of a culture provides the structure within which **enculturation,** or the process whereby children acquire knowledge and internalize values and attitudes about life events, occurs. A child learns by watching adults and other children while they make inferences about what is appropriate behavior. The resulting values tend to persist for life.

As individuals experience enculturation, they tend to become **culture-bound,** meaning they become limited to their own view of reality and are unable to consider the views of other cultures or persons, unable to alter their own beliefs and values, and unable to learn from others. Nurses are culture-bound when they insist that the scientific method or nursing process is the only way to solve problems, whereas clients may feel some of their problems can be solved in other ways.

Ethnocentrism refers to the belief that one's own lifeway is the right way or is at least better than another. The outcome of ethnocentrism is cultural imposition. The nurse, for example, might impose her beliefs and values on the client. The client, in turn, might perceive such ethnocentrism as demeaning, possibly resulting in client dysfunction, noncompliance, anger, and/or feelings of inferiority. Such outcomes can be avoided when the nurse has an attitude of openness and the desire to learn from others.

Homogeneity is the assumption that all persons from a particular ethnic group or culture share the same beliefs and values. Variations within a culture or family occur because of age, religion, dialect or language, gender identification and roles, socioeconomic status, geographic location, history of the subcultural group, amount and type of contact between younger and older generations, and degree of adoption of values by the subgroup. It is necessary, therefore, to instead assume that each individual person holds unique beliefs, values, and health care practices.

Ethnicity refers to a group whose members share a common social and cultural heritage passed on to successive generations. Members of an ethnic group feel a bond and a sense of identity. **Race** implies biological characteristics, such as skin color and bone structure, that are genetically transmitted from one generation to another. **Minority** is a label applied to race, ethnicity, religion, occupation, gender, or sexual orientation. The term carries a variety of potential meanings but in general implies fewer in number than the general population. It may, however, refer to those who lack power or have characteristics perceived as undesirable by those in power.

Acculturation refers to the change of cultural values over time when the influence of another culture is experienced. In the United States, many cultures are represented, and people are influenced by each other. This process accounts, to a large extent, for the great variety of cultural beliefs and practices within any group of people.

The Leininger and the Giger and Davidhizar models provide frameworks for assessing cultural issues involved in nursing relationships where value conflicts exist (see also Chapter 8 on transcultural communication).

CULTURAL BELIEFS AND VALUES OF PROFESSIONAL NURSING AND THE NURSE

Cultural awareness and understanding applies not only to the cultural beliefs and practices of the client but also to those of the nurse. Self-awareness and careful identification of one's own values as cultural phenomena facilitate understanding in transcultural settings and relationships. The values the nurse may explore include those shared with the culture of the nursing profession, those shared with the dominant culture, ethnic values shared with family, and individual values shared with select peers and friends.

Cultural Beliefs and Values of Professional Nursing

Value conflicts often occur between clients and nurses and/or between clients and others who work in health care. A look at some of the shared beliefs held not only by nurses but also by others within the health care system may be helpful. These beliefs are related to a standardized definition of health and illness and to the omnipotence of technology. Persons are usually considered ill only when medical diagnostic tests indicate disease. Certain procedures are used during birth and death, and rituals surround events such as the physical examination, surgical procedures, and visitors and visiting hours in institutions (Spector, 1996).

Disease prevention is encouraged via the use of immunizations and annual physical examinations involving certain diagnostic procedures. A systematic approach and problem-solving methods are valued. Health promotion activities are linked with diet, exercise, and stress management. As a rule, health care professionals approve of clients who are prompt, neat, clean, and organized and who have a high degree of compliance. More significance is placed on biological processes than on psychological or social processes. The U.S. culture values independence and self-responsibility. Financial dependence on others for health care is therefore met with a certain attitude of disapproval on the part of care providers and shame or embarrassment on the part of indigent care receivers.

Disease is a condition clearly defined in biomedical sciences. Illness, on the other hand, involves a perception of being sick on the part of the person involved. Illness is culturally shaped because it is individually perceived. Human response to perceptions of illness is considered the domain of nursing.

The biomedical approach of contemporary health care has served well but has needed the balance of nursing to promote and nurture positive health and holistic healing. Nursing traditionally has addressed the wholeness of persons. Rogers (1990), an early theorist, defines the person as more than the sum of his or her parts and as "an irreducible, indivisible, multidimensional energy field identified by pattern and manifesting characteristics that are specific to the whole and which cannot be predicted from knowledge of the parts" (p. 7). Furthermore, person and environment are perceived in this paradigm as inseparable, functioning as interpenetrating processes. These notions contrast markedly with the culture of the United States but fit well with many others and tap into a long-standing theme of nursing theory and practice. According to Rogerian nursing theory, organizational patterns of the human–environment interrelationship determine health. Thus, this philosophy or conceptual model for nursing practice uses the term **pattern appraisal** for health assessment.

Nursing theories provide a holistic view of the person that fit with the human need for respect of one's wholeness.

Cultural Beliefs and Values of the Nurse

Exploring one's own beliefs and values is very important in working with those of different cultures. Understanding one's own beliefs and values from a cultural perspective lends clarity to potential value conflicts. Grossman (1994)

Figure 6-3   Developing Cultural Competence

- *Know yourself.* Examine your own values, attitudes, beliefs, and prejudices before trying to help people from other cultures.

- *Keep an open mind.* Look at the world through the perspectives of culturally diverse people by reading books and seeing movies that reflect different cultural perspectives.

- *Respect differences among peoples.* Recognize and appreciate the inherent worth of diverse cultures (including your own), valuing them equally with your own.

- *Be willing to learn.* Learn by getting to know culturally diverse peoples through traveling, reading, attending events held by local ethnic or cultural organizations, and talking with clients and colleagues.

- *Learn to communicate effectively.* Study another language. Be sensitive to the nuances of language and expression, affect, posture, gestures, body movements, and use of personal space. Cultivate trust in your relationships with clients.

- *Do not judge.* Refrain from making judgments about cultural behaviors and practices that seem strange to you.

- *Be resourceful and creative.* Remember that there are many ways to attain the same goal. Tailor your nursing interventions to fit people of different cultures.

Adapted from "Enhancing Your Cultural Competence" by D. Grossman, 1994, American Journal of Nursing, July, pp. 58–62. Copyright 1994 by D. Grossman.

---

suggests ways to develop cultural competence, as outlined in Figure 6-3. Leininger (1978) identifies the values and preferences of U.S. culture: independence; equality; individuality; justice; privacy; materialism; competition; efficiency; and freedom of speech, enterprise, action, and worship. These values, as dear as they are to many in the United States, are often in direct opposition to the values held by other cultures. For example, independence among family members—a valued trait in white, middle-class America—may be viewed negatively in a culture that values cooperation among group members.

FAMILY FOLK HEALTH PRACTICES

Although variation in health beliefs and practices exists among people of any culture, there are many shared beliefs and practices within any given culture and also across cultures. This section outlines some beliefs and practices (grouped according to stage of development)

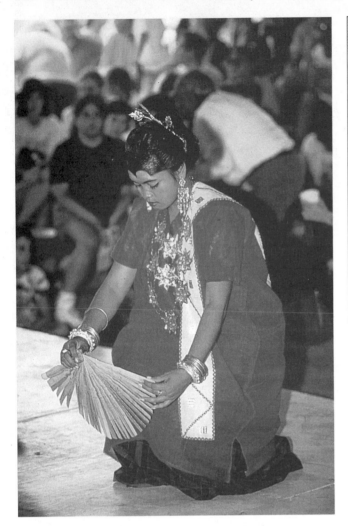

Respect for and interest in the client's cultural background are very important in transcultural assessment. Photo courtesy of Smithsonian Institution.

that, though often unfamiliar to the nurse, the nursing profession, and the dominant culture being served, are found in many cultures.

Pregnancy, Birth, and the Postpartum Period

In all cultures, many beliefs and practices exist that are related to pregnancy, birth, and the postpartum period. Figure 6-4 offers examples of cultural beliefs about pregnancy.

Beliefs surrounding birth have to do with whether the culture defines the birth process as an achievement, a defilement, or a state of pollution necessitating ritual purification. Differences also exist with regard to whether the partner should be present at the birth. In some cultures (Mexican American, Cambodian, Native American), the partner is expected to be present in the birthing room. Other cultures (Orthodox Jewish, Islamic, Chinese, and Asian Indian backgrounds) have prohibitions against the man's viewing the woman's body or require the separation of the husband and wife once the bloody show or

---

Figure 6-4   Family Folk Practices about Pregnancy

Prescriptive Beliefs

• Remain active during pregnancy to aid the baby's circulation (Crow Indian).

• Remain happy to bring the baby joy and good fortune (Pueblo and Navajo Indians, Mexican, Japanese).

• Sleep flat on your back to protect the baby (Mexican).

• Keep active during pregnancy to ensure a small baby and an easy delivery (Mexican).

• Continue sexual intercourse to lubricate the birth canal and prevent dry labor (Haitian, Mexican).

• Continue daily baths and frequent shampoos during pregnancy to produce a clean baby (Filipino).

Restrictive Beliefs

• Avoid cold air during pregnancy (Mexican, Haitian, Asian).

• Do not reach over your head, or the cord will wrap around the baby's neck (African American, Hispanic, Caucasian, Asian).

• Avoid weddings and funerals or you will bring bad fortune to the baby (Vietnamese).

• Do not continue sexual intercourse, or harm will come to you and the baby (Vietnamese, Filipino, Samoan).

• Do not tie knots or braid or allow the baby's father to do so because it will cause difficult labor (Navajo Indian).

• Do not sew (Pueblo Indian, Asian).

Taboos

• Avoid lunar eclipses and moonlight, or the baby may be born with a deformity (Mexican).

• Do not walk on the streets at noon or five o'clock because doing so may make the spirits angry (Vietnamese).

• Do not join in traditional ceremonies such as Yei or Squaw dances, or spirits will harm the baby (Navajo Indian).

• Do not get involved with persons who cast spells, or the baby will be eaten in the womb (Haitian).

• Do not say the baby's name before the naming ceremony, or harm might come to the baby (Orthodox Jewish).

• Do not have your picture taken because it might cause stillbirth (African American).

From Transcultural Nursing Care of the Childbearing Family by J. Lauderdale & D. Greener (1995). In M. M. Andrews & J. S. Boyle (Eds.), Transcultural Concepts in Nursing Care (2nd ed., pp. 99–122), Philadelphia: J. B. Lippincott. Copyright 1995 by J. B. Lippincott. Adapted with permission.

---

cervical dilation has occurred. Thus, the nurse cannot assume that a partner is uninvolved or uninterested in the birth process just because he is absent from the birth (Lauderdale & Greener, 1995).

Many cultural groups have beliefs that postpartum vulnerability is due to *imbalance* (disharmony caused by the processes of pregnancy and birth) or to *pollution* or *being unclean* (bleeding at birth and in the postpartum period). Restitution of balance and purification are achieved through certain behaviors. These include dietary restrictions or prescriptions, ritual baths, seclusion, activity restriction, or other ceremonial events (Andrews, 1995). If the nurse does not understand certain observed behaviors, it is important to inquire about them to ascertain their relevance to the client's situation. For instance, pregnancy is considered a "hot" physical state in the theory of hot/cold practiced by Hispanics and African Americans and in the yin/yang theory practiced by the Chinese and some other Asian cultures. Heat is thought to be lost during the birthing process, so postpartum practices focus on restoring the balance between cold/hot or yin/yang. To this end, clients will eat foods that are considered hot but not those that are considered cold. When providing nutritional information in such instances, the nurse should find out which foods will be acceptable to the client and her family (Andrews, 1995; Spector, 1996).

Infants and Small Children

In many Middle Eastern cultures, children are covered with multiple layers of clothing even in warm temperatures, because it is believed that young children become chilled easily and die from exposure to the cold.

Mal ojo (evil eye) is feared throughout much of the world, and it is believed to be caused by "an individual who voluntarily or involuntarily injures a child by looking at or admiring him or her. The individual has a desire to hold the child, but the wish is frustrated, either by the parent or the infant or by the reserve of the individual" (Andrews, 1995, p. 143). Several hours after this experience, the child cries and develops symptoms of fever, vomiting, diarrhea, appetite loss, eyes rolling back in the head, and listlessness. Mal ojo can be prevented by "touching or patting the child when admiring him or her" (p. 143). The services of a *curandera* (traditional healer) are usually sought, to pray and to massage the child with oil. An unbroken raw egg may first be passed over the child's body and then cracked and placed in a bowl of water under the crib. This process is believed to draw the fever from the child and to poach the egg (Andrews, 1995). From the nurse's perspective, the child's symptoms are indicative of dehydration. Without interfering with the curandera's treatment, however, nurses can teach the family how to treat and prevent dehydration.

In most cultures, symptoms are identified in a culturally unique way. In the Hispanic culture, *susto* (nervousness, loss of appetite, and loss of sleep) is believed to be caused by a frightening experience. Treatment is relaxation. *Pujos* (grunting sounds and protrusions of the umbilicus) is believed to be caused by contact with a woman who is menstruating or by the infant's own mother if she menstruated before 40 days after delivery. The cure is achieved by tying a piece of fabric from the woman's clothing around the baby's waist for three days (Andrews, 1995; Spector, 1996).

Caida de la mollera (fallen fontanel symptoms include crying, fever, vomiting, and diarrhea) is believed to be caused by a variety of things such as falling on the head, abrupt removal of the nipple from the infant's mouth, and failure to place a cap on the infant's head. People of many cultures see it as synonymous with deshidratacion (dehydration), with which the symptoms correspond. Families do not always recognize the need to seek medical help, so the nurse's assessment is very important (Andrews, 1995; Spector, 1996).

Children

Female genital mutilation, a ritual found primarily in many African countries, is potentially devastating and is viewed with disdain by many people outside the countries where it is practiced. This ritual is carried out on girls between 4 and 12 years of age. The procedure ranges from *clitoridectomy* (cutting away part or the whole of the clitoris), to *excision* (amputation of the clitoris and the inner lips of the labia), to *infibulation* (removal of the clitoris and the labia minora, with the labia majora being stitched together and a small opening being created for the passage of urine and menstrual flow). This procedure results in lifelong physical, sexual, and psychological problems. The practice continues because it is believed to be necessary for cleanliness and for becoming a real woman. It is also believed that a woman cannot be married without the completion of the ritual (Touba, 1995). In these countries, being unmarried is an economic calamity. Although outlawed, this ritual continues to be practiced not only by those in the home countries but also by families who have emigrated to the United States or other countries. In addition to the extreme physical danger in which this practice places the female child, marital and childbirth problems continue throughout life.

Empacho (stomach pains and cramps) is believed to be caused by a ball of undigested food clinging to some part of the gastrointestinal tract or by lying about the amount of food eaten. Treatment is to rub and gently pinch the spine. This treatment can be problematic if the cause of symptoms is something serious such as appendicitis (Andrews, 1995; Spector, 1996).

A health treatment used by many Chinese to treat mumps or convulsions is *moxibustion*. The moxa plant is ignited and placed near specific areas of the body. After this treatment, tiny craters can be observed on the skin. Similarly, *skin scraping* (applying special oil to a symptomatic area and rubbing the area with the edge of a coin in a firm, downward motion) may be used for treating colds, heatstroke, headache, and indigestion, and *cupping* (creating a vacuum inside a cup by burning a special material in the cup and then placing the cup immediately on a selected area and keeping the cup there until it is easily removed) may be used for treating headaches, arthritis, and abdominal pain. Skin scraping can result in multiple bruises on the skin, and cupping results in "circular, ecchymotic, painful burn marks two inches in diameter" (Giger & Davidhizar, 1991, p. 369) on the skin. The nurse must understand these practices in order to assess whether they are harmful, neutral, or beneficial to the client. Education can be directed toward supporting beneficial and neutral practices and finding alternatives to those that are harmful. It is important to assess the intention of the family. Practices such as those just described may cause slight physical damage but should not be construed as intentional child abuse.

All Ages

Herbal Remedies

Other beliefs are related to natural healing and herbal practices. Some Chinese families believe in using certain herbs for particular illnesses while also making use of Western medicine (Giger & Davidhizar, 1995). Native Americans use herbs because they believe the basis of therapy lies in nature. Only proper plants are picked, and specific rituals are followed meticulously. Some herbs that have the same effects as pharmaceuticals could result in harmful interactions or overdoses if used along with certain pharmaceuticals. It therefore is important for the nurse to identify all drugs and herbs being used by the client so that potentially harmful results can be avoided.

Traditional Practitioners

Many families are likely to use traditional practitioners prior to or in conjunction with Western medicine. Native Americans have tribal practitioners who use their knowledge of prevention, health maintenance, and treatment and who interweave religious beliefs and healing practices to attain total healing of the mind, body, and spirit. Clients of Hispanic descent may use the services of a curandera. For many African Americans, the church serves as a support, with the minister helping to reinforce health beliefs and practices. Other cultural healers in African American culture are "older women who have herbal knowledge, the spiritualist who has received the gift of healing from God, the voodoo priest or priestess, and the root doctor" (Boyle, 1995, p. 249). In the dominant North American culture, many religious groups incorporate religious leaders into healing practices.

Treatments

Clients may use a wide variety of folk remedies prescribed or administered by family members or folk healers. Some clients, for example, treat respiratory congestion by rubbing the chest with warm, camphorated oil and wrapping up in a warm blanket. They may also apply poultices to painful or inflamed areas to draw out the cause of the infection.

The nurse must not forget that the dominant U.S. culture, composed of Caucasians of European descent (primarily German, Irish, English, Italian, French, Polish, and Dutch), has family folk health beliefs of its own. Some

DECISION MAKING

Family Health Beliefs

You are visiting a Hispanic family who has lived in the United States for six months, having moved here from Mexico. When you enter the home, Leticia, the mother, is rubbing the stomach of her crying, one-month-old child, Roberto. She tells you he has empacho.

• How would you begin a discussion about combining a medical perspective with Leticia's cultural perspective?

• How would you identify a possible cause of the problem from your perspective and at the same time respect Leticia's perspective?

• How can you work with Leticia to teach her how to manage the situation and also respect her health beliefs and practices?

such beliefs are: applying a bag of camphor around the neck prevents the flu (Irish); drafts cause irritation that can lead to a cold and then pneumonia (Italian); sleeping with the windows open prevents illness (German); illness is caused by poor diet (Polish) (Spector, 1996). These and many other beliefs are held by families throughout the United States, prompting health behaviors that may be different from those of the nurse. Each country has its own predominant health beliefs that are powerfully meaningful to the people who practice them. It is important for the nurse to consider the intent behind related behaviors and to work with families in the best interests of positive health outcomes.

ALTERNATIVE/ COMPLEMENTARY THERAPIES

The social emergence of **holistic healing therapies** began during the 1970s and has continued over the past 30 years or so. These therapies are based on the belief in unity of body, mind, and soul (including spirit) and on **ethnomedicine,** the study of traditional healing systems within the field of medical anthropology (Duggan, 1996). The term **holistic health** refers to integration of the whole being and implies feelings of well-being, positive attitudes, a sense of purpose, and spiritual development— variables that cannot be objectively observed, measured, or tested. **Holistic medicine** views illness as an opportunity for learning, personal growth, and transformation.

Holistic therapies are based on the assumption that healing occurs as the body–mind–spirit regenerates itself. On the whole, these therapies have emerged as folk therapies outside the realm of medical science. These modalities have been of interest to many nurses because the underlying purpose is to promote health and healing, an aim synonymous with that of nursing. Most of these therapies assume that human beings, like all of creation, are patterns of energy and that these patterns may be influenced and manipulated in various ways by consciousness and/or the hands to harmonize and balance the energies to promote health and facilitate healing. Some of these therapies have been used for centuries or millennia but have been rejected by Western science because they do not fit with the Western worldview of nature and science.

Recognition of the limits that Western science has placed on the study of holistic phenomena is concomitant with advances in the philosophy of science, which honors different points of view about scientific study of natural phenomena. Advances in the philosophy of science provide support for development of research methods that fit with the study of organizational patterns reflected in health and healing phenomena.

National Interest in Alternative Health Care

In 1992, the U.S. Congress created the Office of Alternative Medicine (OAM) in the National Institutes of Health (NIH) to study medically unrecognized therapies being used by people in the United States. Senator Tom Harkin, a strong advocate of preventive health care and the Chairman of the Senate Appropriations Subcommittee, which oversees the funding of the NIH, and Berkeley Bedell, a retired congressman who used alternative medicine therapies in the successful treatment of Lyme disease and recurrent prostate cancer, promoted establishment of the OAM. Joseph Jacobs, MD, a Native American of Mohawk and Cherokee descent, served as the first OAM director (McDowell, 1994). The OAM has characterized alternative medicine in the United States as any medical intervention that has insufficient documentation in the United States to show it to be safe and effective against specific diseases and conditions, that is not generally taught in medical schools, and that is generally not reimbursable via third-party insurance billing.

During the time that the OAM was being established, Eisenberg, Kessler, and Foster (1993) published an article in the *New England Journal of Medicine* demonstrating a tremendous interest on the part of the people in this country in alternative health care. Their study revealed that one-third of Americans used alternative health care practices on a regular basis for both minor and major problems. There were more visits to alternative care practitioners than to primary care physicians during the year they studied, and people had paid approximately $14 billion for these services ($10 billion out of pocket), which is about half of what people pay privately for hospital service annually. They also found that clients were not telling their conventional medical practitioners about the alternative care, even if the clients were being treated for the same problem in both settings.

Jonas (1996), current director of the OAM, uses the World Health Organization's estimate that 80% of the world's population, or approximately 4 billion people, use traditional medicine as their main, primary health care management system. When traditional medical practices enter the United States or the Western world, they are considered complementary or alternative medicine or health care. McDowell (1994) notes development of an international network of research scientists that may serve as a resource for the OAM and be involved in collaborative research efforts.

A vast amount of information about alternative approaches is available through Medline and the Internet, but relatively little actual research on alternative approaches exists as compared with that on conventional medicine. The OAM was created to help rectify this problem. Ten research centers have been created by the OAM to evaluate alternative treatments for many chronic health conditions. Plans have been made for research scientists and alternative health care practitioners to collaborate on research projects. Results are to be published in the scientific literature and disseminated to the public (Office of Alternative Medicine [OAM], 1995).

Dossey (1993) reflects on the fact that the OAM was created not by developments within the medical field but by pressures outside the health professions. Ongoing health care reforms, including health insurance reform, are also being driven by the people of the United States to decrease costs, enhance quality, and expand access. Studies involving alternative therapies indicate cost effectiveness and high quality of care (Duggan, 1996). Several health maintenance organizations are now offering alternative treatments to their members, and many states now require insurers to cover chiropractic care and acupuncture treatments. The Washington state legislature has mandated that insurers must provide coverage for an array of alternative medical procedures, and other states are expected to follow suit.

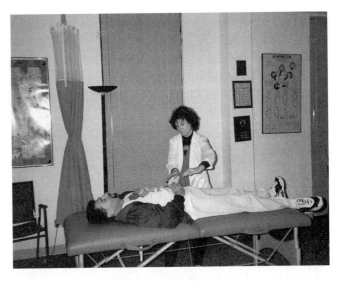

A nurse administering therapeutic touch to a client

Nursing Interest in Alternative Therapies

The American Holistic Nursing Association (AHNA) and the Nurse Healers–Professional Associates, Incorporated (NHPA) are two nursing organizations involved in the promotion of alternative and complementary therapies in nursing. The AHNA offers a course of study with a certificate in holistic nursing practice. The NHPA, an international organization, supports Therapeutic Touch education, research, and practice.

Knowledge of alternative therapies is important to the community health nurse because many clients use holistic therapies; clients may inquire about those holistic therapies being used in the nurse's area of expertise; dialogue among health care professionals about the efficacy of such treatments is increasing; and holistic therapies provide additional tools for community health nursing in various settings. The therapies may be directly applied in certain situations and taught as self-help techniques in others.

Martha Rogers' (1990) nursing theory, Science of Unitary Human Beings, provides a conceptual model for holistic healing as an evolutionary process of the person and for the use of holistic healing therapies in nursing practice. With this theoretical support, community health nurses have entered the private sector as nurse entrepreneurs and have implemented programs using alternative therapies in institutional settings. Community health nurses

who make home visits to individuals and families for public health agencies, home health care agencies, and hospices and those who work in settings where injury is central or more likely, such as occupational health settings or schools, have many opportunities to use complementary care therapies. Family members and friends can be taught to use simple touch therapies to provide comfort, to relieve anxiety, and to facilitate healing. Interested groups in the community may ask the community health nurse to teach self-help classes.

Schubert (1989) interviewed 12 nurses in private community health nursing clinics and 18 of their clients. The nurses used the following holistic healing therapies: a variety of touch therapies (Therapeutic Touch, Jin Shin Jyutsu, massage, and Reiki), guided imagery, health counseling, and holistic health teaching. Their homes or offices served as community health clinics for their neighborhoods, and they taught classes and led groups for people with chronic mental and physical health problems. They also served on community health boards and provided other services to their communities.

Touch therapies are used by many nurses to balance the human energy field by using the hands on the body or near it. Table 6-1 lists a variety of touch therapies of interest to nurses and identified and described by Keegan (1994).

Jin Shin Jyutsu, discussed in Chapter 9, is a self-help approach to health promotion. Many of these therapies are on the OAM's list of alternative/complementary care

Table 6-1　Touch Therapy Modalities

TECHNIQUE	RATIONALE	PRACTICE
Acupressure	Ancient Chinese technique based on the principles of acupuncture.	Practitioners use finger pressure on specific points along body meridians.
Alexander	Based on the idea that poor posture is responsible for energy imbalance and distortion of energy flow.	By way of hands-on guidance and verbal instruction, practitioners teach simple, efficient movements designed to improve balance, posture, and coordination and to provide symptomatic relief.
Feldenkrais	To help create freer, more efficient movement via "functional integration" and "awareness through movement."	Combines movement training, touch, and discussion to improve the client's breathing and body alignment and to help the client relearn proper body movements.
Infant Massage	Designed to enhance bonding between parent and child.	Taught to new parents as preventive therapy and as an aid to relaxation for both infants and parents.
Jin Shin Jyutsu	Based on the belief that attitudes of anxiety, fear, anger, depression, and pretense can create tension, fatigue, and illness by blocking the energy flow through the body.	Practitioners hold their hands lightly on two of the "safety energy locks" simultaneously to open the energy flows and thereby restore harmony and balance. There are 26 pairs of these points on the body.
Massage Therapy	A general term for a range of therapeutic approaches with roots in both Eastern and Western cultures.	Kneading or otherwise manipulating the client's muscles and other soft tissue.

Continued

Table 6-1 Touch Therapy Modalities (Continued)

TECHNIQUE	RATIONALE	PRACTICE
Reflexology	Specific points on the hands and feet correspond to organs and tissues throughout the body.	With fingers and thumbs, the practitioner applies pressure to these points on the hands and feet to treat a wide range of stress-related conditions.
Reiki	This ancient Tibetan healing system channels healing energies to the recipient to treat chronic or acute emotional and mental distress and to assist the client in achieving spiritual focus and clarity.	Practitioners vary widely in technique and philosophy but generally use light hand placements in treatment.
Rolfing	Used to restore the body's natural alignment, which may become rigid by way of injury, emotional trauma, and inefficient movement habits.	Deep manipulation of the fascia is used in a process involving 10 sessions, each focusing on a different part of the body.
Shiatsu	A form of Japanese acupressure that has been used for more than 1,000 years and that stimulates the vital energy.	Practitioners use a series of techniques to apply rhythmic finger pressure at specific points on the body.
Therapeutic Touch	Based on the premise that the body is an open system of energies in constant flux and that illness is caused by a deficit or imbalance in these patterns.	The practitioner "assesses" where the client's energy field is weak or congested and then uses the hands to direct and balance the energy field.
Trager	Used to loosen joints and to ease movement, to retrain the body's old patterns of movement, and to prevent problems from recurring.	The practitioner uses rocking and shaking motions while cradling and moving the client's still limbs.

Adapted from The Nurse as Healer *(pp. 135–138) by L. Keegan, 1994, Albany, NY: Delmar Publishers. Copyright 1994 by Delmar Publishers. Adapted with permission.*

practices and are classified as manual healing modalities (OAM, 1997). Therapeutic Touch has been selected for discussion here because it is better known in the nursing profession and has a body of research.

Therapeutic Touch in Community Health Nursing

Therapeutic Touch (TT) was developed in the early 1970s by Dolores Krieger, PhD, RN (1979, 1993), Professor of Nursing at New York University, and Dora Kunz, a noted healer who believed that anyone with the capacity to care for others could be a healer. The practitioner uses the hands in a consciously directed process of energy exchange to facilitate healing (Nurse Healers–Professional Associates [NHPA], 1994). Krieger and her students continue to provide TT workshops in communities, universities, and places of work in North America and internationally. Consequently, TT is gaining in use as a nursing intervention for providing comfort and facilitating healing. Figure 6-5 lists the basic assumptions underlying TT practice.

Indications for the use of TT include promoting relaxation, altering the perception of pain, decreasing anxiety, accelerating healing, and promoting comfort in the dying process. Treatments are done with the client fully clothed and in a comfortable position—usually sitting or lying down, whichever is better for the client. Lionberger (1986) summarizes the phases of TT (see Figure 6-6).

Centering, the core of the TT process, is also a very helpful tool in living one's personal and professional life. **Centering** consists of bringing body, mind, and emotions to a quiet, focused state of consciousness. It brings about an inner sense of quieting the body, mind, and emotions as well as a feeling of being in harmony with the client and "attuning with his or her well-being, inner strength,

Figure 6-5 Basic Assumptions Underlying Therapeutic Touch Practice

- Human beings are open, complex, and pandimensional energy systems (Rogers, 1990).

- In a state of health, life energy flows freely through the organism in a balanced, symmetrical manner (Kunz, 1991).

- Human beings are capable of both transformation and transcendence (Krieger, 1993).

- Healing is an intrinsic movement toward order that occurs in living organisms and can be facilitated by practitioners. Life energy follows the intent to heal (Kunz, 1991).

Adapted from Therapeutic Touch Teaching Guidelines: Beginner's Level Krieger/Kunz Method *(p. 1) by Nurse Healers–Professional Associates, Inc. (NHPA), 1992, New York: Author. Copyright 1992 by Harriett Lionberger. Adapted with permission.*

Figure 6-6 Phases of Therapeutic Touch

1. Centering oneself physically and psychologically; that is, finding within oneself an inner calm focus of attention;

2. Using the tactile sensitivity of the hands to assess the energy field of the client for cues to differences in the quality of energy flow around the body;

3. Mobilizing areas in the client's energy field that the nurse may perceive as sluggish, congested, or static: that is, lacking in effective energy flow;

4. Consciously influencing body energy through the use of the hands, to assist the client to repattern his or her own energy; and

5. Reassessing the field and eliciting feedback from the client and giving the person an opportunity to rest and integrate the process.

From Therapeutic Touch Teaching Guidelines: Beginner's Level Krieger/Kunz Method (pp. 2–3) by Nurse Healers–Professional Associates, Inc. (NHPA), 1992, New York: Author. Copyright 1992 by Harriett Lionberger. Reprinted with permission.

Figure 6-7 A Centering Exercise

1. Sit comfortably and close your eyes.

2. Inhale and exhale deeply.

3. Focus your mind on some image in nature, such as a tree or a mountain, that brings you a sense of peace. If you become distracted, gently bring your mind back to your image of peace. Remember not to tighten up or try to force your mind to be still. Just maintain a calm but firm center to keep focused on the image.

From Therapeutic Touch: A Practical Guide (p. 24) by J. Macrae, 1987, New York: Alfred A. Knopf.

and peace; being nonjudgmental" (NHPA, 1992, p. 2). Centering is a valuable tool in any situation, from enhancing work to enhancing health. Figure 6-7 offers a centering exercise.

Therapeutic Touch Research

An extensive body of research on the effects of TT has accumulated over the past 25 years, offering evidence that TT promotes relaxation, decreases pain, and reduces anxiety (NHPA, 1992; Quinn, 1992; Hover-Kramer, 1993). It also seems to accelerate wound healing (Wirth, 1990) and to contribute to positive psychoimmunologic changes (Quinn & Strelkauskas, 1993).

Lionberger (1985) undertook an interpretive study to describe the experiences and perceptions of users and to identify elusive aspects of the technique, to illustrate shared meanings, and to interpret findings in terms of common meanings in nursing. Results indicated that participants' practices differed from the standard set by Krieger (1979), specifically, by varying the emphasis on the several phases. Quinn and Strelkauskas (1993) address this issue in their more recent pilot study.

Despite the scientific research and strong clinical evidence accumulated over the past 25 years, we do not know precisely how TT works, as is the case with many other commonly used nursing therapies. Rogers' Science of Unitary Human Beings, however, provides theoretical support, and scientific research and lived experience provide evidence of its effectiveness.

Therapeutic Touch is a spiritual process but is not associated with any particular religion. This therapy seems to facilitate personal growth and resolution of life problems over time, although changes in the presenting symptoms may or may not occur. Because holistic healing occurs in myriad ways, problems arise in scientific study of outcomes, where specific results are expected.

Social Issues Related to the Study of Alternative Therapies

Therapeutic Touch is not the only therapy faced with a problem when it comes to outcomes study, because all holistic therapies address the evolution of human potential—spiritual, mental, emotional, and physical. Duggan (1996) addresses this problem, emphasizing that alternative therapy philosophy is not one of curing but one of enhancing health. He tells the following story:

A few years back a practitioner introduced a [client] to a colleague and expressed regret that she had not fully succeeded in removing the client's painful premenstrual symptoms. The [client], on the other hand, expressed great joy at the treatment she was receiving and at how much her life had changed since she had started acupuncture. About 20 minutes into the conversation, the [client] revealed that she had experienced no premenstrual symptoms for many months but had been afraid to tell the practitioner because she thought she couldn't continue treatment without a symptom. She had found the regular treatment an effective way of caring for her health (p. 9).

Critical questions related to social values arise with the emergence of alternative health care in society. Illich (1977), philosopher and social historian, points out that a culture that bases its medical outcome values on opposition to death and pain is doomed to spend itself out of existence in the attempt to avoid suffering and death. In the 20 years since Illich challenged the underlying values of our mainstream health care paradigm, we have seen national health costs rising astronomically. Costs have skyrocketed as we have pursued high-tech efforts to prevent suffering or delay death. Most reports indicate that at least 20% of our national health expenditures occur in the last six months of life (Duggan, 1996).

REFLECTIVE THINKING

Spirituality and Philosophy of Nursing

- What is your philosophy of nursing?
- How would you define spirituality as it is reflected in your philosophy?

SPIRITUALITY: A UNIVERSAL NEED

Nagai-Jacobson and Burkhardt (1989) conclude from their review of the literature that spirituality is the cornerstone of nursing practice. They found consensus that spirituality is a broader concept than is religion; involves a personal quest for meaning and purpose in life; is related to the inner essence of a person; is a sense of harmonious interconnectedness with self, others, nature, and an ultimate reality, and is the integrating factor of the human personality. Nursing has traditionally held the position that spirituality is at the core of health and healing, the nature of person and environment, and the nurse–client relationship.

Conceptual Foundations for Spiritual Assessment

Spiritual assessment, the collection, verification, and organization of data regarding the client's beliefs, feelings, and experience related to life meaning and purpose, goes beyond inquiring about a client's membership in a particular religion and taps deeper beliefs and feelings about the meaning of life, love, hope, forgiveness, and life after death. Connectedness is an important part of spirituality, including being connected with one's inner self and understanding one's values, being connected with others in meaningful relationships, and being connected with a larger purpose in life. Religious or philosophical beliefs, such as commitment to humankind or trust in God, put life in perspective and provide a reason for living (Pender, 1996).

Newman (1994), who defines health as the expansion of consciousness, assumes that individuals grow personally and spiritually as they experience disease, disability, and death. These conditions, then, are included in one's experience of health.

In Schubert and Lionberger's (1995) view of the person, healing is the process of self-transformation during which one experiences a sense of becoming, or movement toward one's realization of potential. Figure 6-8 depicts this potential as emerging from within as tension and conflict are released. Whereas symptoms of physical or mental distress, at the base of the triangle, are often the presenting problem, healing responses usually involve other aspects of the self. The phases of healing may occur in any order and may overlap. The lines of demarcation

in the figure are included only to help the reader grasp the complexity and general direction of the process. Nevertheless, there seems to be a general pattern of experience.

According to Travelbee (1971), the purpose of nursing is to assist the individual, family, or community to prevent or cope with illness and suffering and, if necessary, to find meaning in these experiences. Nurses' perceptions of the ill individual and their beliefs about human beings are related directly to the quality of care that the client receives. The result is healing through the experience of caring and finding meaning regardless of whether curing occurs.

Frisch and Kelley (1996) note that nurses often have difficulty distinguishing between spirituality, religion, and the psychosocial dimension. It may often be easier to focus on the concrete aspects of religious needs than on abstract spiritual needs.

Spiritual Health Indicators

Spirituality is basic to an understanding of health as a state of wholeness. According to Pender (1996), spiritual health is

the ability to develop one's spiritual nature to its fullest potential, including the ability to discover and

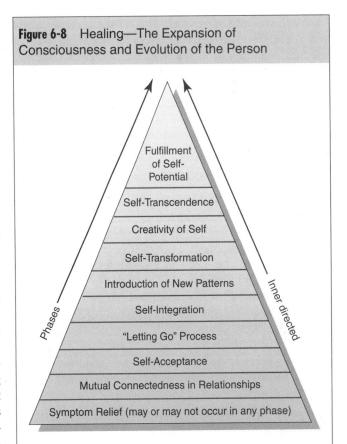

Figure 6-8 Healing—The Expansion of Consciousness and Evolution of the Person

Phases / Inner directed

- Fulfillment of Self-Potential
- Self-Transcendence
- Creativity of Self
- Self-Transformation
- Introduction of New Patterns
- Self-Integration
- "Letting Go" Process
- Self-Acceptance
- Mutual Connectedness in Relationships
- Symptom Relief (may or may not occur in any phase)

From "Mutual Connectedness: A Study of Client–Nurse Interaction Using the Grounded Theory Method" by P. Schubert & H. Lionberger, 1995, Journal of Holistic Nursing, 13(2), pp. 102–116. Copyright 1995 by Schubert and Lionberger. Reprinted with permission.

articulate one's basic purpose in life, to learn how to experience love, joy, peace, and fulfillment, and how to help ourselves and others achieve their fullest potential (pp. 129–130).

Burkhardt (1991) identifies common characteristics of spirituality as they are identified in nursing and health-related literature:

- A unifying force within persons
- A source for discovering and struggling with meaning and purpose in life
- Relatedness to and connectedness or bonding with all of life, which includes self, others, nature, and, frequently, God or a Higher Power
- A sense of peace and harmony with the universe
- Awareness, consciousness, and inner strength (p. 32)

Life Meaning and Purpose

Frankl (1959), a psychiatrist who survived the Nazi concentration camps of World War II, notes that those who could find reasons for living beyond the experience were better able to cope and survive. He developed an approach to help people identify meaning and purpose in their lives, because he found this to be critical to health.

Frankl believes that it is possible to preserve spiritual freedom even under terrible conditions and that spiritual freedom allows the person to make choices about how one perceives any experience. The power to choose how one perceives an experience provides the inner way of strength, courage, love, wisdom, and understanding. He writes, "Meaning is something to be found, rather than given; man cannot invent it but must discover it" (Frankl, 1959, p. 51). Thus, a concern for, and even despair over, the question of *worthwhileness* is a spiritual distress and can therefore engage us in our lives.

Sense of Connectedness

Spirituality is both deeply personal and interrelational in nature. The depth of connectedness to one's inner self, to one's God, or however one names and defines ultimate reality, and to others is reflected in being connected to one's own values, being in meaningful relationships with others, and being committed to God and humankind in a way that provides a reason for living. These relationships are grounded in expressions of love, forgiveness, and trust (Stoll, 1989). Chapman (1987) suggests that spiritual assessment includes relationship with a higher being, relationship with self, and relationship with others. See Figure 6-9 for Chapman's relationship assessment guide.

Sense of Joy, Peace, Inner Strength, and Love of Beauty

Feelings based in a sense of joy, peace, inner strength, and love of beauty are reflections of spiritual health. A nurse's sense of peace is very helpful to recipients of care. Kunz (1992) states, "It is far more important to send peace

REFLECTIVE THINKING

What Gives Life Meaning and Purpose?

- What is the meaning of life for you?
- What gives your life meaning and purpose?
- What do you do to stay in harmony with yourself, with others, and with nature?
- How do these activities affect your state of health and/or facilitate your healing processes?

to someone than to send thoughts that you love them." The thoughts of a man with AIDS as he struggled with the disease are represented in Figure 6-10.

Human beings are spiritually nourished by the beauties of color, sound, and form found in both nature and created art forms (music, sculpture, and painting). Beauty, although culturally defined, is often enjoyed across cultures by those who are spiritually inclined. Religious rituals and art forms reflect beauty as it is perceived by various cultures as well as the shared consciousness of the many people who long for the spiritual. Peace, joy, inner strength, and life harmony are characteristics that seem to be nurtured by the beauty of sound, color, and form.

Figure 6-9 Spiritual Assessment of Connectedness

Relationship with a Higher Being
- The importance of God or a higher being in the client's life
- Use of prayer and spiritually oriented readings as a means of dealing with life situations
- Belief in life after death or continuing spiritual existence
- Participation in individual or group worship activities

Relationship with Self
- Existence of personal life goals that give meaning to life
- Spiritual beliefs that engender hope and zest for living
- Awareness of life priorities
- Commitment to spiritual growth

Relationship with Others
- Extent of concern about the spiritual well-being of others
- Openness to sharing thoughts, feelings, and spiritual beliefs with others
- Respect for other individuals as spiritual beings

Adapted from "Developing a Useful Perspective on Spiritual Health: Love, Joy, Peace and Fulfillment" by L. Chapman, 1987, American Journal of Health Promotion, pp. 12–17.

Figure 6-10   An Experience of Holistic Healing

Finding Peace and Inner Strength

I am much more at peace and much healthier when I listen chiefly to my own body signals and hardly at all to the messages from the media, medical experts, or even social activists and alternative healing groups. . . . One of my first acts when in danger is to reach out for help to mother or father, to doctors, to friends, to pills and potions, to books, anything to hold on to or lean upon, like the drowning man to straws. The real source of my strength and healing is from within and it is important for me to go there, stay there, live there, see from there, meet and make peace with whatever comes from there and do my reaching from there from my body. I think when some of my friends got sick, the fear and desperation took them a long way out from their bodies in search of a cure. So much of their hope was invested in external possibilities that they almost abandoned their bodies—as if they could flee what is happening inside. I think it is necessary to go back down and deep within yourself to face and feel and own your own experience. I realize I can't send something else down to do battle in my place. No miracle, no surgeon's knife, no megavitamin, no medicine or macrobiotic diet, no crystal energy, no faith healer's touch, or shaman's prayer—nothing is of any value at all unless I am there fully present . . . without one foot in the past, the other in the future. I think of healing a little differently than I used to—it's not about living forever or curing disease. It is about living and feeling fully the whole spectrum from joy to sadness, however long that is, dying with a sense of peace, whenever that comes.

Anonymous.

Signs of Spiritual Distress

Spiritual distress (distress of the human spirit) is defined by the North American Nursing Diagnosis Association (NANDA, 1999) as "a disturbance in the belief or value system that provides strength, hope, and meaning in life" (p. 852). Causes of spiritual distress include concerns about the meaning or purpose of life, death, and suffering; conflicts in beliefs and values; and participation in religious rituals. Signs of distress may include feelings of hopelessness as well as mood and behavioral changes (Frisch & Kelley, 1996). Families and communities may suffer spiritual distress as a result of disasters. Interventions include helping the client (individual, family, or community) to find hope and to mend disrupted relationships.

Spirituality and Health and Healing Practices

Arrien (1993), in her studies of health beliefs across cultures, found several universal agreements regarding behaviors that support health and healing. One such agreement

is that food and its rituals sustain health and well-being. Gathering the food, cooking, sitting down, breaking bread, communing with each other, and celebrating life together are as important as are the food nutrients. The foods eaten as children in our own families and cultural traditions are found to be the most healing for us throughout our lives.

All cultures utilize some form of communication with a God-force: that is, meditation, prayer, contemplation, or ritual. Music, singing, and dancing also are important in all cultures. Native Americans believe that when one does not sing, one loses life and experiences soul loss. Hindus use mantras and sonics to waken the **chakras** (energy centers within the energy fields) and elevate consciousness. The universal instruments of drums, bells, rattles, and silence are used in rituals to honor Spirit (Arrien, 1993).

All or most cultures hold the following to be essential for good health and healing: positive affirmations, imagery, and avoidance of negative thinking or judgments; being with nature; beauty and order in the home; and being in right relationship with self, family, friends, and community.

Nagai-Jacobson and Burkhardt (1989) suggest that both client and nurse explore the question "Who am I?" in all its ramifications. The nurse is encouraged to view the myriad assessment data (physical, mental status, and laboratory) within the context of beginning to know the client and to promote the client's self-knowledge. In this way, the nurse helps the client make sense of all the information in terms of personal meaning. Figure 6-11 is Nagai-Jacobson and Burkhardt's guide for self-assessment for the client.

Figure 6-11   A Guide for Spiritual Self-Assessment

Clients may be encouraged to ask themselves:

- What is most difficult about this experience for me and my loved ones?
- What and who helps me, from within myself and from outside?
- With whom can I most easily be myself and share what this experience means to me?
- What are my fears?

The nurse is encouraged to consider the following questions:

- What is sacred to this client?
- What connections are most significant to this client?
- In what or whom does this client place trust?
- Is this client's life marked by joy? Fear? Caution? Creativity?
- How does this client understand God? Ultimate Other? Universe?

Adapted from "Spirituality: Cornerstone of Holistic Nursing Practice" by M. G. Nagai-Jacobson and M. A. Burkhardt, 1989, Holistic Nursing Practice, 3(3), p. 23. Copyright 1989 by Aspen.

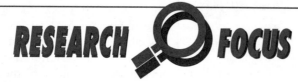

RESEARCH FOCUS

The Lived Experience of Staying Healthy in Rural African American Families

STUDY PROBLEM/PURPOSE

To reveal the meanings of staying healthy within rural, poor African American families. This population has a high incidence of diseases that are considered amenable to prevention-and-protection strategies, such as stroke, diabetes, and infant death. Phenomenological methods were chosen to help nurses understand the meaning of staying healthy for this population and to give culturally competent care. The research question for this study was: What is the meaning of staying healthy in the low-income, rural African American family?

METHODS

Participants for this study were recruited from families with children enrolled in a Head Start program in a rural southern community. They identified themselves as being African American, having annual incomes below $15,000, residing within the same community, and having families who were staying healthy. Ten families with a total of 21 adult members (that is, over 14 years of age) participated. Families met in their homes with the researcher for the interviews. The eliciting question was: When you identified your family as one that is staying healthy, what thoughts or feelings did you have that made you decide that this is true? No attempt was made to guide the types of situations described. Exploratory questions were used only to promote description. Situations discussed included how staying healthy was different from other health-related experiences. A second interview was conducted for the families to add to or clarify what they had described in the first session.

Interviews were taped, the data transcribed, and the data reflecting meaning were isolated for phenomenological analysis. Central themes for the isolated phrases or sections were explored in terms of the central question, "What does this statement tell me about staying healthy?" Ten different statements or descriptions that characterized the universal structure of meaning for staying healthy in these families were identified. A second researcher listened to the tapes and verified the findings.

FINDINGS

The collective description of what staying healthy means in these families provided knowledge of their cultural beliefs about health. Staying healthy for them meant being active, living according to their rules, and maintaining a sense of tranquility. They relied heavily on a sense of what is right and beliefs about the purpose of life. Activity reinforced their feelings of being in control and strong, necessities for staying healthy. Hard work, play, and interaction with persons inside and outside the family demonstrated and protected health. Ignoring physical signs of discomfort helped one remain active. Staying healthy also meant having knowledge about health and the ability to learn from others or from trusted networks. Tranquility was maintained by avoiding causes for worry: avoiding persons who might cause self-doubt or shatter one's sense of being right or in control.

IMPLICATIONS

The findings of this study supported Newman's (1994) view that the process of the evolution of consciousness and the process of health are one and the same. The families in the study continually "sought a sense of wholeness as they experienced alterations in life patterns and looked for rules that could help them transcend their experiences" (p. 20).

Smith used Newman's (1994) theory, which indicates that nurses help clients gain insight (or pattern recognition) and synthesize life experiences into a meaningful pattern of being healthy. Nursing research, then, helps the nurse find ways to interact with the client and to enhance the client's movement toward expanding consciousness. Health values, beliefs, and practices provide context not only for nursing practice but also for nursing research.

SOURCE

From "The Lived Experience of Staying Healthy in Rural African American Families" by C. Smith, 1995, Nursing Science Quarterly, 8(1), pp. 17–21. Copyright 1995 by Chestnut House.

RELIGION AND THE SEARCH FOR LIFE MEANING AND PURPOSE

The search for the meaning of life has provided the impetus for the formation of religion. Every religion has three aspects: philosophical, mythological, and ritualistic. Among the various religions, the fundamental philosophical principles are very much alike; the mythology is in some ways similar and in some ways different; and the rituals and practices are quite different (Viswananda, 1938/1992). All religions purport that there is an ultimate being who is creator, and most purport that the ultimate being has sent at least one (and, in some cases, several) great teacher to the earth to help humankind in some way. Some believe their religion to be the only true way, and others believe that all of the world's great religions lead to truth.

A common theme in religious mythology is that, in the beginning, a great sea of unfathomable chaos—a profound darkness—covered a vast potential having no beginning and from which emerged the One from which all creation is manifested. These mythological stories purport to reveal the origin of the world. Though the stories differ from culture to culture, the sacred theme reveals the underlying search for the meaning and purpose of life and death. Stories, symbols, and rituals provide guidelines for happy and productive lives. When the inevitable suffering occurs, the legends guide the search for meaning. These stories form the foundation for the cultural beliefs from which individuals derive meaning. The quest for this spiritual understanding is as universal as are these stories and can be seen as guiding the unfolding of our lives.

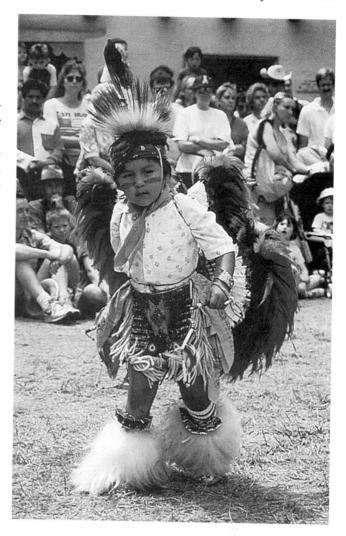

This young Native American celebrates an ancient tradition. Photo courtesy of Smithsonian Institution.

Religious Beliefs of Indigenous Peoples

The indigenous peoples of the world—Australian Aborigines, native peoples of New Zealand, Peru, Africa, Oceania, North and South America, Canada, and Asia—are the carriers of the ancient traditions. Members of these groups believe that one life pervades all form, that all are one, and that all life is sacred. The life goal of these peoples is to live in constant consciousness with the sacred. A dynamic sense of harmony with the earth and her cycles permeates all life, and a spiritual force surrounds art, ritual, and ceremony (Heinberg, 1989).

The Major World Religions

In this section the major religions of the world are briefly described. The purposes of the discussion are to promote understanding and appreciation for the similarities in their philosophical positions and to foster awareness of the great variances in health care practices and rituals within

each religion, branch, denomination, group, or practicing family.

Hinduism

The Hindu religions are thought to be the oldest of the world religions. Hinduism reflects a metaphysical understanding and way of life—defining morals, customs, medicine, art, music, and dance—and comprises a vast range of beliefs and practices. The one guiding philosophy for all Hindus is that all is Brahman (the supreme being) (Ross, 1966). Hindus believe that the universe is in constant change but there is order and meaning in which one must participate for health and well-being. The purpose of life is seen as attainment of enlightenment through union with Brahman or God. Although one may not reach Oneness or God-realization in this life, any spiritual development attained is not wasted but, instead, is brought back for use in the next life.

Health practices in the Hindu culture are based on an understanding of prana, the life force energy of the human being. Chakras (energy centers) are associated with consciousness and body function. Health results when these primary forces are in harmony. Disease or illness is thought to result when there is a break in this system. Disease reflects the whole of one's life; so diet, relationships, environment, season, thoughts, attitudes, and lifestyle are considered in diagnosis and treatment. Treatment is directed toward reestablishing balance among the humors—air, fire, earth, and water—and releasing toxins by means of diet, fasting, enemas, purgatives, and massage (Lad, 1984). Rituals often include elaborate use of fire, water, light, scents, sounds, flowers, postures, gestures, and mantras.

Buddhism

The Buddha, born Siddhartha Gautama in 563 B.C. in present-day Nepal, was thought to be the reformer of Hinduism. Known as the Enlightened One, or Awakened Being, he could show the way to Enlightenment, but it was up to each person to practice a way of life that emphasizes compassion, mind control, transformation of negative thought, and attainment of ultimate wisdom (Blofeld, 1970).

Many schools of thought and numerous sects exist within the Buddhist religion. Yet, certain core beliefs unify this culture. There is no supreme, single, personalized, great Being whose word must be followed but, rather, an accumulation of wisdom to which each generation is free to add its understandings (Ross, 1966, 1980).

Health practices and beliefs are one and the same. Disease is considered a resource in the search for enlightenment, and suffering the plea for help. Healing is the elimination of the causes of suffering—lust, anger, and delusion. Buddhist tradition includes meditation and mind control, the four requisites (proper clothing, food, lodging, and medicine), emetics and purging, oils and ointments, drugs and herbs, and surgery (Birnbaum, 1979).

Judaism

Judaism is best understood through the historical experience of the Jewish people, because this experience designates the Jews as an ethno-socio-cultural group. According to Judaism, the divine covenant with God can never be broken, and the Jewish people must for all time follow the Law as set forth in the Bible as the Ten Commandments. In the Jewish tradition, God has promised a vision of a new heaven and a new earth, which are to be ushered in by the Messiah, yet to come (Griffiths, 1984).

The core beliefs of Judaism are that there is but one God and that only the sins of humankind separate people from the divine. Central to Jewish faith is that humans are to love, praise, and serve God above all else. The Torah holds the laws and sacred traditions (Steinberg, 1974).

The family is seen as the basic unit of society; it has sacred obligations to maintain integrity and purity in relationship with God. The Sabbath is the central day of the week. There are regulations regarding permitted and forbidden foods, including regulations against eating flesh

---

🌀🌀 REFLECTIVE THINKING 🌀🌀

Honoring a Jewish Family's Death Rituals

How can you show respect for a Jewish family at the time of death?

• The rituals surrounding death are complex and important aspects of Jewish tradition. How would you learn about these rituals?

• How would you provide support to the family as they honor their traditions?

• How would you share in these traditions if you are Jewish? If you are not?

---

cooked with milk, certain animal parts, an animal that has not been killed in accordance with the law, and the like (Steinberg, 1974). Many laws regulate caring for the sick and dying. Specific prayers are uttered while loved ones lie on their deathbeds and at synagogue services for 11 months after death. Spirit and body are considered separated at death, with the spirit entrusted to God and the body returned to the earth.

Christianity

Christianity emerged with the birth of Jesus around the year A.D. 5. Jesus Christ, the healer-teacher-visionary and the revealer of God's laws, came to fulfill and transform the old laws of Judaism. Christianity teaches of one God consisting of a trinity: the Father, the Son, and the Holy Spirit—the spirit of love and grace that descends upon humanity for relief of suffering. God is found within, and the search provides the purpose and meaning of life.

Christianity is divided into many different churches or denominations, with each group having a set of beliefs, practices, and rituals. Even the beliefs surrounding the role of Jesus on the earth vary from group to group. Health beliefs and practices vary widely. The Bible is the source of inspiration for Christians, although interpretation and understanding vary.

The writings about Jesus contain many examples of his healing the sick through laying on of hands, faith healing, and releasing demons. These practices continue in certain Christian churches. Common to most denominations, if not all, is the use of prayer in support of those who are ill or suffering (Mitchell, 1991).

Islam

The prophet Muhammad was born in Mecca around A.D. 570 and became the channel through which the nature of God as the Absolute was made known. In his middle years, after being married and raising a family, Muhammed spent his time praying in a cave. In the silence,

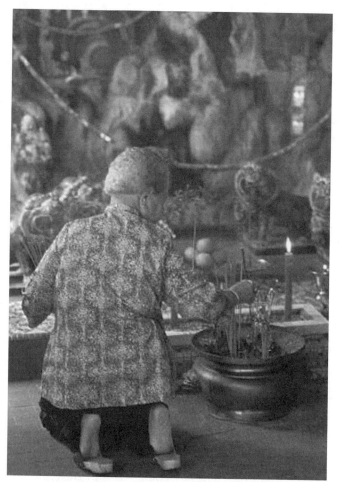

A community health nurse must be accepting and understanding of the different religions and cultures of her clients. Photo courtesy of Adam Woolfitt/Corbis.

DECISION MAKING

Cultural Conflict

You are case manager for an elderly woman with breast cancer who has been told that her condition is terminal. Family members tell you of a plan to take their dying mother on a pilgrimage to Mecca against medical advice.

- How would you proceed?

- What resources would you use?

- How would you evaluate the client's wishes in this matter?

- What goals of care would influence your intervention?

- What factors of care and prognosis would you consider most important?

of ultimate reality and for others. It is important to note that extremists of any religion do not reflect the mainstream and, as such, may be dangerous and oppressive to others (Viswananda, 1938/1992).

Although religion does not provide specific information about health care practices, it does provide a basis for understanding people and their behaviors. Other cultural health care practices may be specific to a certain locality or ethnic group, but even these practices can vary greatly with education, acculturation, and social contacts.

PRACTICE APPLICATIONS IN TRANSCULTURAL NURSING

Culturally diverse nursing care is characterized by variability in nursing approaches. Because intercultural differences in care beliefs, values, and practices do exist, nursing practice must reflect these differences. Nurses must provide clinically appropriate care while supporting health behaviors based on the client's beliefs, religion, and cultural practices. The nurse is thus required to step back, see the client's perspective, and work to bring the best of both the professional system's and the folk system's approaches to the situation. Case management can provide a framework for facilitating culturally appropriate care. In this way, the nurse can meet the needs of each client by marshaling resources, interventions, activities, and services.

Assessment Tools for Transcultural Nursing Practice

A variety of assessment tools help uncover the meaning of health behaviors. Leininger (1978) defines cultural

he heard the revelation "Thou art the messenger of God, and I am Gabriel" (Azzam, 1964, p. 30). The teachings channeled through Muhammad by the archangel Gabriel while Muhammed was in the cave are recorded in the Koran. Central to this book are the covenant between God and Man, the gift of intelligence, and the freedom to choose within the context of all opportunities and dangers. The Koran is central to Islamic life, and portions of this book are chanted at births, weddings, and deaths.

The Koran proclaims repeatedly that there is no God but Allah and warns against worship of idols (Nasr, 1975). Muhammad established a political, social, and religious structure based on his understandings of the teachings.

Like all world religions, the Law of Islam orders that one do good and reject all that is reprehensible. Rituals of faith associated with Islam are prayer, giving of money or food, fasting, and making the pilgrimage to Mecca at least once in one's life. Specific rules govern the way of death and proper burial.

All these religious traditions have similar belief systems and contain a strong message of love for a divine nature

Perspectives...

Insights of a Community Health Nurse

I work for a public health department, providing care to people who have communicable diseases. This work has given me a lot of field experience teaching people about bacteria and "bugs." Sometimes, my teaching falls on deaf ears. The population we serve is culturally diverse: Vietnamese, Laotian, Cambodian, Eretrian, Filipino, Korean, Japanese, and Spanish-speaking. I am bilingual in Spanish and English, so much of the teaching I do is with the Spanish-speaking community.

Our staff of public health aides reflects a smattering of our client population, and they are super-helpful to we Caucasian nurses regarding the culturally sensitive issues of our clients. Even so, my interventions are not always heeded, and I get disappointed. I tell myself not to have expectations—to go with the flow—but it is easy to assume that people will act how I think they should . . . and when they do not, I get really disappointed. Other times, I think the people are a certain way—so I think they live in a certain kind of house, and it ends up different than what I expected. So I am often surprised because I have expectations, and things are often different than what I think they will be. I will give you a couple of examples.

A Vietnamese public health aide helped us to understand why a young Chinese woman refused to have blood drawn around the time of the Chinese New Year. He explained that it is a bad omen to take blood out of the body at any time, but especially at the New Year. We could, then, understand why—no matter how easy we made it for this educated Chinese student—she did not follow through with our instructions. One nurse was able to use a lot of coaxing to get her to do her blood test.

Another time, I was doing follow-up on an active TB case who was Hispanic. I went to a lumbermill where the contact was the only woman who worked in the mill, a middle-aged Caucasian woman who does cleanup. She wore a hard hat, flannel jeans, work pants, and boots, and even after washing her hands, they looked dirty. The dirt was embedded in her skin. When she came to clinic appointments, she dressed the same, except without the hard hat. Her 12-year-old daughter (who could not stop talking) was also a contact. The girl was given a PPD test at the clinic and came back three days later to have it read. When the repeat PPD was done three months later there were transportation problems. I ended up taking the mom home from the clinic so I could read the girl's skin test. My expectation (I cannot get away from them) was that they would live in some sort of shack or very low-income apartment or cottage. As I pulled up to this large, modern, ranch home, I was surprised. The home was very much one you would find in any middle-class suburb. The furnishings were simple and plain.

—*Anonymous*

nursing assessment as a "systematic appraisal or examination of individuals, groups, and communities as to their cultural beliefs, values, and practices within the cultural context of the people being evaluated" (p. 86). Tripp-Reimer, Brink, and Saunders (1984) note that cultural assessments elicit shared beliefs, values, and customs that have relevance to health behaviors. Table 6-2 presents an overview of cultural assessment components (Boyle, 1995). These components can be used to assess diverse cultural groups within a community. Boyle (1995) notes that the concept of culture may be more easily applied to a community or group of persons than to an individual. Cultural and spiritual assessments are a part of the nurs-

REFLECTIVE THINKING

Solving a Dietary Problem

Suppose your cultural assessment reveals that a (child) client is diabetic and the family is unwilling to provide a prescribed diet.

• Which cultural standard is most likely to be met?

• How could you discover a potentially successful intervention?

• Is there a way you could alter the health care system's standard in this case?

Table 6-2 Components of the Cultural Assessment

CULTURAL COMPONENT	DESCRIPTION
Family and kinship systems	Is the family nuclear, extended, or "blended"? Do family members live nearby? What are the communication patterns among family members? What are the role and status of individual family members? By age and gender?
Social life	What is the daily routine of the group? What are the important life-cycle events such as birth, marriage, death, etc.? How are the educational systems organized? What are the social problems experienced by the group? How does the social environment contribute to a sense of belonging? What are the group's social interaction patterns? What are its commonly prescribed nutritional practices?
Political systems	Which factors in the political system influence the way the group perceives its status vis-à-vis the dominant culture: that is, laws, justice, and "cultural heros"? How does the economic system influence control of resources such as land, water, housing, jobs, and opportunities?
Language and traditions	Are there differences in dialects or language spoken between health care professionals and the cultural group? How do major cultural traditions of history, art, drama, etc. influence the cultural identity of the group? What are the common language patterns with regard to verbal and nonverbal communication? How is the use of personal space related to communication?
Worldview, value orientations, and cultural norms	What are the major cultural values about human nature and humankind's relationship to nature and to one another? How can the group's ethical beliefs be described? What are the norms and standards of behavior (authority, responsibility, dependability, and competition)? What are the cultural attitudes about time, work, and leisure?
Religion	What are the religious beliefs and practices of the group? How are these related to health practices? What are the rituals and taboos surrounding major life events such as birth and death?
Health beliefs and practices	What are the group's values, attitudes, and beliefs regarding health and illness? Does the cultural group seek care from indigenous health (or folk) practitioners? Who makes decisions about health care? Are there biological variations that are important to the health of this group?

From *Alterations in Lifestyle: Transcultural Concepts in Chronic Illness* by J. S. Boyle (1995). In M. M. Andrews & J. S. Boyle (Eds.), *Transcultural Concepts in Nursing Care* (2nd ed., pp. 237–252), Philadelphia: J. B. Lippincott. Copyright 1995 by J. B. Lippincott. Reprinted with permission.

ing process and are performed to identify patterns that may assist or interfere with a nursing intervention or planned treatment regimen.

Questions related to spiritual assessment are best asked toward the end of the interview, when the client and nurse are more at ease with each other. Clients should be informed that assessing their spiritual well-being is integral to evaluating their overall health (Pender, 1996).

CARING AND CULTURAL DIVERSITY

In a study of 30 cultures, Leininger (1978, 1984) found a universal desire for and expression of caring, respect, and cherishing, even though caring practices varied from culture to culture. She notes that caring for oneself and for others seems to be significant to the survival of a culture. Indeed, care values, behaviors, and beliefs are considered essential to human growth, living, and survival. Human beings across time have sought ways to care and be cared for, to relate, and to express caring. These same needs are reflected in today's world.

Ethnocentrism often creates barriers in client–nurse relationships and is a deterrent to effective health care. Chinn and Wheeler (1991) present a model for transforming real or potential conflict into unity and wholeness through caring and creativity. The constructive power of diversity increases as alternative views are valued. Diversity is honored when we:

- stop to consider another's point of view, especially when our immediate response is to reject it, and
- take deliberate action to keep ourselves open to differences.

Caring is the spiritual process through which we seek to understand our individual place within the whole of our society. Suffering is a human given; caring is the antidote. Found within one's culture are the supports for emergence to wholeness (Arrien, 1993).

COMMUNITY NURSING VIEW

Nancy is a 19-year-old Native American woman who grew up on the reservation in a family of alcohol- and drug-addicted relatives. Physical and sexual abuse started early in her life, and she became an alcohol abuser at age 14. She moved to the city at age 16, lived with a boyfriend who battered her, and was a member of a gang in which relationships were violent. The nurse first saw her after Nancy had been raped by a stranger. She had kept the shame to herself and had told no one. Pattern appraisal (a Rogerian nursing assessment) revealed isolation, hopelessness, low self-worth, feelings of powerlessness, and no future goals except to have a baby. She had been trying to have a baby for three years. The nurse started slowly teaching her about addiction, domestic violence, choices, and basic human rights, including suggestions to help maintain her safety. In addition, the nurse provided counseling support and Therapeutic Touch treatments that were consistent with Nancy's cultural beliefs.

Each time the nurse saw her, Nancy's expressions of health and self-confidence had grown. As her interests and social patterns grew more diverse and her self-esteem increased, she started making plans to return to school and work. She retold her life experiences with insight and expanding awareness. She was making changes for the better, at her own pace.

Her action plan included incorporating traditional Native American spirituality, healing, and ritual. Nancy and the nurse explored the female aspect within the Native American culture. In the past, Nancy's personal role models had included only women from her family who reflected a picture of subservience, chemical addiction, and domination by male partners. These role models were in direct conflict with traditional Native American female characterizations. She found that, actually, women had always been the power figures and leaders of tribal spirituality and law. Each visit included discussion of a role model chosen from among

her women ancestors to emulate and an exploration of available choices.

The nurse stated that she believes that when she sees one person from the Native American community, she is working with at least 50 people. Discuss the following questions regarding the client–nurse relationship and what you would do if you were the community health nurse in this situation.

Nursing Considerations

ASSESSMENT
• What would be your plan for cultural assessment?
• How would you know whether the client has decided that she can trust you?

DIAGNOSIS
• What is the relevancy of a pattern-appraisal perspective for nursing diagnosis in this situation?

OUTCOME IDENTIFICATION
• Give one expected treatment outcome identified by the client.
• Give one expected treatment outcome identified by you, the nurse.
• Is it possible to identify expected outcomes in a way that is philosophically consistent with the Rogerian concept of pattern appraisal?

PLANNING/INTERVENTIONS
• How would you involve Nancy in a mutual planning process for her treatment?
• On the basis of your knowledge of Native American cultural beliefs about health and healing, what interventions might be appropriate for Nancy?

EVALUATION
• How would you evaluate Nancy's progress?
• What do you think the nurse meant when she said, "When I work with one person, I believe I am working with at least 50 people"?

(ROSZE BARRINGTON, 1997)

〜 Key Concepts

- Increased cultural diversity demands that nurses expand their views of health, illness, and nursing care.

- Transcultural nursing involves understanding and supporting different meanings among diverse health values and beliefs.

- Ethnocentrism presents barriers in the client–nurse relationship and is a deterrent to caring practice.

- Nurses should encourage cultural health practices unless such practices are known to be dysfunctional.

- Western culture is moving toward a paradigm or worldview that acknowledges interrelationship structures and wholeness, a view compatible with alternative and complementary therapies.

- Spiritual assessment focuses on the client's inner strength, awareness of life meaning and purpose, and sense of peace and harmony with the universe.

- Culture represents the infinite variety of beliefs and lifeways reflected in our differences.

- Cultural assessment tools help the nurse understand the meaning of client health behaviors.

- All cultures express caring, but in different ways.

Environmental Perspectives

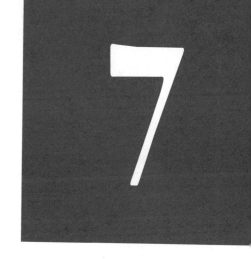

Phyllis Schubert, DNSc, RN
Harriett Lionberger, DNSc, RN

What nursing has to do . . . is to put the patient in the best condition for nature to act upon him. Generally, just the contrary is done. You think fresh air, and quiet and cleanliness extravagant, perhaps dangerous, luxuries, which should be given to the patient only when quite convenient, and medicine the sine qua non, the panacea. If I have succeeded in any measure in dispelling this illusion, and in showing what true nursing is, and what it is not, my object will have been answered.

—Nightingale, 1860/1969, p. 133

COMPETENCIES

Upon completion of this chapter, the reader should be able to:

- Discuss environmental hazards—those related to air, water, and soil—and concomitant health effects to communities.
- Discuss the Institute of Medicine's recommendation that nurses address environmental concerns in nursing practice, education, and research.
- Identify five dimensions of environment and their significance to a method for applying the nursing process to environmental problems.
- Consider how five human responses interact with the five dimensions of environment.
- Review the characteristics of a healing environment and how they are related to caring.
- Examine the works of nurse theorists to understand the person–environment relationship and its impact on health.
- Summarize ways to apply the systematic nursing process to environmental issues and concerns.

As we enter the new millennium, there is cause for grave concern; environmental issues are threatening the life of the earth, at least life on the earth as we know it. Because life essentially depends on air, soil, and water, human health and the **environment**, that which is perceived as being outside the self, are inextricably woven, and because nursing is involved with human health, environment is central to nursing. Conceptually, health can be thought of as the manifestation of the **person–environment interrelationship**, the whole of interpenetrating, inseparable process that makes up the person and environment.

137

ENVIRONMENTAL CONCERNS BY SETTING

Although all dimensions of environment in various settings where human beings live and work—homes, workplaces, schools, communities, and the world at large—are addressed conceptually in this chapter, the major focus is community concern related to the need for clean air, water, and soil. Environmental concerns related to the home are addressed more fully in Chapters 15 and 18, and global concerns in Chapter 28.

Environmental Concerns in Homes and of Families

Economically disadvantaged people, most often served by community health nurses, are at increased risk for exposure to hazardous environmental pollutants. Low-income and minority populations often live near or work in or near heavily polluting industries, hazardous-waste dump sites, or incinerators. Such populations live in substandard houses with friable asbestos and deteriorating lead paint and have contaminated soil in their yards. They may be exposed to toxic chemicals through diets of seafood or fish taken from local waters designated unfit for swimming and fishing. Nurses serving these populations must serve as educators to and advocates for the people to solve these problems (Institute of Medicine [IOM], 1995).

The U.S. Environmental Protection Agency (EPA) reports that more than 40 million people live within four miles of **Superfund sites**, known hazardous waste dumps designated by the EPA as threats to human health, and approximately 4 million people reside within one mile of such sites. In addition, home environmental hazards that carry documented health risks include "radon, environmental tobacco smoke, pesticides, carbon monoxide and airborne particulate from wood-burning stoves, nitrogen dioxide from natural gas stoves, formaldehyde and other chemicals . . . from new carpets, blown-in foam insulation, and the synthetic materials that cover the indoor surfaces of many mobile homes" (IOM, 1995, p. 25).

Because they work in homes, workplaces, schools, and various community settings, community health nurses have repeated opportunities to detect possible environmental disease and underlying etiology. Residents seek counsel from the nurse about birth-defect risk, drinking-water safety, cancer risk from chemical exposure in the workplace, the effects of residential lead or radon, workers' compensation claims, and the costs of rectifying such problems. The Institute of Medicine (IOM) (1995) recommends that nurses be aware of environmental hazards and work as investigators, educators, and advocates for individuals and the community at large to identify environmental disorders and to eliminate the causes.

Environmental Concerns in Workplaces

Occupational safety is one of the 22 priority concerns (see Appendix A) of the *Healthy People 2000* project (U.S. Department of Health & Human Services [USDHHS], 1992a). Work stress is an issue because of expanded duty hours, compressed workweeks, shift work (where the employees' hours vary), and longer work periods without breaks. These factors challenge efforts to prevent disease, injury, and death.

Exposure to toxic chemicals and other environmental hazards in occupational settings is well documented. The U.S. Department of Labor (Bureau of Labor Statistics, 1995a) reports 2.25 million work-related illnesses and injuries having occurred in 1993. Sprains and strains predominantly involving the upper body were the most frequent injuries. High-incidence work-related illnesses included repetitive motion injuries and long-term latent diseases, such as skin cancer following exposure to arsenic or to the transfer of energy via electromagnetic waves or subatomic particles, which is known as **ionizing radiation**. A total of 6,271 fatal work injuries occurred in 1993, the most common work-related deaths being traffic accidents and homicides (Bureau of Labor Statistics, 1995b).

Healthy People 2000 (USDHHS, 1996) reports progress since 1992 in the decrease of hepatitis B and occupation-related lung disease but a dramatic increase in cumulative trauma disorders such as **repetitive motion injuries (RMIs)** and occupational skin disorders. Homicides in the workplace have become a major area of concern since the original document was developed.

Regional, National, and International Concerns

There are a number of issues requiring global attention. These include burning of fossil fuels, which causes air pollution and global warming along with other climatic changes; use of chlorinated compounds that do not decay **(biopersistent)** and tend to accumulate as a result of their nondecaying nature **(bioaccumulative)**, thereby disrupting endocrine and immune functioning; mining and distribution of uranium and its by-products, resulting in radioactive waste; and overdevelopment, which diminishes **biodiversity**, the variety of life that now exists, thereby destabilizing the **ecological balance**, the relationship among living things and between a specific organism and its environment, and creating unknown consequences (Tiedje & Wood, 1995).

Environmental Concerns of Local Communities and of Cities

Environmental hazards affecting communities and cities are generally classified as chemical, physical, biological, or psychosocial. The first three types may occur naturally, such as radon emitted from materials of the earth and ultraviolet light emitted from the sun, or they may be man-made, such as particulates and gases released into the environment as exhaust fumes from automobiles, industrial waste, or tobacco smoke (IOM, 1995). Psychosocial hazards, including racism, prejudice, crime, and violence, are addressed later in this chapter as well as in Chapter 24.

The *Healthy People 2000* (USDHHS, 1992a) project of the United States set priority goals and objectives to achieve a healthier nation by the year 2000. These objectives must be met at the local community or city level but are supported by and fit within the structure of state and federal environmental programs and funding. Lead agencies charged with the responsibility of meeting these goals are the Centers for Disease Control and Prevention (CDC) and the National Institutes of Health (NIH). These agencies agree that substantial efforts to meet these goals must be made by federal, state, and local health and environmental agencies; private citizens; professional organizations; and community leaders if the goals and objectives are to be met. Appendix A offers a full list of priorities. A lengthier discussion of Healthy People 2000 can be found in Chapter 9.

Healthy People 2000: Midcourse Review and 1995 Revisions (USDHHS, 1996) evaluates progress made toward meeting the objectives at mid-decade. Appendix A includes a summary of these findings. The report indicates that substantial progress had been made in certain areas (specifically, blood lead levels, air pollution, household hazardous-waste collection, and release into the soil, water, and air of those chemical carcinogens listed by the USDHHS and the Agency for Toxic Substances and Disease Registry [ATSDR]). Areas where lack of progress or a worsening of problems exists include waterborne diseases, solid waste per person per day, safe drinking water, and impaired surface water (most noticeably, lakes).

ENVIRONMENTAL HEALTH: A NEW ROLE FOR COMMUNITY HEALTH NURSING

Environmental health efforts present critical challenges at this time. The IOM (1995) challenges nurses to take responsibility for serving aggregates and populations and working to create healthy environments. The IOM report encourages more population-focused practice, education, and research by the nursing profession. Given that there are an estimated 2.2 million nurses in the United States, the nursing profession could have a tremendous influence on the environmental health of this nation and the world. Chapter 10 addresses population-focused practice.

Neufer (1994) states that although environmental health issues are central to the historical and theoretical perspectives of nursing, application has been limited to individuals and families. However, the critical state of

environmental health now requires that community health nurses adapt their assessment and diagnostic skills and play a proactive role in the treatment of environmental health hazards.

Community health nursing has historically merged public health and nursing in applying the nursing process to primary, secondary, and tertiary situations that involve individuals, families, and communities. At this time, nurses are being asked to take more responsibility for assessing environmental health risks and serving in the roles of investigator, educator, and advocate for those at risk. Nurses with graduate preparation are expected to assume leadership positions in environmental health.

School nurses, occupational health nurses, and public health nurses must work to improve environmental health conditions in schools, workplaces, and the general community, respectively. All nurses, in fact, are being encouraged to address environmental health factors in their work with individuals and families (IOM, 1995). Public health functions identified by the Public Health Service (1994) are given in Figure 7-1. All can be seen as within the realm of nursing.

Community health nursing has traditionally been considered a synthesis of the public health perspective and nursing perspectives. What the public health perspective brings to nursing is a focus on prevention as opposed to one on illness, the focus inherent in traditional care-and-cure models. Although the nursing discipline deals with environment and health, most nurses are unprepared to deal with such issues except on an individual basis. The IOM (1995) report states:

Public health issues must be approached from a population-based, primary-prevention perspective. Yet, most nurses practice their profession from a curative perspective that focuses on ill individuals. This mismatch creates conceptual and practical difficulties for nurses involved with environmental health issues. They may feel that they lack the authority to take a public health approach or that they lack the skills to analyze health issues in population-based terms. . . . In light of the controversy that sometimes surrounds public health issues, nurses may feel safer caring for individuals because this is the task with which they

---

Figure 7-1 Public Health Functions

- Prevent epidemics and the spread of disease.
- Protect against environmental hazards.
- Prevent injuries.
- Promote and encourage healthy behaviors.
- Respond to disasters and assist communities in recovery.
- Ensure the quality and accessibility of health services.

From Public Health in America *by Public Health Service, 1994, Washington, DC: Author.*

are more familiar; caring for individuals allows nurses to stay solidly within the boundaries of the health care system without stepping into the social, legal, and political arenas important for disease prevention (p. 18).

Many nurses, though, do have the skills and knowledge required to assess and assist individuals, families, and communities in primary, secondary, and tertiary prevention of environment-related illness. They are able to elicit an environmental health history, conduct a community assessment, educate, and serve as advocates. Application of these skills in social, legal, and political arenas is a challenge that nurses can meet.

A CONCEPTUAL FRAMEWORK FOR ASSESSING ENVIRONMENTS

A model for applying the nursing process to environmental issues is proposed in this section. The process involves assessing the five **dimensions of environment**—physical, organizational, social, human aggregate, and internal—identifying **human responses** to environmental issues, and proposing an intervention that will alter the environment in a health-promoting way.

The model provides a conceptual framework for assessing environmental issues and is not intended to provide the student with all that needs to be known about environment, but, instead, with one way of thinking about the person–environment interrelationship.

Although this model provides a broad look at environmental concerns in all five dimensions, particular emphasis is placed on the physical dimension of the community aggregate. The nurse is encouraged to use this model conceptually and creatively for assessment at all levels and dimensions of environment.

Kim (1983) suggests the use of **subenvironments** to approach analysis of the whole and to draw boundaries around specific areas of study for nursing intervention. Five structural dimensions of environment—physical, organizational, social, human aggregate, and internal—similar to Kim's concept of subenvironments are derived primarily from the work of Moos (1979) and are adapted by Puntillo (1992) to assist with the assessment phase of the nursing process.

Physical Dimension

The **physical dimension** of environmental health includes the elements of architecture design, climate, sound, lighting, cleanliness, and adequacy of water, air, and food supply. Concerns related to the physical dimension of the environment at the community aggregate level are, primarily, those related to contamination of air, water, soil, and food supply. The physical environmental hazards

are commonly classified, and are discussed here, as physical, chemical, or biological.

Physical Hazards

Common physical hazards to the air, water, soil, and food supply include ionizing radiation, lead and other heavy metals, mechanical hazards, and noise. Ionizing radiation can result from natural processes occurring inside and outside the earth or from artificial processes created by human beings, such as those associated with medical x-rays or nuclear events. Radiation has both positive and negative outcomes.

Ultraviolet radiation, a natural by-product of sunlight, helps to produce vitamin D when the skin is exposed to the sun but also causes sunburn and acts as a causal factor in basal- and squamous-cell carcinomas and malignant melanomas. The ozone layer of the atmosphere protects against this radiation, but with the loss of this layer as a result of chemicals' being released into the atmosphere, skin cancer is increasing significantly.

Infrared radiation, produced by the sun and molten metals, causes burns to the skin and eyes, potentially causing cataracts. Radon occurs naturally in the materials of the earth; when inhaled as dust, radon can damage lung tissue. Electrical and magnetic fields—created by high-voltage electric power lines, electric blankets, toasters, microwave ovens, hair dryers, televisions, and video display terminals—may have deleterious health effects (Chivian, McCally, Hu, & Haines, 1993).

Lead and other heavy metals (mercury, arsenic, and cadmium) contaminate air, water, and soil. Sources of lead are vehicle emissions, burning of coal, industrial processes, lead-based paint, and solid-waste decomposition. In the United States, much progress has been made by using unleaded gasoline and removing the lead from paint. There remain, however, old houses that still have lead-based paint on their walls. Approximately 74% of all houses built before 1980, in fact, were painted with lead-based paint (Lum, 1995); thus, community health nurses working in older residential areas still encounter many

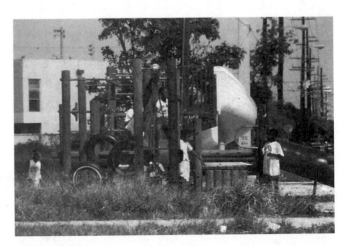

Review this photograph. List positive and negative aspects of this children's playground environment.

children who have ingested lead. Such children put things that are covered with lead paint in their mouths or breathe lead-contaminated dust. Neurological, behavioral, and learning deficits are some signs of lead absorption. See Table 7-1 for information regarding other hazardous agents, including sources, exposure pathways, and body systems affected.

Noise can cause a variety of symptoms, not the least of these being loss of hearing. Other potential health effects of persistent or excessive noise include anxiety, stress, nausea, headaches, sexual impotence, insomnia, hypertension, cardiac disrhythmias, and increased accidents (Chivian et al., 1993).

Mechanical hazards occur most often in the workplace and include vibration, repetitive motion, and lifting in var-ious cumulative-trauma situations. Repetitive motion and lifting cause injuries over time and tend to affect the upper body: that is the neck, shoulders, arms, and hands (USD-HHS, 1996).

Chemical Hazards

Chemical and gaseous hazards constitute another category of toxins that harm body tissues and are found in the air, water, and soil. Insecticides, herbicides, fungicides, and rodenticides all contain chemical poisons. Health effects of pesticide poisoning include dizziness, nausea, lymphoma, leukemia, bladder cancer, and neurotoxicity. Exposure occurs when working with the chemicals or by ingesting them through food and water. Another environ-

Table 7-1 Agency for Toxic Substances and Disease Registry 1993 Priority List of Rank-Ordered Top 10 Hazardous Substances			
HAZARDOUS AGENT	**SOURCES**	**EXPOSURE PATHWAYS**	**SYSTEMS AFFECTED**
Lead	Storage batteries; manufacture of paint, enamel, ink, glass, rubber, ceramics, chemicals	Ingestion, inhalation	Hematologic, renal, neuromuscular, GI, CNS
Arsenic	Manufacture of pigments, glass, pharmaceuticals, insecticides, fungicides, rodenticides; tanning	Ingestion, inhalation	Neuromuscular, skin, GI
Metallic mercury	Electronics; paints; metal and textile production; chemical manufacturing; pharmaceutical production	Inhalation, percutaneous and GI absorption	Pulmonary, CNS, renal
Benzene	Manufacture of organic chemicals, detergents, pesticides, solvents, paint removers	Inhalation, percutaneous absorption	CNS, hematopoietic
Vinyl chloride	Production of polyvinyl chloride and other plastics; chlorinated compounds; used as a refrigerant	Inhalation, ingestion	Hepatic, neurological, pulmonary
Cadmium	Electroplating, solder	Inhalation	Pulmonary, renal
Polychlorinated biphenyls	Formerly used in electrical equipment	Inhalation, ingestion	Skin, eyes, hepatic
Benzo(a)pyrene	Emissions from refuse burning and autos; used as laboratory reagent; found on charcoal-grilled meats and in cigarette smoke	Inhalation, ingestion, and percutaneous absorption	Pulmonary, skin, eyes (BaP is a probable human carcinogen)
Chloroform	Aerosol propellants, fluorinated resins; produced during chlorination of water; used as a refrigerant	Inhalation, percutaneous absorption, ingestion	CNS, renal, hepatic, mucous membrane, cardiac
Benzo(b)-fluoranthene	Cigarette smoke	Inhalation	Pulmonary

From Nursing, Health, and the Environment *(pp. 36–37) by Institute of Medicine, 1995, Washington, DC: National Academy Press. Copyright 1995 by Institute of Medicine.*

Note: *CNS = central nervous system; GI = gastrointestinal.*

RESEARCH FOCUS

Exposure to Styrene and Mortality from Nervous System Diseases and Mental Disorders

STUDY PROBLEM/PURPOSE

Styrene, an aromatic hydrocarbon used in the manufacture of plastics, latex paints, synthetic rubbers, polyesters, and coatings, is produced in large quantities throughout the world (14,000 tons in 1992). Styrene is known to be absorbed through the lungs and the skin; to cause irritation of the skin, eyes, throat, and respiratory tract; and to cause acute disturbances of the central and peripheral nervous systems.

The purpose of this study was to determine whether exposure to styrene contributes to mortality from chronic diseases of the central nervous system.

METHODS

Manufacturing plants from six countries (Denmark, Finland, Italy, Norway, Sweden, and the United Kingdom) and 32,802 exposed workers participated in this longitudinal study. The participants entered the study when they started employment. During 1945–1991, 406 person-years were accumulated, with an average of 12.4 years per person of follow-up study. Indicators of exposure were reconstructed through job histories and environmental and biological monitoring data, and exposure was assessed through determination of styrene metabolites in the urine. Underlying causes of death for deceased cohort members were retrieved from national death certificate records.

FINDINGS

The only areas in which exposed workers had higher mortality rates than those of the general population were suicide, self-inflicted injury, and death from other violent causes. Because the mortality rate for these causes was greatest during the first year of employment and decreased over time, it was thought that this finding was due to lifestyle factors.

Within the cohort, mortality from diseases of the central nervous system increased with time since first exposure; duration of exposure; average level of exposure; and cumulative exposure to styrene. Mortality from epilepsy increased with styrene exposure indicators, as did associations with degenerative diseases of the central nervous system, although not as much.

IMPLICATIONS

Assuming that only healthy individuals were hired for employment, it may also be assumed that the cohort was considerably healthier than the general population (the "healthy worker effect"). Given that many people in the general population who have chronic disabling diseases die of neurological problems, it can probably be assumed that the association between styrene and central nervous system mortality may be even stronger than suggested in the analysis. It is unknown whether the increased rate of suicide and mental disorders during the first year of employment was due to stress and lifestyle factors or to acute response to styrene toxicity. Epilepsy was among the most frequent causes of death from central nervous system diseases in this population and was positively associated with all exposure indicators. Findings indicate that in addition to acute responses to styrene toxicity, exposure may also contribute to chronic disease of the central nervous system.

SOURCE

From "Exposure to Styrene and Mortality from Nervous System Diseases and Mental Disorders" by E. Welp, M. Kogevinas, A. Andersen, T. Bellander, M. Biocca, D. Coggon, J. Esteve, V. Gennaro, H. Kolstad, I. Lundberg, E. Lynge, T. Partanen, A. Spence, P. Boffetta, G. Ferro, & R. Saracci, 1996, American Journal of Epidemiology, 144(7), pp. 623–633. Copyright 1996 by Johns Hopkins University.

mental hazard is accidental poisoning of children who ingest household chemicals. The community health nurse should always check for these hazards on the home visit (see Chapter 15).

Pesticide residues on fruits and vegetables and the bioaccumulation of chemicals and other pollutants in fish and seafood are other areas of concern. Community health nurses can educate people regarding eating fish from contaminated waters and proper cleaning of fresh vegetables and fruits (IOM, 1995). See Chapter 9 for specific suggestions.

The diseases and conditions known to have strong links to the physical environment are cancer, reproductive disorders such as infertility and low birth weight, neurological and immune system impairments, and respiratory conditions such as asthma. A major focus of attention at present is breast cancer, the second leading cause of cancer death in women. This disease results from a complex interaction of genetics, hormonal, and, possibly, environmental factors. Environmental hazards currently being studied—including pesticides, radiation, and toxic chemicals—enter the body through air, water, and food. These hazards are being evaluated to determine whether they do in fact contribute to disease or other disruptions in health (USDHHS, 1996).

Authors of the *Healthy People 2000* project (USDHHS, 1992b) recognize the interrelationship between human beings and environment. They state, "The most difficult challenges for environmental health today come from uncertainties about the toxic and ecological effects of the use of natural and synthetic chemicals, fossil fuels, and physical agents in modern society" (pp. 11–12). Approximately 82% of major industrial chemicals have not at this time been tested for toxic properties and links to specific diseases, and only a small proportion of chemicals have been adequately tested for ability to cause or promote cancer. Health concerns play a huge part in the efforts of the U.S. government to foster a safe physical environment.

Nursing research on environmental health is rare, but nurses may turn to related research carried out in other health disciplines, for instance, epidemiology. The accompanying research box demonstrates some of the problems of epidemiological research.

Biological Hazards

Biological hazards in the environment include infectious agents, insects, animals, and plants. Infectious agents are most often found in water. Waterborne diseases are occurring more often in the United States (USDHHS, 1996) but are a serious problem in many areas of the world. Contamination of the water supply generally results from problems related to sewage and to solid-waste–disposal methods. Rainwater that runs through waste-disposal sites carries organisms into water-supply systems. Waste water must be carefully monitored because it is often recycled for irrigation and may contaminate fruit and vegetable produce. Improper disposal of medical supplies such as needles and syringes that have been contaminated with human blood or other body fluids constitutes another major biological hazard. Infectious organisms are also transmitted in the air, including indoors, by unclean air-conditioning and heating systems, which serve as breeding grounds for pathogenic organisms (Chivian et al., 1993).

Insects and animals breed in solid-waste and spread communicable diseases. Feces provides a breeding ground for insects that transmit disease. Plants also pose a biological hazard because some are poisonous when ingested or touched, and some are allergens.

In addition to these physical environmental hazards, assessment of any setting requires a careful look at its structures and neighborhoods and how they function. The community health nurse, upon entering a home, school, or workplace, checks for adequate heating and cooling systems with vents to prevent air poisoning, adequate food and water supply, a functioning sewage system, appropriate clothing, and other physical things needed for health. Community assessment requires many of the same observational skills but involves more input from and involvement with other community workers in assessment, planning, intervention, and evaluation. The nurse

---

REFLECTIVE THINKING

Physical Environmental Hazards

There are three common categories of physical environmental hazards: physical, chemical, and biological.

- Think about recent news reports regarding any of these three types of hazards in the community.

- How might you, as a nurse, have become involved in the events?

- How might you have worked to prevent one of the events?

---

must be aware of the total community and how its structure affects the well-being of individuals, families, schools, workplaces, and the general community.

All systems of community—from individual and family to local, state, national, and international—have a physical dimension that affects health. Nurses are involved in all these levels of community. Many examples are discussed in later chapters.

Organizational Dimension

Assessing the **organizational dimension** of environmental health involves looking at the structural and functional effectiveness of any particular person, family, community, or population. A careful family assessment will certainly reveal how community organization has affected the family at hand. Community organization comprises all the various community structures—political, economic, public assistance, legal and judicial, health care, schools, transportation, housing, and recreational.

Organizational patterns may be formal (officially recognized by those involved) or informal (not officially part of the organizational plan). Informal patterns are often more powerful than formal ones—and more difficult to change. If the community health nurse finds that families are having difficulty because of a problem in community organization, the nurse may serve as an advocate and take action to change the organizational system of the community. (See Chapters 3 and 4 regarding health care delivery and health care economics, respectively.)

Salmon (1995) maintains that the **policy framework** (policies structured to meet the needs of society and individuals within that society) for health care delivery is a **health determinant** that either enhances or detracts from the health of the people. Assessment of that policy framework indicates that the United States is "rich in knowledge and technology but currently poor in the public health policies that mobilize these assets on behalf of the public's health" (p. 2). She advocates a system in which public health rather than illness, individual medical care, and technology is the foundation, pointing out that in 1993, less than 1% of the aggregate amount for all health care in the United States was spent on population-based public health activities. Public policy provides the organizational aspect of environment, which affects health at the local, state, and national levels.

Just as the organizational structure of the family is assessed by the community health nurse (see Chapters 15 and 18), community structure and organization are the focus of community assessment (see Chapter 12).

Social Dimension

The **social dimension** of the community environment comprises the attitudes of various groups and cultures regarding age, race, ethnicity, religion, socioeconomic status, and lifestyle. Prejudice affects the health of individuals, families, the group being attacked, and the community as a whole.

The social dimension of environment embodies relationships among people within a setting, personal growth or goal orientation, and variables related to system maintenance or system change. The quality of the relationships among immediate family members, extended family members, friends, neighbors, community groups, and health care workers all contribute to **social support**, a perceived sense of support from a complex network of interpersonal ties and from backup support systems for nurturance. Social support is a necessary ingredient of a healthy and healing environment.

Theory and research regarding social support and its relationship to health have been a part of nursing science since 1976 (Powers, 1988). The role of self-esteem in health status emerged in several studies. In 1981, the California Department of Mental Health undertook a major educational project to encourage its citizens—in the name of improving their health—to strengthen their social support systems. This project was based on numerous stud-

ies indicating that social support improved physical and mental health.

Human Aggregate Dimension

The **human aggregate dimension** refers to certain composite characteristics of people within a specific environment—age range, educational level, areas of knowledge, values, culture, communication style, and self-care practices. The human aggregate dimension of environment is addressed from the perspective of the group as a whole and from the personal perspective of the involved individuals. Community assessment includes a description and analysis of the human aggregate (as outlined in Chapter 12). Program planning is determined by this description and analysis (see Chapter 13).

Cultural values held by the human aggregate constitute a significant factor in environmental health issues and all public health concerns. Cultural values in the United States have played a significant part in the efforts to reform health care (Lum, 1995; Williams, 1995). A report by an interdisciplinary group at the Center for Biomedical Ethics (1992) at the University of Minnesota offers the perspective that cultural values prevent the United States from building a health care system that would provide universal access to health care and make a serious commitment to the mission of public health. Data indicate that the United States, although sharing similar culture, philosophy, democratic tradition, and demographics with other Western countries, stands alone as a country lacking universal access to health care and a commitment to public health. The group concludes that "the United States stands alone with its non-universal, patchwork health care

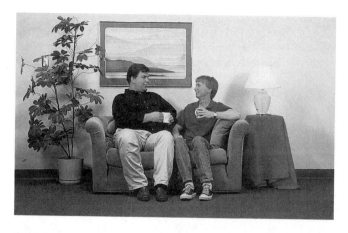

Social support is an important part of a healthy and healing environment.

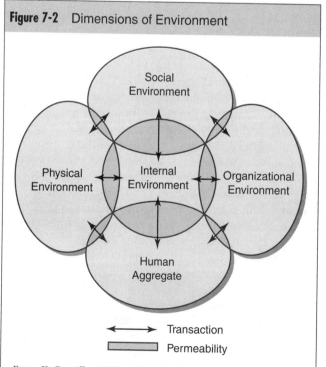

system, in part, because of its embrace of individualism, its establishment of provider autonomy as the preeminent value, and its neglect of community oriented values" (Center for Biomedical Ethics, 1992, p. 15). Williams (1995) states that recognition of these underlying cultural values is important and that acknowledgment simply clarifies the nature of the challenges related to values and political context.

Lum (1995) also recognizes the difficulties involved in building a strong environmental health and public health program. He encourages nurses to serve as educators of the public and emphasizes the importance of **cultural competence** (the ability to communicate with people of various cultures, beliefs, and values to promote a positive outcome) and of **health risk communication** (informing people about environmental health hazards and health risks) in bringing about exchange of information and clarification of values.

Internal Dimension

The **internal dimension** of environment comprises the biological, psychological, and spiritual attributes of the person. Modern psychology supports the notion that perception determines boundaries of person and environment and that perception changes with developmental processes and consciousness. For example, the infant perceives its mother and itself as one being. The growing child learns to differentiate the self and the mother, to perceive the body as the self and everything outside the body as separate. Further into adulthood, the person may perceive the body as environment for the self. At some point, the perceived outer environment may include aspects of **consciousness**, such as thoughts and feelings, in which case the self is equated with the soul or spirit, and thoughts, feelings, and perceptions are experienced as environment. These aspects of consciousness, then, are considered to be one's internal environment. Consciousness, therefore, plays a profound role in this relationship and in health or healing. This model treats the outer environment as that which is outside the mind and body.

The internal dimension of community environment is considered here as the individual inner experiences of the people within the community. Although the sum of these experiences makes up the human aggregate, the internal dimension speaks to the individual and to the individual's attitudes, beliefs, values, and internal experiences.

An assessment of internal environment addresses the biological, psychological, and spiritual attributes of individuals and the unique ways individuals relate to the outer environment. The internal and external environments are interrelated and are involved in constant interaction, influencing and being influenced.

Figure 7-2 depicts both process and structure within the environmental model, with the structure comprising the five dimensions described previously. The process

Figure 7-2   Dimensions of Environment

Social Environment

Physical Environment

Internal Environment

Organizational Environment

Human Aggregate

← → Transaction

▭ Permeability

From K. Puntillo, 1992, A Model of Environment, *unpublished paper for class syllabus, Rohnert Park, CA: Sonoma State University.*

components are permeability and transaction. Permeability, denoted by overlapping of the circles, refers to the inseparability of person and environment. Transaction, denoted by bidirectional arrows, refers to an integrative relationship between person and environment and between dimensions—that is, person and environment affect and are affected by each other, and both change as a result of an encounter.

The nurse is required not only to assess each of these dimensions of environment for health hazards and strengths but also to determine the human response to the myriad environmental factors in these dimensions. Remember, the aim of nursing has been identified as the study of human responses to health and illness (American Nurses Association, 1995).

❧ REFLECTIVE THINKING ❧

The Human Response of a Community

When a child is kidnapped or missing, the pain and loss can be felt at many levels of community. Consider the case of Polly Klass, a California youngster who was kidnapped and later found murdered.

• What levels of community might experience response to such an event?

• How might you be involved as a community health nurse? If you knew Polly, how would that fact affect your ability to focus?

• In what dimensions of environment might you consider intervention?

HUMAN RESPONSES

Human responses to environment are often determined during health assessment of individuals and families. Problems are identified and interventions devised on the basis of those findings. Among the many common examples of human responses that may indicate a need for nursing intervention are failure to thrive, altered immunocompetence, loss, conflict, pain, illness, injury, disability, and technology dependence. Human response phenomena cross clinical sites and conditions and are balanced by varying strengths that facilitate self-sufficiency.

Physical findings may provide clues to environmental health hazards in the person's life. Epidemiologic studies using morbidity and mortality statistics and investigation of possible causes help identify environmental factors involved.

Human responses, however, are numerous and may be determined in large part by the internal dimension of the environment. The very young, elders, and those who are in weakened conditions may be more dramatically affected by environmental health hazards than are members of the general population. For instance, children are especially vulnerable to lead poisoning because of rapid growth and cell division, high metabolic and respiratory rates, and dietary patterns that differ from those of adults (National Research Council, 1993). Elders tend to experience progressive deterioration in cardiac-, renal-, pulmonary-, and immune-system function and in the ability to detoxify chemicals. Studies of drug therapies for the aged, in fact, reveal a decline in blood flow to both liver and kidney, making it increasingly difficult for the aged to rid the body of drug residues and, most likely, environmental toxins (IOM, 1995).

In practice, individuals' responses are often analyzed and treated as the focus of intervention, yet a shift of focus toward environment can often provide a more appropriate approach to relieving certain responses. For example, pain might be lessened by increased social support, or immunocompetence may be strengthened by lessening

environmental stress in some way. Studies in the field of psychoneuroimmunology indicate that attitudes affect the ability of the body to deal with stressors (Schmoll, Tewes, & Plotnikoff, 1992). Depression and despair weaken the immune system and increase vulnerability.

Community Responses

Human responses can be understood as community as well as individual phenomena. Thus, mental health teams respond to communities where earthquakes, floods, and other disasters occur, helping these aggregates deal with their losses, regroup, and move on with their lives as quickly as possible. In this way, the severity of the response is mitigated. On an even larger scale, the Chernoble nuclear disaster had worldwide effects—loss, pain, and conflict felt at many levels of community. Certainly, technology dependence and altered immunocompetence have been results, and, years later, communities worldwide continue to act in response to the event.

Societal Responses

Human responses to factors related to the social dimension of environment are addressed as indicators of social health. Social health in the United States has been measured using the Index of Social Health, developed by researchers at Fordham University in New York City (Social Health, 1996). Indicators include 16 measures of well-being, and data have been collected and analyzed from 1970 to 1993. Miringoff (1995) examined measurement of economic well-being as reflected by the gross domestic product (GDP), generally used as the indicator of progress, and measurement of well-being as reflected by the Index of Social Health. The Index of Social Health accounts for well-being during different stages of life.

Figure 7-3   Fordham Index of Social Health and GDP: 1970–1983

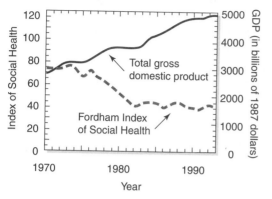

From 1995 Index of Social Health: Monitoring the Social Well-Being of the Nation by M. L. Miringoff, 1995, Tarrytown, NY: Institute for Innovation in Social Policy, Fordham Graduate Center. Used with permission.

Each measurement is compared with a standard, the highest measurement achieved in that particular area since 1970.

Figure 7-3 shows the total GDP steadily rising and the Fordham Index of Social Health steadily falling. Since 1970, 11 measures have declined and 5 have risen. Improvements have been seen in infant mortality, drug abuse, high-school dropout rate, poverty among those over age 65, and food-stamp coverage. Indicators that have worsened over time are children in poverty, child abuse, teen suicide, unemployment, average weekly wages, health insurance coverage, out-of-pocket health costs for those over age 65, homicide, alcohol-related highway deaths, housing, and the gap between the rich and the poor. The results indicate that social health in the United States has fallen from 73.8 out of a possible 100 points in 1970 to 40.6 points in 1993, a 45% decrease.

The Human Response to Disaster

Although the human spirit is strong, certain events can be so overwhelming that people lose hope and sink into despair. When disaster strikes and others come with help, people are better able to cope and rebuild their lives. When a whole community or country falls, as in a war or other devastating act of violence, the resulting despair can render people helpless and unable to go on. At such times, help is essential but often difficult to find. Agencies such as the Red Cross help by furnishing necessary items to sustain physical life and nurture the human spirit.

Natural disasters, such as floods, earthquakes, or hurricanes, often cause great stress in all dimensions of environment. Nurses are often involved in community efforts to provide needed assistance and to help people find the strength and ability to cope in such situations. The nursing model described in this section provides a framework for disaster nursing in the community. Application of the nursing process to the environment requires assessment of each dimension of environment and the associated human responses. The base of the triangle in Figure 7-4 represents the five dimensions of environment to be assessed; the left side depicts the human responses to the environment. Planning for intervention requires linking these two sets of concepts with a third set—creating a caring environment (one that supports health and healing)—in order to alter the environment to increase its propensity to promote health and healing.

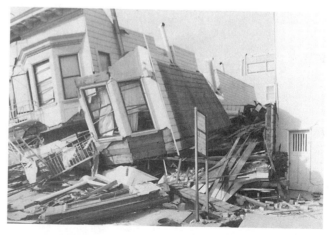

The community health nurse can provide assistance and help people cope with difficult situations.

Perspectives...

Insights of a Community Health Nurse

I work as a public health nurse in a county where a major river floods every few years, leaving at least one small town, hundreds of homes, and highways and roads under several feet of water. The flood relief plan is put together by the county EMS (emergency medical services). That agency is an umbrella group for coordinating with county departments—the Red Cross and other flood relief agencies. The EMS assists in setting up shelters at county veterans' buildings. In Guernville, the old and defunct Bank of America is used as a center where agencies set up tables and send their workers to help people of the community get what they need to cope with the flood and to restore their homes and lives. So, flood victims can do "one-stop shopping" at the center.

At the center, one can apply for emergency Aid to Families with Dependent Children (AFDC), Medicaid, and delay of tax payment and can get a free lunch, cleaning supplies, water, and other basic supplies from the Red Cross.

I help answer telephone calls that the other agencies cannot help with and vice versa. I assist the Red Cross volunteers, do triage, and teach hand washing, food handling, and kitchen precautions to prevent the occurrence and spread of infection. I offer advice, assist victims with finding resources, and give tetanus shots.

Workers represent agencies such as social services, the Red Cross, the county tax department, and county environmental health inspectors. The mental health department offers resources and crisis counseling. Mental health and social service workers are available to clients.

The public health nurse in this setting works the shelters and the centers where flood victims seek help. I am involved in all multidisciplinary meetings, and I help with planning. Meetings are held at the start and end of the day. I am able to share my knowledge and expertise regarding the community with my colleagues.

—Susan Miller, PHN

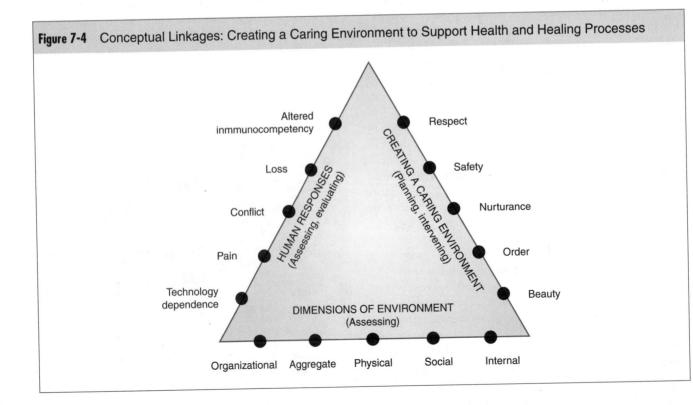

Figure 7-4   Conceptual Linkages: Creating a Caring Environment to Support Health and Healing Processes

CREATING A CARING ENVIRONMENT

Using qualitative research methods, Schubert (1989) identified five elements provided by nurses in creating an environment supportive of health and healing processes: respect, safety, nurturance, order, and beauty. The nurses' efforts were grounded in both science and their intuitive knowledge of natural healing processes. Thus, the right side of the triangle in Figure 7-4 can serve as a goal for proposal development and nursing intervention related to environment.

Caring in modern nursing can be applied through the nursing process to create environments that promote health and healing. The idea of using the nursing process to create healthy and **healing environments** that are safe, nurturing, respectful, orderly, and beautiful is applicable to the world, nations, populations, communities, families, and individuals. Communities, however, are where grassroots actions take place—where families and individuals who are touched by environmental problems and feel strongly about these issues demand action. None of these entities operates independently of the others because each either comprises or is a component of other levels, or both.

Caring with intent to promote health and healing is the motivational force that provides guidance as the nurse identifies appropriate environmental health interventions. It is the integrative force that underlies safety, nurturance, respect, order, and beauty in an environment that supports natural healing processes. Focused intention to help and to facilitate healing provides direction for nursing activities related to environment. Thus, nursing practice is extended to issues of environmental health in all dimensions, levels, and settings.

Safety

Client safety can be classified as physical, mental, emotional, or spiritual. **Safety** is that component of environment that protects and keeps a person secure, unharmed, and free from danger. Nursing commonly involves protection of clients from external forces, but it also involves protection from internal forces, as in the case of suicide attempts and self-abuse. Specific safety issues vary with the setting. Safety issues in various settings are discussed in the following sections.

Safety in the Home

It is sometimes easiest for nurses to see the client's safety as a concern at the individual level. When working with families in the home, the nurse would likely be especially aware of the presence or absence and the appropriate placement and maintenance of fire alarm units, as well as avenues of escape in case of emergency. In both individual and family care, safety concerns tend to center on an identified problem. For example, in providing care to clients with diminished ability to walk, a concern might be obstacles to safe movement around the home. Climbing stairs or performing other types of physical exertion may be of concern for the client who has circulatory or respiratory problems.

Similarly, a visit to a family with a member who is experiencing allergies includes a search for allergens in the environment. In the case of food allergies, the concern is foods, items used in meal preparation, and sources of products used; in the case of allergies related to inhalation, sources of dust, animal dander, fibers, and pollens are investigated, as is evidence of efforts to restrict levels of these allergens.

Safety in Communities

We can carry the example of an allergy related to inhalation a step further. Some communities have higher-than-average levels of air pollution. Efforts to intervene might include involvement in a community-action group aimed at controlling either emissions from local industries or by-products of community waste-disposal systems.

Safety in Populations

Both damaging emissions and rising consumption leading to waste-disposal problems can be seen as results of growing populations' making ever greater demands on the environment (Kennedy, 1993). Because of this, populations constitute an important stratum in the environmental impact on health. Obviously, when such broader-reaching strata are involved, it no longer makes sense to limit health advocacy to narrow concerns. With this recognition, some individuals in various populations—for example, different countries or varying segments of communities—band together and begin to work toward change. As is the case with other groups, some nurses will become political activists and some will not, but it is important that all nurses be aware of the broader implications. Membership in state, national, and international nursing organizations is one way that individuals can support interventions in the larger context.

Even in smaller communities, populations may constitute a stratum of concern when minority aggregates are at risk for certain health problems or have less access to health care than do other community members. Frequently, these groups are also less likely to be in a position to advocate change. It then becomes the responsibility of health care professionals to identify the problems and seek solutions.

Safety in Nations

Often when we think of populations, we think at the national level. With the emergence of rapid-communication systems, it has become easier than in the past to share information about health care, whether that information concerns disease-specific treatments, common habits or activities that affect health, or conditions that threaten the quality of air, water, housing, and the like. Many threats to health must be confronted at the national level, simply because local measures lack sufficient scope to maintain healthful conditions, even locally. Air quality is one example; whatever changes are instituted locally, the problem is likely to be aggravated by conditions beyond local control.

Safety in the World

Some threats to individual safety are being recognized as so far-reaching that only international interventions can be expected to reduce the danger. Among the global issues identified by Kennedy (1993) and Harrison (1992) as posing the severest environmental crisis in history are rising consumption and damaging technology. We have only a few decades' worth of oil supplies left, the world's rain forests are shrinking, species are being extinguished at a rapid rate, and much of the world's farmland is deteriorating. Air pollution, acid rain, ozone depletion, and rising carbon dioxide concentrations are destroying the atmosphere.

The community health nurse can have an impact on all levels of physical safety by increasing consciousness of the issues through example. By contributing to others' awareness, the nurse may influence individual and group attitudes, leading indirectly to healthier environments.

Mental, Emotional, and Spiritual Safety

Mental safety related to values and beliefs was discussed in Chapter 6 and will not be explored at length here. Beliefs and values stem primarily from culture and religion and are sometimes altered by experience and education. Freedom and individual responsibility are important values in the free world, where it is generally assumed that safety to believe as one chooses is a right as long as behavior does not threaten the safety of oneself or of others. Again, the student is reminded that respect for various beliefs and values contributes to environmental safety.

Tending to mental and emotional safety often begins

with the nurse's attitude when addressing physical issues. Knowing that someone cares and will listen seriously to one's problems can make it easier for the client to think clearly and can reduce client stress related to uncertainty. Treating the client as a partner in health promotion enhances this feeling. As clients take more responsibility for their feelings, they will be more in control and will perceive less threat in the relationship with environment. Clients learn to think more positively about themselves while progressively feeling safer in their respective environments. Specific issues vary with the setting and the client's basic needs.

It is sometimes necessary to make clients aware of how the nurse's activities will promote safety, reassuring them that their safety is a concern. Families often feel threatened when visited by someone in an official capacity, such as a community health nurse, but when the nurse's attitude is one of genuine caring, the client usually is able to enter into a working partnership.

Spiritual safety can also imply confidence to follow one's religious beliefs or spiritual discipline without criticism or persecution. More subtly, it can imply an environment that allows clients to repattern the energy of fear engendered by feelings of being physically or emotionally unsafe. Fears may occur in response to external or internal stimuli and might include fear for physical safety, fear of rejection, or fear of being judged as incompetent or as having little value, among other fears. Such fears may be traced to ideas about oneself, as in suicidal ideation, or to one's perceptions of others' judgments, as in low self-worth.

Respect

Respect is an aspect of caring (see Chapter 1) and has also been identified by Schubert (1989) as a crucial element of environments that support health and healing. Respect includes consideration and concern for others, as well as trust in others' capability and potential for growth and healing. A respectful environment provides support as the individual or aggregate experiences increasing order, organization, and ability to be interactive, independent, and interdependent. As indicated in Figure 7-5, the client may make mistakes and learns from those mistakes.

❧ REFLECTIVE THINKING ❧

Environmental Health Behavior

• Why is nursing concerned with recycling? Waste disposal? Air pollution?

• At what environmental level or levels might these issues trigger concern?

• At what level or levels would intervention be appropriate?

• Who or what might the client be?

Figure 7-5 Characteristics of a Respectful Environment

• The client identifies the problem.

• The nurse plays a supportive role as the client learns, develops, and fulfills the solution to the problem.

• Problems are opportunities for learning and growth.

• The nurse acknowledges the client's ability to take advantage of the opportunity.

• The nurse cannot independently solve the problem.

This attitude toward the client requires the nurse to encourage each person, family, or group to assume self-responsibility. The nurse supports the client's efforts but does not take over and try to *fix* the problem. Within a relationship of mutuality and partnership, the nurse exhibits patience as the client learns to take charge.

Colodzin (1993) suggests that in environments where disrespect is the rule, it becomes a habit and is taken for granted. If the opposite is also true, we can assume that when nurses model and teach caring at all practice levels, they contribute not only to a more balanced society but also to a world that can more effectively promote and protect health.

Nurturance

Nurturance is the provision of materials discussed by Nightingale (1860/1969), such as nourishing food, proper temperature, quiet, light, fresh air, cleanliness, and shelter. To this list, the authors would add respectful touch.

Nurturance in the Home and Family

The home and family are major sources of nurturance in all cultures. The family provides shelter and protection from the weather, food, furnishings for comfort, and affection and respectful touch. When families fail to provide nurturance, the deprivation is destructive to physical and emotional health. Their young members may suffer from addictions, nutritional disorders, or physical or mental chronic illness. The community nurse works to strengthen the family's ability to provide nurturance and, thus, to prevent these problems.

Nurturance in the Community

The family and community share resources to provide individuals with food, clothing, shelter, and necessities for health and healing. When the family and community are both strong, mutual sharing occurs; when the family is in some way weakened, the community must absorb more responsibility for the family. For example, if a parent becomes jobless, extended family, friends, churches, and other organizations that provide food, clothing, and shelter may become involved. When the specific community is significantly weakened and these resources become unavailable, malnutrition, homelessness, and disease bring suffering. In such a case, agencies, both governmental and private, often assume responsibility for helping those in distress.

Ingenuity and creativity are useful in finding community resources for a family. The nurse serves as client advocate in approaching organizations designed to help in certain circumstances. The nurse can identify available services and help the client contact resources. The nurse can sometimes help by guiding the family back to lost social supports such as extended family, friends, and church groups.

DECISION MAKING

A Respectful Environment

Imagine that a family in the small, rural community where you work as a community health nurse is one of three African American families in the community. One of the children has been hurt in a fight on the way home from school. Use the triangle in Figure 7-4 to assess the situation by considering the following:

- The various dimensions of environment
- The human responses
- Those characteristics, if any, that need work

How would you intervene?

Nurturance in World Populations

Nurturance is a major problem for the world at large. Much of the problem can be traced to exploding population, growing at the staggering rate of 100 million people each year and thereby doubling the earth's population every 40 years (Ehrlich & Ehrlich, 1990).

This population explosion is fostering disparities between the rich and the poor, both within and outside the United States. Income per person in developed countries is approximately 30 times that in the poorest countries. The worst devastation related to this poverty is starvation and malnutrition. Ehrlich and Ehrlich (1990) indicate that starvation kills as many people every four months as did the Holocaust.

These problems create great concerns for community nurses who work to provide a nurturing community and world environment. Nurses are joining the ranks of policymakers and international health workers who attempt to guide the world's population to greater health by working to create an environment that supports health and healing.

Order

Order, or the methodical and harmonious arrangement of time, space, and objects in one's life, is another aspect of a healing environment. Its presence or relative absence can be observed in physical, psychological, time-related, or other aspects of a client's situation. The harmony and rhythmic patterns of a productive nurse–client interaction require creative sensitivity and can themselves contribute to order—an esthetic quality of the environment. For example, the sensitivity of the nurse to the client's time and activity schedule is important, and, in the United States, the client is apt to feel disrespected if the nurse does not keep appointments on schedule. This is true whether the nurse is visiting a family at home or has a speaking engagement at a community-service group meeting.

Individuals and organized groups have varying degrees of tolerance for the unexpected, and when a client experiences dislocation for any reason, the nurse's assistance may be necessary to help bring about or guide and support the process of restoring order. Sorrell (1994) describes esthetic knowing as an aspect of the art of nursing that includes synthesis of scattered details of perception into a coherent whole. The understanding that emerges from this synthesis is what helps the nurse work with discordant issues that arise in the community.

The structure of time and activity and the arrangement of things in the home, workplace, school, or other community setting very definitely influence ability to function, whether the focus is the individual, the family, or a larger aggregate. In the home involved, individuals may need the nurse's assistance to regain order and the ability to function. In society, more people and planning are required to restore the infrastructure and the organizational structures that establish and maintain optimum order.

A word of caution is necessary here. Just as lack of order may interfere with one's ability to function, so may an overemphasis on maintaining order. On one hand, order is a friend and facilitates living processes; on the other, an obsession with order may interfere with functioning. Individuals, families, or groups who cannot tolerate disorder may stifle activity and functioning. For example, a home or classroom that is never cluttered may be the setting for a family or group of students whose creativity and freedom to grow and develop according to their human potential are stifled and limited.

Human attempts to control the forces of nature seem to have created more disorder in the world; cooperation with and respect for natural forces could potentially promote more order and less destruction. Order, as a characteristic of a healthy and healing environment in communities and the world, is influenced by natural forces. Nature also provides the beauty of color, sound, form, and rhythm, which support health and healing.

from deep emotional and spiritual wounds. Artistic self-expression through movement and other art forms demonstrates healing in the interpenetrating processes and pattern reorganization of the person–environment interrelationship. Many cultures use the beauty of dance to restore balance and harmony and to promote health and wholeness.

Certain sounds, such as those of ocean waves, a waterfall, or a breeze in the trees, can restore a sense of balance and harmony for some individuals. A Bach fugue, with its interweaving and integration of parts, can be very healing for others who feel confused and helpless. Clients themselves are the best sources of ideas regarding those things that enhance their sense of beauty.

Color is used by some nurses to stimulate healing. Perhaps the wave frequencies of colors promote healing for persons of different energy patterns or resonances. Appreciation of beauty depends on one's ability to perceive it and on one's level of awareness, but these are difficult to assess. Maslow (1962) referred to appreciation of beauty as a self-actualizing process. It is unlikely, however, that only those persons whose basic needs have been met can respond therapeutically to beauty, as Maslow's hierarchy of needs might suggest.

Beauty in Communities

Beauty in larger communities can be achieved through order, discussed previously, and through development of the resources of the community itself. These resources are both material and personal. In relatively rare cases, the nurse may be involved in planning or implementing the aesthetic aspects of a physical community. Nevertheless, all of the work that community health nurses do at the level of larger communities can be seen as addressing beauty in some way. One such example is the harmony that grows out of a community's increasing understanding of itself and its responsibilities.

Beauty

Aesthetic **beauty** is experienced through the senses and either exists naturally in or is developed as a part of the environment. The components of beauty are sound, color, and form. Form is expressed as patterns or rhythms of matter and energy and often is intimately associated with sound and color. Those forms found in nature seem to have healing qualities. At the same time, each person manifests his own unique pattern such that not everyone experiences the same form of beauty as healing.

Gardens, beaches, and forest walks may be used when possible for nurse–client interaction and as an environment for health and healing. In addition to benefiting from the incredible beauty found in nature, persons need to create things of beauty. Artistic creation and the enjoyment of others' work can serve as media for inner healing

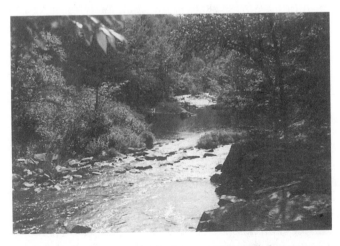

The sights and sounds of a flowing stream may bring about healing to a client. What enhances your sense of beauty?

Proposals for Creating Healthy and Healing Environments

The triangle in Figure 7-4 may be used in the development of proposals for creating and maintaining healthy and healing environments. For instance, a problem found in the assessment of the physical dimension and indicating the presence of an environmental hazard associated with the human response of a related skin disorder indicates a possible physical safety issue. Thus, the nurse would design her proposal to increase safety in the questionable dimension of environment and would protect the client through education and appropriate treatment to prevent further disability. Primary, secondary, and tertiary prevention are applied, then, not only to the person involved but also to the environment.

Josten, Clarke, Ostwald, Stoskopf, and Shannon (1995) encourage development of the public health specialist role, wherein nurses with graduate degrees would work to create healthy environments in the community and to educate and guide the populace toward positive health behavior. In this model, community health nurses participate in activities to create healthy environments; at present, however, the major focus of the community health nurse is providing individual or family care in community settings such as a home or a workplace.

PERSON–ENVIRONMENT THEORIES

More than any other nurse theorist, Florence Nightingale (1860/1969) emphasized the importance of environment to health and healing. She clearly established that it is within the realm of nursing to create a healing environment. Her work in lowering morbidity and mortality rates in hospitals demonstrated the strong link between environment and health and healing. These events firmly established environment as a central concept of nursing theory. Nurse theorists have continued to study and to increase understanding of the conceptual linkages among health, environment, person, and nursing.

Einstein's Theory

Since Nightingale's time, scientific breakthroughs have changed our understanding of the nature of the person–environment relationship. Einstein's work during the early 1900s challenged the idea that the world of nature, including human beings, consists of parts that fit together in a machinelike manner. Conventional wisdom had been that we could understand the whole by studying the parts in isolation from the rest and that, in learning about the parts, the whole would become known. Applied to health, the belief was that we could study health and illness separately and could understand environment apart

from its relationship to persons. Within this understanding, the whole was thought to be the sum of the parts. Einstein's work, however, refuted those notions of separateness and, instead, proposed ideas of process, relationship, and organizational pattern as significant areas for the study of nature.

Einstein's work in **quantum mechanics**, that branch of physics concerned with the energy characteristics of matter at the subatomic level, is now approximately 100 years old, yet there is still little general understanding or acceptance of how this work applies to health and healing. Some theorists believe that when Einstein's work is interpreted to apply to the nature of the human being, activities to promote health and healing will change dramatically (Herbert, 1987).

Systems Perspectives

Influenced by Einstein, von Bertalanffy (1968) attempted to apply Einstein's ideas to social systems. He developed **general systems theory**, in which he supported the view of system theorists that the whole is more than and different from the sum of the parts. This work has greatly influenced nursing theory and understanding of the human–environment interrelationship. General systems theory has served as a foundation for organizational knowledge used in working with families, communities, and environmental health. See Chapter 18 for more on systems theory and its application to family processes.

Whitehead (1969), a contemporary of Einstein, argued not only that the whole is more than and different from the sum of the parts but also that all consist of **interpenetrating processes** of energy patterns that are totally inseparable from all else. His work and that of others provided a foundation for understanding the oneness of person and environment, leading to the study of consciousness and caring in health and healing. Today, physicists, theologians, philosophers, and scientists of many disciplines are studying what mystics of both the East and the West have taught for ages. This is part of the shift toward understanding patterns of wholeness as related to health and healing (as discussed in Chapter 6).

Nursing Theories

The work of Nightingale, Einstein, Whitehead, and von Bertalanffy greatly influenced Martha Rogers, a major nurse theorist. In the 1970s, she argued that humans and environment are inseparable and brought about renewed interest in environment as a central phenomenon of nursing (Newman, 1994).

Rogers (1990) uses Einstein's theory to define the universe as an energy field in which person–environment fields are identified by pattern and organization. Her descriptors of resonancy, helicy, and integrality characterize these field patterns and their related principles.

Resonancy refers to a continuous change from lower- to higher-frequency wave patterns (the evolutionary principle); **helicy** refers to the unpredictability, diversity, and innovation of human and environmental field patterns (the complexity principle); and **integrality** refers to the continuous mutual process of these field patterns (the spirituality principle). In Rogers' construct, **human field patterns** are irreducible, indivisible, and pandimensional. They are identified by characteristics specific to the whole and cannot be predicted simply from knowledge of the parts.

Newman (1994) was influenced by physical scientist David Bohm's (1980) work concerning quantum realities. Newman defines health as the expansion of consciousness and consciousness as the informational capacity of the person–environment system. Components of this system include the nervous system, the endocrine system, the immune system, and the genetic code, to name a few. Knowledge of these systems indicates the inherent com-plexity in the person–environment response (Newman, 1994).

Mutual Connectedness Theory utilizes concepts of caring and consciousness to address client–nurse relationships within healthy and healing environments (Schubert & Lionberger, 1995). Both the client and the nurse experience health and healing in such a relationship. Caring in practice requires a balance of many responsibilities in demonstrating caring for the nurse's self and family, clients and their families, the community, the country, and the world. Expanding consciousness parallels an increasing sense of responsibility (see Figure 7-6); being centered and at peace with oneself requires the nurse to focus attention on what is at hand while maintaining an awareness of the whole. The admonition, thus, is to *think globally but act locally.*

Caring and concern for the well-being of people and environment must be balanced with caring for oneself. Staying centered helps one practice caring within the lim-

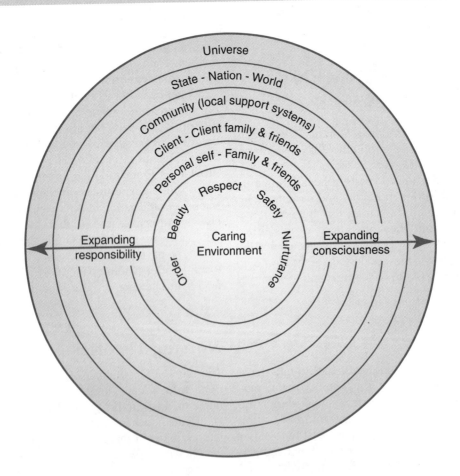

Figure 7-6   Expanding of Caring, Consciousness, and Responsibility in the Creation of Healthy and Healing Environments

From "Mutual Connectedness: A Study of Client–Nurse Interaction Using the Grounded Theory Method" by P. Schubert & H. Lionberger, 1995, Journal of Holistic Nursing, 13*(2), pp. 102–116. Copyright 1995 by P. Schubert and H. Lionberger. Reprinted with permission.*

its of what is possible for one human being to accomplish. Dass (1993) provides some additional guidelines that can help community nurses avoid overextending themselves and becoming exhausted from too much responsibility and overwork. He suggests that the helper act from deep intuitive appreciation of what is appropriate in the moment by asking whether each act undertaken:

- Is in harmony with the helper's personal values,
- Uses the helper's particular skills, talents, and personality characteristics,
- Makes use of opportunities,
- Acknowledges liabilities as well as assets,
- Takes into account existing responsibilities, and
- Honors the diverse roles the helper is called on to fulfill in the moment.

Figure 7-7   Questions to Assess Exposure to Potential Environmental Hazards

- What are your current and past longest-held jobs? (For children and teenagers, the question can be modified to, "Where do you spend your day, and what do you do there?")
- Have you had any recent exposure to chemicals (including dusts, mists, and fumes) or radiation?
- Have you noticed any (temporal) relationship between your current symptoms and activities at work, home, or other environments?

From Nursing, Health and the Environment, *(p. 45) by Institute of Medicine, 1995, Washington, DC: National Academy Press. Copyright 1995 by Institute of Medicine. Reprinted with permission.*

APPLICATION OF THE NURSING PROCESS TO ENVIRONMENT

The nursing process—assessing, diagnosing, planning, implementing, and evaluating—is a deliberate, logical, and rational problem-solving process whereby the practice of nursing is performed systematically. Assessment of potential environmental hazards in the lives of individuals and families should include questions about exposure to chemical, physical, or biological hazards and about temporal elements between environmental events and symptoms (see Figure 7-7).

Although the nursing process was developed for use in the care of individuals, it has been expanded for use in the care of families, communities, and larger populations. The IOM (1995) report suggests that new methods may be required for application of the nursing process to environmental health issues. The nursing process is compatible with the California Public Health Foundation (1992) framework, an approach utilizing investigator, educator, and advocate roles to address environmental health

issues. The **investigator role**, the gathering of data and formulation of a nursing diagnosis, is equivalent to the assessment and evaluation phases; the **educator** and **advocacy roles** constitute the intervention phase. The educator role involves helping others gain knowledge, skills, and characteristics needed for good health; the advocacy role involves speaking or acting in behalf of those who are unable to do so for themselves. Policy making and program planning are among the skills needed for the intervention phase.

An aggregate focus for community health nursing requires additional skills and reinterpretation of the nursing process. Neufer (1994) offers a method for application of the nursing process to aggregates when environmental issues are concerned. First, data from federal, state, and local resources are collected (see Table 7-2). Major federal resources are the Environmental Protection Agency (EPA); the ATSDR; the national priorities list (NPL), which includes identified hazardous toxic waste sites; and the toxic chemical release inventory database, which lists all reported substances by city, county, or zip code. Environmental laws are available through the EPA and other

---

Table 7-2   Sources of Environmental Health Data

FEDERAL	STATE	LOCAL
EPA studies and ATSDR public health assessments for NPL sites	State environmental agencies (priority lists, environmental monitoring data, other studies)	Community health concerns
ATSDR public health assessments, consultations, studies	State health agencies (health advisories, disease registries, epidemiologic studies or surveys)	Community action groups
Toxic chemical release inventory database		Health screening programs and surveys
		Local health departments

From "The Role of the Community Health Nurse in Environmental Health" by L. Neufer, 1994, Public Health Nursing 11*(3), p. 157. Copyright 1994 by Blackwell Science, Inc. Reprinted with permission.*

COMMUNITY NURSING VIEW

A public health nurse works as an environmental scientist at ATSDR, assisting communities affected by hazardous-waste releases. ATSDR is contacted by an activist group concerning a creek in the group's local area, and the resulting report is forwarded to the PHN for follow-up. The report indicates that the creek is grossly polluted with dangerous industrial wastes. The group is especially concerned because, although there are warning signs posted, children and adults continue to play and fish in the creek (Phillips, 1995).

Nursing Considerations

ASSESSMENT

• Where would the nurse look for clues of potential sources of pollution?
• What steps would the nurse take to determine the level of contamination?
• What other factors besides the contaminated water would the nurse consider when formulating the assessment?
• What resources would the nurse have to use to obtain assessment data?

DIAGNOSIS

• Who in the community may be at risk?

• Can a significant potential for injury be identified?
• What are the host and environmental factors related to diagnosis?

OUTCOME IDENTIFICATION

• What outcomes would be identified for people who have already been exposed to the creek? For those who have potential for exposure?

PLANNING/INTERVENTIONS

• What interventions would the nurse employ to minimize further exposure to the creek?
• How would the nurse identify those who have been exposed?
• What type of educational programs would the nurse devise to encourage full community awareness of treatment methods for those already exposed?
• What types of agencies would the nurse notify to aid in cleanup efforts?

EVALUATION

• What factors would indicate that the nurse's plan is successful?
If the plan were not successful, what amendments could be made?

---

state and local agencies. Applicable state and local agencies and groups vary. Data gathering should involve consultation with environmental activists and experts on specific topics as well as with the people at risk.

Figure 7-8 Formulating Nursing Diagnoses for an Environmental Health Assessment

Nursing diagnosis in an environmental health assessment provides answers to the following questions:

• Who in the community is at highest risk?

• Can a significant potential for injury be identified?

• What are the host and environmental factors related to the diagnosis?

• Do data substantiate the nursing diagnosis?

From "The Role of the Community Health Nurse in Environmental Health" by L. Neufer, 1994, Public Health Nursing 11(3), pp. 155–162. Copyright 1994 by Blackwell Scientific Publications. Reprinted with permission.

Next, an environmental health nursing diagnosis should be formulated (see Figure 7-8). This diagnosis identifies the potentially unhealthful response for a community. It is aimed at a specific aggregate of people, a "collection of individuals who are not part of an interdependent group, but who share some health risk or health-seeking behavior" (Neufeld & Harrison, 1990, p. 252). When the aggregate has been identified, the potential for injury and the factors (both host and environmental) related to the health problem are determined. Data gathering should continue to monitor results.

Key Concepts

• Community health nursing perspectives include both public health and the environmental focus of nursing.

• The Institute of Medicine report recommends that nurses address environmental health concerns.

• Assessment of the environment can be facilitated by analyzing the various dimensions of the environment and the human responses of the client.

- Proposals for intervention link assessment data from the various dimensions of environment and the human responses of the client with actions to enhance health or healing qualities of the environment.

- A healthy and healing environment reflects caring and is characterized by safety, nurturance, respect, order, and beauty.

- Nurse theorists since the time of Florence Nightingale have emphasized the creation and maintenance of healthy and healing environments as the goal of nursing.

- The nursing process—assessing, planning, intervening, and evaluating—can be applied to the environment to promote client health and healing.

Caring Communication and Client Teaching/Learning

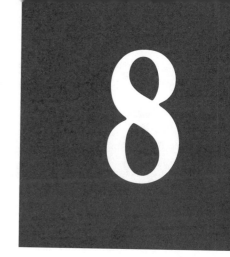

Phyllis E. Schubert, DNSc, RN, MA
Janice Hitchcock, DNSc, RN
Harriett J. Lionberger, DNSc, RN

Talking with [clients] is easy when the nurse treats the [client] as a chum and engages in a give-and-take of social chitchat. But when the nurse sees her part in verbal interchanges with [clients] as a major component in direct nursing service, then she must recognize the complexity of that process. Social chitchat is replaced by the responsible use of words which help to further the personal development of the [client].

—Peplau, 1960, p. 964

COMPETENCIES

Upon completion of this chapter, the reader should be able to:

- Name one factor that sets health care models apart from other models of communication.
- List at least five concepts defined in nursing communication theory.
- Describe and explain two possible levels of client responsibility in developing the nurse–client relationship.
- Demonstrate four forms of active listening.
- Compare and contrast information sharing and therapeutic interviews.
- Identify the phases of group development.
- Identify a goal of Healthy People: 2000 that is related to health education and describe how the characteristics of andragogy can be used to help meet the goal.
- Identify nine factors that are important to the physical learning environment.
- Describe the five components of the learning process.
- Describe the three stages that form the basis of an empowering community-education program.
- Identify elements of a win-win conflict-management strategy.

Communication, the process of using a common set of rules in order to share information, is the core of client–nurse work, dictating its quality and effectiveness. Communication is required of nurses in all situations, especially in the home and community settings, and may take the form of information gathering, therapeutic communication, or teaching. **Information gathering** is obtaining information necessary to carry out the nursing process. **Therapeutic communication** helps the client cope with stress, get along with other people, adapt to situations that cannot be changed, and overcome emotional and mental blocks that prevent evolution of one's potential. **Teaching** is helping another gain knowledge, understanding, or skills by instructing, demonstrating, or guiding the learning process. Whether the job at hand is teaching parenting skills, completing an infant health assessment, counseling a discouraged or rebellious adolescent, or planning and implementing a health-education program, the nurse must be able to communicate caring in a way that is helpful to clients.

Efficient and effective communication is also a necessity in professional relationships, whether one is making referrals, reports, or suggestions; leading groups; chairing meetings; or participating in conflict-resolution activities. This chapter focuses on health care communication skills, adult learning theory, and teaching skills and how these apply in the helping relationship.

HEALTH-RELATED COMMUNICATION

Health communication is communication centering on health-related issues of individuals and groups. It encompasses feelings and attitudes as well as information and is carried out by the use of symbols and language. Transactions are verbal or nonverbal, oral or written, personal or impersonal, issue oriented or relationship oriented.

Contexts for community nurses' communication include **intrapersonal systems, interpersonal systems,** and **social systems,** the latter including small-group, organizational, and public systems. The intrapersonal context is our inner thoughts, beliefs, and feelings, as well as our "self-talk" about issues that influence our health-directed behaviors and attitudes toward our clients and colleagues. Interpersonal contexts include client–nurse, nurse–nurse,

and nurse–other professional situations. In small groups, nurses are involved with client family constellations and in group teaching, treatment or education planning, staff reports, and health-team interactions. Organizational health communication occurs in contexts such as administration, program planning, staff relations, and dialogue with institutions involved in a client's care. Public communication encompasses presentations, speeches, and public addresses made by individuals on health-related topics such as national and world health programs, health promotion, and public health planning.

Carl Rogers' Client-Centered Model

Carl Rogers (1951), a psychologist, set the stage for therapeutic models of communication, which emphasize the important role that relationships play in assisting clients to adjust to their circumstances, move toward health and away from illness, or learn to cope with the illness. When used by health professionals, therapeutic communication can be defined as a skill that helps others find the strength to do what they need to do. It is used to help clients learn to deal with stress, get along with other people, adapt to situations they cannot change, and overcome emotional and mental blocks to achieving their potential.

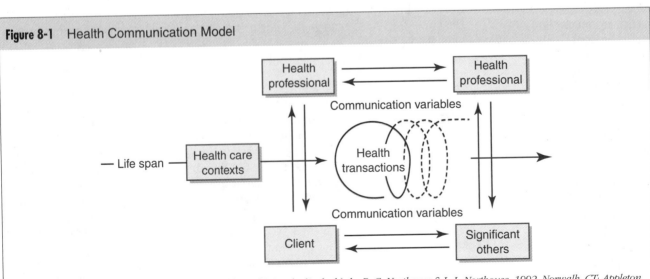

Figure 8-1 Health Communication Model

From Health Communication: Strategies for Health Professionals *(2nd ed.), by P. G. Northouse & L. L. Northouse, 1992, Norwalk, CT: Appleton & Lange, p. 16. Printed with permission by Appleton & Lange.*

Health Communication Model

The Health Communication Model (HCM) (Northouse & Northouse, 1992) focuses specifically on transactions between health care participants about health-related issues. Figure 8-1 shows the variables and directions of communication in this model. The focus is communication that occurs in various kinds of relationships in health care; the three major variables of the health-communication process are **relationships, transactions,** and **contexts.**

Relationships are of four major types: professional–professional, professional–client, professional–significant other, and client–significant other. Transactions are interactions between participants in the health-communication process over the life span and involve both content and relationship dimensions. The spirals in the model reflect the ongoing, transactional nature of the process. In community nursing, the context is usually outside the hospital, typically in homes, clinics, schools, and workplaces. The nature of these settings and the number of people involved also affect health communication.

NURSING-INTERACTION MODELS

Nursing scholars have developed a progression of theories to account for the unique focus of nursing as it applies to interactions with clients and to other health care disciplines. These efforts began when Peplau (1952) identified communication and nurse–client interaction as nursing concerns. The following is a discussion of the nursing theories that ultimately served as the basis for Schubert's Theory of Mutual Connectedness, a practice model emphasizing the importance of communication.

Peplau defines nursing as a therapeutic, interpersonal process requiring supportive communication, including **nonverbal behaviors** which communicate attitudes, meaning, or content to another, either intentionally, through gestures, or unintentionally, through body language). She defines supportive communication as being characterized by **clarity** and **continuity;** that is, the meaning is understood and agreed upon by sender and receiver, and the nurse picks up on threads of the client's meaning in the process of conversation.

Influenced by Peplau, Orlando (1961, 1972) identifies the nursing process as consisting of three basic elements: client behavior, the reaction of the nurse, and nursing actions designed for the client's benefit. Into this framework, Travelbee (1963, 1964, 1971) introduces the concept of **empathy** (understanding the subjective world of another and then communicating that understanding) and the importance of the nurse's caring for the client.

King (1981) depicts nurse–client interactions as acknowledging the influence of perceptions, responsibility for sharing information, and the client's right to participate in decisions influencing his or her health. King places the nurse–client interaction in an open-systems framework

(**open systems** are systems, such as human beings, that exist in interrelationship with their environment, taking in and assimilating energy and eliminating waste).

Rogers' Science of Unitary Human Beings (Rogers, 1990) is based on the premise that human beings and environment are inseparable open systems. This premise enables us to see the nurse as one aspect of the client's environment and vice versa. Thus, anxiety, fear, anger, or nonjudgmental acceptance, for example, is expressed in the nurse's **energy field** (the whole of a person's being as seen in one's presence through observation, sensing, and timing) and is communicated to the client. The reverse is also expected, with the nurse able to sense changes in the client's field, especially when the nurse has sensitized herself to perception of energy (Krieger, 1993).

Rogers' energy field is one way of understanding the phenomena that are at the heart of interpersonal theories of nursing. Empathy, for example, increases awareness of feelings in the other person and communicates a healing atmosphere. With her notions of energy exchange, Rogers' theory complements traditional definitions of interpersonal interaction. On this foundation, Schubert (1989) built a nursing practice theory, as described in the accompanying research focus.

INFLUENCES ON NURSE–CLIENT COMMUNICATION

King's (1981) model, mentioned earlier, introduces the concepts of mutual goal setting and goal attainment in the client–nurse relationship. Schubert's model (Schubert & Lionberger, 1995) emphasizes the importance of communication in implementing these concepts. Before discussing communication skills themselves, one must understand the three aspects of the nurse–client relationship that influence communication in modern nursing: namely, mutual problem solving, the client's evolving level of responsibility in that process, and shifting roles in the client–nurse relationship.

Mutual Problem Solving in the Client–Nurse Relationship

Mutual problem solving depends on the use of validation (Smith, 1992). **Validation** is consciously seeking out the client's opinions and feelings at each step and phase of the nursing process. Implicit in validation are unearthing questions or concerns about plans for health care and securing understanding and willingness to proceed to the next step (see Figure 8-3).

Contracts or agreements between the client and nurse constitute useful tools in the mutual problem-solving process. The contract outlines the activities and responsibilities for which each will be accountable.

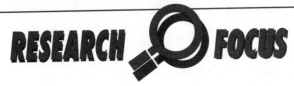

Mutual Connectedness: A Qualitative Study of Caring in the Client–Nurse Relationship

STUDY PROBLEM/PURPOSE

To generate a grounded theory of caring in client–nurse interaction.

METHODS

The setting under study was independent private practice in the community (Schubert, 1989). This practice was described as providing counseling, teaching, imagery, and touch therapies within a setting and interpersonal environment created with the goals of caring and the promotion of health and healing. Because it required nurse autonomy and depended heavily on the client–nurse interrelationship, the setting was considered an exemplar for healing through caring.

Nurses in private practice (n=12) and their new clients (n=18) participated in the study. Data were obtained through one face-to-face taped interview with each nurse prior to the nurse's meeting the client participants and three interviews with each client over a three-month period. Information was elicited from the nurses to discover (1) whether they met the predetermined criteria of using counseling, teaching, imagery, and touch therapies and (2) their interactional stances. Clients described their respective experiences; perceptions of and responses to the nurses' behavior in the relationship; and any perceived changes in their own health status or lifestyle. Grounded theory strategies were employed.

FINDINGS

The Theory of Mutual Connectedness emerged through analysis of the interactional data. Major concepts that surfaced were intimacy, mutual connectedness, nursing therapies, and healing. In a secondary analysis (Schubert & Lionberger, 1995), the concept of caring environment replaced intimacy, and intimacy became the outcome of the caring environment category. Figure 8-2 illustrates the develop-

ment of mutual connectedness, which seemed to vary with the conditions of nurse readiness and client decision to trust (Figure 8-2).

Conceptual linkages for theory development were as follows: Mutual connectedness served as the context for nursing therapeutics and occurred under conditions of a caring environment; nursing therapies served as strategies for facilitation of healing by aiding letting-go processes and self-transformation.

This theory provides an explanation of interactional processes that either facilitate or deter healing in the client–nurse relationship. Table 8-1 indicates the linkages of the major categories and concepts (Schubert & Lionberger, 1995). The table is best understood by reading from top to bottom and left to right. The Properties cells represent identified qualities of the concept being addressed. The Conditions cells represent readiness for beginning strategies. Conditions acted on by strategies produce outcomes. Outcomes for each of the first three major categories become conditions for the next. This undulating movement builds across the table, triggered by properties of each major category (Schubert & Lionberger, 1995).

IMPLICATIONS

The descriptive and explorative study provides beginning knowledge and understanding of caring in this community nursing role. It further suggests the importance of communication skills in optimizing the nurse–client relationship in community nursing.

SOURCE

From Mutual Connectedness: Holistic Nursing Practice under Varying Conditions of Intimacy by P. Schubert, 1989, doctoral dissertation, University of California, San Francisco, Dissertation Abstracts International, 50, *p. 4987B. Copyright 1989 by P. Schubert.*
From "Mutual Connectedness: A Study of Client–Nurse Interaction Using the Grounded Theory Method. by P. E. Schubert and H. J. Lionberger, 1995, Journal of Holistic Nursing, 13, *pp. 102–116. Copyright 1995 by P. Schubert & H Lionberger.*

Client's Evolving Level of Responsibility

In all interactions with a client, the nurse must be alert for indications of how much responsibility the client wants or is willing to assume. The nurse's communication skills are crucial as changes occur. Clients who have a clear understanding of their health problems and those things that they and their nurse can do about those problems will expend less energy worrying and more energy doing something constructive. Having clarity regarding nursing diagnoses and having a say in the best ways to handle the diagnoses give clients a sense of control.

Consumers today are speaking up, asking questions,

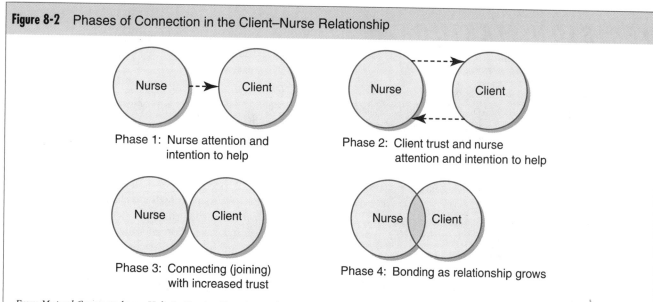

Figure 8-2 Phases of Connection in the Client–Nurse Relationship

Phase 1: Nurse attention and intention to help

Phase 2: Client trust and nurse attention and intention to help

Phase 3: Connecting (joining) with increased trust

Phase 4: Bonding as relationship grows

From Mutual Connectedness: Holistic Nursing Practice under Varying Conditions of Intimacy by P. Schubert, 1989, doctoral dissertation, University of California, San Francisco, Dissertation Abstracts International, 50, *p. 4987B.*

Table 8-1	**Theory of Mutual Connectedness: Categories and Conceptual Linkages**			
MAJOR CATEGORY	**CARING ENVIRONMENT**	**MUTUAL CONNECTEDNESS**	**NURSING THERAPY**	**HEALING**
Properties	Safety Nurturance Respect Beauty	Trust Compassion Shared consciousness	Identification and enhancement of health patterns	Inner directed Unpredictable Nature's time frame
Conditions	Nurse readiness Client comfort with intimacy	Intimacy and trust become bonding	Works roles formed	Releasing old and introducing new patterns
Strategies	Nurse centering Client inner negotiation for trust	Both parties listening and opening	Counseling Teaching Touch therapies Imagery	Self-acceptance worked on by each party
Outcomes	Intimacy Client decision to trust and bond	Roles formed for further work	Releasing old and introducing new patterns	Transformation Evolution of self-potential Creativity

From Mutual Connectedness: A Study of Client–Nurse Interaction Using the Grounded Theory Method by P. Schubert & H. Lionberger, 1995, Journal of Holistic Nursing, 13, *pp. 102–116. Copyright 1995 by P. Schubert and H. Lionberger. Reprinted with permission.*

seeking second opinions, demanding alternative health care options, and forming self-help groups. This assertiveness and independence reflect the true meaning of the label "client"—one who claims the rights and privileges of partnership in health care (Balzer-Riley, 1996). Figure 8-4 lists client privileges.

Smith (1992) encourages nurses to transform all client–nurse relationships into relationships of mutual problem solving and participation by calling on the strengths of the clients and inviting—even requesting—their full participation as partners in the process. Active listening, discussed below, is a useful tool for accomplishing this goal.

Shifting Roles in the Client–Nurse Relationship

The importance of communication skills is evident in Schubert's (1989) study of private community nursing clients. Interviews revealed diverse and shifting patterns of roles taken by the nurse and client over time. Clients reported a parent–child or a teacher–student relationship, a partnership, or they saw the nurse as serving as the catalyst for growth. Some nurses were particularly adept at shifting their roles as their clients were able to take more responsibility for their health and healing. These roles

DECISION MAKING

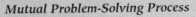

Mutual Problem-Solving Process

The school principal has referred fourteen-year-old Juan to the clinic where you work. The principal says the boy complains of stomachaches every day and refuses to participate in physical-education activities. You interview Juan and learn that there are many problems. First of all, he has received major orthodontic treatment and has braces on his teeth. This work was financially supported by a migrant health program provided by the school nurses in the area. Juan says the orthodontist told him not to get hit with a ball. Juan had imagined that if he got hit anywhere on his body, his teeth would fall out. You reassure him and explain the dentist's instruction. You ask Juan about his family, and, as you ask questions and he hesitantly answers, you get an idea about the family. There are nine children, of which he is the third; his father is out of work; they have no money to buy food; and Juan is afraid his father is going to kill a neighbor.

As you talk about all of Juan's concerns you ask, "What is your biggest worry?" He responds, "I do not know how to work my combination lock at school. I have to find someone to help me all the time, and I am always late for class. The teachers are mad at me."

• What would you do first?

• Develop a plan including support for Juan at school, a home visit, and potential community resources for the family.

were experienced in alternating rhythms by both nurses and clients as clients took more or less responsibility in the different areas of their lives.

COMMUNICATION SKILLS

A nurse's abilities to comprehend the client's needs and to successfully exchange information are always crucial. In community health nursing, the process is complicated

෨෨ REFLECTIVE THINKING ෨෨

Passive or Active Client Role?

• Put yourself in the role of a person seeking health care. Would you choose a passive role or a more active and responsible role as client? Why?

• As the nurse, how might you support your client in taking a more active and responsible role in the relationship?

Figure 8-3 The Mutual Problem-Solving Process

• Collect data.
• Analyze data.
• Validate your interpretation of data with the client.
• Identify actual or potential problems in collaboration with the client.
• Validate the nursing diagnoses with the client.
• Set priorities for resolution of identified problems in collaboration with the client.
• Determine expected and desired outcomes of nursing actions in collaboration with the client.
• Decide on the nursing strategies to achieve those outcomes in collaboration with the client.
• Implement nursing actions with assistance from the client.
• Encourage client participation in carrying out nursing actions.
• Evaluating the outcomes of nursing care in consultation with the client.

From Communications in Nursing: Communicating Assertively and Responsibly in Nursing: A Guidebook (3rd ed., p. 42) by J. Balzer-Riley, 1996, St. Louis: Mosby. Printed with permission by Mosby-Yearbook.

Figure 8-4 Client Privileges in the Helping Relationship

Clients, as consumers of our health care services, have a right to:

• Expect a systematic and accurate investigation of their health concerns by a thorough and well-organized nurse.

• Be informed about their health status and have all their questions answered so that they clearly understand the information communicated by the nurse.

• Receive health care from a nurse who has current knowledge about their diagnoses and is capable of providing safe and efficient care.

• Feel confident that they will be treated courteously and that the nurse will show genuine interest in them.

• Trust that confidentiality will be respected.

• Be informed about any plans of action to be carried out for their benefit.

• Refuse or consent to nursing treatments without jeopardizing the relationship with the nurse.

• Secure help conveniently and without impediments.

• Receive consistent quality of care from all nurses.

Adapted from Communications in Nursing: Communicating Assertively and Responsibly in Nursing: A Guidebook (2nd ed., pp. 27–28) by S. Smith, 1992, St. Louis: Mosby. Printed with permission by Mosby-Yearbook.

by the variety of situations wherein communication occurs. In every instance, active listening enhances the process. A discussion of this skill is followed by discussions of a number of applications including interviewing, group process, teaching, conflict management, translating in cross-cultural communication, and public speaking.

Active Listening

Active listening, also called reflective listening, focuses on feelings and thoughts, demonstrating the inherent value of the client's needs as compared with those of the health care world. The nurse focuses attention first on the client and then shifts the focus back to processing knowledge of the client's feelings in order to develop a plan of things to say or do that will be in the client's best interest.

In active listening, the nurse verbally reflects as closely as possible the content of the client's statement, any feelings heard or observed, the nuance and strength of those feelings, and the reasons for those feelings. Four kinds of reflection are commonly used: paraphrasing, feelings reflection, meanings reflection, and summative reflection.

Parroting the same words back is irritating and implies lack of understanding. **Paraphrasing,** on the other hand, lets the client know how much has been understood and invites clarification if the nurse has missed an important part of the message. The following is an example of this skill:

Client: We get a little further behind financially every month. I'm thinking about taking a job helping to serve lunches at school, but it will take almost all the free time I have now. And I don't know what I'll do if one of the kids gets sick.

Nurse: You want to help out by earning some extra money, but you are not clear yet how getting a job will affect your responsibilities at home.

Sometimes a client's difficulties are related more to his or her feelings about a situation than to the situation itself. Words or body language, or both, may alert the nurse to such a situation, especially if the two are incongruent. In such a case, **feelings reflection** can be used to help the client recognize and deal with feelings. The nurse might say, for example, "You seem tense as you talk about that," giving the client an opportunity to clarify.

In feelings reflection, the words chosen by the nurse must match the feelings expressed by the client verbally or otherwise. For any given feeling, the nurse may have many corresponding words from which to choose. For instance, the corresponding empathic word for *feeling afraid* might be any of the following: *afraid, agonized, alarmed, anxious, apprehensive, cautious, concerned, disturbed, in dread, fearful, fidgety, frightened, hesitant, ill at ease, in a cold sweat, jittery, jumpy, nervous, on edge, panicky, petrified, quaking, quivering, restless, scared, shaken, tense, terrified, trembling, troubled, uncomfortable, uneasy, wary,* or *worried* (Smith, 1992).

Figure 8-5   Characteristics of the Effective Helper

Warmth: Showing warmth to others means conveying that you like to be with them and accept them as they are. It is usually displayed nonverbally by subtle facial expressions, body language, and gestures. Culturally prescribed rules for displaying warmth are related to factors such as the need, occupation, status, role position, and gender of the people involved.

Respect: Respect means accepting others for who they are rather than on condition of certain behaviors or characteristics. Behaviors characteristic of respect are looking at the client, giving undivided attention, maintaining eye contact (in some cultures), moving toward the client, determining how the client likes to be addressed, making contact by handshaking or gentle touching, making it clear who you are and what your role is, and being clear about how you can help. In some situations, a deeper respect based on belief in the client's ability to learn and to change requires that the nurse challenge the client in different ways.

Genuineness: Genuineness is behavior congruent with thoughts and feelings. If we pretend our thoughts and feelings are different from what they are, we say things we do not believe. If we act on thoughts and feelings we do not have, we give the wrong impression about ourselves. We tend to lack genuineness when we feel at risk for rejection.

Specificity: Being specific involves giving concrete details so that communication is focused, clear, and logical. When the nurse helps the client to address concerns specifically, clarity and self-understanding are increased for both parties.

Empathy: Empathy is the act of communicating understanding of the client's feelings (see active listening discussion) and is nonjudgmental and accepting. The benefit to the client often is tremendous relief because the need to struggle to be heard or to justify reactions is eliminated.

Self-disclosure: Self-disclosure is one's willingness to be known to others. Thoughts, feelings, and experiences should be revealed only for the sake of the client. The nurse self-discloses to show understanding that derives from similar thoughts and experiences. Consider two questions before self-disclosing: Is the disclosure likely to demonstrate understanding? Will I feel safe from repercussions and embarrassment—that is, legally, morally, and emotionally secure—if I reveal this information to my client? Each question should get a clear affirmative answer before proceeding with self-disclosure.

Confrontation: Confrontation is pointing out incongruities or discrepancies between beliefs, attitudes, thoughts, and behaviors. It is an invitation for persons to examine their behavior honestly when that behavior invades the rights of the nurse or others or is destructive to the client or others. Confrontation encourages change by placing respectful emphasis on positive outcomes

Adapted from Communications in Nursing: Communicating Assertively and Responsibly in Nursing: A Guidebook. (3rd ed.) by J. Balzer-Riley, 1996, St. Louis: Mosby. Printed with permission by Mosby-Yearbook.

Meanings reflection is a response that addresses meanings and facts together in one phrase. Suppose, for example, that a client describes satisfaction regarding a new job that a family member has just found in another town but at the same time is frowning and is hunched in the shoulders. Upon hearing the information being communicated and witnessing the incongruent body language, the nurse might respond, "You're proud of your child's success but a little fearful about being separated for the first time."

A **summative reflection** groups the topics discussed in a foregoing conversation into several categories so that the client and nurse can have a clear idea of those things that have been accomplished and those things that remain to be done. For example:

> We have talked about how you are caring for your colostomy and how your relationships have been affected since the surgery. You asked about relaxation exercises and whether they might help with your nervousness about what is happening; so, unless you have some other questions, we can do some work on that before I go.

The community nurse's use of active listening can facilitate some of the client privileges listed in Figure 8-4. Figure 8-5 lists some characteristics of effective helpers that either enhance or are enhanced by active listening. Although this significant body of work was originated by Truax and Carkhuff (1967) for the counseling profession, it provides a theoretical foundation for all the helping professions today. In fact, effective helping theory is currently being used to teach communication skills to nurses (Balzer-Riley, 1996). The characteristics and associated skills are applicable whether the nurse is teaching or counseling individuals, families, or groups; facilitating or participating in committee- or work-related meetings; engaging in public speaking; or presenting educational materials for mass media.

INTERVIEWING

Northouse and Northouse (1992) define the interview as purposeful and serious interpersonal communication, usually involving questions and answers, with the goal of sharing information or facilitating therapeutic outcomes. Effective questioning saves time and elicits pertinent and useful information. Figure 8-6 lists guidelines for asking questions. Helping interviews are of two types: information sharing and therapeutic.

Information-Sharing Interviews

Information-sharing interviews center on the request for and provision of information, with the focus being on content rather than on relationship or feelings. This type of interview is useful for admission and history taking,

---

Figure 8-6 Guidelines for Asking Questions

- The client is the best person to interview, when possible. If it is helpful to ask questions of family members, this should be done in the presence of the client or with the client's permission. There are, of course, times when clients cannot answer questions, and the nurse will have to find the appropriate persons from whom to obtain the necessary information.

- Find an appropriate place and time within the home, clinic, or other community setting where and when there is privacy to ask questions without interruptions.

- Be sure both you and the client know why you are asking a question. When clients understand your purpose for asking they are more likely to be open and to reveal information.

- Respect your client's privacy. Explain confidentiality. What will be kept confidential? With whom will you share this information? There is no way to know what areas may be sensitive for the client, so the nurse must assume that all the questions may touch on sensitive issues.

- Be sure the client has time to respond unhurriedly. Allow the client to answer one question before asking another, and give clients plenty of time to offer their thoughts about a question before you jump in with your opinions, beliefs, and advice.

- Consider what you will ask and how you will phrase your question so that your client will want to respond. Phrase questions clearly and present them in a logical progression.

- Avoid asking "why" questions because they tend to be threatening or intimidating.

- Avoid using medical jargon. Instead, use language the client understands.

- Keep the client informed by giving feedback on the data collection or the problem-solving process.

Adapted from Communications in Nursing: Communicating Assertively and Responsibly in Nursing: A Guidebook (2nd ed., pp. 127–139) by S. Smith, 1992, St. Louis: Mosby.

---

relies primarily on closed questions, and assumes a **directive approach**, meaning that the nurse defines the nature of the client's problem, prescribes appropriate solutions, and provides specific, concrete information needed for problem solving. **Closed questions** restrict the client to providing specific information; **open questions** (addressed in the discussion of therapeutic interviews, below) do not restrict the client's responses. Closed questions, used in health care to gather demographic data, medical histories, or diagnostic information, often ask for a "yes" or "no" answer. For example:

"Have you ever had surgery?"

"Is there a history of heart problems in your family?"

The directive approach is efficient; interviews focus on the problem and take less time than other approaches. There are, however, disadvantages, to the directive approach. Assessment information known only to the client is missed. The nurse may then, in turn, give the client erroneous information or make decisions before getting necessary information about the client's situation. Ineffective or misdirected solutions may in turn result.

Conversational Interviews

Brown (1995) suggests, as an alternative to the information-sharing interview, the **conversational interview,** which combines elements of the information-sharing interview with a more personal style. This approach is more flexible and client focused than the directive approach. Rather than having the client answer a lot of questions, the nurse encourages the client to tell his or her story without interruption, eliciting information about the client's feelings regarding his or her health or illness situation. Consistent with the active role of clients, this approach provides more complete data on which to base a nursing diagnosis, allows for a more comfortable health care–assessment encounter, and affords the client more control during the encounter. As a result, clients often disclose more, feel freer to ask questions, and more readily reveal their concerns and levels of knowledge.

Therapeutic Interviews

Therapeutic interviews are designed to help clients identify and work through personal issues, concerns, and problems. Clients feel free to express their personal thoughts and feelings, gain new insights, develop new problem-solving strategies, and find better ways of coping with their experiences. Therapeutic interviews frequently involve open questions and either a directive or a nondirective approach. A **nondirective approach** encourages clients to seek solutions to their own problems and to express thoughts and feelings.

Open questions do not restrict the client's responses; rather, they allow extended and unlimited answers. Open questions are a means of providing an opportunity for clients to freely disclose their situations and problems. For example:

"You seem concerned. Tell me what is bothering you."

"Describe what you think might happen to you."

"How do you think we are doing in meeting our contract?"

The nondirective approach is based on the assumption that the client is the person best able to identify and resolve his or her problems. Advantages of this approach are interrelated. Inherent in the nondirective approach is acknowledgment of the client's potential for identifying and solving problems; thus, one advantage is increased opportunity of identifying and therefore addressing the problem experienced by the client. Furthermore, the enhanced sense of control associated with being an active participant increases probability of client follow-through on making necessary changes.

Phases in the Interview Process

Interviews take place in clinics, homes, schools, meeting houses, hospitals, public places—every place that people go and live. The length of an interview depends on the goal of the interview, the severity of the client's problem, the skills of the clinician, and the number of problem areas that emerge. Less time is needed when the goal is information sharing rather than therapeutic change, when the client's personality is well integrated as opposed to severely disorganized, and when there is a single problem rather than several. In the following discussion, Northouse and Northouse's (1992) interview phases for health professionals are adapted for community health nurses.

The Preparation Phase

The preparation phase involves anticipating and planning for the interview. In a community health setting, a nurse who receives a referral from another agency may have considerable information about the client before the initial meeting with the client. Likewise, the client often seeks information about a nurse before the initial meeting by consulting with friends, relatives, or other professionals. Nurse preparation may include researching recent treatment advances, preparing assessment forms and educational materials, or locating an appropriate place to meet. The nurse also arranges for a comfortable setting by, for example, ensuring that there are enough chairs to accommodate a family.

A second task of this phase is self-assessment (Stuart & Laraia, 1998). Self-assessment means that the nurse sorts through personal feelings and biases and, if necessary, seeks help in resolving personal anxieties related to problem areas. **Centering** oneself in the present moment and focusing attention on the well-being of the client is another part of preparation. It can be accomplished by sitting quietly and taking a breath or two while drawing one's attention inward and focusing on the task at hand.

The Initiation Phase

The initiation phase begins with the first face-to-face client–nurse contact. After reconciling initial expectations of each other, the first task is to establish a therapeutic, nonthreatening climate that will foster trust and understanding. A brief period of commonplace talk gives participants time to adjust to the setting and to each other (e.g., "Did you have any trouble finding the clinic?" or "Your directions were excellent; I had no problem finding you").

The next task is to clarify the purpose of the interview. A community health nurse on a first home visit, for example, might say, "We talked on the phone about my coming to share ideas on home care for your baby when your baby comes home from the hospital next week" or "I know you have some concerns about caring for the colostomy. We can talk about those concerns today and tomorrow I can come back to teach you how to do colostomy care." At this point, the contract can be formulated and mutual goals established. Northouse and Northouse (1992) identify common initiation-phase errors: a vague explanation of the interview purpose by the nurse, a premature attempt to elicit personal information from the client, or a drifting on the part of either party into social conversation to avoid feelings of discomfort.

The Exploration, or Working, Phase

The exploration phase is the time to confront, analyze, and work on the client's problems. The nurse tries to help clients master anxieties, increase their sense of independence and responsibility, and acquire new coping abilities (Stuart & Laraia, 1998). Clients often will first introduce a lesser problem and decide whether to trust the nurse with a more important problem on the basis of how the lesser problem was handled. A second task in this phase is to help clients manage feelings generated by the discussion of issues. In an atmosphere of acceptance and support, the nurse can help clients manage and express their feelings.

Common errors by nurses in this phase are loss of focus and changing the topic or giving insufficient feedback to help the client continue the discussion. Other errors include giving inappropriate advice, approval, or reassurances and responding in stereotyped ways such as the overuse of reflective statements.

The Termination Phase

The termination phase is a time to acknowledge that the purpose for the interview has been met and that it is time to end a meaningful relationship. Termination is often difficult because, along with the feelings of joy associated

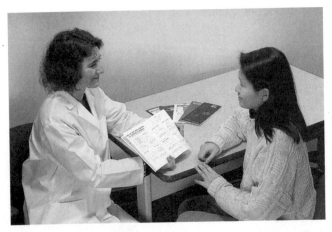

The exploration phase is the time to confront, analyze, and work on the client's problem.

with meeting goals, termination can evoke feelings of sadness, fear, or uncertainty. The major task, thus, is to plan for closure. This is a part of the contract and should therefore be a part of the discussion throughout the entire interview or set of interviews. Finally, the nurse helps the client express feelings about termination. Feelings are often mixed; although termination may be desired, it is common for the client to also feel sadness, anger, abandonment, guilt, and helplessness (Northouse & Northouse, 1992).

Community nurses who make home visits to families over a period of time often find it very difficult to simply say goodbye to their clients and sometimes instead say things like "I will stop to see you now and then" or "I will call to see how you are." These ways of saying goodbye leave expectations that often go unfulfilled, causing unnecessary pain and disappointment. At the other extreme, nurses must guard against feeling uncertain and quickly terminating the interaction. They may allow too little time to deal with the feelings, bring up emotional issues that should have been dealt with earlier, or avoid termination issues, feeling that they have not been helpful to the client. It is useful to anticipate these feelings in order to effectively negotiate them.

COMMUNICATION BARRIERS

Communication barriers are responses that affect communication in a negative way. Gordon (1970) identifies three general categories of barriers: judgment, sending solutions, and avoidance of others' concerns. Most likely to be destructive when one or more involved persons are interacting under stress, barriers can diminish self-esteem and trigger defensiveness, resistance, and resentment. Barriers can also lead to withdrawal, dependency, and feelings of defeat or inadequacy, and they can decrease the likelihood that the client will find a solution to the problem. Further, each barrier can reduce the probability that all parties will constructively express their true feelings. Over time, these negative effects can cause permanent damage to relationships.

GROUP MEMBERSHIP AND LEADERSHIP

During the past decade, groups have been used for many discussion and therapy functions that once were performed on an individual basis (or not at all). The number of self-help groups has increased dramatically in recent years, and many other types of groups are now being formed to teach clients how to maintain health and to overcome or cope with illness. There are fitness groups, relaxation groups, nutrition groups, health-education groups, and support groups. Groups among health professionals are also more plentiful. Interdisciplinary groups, advisory groups, task forces, management groups, stress-reduction groups, and care-for-the-caregiver groups are some of these professionally oriented groups (Northouse & Northouse, 1992).

The community nurse is often called on to be a group member or leader in one or several such groups. It is imperative, therefore, that the nurse understand how groups work and how members communicate within groups. Communication is the process that connects members to one another and enables them to work interdependently.

Small-group communication refers to the verbal and nonverbal communication that occurs among three or more individuals who are interdependent to some degree. **Content-oriented groups** focus on tasks and goals. **Process-oriented groups** focus on relating to and getting along with people. **Midrange groups** focus on a blend of process and content or tasks (Loomis, 1979). Some major components of groups are goals, norms, cohesiveness, leader behavior, member behavior, and curative factors that influence group functioning. Because they are concerned with how the group works, the first three components are considered here under the general heading of group behaviors. The last three components are treated separately. The phases of group development are then reviewed. It should be noted that these discussions are necessarily brief and that the student is encouraged to seek more in-depth training in small-group leadership.

Group Behaviors

Its goals provide the reason for the existence of the group. Group goals and individual goals exist simultaneously in any group and must be compatible in order for the group to succeed. Norms are the rules of behavior established and shared by group members. Overt norms are those verbally agreed-on rules known to the members; covert norms are not usually verbally acknowledged by the group members. An example of a covert norm might be that when one person talks, the others listen. Cohesiveness is a sense of "we-ness," the cement that holds groups together. High cohesiveness is frequently associated with increased participation, consistent attendance, and high member satisfaction.

Leader Behaviors

Leadership is the process whereby one person attempts to influence others in order to attain some mutually agreed-on goal. In groups, leader behavior has a strong effect on member interactions. An effective leader selects communication methods that are likely to have a positive impact on followers and will move the group toward its goals. Emergent leaders are verbally active and fluent and express their thoughts articulately in group interaction.

Figure 8-7   Constructive Group Member Behaviors

- **Initiator-contributor:** Suggests new ideas or a new way of viewing the group task.
- **Information seeker:** Asks for clarification or for additional information about the problem being discussed.
- **Opinion seeker:** Asks for clarification of values that may be involved in the goal or task that the group is discussing.
- **Information giver:** Offers facts or personal experiences that are related to problems being discussed by the group.
- **Elaborator:** Expands on ideas being discussed by offering an example or the rationale for a suggestion.
- **Coordinator:** Pulls together various ideas and suggestions made by group members or tries to coordinate group activities.
- **Orientor:** Defines the present position of the group in relation to its goals or raises questions about the direction in which the discussion is moving.
- **Evaluator-critic:** Considers the practicality or logic of suggestions offered in the group.
- **Energizer:** Stimulates the group toward an action or a decision.
- **Procedural technician:** Assists group movement by carrying out routine tasks for the group.
- **Recorder:** Writes down suggestions or activities decided on by the group.

Adapted from Health Communication: Strategies for Health Professionals by P. G. Northouse & L. L. Northouse, 1992, (2nd ed., pp. 195–197) Norwalk, CT: Appleton & Lange. Printed with permission by Appleton & Lange.

They initiate new ideas in conferences, seek opinions from others, and express their own opinions with firmness but not rigidity (Northouse & Northouse, 1992).

Member Behaviors

Member behavior is just as important as leader behavior. Some member behaviors are constructive to the group process, and some are destructive. Roles of group members are classified into three broad categories: group-task roles, group-building and group-maintenance roles, and individual roles (Northouse & Northouse, 1992).

Group-task roles are identified as follows: initiator–contributor, information seeker, opinion seeker, information giver, elaborator, coordinator, orientor, evaluator–critic, energizer, procedural technician, and recorder (see Figure 8-7). Group-building and group-maintenance roles promote cohesiveness among group members. The role names reflect constructive participation in the work of the group. They are: encourager, harmonizer, compromiser,

Figure 8-8   Destructive Group Member Behaviors

- **Aggressor:** Attacks or disapproves of others' suggestions, feelings, or values.
- **Blocker:** Resists, without good reason, or becomes extremely negative to others' suggestions.
- **Recognition seeker:** Calls attention repeatedly to own accomplishments and diverts the group's attention.
- **Self-confessor:** Uses the group's time to express personal, non-group-oriented feelings or comments.
- **Playboy/playgirl:** Plays around and displays other behavior that indicates that he or she is not involved in the group process.
- **Dominator:** Tries repeatedly to assert own authority and often interrupts other group members.
- **Help seeker:** Tries to elicit sympathy from other group members.
- **Special interest pleader:** Speaks for a particular group or person (e.g. the union, the unemployed, the American people) but is really using the group to meet personal needs and to cloak personal biases and prejudices.

Adapted from Health Communication: Strategies for Health Professionals by P. G. Northouse & L. L. Northouse, 1992, (2nd ed., pp. 195–197) Norwalk, CT: Appleton & Lange. Printed with permission by Appleton & Lange.

gatekeeper, standard setter, group observer, and follower. Some of the related effects of these various roles are cited in the discussion of curative factors, below.

Individual roles are those roles that are not helpful to the group. Named for behaviors reflecting the participant's psychological needs rather than the needs of the group, these roles are: aggressor, blocker, recognition seeker, self-confessor, playboy/playgirl, dominator, help seeker, and special-interest pleader (see Figure 8-8).

Curative Factors

Curative factors exert a therapeutic influence on the group members. Yalom (1983) identifies these positive factors as

✺✺ REFLECTIVE THINKING ✺✺

Group-Membership Roles

- Which group-task roles do you usually play?
- Which group-building and group-maintenance roles do you usually play?
- Which of these roles do you need to practice?
- Do you play an individual role in groups?

(1) instillation of hope as members realize others have succeeded or overcome similar issues; (2) universality, with the realization that one is not alone; (3) information sharing with each other; (4) altruism as members help each other; (5) corrective recapitulation of the primary family group as parallel relationships occur in the group and in the member's family; (6) development of socializing techniques or development of needed social skills; (7) imitative behavior as the leader and other members model desirable behavior; (8) interpersonal learning as members provide one another with feedback regarding interpersonal behavior; (9) catharsis as members learn to express feelings appropriately coupled with interpersonal learning; and (10) existential factors as members realize that life is sometimes not fair and we must take responsibility for the way we live our lives.

Phases of Group Development

One popular version of group development phases is presented by Tuckman (1965): forming, norming, storming, and performing. Yalom (1975) conceives of these phases as orientation, conflict, cohesion, and working and adds termination. Short-term and ad hoc groups may move through these phases in a single session, whereas long-term groups may spend weeks in a single phase.

Orientation

In the orientation period, the task is to assess the members' purposes for joining the group and to figure out where they fit in the group. Communication during this phase is often stereotypic and restricted. Leadership during this phase is directed toward helping members satisfy their needs for belonging. This involves helping them to feel a part of the group but also to feel a sense of privacy and independence. In addition, the leader provides structure, establishes group guidelines, shapes norms, and assists members in understanding their roles in the overall functioning of the group.

Conflict

The conflict phase occurs as members become interested in control issues such as how they are influencing the group. Each wants to be perceived by others as a competent group member with something to offer. Conflicts arise in this struggle for control, and the work of the leader is to help the members accept and work through group conflicts. As members satisfy their needs for control, conflicts lessen, and the group moves on.

Cohesion

The cohesion phase occurs as members realize that time is moving on and work needs to be done; they become more understanding and accepting of one another, and there surfaces a desire to move closer to one another but not too close. The leader has only to provide guidance and direction as needed and, thus, plays a lesser role during this time.

Working

The working phase is similar to the cohesion phase but is longer. The members actually perform the work they set out to do. Group spirit and a feeling of unity among members are often high during this time. The work of the leader is similar to that in the cohesion phase.

Termination

The termination phase occurs when the work has been completed or the allotted time is running out. The end of the group is a loss, and this phase is a time for sharing the whole range of emotions, from guilt to fear, depending on each person's experience with termination. The leader must summarize the work of the group, emphasize goals that have been achieved, and help group members find a sense of closure as they confront their feelings about the approaching end of the group meetings and member relationships.

TEACHING/LEARNING

The **teaching/learning process** involves all the communication skills described previously and is a part of almost every nursing intervention, whether with individuals or groups. As hospital stays become shorter and nurses increasingly care for clients in ambulatory and home settings, the importance of the nurse's role in assisting clients to understand their health care needs and to care for themselves takes on additional importance.

The mandate from Healthy People: 2000 emphasizes aggregate client education (see Appendix A) (U.S. Department of Health and Human Services, 1996). Health education is a key component of health-promotion programs and is emphasized as the major strategy for achieving the global target of health for all by the year 2000.

Adult-Learning Theory

Whereas traditional teaching/learning methods (**pedagogy**) tend to emphasize passive learning (often through short-term lecture methods), current thinking is that **andragogy** is a more appropriate approach to health education. Andragogy, which addresses the learner's need to be a part of the process rather than a passive recipient, fits well with teaching self-care. Table 8-2 clarifies the differences between the two approaches. Tones, Tilford, and Robinson (1990) believe that the **client-centered** approach is self-empowering for the learner.

Knowles (1990) delineates four variables of teaching behavior: warmth, indirectness, cognitive organization, and enthusiasm. **Warmth,** as defined in Figure 8-5, conveys to someone that he or she is liked and is accepted. **Indirectness** means guiding the learner to find his or her own way rather than supplying pat answers to problems. Knowles notes, however, that the andragogical model, while espousing active learning, does allow for the provision of directed information when necessary. For instance, it is appropriate to give a mother instructions about how to change her daughter's dressing as long as time is provided for her to practice the skill and ask questions about the procedure.

Cognitive organization refers to an intellectual grasp of the material required of any effective teacher, and **enthusiasm** refers to interest and excitement about the subject being taught. These teaching behaviors are congruent with the nursing profession's concept of caring.

Table 8-2 **Comparison of Pedagogy and Andragogy**	
PEDAGOGY	**ANDRAGOGY**
1. Learners must learn what the teacher teaches—not how it applies to learners' lives.	1. Learners need to know why they need to learn.
2. Learner's concept of self reflects teacher's concept of learner—that of a dependent personality.	2. Learners have self-concept of being responsible for own decisions and lives.
3. Learner's experience of little worth. What counts are the individual experience of the teacher and the media used for teaching.	3. Quality of experience: individual differences, life experiences, biases, self-identity derived from experiences.
4. In order to pass, learners become ready to learn what the teacher tells them to learn.	4. Ready to learn what they need to know to cope with life situations.
5. Subject-centered orientation: learning is acquiring subject-matter content.	5. Life-centered (or task-centered or problem-centered) orientation to learning.
6. Learners motivated to learn by external motivators.	6. Most potent motivator is internal pressure to learn.

Adapted from The Adult Learner *(4th ed., pp. 54–63) by M. Knowles, 1990, Houston: Gulf.*

Approaches to Client Education

Three dimensions of client education must be considered. They are client-education models, types of teaching, and modalities for teaching.

Models

Client-education models provide frameworks that help the nurse understand client motivation for participating in health care practices that promote healthier lifestyles. Two such commonly used models are the Health Belief Model and Pender's Health Promotion Model (see Chapter 9). They represent compliance models focusing on the variables that motivate clients to follow or not to follow recommended behaviors that facilitate health. These models tend to emphasize professional, rather than personal, health expectations. Tones et al. (1990) call these models the Preventive Models and note that the emphasis on client compliance has a blaming-the-victim quality.

On the other hand, the Self-Regulation Model (also discussed in Chapter 9) suggests that personal meanings and responses to illness may be the critical factors in client decision making related to health (Rankin & Stallings, 1996). It does not, however, address how emotions and social activities are affected or how "valued social activities affect emotional adjustment to illness, health definitions, and health practices" (p. 48). Snyder (1993) notes that, congruent with the Self-Regulation Model, in order to provide consumer-focused care, nurses must "develop critical thinking skills that utilize logical/analytical and intuitive/creative approaches to solving problems" (p. 206). **Critical thinking** involves looking at a situation from multiple perspectives. The purpose is to help clients make use of the knowledge they already have and be able to reason through difficult problems.

Empowerment education, another approach that reflects **self-efficacy** (the power to produce effects and intended results on one's own health and in one's own life), is particularly applicable to community health education. **Empowerment education** is based on Freire's (1983) ideas. Wallerstein and Bernstein (1988) describe this process as "the collective knowledge that emerges from a group sharing experiences and understanding the social influences that affect individual lives" (p. 382). The purpose of empowerment education is human liberation so that learners are a part of their own destinies. Freire's ideas are similar to health education's guiding principles; that is, start with the community's concerns, use active learning methods, and engage clients in determining their own needs and priorities. It is up to the group to raise its themes for mutual reflection and for the health educator to contribute information afterward.

Three stages to establishing an empowering education program are as follows:

1. Listen so as to understand the felt issues or themes of the community. Community members and health providers are equal partners in identifying problems and determining priorities. Community members are active in all program stages.

2. Institute a problem-posing dialogue about issues. This process is called *problem posing* rather than *problem solving* because the problems explored through this process are complex, do not have immediate solutions, and, in any case, are slow to change. Problem posing reflects the recognition of the complexity of the problems and of the time needed for solutions. "Problem posing can be a nurturing process with people exploring visions as they work on problems" (Wallerstein & Bernstein, 1988, p. 383). The group describes those things that they see and feel, defines the many levels of the problem, shares similar experiences from the individual members' lives, questions why the problem exists, and develops action plans to address the problem.

3. Take action toward positive changes that people envision during their dialogue. Solutions emerge from an exploration of the problems in the real world. This action provides new information that leads to further reflection on the problem at a deeper level, enabling people to "learn from their collective attempts at change and to become more deeply involved to surmount the cultural, social, or historic barriers" (Wallerstein & Bernstein, 1988, p. 383).

All of these models contribute information about client variables and dynamics that is important to health education. Nurses must consider which models are most appropriate to their particular teaching needs. The critical challenge is to remember that the client is the center of the health care team and "it is the responsibility of all of us in the health care professions to legitimatize that role" (Weaver & Wilson, 1994, p. 483). Further, it is the responsibility of the health professional both to work with people in the community to facilitate their abilities to identify their problems and solutions and to create the conditions under which professionals and communities can collaboratively engage in empowering practice (Wallerstein & Bernstein, 1994).

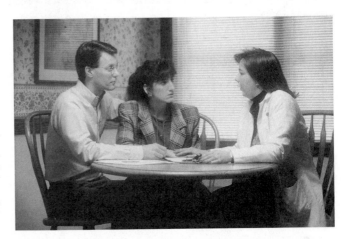

This nurse is using a private setting to teach this couple about their birth control options. *Photo courtesy of Bellevue... The Woman's Hospital, Niskayuna, NY.*

Types of Teaching

Teaching may be formal or informal. **Informal teaching** occurs during interactions with individual clients and families in spontaneous, one-to-one teaching sessions or family conferences (Arnold & Boggs, 1995). **Formal teaching** usually occurs in a group setting or at a pre-arranged individual or family appointment. For instance, during a family visit, a nurse might schedule another visit specifically to discuss parenting skills with a mother and father. Another example would be a weekly seniors group in a day care center wherein various health topics are discussed.

Modalities

Hartmann and Kochar (1994) suggest a variety of modalities for teaching: workshops, lectures, support groups, computer-assisted instruction, self-help groups, and interactive videotapes. In general, learning is enhanced when more than one modality is used, for instance, by including media as part of a workshop or lecture. In addition to using these formats, nurses also create educational videotapes, information pamphlets, or other written or spoken material to be distributed to the public. Nurses also participate at local, state, national, and international levels in the development of broad-based education programs that use all of these modalities.

The Teaching/Learning Environment

Babcock and Miller (1994) identify several factors of physical learning environments that affect the teaching/learning experience. These factors include space; temperature; visual, auditory, and olfactory stimuli; equipment; resources; furniture arrangement; physical comfort; and time. If the space in which the teaching is to take place is too small, clients may find the closeness uncomfortable, or, if instruction is to occur in a public place, such as a waiting room, privacy may be lacking and noise intrusive. In the latter case, it would be important to find a room that has fewer distractions and would therefore facilitate confidential discussion. An environment that is too hot or too cold would constitute a distraction in the form of the related physical discomfort. Likewise, the visual, auditory, and olfactory distractions could impede learning in a home where the television is on and dinner is cooking.

In groups or at home, if a VCR is available, the nurse may use a videotape that illustrates a procedure. Written material can explain or reinforce aspects of the teaching. Audiotapes (and, at times, videotapes) may be left with clients to reinforce learning but should not take the place of nurse–client interaction. Such materials are supplemental and must be discussed with the individual, family, or group so that the clients understand and can use the information.

When teaching a group of people, arranging chairs in a circle rather than in rows will facilitate interaction

DECISION MAKING

Teaching/Learning Environments

You are visiting a family for the second time. Your plan is to discuss parenting skills with the mother and father as they had requested during your first meeting. When you enter, the two children are watching television in the room where you will be meeting, and the father is not home. The mother says she will tell him about what is discussed.

- Can you continue with your teaching plan?
- How do you deal with the children and the television?
- How do you address the issue of the absent father?

among group members. If a meeting with a family takes place in the home, part of the assessment is to notice where family members arrange themselves in relation to one another. For instance, do they line themselves up to face the nurse (thereby facilitating interaction with the nurse rather than among each other), sit facing one another (thereby facilitating family interaction), or keep a distance between one or more family members (thereby suggesting barriers to family interaction)?

In today's health care system, time is often limited. Teaching should be planned so that there is not too much content relative to the time available. More than one session may be necessary to convey the necessary information. Written, audio, or visual material may reinforce a verbal presentation and discussion of the subject, particularly if the information can be studied by the learners at their leisure.

The nurse can solicit the help of the client in creating a suitable learning environment, for instance, by asking a group to put their chairs in a circle or asking a family member to turn off the television. Explaining the reasons for such a request itself constitutes an element of teaching. Creativity and flexibility are needed to provide an optimal environment.

THE LEARNING PROCESS

Regardless of where the teaching/learning takes place, the learning process is the same. That pattern is discussed next.

Phases of the Learning Process

The **learning process** parallels the nursing process in that both are based on the problem-solving model. Learning involves cognitive, affective, and psychomotor com-

Perspectives...

Insights of a Public Health Nurse

I am a public health nurse and receive referrals for 13- to 14-year-old (and sometimes younger) pregnant girls and substance-abusing women in their twenties. I make home visits, connect individuals and families with care providers and community resources, and serve as an advocate when needed. I take weights and measures, teach child development and infant and child care, promote bonding, and give emotional support.

The child mothers are in a developmental crisis and need extra support. Actually, they are in this situation because they need attention and affection. The mothers turn to their babies to get their needs met. They give their babies adult characteristics. For instance, the mother tends to interpret the baby's crying as rejection of herself, as illustrated by remarks such as "She doesn't like me" or "He doesn't want me." When the baby cries to eat every little bit, the mother often says, "She is greedy," or when the baby watches her with normal curiosity the mother may say, "She is so nosy."

I enjoy my work even though I often feel frustrated and overwhelmed. In the beginning, I did a lot more for clients. Now I do more teaching. The mothers are actually strengthened and empowered when they learn to do things themselves. When they learn to care for their babies, they do not abuse or neglect their babies; when they learn about normal developmental milestones, they do not abuse their children later on; and when they get appropriate emotional support, they do not reject their babies.

—Paula, PHN

---

ponents. In some cases, assessment and diagnosis are treated as one step. Here, assessment, diagnosis, planning, implementation, and evaluation are each presented as they pertain specifically to the learning process.

Assessment

The assessment determines the health-related needs of the client by way of identifying health problems, those things that the client knows about or wants to know about these problems, and the client's readiness to learn (Whitman, 1998). Additional factors to assess are the most acute needs to be met, unmet **learning needs** (the gaps between the information an individual knows and the information the individual needs to know in order to perform a function or to care for himself), and life-threatening problems (Rankin & Stallings, 1996). It is always important to consider the degree to which an individual's, family's, or group's cultural practices may influence client teaching. Some considerations are (1) immigration issues, including recency of immigration, whether it was forced, how different the client's culture is from that of the United States, and whether the client came from an urban or a rural area; (2) cultural norms and behaviors, such as whether religious, social, and recreational activities are within the cultural group, whether the client maintains traditional dietary habits and dress and speaks the native language exclusively or only in the home, and whether the client stays within the neighborhood; (3) support systems—specifically, whether the client's friends are from the same ethnic group and whether the client lives in an ethnoculturally diverse or homogeneous neighborhood; (4) use of folk medicine or traditional healers; and (5) existence of discrimination against the client's ethnocultural group that may make acculturation more difficult (Rankin & Stallings, 1996). Such information will help direct the nurse in identifying learning needs and determining teaching methods.

The client's education and reading levels must also be assessed. Literacy levels are usually three to four grades below the grade completed in school (Davis, Crouch, Wills, Miller, & Abdehou, 1990). If material is hard to read or is not understandable to the client, no learning can take place. One assessment tool that has been developed and is being used in a preventive medicine clinic at Louisiana State University Medical Center in Shreveport is called Rapid Estimate of Adult Literacy in Medicine (REALM). In this test, clients are asked to read a series of 66 common medical words that become progressively more difficult. Testing of the tool has shown that the scores can be interpreted as estimates of literacy; as such, the scores can be used to identify clients who are nonreaders and those who have trouble reading medical words. Although this test focuses on reading recognition rather than on reading comprehension, it alerts health care providers to clients who have limited reading skills and will probably have difficulty comprehending most client-education materials (Murphy, Davis, Long, Jackson, & Decker, 1993). Unfortunately, the test has been proved useful only for English-speaking clients. For clients who do not speak English, the nurse must perform reading comprehension tasks, such as observing whether clients have difficulty reading and understanding medical instructions (Nurss, Baker, Davis, Parker, & Williams, 1995).

As in all communication, active listening and observation of nonverbal language are critical. Watching and listening to family and friends as well as to the client are vital. Individuals or groups with whom the client routinely interacts can be supportive or may create barriers to learning and applying new behaviors. Family feedback is also important in evaluating teaching effectiveness.

Arnold and Boggs (1995) provide a framework for the kinds of information the nurse must obtain to complete an assessment (see Figure 8-9). They note that it is best to begin with the least threatening questions and to move to more sensitive topics only after **rapport** (a close, harmonious relationship between or among human beings) is established. Sample questions might be:

"What has this illness been like for you?"

"Have you had any previous experiences or heard any information about other people with similar health problems?"

"Can you tell me what your doctor has told you about your treatment?" (p. 384)

A summary of significant points identified during the assessment serves two purposes: it helps clients identify critical factors relevant to their learning, and it illuminates misinformation the nurse may have about any of the collected data (Arnold & Boggs, 1995).

DECISION MAKING

Planning and Implementing a Teaching Strategy

You are visiting a 65-year-old woman in her home. She is hypertensive and lives with her husband, who is diabetic. As you are talking with her in her kitchen, you notice the groceries on her shelves. They include several cans of soup, chocolate cereal, fruit, and hot dog rolls.

• What nursing diagnoses might you consider regarding the family's educational needs about nutrition?

• How would you initiate a discussion with her about your concerns?

• Would you include her husband in your discussion? Why or why not?

Nursing Diagnosis

The most common NANDA nursing diagnoses in relation to learning needs are likely to have to do with a knowledge deficit or with ineffective coping. It is not enough to simply identify the deficit or the coping problem; it is most meaningful to know (*not* to assume) the reasons behind the problem. For instance, a knowledge deficit may be "related to a lack of exposure or experience, cultural values, misinformation, lack of interest or motivation, organic deficits, unfamiliarity with support resources in the community, or lack of confidence in the health care system" (Arnold and Boggs, 1995, p. 385).

Planning

With the assessment performed and learning diagnosis determined, teaching tools and objectives can be established, priorities identified, and content and teaching methods selected. It is important to organize the content in manageable amounts appropriate to the time available. All such activities are subject to the basic rules of teaching: for instance, developing measurable objectives, structuring the environment to foster learning, considering the client's readiness and motivation to learn, identifying the client's learning style (see Table 8-3), and selecting strategies that meet the needs of the client. The reader is referred to any basic client-education text for more detail regarding these components of teaching.

Teaching strategies that help strengthen teaching and that encourage client involvement include set induction, stimulus variation, reinforcement, use of examples and models, questioning, and closing. Definitions, specific purposes, and examples of these strategies are listed in Table 8-4. By planning ahead for the use of these strategies, the nurse prepares for a focused and meaningful learning experience.

Figure 8-9 Assessment Framework

• What events in the client's life are related to this situation?

• What does the client already know about his or her condition and treatment?

• In what ways is the client affected?

• In what ways are those intimately involved with the client affected?

• Is the client willing to take personal responsibility for seeking solutions?

• What goals would the client like to achieve?

• What will the client have to do in order to achieve those goals?

• What resources are available to the client and family?

• What barriers to learning exist?

Adapted from Interpersonal Relationships *(2nd ed., p. 391) by E. Arnold & K. Boggs, 1995, Philadelphia: W. B. Saunders. Reprinted with permission by W. B. Saunders and Company.*

Table 8-3   Characteristics of Different Learning Styles

VISUAL	AUDITORY	KINESIC
Learns best by seeing.	Learns best with verbal instruction.	Learns best by doing.
Likes to watch demonstration.	Likes to walk through things.	Likes hands-on involvement.
Organizes thoughts by writing them down.	Likes to have ideas explained or to explain.	Needs action and likes to touch, feel.
Needs detail.	Detail not as important.	Loses interest with detailed instruction.
Looks around and examines situations.	Talks about situations—pros, cons.	Tries things.

Adapted from Interpersonal Relationships *(2nd ed., p. 391) by E. Arnold & K. Boggs, 1995, Philadelphia: W. B. Saunders. Printed with permission of W. B. Saunders and Company.*

Teaching people with low literacy skills requires special approaches and planning. Written, audio- or videotaped, or other materials and verbal strategies must be simple and clear and must be presented in an orderly, logical sequence that allows time for the client to process the information. The message should be short, direct, and specific because clients with low literacy skills tend to have short attention spans (Rankin & Stallings, 1996). Dixon and Park (1990) have developed guidelines for nurses' use in providing information to their clients as follows:

- Use clear titles, headings, and subheadings to summarize main points.
- Emphasize important information in bold type.
- Highlight important points with questions or a box format.
- Use a list format whenever appropriate and possible.
- Print matter in an 8- or 10-point type size.
- Test material on a random sample of clients for feedback.
- Use large, boldface print to accommodate clients with special needs, such as diabetic or cataract clients (p. 281).

Audiotape instruction is useful for clients who are visually impaired or who learn better by listening than by reading (Boyd, 1998). It is also useful for standardized or introductory material and in cases of a foreign-language or dialect problem (if the tape can be made in the language or dialect in question). Audiotapes can also be used in conjunction with written material or pictures.

Implementation

Nurses must have knowledge about and confidence in the content they are teaching. However, mastery of content is useful only in concert with good communication and assessment skills to identify client-learning needs. In addition, the nurse must be able to engage the client in learning by working in partnership with the client (Rankin & Stallings, 1996).

The content being taught is often emotionally charged, as when discussing prenatal care with a pregnant teen and her family or when presenting a class at a senior citizens' center about how to care for a family member diagnosed with Alzheimer's disease. Such situations require a combination of teaching and support. It is important to acknowledge the client's anxiety and to support needs if learning is to take place (Rankin & Stallings, 1996). For example, a nurse who is giving information to a family about community resources available for a family member who has Alzheimer's disease may note reluctance on the part of the family to consider these options. In this case, the nurse should take the time to explore with the family their concerns and their sense of inadequacy in providing the necessary care. This discussion might reveal some knowledge deficits about the course of the disease, in which case the nurse would provide needed information and clarification with the goal of reducing the family's worries and thereby facilitating the family's emotional

DECISION MAKING

Developing Teaching Strategies

You are working in a clinic that serves homeless men and women. You have found that many of the clients have severe foot problems and little understanding of how to identify symptoms and the need to seek treatment early.

- How might you go about planning a group to teach foot care?

- How would you facilitate the clients' readiness and motivation to learn?

- What teaching strategies would you consider using to facilitate learning? Why?

Table 8-4   Selected Teaching Strategies

STRATEGY	PURPOSE	EXAMPLE
1. SET INDUCTION Sets the tone for the session.	• Prepare for what will be learned • Provide framework for organization of teaching • Create curiosity and readiness to learn	• Begin teaching by reading a poem pertinent to the subject to be presented. Use the ideas from the poem to show connections to the ideas to be taught.
2. STIMULUS VARIATION Different types of learning activities and approaches to teaching are used.	• Keep students interested in the subject • Increase attention span	When teaching a family the components of a diabetic diet: • show models of portion size of selected foods, • provide written information about the subject, • show a short videotape that demonstrates how to measure food amounts.
3. REINFORCEMENT Instructor or student, or both, repeat information verbally or through actions.	• Strengthen learning	When demonstrating how to bathe a baby at home: • ask the mother to return the demonstration. • Also, provide written material or a videotape that shows the steps of bathing.
4. EXAMPLES AND MODELS Provides an illustration to explain content verbally and visually.	• Foster a common language between teacher and learner	• Example: When explaining the mechanism of the heart, compare it to something familiar to the student, such as a car motor. • Model: When discussing the various forms of birth control with a group, provide samples of each type for the group members to look at and touch.
5. QUESTIONING Raises issues about content for learner to think about.	• Encourages learner to pay attention • Encourages critical thinking • Clarifies issues • Refocuses or redirects discussion	• When teaching about any health topic, ask the students to tell you what they know about the subject before giving any information. • During the teaching, ask students to problem solve a situation. For instance, what are the symptoms of an infected incision, and what would they do if they had these symptoms?
6. CLOSING Reviews or summarizes content; can include application to similar or new situations.	• Facilitates retention of content • Organizes content through review of major points and application to situations	• Summarize, or have the client review with you, the major points of the session. • Point out how this information can be used in other situations as well as in the one discussed.

Hitchcock, J. from unpublished class notes, Sonoma State University, Rohnert Park, CA. Based on Detornyay, R. (1971), Strategies for Teaching Nursing. *NY: John Wiley & Sons.*

Figure 8-10 Strategies for Teaching People Who Are Partially Fluent in English

- Speak slowly and plan for the teaching session to last at least twice as long as a typical session.

- Use simple sentence structure. Use active, not passive, voice, and use a straightforward subject-verb pattern (e.g., say *bathe the baby every day* rather than *the baby is to be bathed every day*).

- Avoid using technical terms (e.g., use *heart* rather than *cardiac*), professional jargon, and American idioms (e.g., *red tape*).

- Provide instructional material in the same sequence in which the patient should carry out the plan.

- Do not assume you have been understood. Ask the patient to explain the protocol; optimally, if appropriate, ask the patient to demonstrate.

Adapted from "Cross-Cultural Perspectives on Patient Teaching" by Tripp-Reimer, 1989, Nursing Clinics of North America, 24, *p. 614.*

⚉⚉ REFLECTIVE THINKING ⚉⚉

Assessing the Problem

You are visiting Mrs. Sayer, a 70-year-old woman with severe emphysema, and her husband. Mrs. Sayer is continuously on oxygen. On her table, you notice an ashtray holding several half-smoked cigarettes.

- What is your first reaction to this observation?

- What issues of your own must you address before approaching the client regarding this observation?

- How would you develop your teaching goal? Why?

- How would you include Mr. Sayer in your teaching?

readiness to consider the community supports initially described to them by the nurse.

Other persons who must be included in the teaching have to be identified. For instance, McMaster and Connell (1994) explain that when a health care worker is teaching Native Americans, identifying incongruities between the health beliefs and practices of the Native American culture and of the health provider's culture is not enough to ensure cultural relevance. They caution that the tribal authority and other members of the community must be involved in securing approval for the intervention.

Accessing knowledge by reasoning through problems is particularly difficult when teaching people who are partially fluent in English. Tripp-Reimer (1989) recommends strategies for doing so when no bilingual persons are available to facilitate communication (see Figure 8-10).

When a client is being taught in the home, reimbursement mechanisms usually require that visits be time limited. Thus, the nurse must be well organized to ensure that necessary teaching for both the client and caregivers as well as other necessary activities are performed (Graham & Gleit, 1998). Teaching the elderly client requires slower presentation of information, careful observation for tiring or for lapsed attention, and accommodation to sensory deficits. Follow-up evaluation of learning outcomes is always crucial.

Evaluation

Evaluation is linked to assessment and to the learning objectives, and it is ongoing. With the learning objectives as a guide, the nurse can judge the results of teaching. How have the objectives been met? Determining the

answer to that question can be difficult. Some change in behavior is usually the desired outcome. Thus, the nurse may ask clients to describe their behavior or may question clients about their knowledge and activities (Babcock & Miller, 1994). Figure 8-11 lists suggested questions to guide the nurse in the evaluation process.

Another aspect of evaluation is to review the teaching module itself. How effective was it? How could it be changed to be more effective? Is the source of a given problem the client, the teacher, or the teaching plan?

Figure 8-11 Questions to Ask During the Evaluation Phase

- What effect did the regimen negotiated by you, your medical colleagues, and the client have on the outcome for the client?

- Did the client get better because of following your recommendations?

- Did the client get worse because of following your recommendations?

- Did the client get better despite your advice?

- Did the client actually comply? How do you know?

- What factors were actually involved in the client's improved condition? According to whose perceptions?

- How does the client perceive the effectiveness of your health interventions?

- Is there something you missed during the assessment step that you have now discovered that affected the client's compliance?

- Did you miss some cues that would have spared you useless effort or that would have increased your chances of obtaining client cooperation?

Adapted from Client Education: Theory and Practice, *(p. 252) by D. E. Babcock & M. A. Miller, 1994, St. Louis: Mosby-Yearbook.*

Child As Learner

When the learner is a child, the learning process is the same as for an adult except that the level of educational readiness must be assessed. In the case of preschool-aged children, teaching is usually done through the parent or caretaker. With school-aged children and adolescents, the school nurse plays an important part in teaching. The nurse providing care in a clinic or home setting will also have many teaching opportunities. School-aged children are ready for direct, formal teaching, and they welcome basic factual information (Babcock & Miller, 1994). They can learn those things to do to promote their well-being, and, if they have a chronic illness, they can be well informed about both the illness itself and the things they must do to care for themselves.

Teaching adolescents is sometimes more difficult than teaching younger children. It is vital to gain their trust as well as to gain an understanding of their language by asking them to explain unknown words and phrases. **Peer education** (using peers of the target group to provide education in either a one-on-one or a group situation) can be very effective in that teens benefit from talking with others who are like them and who are dealing with similar issues. The teen should be afforded as much control as possible. Developing trusting relationships is imperative before discussing issues surrounding sex, alcohol, and other drugs. In addition, the nurse, as in any other situation, must be comfortable discussing such issues. Only when the nurse is comfortable and a trusting nurse–client relationship has been established can such sensitive issues be freely discussed between nurse and teenager (Babcock & Miller, 1994).

RELATED HEALTH-EDUCATION AND COMMUNICATION ISSUES

The focus of community health education is on health promotion for population aggregates. Such education may take place at the local, state, national, or international level. People of all ages and socioeconomic and sociocultural backgrounds are included. Education occurs in such places as schools, clinics, prisons, occupational settings, homeless shelters, and community forums. Education programs may be directed toward a specific population, such as diabetic pregnant women, or toward a specific community, such as a village in Cambodia where people want to learn about immunizations. Programs may range from one-time presentations to long-term, state-initiated, multifaceted programs that involve the cooperative planning of health, governmental, environmental, and other community systems.

The same process of assessment, diagnosis, planning, implementation, and evaluation used in individualized teaching is used in large community health education programs. There are additional considerations, however.

DECISION MAKING

The Child As Learner

Ann Parlo is a 14-year-old newly diagnosed diabetic who has just returned home from a one-week course on how to manage her diabetes. Her parents and her 12-year-old sister participated in a one-day seminar for relatives of diabetics. Her mother tells you that the whole family is still trying to absorb all they have learned. She is worried that she will not cook the right foods, and Ann still finds it difficult to self-administer her insulin, so the mother has been doing it for her.

Consider the following in developing a teaching plan with the family:

• What goals and objectives would you want to develop with the family?

• What assessment data do you need?

• What is your learning diagnosis?

• What plan would you want to make? What teaching strategies would you use? What environmental considerations would be relevant?

• How could you evaluate the outcome of your teaching?

In large programs, many people and departments are involved. Thus, the nurse must use good communication, group-process, and community-organization skills to coordinate the various components of program planning. Furthermore, a large project requires time to arrange and to obtain community support. It also involves working with different cultural groups and with people with opposing interests. Political and legal influences are other significant factors to be considered. Decision makers, such as legislators or special groups, with interests in such things as tobacco or drugs can influence the direction of a program by effecting legislation that addresses these issues or by providing money for programs that promote their interests but not necessarily the needs of the community. Rankin and Stallings (1996) have summarized the factors that affect health-promotion programs. These include socioeconomic status, educational level, culture and language, formal and informal power structures, occupation, and marketing forces.

Conflict Management

Conflict arises when persons hold seemingly incompatible ideas, interests, or values (Cushnie, 1988). Conflict is inevitable in any relationship; in fact, it has been said that without conflict there is no relationship. Although conflict is inevitable, it is also rich with opportunity for mutual gain arising from cooperation and collaboration. Cushnie identifies four categories of conflict: intrapersonal, interpersonal, intragroup, and intergroup.

There are three ways to approach **conflict resolution** (efforts to resolve conflict by expressing concerns and differences of opinion until clarity and resolution are achieved); one is constructive and two are destructive. The **win–win approach** is constructive and requires self-assertion and responsibility. This approach results in a solution with which all participants are satisfied. **Conflict management** is those efforts to work together while at the same time recognizing and accepting the conflicts inherent in the relationship. See Figure 8-12 for the steps involved in an integrative problem-solving approach, a win-win conflict-management strategy recommended by the American Nurses Association (1995). In the **lose–win approach** to conflict resolution, one person allows resolution of the conflict at his or her own expense. This approach is nonassertive and nonresponsible. The **win–lose approach** is the opposite; one person resolves the conflict in a way satisfying to him- or herself but in the process "bulldozes" the rights of the others. This is an aggressive and irresponsible approach.

Translating/Interpreting in Cross-Cultural Communication

Discussion of and guidelines for cross-cultural communication were presented in Chapter 6, with the exception of issues regarding the use of an interpreter for translating from one language to another. In many countries, and certainly in the United States, community nursing often requires proficiency in more than one language as well as the use of interpreters. It is not uncommon for a given community to have or for a public health nurse to be working with a caseload of families from several cultures who speak several languages.

Carol (1989) recommends the use of an interpreter unless the nurse is thoroughly fluent and effective in the

client's language. Family members should not be used as interpreters, especially young children, even those fluent in English. When family members are used as translators, confidentiality—so important, especially in matters of intimacy and serious illness—is difficult to maintain. Written instructions must be given in the client's language. The nurse must be patient when working with an interpreter because careful interpretation is time consuming and tedious. It is important to meet regularly with the interpreter and to develop a harmonious working relationship.

Hatton and Webb (1993) found three different types of interaction styles among nurses, interpreters, and clients: voice box, excluder, and collaborator. In the **voice box** style, the interpreter attempts to translate word for word. In the **excluder** style, the interpreter takes over the provider–client interaction, excludes the nurse from the conversation, and explains to the nurse after the completion of the interaction what was said during the interaction. The **collaborator** style is a combination of the other two; the nurse and interpreter work as colleagues and engage in interaction with the client as appropriate to the situation.

Interpretation is complex. Andrews (1995) identifies a number of points that must be considered. One must be aware of the compatibility of the client and interpreter. For instance, they should not be from rival tribes, states, regions, or nations. It is preferable that the interpreter be older and more mature than and of the same sex as the client. Socioeconomic differences may be a factor. Interpreting can be time consuming and one of the greatest challenges in cross-cultural communication.

Public Speaking

Throughout this chapter we have discussed intrapersonal communication, or "self-talk" in the process of self-awareness, and interpersonal communication, or interacting and sharing information with others. **Public speaking** is the act of using spoken words to communicate with many individuals at one time. Nurses can expect to be involved in this activity, particularly with regard to community education and to involvement in community-health issues.

The goals of public speaking with regard to health teaching are to reach large numbers of people with infor-

---

Figure 8-12 Win–Win Conflict Management Strategy

- Identify the problem (including values, purposes, goals).
- Encourage free exchange of ideas, feelings, attitudes, and values in an atmosphere of trust.
- Search for alternative ways to resolve the problem.
- Ask for help from outside sources as needed.
- Set up means for evaluation of solutions.
- Keep interacting until all members want and value the solution.

Adapted from What You Need to Know about Today's Workplace: A Survival Guide for the Workplace *by American Nurses Association, 1995, Washington D.C.: Author.*

COMMUNITY NURSING VIEW

A 17-year-old girl who is six months pregnant and living in a temporary shelter for homeless women has been referred to you. The referral states that she must leave in four weeks and that she has not made any effort to find another place to live. Further, she made one prenatal visit to a local clinic but has missed the last three appointments. You make a home visit to the shelter to interview the girl and to assess the situation. She seems friendly and receptive to you and your visit. She appears to be underweight and states that she has gained only five pounds since she got pregnant and just does not feel like eating. She is worried because she does not want to get fat. When you encourage her to eat, explaining why it is so important, she responds by saying that she will try to eat more. You express your concern that she must get prenatal care and find another place to live. She says the most important thing for her to do is get a job. You make an appointment for a follow-up visit in two days to do a physical assessment, get a complete health history, formulate a treatment plan, and make a contract with her. When you arrive at the designated time, she is not home. A staff person says she went out to look for a job.

Nursing Considerations

ASSESSMENT
• How will you assess her physical condition? Where will you do the examination? What equipment will you need? What records will you keep?

• The psychosocial situation indicates serious problems. What questions will you ask to gain further information about her situation? How will you assess strengths in her environment? Why is it important to assess for potential support systems (i.e., family, church, friends, or groups)?

• What are her inner strengths? Beliefs? Values? Cultural health care practices?

DIAGNOSIS
• What diagnoses would be appropriate for her?
• What issues are related to the diagnoses?

OUTCOME IDENTIFICATION
• What behaviors could serve as indicators of progress?
• What psychological indicators might reflect positive treatment outcomes?
• What psychological outcomes could reflect positive treatment outcomes?

PLANNING/INTERVENTIONS
• When will you make a return visit? Will you notify her of your intention to visit? If so, how will you notify her?

• What is your plan of action for when you do next meet with her? How will you learn what she is willing to do for herself? How will you address your concerns for her?

• Do you think a contract might be helpful? Would you do it verbally, or would you put it in writing complete with signatures?

• What information does she need to empower her to take more responsibility for herself and her unborn child? How will you know when she is actively participating in the teaching/learning process? Is she interested in learning some relaxation techniques for stress management and for labor?

• How does your listening help motivate her to do what she needs to do for herself?

• What referrals may be appropriate? How can you serve as an advocate for her?

EVALUATION
• How will you evaluate the success of your plan and interventions? Will you measure success against physical findings? Her keeping of appointments? Her follow-through on contracted responsibilities?

Figure 8-13   Ten Steps to Making a Public Speech

1. Select a topic that interests you and will hold the interest of your audience.

2. Create an outline that has an introduction, a body, and a conclusion.

3. Organize your thoughts and public remarks with the following in mind: your personal experience, what you bring to the topic, what your audience knows already and what you can tell them.

4. Give special attention to how you are going to start your speech (the introduction) and how you are going to finish your speech (the conclusion).

5. Outline the major points you wish to make in the body of your speech along with appropriate supporting statements for those points.

6. Rehearse your speech *aloud* and use a tape recorder, or a VCR if possible, for feedback.

7. Do not worry about gestures; concentrate on making your ideas clear to the audience.

8. Use your outline as notes (one page at most). Rehearse with the outline so that you are not tied to it and can look at the audience.

9. Do not use profanity or vulgar language unless you have a definite reason for doing so and are aware of the possible negative consequences.

10. Wear clothing that you think complements your appearance but does not call attention to itself.

Adapted from Public Speaking, *pp. 24–26 by F. E. X. Dance & C. C. Zak-Dance, 1986, New York: Harper & Row.*

---

mation about health topics that affect the community and to urge adoption of healthy behaviors. Public speaking is a powerful tool, the necessary skills of which take time and effort to develop. Great speaking skills are respected and, in general, are a mark of successful men and women. For a summary of 10 steps to making a public speech, see Figure 8-13.

Key Concepts

- Communication is the core of client–nurse work in the community, dictating its quality and effectiveness in serving the best interests of the client.

- The interactionist nurse theorists emphasize the nurse–client relationship, particularly with regard to its serving to meet the health needs of the client.

- Client–nurse communication embodies the sharing of information, feelings, thoughts, beliefs, values, and behaviors related to client health and healing processes as the client assumes increasing responsibility.

- Active listening, a powerful tool in communicating empathic understanding, calls for the qualities of effective helping: warmth, respect, genuineness, specificity, empathy, self-disclosure, and confrontation.

- The contract is often helpful as a tool for goal attainment in the therapeutic process, defining nurse and client responsibilities in solving a problem.

- All groups follow a predictable developmental pattern, whether their goals are related to work planning or the therapeutic process.

- Education is necessary in meeting many of the Healthy People: 2000 objectives, and andragogy is the most appropriate approach because it emphasizes client self-efficacy.

- Various factors including space; temperature; visual, auditory, and olfactory stimuli; equipment; resources; furniture arrangement; physical comfort, and time affect the teaching/learning environment.

- The learning process uses the same steps as the nursing process; a child's learning process differs from an adult's only with regard to level of educational readiness.

- Empowerment community education encourages the community to find solutions to its own problems by starting with the community's concerns, using active-learning methods, and engaging clients in determining their own needs and priorities.

- Conflict is inevitable in any relationship, and resolution can bring about closeness and shared understandings.

Health-Promotion and Disease-Prevention Perspectives

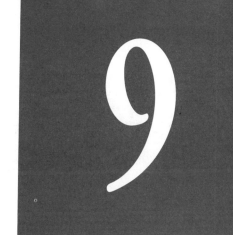

Phyllis E. Schubert, DNSc, RN, MA
Mary Jo Starsiak, MSN, RN
Joan Heron, RN, PhD

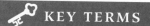

KEY TERMS

aerobic conditioning
community nursing
  centers
complementary care
  therapies
created-environment
deep relaxation
degenerative disease
disease prevention
energy
guided imagery
health behaviors
health education
health promotion
health protection
imagery
integrative models of
  health
interactive guided
  imagery
Jin Shin Jyutsu (JSJ)
lacto-ovovegan diet
lactovegan diet
ovovegan diet
paradigm
primary prevention
psychoneuroimmunology
rehabilitation
risk factors
safety energy locks
secondary prevention
self-esteem
social support
story telling
stress
stress response
stressors
tertiary prevention
touch therapy
vegans
vegetarian diet
visualization
wellness

Life is . . . .

To endure
The ebb and tide of keeping life's balance,
To care . . . .
Not just to procure.
Disease or illness is . . . .
To prevent with the power of knowledge,
To accept things that cannot be altered,
To travel the road with leverage.
Death is . . . .
To accept transition . . . .
To respect the rose with petals falling,
To ease the change of time or place . . . .
Not just to say good-bye, but to heed the calling.
—Starsiak

COMPETENCIES

Upon completion of this chapter, the reader should be able to:

- Trace the recent history of the efforts to move national and international health care toward a focus on disease prevention and health promotion in addition to treatment of disease.
- Discuss theoretical perspectives related to health promotion, disease prevention, health behavior choice, and health education.
- Discuss moral and ethical issues related to social and individual responsibilities for health.
- Recount recommendations related to diet, exercise, sleep, and stress management.
- Discuss philosophical issues related to research in the areas of health promotion and disease prevention.
- Explain a conceptual model for application of caring in the clinical practice of health promotion.
- Introduce alternative/complementary therapies to primary, secondary, and tertiary community health nursing practice.
- Discuss clinical application to nursing practice of disease prevention and health promotion in the community.

The definition of health as living a long life or as the absence of disease dates back to the 12th century A.D., when lives were short and people were fortunate to be free of disease (Byer & Shainberg, 1995). The definition of health has been evolving since 1974, when the World Health Organization (WHO) stated that "health is a state of complete physical, mental, and social well-being and not merely the absence of disease and infirmity." In 1981, Smith categorized health as: (1) clinical absence of disease or illness, (2) maximum social role performance, (3) flexible adaptation to environment to maximum advantage, and (4) eudaimonistic or exuberant well-being.

Pender (1996) integrates stabilization and actualization in a definition of health:

> Health is the actualization of inherent and acquired human potential through goal-directed behavior, competent self-care, and satisfying relationships with others while adjustments are made as needed to maintain structural integrity and harmony with relevant environments (p. 22).

Because health is reflected in the context of the person–environment relationship, environmental influences are pivotal in health processes. Figure 9-1 reflects many influences on health status.

Health is increasingly being viewed as a cultural concept defined in various ways according to cultural beliefs. Although **health behaviors** (behaviors exhibited by persons that affect their health either constructively or destructively) are culturally determined, increasing numbers of people are seeking **wellness** (a state of health accompanied by a sense of exuberant well-being) through commitment to lifestyles that promote health and, thereby, reduce risk of premature death and disability.

Although the same positive health behaviors are employed for both **health promotion** and **health protection** (**disease prevention**), definitions of these terms differ. Pender (1996) defines disease prevention as health protection:

> Health protection is directed toward decreasing the probability of experiencing health problems by active protection against pathologic stressors or detection of health problems in the asymptomatic stage. Health protection focuses on efforts to move away from or avoid the negatively valanced states of illness and injury. . . . Health promotion is directed toward increasing the level of well-being and self-actualization of a given individual or group. Health promotion focuses on efforts to approach or move toward a positively valenced state of high-level health and well-being (Pender, 1996, p. 34).

The purpose of this chapter is to explore nursing issues and implications related to national and international political efforts to promote health and prevent disease. Because both individual responsibility and social responsibility are required in these efforts, a synthesis of individual health behavior choice and societal efforts to provide a healthy environment for all is emphasized. (Application of these concepts to populations is more fully developed in other chapters, with population-focused strategies for health promotion and prevention serving as the major focus of Chapter 10.) The material related to individuals may serve as content for health-education programs. **Health education** is defined as obtaining self-awareness, information, and support for changing problem health behaviors through the teaching/learning process. Because to a large extent health behavior is taught via modeling, some features in this chapter focus on the health behavior of the nurse. A brief overview of theoretical perspectives related to health promotion and wellness, disease prevention, health education, and health behavior choice is also included. These models provide a basis for research and the application of health education and clinical programs.

HEALTHY PEOPLE 2000: A NATIONAL PLAN

Theoretical frameworks and research have long indicated the need for emphasis on health promotion and disease prevention in order to reduce health care costs and to improve the quality of life internationally and nationally. In 1978, the Declaration of Alma Ata (World Health Organization [WHO], 1981), which addressed worldwide concerns about health and health care, emphasized the need to shift from a disease-care focus to a focus on health. Health for All (HFA) by the Year 2000 became the guiding slogan for the work at the WHO conference in Ottawa, Canada, where the historic Ottawa Charter for Health Promotion (WHO, 1986) was developed. This charter identified the factors fundamental to community health: peace, shelter, education, food, income, a stable ecosystem, sustainable resources, social justice, and equity.

ଚ⊘ REFLECTIVE THINKING ଚ⊘

How Is the Health Behavior of the Nurse Significant?

Given that role modeling is a powerful teaching tool (see Chapter 8) and self-care is necessary not only for the client but also for the nurse:

• Reflect on the circle of influence in your own environment (see Figure 9-1). Start by examining your responsibility to yourself and expand your examination to include your responsibility to your family, peers, clients, communities, nation, world, and universe.

• How does your choice of health behaviors affect your client?

Figure 9-1   Factors That Influence Health Status

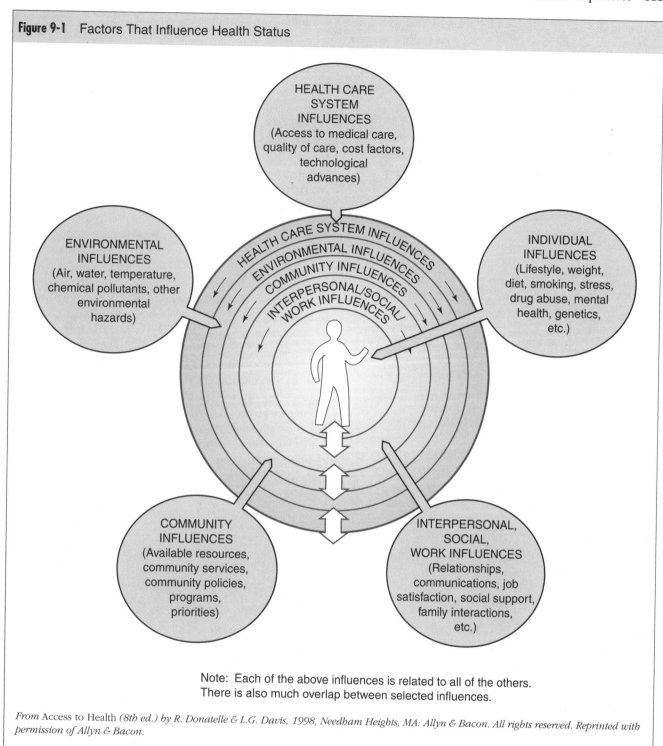

HEALTH CARE
SYSTEM
INFLUENCES
(Access to medical care,
quality of care, cost factors,
technological
advances)

ENVIRONMENTAL
INFLUENCES
(Air, water, temperature,
chemical pollutants, other
environmental
hazards)

INDIVIDUAL
INFLUENCES
(Lifestyle, weight,
diet, smoking, stress,
drug abuse, mental
health, genetics,
etc.)

HEALTH CARE SYSTEM INFLUENCES
ENVIRONMENTAL INFLUENCES
COMMUNITY INFLUENCES
INTERPERSONAL/SOCIAL/
WORK INFLUENCES

COMMUNITY
INFLUENCES
(Available resources,
community services,
community policies,
programs,
priorities)

INTERPERSONAL,
SOCIAL,
WORK INFLUENCES
(Relationships,
communications, job
satisfaction, social support,
family interactions,
etc.)

Note: Each of the above influences is related to all of the others.
There is also much overlap between selected influences.

From Access to Health *(8th ed.) by R. Donatelle & L.G. Davis, 1998, Needham Heights, MA: Allyn & Bacon. All rights reserved. Reprinted with permission of Allyn & Bacon.*

In the United States, a need for emphasis on the promotion of health rather than on the treatment of disease was also being addressed. According to the U.S. Department of Health and Human Services (1992), a federal health strategy was initiated by the U.S. Department of Health and Human Services (USDHHS) with the publication of *Healthy People: The Surgeon General's Report on Health Promotion and Disease Prevention* in 1979. This document identified public health goals for 1990, including targeted decreases in mortality for each age group. In 1980, *Promoting Health/Preventing Disease: Objectives for the Nation* set forth specific objectives for improving health status, reducing health risks, expanding professional and public awareness, providing service provisions, and surveillancing and evaluating techniques (p. 4). These works were forerunners to *Healthy People 2000: National Health Promotion and Disease Prevention Objectives*, released in 1990. The goal of this work was to achieve a healthier nation by the year 2000, with recognition that success depends on all levels of government, the media, health professionals, communities, families, and individuals. Thus, it was recognized that full achievement of the goals and objectives could not be attained by government alone; rather a combination of individual health behavior and government working to establish and protect environmental resources was required. Individual responsibility for personal health was considered equally important to the responsibility of social organizations.

Twenty-two health-promotion priorities with goals and objectives related to behavioral concerns were identified in the Healthy People 2000 documents and assessed in the *Healthy People 2000: Midcourse Review and 1995 Revisions* (U.S. Department of Health and Human Services [USDHHS], 1996). The *Midcourse Review* provides an assessment of U.S. progress in attaining its objectives at the midpoint of the decade.

The overall goals of Healthy People 2000 are to (1) increase the span of healthy life in the United States; (2) reduce health disparities among citizens, especially those who are economically, educationally, or politically disadvantaged; and (3) ensure access to preventive services for all. The objectives were designed to meet the goals of the plan and to address specifically those high-risk groups who bear a disproportionate share of disease, disability, and premature death compared with the total population. The establishment of surveillance and data systems is a necessary component of the program to measure progress toward attainment of these goals by the year 2000.

The *Midcourse Review* (USDHHS 1996) reports that progress toward meeting the established goals is being made in more than two-thirds of the stated objectives for which data are now available, but in some (obesity among all ages and substance abuse and violence among young people), movement is in the reverse. These areas are causing great concern and a sense of alarm.

religious institutions, and voluntary organizations—can become more actively engaged in promoting health. Employers can make worksites healthy (USDHHS 1996, p. 5).

In Chapter 7, Schubert and Lionberger propose that responsibility starts with providing the best environment possible for oneself to be healthy or to heal. As health and expanding consciousness occur and awareness regarding needs at various levels of environment—family, local, state, national, international, planetary, and universal—increases, social responsibility for the world at large also increases. With heightened awareness and responsibility, people can make decisions appropriate to their situations, whether that means recycling waste in the home or making proposals on the floor of the U.S. Senate or in the WHO.

This perspective also presumes a caring environment for growth and development of human potential, health, and healing. When an individual, family, or community is in a situation where basic needs cannot be met, help and assistance are essential until caring, nurturance, respect, safety, and order (beauty) can be reestablished. Obviously, caring for others and oneself requires services necessary for disease prevention and health promotion. Health-promotion activities depend on acceptance of oneself and others, with each person being viewed as whole and as perfect in the present phase of spiritual growth and development. Then, and only then, can helping serve the needs of both the giver and receiver.

BALANCING SOCIAL AND INDIVIDUAL RESPONSIBILITY FOR HEALTH

The Centers for Disease Control and Prevention (CDC) (1994) has estimated that nearly 47% of premature deaths among Americans can be prevented by way of changes in individual behaviors, and another 17% via reduced environmental risks. In contrast, an estimated 11% of premature deaths among Americans are deemed preventable through improvements in access to medical treatment.

Healthy People 2000 reports call for commitment at all levels to improve health in this nation.

Leadership must come from institutions and individuals throughout the nation. Each person makes decisions about how fast to drive, whether to wear a safety belt, what to eat, and how much alcohol to drink. In families, parents have the opportunity to promote health and encourage healthy habits for their children. Community organizations—schools,

⦿⦿ REFLECTIVE THINKING ⦿⦿

Individual Versus Social Responsibility for Health

In the United States, third-party payment most often extends to those who need medical care: for example, those who are hospitalized for drug therapy or surgery. Educational programs for those with addictions and destructive health behaviors are less often funded. Drug rehabilitation programs have long waiting lists. Emphasis on nutrition, sleep, and exercise is seldom a part of prevention and treatment programs, and health-promotion programs are almost nonexistent.

• What changes would you make to provide a more economical, effective, and efficient system?

• Give examples of appropriate individual responsibility for health promotion.

• Give examples of appropriate societal responsibility.

• How would you avoid a "blame the victim" perspective and still require individual responsibility for health behavior choice?

THEORETICAL PERSPECTIVES OF HEALTH AND WELLNESS

Nurse theorists and authors on the whole conceptualize health as adaptation, self-actualization, or some combination thereof, and address health as either a state of being or a process of evolving potentiality. The Neuman Systems Model (Neuman, 1990) is one nursing theory that addresses health as a process of adaptation and achievement of equilibrium. Neuman's model focuses on the concepts of energy and created-environment. **Energy** is defined as "the pervasive force within the client that empowers and regulates all systemic functions from cellular to motor" (p. 129). Energy, then, may be thought of as a resource for system empowerment and achievement of wellness. A state of health or wellness is facilitated by conservation of energy through increasing awareness of environmental stressors as risk factors that threaten or challenge health and by increasing or strengthening existing client strengths.

The **created-environment** is the protective, unconsciously derived environment that exists for all clients. Energy is used to develop and maintain the created-environment. This mechanism often is destructive, and the nurse or caregiver provides support while changes are made toward a more constructive way of being. When the created-environment changes and bound energy is released, the nurse must find ways to help the client or system integrate and adjust to the change. For Neuman, then, health is a living energy process with a goal of creating and maintaining equilibrium.

Rogers (1990) and Newman (1994) are among those nurse theorists who view health as the process of emerging human potential. Newman uses Rogers' Theory of Unitary Human Beings as a **paradigm**, or way of understanding the nature of things, in building her theory of health as a process of expanding consciousness. Because all nursing theories reflect health as being determined by the person–environment relationship, all provide strong foundations for health-promotion programs.

Pender's (1996) model of health promotion encourages the use of **integrative models of health**, which take a broad biopsychosocial view of human health phenomena. Clinical indicators in such models are numerous and include interpersonal behavior, social support, socioeconomic status, mood state, cognitive efficiency, symptom complaints, hormone levels, neurotransmitter breakdown products, neurochemical substrates, immunoglobulin status, or any combination of the preceding. Human response patterns may be identified to determine predictors of healthy or unhealthy outcomes. The scope of therapeutic options for treating health problems or responses to health problems in such models will undoubtedly enlarge.

Although health behavior choice is only one of the many complex factors that determine health status, it is a significant determinant. Because health-education programs are established to influence health behavior choice, and because nurses develop and teach such programs, some potentially useful conceptual frameworks are presented next.

Pender's Health Promotion Model

Pender's (1996) model of health promotion (see Figure 9-2) is a modification of Rosenstock's Health Belief Model, developed by Rosenstock (1966) to predict the use of preventive health actions such as going to a clinic for screening procedures and modified by Becker (1974) to predict other preventive behaviors. Pender's (1996) model provides a tool for "exploring complex biopsychosocial processes that motivate individuals to engage in behaviors directed toward the enhancement of health" (p. 51). Whereas in the Rosenstock model, perceived threat was viewed as a motivator, Pender argued that although immediate threats to health may serve to motivate action, threats in the distant future lack the same motivational strength. Because adolescents and young adults tend to see themselves as invulnerable to illness, perceived threat has been replaced in Pender's model by perceived potentiality. And given that the Pender model relies on perceived potentiality as a motivator for health behavior choice, the model has applicability throughout the life span.

Pender's efforts to test and refine the Health Promotion Model strengthen nursing science by broadening knowledge of health and health behavior choice. Refinement increases the model's potential use in prediction and intervention with regard to health behavior choice.

Travis's Wellness Model

Travis (1977) addresses a continuum of health, ranging from high-level wellness at one end to premature death at the other end. In the middle of the continuum (see Figure 9-3) is a state void of physical signs and symptoms *and* of a sense of well-being. He observes, "Many people lack physical symptoms but are bored, depressed, tense, anxious or generally unhappy with their lives. These emotional states often lead to physical disease through the lowering of the body's resistance." (p. 2).

Travis's illness/wellness continuum was adapted by Donatelle and Davis (1998) to reflect differences between illness- and wellness-oriented care. As the client moves to the right of the neutral point, increasing levels of health and well-being are experienced; as the client moves toward the left, decreasing health and disease-oriented care are experienced (Donatelle & Davis, 1998).

It is important to realize that many people, especially elders and those who are disabled, live in states of wellness yet are physically handicapped, chronically ill, or dying. Thus, wellness does not depend solely on physical functioning. In wellness-oriented care, the focus is on awareness, education, and growth, whereas in disease- or illness-oriented care, the focus is on treating signs, symptoms, and disability. Although the wellness model

Figure 9-2 Pender's Health Promotion Model

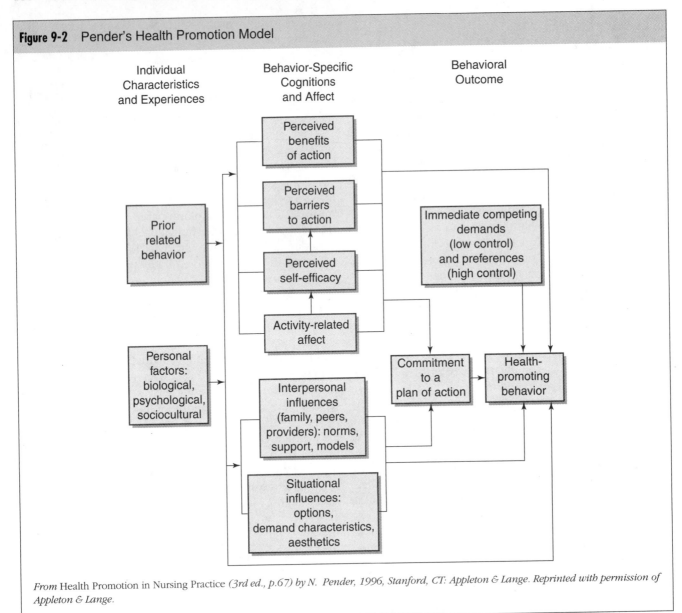

From Health Promotion in Nursing Practice (3rd ed., p.67) by N. Pender, 1996, Stanford, CT: Appleton & Lange. Reprinted with permission of Appleton & Lange.

does take symptoms into account, the overall perspective is one of education, healing, and wholeness. This model is frequently used as a conceptual model for health-promotion services.

The haiku in Figure 9-4 reflects an understanding of health as the total experience of life and living.

Mutual Connectedness Model

The Mutual Connectedness Model (Schubert, 1989; Schubert & Lionberger, 1995) for clinical practice (see Chapter 32) provides a conceptual perspective for nurses and clients interested in wellness and health-promotion approaches. In this model, health is treated as the integration of body, emotions, mind, and spirit through consciousness within a caring environment that is dynamic in nature and is in harmonious interrelationship with the person (see Figure 9-5). Although the model focuses on

the individual within the family, group, or community, it may be adapted for application to clients of all dimensions (families, groups, populations, communities) within their environmental contexts.

Figure 9-5 indicates a pattern of wholeness—a dynamic, moving, constantly changing evolutionary process of being and becoming wherein a caring environment supports integration and healing. Persons establish their reality through integration of self within the context of these processes as their worlds are continuously reshaped by new meanings and relationships. Changes in health behavior accompany expansion of consciousness, the specific changes being dictated by inner-directed healing processes.

The pattern of the whole reflects one's state of health. Although separation of these aspects is artificial, Figure 9-6 represents some of the needs likely to be inherent in an individual's physical, emotional, mental, and spiritual aspects. The model can be used as a tool to help clients assess their overall health needs and to make health

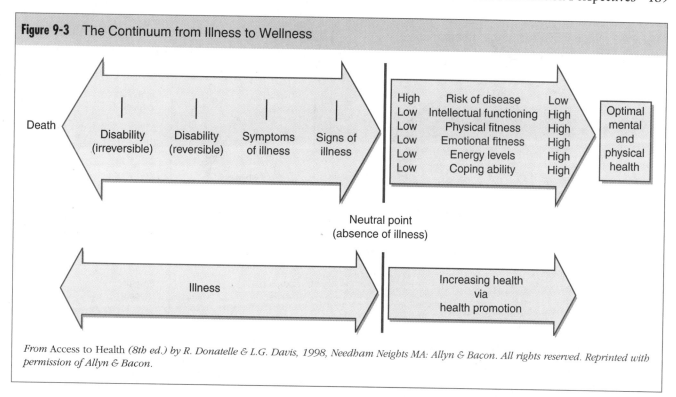

Figure 9-3 The Continuum from Illness to Wellness

behavior choices. The nurse can then plan strategies with the client to implement those choices.

The sides of the triangles in Figure 9-6 represent areas of need affecting health behavior choice. Clients are able to look at the various needs represented and determine areas of concern. The base of each triangle represents that aspect's area of creative expression in the person—environment interrelationship.

Physical Aspect

The three sides of the physical-aspect triangle represent needs for biochemical balance, sleep and rest, and movement and sensing. Despite the fact that there is no real way to separate these needs (because every health variable affects every other health variable), a brief discussion of each is presented here.

Biochemical balance encompasses a variety of factors including nutrition intake via food and supplements; metabolism; environmental factors such as air, water, and pollutants or toxic substances; and medications. Nutrition is discussed later in this chapter.

Nature, including the human body, has a strong urge toward health and healing. The body, given the nutrients and periods of deep rest and sleep it needs, has a great capacity to maintain health and to heal itself. Relaxation, as a way to provide brief periods of deep rest, and sleep are briefly discussed later in this chapter.

Figure 9-4 Health: A Haiku

Health is well-being,
Self-actualization,
Ever-unfolding.

Health is potential,
Soaring to greater heights,
Becoming one's best.

Health is energy,
Dynamic and ongoing,
Continuous flow.

Health is fulfillment,
Ability to perform,
Aggregate powers.

Health is adapting,
Balance with environment,
Equilibrium.

Health is expression
Of one's source and direction,
Of values and goals.

Health is here and now,
Yesterdays and tomorrows,
Time continuum.

Health is holistic,
Integration of oneself,
Higher awareness.

Health is one's wholeness,
A process of functioning,
A state of being.

Figure 9-5 Model of Health: Interrelatedness of Caring and Consciousness

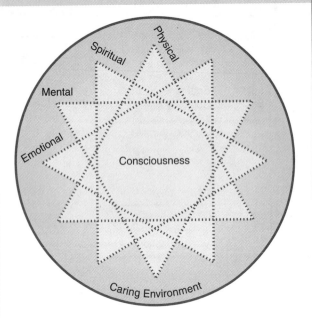

From "Mutual Connectedness: A Study of Client–Nurse Interaction Using the Grounded Theory Method" by P. Schubert & H. Lionberger, Journal of Holistic Nursing, 13, 1995, p. 105.

Figure 9-6 Aspects of Health and Multidimensional Needs Affecting Health Behavior Choice

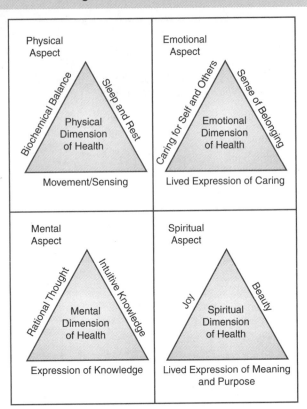

From "Mutual Connectedness: A Study of Client–Nurse Interaction Using the Grounded Theory Method" by P. Schubert & H. Lionberger, Journal of Holistic Nursing, 13, 1995, p. 105.

Movement refers to the experience of internal rhythms and to the integration of body–mind and person–environment. Sensing—sight, hearing, taste, smell, and touch—also are a part of this experience. When one sense is missing, others become more acute. Physical exercise is addressed later in this chapter, and the student is encouraged to pursue further study in the area of expressive arts and dance for understanding of body–mind integration.

Emotional Aspect

Emotions affect the physical body, mental capacity, and spiritual development. Health behavior choice involves one's relationships with self and others. The emotional aspect of health includes caring for and being cared for by others and a sense of belonging. **Social support** (resources provided to a person by others, such as affection, indications of belonging, emotional support, and actual material goods, when needed) has been shown to be fundamental to health (McCuen, 1993).

Holding oneself and others in high esteem is a hallmark of good emotional health. **Self-esteem** (feelings about oneself and how one measures up to that which one expects) is important in health behavior choice; in fact, lack of self-esteem is a major motivating factor in self-destructive behaviors. The need to belong—to be a part of a couple, a family, or a group—is also key. Feeling isolated, alone, and without social support contributes to both physical and mental illness.

Expression of caring is necessary for harmony and bal-

ance in the person–environment interrelationship. Lack of such expression creates conflict and disharmony in relationships. An open heart reveals qualities of caring and nourishes relationships as well as one's own health and the health of others.

Mental Aspect

The mental aspect refers to a person's need to learn and to express knowledge gained from the person–environment experience. Knowledge is gained through both intuition and rational thought processes. Knowledge also seeks expression in the person's lived experience. The mental aspect shapes information provided by the physical, mental, emotional, and spiritual aspects into thoughts, beliefs, values, and understandings that shape belief systems upon which lives are built.

Intuitive knowledge refers to the direct knowing or learning of something without the conscious use of rational thought or reasoning. Much knowledge from the everyday world is obtained in this way. Although some of this knowledge is tested by logical, rational thought, more goes unquestioned because it is simply recognized and accepted.

Rational thought is based on reasoning. For example, careful consideration is given to the events leading to an unexpected outcome in order to determine the thing or things that change the expected outcome. This kind of careful consideration of cause and effect is highly valued in science and in Western culture as a whole. Although scientific thought is based in reason, reasoning is limited to a single cause and effect. In an orientation to integrated wholeness, such thought becomes increasingly difficult because there are limitless variables in the life experience. Reason is also valued highly in Eastern cultures, but in these cultures, reasoning involves the holistic, or integrated, perspective that allows for many causes and effects.

Critical thinking requires both intuitive and rational skills. All information obtained from any source is considered. Intuition and reasoning are equally important, with each providing a valuable means of testing knowledge and understanding.

Because knowledge is shared through activities such as building, teaching, communicating, sharing, and writing, expression of knowledge is also valued as a means to interrelatedness and person–environment integration.

Spiritual Aspect

Spirituality lifts daily experience into a higher dimension of consciousness. (See Chapter 6 for a more in-depth discussion of the spiritual aspect and its related needs.) Emotional aspects of health, discussed previously, nurture one's spiritual growth through the lived experiences of caring, compassion, and belonging as they lead to an experience of unity.

Spiritual health is reflected in a sense of deep joy and peace that may or not be related to external events. Faith in a higher order, a sense of oneness with all that is good or divine, and a belief that there is purpose in this life and that the individual's life is in harmony with that purpose are characteristic of the spiritual aspect. Joy, beauty, and life meaning and purpose seem to be areas of need experienced by all persons regardless of belief in a Supreme Being.

The Mutual Connectedness Model for clinical practice seems to be consistent with the assumptions and conceptual frameworks of Martha Rogers (1990) and Margaret Newman (1994). These models encourage intervention strategies wherein the nurse gives appropriate support and assistance to the client as the client sets his or her own goals and works to meet them. The nurse who views health as a developmental process is less apt to rely on the practice of giving advice and information and instead will emphasize caring support and encouragement. The client is thus empowered, and creativity is strengthened.

Creativity is the expression of one's unique way of being in the world. The expression of one's totality—of one's blueprint of experience—is reflected in the creative act. Creativity is not limited to art, music, poetry, sculpture, or pottery. It means drawing upon one's own resources, capacities, and roots. It means facing life directly and honestly, courageously searching for and discovering grief, joy, suffering, pain, struggle, conflict, and inner solitude.

RESEARCH IN HEALTH-PROMOTIVE BEHAVIORS

Far more concern and, consequently, research has been directed toward the phenomenon of disease than toward either health or healing. Many unknowns exist with regard to health promotion and healing, and agreement is lacking in many (if not all) areas of health behavior and its effect on health-status outcomes.

Some philosophical issues make currently available research methods difficult to use in the areas of health and healing. First, research methods accepted in the scientific world today do not seem to be philosophically suitable for the study of holistic processes such as health and healing. Required are methods that address changing human energy patterns as evolving processes affected by consciousness. An unlimited number of factors affect these phenomena. Qualitative research methods deal with numerous factors and individual responses, but these methods do not lend themselves to measurement and statistical analysis as those in program planning and decision making would prefer. On the other hand, quantitative research methods ordinarily used in health studies depend on isolation of one or several variables that can be measured and analyzed statistically.

Secondly, guidelines for health behavior choice have been developed for application to whole populations and large numbers of people, even though individuals differ in their responses to any variable or set of variables. In this sense, each person is his or her own experiment in health and healing. For example, whereas most persons seem to do well by eating whole-grain products, others who have allergic responses to gluten or to a certain grain do poorly.

DECISION MAKING

Clinical Application of Health and Wellness Models

You are working with a client, a 43-year-old Caucasian male who became quadriplegic as a result of a diving accident 10 years ago. He lives with his wife and two adolescent boys. He has been referred to you because of irritability, sleeplessness, and frequent respiratory infections.

• Select one of the wellness and health-promotion models described in this section to develop an appropriate plan for application of the nursing process.

Thoughtful and creative use and development of research methods are needed, especially in the areas of health promotion and healing. Personal experience and anecdotal evidence indicate that a positive attitude, playing, having fun, practicing deep relaxation, exercising, and other such activities have a positive effect on health and stimulate healing. On the other hand, depression, guilt, anger, fear, worry, and pretense negatively affect health and healing. Research in this area is currently being conducted in **psychoneuroimmunology** (Friedman, Thomas, Klein & Friedman, 1996), a new field focusing on the manufacture of neurotransmitters, specifically endorphins and enkephalins, by the brain. Studies have shown that these brain hormones increase with certain behaviors such as laughing, running, meditating, and hugging and that increased hormone levels are accompanied by feelings of well-being and peace (Hardman, Limbrid, Molinoff, Rudder, & Goodman-Gilman, 1996). These findings are rich in potential for application to health promotion and healing.

HEALTH BEHAVIORS FOR HEALTH PROMOTION AND DISEASE PREVENTION

Individuals' health behavior choices with regard to nutrition, exercise, sleep, and stress management play a large part in the promotion of health and the prevention of disease. Healthy People 2000 objectives related to nutrition and exercise for U.S. citizens are included in Appendix A.

Nutrition in the American Diet

Nutrition includes all the processes by which food is ingested, assimilated, and utilized to promote health and prevent disease. Eating habits affect almost every aspect of one's life—appearance, energy, stamina, resistance to illness, mental outlook, stress level, and academic and social success. Healthy eating, then, requires not only knowledge of nutrition but also an understanding of oneself and an awareness of how different foods affect one's sense of wellness. Dysfunctional eating may be the result of social, emotional or educational barriers. Chapter 26 focuses on nutritional diseases and disorders, including hunger and malnutrition due to poverty and lack of food supply.

Although a nutritionally adequate diet is not difficult to accomplish for most people in the United States, many who have the necessary resources to do so just do not get the nutrition they need. This seems to be a cultural issue in that people do not plan their meals for adequate nutrition. Americans tend to eat whatever is fast, convenient, and affordable, even though this diet is associated with heart disease, hypertension, tooth decay, obesity, and cancer of various organs.

The National Research Council (1989) figures reveal that the average diet in the United States comprises 42% total fat, 10% saturated fat, 25% complex carbohydrates, 21% simple sugars, and 12% protein. This compares with the recommendations of 50% to 55% complex carbohydrates; less than 30% total fat; less than 10% saturated fat; 12% protein; and less than 10% simple sugars.

Data currently available (USDHHS, 1996) indicate increases in obesity at the same time that other data show improvement in areas such as availability of reduced-fat foods and of low-fat, low-calorie food choices in restaurants. And while more worksite nutrition/weight-management programs and education are available, only 1% of schools offer school lunches that fit the less than 30% fat recommendation.

The U.S. Department of Agriculture (USDA) and the USDHHS's report on nutrition monitoring in the United States (1995) was released with this summary:

- Americans are slowly changing their eating patterns toward more healthful diets.
- Approximately one-third of adults and one-fifth of adolescents in the United States are overweight.
- Despite significant progress, 20% of Americans still have high serum-cholesterol levels.
- Hypertension remains a major public health problem in middle-aged and elderly people.
- Many Americans are not getting the calcium they need to maintain optimal bone health and prevent age-related bone loss.
- Fewer than one-third of American adults meet the recommendation to consume five or more servings of fruits and vegetables per day.
- While the availability of food, on a per capita basis, is generally adequate to prevent undernutrition and deficiency-related diseases, data show that some Americans report not always getting enough to eat.

In 1995, the USDA and USDHHS updated their Dietary Guidelines for Americans and encouraged positive behavior choices, as summarized in Figure 9-7.

Figure 9-7   Nutritional Advice for the U.S. Public

In 1995, the USDA updated and summarized the Dietary Guidelines for Americans and advised:

- Eat a variety of foods.
- Balance a diet with plenty of vegetables, fruits, and grain products.
- Choose a diet low in fat, saturated fat, and cholesterol.
- Choose a diet moderate in sugars.
- Choose a diet moderate in salt and sodium.
- If you drink alcoholic beverages, do so in moderation.

From Dietary Guidelines for Americans, *December 1995, USDA & DHHS.*

Figure 9-8 The Eat Right Pyramid

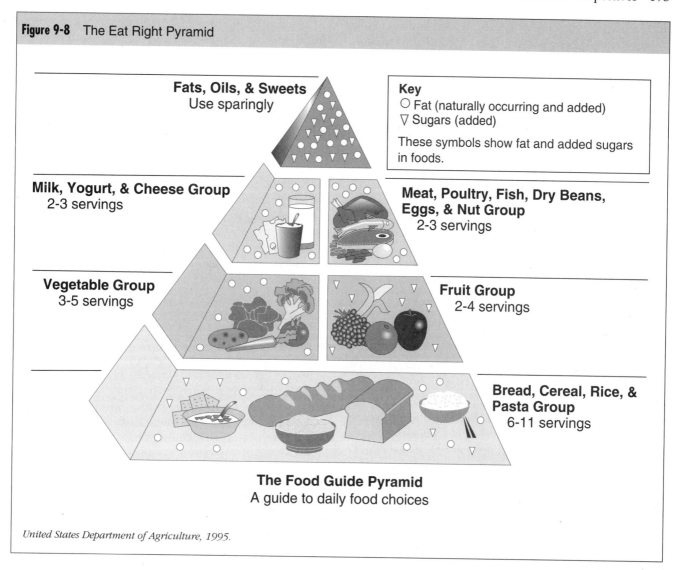

Fats, Oils, & Sweets
Use sparingly

Key
○ Fat (naturally occurring and added)
▽ Sugars (added)

These symbols show fat and added sugars in foods.

Milk, Yogurt, & Cheese Group
2-3 servings

Meat, Poultry, Fish, Dry Beans, Eggs, & Nut Group
2-3 servings

Vegetable Group
3-5 servings

Fruit Group
2-4 servings

Bread, Cereal, Rice, & Pasta Group
6-11 servings

The Food Guide Pyramid
A guide to daily food choices

United States Department of Agriculture, 1995.

Included in the guidelines was the Food Guide Pyramid developed in 1992 (Figure 9-8). The USDA guidelines and corresponding pyramid encouraged consumption of more grains and fewer meats, sweets, and fats, with a broad area representing grains and a narrow area representing sweets and fats to emphasize the relative importance of those foods and the others that were placed between them on the pyramid.

The Daily Food Guide used in Canada takes the form of a rainbow but conveys essentially the same information as that on the Food Guide Pyramid. Both the Daily Food Guide and the Food Guide Pyramid can be easily adapted to include foods from different cultures. (Although fruits, vegetables, and grains as well as the way foods are prepared may vary across cultures, they still correspond to these food guides.)

Vegetarian diets (those composed mainly of grains, vegetables, and fruit) were declared healthful as long as attention was paid to obtaining adequate amounts of iron, zinc, and the B vitamins most commonly found in meat. **Vegans** (persons who choose to eat no meat, eggs, or dairy products) were advised to supplement their diets with Vitamin B_{12} (See the section on vegetarian diets, fol-

lowing.) Also recommended was moderate use of alcohol—no more than one drink per day at mealtime for women or two drinks per day at mealtime for men. A drink was defined as 1.5 oz. of hard liquor, 12 oz. of beer, or 5 oz. of wine.

Vegetarian Diets

A planned vegetarian diet can easily provide the body's nutritional needs. There are four types of vegetarian diets: a **lacto-ovovegan** diet, which includes both dairy products and eggs, a **lactovegan** diet, which includes dairy products but no eggs, an **ovovegan** diet, which includes eggs but no dairy, and a vegan diet, which consists solely of grains, legumes, nuts, seeds, fruits, and vegetables and must be supplemented with vitamin B_{12}.

People choose to be vegetarians for various reasons, including:

- Religious and philosophical concerns related to killing or abusing animals.
- Environmental concerns. It takes approximately 10 pounds of livestock feed to produce 1 pound of meat.

Thus, the food it takes to make 1 pound of meat would serve several people in this time of world hunger being so great.

- Health concerns. Studies show that vegetarians tend to live longer and to experience less disease. In fact, evidence of a positive relationship between consumption of a plant-based diet and prevention of certain diseases is increasing (Keegan, 1996). The latest *Dietary Guidelines* (USDA & USDHHS, 1995) addresses these data in its recommendations. Vegetarians also tend to live healthier lifestyles in nondietary ways.

Vegetarian diets rely mainly on plant foods: grains, vegetables, legumes, fruits, seeds, and nuts. Vegetarians can use food guides but must select meat alternates to fulfill meat requirements (i.e., legumes, seeds, nuts, and tofu). Soy products provide nutrients similar to dairy products, especially if they have been fortified with calcium, vitamin D, and vitamin B_{12}. A vegetarian diet requires the use of vegetable protein sources, such as soybeans and grains, to prevent protein deficiency (Health and Welfare Canada, 1992).

Advantages of a vegetarian diet are: (1) increased fiber, which helps prevent colon cancer and diverticulitis; (2) decreased daily caloric intake and, thus, obesity, because vegetables tend to be low in calories; (3) decreased total fat, saturated fat, and cholesterol intake, which decreases the risk of many diseases including heart disease, stroke, and cancer; and (4) financial economy, because vegetables, fruits, and grains are much less expensive than meat (Messina & Barnes, 1991).

Nutritional Supplements

A controversy surrounds the supplemental use of vitamins and minerals generally provided by fruits, vegetables, and whole grains. Conventional wisdom holds that a well-balanced diet consisting of plenty of whole foods—whole-grain breads, fresh fruits, and vegetables—supplies the necessary variety and amounts of vitamins and minerals. In this view, supplementation should be necessary only for those people who primarily eat processed foods, in which vitamins and minerals have been destroyed.

Many nutritionists and researchers, however, believe that the recommended dietary allowances (RDAs) for many vitamins and minerals are too low and that it is probably wise to take a well-balanced daily vitamin supplement in addition to following a well-balanced diet. They furthermore contend that other supplements may be needed for treatment and prevention of health problems. Use of nutritional supplements for treatment purposes seems to be increasing, and ongoing research will continue to add to the knowledge base.

As people seek more natural ways of managing their health, herbal remedies are seeing increasing use. Herbs have been used for medicinal purposes in all cultures since ancient time. Many herbs continue to be used in modern prescription and nonprescription drugs (e.g., aspirin, Listerine, Metamucil) and in our everyday lives as stimulants (coffee) or gastrointestinal aids (mints).

Herbal remedies are used by many in place of medication or in addition to medication. Health professionals concerned with the potential dangers of herbal remedies are engaged in a political struggle with those who demand the right to purchase and consume herbs of their choice. While most herbal remedies are probably harmless, there is concern that some may be dangerous, especially when in combination with other prescribed medications or drugs. Consumers are often hesitant to tell their physicians about using herbs, but physicians should know about such use before prescribing medications.

The nurse will find a good reference book on the use of herbs for health purposes a valuable resource in understanding a client's herbal practices. Further, a good reference book on herbal practices will provide information on the undesirable qualities associated with the various herbs (Castleman, 1991).

Substances to Avoid

Other nutritional and lifestyle factors to be considered are the use of alcohol and caffeine. Alcohol use is generally considered addictive, habituating, and diuretic. It also depletes the body's stores of B vitamins and folic acid, inducing fatigue, uncomfortable menstruation, more severe premenstrual syndrome, headaches, and dehydration. Caffeine is also a diuretic and causes the body to excrete needed nutrients and causes the stomach to produce irritating excess gastric acid and enzymes. Decaffeinated coffee and tea pose other health risks in that the solvent most often used to remove the caffeine is a suspected carcinogen.

Additives

American food manufacturers use thousands of artificial colorings, preservatives, flavorings, and emulsifiers in their products to make foods less expensive, safe to eat, more visually appealing, and easier to store. Certain additives help prevent food poisoning. Whereas some additives may be safe, others have not yet been sufficiently tested. Some are associated with allergic reactions and increased risk of cancer. The National Research Council (NRC) reports that in the United States, nearly 3,000 substances are intentionally added to foods during processing. Reducing the risk of these substances means using fresh and/or organic produce and simple, unprocessed foods. Reading all labels of packaged foods is essential (NRC, 1989).

Environmental Pollutants of Food

Part of Chapter 7 was devoted to a discussion of environmental pollution and its effect on the food supply. Synthetic pesticides are subject to the approval of the Environmental Protection Agency (EPA) and are applied to fruits and vegetables to kill insects that could damage the crops. Fungicides, the class of pesticides of greatest concern, are applied to extend shelf life and to make produce picture-perfect. The EPA sets tolerance levels for

Figure 9-9 Protection from Pesticide Residue

- Use organically grown produce.
- Use domestically grown produce.
- Buy in season.
- Wash all fresh produce with water only.
- Peel or remove the outer layers of lettuce, cabbage, and other leafy vegetables. Peel waxed coatings from cucumbers and apples.
- Grow your own fruit and vegetables. Join an organic gardening cooperative.
- Select fresh meat and poultry with a nonslimy appearance.
- Trim all visible fat from meat and skin from poultry prior to cooking.
- Cook meat and fish thoroughly.
- Rinse all meats with water before cooking.
- Become a vegetarian and eliminate meat, poultry, and fish from your diet.
- Keep food cold.
- Clean everything thoroughly.

National Research Council, 1989.

pesticide residues, and the Food and Drug Administration (FDA) enforces the residue-monitoring program.

Environmental activists such as the National Resource Defense Council (NRDC) and the Americans for Safe Food (AFSF) claim that governmental agencies are too lax in their approval processes, regulations, and monitoring with regard to pesticides. The degree of risk is controversial at this time. Figure 9-9 lists safeguards for those who are concerned about pesticide residue in foods.

Consumers concerned with wellness and health promotion often advocate a simple diet of vegetables, fruits, nuts, seeds, grains, and fish. Foods that are "enriched" and "preserved" with additives are believed to stress the liver in its attempts to break down, detoxify, or store those substances that do not metabolize. Junk foods are discouraged because they decrease the appetite for nutritious foods.

The community health nurse must have in-depth knowledge not only of nutritional processes but also of human responses to the many psychological and cultural issues surrounding food and eating. Because nutrition is a major factor in health and healing, the nurse uses such knowledge daily, when teaching and counseling individuals, families, and groups. Because much is still to be discovered, the nurse's educational process with regard to nutrition should be lifelong.

Sleep and Health Behavior Choice

Adequate sleep is known to enhance attentiveness, concentration, mood, and motivation. Lack of sleep impairs judgment and makes one irritable. Research has shown that sleep deprivation may also play a major role in some chronic conditions (Cridland, 1993).

Sleep researchers believe that to make more time for other things that crowd their lives the majority of Americans sleep 60 to 90 minutes fewer a night than is necessary for optimum functioning. Sleep is considered expendable, and less sleep is culturally valued as a sign of ambition and drive (Edlin & Golanty, 1992).

While cultural beliefs and values influence the quantity of sleep people allow themselves, other sleep problems arise from overeating, sickness, jet lag, anxiety, excitement, or losing a loved one. These problems, however, tend to resolve quickly.

The majority of people with long-term sleep problems have insomnia. They have trouble falling asleep or staying asleep, or they awaken after a few hours and cannot go back to sleep. The results are fatigue, desire to nap, inability to concentrate, impaired judgment, and a lack of interest in life. Such sleep problems are usually due to disease, chronic pain, depression, addictions, or other mental health disorders. Although sleep disorders may occur because of damage to the sleep centers in the brain, most represent some form of disharmony within the self or with one's surroundings. Restoring inner harmony is a way to return to one's natural rest–activity cycle (Edlin & Golanty, 1992).

Cridland (1993), a family practice physician and specialist in health promotion, recommends eight or nine hours of sleep per night as part of a healthful lifestyle. Sleep enables healing as well as recovery from everyday wear and tear. If sleep is insufficient, this wear and tear accumulates until symptoms of degenerative changes surface. Cridland maintains that sleep is essential for normal functioning and to maintain health over a lifetime.

When body energy is low and the nervous system is fatigued, the immune system is affected, resulting in more infections and allergies and impaired cognitive functioning and coping ability. The nurse can promote the client's health by teaching and encouraging constructive sleep behavior. Figure 9-10 lists suggestions by Castleman (1996) for addressing sleep problems.

◎◎ REFLECTIVE THINKING ◎◎

How Could You Improve Your Nutrition?

- Think about your own food intake in recent years. How does it fit with the recommendations cited in this section? Which recommendations do you follow consistently? Which ones are more difficult for you?

- Name some small changes you can make now.

- Make a plan to implement one change you would like to make in your food patterns.

- Why are your own eating habits important to your role as a community health nurse?

Figure 9-10 How to Get a Good Night's Sleep

- First, see your physician to rule out diseases that can cause disrupted sleep: depression, epilepsy, chronic pain, Parkinson's disease, and other conditions. Review with the physician all medications you are taking, including over-the-counter medications.
- Reduce consumption of such stimulants as coffee, tea, cocoa, chocolate, and soft drinks.
- Limit alcohol (often causes troubled sleep).
- Quit smoking; nicotine is a powerful stimulant.
- Do not eat near bedtime; digestive processes disturb sleep.
- Take vitamins and minerals; deficiencies in the B vitamins, calcium, copper, iron, magnesium, or zinc can contribute to sleep problems.
- Sleep in a large enough bed. Couples should have a queen or king size bed or sleep separately if differing sleep patterns create sleep problems for either partner.
- Wear ear plugs to keep things quiet and use double-paned windows.
- Make the room dark by using blackout drapes, blinds, shades, or a sleep mask.
- Get out of bed when it is time to get up even if you have not slept well.
- Go to bed and wake up at the same time every day, including on weekends.
- Try deep relaxation to help minimize the stress that contributes to sleep problems. Try meditation, massage, or listening to soothing music.
- Keep a *To Do* list if you stay awake worrying that you might forget to do something. Before going to bed, jot down all concerns that might keep you awake.
- Try herbal sleep aids, such as balm, catnip, chamomile, passionflower, skullcap, or valerian.
- Try melatonin, a hormone that is produced by the pineal gland and helps many people fall asleep and stay asleep (suggested dosage: 0.1 to 3.0 mg).

From Dead Tired by M. Castleman, 1996, San Francisco Focus, October 1996, p. 136. Adapted with permission of Michael Castleman.

Physical Exercise

Epidemiologic studies show that approximately 250,000 deaths per year in the United States result from lack of regular physical activity. Regular physical activity reduces the risk of many diseases including heart disease, hypertension, cancer, osteoporosis, and diabetes mellitus. In addition, physiological evidence shows that physical activity improves many biological measures associated with health and psychological functioning. It is therefore essential that our society move from being a sedentary one to one that is more active.

At the same time that more and more people are sitting in front of computer screens at work and at schools,

schools and universities are cutting back on their physical education programs because of financial cutbacks. Communities have less money to build and staff parks, recreational areas, and playgrounds. Children and youth find it easier to watch television or play video games than to engage in individual or group physical activity (USDHHS, 1996). One of the greatest challenges encountered by the Healthy People 2000 project is getting people to exercise. Although more worksites have workout rooms and exercise programs, the exercise objectives with regard to children and youth are losing ground. See Appendix A for the list of objectives developed for the fitness priority.

The USDA and the USDHHS (1995) included exercise guidelines as part of their dietary recommendations. Exercise was stressed in this way because of its role in weight management. An increase in physical activity allows for greater caloric and nutrient intake without weight gain. People are encouraged to apply the principles of variety, balance, and moderation in their selection of activities. Participating in many different physical activities exercises many muscles. The activities chosen should provide an exercise balance, focusing on cardiovascular endurance,

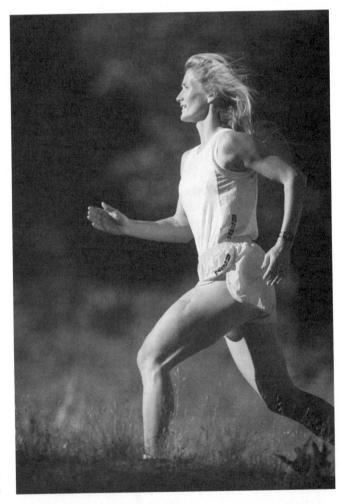

Regular physical activity coupled with proper nutrition and adequate sleep promotes wellness. Examine your own activity, nutrition and sleep patterns. How could you improve them?

muscular strength, bone strength, and flexibility. One should exercise to stay fit without overdoing. Thirty minutes or more of moderate daily exercise most days of the week is generally advised.

Culture is a major determinant of the quantity and quality of exercise. In the past, hunting for food and traveling met this human need in some cultures and civilizations. In more recent times, work on farms and in industrial settings required physical exercise. Recreational activities often involve movement and exercise. Culturally based dances have traditionally offered rich opportunities to be physically active while enjoying the spiritual benefits of dance rituals. African dance, for example, can be aerobic, work upper body muscles, and improve coordination.

In the Western European cultures, walking, jogging, running, bicycling, dancing, and aerobic workouts have become favorites of the middle class. Aerobic exercise practiced according to cardiovascular training principles provides an efficient and effective way to achieve the exercise needed for optimum health.

The best known benefit of physical exercise is **aerobic conditioning**, wherein the heart and lungs are subjected to a *planned* series of exercises that forcefully cause heart and respiration rates to rise rapidly and thus deliver large volumes of blood and oxygen to the cells of the body. See Figure 9-11 for beneficial outcomes of regular aerobic exercise.

People who exercise regularly often report psychological and spiritual benefits such as reduced anxiety, tension, and fatigue and increased vigor and ability to cope with stress. Regular exercise also tends to eliminate depression, improve self-image and self-esteem, and promote a sense of calmness (Edlin & Golanty, 1992).

Coping with Stress

Stress is the body's reaction to any stimulant. **Stressors** are the environmental pressures that activate one's **stress response**. These pressures can be either desirable, thereby providing opportunity, or undesirable, thereby posing obstacles to progress. The stress response presents as behavior changes and changes in the autonomic nervous and immune systems. Chronic stress response may precipitate a variety of physical disorders.

Stress has been shown to lead to illness in three different ways: by directly damaging tissues, by leading to self-destructive habits as means of coping (e.g., drug and alcohol use), and/or by fostering denial such that necessary lifestyle changes or need for appropriate assistance is ignored. During stress, tissue function is altered and neurohormonal changes occur. Tissue changes associated with short-term stress are temporary. Alterations in tissue resulting from long-term stress are often permanent.

Plotnikoff, Faith, and Murgo (1991) have contributed greatly to the understanding of how stress affects the body and how certain coping behaviors alter stress and its effects. The positive health behaviors discussed here and in other chapters have been found to improve coping ability. These behaviors include a healthy diet; exercise; **deep relaxation** (a state intentionally induced to promote inner-healing processes and rejuvenation) and sleep; conflict resolution; enjoying the beauty of nature; living creatively with joy, meaning, and purpose; and maintaining a strong support system. See Table 9-1 for a comparison of personal characteristics that make one less prone or more prone to stress.

Figure 9-11 Benefits of Regular Exercise

Aerobic workouts are used by many to accomplish their fitness goals. Short of planned aerobic workouts, Donna Shalala, Secretary of U.S. Health and Human Services (1995), encouraged citizens to garden, play golf, walk briskly, and use the stairs instead of elevators. These activities can help control weight, improve health, and prevent disease.

The benefits of a regular exercise program include:

- A healthy heart and blood vessels.
- Maintenance of body weight within generally accepted normal limits.
- Prevention and alleviation of chronic low-back pain.
- Improved sleep.
- Greater energy reserve for work and recreation.
- Improved posture, which leads to improved physical appearance and the ability to withstand fatigue.
- Greater ability of the body to cope with illness or accidents.

From Nutrition and Your Health: Dietary Guidelines for Americans (4th ed) *by U.S. Department of Agriculture and U.S. Department of Health and Human Services, 1995, Washington, D.C.: Author.*

ꙮ ꙮ REFLECTIVE THINKING ꙮ ꙮ

Stress

- How do you experience stress?

- Which stressful situations in your life can you influence so that they are less stressful?

- Which stressful situations do you believe cannot be changed? How can you better cope with these situations?

- Are you aware of a time when you became ill due to stress? What early signals might you have noticed? What might you have done differently to alter your stress level or your ability to cope?

- How can you distinguish between stress sufficient to provide a challenge for growth and stress sufficient to make you ill?

Table 9.1 Personal Characteristics As Indicators of Proneness to Stress Response	
LESS PRONE	**MORE PRONE**
• Believe they can control their environment	• Believe they lack control
• Perceive life changes to be opportunities for growth	• Feel helpless in the face of change
• Ready and willing to respond to challenges	• In the face of challenges, hold little hope for favorable outcomes
• Optimistic about their ability to succeed	• Seek permission from others prior to acting

Adapted from Health and Wellness: A Holistic Approach *(4th ed., p. 216) by G. Edlin & E. Golanty, 1992, Boston: Jones & Bartlett. Copyright 1992 by Jones & Bartlett.*

A good social support system depends on the availability of other people who offer care and support, positive social climate (absence of prejudice, racism, and expectations), and institutional support and services. Necessary resources for those who seek help in stressful situations include appropriate income, food, and shelter; access to information and helping services; and, perhaps, tools and equipment. These are all resources the nurse may be able to offer.

Behavior Choice and Prevention of Disease and Disability

Behaviors related to nutrition, exercise, sleep, and stress management are significant in preventing disease and disability. Because accidents often happen when people are stressed or sleep deprived, preventive behaviors also include those that address safety. Stressed people are often hurried and distracted and may ignore safety precautions and regulations made by society to protect

✪ REFLECTIVE THINKING ✪

Social Support

• List the people you have warm feelings for, feel comfortable with, and who nurture you. Think of long-standing friends—friends from school, work, classes, churches, and social or political groups.

• Look at your list of friends. Are there some with whom you would like to reconnect, even in the form of a long-distance relationship?

• Some names may trigger a feeling of wanting to do something for those people—to send a card, a note, a tape, a gift. Note these feelings on another list.

• Make your lists into a diagram—or place the names of the people on a map of the world wherever the people live.

• Put this map in a prominent place. When you glance at it, imagine those people and send them a warm thought or a beautiful color. Do not be surprised if you hear from someone on your list.

human health. A distracted mind and a lack of concentration or mindfulness in the present may also contribute to accidents. The practice of meditation helps to focus the mind, develop concentration, and promote calmness.

ALTERNATIVE/COMPLEMENTARY THERAPIES USED FOR HEALTH PROMOTION

Alternative therapies to facilitate holistic healing processes were discussed in Chapter 6 and include those that are used by consumers in place of or in addition to traditional medical care. These approaches are also used for health promotion and disease prevention by clients and care providers. Many therapies are currently in use; those selected for discussion here are deep relaxation and **imagery** (a quasiperceptual event of which we are self-consciously aware and that exists in the absence of stimuli that produce genuine sensory or perceptual counterparts) and Jin Shin Jyutsu, a **touch therapy** to promote energy balance and harmony. The techniques presented here are simple to use, and further training is available as continuing education for nurses.

Deep Relaxation

Deep relaxation and imagery are used together to influence a person's physiology, mental state, and behavior. Such therapy can counter chronic distress and promote more positive self-perceptions and a stronger sense of well-being. Chronic distress can precipitate physiological damage resulting in heart disease, ulcers, and other disorders, or it may manifest as emotional difficulties such as depression and chronic anxiety (Bresler, 1991). It seems that when the body/mind is deeply relaxed, a healing process inherent in nature is triggered.

As is evident in the following discussion, relaxation strategies incorporate imagery without always identifying it as such. Conversely, imagery strategies employ relaxation techniques, and their outcomes result in part from the relaxation response, although the imagery may make the intervention more meaningful to the individual.

Clearly, the two strategies potentiate each other; yet, each has value in its own right, and they are usually defined separately. Discussion here begins with relaxation.

Relaxation as a state is usually defined as the absence or lessening of tension. It affects heart rate, respiratory rate, and blood pressure and reflects psychological and physiological conditions such as anxiety and muscle tension. The concept came into general use as an intervention when Benson (1975) coined the term *relaxation response* to denote the state produced by an exercise that came to be known as a technique. Others later developed variations on the exercise, and it became an integral part of guided imagery experiences (Shames, 1996). In **guided imagery**, the guide (or nurse) makes suggestions to help guide the client's experience. In **interactive guided imagery**, dialogue is ongoing between the nurse and client, with the suggestions made by the nurse depending on the client's responses.

Benson (1975) identified four essential ingredients of a technique to bring about the relaxation response: decreased environmental stimuli; a mental device such as an object on which to dwell (a word, sound, object, or feeling); a passive attitude; and a comfortable position requiring minimal muscular work. His relaxation exercise incorporated these qualities in a systematic manner (see Figure 9-12).

Relaxation exercises are often employed as adjuncts to other therapies and are used in a variety of settings. They are particularly appropriate for use in home visits, hospice, and private practice, where community health nurses often work with clients who are experiencing stress. Pain and other symptoms that result from muscle tension and insomnia caused by emotional stress are often relieved by relaxation exercises. In general, application opportunities are similar to those for guided imagery, discussed next.

Guided Imagery

Imagery involves mental pictures, as in visualization, and/or mental representations of hearing, touch, smell, taste, and movement. Such representations may be of reality, fantasy, or both. The body responds physiologically to imagery in the same way as to an external event. In our minds, "We can hear the sound of our child's voice, see a loved one's face, smell a fish, taste a lemon, feel our feet buried in warm sand, and sense our bodies swimming in cool water" (Zahourek, 1988, p. 53). Imagining any of these stimuli can evoke noticeable responses.

In imagery as a health care intervention, our ability to visualize and form other mental images is put to use to benefit well-being. Mental images can have a profound effect on physiology and view of self. The nurse may guide the client in using the imagery process to facilitate natural healing processes and may teach the client to use the process at other times to enhance the overall healing effect.

Rew (1996) notes that a number of nursing research studies have indicated that imagery promotes the healing process. She finds imagery appropriate for nursing because it is noninvasive and always available for use and "demonstrates the application of esthetic knowledge in healing" (p. 79). Moreover, clinical reports show that imagery helps clients work with a wide range of conditions including chronic pain, allergies, high blood pressure, irregular heartbeat, autoimmune diseases, cold and flu symptoms, and stress-related gastrointestinal, reproductive, and urinary complaints (Rossman, 1993). Imagery also seems to help speed healing after injuries such as sprains, strains, or broken bones. Much of the benefit is probably due to the client's becoming deeply relaxed and learning to cope with stress.

Because of a desire to provide noninvasive and non-chemical support to clients seeking help for physiological or psychosocial difficulties, nurses' interest in imagery has grown in recent years. Current research in the area of psychoneuroimmunology reinforces the idea that what occurs in the mind affects the body (Shames, 1996).

Visualization, the most common form of imagery, is based on the ability to see an image in the mind's eye, although all the senses may be involved. One might imagine lying on the beach, feeling the warm sand, listening to the ocean, and smelling the sea air. Try the exercise in Figure 9-13 to experience visualization. Rossman (1993) suggests that persons who are unable to visualize "may be able to relax by imagining the warmth of the sun, recalling a favorite tune, or conjuring up the aroma of brewing coffee or the taste of freshly baked bread" (p. 12). Often, a person who is not ordinarily aware of visual images will experience them when doing an imagery exercise.

Figure 9-12   Benson's Relaxation Technique

1. Sit quietly in a comfortable position.

2. Close your eyes.

3. Deeply relax all your muscles, beginning at your feet and progressing up to your face. Keep them relaxed.

4. Breathe through your nose. Become aware of your breathing. As you breathe out, silently say the word "one" to yourself. Breathe easily and naturally.

5. Continue for 10 to 20 minutes. You may open your eyes to check the time, but do not use an alarm. When finished, sit quietly for several minutes, at first with your eyes closed and later with your eyes opened. Do not stand up for a few minutes.

6. Do not worry about whether you are successful in achieving a deep level of relaxation. Maintain a passive attitude and permit relaxation to occur at its own pace. When distracting thoughts occur, ignore them by not dwelling on them and return to repeating "one." With practice the response should come with little effort. Practice the technique once or twice daily, but not within 2 hours after any meal.

From The Relaxation Response *by H. Benson, 1975, New York: William Morrow.*

Figure 9-13   A Relaxing Imagery Exercise

- Keep your eyes closed while taking a few deep, easy breaths and imagining yourself in the most peaceful, beautiful, serene place possible. Think of a time when you felt relaxed and peaceful—perhaps during a walk in the park, a day on a sunny beach, or an evening at a concert—and focus intently on the sights, smells, and physical sensations associated with that event. Focus on this image for approximately five minutes.

- Reorient to everyday reality and take notice of how you feel. You may feel calmer, more alert, and refreshed—as if you had had a longer rest.

Training in interactive guided imagery (Rossman & Bressler, 1994) is also available to nurses. In this form of guided imagery, the nurse and client work together, with the nurse providing the structure and the client directing the interaction. The client is thus self-empowered by using unconscious processes to direct and guide the therapeutic intervention, and the nurse honors the client's inner guidance by accepting whatever comes and providing support as the client explores the images for meaning.

Jin Shin Jyutsu

Jin Shin Jyutsu® (JSJ) uses hand contact at specific points on the body to promote energy flow and thus improve health and well-being. An ancient art rediscovered in the 20th century by Jiro Murai in Japan, JSJ has been taught in the United States by Mary Burmeister since the 1950s. Her students now lead workshops throughout the United States and around the world.

According to this therapy, there are 26 JSJ **safety energy locks** located on each side of the body (see Figure 9-14), so called because each is understood to lock as a safety mechanism when it becomes overloaded by such factors as lifestyle excesses, tensions, habits, emotional anxieties, accidents, or hereditary characteristics (Burmeister, 1994). Resulting alterations in energy flow produce discomfort, letting us know when attention must be paid to the body.

The goal of a JSJ session is to facilitate harmony and balance in the client's energy patterns. The role of the practitioner is to use the hands to help restore the natural flow and rhythm of the universal revitalizing energy along the client's energy circulation pathways. Comparing the relationship between the universal energy source and one's body to that between a battery and a car, Burmeister (1994) speaks of using the hands as "jumper cables" (pp. 5–6). According to Burmeister, unlocking one or more of the 26 safety energy locks can relieve the tensions that cause imbalances, restoring proper functioning of the body. During a JSJ treatment, hand contact (jumper cabling) is used at two safety energy locks to promote energy flow.

Clients are encouraged to participate in their care and become independent from the practitioner by learning to maintain energy balance on their own through JSJ self-help flow patterns. Self-help flow patterns differ from those performed by one person to help another in that they are brief and simple. For example, one set of safety energy locks may be used, or a finger of one hand may be held with the other hand. One of the authors recently helped a fellow passenger on an interstate airline flight to ease severe pain simply by using a self-help flow, which she demonstrated and for which she offered support as it was used.

A regular JSJ self-help program may be practiced by those interested in following a lifestyle of health promotion. Figure 9-15 offers a basic self-help flow that can be done regularly to help maintain balance and harmony, the goal of many **alternative** and **complementary therapies**, those therapies used in place of or in addition to standard medical interventions.

Clinical Application of Alternative Therapies in Community Health Nursing

Alternative therapies may be used for direct intervention in community health nursing. These tools are intended to support healing processes inherent in nature and to help provide an environment in which the person can either heal or experience optimum health.

Tools such as Therapeutic Touch (introduced in Chapter 6), JSJ, deep relaxation, and guided imagery may be used along with counseling and teaching as direct services in primary, secondary, and tertiary situations. These tools also provide self-help mechanisms that can be taught in a myriad of situations unique to the individual or family. For example the nurse who goes into a home and finds someone in physical, emotional, mental, or spiritual pain may decide to offer Therapeutic Touch (TT). A few minutes of TT during each visit to an expectant mother experiencing a high-risk pregnancy may provide the comfort, support, and relaxation needed. A treatment of TT for someone dying of a painful illness may help to bring peace and comfort in that process.

A host of JSJ self-help techniques can be applied by the client or by family members. These tools can help people who are dealing with addictions and other psychological stressors. Family members who are taught to do the treatments may, in turn, find comfort in their own abilities to help their loved ones. These and other health enhancers are brought to larger populations through presentations at established facilities in the community, such as senior centers and youth programs.

The nurse speaking in the accompanying perspectives box, who works as the coordinator for HIV/AIDS/hepatitis B services in a county health department, uses alternative methods in her approach to self-care.

Figure 9-14   Location of 26 "Safety Energy Locks" Used in Jin Shin Jyutsu®

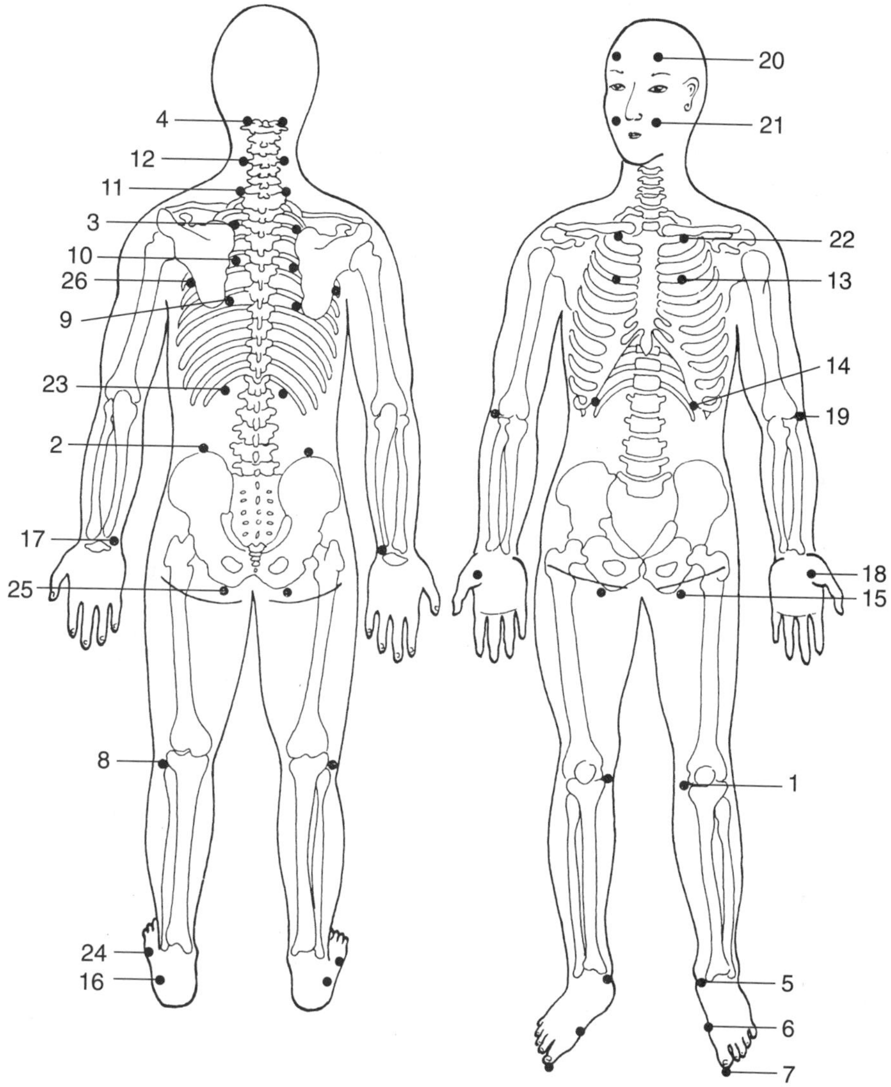

From Introducing Jin Shin Jyustu, Book I *(6th ed., p.14) by M. Burmeister, 1994, Scottsdale, AZ: Jin Shin Jyutsu, Inc. Copyright 1985, 1994. Reprinted with permission of Jin Shin Jyutsu, Inc.*

Figure 9-15   Jin Shin Jyutsu® Self-Help Flow: Main Central

Right hand on top of head

Left hand between eyebrows

Left hand on tip of nose

Left hand between the breasts

Left hand at base of sternum

Left hand on top of pubic bone

Right hand at base of spine (coccyx)

Hold fingers of the right hand on top of the head and hold fingers of the left hand between the eyebrows. Hold the two areas for a minute or two or until a pulse is felt in both hands and comes into its own harmony. Continue to hold the right hand on top of head while you hold each of the other areas listed above. Move your right hand to the coccyx while keeping your left at the top of the pubic bone to complete the flow. Do this flow every day to feel a difference in your well-being.

From Introducing Jin Shin Jyustu, Book I *(6th ed., p.14) by M. Burmeister, 1994, Scottsdale, AZ: Jin Shin Jyutsu, Inc. Copyright, 1985, 1994. Reprinted with permission of Jin Shin Jyutsu, Inc.*

Perspectives...

Insights of a Public Health Nurse

My success as a public health nurse depends on the choices I make to keep my body, mind, and spirit in balance. If I am to serve as an effective catalyst, I must create a balance of family dynamics and work issues and actively participate in my own well-being. Only then can I raise my consciousness and be a catalyst for change.

I have a responsibility to give information to my clients that will help them function at a higher level. They will not use the information to improve or learn new skills unless they are receptive and choose to do so. Trust and acceptance are built by my listening and being nonjudgmental. The family begins to heal on its own when listening is my instrument.

I am unable to provide a healing environment for myself or others when I allow negative thoughts and attitudes to enter my mind. During these times, I depend on my intuition and take time out to restore my body, mind, and spirit. I may use pleasant aromas, sounds, or tastes or take time to experience some form of healing to align myself with the Higher Spirit.

I typically begin my day with a few deep breaths and stretches, a dip in the hot tub, a few minutes of meditation to erase negative thoughts from my mind, a cup of herbal tea, and some music for my soul. I try to eat a balance of organic fruits, vegetables, and grains and to drink purified water to nourish my body.

My commute to work is often a challenging experience, but with the help of classical music or inspirational words on tape, I usually arrive with a positive attitude and feeling refreshed. Throughout the day, I seek ways to practice acts of kindness. I believe that the goodness that is put out to the universe comes back in return.

I apply the principles of Feng Shui to create a harmonious environment in my office. Feng Shui is an ancient art of arranging the environment to create a state of well-being. I have a small water fountain on my desk, a broad-spectrum light, and a healing corner with herbal teas, linaments, herbal remedies, and some green plants. I use a headset to prevent neck and shoulder pain when using the phone, use an ergonomically correct chair to prevent back strain, and walk a mile at least once a day.

When a client or coworker is experiencing headache, back pain, menstrual cramps, or some other discomfort, I spend a few minutes listening and then, if he or she is willing, apply some healing energy in the form of acupressure or Therapeutic Touch.

I do Chi Gong energizing movement exercises or some form of self-massage when I feel my energy is being depleted. Chi Gong is a series of movements to enhance the energy flow of the body, calming the mind and deepening the breath. I wear stones and crystals to help me feel grounded, and I take supplements to maintain my vitality. If I am in an environment where illness is present, I stimulate my immune system by using herbs such as echinacea and astragalus.

When I approach families and individuals who are in emotional or physical pain, I visualize a protective white light surrounding my body. Illness and wellness are all part of the life–death cycle, and it is my work to stay in balance.

—*Lynn Whitney, RN, CHN*

CLINICAL IMPLICATIONS

Health promotion is not a primary focus in most nursing settings. Primary prevention is the major emphasis of health-education programs. Community health nurses in certain settings such as schools and workplaces do have opportunities to teach individuals and groups in health-promotion efforts. Creative, energetic, and entrepreneurial nurses in private practice can experiment with alternative/complementary therapies and practice health promotion. See Appendix C for a Lifestyle Assessment Questionnaire (National Wellness Institute, Inc. 1997). This assessment tool reflects a picture of health in many aspects.

Preventive work often is done by nurses in homes, schools, workplaces, and community clinics. Community health nursing practice is primarily based on the prevention model. Activities involve primary, secondary, and tertiary care work. This work includes identifying health risks, screening for potential health deviations, providing updated information and general health education, and counseling to gain participation. Although health-education programs are multidisciplinary, the community health nurse is crucial to prevention programs.

Community nursing centers (CNCs), a recent development, are places where clients are observed, screened, and treated. Key management and staff positions are filled by nurses with graduate and baccalaureate degrees. Two-thirds are certified for advanced nursing practice (Barger & Rosenfeld, 1993). These centers generally serve older individuals and young families with lower incomes; one-half of the clients served are members of minority groups. The populations reached by these centers are those typically neglected or underserved. These nursing centers may take a larger role in health care delivery of the future and are discussed further in Chapter 32.

Primary Prevention

Primary prevention is those activities carried out to prevent disease, disability, and injury. Health education is a major strategy in primary prevention. Research has indicated that health education affects health behavior choice and change (Niknian, Lefebvre, & Carleton, 1991). Multifaceted programs are needed to address varied needs. Colorful, fast-moving, and interactive presentations appeal to a public accustomed to television and telecommunication. Learning within the context of a caring relationship, though, is important because health behavior is personal. Chapter 8 discusses effective social environments for learning.

Community health nurses are seeking ways to be increasingly creative in their approaches to health education. Some ideas are offered here to stimulate imaginative and creative strategies to make teaching and learning fun for clients and groups of clients.

The therapeutic use of story is an enjoyable and effective tool in health-education programs. **Story telling** is the sharing of stories from one person to another. Clients naturally tell their stories as they give their life histories, and nurses convey stories of how other clients have coped or experienced success with challenges they have faced. Stories also provide myth and metaphor for the unconscious mind as it seeks healing through symbolic meanings. People create their own meanings in relation to the stories they hear, making stories powerful tools for healing. Appreciation of cultural diversity and cultural understanding is effectively taught through story telling, and these stories seem to "burst for the telling" (Takaki, 1993).

Television offers a powerful tool for education of the general public. There has been grave concern in recent years that children are being taught to value violence through television's use. It seems likely that life-affirming values could also be taught on television. Such values might be equally influential in society and help to teach positive health behaviors. To this end, creative and artistic nurses can offer educational programming for health education.

Local television stations offer opportunities for innovative programming. Nurses can take advantage of such opportunities to deliver primary prevention to large and targeted populations. A children's puppet show, for example, could tell the tale of Cindy's strep throat, or a health-education program could include a community health nurse and a primary physician or nurse practitioner as cohosts. Because many families have access to video cassette recorders (VCRs), video production also provides opportunities.

The nurse may also use creative abilities to write for magazines or develop pamphlets, comic books, television scripts, or plays. For example, Kaiser Foundation Health Education in California developed a play in which teens demonstrate how lack of openness and knowledge can contribute to the spread of sexually transmitted diseases.

Computer communication is an increasingly valuable resource for health education as more and more people acquire this technology. The computer-savvy nurse can write educational computer programs and use graphic design software to develop visual teaching aids. The opportunities for community health education are great. Community health nurses must continue working with public health and volunteer agencies such as the American Cancer Society, the American Heart Association, American Lung Association, the American Red Cross, and the American Diabetes Association to reach people at health fairs, classes, and counseling. At the same time, nurses must address the technological influences in society through creative development of educational programs using today's technology.

Finally, nurses teach by modeling healthy behavior; exhibition of destructive health behaviors undermines credibility of the teacher. Modeling is a powerful tool, as the nurse goes beyond "illness" or "disease" care and guides clients to health and high-level wellness. This extension is necessary as social awareness shifts from a disease orientation to one of health and wellness and as costs of disease care rise (Swinford & Webster, 1989).

Secondary Prevention

Secondary prevention is those activities related to early detection and treatment. It focuses on clinical screening to detect disease in its early stages and involves in-depth interviewing, history taking, and physical examination. While engaged in these processes, the well-educated, alert, psychologically astute, and culturally sensitive nurse uses observational skills to detect persons who are either at risk or show early signs of disease. Identification of **risk factors** (precursors to disease that increase one's risk of the disease) is a crucial aspect of community health nursing practice.

History taking provides the foundation for identification of risk factors, and this process continues for the length of the nurse–client relationship. With the deepening of

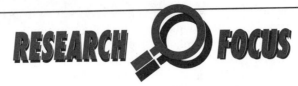

Are People More Health Conscious? A Longitudinal Study of One Community

STUDY PROBLEM/PURPOSE

The purpose of this study was to test the assumption that people will make decisions to adopt recommended health behaviors if provided with the information and motivation to support those decisions.

METHODS

Innovative television programming was introduced at the Pawtucket Heart Health Program in New England as part of its health-education program. Twelve hundred and fifty participants between ages 18 and 65 and from randomly selected families (one member from each family) were interviewed yearly over a period of five years to document awareness, knowledge, and behavior changes over time and to determine health behavior trends. Physical assessment and laboratory testing were used to measure height, weight, pulse, blood pressure, cholesterol (with HDL/LDL ratios), and triglyceride levels. Members of another similar town without the television intervention served as a control group.

FINDINGS

The participants from the town that used the television media as part of the program made the most change. Statistical regression analysis techniques were employed to rule out confounding data related to age, gender, education level, and employment status.

Because a high proportion of respondents spoke a foreign language at home, questions were raised about the influence of culture on health behavior change. The data indicated that the more homogeneous, affluent, and well-educated the people, the more the change in awareness, knowledge, and behavior.

IMPLICATIONS

Results indicated that important changes are emerging in cardiovascular health awareness, knowledge, and behavior and that such changes are *not* due to the increased presence of prevention programs at either worksites or religious or social organizations but, instead, are likely attributable to programs mediated through electronic and print mass media (p. 206).

The findings support the use of electronic and mass media in health education and further validate the idea that nursing should develop new teaching roles in health education. Creative domains such as theater, television drama, computer interaction, and virtual reality media may provide powerful opportunities for health education. Nurses are encouraged to use electronic and mass media to address lifestyle issues inherent in a world of many cultures and changing social mores.

SOURCE

From "Are People More Health Conscious? A Longitudinal Study of One Community" by M. Niknian, C. Lefebvre, & R. Carleton, 1991, American Journal of Public Health, 81 *(2), pp. 205–207. Copyright 1991 by American Journal of Public Health.*

---

relationship, client comfort increases. Concomitant sharing of private health beliefs and lifestyle facilitates continued revelation of risk factors. Ignorance of risk factors greatly increases the risk of developing certain diseases (Thibodeaux & Patton, 1997). When a client is identified as being at risk, appropriate laboratory tests are then conducted. Data from the history and laboratory tests are then combined to determine the need for further intervention or referral. When a client is found to have a subclinical communicable disease, a case-finding interview to determine the number and type of contacts provides information leading to new cases.

Tertiary Prevention

Tertiary prevention is directed toward preventing chronicity and disability in the light of full-blown disease. It is appropriate in acute diseases such as pneumonia and

in **degenerative diseases**, such as diabetes, which can lead to breakdown of organ systems and other body tissues and, thus, impeded performance and functioning (Memmler, Cohen, & Wood, 1996). Degenerative diseases can be caused by genetic factors (cystic fibrosis), continuous infection (chronic ear infections), toxins (lung cancer and smoking), repeated injuries (arthritis), and/or aging, or the "normal" wear and tear of life (decreased muscle size and bone density).

Nursing activities include health education related to taking medication, receiving or self-administering treatments and procedures, and follow-up care. In counseling and educative roles, the nurse reexplains, reinforces, and redirects health promotion as well as **rehabilitation**, or limiting disability to the lowest possible level. Assessment of temporary and permanent damage guides appropriate interventions. Rehabilitation addresses not only the physical but also the spiritual/psychological need to become

COMMUNITY NURSING VIEW

Eiswari Osler is a divorced, 57-year-old woman. Her two daughters are grown, live in distant cities, are busy with families of their own, and call their mother approximately once a month. Eiswari works in a very busy accounting office, shouldering heavy responsibilities and working long hours. She is also active in several community organizations, filling her time with activities.

Eiswari attended a community nursing clinic for a routine physical because one of her friends worked there as a nurse. She completed a computerized health-risk appraisal and was interviewed by the nurse, who took a thorough health history. The nurse identified and recorded the following lifestyle factors that placed Eiswari at risk for certain health conditions.

Physical: Walks one block each morning from her car to the office. She has a very full schedule and has not planned for further exercise. She says she enjoys these brief walks and enjoyed swimming when she was younger.

Psychological: Feels intense pressure from being in a middle-management position at work. States she feels angry a lot but tries not to lash out, and she does not have a good way to express her anger. States she has been thinking about joining a support group for women in management positions.

Sociological/physical: Has four or five female friends who exchange phone calls and meet her for lunch from time to time. Attends many social events associated with work and her community-organization activities. Tends to eat fatty, salted foods with others at work and at social events because these snack foods are always available. Smokes one pack per day, drinks scotch and water after work and at social events. Takes Valium three or four times a day for stress.

Spiritual: States she has not identified her life meaning or purpose. She simply wants to save enough money for her older years so that she will not be a burden to her children.

Environmental: Lives in the inner city and states she is concerned about traffic and safety in the streets. She carries a beeper that makes a loud noise in her purse in case of attack.

Nursing Considerations

ASSESSMENT
• You find that her physical examination is essentially negative. What, if any, tests (other than physical) might be indicated in her assessment?

DIAGNOSIS
• Based on the information you have, what nursing diagnoses might you identify?
• What risk factors are inherent in Eiswari's situation.
• For what diseases and/or conditions would you expect her to be at risk?

OUTCOME IDENTIFICATION
• What are the client's goals for health behavior change?
• How can you help her set realistic goals?
• What are signs of accomplishment? Discouragement?
• How can you encourage and support her progress?

PLANNING/INTERVENTIONS
• What strategies would you use for building a therapeutic relationship with Eiswari?
• How might you initiate development of a treatment plan and a contract with her?
• What is she choosing to work on?
• Does she wish to change any of her health behaviors?
• How will you introduce your concerns, or will you introduce them? (Refer to Chapter 8 for the mutual problem-solving process nursing checklist and follow the suggestions there.)
• What specific nursing therapies could you use?
• How would you use teaching? Counseling? Deep relaxation or guided imagery? Touch therapies?
• Where would you start with an educational program?
• What medical or community health programs might be appropriate referrals for Eiswari?

EVALUATION
• What indicators might help you determine whether the plan is working for Eiswari?
• How will you know whether the plan is successful?

whole again. Rehabilitation and wellness efforts might include meditation and biofeedback techniques, healthful nutrition, exercise, and psychological/spiritual healing. Prostheses and equipment may be necessary, and self-help support groups, such as Special Olympics for physically and mentally disabled persons, may provide a social tie and reduce feelings of victimization.

Using an integrated model of health promotion, the community health nurse can help the client identify particular health needs. What are the nutritional needs? Is equipment needed for movement or sensing? Is a stronger support system needed? Is there life meaning and purpose? A need for expression? And how can all these needs be met? The client and nurse work together to promote health and healing within a safe, nurturing, caring, and orderly or aesthetically pleasing environment. The aim is to help the client experience higher levels of wellness even when disease is progressive.

〰 Key Concepts

- A shift is occurring in health care policy that could change the health care delivery system from one focused on disease care to one focused on prevention and health promotion.

- Health promotion is more than the prevention of disease; its focus is to expand consciousness and human potential.

- Lifestyle issues and health behavior choice are major responsibilities of individuals in society.

- Environmental issues and social policy are areas of social responsibility for disease prevention and health promotion.

- Core lifestyle issues and health determinants are related to nutrition, exercise, sleep, and stress management.

- Current methods for health-related research are challenged by the definition of health as a process.

- Health-promotion and disease-prevention research is limited because current quantitative methods are designed to measure intervention outcomes based on single cause and effect rather than on processes of organization or dynamic wholeness.

- Community health nurses work to help enhance the health status of clients who may fall anywhere along the illness/wellness continuum.

- Nurses may use alternative/complementary care therapies as tools to promote health and prevent disease.

- Nursing serves as a critical link in community health-education programs and provides much-needed services to help individuals, families, and populations meet their health needs.

Caring for the Community

The primary aim of community health is to serve aggregate populations. This emphasis on the total population, while challenging, does reinforce the necessity to consider aggregate needs. This includes the considerations of distribution of resources, community involvement, a multisectoral approach, and an emphasis on primary health care. These considerations are discussed in Unit IV.

UNIT

IV

Population-Focused Practice

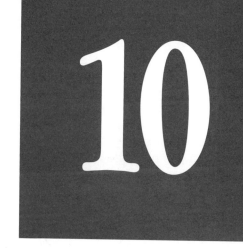

10

Eileen M. Willis, BEd, MEd
Anne L. Biggins, RN, RM, Psych, BN, MPHC
Jenny E. Donovan, RN, RM, MCHN,
 DipApp/Sci, BN, MSC

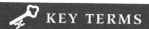 **KEY TERMS**

assessment
assets assessment
assurance
empowerment
health promotion
intersectoral
 collaboration
needs assessment
policy development
population approach
population-focused care
primary health care

*Give a man a fish, and you feed him for a day. Teach a man to fish,
and you feed him for a lifetime.*

—*Chinese proverb*

COMPETENCIES

Upon completion of this chapter, the reader should be able to:

- Discuss the history of population-focused health care.
- Identify the key concepts contributing to a theoretical understanding of a population approach: e.g., primary health care, intersectoral collaboration, multidisciplinary teamwork, new public health, equity in health, and sustainable health care.
- State the mission and core functions of public health as a population-focused practice.
- Examine the issues surrounding population-focused health care.
- Discuss social science theories that provide insights into population-focused nursing care.
- Examine key practice approaches to population-focused health care.
- Discuss population-focused practice as the foundation for community/public health nursing.
- Consider the practical benefits and political implications of community participation and collaboration in health care.

The landmark Ottawa Charter for Health Promotion (World Health Organization, 1986) identified the prerequisites for Health for All as peace, shelter, education, food, income, a stable ecosystem, sustainable resources, social justice, and equity. This is a change in the definition of health from a traditional focus on the absence of disease to a social model of health and calls for a shift in health care practice (World Health Organization and Commonwealth Department of Community Services and Health, 1988). It is a recognition that the struggle for better health happens primarily outside of the medical care, or sick care system as it is sometimes called. This shift also has implications for nursing practice and is a shift to promoting health for all.

Health promotion is the process of enabling individuals and communities to increase control over the determinants of health and thereby improve their health (Nutbeam, 1986, p. 114). Health promotion facilitates the development of people's personal and social skills and enables them to recognize their own health needs. It facilitates strategies for self-care through empowerment and participation. Health needs are understood to be those states, conditions, or factors in the community that, if absent, prevent people from achieving optimum physical, mental, and social well-being (Hawe Degeling, Hall, & Brierley, 1990, p. 17).

A **population approach** to health promotion requires a shift from a focus on individuals to a focus on communities or aggregates of populations. It is an approach that builds on sound epidemiologic research, needs assessment, program planning, and evaluation. A population approach to health care is about sound management and service provision to communities, regions, nations, and the international community. A population approach focuses on strategies for health promotion, health maintenance, and disease prevention, taking into account the sociopolitical context in which community problems exist and are resolved.

ORIGINS OF POPULATION-FOCUSED CARE

The term **population-focused health care** can have many different meanings depending on the contextual framework within which it is being used. At the global level the World Health Organization (WHO) has discussed population-focused health care as a concept in a number of documents and international conferences on health promotion. Action by the WHO has tended toward selective population primary health care such as EIP (extended immunization program) and GOBI (growth, oral rehydration therapy, and breast feeding). These programs tend to focus on specific population groups or specific conditions and attempt to eradicate the condition through technical and medical intervention. Comprehensive population-focused care, on the other hand, deals with social, political, and environmental issues. The difference between these two approaches is discussed later in the chapter.

The documents, conferences, and programs related to health promotion that give shape to what the World Health Organization understands by population-focused health care are presented in its Global Strategy of Health for All by the Year 2000 (World Health Organization, 1993). This section examines the strategies recommended and provides an overview of primary health care and health promotion as population-focused principles and strategies.

The Global Strategy of Health for All by the Year 2000

The idea for a global strategy of Health for All by the Year 2000 arose from a study conducted by the World Health Organization, released in 1973 (World Health Organization, 1978b). This study identified universal worldwide dissatisfaction with health services and a correlation between the health status of the population and the social and economic development of a country. With that study, health became recognized as more than the provision of health services (Newell, 1988).

The World Health Organization initiated a global strategy of "Health for All by the Year 2000" at the 30th World Health Assembly in 1977. The target of Health for All set by WHO for governments and member nations was defined as: "The attainment by all citizens of the world that will permit them to lead a socially and economically productive life" (World Health Organization, 1978b, p. 3).

The seven principles of Health for All outlined by the World Health Organization are:

- The right to health
- Equity in health
- Community participation
- Intersectoral collaboration
- Health promotion
- Primary health care
- International cooperation (Bastian, 1989, p. 15)

These seven principles are seen as a framework for guiding health care workers working with groups of people whether at an international level or at the level of an individual country or community. The global strategy of Health for All by the Year 2000 was adopted by WHO in 1991. The very term "Health for All" suggests a focus on the total population rather than on individuals.

Table 10-1 provides an overview of the Health for All movement. Different phases of the movement are identified, beginning with the primary health care phase; the

Table 10-1 Overview of the Health for All Movement: Initiatives and Phases		
YEAR	**INITIATIVE**	**PHASE**
1977	Target of Health for All by Year 2000	Primary Health Care Phase
1978	Alma Ata Declaration on Primary Health Care	
1979	WHO Global Strategy	
1981	European Lifestyle Movement	Lifestyle Phase
1984	Canadian Health field concept	New Public Health Phase
1986	WHO Charter for Health Promotion WHO Healthy Cities symposium	
1987	Report of World Commission on Environment and Development	
1988	WHO Healthy Public Policy Conference	Ecological Public Health Phase
1989	Ecology of Health	

From: *Model of the Health for All Movement* by P. McPherson, 1992. In H. Gardner (Ed.), Health Policy: Development, Implementation, and Evaluation in Australia, *Melbourne, Australia: Churchill Livingstone.*

Dissatisfaction with Health Services

Governments throughout the industrialized and developing countries have expressed dissatisfaction with health services. Many countries are grappling with the escalation of costs linked to expensive and complex medical technologies and an increase in the population's expectation to have access to these expensive medical technologies. Is the problem unrealistic expectations by the majority of the population? Consider the following questions.

- Australia spends approximately 8% of its gross domestic product on health care while the United States spends approximately 15%, yet both governments are dissatisfied with existing health services. Is the problem primarily the "amount" allocated to health care by governments? Explain your answer.

- In some countries health care is seen as a social right; in others it is viewed as a commodity to be purchased. However it is viewed, consumers and clients wish to have more say. Is this dissatisfaction simply a matter of consumer control? Do we accept the argument that the sick person who pays has more say? Explain your answer.

- The United States and South Africa are the only two nations in the Western world that do not have some form of national health care system. Could dissatisfaction be overcome by providing universal health care coverage? Explain your answer.

- From your knowledge of health care issues, identify the dimensions of dissatisfaction with the health care service in your country.

lifestyle phase based on the European lifestyle movement; the new public health phase, which is discussed in this chapter; and the ecological public health phase, which focuses on creating and maintaining sustainable environments through healthy public policy. These various initiatives provide the framework for the current Health for All movement.

In order to take positive steps to maintain and improve the health status of populations, the WHO recognized the need for implementation strategies. If the target was to be reached, national and international actions at both operational and policy levels were required. Part of the challenge was to make widespread the recognition that health is a fundamental right for all people and includes the right and duty to participate in the planning as well as implementation of health care. Including other sectors that impinge on health such as welfare, transportation, and education was understood as an important feature of the strategy. This planning strategy has been termed **intersectoral collaboration.** The role that the individual, fam-

ily, and community could play in health development was also emphasized (World Health Organization, 1978b, p. 6).

In 1993, the World Health Organization released an evaluation report that analyzed the progress of the Health for All strategy in 151 of the 168 countries involved in the strategy (World Health Organization, 1993, p. 1). The report identified trends and challenges for a new framework for sustainable development and argued for the following:

- Mobilizing resources for high-priority population groups and health needs
- Ensuring equity in health through more effective collaboration and intersectoral health promotion and protection
- Pursuing equality in access to primary health care

The Health for All global strategy continues to emphasize the importance of a population-focused approach at all levels but has begun to be more selective in the way in which the strategy targets specific population groups. Two strategies emphasized in the document are those of primary health care and health promotion, both of which have a population focus.

Primary Health Care As a Strategy toward a Population Approach

In 1978 in Alma Ata, in the former Soviet Republic of Russia, the World Health Organization proclaimed primary health care as the strategy to achieve the target of Health for All by the Year 2000. The Alma Ata Declaration defined **primary health care** as health care that is

> based on practical, scientifically sound and socially acceptable methods and technology made universally accessible to individuals and families in the community and at a level the country can afford to maintain at every stage of their development in the spirit of self-reliance and self-determination (WHO, 1978a, p. 3).

Primary health care includes a comprehensive range of services, such as public health, prevention, and diagnostic, therapeutic, and rehabilitative services. Primary health care was endorsed by the international community. A number of governments and many health professionals saw it as the answer to the health problems of both developed and developing nations. The use of this model of health care, which epitomized a social view of health, however, required changes in the way governments and communities understood and implemented health care.

The Alma Ata Declaration viewed the health problems in terms of inequalities in health care between nations and between individuals within nations. The Health for All strategy was the approach selected to overcome this inequality. Consequently, primary health care was seen not only as the first level of care but also as an approach to health care, incorporating the following principles:

- Building self-reliance at personal and community level
- Supporting community participation in the development of health care programs

- Intersectoral collaboration in working to establish environments that are supportive for health and in which "healthy choices are the easier choices"
- Integration of health services to facilitate continuity of care and efficiency in resource use
- Providing special attention to high-risk and vulnerable groups, as a precondition for equity in health outcomes and health care access
- Use of appropriate technology (World Health Organization, 1985)

As Baum, Fry, and Lennie (1992) note, primary health care was viewed both as a level of health care and as an approach. As an approach, it is a reorientation of the health care system from its present concentration of expensive late-stage, high-technology hospital services to community and preventive services. It is in effect a framework for policy development. Primary health care, as a policy approach, goes beyond policies directed specifically to health promotion and disease prevention to consider how the principles can be applied to the acute care sector. It calls into question approaches to health financing, management of services, and health evaluation (National Centre for Epidemiology and Population Health, 1991).

Health Promotion and a Population Approach

The concept of a population approach was formally endorsed in 1986 at the first International Conference on Health Promotion, held in Ottawa, Canada. A focus on the health of the public is not new; however, the processes are. At Ottawa, a shift was made from focusing on primary health care to including healthy public policy, and the term "new public health" emerged. The new public health concept builds on the traditional or the "old public health" concerns that had begun to focus mainly on physical environments. The intention was to broaden this to include environmental, political, social, and economic factors in analyzing and devising strategies to deal with public health issues (Ashton & Seymour, 1988).

The original public health movement of the 19th century had a strong political and social focus, but by the 1970s the medical model, which focused on cure of illness, became paramount. Public health was often associated with "sewerage, rats and adulterated food" (Baum et al., 1992, p. 304). Public health was seen to be a poor cousin of high-status acute care in clinical hospital settings. According to Baum, Fry, and Lennie (1992), the new public health sought to involve citizens, as well as health professionals and government, in policy development in all sectors that had implications for health and illness.

Primary health care came to be seen as the operational tool by which improvements to the health status of the community at the local level could be achieved. Creating healthy public policy became the strategy for regional and national organizations, with primary health care as the means of operationalizing public policy. Five health promotion action areas were advocated at Ottawa: building healthy public policy, creating supportive environments, strengthening community action, developing personal skills, and reorienting health services (Gardner, 1992).

Subsequent conferences following the international conference in Ottawa have reiterated the commitment to equity, access, development, accountability, and the forming of health alliances between countries and populations (World Health Organization and Commonwealth Department of Community Services and Health, 1988), creating supportive environments, sustainability, and empowerment (World Health Organization, 1991). The concept of a population focus is thus concerned with three levels of action:

- Policy development
- The community or local level
- The individual

REFLECTIVE THINKING

Socioeconomic Status Effects

One of the guiding principles of the focus on populations in health care is the recognition that the health status of individuals and of nations is linked to socioeconomic status.

- In what way does your socioeconomic status affect your health?
- Does your socioeconomic status affect your health behavior? Explain.
- Does your socioeconomic status prevent you from changing behaviors that are not health promoting? Explain.
- Can you think of examples of social or cultural groups whose health status is clearly linked to their economic status?
- Do you think culture or class is the best indicator of health status? Why?

DEBATES SURROUNDING THE HEALTH FOR ALL MOVEMENT AND POPULATION-FOCUSED HEALTH CARE

Challenges to the Health for All movement and the strategies that inform population-focused health care come from a variety of sources. The Alma Ata Declaration itself is not without its critics. The Alma Ata Declaration argues that primary health care should be defined in a manner that is specific to each country's health needs and that reflects the sociopolitical and cultural requirements of that particular society (Petersen, 1994; Cheek & Willis, 1998). This attempt to be politically and culturally sensitive is problematic. If primary health care is to be used as the strategy for reframing health care services globally then it needs to be both a cultural and political agent of social change at all levels of health care (globally, nationally, and locally). Some cultural practices are detrimental to a social model of health: for example, cultural beliefs that hinder women from attaining literacy skills. But whether and how community health nurses should challenge such beliefs and practices is another question.

Further, resources are not distributed equally, and equity is not universal. Questions need to be asked about what resources are available in each country and how wealthy nations participate in the redistribution of resources so that the world population has acceptable and accessible health care. In dealing with these issues, the international community has yet to come to terms and work with the fact that nations come to the negotiating table with different political and sociocultural knowledge and that the questions address the core of the economic systems.

Population-Focused Care and Risk

McPherson (1992) argues that initially the primary health care concepts of self-reliance and community participation had a narrow focus that concentrated on primary prevention. This focus, as McPherson suggests, occurred when the Health for All movement joined with the "lifestyle movement" in the early 1980s. During this phase health was seen to be determined by the individual, plus social factors related to interpersonal behavior. Ill health, therefore, resulted from faults in either or both of these two factors and was the responsibility of the individual. Prevention depended on reducing identified health risk factors at the individual level and in changing individual behavior. The role of health education was to help people identify their risk factors and modify their "faulty" behavior. The problem with this approach was that there was a potential for blaming the victim, with little recognition of the social, political, environmental, and economic forces that act on individuals and are outside their control.

More recent interaction between social scientists and health professionals has resulted in a realization that many risk factors are outside the control of individuals. Risk is now viewed as a part of the local, national, and global food chains, the atmosphere, and political systems. Decisions on environmental toxins made in one country, for example, affect citizens in another. These issues call for multisectoral, international collaboration (Beck, 1989).

Selective versus Comprehensive Approaches

In 1988 the international journal *Social Science and Medicine* published a series of articles by Warren, Wisner, Mosley, and Walsh debating the topic selective versus comprehensive primary health care. The crux of the debate was that the approach to health care taken with particular populations should be comprehensive rather than selective. Proponents of comprehensive primary health care argued that health programs should involve the entire population in health-promoting activities utilizing community development approaches that work on identifying health problems and solutions in conjunction with the population concerned. This approach was argued to be truly participatory, with ideas and solutions emerging from within the entire population. Further, solutions developed within the group would be culturally congruent, and the technologies and skills needed would be affordable. In this approach the underlying cause of ill health was seen to be economic and social inequality. Improvements in health care called for structural, political, cultural, social, and economic reform, including democratic forms of health service management.

Those representing the case for selective primary health care argued that the WHO and UNICEF had had a number of successes in eradicating specific diseases, such as smallpox, by dealing with these diseases exclusively or by identifying specific at-risk groups within populations, such as women or people with disabilities, and concentrating resources on those groups. Comprehensive primary health care was not viewed as cost effective or efficient. The debate regarding comprehensive versus selective primary care continues as we move toward the 21st century.

Consider the following example in light of the discussion on selective versus comprehensive population care. The Australian and U.S. responses to the World Health Organization's call for Health for All by the Year 2000 show a similar pattern. Australia became a signatory to the global Health for All by the Year 2000 strategy in 1981. The initial report *Looking forward to Better Health* was released in 1986 and *Health for All Australians* in 1988. The two major principles were improving the health status of Australians and decreasing the inequalities in health status between subgroups such as migrants, aboriginal people, and the elderly. Goals and targets were identified in the following areas: hypertension, nutrition, injury prevention, the health of older people, and preventable cancers of the lung, skin, and breast. Although inequalities in the social system and in the health care system were recognized, the target remained illness prevention.

The *Healthy People 2000* report published in the United States (U.S. Department of Health and Human Services, 1991) had three goals: increasing the span of healthy life, reducing health disparities, and achieving access to preventive services for all Americans. Twenty-two priority areas from 300 measurable objectives, plus additional ones for at-risk groups, were identified and organized under three categories: health promotion, focused on lifestyle choices; health protection, focused on regulatory measures for occupations, health, food, etc.; and preventive services, focused on screening services, immunizations, etc.

As do the Australian responses, the U.S. objectives remain focused on illness prevention and the physical, affective, and mental factors associated with the consumers of health care. A comprehensive health service system based on the principles of social health has yet to be operationalized in either country.

PUBLIC HEALTH PRACTICE: HEALTHY PEOPLE IN HEALTHY COMMUNITIES

Public health practice in the United States, as well as in most other industrialized nations, has significantly improved the health status and life expectancy of the population over the past 200 years (Keck & Scutchfield, 1997). Most of these improvements have come from measures used to protect the public from environmental hazards (for example, food supply, water safety, sewage disposal, injury control) and to pursue health promotion activities (for example, changes in tobacco use, hypertension control, dietary patterns, injury control, automobile safety restraint). The public, however, has been largely unaware of the many contributions of public health. In the Institute of Medicine (1988) report to the United States, *The Future*

of Public Health, the Institute's Committee for the Study of the Future of Public Health described agreement across the United States that "public health does things that benefit everybody" and that "public health prevents illness and educates the population" (p. 3).

In an effort, however, to further clarify the role of public health's population-focused services, the Institute of Medicine committee proposed a public health mission statement and a set of core functions. The committee defined the mission of public health as "fulfilling society's interest in assuring conditions in which people can be healthy" (Institute of Medicine, 1988, p. 7). The core functions of public health agencies at all levels of government were identified as "assessment, policy development, and assurance" (p. 7). **Assessment** refers to systematic data collection on the health of the community; monitoring the population's health status, health needs, and health problems; and making information available on the health of the community. **Policy development** refers to the provision of leadership in developing comprehensive public health policies, including the use of a scientific knowledge base in decision making about policy. **Assurance** refers to the role of every public agency in assuring that high-priority personal and communitywide health services

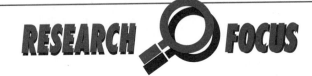

U.S. Mortality by Economic, Demographic, and Social Characteristics: The National Longitudinal Mortality Study

STUDY PROBLEM/PURPOSE

Socioeconomic conditions play a significant role in morbidity and mortality, as well as the demographic variables of age, sex, and racial characteristics. To describe the effects of different economic, demographic, and social characteristics on mortality, studies require large and diverse populations. The primary purpose of this longitudinal study was to describe the effects of race, employment status, income, education, occupation, marital status, and household size on mortality.

METHODS

Approximately 530,000 persons 25 years of age or older were identified from selected Current Population Surveys between 1979 and 1985. These individuals were followed for mortality through use of the National Death Index from 1979 through 1989.

FINDINGS

Higher mortality was found in African Americans than in Caucasians less than 65 years of age; in per-

sons not in the labor force, with lower incomes, with less education, and in service and other lower level occupations; and in persons not married, living alone. With occasional exceptions, in specific sex and age groups, these relationships remained statistically significant ($p < .01$) when each variable was adjusted for all of the other characteristics. The relationships were generally weaker in individuals 65 years of age or older.

IMPLICATIONS

Employment status, income, education, occupation, race, and marital status all have substantial associations with mortality. This longitudinal study identified segments of the population in need of public health attention and concerted action by public health professionals. The study demonstrated the importance of including these variables in morbidity and mortality studies.

SOURCE

From "U.S. Mortality by Economic, Demographic, and Social Characteristics: The National Longitudinal Mortality Study by P. D. Sorlie, E. Backlund & J. B. Keller, 1995, American Journal of Public Health, 85 *(7), pp. 949–956.*

are available, which may include the direct provision of high-priority personal health services for those who are not able to afford them. Assurance also refers to making sure that a public health and personal health care work force is competent and available.

The proposed mission statement and core functions generated a great deal of discussion and action in the United States, with positive responses received. In the state of Washington, for example, the Washington State Department of Health and its core governmental Public Health Functions Task Force developed a definition of the Institute's core functions and the role they play in improving a community's health. Following this activity, the state's Public Health Improvement Plan Steering Committee developed in 1994 a "Public Health Improvement Plan" intended to improve the health status in the state through prevention and improved public health services delivery (Washington State Department of Health, 1994).

In July 1994, the National Association of County Health Officers (NACHO) (1994) published its *Blueprint for a Healthy Community: A Guide for Local Health Departments*, in which it examined the core public health functions in terms of the services needed to create and maintain a healthy community. Health departments are charged with the responsibility of assuring that 10 essential elements are provided by some community-based agency or program. The 10 essential elements identified by NACHO included:

1. Conduct a community diagnosis—analyze data for the purpose of information-based decision making.

2. Prevent and control epidemics and injuries.

3. Provide a safe and healthy environment—clean and safe air, water, food, and facilities.

4. Measure performance, effectiveness, and outcomes of health services.

5. Promote healthy lifestyles—provision of health education to individuals and communities.

6. Provide laboratory testing—identify disease agents.

7. Provide targeted outreach and form partnerships—assure access to services for vulnerable populations and the development of culturally congruent care.

8. Provide personal health services ranging from primary and preventive care to specialty and tertiary treatment.

9. Promote research and innovation.

10. Mobilize the community for action—initiate collaborative efforts and provide leadership to improve the community's health.

Because of public health's importance in influencing population health and in providing a foundation for the health care system, the U.S. Public Health Service and other groups are advocating a renewed emphasis on population-focused services. To ensure that all citizens will receive the effective services they need in the future, public health departments in the United States will need

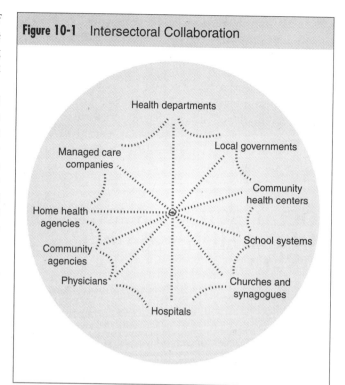

Figure 10-1 Intersectoral Collaboration

to build collaborative public-private partnerships with other community health agencies and with the illness care systems in the community, including other health departments, other departments of local governments, community health centers, school systems, churches, and other community agencies. Such collaboration is imperative for

DECISION MAKING

Community Experience

What is your own experience of community? Consider this experience in terms of class, ethnicity, race, religion, gender, geography, age, sexual preference or interest.

• What issues brought this community together, and how did they come together?

• What were the beliefs, practices, and values of this community?

• How were decisions made in this community?

• Can you think of specific health interests and needs of this community?

• If you were a community health nurse working in this community, whom would you approach to discuss the identified health needs?

• Can you think of an environmental issue in your town that a community health nurse could work on that would generate a community of interest?

effectively improving population health not only in the United States but in other industrialized nations as well. Service and referral linkages with hospitals, physicians, home health agencies, managed care companies, and other illness-based services are necessary also in order to provide a seamless system of services that promote population health, prevent illness, diagnose disease early, and provide treatment within a culturally sensitive, caring, healing environment. See Figure 10-1 for an illustration of intersectoral collaboration.

SOCIAL SCIENCES AND POPULATION-FOCUSED CARE

The shift from a health care system that primarily focuses on acute hospital-based services to one of preventive and population-based care is a direct result of social science research. The social model of health arises from social epidemiology and sociological research that has established clear links between socioeconomic status and health status (Black, Townsend, & Davidson, 1982). In short, mortality and morbidity rates of countries, and of groups within countries, mirror the socioeconomic conditions of these groups or nations. What is not clear is why or how political, economic, and social factors influence health status. The most debated factors are those in the Black Report (Black, Townsend, & Davidson, 1982) commissioned by the British Labour government in the 1970s. The Black Report argued that inequalities in health are a result of one of four factors: artifact explanations, natural selection, materialist or structural explanations, or cultural or behavioral explanations.

Artifact explanations deal with problems inherent in the research tools that establish the links between morbidity and mortality patterns and the socioeconomic status of the population being studied. The problem of how to measure the relationship between social class and health status remains an issue for social scientists and health planners. One of the difficulties is in defining social class. In the 1980s the *Health for All Australians* (Health Targets and Implementation [Health for All] Committee, 1988) report listed a number of studies in support of a link between social class and health. These studies, however, used different measures or scales. Some scales defined social class as simply a matter of income, or the control an individual had over his or her work. Others sought to incorporate social status, prestige, occupation, and even residence. This measure is often referred to as socioeconomic status and may also include age, disability, gender, and isolation.

Natural selection refers to the suggestion that healthy individuals do well economically in any society, while those who are not healthy or able-bodied will not do well economically (Powles & Salzberg, 1989). This theory was originally based on the belief that some groups in the population were biologically healthier than others. What this fails to explain is why certain morbidity and mortality patterns are found in occupational, ethnic, and gender groups, as well as geographic areas. Lundberg (1991) and Vagero (1991) argue that those born with certain chronic diseases are more likely to have inferior education and fewer employment opportunities. As a consequence they are more likely to be poor and hence lack access to adequate health care resources.

Materialist or structural explanations argue that morbidity and mortality are a result of material conditions. Simply stated, those born into poor families are more likely to live in substandard houses and poor neighborhoods, have inferior health care services or no health care resources at all, have limited access to education and hence fewer opportunities for employment or to be employed in low-skilled, low-paid occupations that are highly dangerous. The cultural explanations have been linked to materialist explanations, suggesting that people who live in poverty have behaviors and cultural beliefs that are illness-producing. An example of this is the high rate of diabetes, hypertension, and renal failure among Australian Aborigines (Anderson, 1996). While it is no doubt true that different groups in a society have different habits and beliefs that may not be health-enhancing, one needs to ask whether these behaviors are based on cultural beliefs or poverty exacerbated by racism. It may be that poverty, rather than cultural beliefs and habits, creates certain unhealthy ways of being in the world.

Cultural explanations place the problem with the at-risk groups, while materialist explanations situate the problems with inequalities in the society, including inequalities in access to health care. The World Health Organization promotes the view that universal free health care is a prerequisite for primary health care. This debate has been further enriched by what is known as the McKeown thesis. Thomas McKeown (1962), a medical researcher, stated that improvements in the health of the population in Britain following the industrialization in the 19th century was not the result of advances in medical science primarily, but was the result of improvements in living conditions. McKeown argued that the decline in the death rate in Britain between 1870 and 1914 was the direct result of improvements in nutrition.

Others have argued that the improvements in the health of the population were a result of improvements in the living conditions of the poor, a direct result of improved working conditions, better housing, and increased wages achieved by working-class people better positioned to negotiate with employers (Blane, 1987). Scheyner, Landefeld, and Sandifer (1981) pointed out that the proponents of the old public health movement had begun the process of reform through the regulation of sanitation, water supply, food control, and town planning. However argued, the McKeown thesis supports preventive health over curative measures and materialist and structuralist explanations over cultural explanations.

More recently, social scientists have offered a post structural critique of health promotion directed at specific populations. This critique is based on the work of the

French social critic Michel Foucault (Foucault, 1980), who addressed both the self-help, individually based behavioral change approach to public health and the more broadly based population-focused campaigns. Foucault's argument was that the rise of medicine coincided with the emergence of the social sciences and that the fundamental aim of both is the control of the population. The old forms of social control such as death and torture gave way to prisons, asylums, and institutions for those who were deemed deviant. Those who were institutionalized came under the control of wardens, psychiatrists, social workers, and nurses. In the late 20th century new forms of social control have emerged. Asylums are no longer necessary to separate deviants from those who are perceived as normal. We do this for ourselves by embracing ideologies of what constitutes normal developmental stages and behaviors or what constitutes appropriate health-enhancing behaviors. We now regulate our own health through diets, exercise, and annual visits to our physician for pap smears, cholesterol checks, and mammograms, for example. At the macro level, the health behaviors of the population are regulated through legislation (e.g., antismoking laws), gathering of disease statistics, and identifying at-risk and high-risk groups. Population-focused health care runs the risk of focusing on control rather than on the concept of empowerment. Empowerment enhances community participation in health promotion efforts, and community health nurses play a vital role in the empowerment process. Empowerment of communities to participate in the process of health promotion is critical.

Clearly these theoretical explanations have implications for nursing actions. Cultural explanations lead to health promotion activities based on individual and group behavioral change, while materialist and structural explanations lead to health promotion activities based primarily on identifying community needs, deficits, or impediments to health. A variety of approaches is needed.

POPULATION-FOCUSED PRACTICE

A population approach suggests that a regional approach to health planning be aimed at providing a comprehensive health service across the three levels of health care: primary, secondary, and tertiary. A population approach provides management with directions for service provisions. Community assessments based on the use of epidemiology and biostatistics, community needs surveys and focus groups, as well as community involvement all help to determine those priorities and subsequent planning of services for the community. Managers provide the directions for services that are consistent with the identified needs. A needs- and assets-based approach also enables the identification of disadvantaged groups who might otherwise be neglected. Chapter 12 includes further discussion of community assessment.

Needs- and Assets-Based Planning

Program planning is essential to meet local, state, and national government mandates for funding, as well as philanthropic organization funding guidelines. Planning programs and planning for program evaluation are two critical activities for community health nurses in order to implement successful programs. These important skills are discussed further in Chapter 13.

There are two key ingredients in the planning process, needs assessment and assets assessment. **Needs assessment** is defined as the systematic appraisal of the type, depth, and nature of health needs/problems as perceived by clients, health providers, or both, in a given community. Prior to implementing any program, a needs assessment should be conducted to ensure that the program is meeting client and not the service provider needs. The data gathered from a needs assessment, as well as an assets assessment, should be the basis and rationale for program planning. It is important to understand the process involved in needs assessment and the different types of needs.

Hawe et al. (1990) outlined the following needs as necessary to identify:

- Normative needs—needs of a community defined by experts who judge what a community needs on the basis of their expert experience.
- Expressed needs—needs that have been expressed by members of the community.
- Comparative needs—those needs that emerge when one community lacks services that are provided in another community.
- Felt needs—those needs that the members of the community say they want, via a community survey, for example.

Hawe et al. (1990) also outlined the following nine steps, divided into two stages, that should be followed to ensure accurate assessment of client needs:

Stage 1: Identification of the health problem/need

Consultation

Data collection

Presentation of findings

Determining priorities

Stage 2: Analysis of the health problem/need

Literature review

Description of the target population

Exploration of the health problem/need

Analysis of factors contributing to the problem/need

Reassessment and strengthening of community resources

Assets assessment is also a very important ingredient in the planning process. The approach was recommended by John McKnight (1986), who argued that health professionals should view communities and populations in terms of the resources (assets) that they possess and that these resources should be acknowledged and utilized. Professionals, he suggests, should abandon the tendency to define communities only by what they lack. By focusing only on need, health professionals lose touch with the rich capability of communities and the people in them. Thus, population-focused practice includes both needs- and assets-based assessment in the planning process.

Population-Focused Practice in Community/Public Health Nursing

Population-focused practice is historically consistent with public health philosophy and is reflected in the 1996 American Public Health Association (APHA) definition of public health nursing (APHA, 1996). Public health nursing is defined as "the practice of promoting and protecting the health of populations using knowledge from nursing, social, and public health sciences" (p. 1). Of particular importance is the APHA statement about public health nursing practice, which "includes assessment and identification of sub-populations who are at high risk of injury, disease, threat of disease, or poor recovery and focusing resources so that services are available and accessible" (p. 4). The APHA goal of public health nursing is "to improve the health of populations through ongoing assessment, coordinated interventions; and care management, working with and through relevant community leaders, interest groups, employers, families, and individuals; and through involvement in relevant social and political actions" (p. 4).

Public health nursing in the United States is viewed as a specialty in the broad field of community health nursing (Williams, 1996). "Public health nurses integrate community involvement and knowledge about the entire population with personal, clinical understandings of the health and illness experiences of individuals and families within the population" (APHA, 1996, p. 2). Public health nurses "translate and articulate the health and illness experiences of diverse, often vulnerable individuals and families in the population to health planners and policy makers, and assist members of the community to voice their problems and aspirations" (p. 2).

Population-level decision making is different from clinical care decision making. At the clinical level the focus is on the individual client—assessing the health status, planning care with the client, and evaluating the effects of care. At the population level, the focus includes, for example, questions that address the incidence and prevalence of health conditions among various age, race, economic, and gender groups in the community. Obtaining information regarding the community's perceived health needs and assets is also included. Planning includes the development of programs in the community through coalition building and partnerships to lower the risk of certain conditions. Program evaluation is also included as part of the process. Table 10-2 outlines some of the distinctions between population-level and clinical care decision making.

The current changes occurring in the health care delivery system, as well as projected changes, will require nursing leaders, in addition to those in the public health nursing specialty, to think in population terms. This focus on populations and preparation in the use of population-oriented methods (e.g., epidemiology, biostatistics, demography, and community building) is necessary to make evidenced-based decisions in program development. There is a need for nurses with skills in population assessment, management, and evaluation. In addition, there is a need for nurses prepared to participate in coalition building and partnership efforts to improve the health of populations.

Community Development

One of the major strategies for health promotion in population-focused health care, which emerged for example in Australia, Canada, and New Zealand, is community development, where the focus is empowerment through participation and equity (Jackson, Mitchel, & Wright, 1989; Labonte, 1990). Currently within community health practice, a tension exists between the perceived value of one-to-one casework and community development with its

Table 10-2 Population-Level Decision Making versus Clinical Care Decision Making	
POPULATION LEVEL	**CLINICAL CARE**
• Consider the incidence and prevalence of health conditions among various age, race, economic, and gender groups within community.	• Focus on individual client. —Assess health status. —Plan care with client. —Evaluate the care.
• Obtain information regarding the community's perceived health needs and assets.	
• Develop programs with the community through coalition building and partnerships that would lower the risk of certain conditions.	
• Perform program evaluation.	

DECISION MAKING

Community Development Continuum

Examine the community development continuum presented in Figure 10-2.

• How helpful do you think this model is for understanding the community development process?

• Do you think the representation of the continuum should be circular, given that in reality people might enter at one or several points?

group action focus. This tension has led some community nurses to situate good practice primarily in group-focused activities. The concept of the community development continuum proposed by Jackson et al. (1989) has attempted to overcome this tension (Willis, 1990). The five points on the continuum defined by Jackson et al. (1989) are:

1. Developmental casework
2. Mutual support
3. Issue identification and campaigns
4. Participation
5. Control of services and social movements

Jackson, Mitchel, and Wright (1989) suggest that health workers can work through the continuum in the course of their work and can be engaged in several points at any one time. As can be seen from the points identified in Figure 10-2, individuals ideally move along the continuum

toward greater levels of control over areas of their own lives, joining with other people who hold similar interests to assume more social and economic power, forming communities of interest. The continuum provides a variety of possibilities for community health nurses in a variety of settings. The continuum supports all nursing actions, including advocacy for a single client, client education as part of continuity of care, comprehensive discharge planning, as well as group work and social action.

Empowerment

Each stage in the community development continuum is characterized by empowerment and an opening to the possibilities of further action along the continuum. **Empowerment** is the process whereby individuals feel increasingly in control of their own affairs. Generally, the process begins with one or more motivational triggers, such as a crisis, frustration, or outrage. In most cases, the motivational trigger leads to change because individuals learn that they have a voice and that there are people who

REFLECTIVE THINKING

Empowerment

• What does empowerment mean to you?

• What do you think about the criteria for empowerment proposed by Labonte?

• How do you experience empowerment both personally and professionally in your own life?

Figure 10-2 The Community Development Continuum

Developmental Caseword	Mutual Support	Issue Identification and Campaigns	Participation	Control of Services and Social Movements
• Casework emphasizing self-help • Liaison and networking • Information collection and dissemination • Referral • Linking to family and friends • Advocacy	• Promoting self-help support groups • Creating mutual support networks • Linking isolated individuals with existing social groups • Strengthening neighborhood networks • Improving social support	• Community education and public awareness • Formation of action groups to deal with the issues • Support of action groups to raise profile of issues to the conscious level • Encouraging critical profile/community action	• Collective participation	• Control • Intensifying advocacy • Participating in policy and legislative changes

Adapted from "The Community Development Continium" by T. Jackson, S. Mitchel, M. Wright, 1989. Community Health Statistics, 13(1).

will listen and understand (Lord & McKillop, 1990, p. 4). The criteria for empowerment identified by Labonte (1990) are: improved status, self-esteem, and cultural identity; the ability to reflect critically and solve problems; the ability to make choices; increased access to resources; increased collective bargaining power; the legitimating of people's demands by officials; and self-discipline and the ability to work with others.

The role of nurses is not to do unto others but to assist others by working with them and functioning as resources, supporting their right to make decisions for themselves. An empowering practice requires that we view clients as equal community members, as persons capable of and responsible for their own empowerment. A critical element in the empowerment process for the individual or family is someone characterized as a "good listener," an "equal," a "guide," and as a person "who really cares" (Lord & McKillop, 1990, p. 5). Stacey (1988) states that "the goal of empowering and enabling must be to make it unnecessary to enable or empower, because people will understand what of value we have to offer" (p. 321).

Empowerment enhances community participation. An essential ingredient for effective population-focused practice is community participation in assessment, planning,

Perspectives...

Insights of a Community Health Nursing Professor

Population-focused care is central to community health nursing practice. A population approach to health care has received a much greater emphasis since the Alma Ata conference, the World Health Organization Health for All initiative, and the publication of the Ottawa Charter for Health Promotion, all previously mentioned in this chapter. This increased emphasis on population health and the building of healthy public policy has required a reorientation of health services as well as changes in the preparation of nurses and other health professionals at all levels of practice.

As a community health nursing faculty member in the United States with practice experience in public health nursing; experience in organizational collaborative efforts at regional, national, and international levels; and experience in teaching and consulting in another country, I have had the opportunity to work with faculty and health colleagues with broad global population perspectives. These various experiences have significantly enhanced my teaching and recognition of the need for those of us with community health nursing experience, those who have had opportunities to work in many different sectors, to assist other faculty and students in expanding their knowledge of population-focused care. Assisting faculty and students to more fully comprehend the vital role that nurses can play in this endeavor is critical, whether the focus is at the local, regional, national, or international level.

Preparing students to think beyond the individual, family focus requires not only community health nursing faculty who are prepared to assist students in this learning process but other nursing faculty members as well. As one of my postregistration students recently stated: "I did not really stop to think about health in broader population terms since my focus has been primarily the care of individual acutely ill patients. I can now see how important it is for nurses to develop the knowledge and skills to participate in population focused-care. We live in a global society and have a very important role to play in the rapidly changing health care environment." A population orientation to health care is an imperative for the future. This change in focus to a broader perspective of health, with a much greater emphasis on health promotion, requires the preparation of students and faculty who will be able to participate in building healthy public policy: creating sustainable, supportive environments that enhance health; strengthening community action through empowerment of clients and community members; assisting others to develop personal skills that promote health; and working with others (health professionals, individuals and community groups, government sectors, and health service institutions) to continue to build health care systems that demonstrate a health promotion direction. As nurses we can make a difference!

—*Sue A. Thomas, RN, EdD*

COMMUNITY NURSING VIEW

In the state of South Australia, the Child Adolescent and Family Health Service, a government-funded service, works with families who have new babies and young children. Under the affirmative action policy, after the birth of a child, some families are visited in their own homes. Others are contacted by phone or letter or are referred directly by interagency contact with the maternity hospital concerned. In rural areas, all new mothers are visited in the local hospital.

At the clinic visit, clients initially experience one-to-one developmental casework, where the professional enables consumers of that service to draw on their own experiences and look for their own solutions (World Health Organization, 1986). This is in contrast to the more traditional approach wherein people depend on the health workers (Jackson et al., 1989). Women and men are supported to make informed choices during their current experiences as new parents; however, few fathers attend the clinics.

In 1989, a universal parent education program was developed for all parents with new children. Topics focused on issues such as pregnancy, birth and homecoming, settling babies and nutrition, when to call the doctor, child development, play ideas, discipline and safety, and self-esteem for parents and their children. The program provided parents with information, support, and the opportunity to network with other parents who were going through similar experiences (Brown, Donovan, & Islip, 1988). Jackson et al. (1989) recognized that people are able to develop greater control over their lives when they are not socially isolated.

Parents gain valuable information about their babies' normal behavior and find that they experience similar issues. They are invited to attend new parents courses or coffee mornings, to see how they might help and support each other. By meeting together, parents establish more realistic, attainable standards that can be adapted to individual preferences and needs. Being accepted as a member of the group is an important factor for many people. Group education has the added bonus of empowering parents, who, while sharing their ideas, discover that their parenting is satisfactory and that their feelings about parenting, both positive and negative, are normal. The participants gradually gain more confidence in themselves and their own ability to make decisions.

Small groups, particularly self-help groups, can be empowering because they normalize people's experience of powerlessness. Once trust and acceptance have been established with others, participants feel more able to contribute and to move on to broader community issues. This is considered to be the successful transition from reliance on one-to-one contact with a professional to recognizing the value of mutual support and being able to build links with each other. Facilitators can enhance the parents' sense of competence and control by assisting them to develop a support network within and outside the group. Research by Telleen, Herzog, and Kilbane (1989) showed the effectiveness of educating parents about the use of social support as a means of coping and enhancing their problem-solving capabilities.

It is intended that the groups be in an environment that is socially, culturally, and geographically acceptable to all clients and that a primary health care focus is maintained. The programs encourage the development of friendships and social networks to bring people together who are dealing with common issues and similar life circumstances. "This point marks the transition from participation for survival to participation to achieve change" (Jackson et al., 1989, p. 70). The program has positive effects on the mothers' attitudes toward their children and reduces the sense of social isolation in their parental role (Parke & Power, 1984; Telleen et al., 1989; Lord & McKillop, 1990).

As parents move from participation for survival to participation to achieve change, collective participation occurs and they take a more active role in assisting others. The outcomes for people moving along the community development continuum are similar to some of the areas identified in the Ottawa Charter for Health Promotion. A supportive environment is created when people form mutual support groups. Community action is strengthened when people identify and campaign for change. By being involved, people

Continued

Continued

are able to develop personal skills such as the ability to work out health-promoting solutions, contribute as an active team member, and encourage others to think about options for change.

Nursing Considerations

Having read the scenario about the community development continuum, consider how empowerment, community development, and community participation were utilized in the example given. Were the strategies of the Ottawa Charter for Health Promotion apparent? What would you have done differently?

ASSESSMENT
• What data would you need to begin to plan a parent education and support program?
• What are some of the barriers that might prevent parents from attending child health clinics or family-centered health centers?
• What might be the contributing factors to these barriers?
• How would you distinguish the needs of parents from differing socioeconomic groups?

DIAGNOSIS
• What should be considered in formulating nursing diagnoses related to parents who participate in a parent program?

PLANNING/INTERVENTIONS
• If you were organizing parent education and support groups for parents, how would you establish them? What process would you use?
• What problems might occur in the process of organizing parent education groups within an organization, given the different needs of clients?
• How might you work collaboratively with parents in program planning?
• How might you work collaboratively with other organizations to maximize the health professionals' input?
• Since the social movement stage of the continuum was not discussed in the scenario provided, what would you suggest that would demonstrate this movement?

OUTCOME IDENTIFICATION
• What expected outcomes would you formulate specific to the development of a parent education and support program?

EVALUATION
• Who should be involved in developing the evaluation process and methods?
• What evaluation methods would you recommend?

and policy development. Active involvement of the people who are affected by health programs and policies is a shift to community responsibility in planning, for either preventive or curative services.

Empowerment provides for the creation of new ways of being, doing, and living. It promotes the creation of caring communities, the possibility of establishing an equitable, just society in which community members have an opportunity to develop their unique contributions regardless of age, race, gender, culture, sexual orientation, or economics.

This chapter discusses population-focused practice and health care, highlighting that a population approach is one element of health promotion. A discussion of the World Health Organization initiatives pertaining to Health for All by the Year 2000 provides the key concepts for the terminology and processes that underpin population-focused health care. A discussion of population-focused practice in community/public health nursing and in public health provides an opportunity to examine strategies that foster the development of healthy communities, strategies such as needs- and assets-based planning, community development, and empowerment.

Key Concepts

• The focus of population-focused health care is the health of communities or aggregates of populations.

• Primary health care as a policy model emphasizes community participation, intersectoral collaboration, integration of health services, and health care access and equity for all.

• Primary health care has a key role to play in reducing the current inequalities in the health status between different sections of the population and in providing equal opportunities for access to health care for the whole population.

• The core functions of public health in the United States are assessment, policy development, and assurance.

• Needs and assets assessment is about collecting information that will give a good indication of the needs and assets of a community, laying the foundation for creating healthy, caring communities.

- Community development is a construct that describes the actions intended to change the aspects of the environment that promote ill health, inequity, poverty, and powerlessness. Community participation promotes the philosophy of the World Health Organization that people have a right and duty to participate in the planning and implementation of health care.

- Empowerment is the process whereby individuals and families feel increasingly in control of their own affairs.

- Strengthening community action with information, education, and support is about empowering communities and individuals to work toward ownership and control of their issues. It is about communities' acting in partnership to enhance opportunities for social change.

- Reorienting health services includes sharing the responsibility for health decisions and services between individuals, community groups, community leaders, health professionals, and governments while working to promote health. Community health nurses have a vital role to play in this process.

- Building healthy public policy by raising awareness beyond the health care system includes acting as advocates at all levels of the health system in cooperation with a wide range of agencies. It includes developing social policies that foster greater equity and access to health care for everyone, aiming to provide the opportunity for people to make choices that will promote health and healing.

Epidemiology

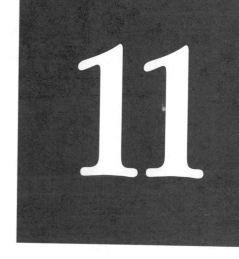

Janice A. Young, RN, MS
Lindsey K. Phillips, RN, MS

The potential for preventing or alleviating illness has grown at an astounding rate. This may be attributed to the rapid pace of discovery, aided by public confidence and willingness to support research, and to the decreasing lags between scientific discovery and its practical application.

—Freeman, 1963, p. 13

COMPETENCIES

Upon completion of this chapter, the reader should be able to:

- Define *epidemiology*.
- Examine the historical development of epidemiology.
- Identify key concepts in the epidemiologic approach.
- Discuss the significance of the epidemiologic approach in community health nursing.
- Describe the types of epidemiologic investigations and study designs.
- Identify key population measures and vital statistics used in epidemiology.
- Discuss the uses and application of the epidemiologic approach in community health nursing practice.

The science of epidemiology is important to community health nurses because its methods provide for the assessment and understanding of health, disease, and injury in a community or target population. **Epidemiology** is a population-focused applied science that uses research and statistical data collection methodology to find answers to the following questions:

- Who in a population is affected by a disease, disorder, or injury?
- What is the occurrence of this health problem in the community?
- Can the causative factors and risk factors contributing to the problem be determined?

The epidemiologic approach provides community health nurses with the methodology and language to describe and analyze health concerns in population-based care. Related community health disciplines such as public health, occupational health, and the environmental sciences also use epidemiology in everyday practice. The use of epidemiologic techniques also alerts community health nurses to the possible etiology of health problems in a neighborhood or district.

This chapter serves as an introduction to the epidemiologic concepts, methods, and measures that enable the community health nurse to examine aggregate health concerns in a neighborhood, community, or township.

KEY TERMS *(Continued)*

physical agents
point prevalence
PRECEDE–PROCEED model
prevalence rate
prevention trials

prospective study
relative risk
retrospective study
risk
sensitivity

specificity
surveillance
therapeutic trials
vital statistics

DEFINITION AND BACKGROUND

Green (1990) describes community health as a triad of applied sciences that includes epidemiology, human ecology, and demography. Community health goes beyond the individual to focus on the health problems of populations. This group focus is the distinguishing difference between community health nursing and clinical nursing, which focuses on the individual or family.

Ecology in community health, according to Green (1990), refers to the interrelationship between the individual and his or her physical, cultural, and social environments. Ecology in this sense, then, may include climate, geography, industry, and religious and cultural factors influencing a community. **Demography** is an analytic tool used to measure a population by recording births, deaths, age distribution, and other vital statistics. Epidemiology is a companion science to demography in that it also uses analytic tools to find causes, frequency, and distribution of health problems in a community. A clear and concise definition of epidemiology is provided by Last (1995): "Epidemiology is the study of the distribution and determinants of health-related states or events in specified populations, and the application of this study to the control of health problems" (p. 42).

Historically, the term *epidemiology* originated from the study of **epidemics** (rapid rises in disease occurrence beyond the expected norm) of infectious diseases such as yellow fever, cholera, and bubonic plague. Contemporary epidemiology focuses on a broad spectrum of health problems including communicable and chronic diseases, injury control, nutrition, and violence (Friedman, 1987).

The use of epidemiologic methods dates back to the 5th century B.C. Hippocrates, a Greek physician and the father of modern medicine, was the first to use observa-

tion and data collection to describe infectious diseases such as tetanus and mumps. Epidemiologic methods were used to investigate and conquer such epidemics as the bubonic plague, which killed 25 million Europeans in the Middle Ages. Into the 17th and 18th centuries, vital record collection and analysis became important tools in determining the impact of the great epidemics on communities by examining age distribution and seasonal changes in the number of deaths. John Graunt (1620–1674) is credited with the first analysis of birth and death records, published in *Natural and Political Observations Made upon the Bills of Mortality* as cited in Hennekens & Buring (1987). During a time when bubonic plague caused deaths to outnumber births, his report contributed to the understanding of the pattern of this disease in the London population.

John Snow (1813–1858) wrote about his epidemiologic investigation of the London cholera epidemic in *On the Mode of Communication of Cholera* as cited in Hennekens & Buring (1987). His important work is considered the first application of epidemiologic methods. Snow investigated an outbreak of cholera in London and linked the cause of the epidemic to a contaminated water supply. He used observational methods, neighborhood interviews, and analysis of death records according to geographic location to show that death rates were higher in a community whose water source was supplied by one particular water company.

In the southern United States, a Public Health Service physician named John Goldberger (1874–1927) conducted a famous epidemiologic investigation on **pellagra**, a deficiency disease causing gastrointestinal, mucosal, neurological, and mental symptoms. Using methods established by John Snow, Goldberger determined the cause of pellagra to be dietary rather than infectious, as was previously believed. The epidemiologic methods used were observing those with and without the disease and interviewing local residents about environmental conditions and dietary habits.

Prior to the discovery of disease-producing microorganisms, many diseases were attributed to poverty, overcrowding, and poor environmental conditions and occurrences. Contemporary epidemiology mirrors the technologic advances of the past century and the changes in life expectancy. During the past century, life expectancy in the United States has increased by nearly 60%. In 1900, life expectancy was 47 years (USDHHS, 1990). In 1990, life expectancy was 75 years and in 1992 was nearly 76 years (USDHHS, 1996). Evolutionary changes of an aging

REFLECTIVE THINKING

Assessing Your Community

• Can you call to mind a particular disease, health concern, or injury that affects your community?

• Can you describe the population in the community that is most affected by this particular problem?

• What factors may be contributing to the problem?

Table 11-1 Ten Leading Causes of Death in the United States, 1900 and 1996, All Ages

1900	1996
Pneumonia/influenza	Heart diseases
Tuberculosis	Cancer
Heart diseases	Stroke
Stroke	Chronic obstructive pulmonary disease
Diarrhea/enteritis	Accidents
Nephritis	Pneumonia/influenza
Cancer	Diabetes
Injuries	HIV/AIDS
Diphtheria	Suicide
Other	Chronic liver disease and cirrhosis

From "Ten Leading Causes of Death in the United States, 1900 and 1996, All Ages" by National Center for Health Statistics, 1997, Monthly Vital Statistics Report 46(1). Hyattsville, MD: Public Health Services.

population linked with the cure and control of many communicable diseases has resulted in the modern epidemics of chronic diseases such as heart disease, cancer, and stroke. Table 11-1 illustrates this evolutionary shift in the leading causes of death in the United States from 1900 to 1996 (when adjusted for age). Applying epidemiology to the study of chronic diseases such as cancer as opposed to that of communicable diseases has required the development of more complex research methods because of the long induction period between exposure to a disease-causing agent and appearance of signs of the disease.

BASIC CONCEPTS OF DISEASE IN THE EPIDEMIOLOGIC APPROACH

The epidemiologic approach is an application of the scientific method and assumes that health, disease, and injury do not occur randomly. The historical development of epidemiologic methods illustrates the necessity of investigating a health problem before everything is known about the disease etiology. For example, prior to the discovery of the microorganism responsible for cholera, John Snow used epidemiologic methods to show that a conta-

🌀🌀 REFLECTIVE THINKING 🌀🌀

Causes of Death

• As a community health nurse, what resource would you use to find data about the leading causes of death in your community?

• What are the leading age-specific causes of death in your community?

minated water source was causing a cholera outbreak in London. Similarly, community health nurses working in health districts and neighborhoods may employ epidemiologic methods to investigate health, social, and environmental problems. This section provides an overview of several key concepts framing the foundation and historical development of epidemiology.

The Epidemiologic Triad: Agent, Host, and Environment

One of the functions of the epidemiologic approach to the study of disease is to determine the etiology, or cause, of the disease or risk factor. Although most of the concepts inherent in the science of epidemiology evolved from the study of infectious diseases, these concepts can be applied to noninfectious diseases and conditions as well (Lilienfeld & Stolley, 1994). The concepts of epidemiology can also be applied to the study of injuries and, more recently, have been applied to the study of health and wellness. In order to study the etiology or causality of a health problem, the epidemiologist systematically views three multifactorial elements: agent, host, and environment.

Agent

The **agent** is a toxic substance, microorganism, or environmental factor, such as radiation or a lifestyle, that must be present (or absent) for the problem to occur. Analytic epidemiology seeks to link the agent to the disease or condition in order to determine causality. In other words, the epidemiologist must examine factors that influence the probability of contact between, for example, an infectious agent and a susceptible person or population, known as a host. To illustrate the concept of an agent linked to the development of a disease or risk factor, consider the relationship between asbestos exposure or smoking and the development of lung cancer or the relationship between Type A behavior and heart disease. According to Lilienfeld and Stolley (1994), disease agents and etiologic factors can be classified into four categories: nutritive elements, chemical agents, physical agents, and infectious agents.

Nutritive elements can be described as excesses or deficiencies within a host, such as vitamin or protein deficiencies. Cholesterol is one example of a nutritive element that can be viewed as an agent of disease, in this case, hyperlipidemia. **Chemical agents** include poisons and allergens. Examples of poisons include pharmaceuticals taken in excess, carbon monoxide, and caustic substances such as lye. Allergens are agents such as ragweed and poison oak and may also include medications or foods. **Physical agents** include radiation, excessive sun exposure, and mechanical agents. Because mechanical agents may be more difficult to conceptualize than are other physical agents, two examples are presented here to clarify this concept.

In the 1950s, when jet aircraft were in the initial stages of development and usage, many of the pilots being trained to fly the new airplanes were found to have hearing loss in some decibel ranges. Upon investigation, it was determined that the high-pitched sounds emitted by the jet engines damaged the ear and caused permanent hearing loss in certain decibel ranges. Since that discovery, pilots and others working around jet aircraft have been required to wear protective ear coverings to block out damaging sounds.

More recently, with the advent of computer technology and the widespread use of computers in the office and home, many people have developed a type of carpal tunnel syndrome. In computer users, this condition has been traced to the position in which the hands are held for long periods of time when working at a computer. Consequently, those who use the computer for many hours a day are now advised to change hand positions often and to take periodic breaks from their work at the computer.

Infectious agents of disease include metazoa, such as hookworm; protozoa, including those causing malaria and toxoplasmosis; bacteria, associated with syphilis, tuberculosis, and other diseases; fungi; and viruses. An example of an infectious agent is one that causes foodborne illness such as salmonellosis; the illness is caused by the bacterial contamination of certain (usually uncooked or undercooked) foods, which are ingested by a susceptible host.

Host

The **host** is the person or population on which the agent acts. Before the host population is examined, the persons composing a population must be looked at individually. In this way, the epidemiologist or community health nurse can determine those factors that individuals possess that might be factors linked to a particular disease or disability. In examining the individual host, the epidemiologist must look at demographic characteristics including age, gender, ethnicity, socioeconomic status, marital status, nutritional and immune status, genetic or familial factors, occupation, physiological or psychological state, preexisting conditions or disease, and lifestyle. Each of these characteristics will have an impact on the development of disease or other conditions as well as on the general health or wellness of the individual host. Although the host is, technically, always an individual, epidemiology is a science that examines the presence of disease or risk factors in populations over time. Thus, epidemiologists examine a group or population of hosts in which a particular agent or risk factor is present. To draw conclusions about disease, injury, or wellness in a population without closely examining individual host characteristics for common factors can lead to misinterpretation of data and, in turn, false conclusions.

Through scientific investigation, we have become increasingly aware of the role played by genetic factors in the development of disease. Sickle cell anemia and hemophilia are two examples of genetically transferred disease. Age is also an important factor; whereas some diseases appear to primarily strike young people, others develop with the aging process. Gender must also be considered,

in that some diseases or conditions are more common among women or among men. For example, although cases of breast cancer are occasionally seen in men, this disease primarily affects women. Some diseases are more common in one ethnic group than in another. The higher rate of sickle cell anemia among African Americans is an example of an ethnically related factor. The psychological or physiological state of the host must also be considered. Pregnancy, obesity, and high blood pressure are among the many physiological states that may place the individual at risk for disease, disability, or injury. Stress, one of many psychological factors, is now recognized as an important factor in the development of some diseases and conditions. Preexisting disease and immunocompetence are also key factors affecting susceptibility and resistance to disease. The development of opportunistic infections such as tuberculosis or toxoplasmosis among persons with AIDS is an example of poor host resistance. Risk factors for disease are increasingly being attributed to lifestyle factors: Amount and type of exercise; elements of diet, including fat and alcohol intake; and smoking habits, among others, are now seen as key risk factors in the development of certain diseases and conditions. Marital status may also be an indicator of the probability of developing a particular disease or of life expectancy. People who are married or partnered, for example, may have a longer life expectancy.

Environment

The third concept inherent in the epidemiologic triad is **environment**. The environment comprises those factors outside of the host that are associated with the development of disease, disorder, or injury. Elements of environment that must be considered when linking agent and host include geographic factors (climate, latitude, and altitude), occupational hazards, and personal and secular trends (changes in lifestyle patterns or environmental risks over years or decades, such as sewage treatment or availability of immunizations).

The interaction of host and environmental factors is very important in tracing the etiology of disease and other conditions. Whether being examined by the epidemiologist or the community health nurse, the importance of individual host characteristics, or factors, cannot be overemphasized.

With regard to the impact of environmental factors (those outside of the host) on disease development, physical environment is important in that certain diseases are more prevalent in a particular climate or geographic location, or even at certain times of the year. Malaria, for example, is a disease that is rare in the United States but indigenous to many parts of Africa. Biological factors are those related to density of populations, sources of food and water, and the presence of disease agents in the area being studied. Whether the host lives in an urban or rural setting may be a factor related to disease development. For instance, people living and working close together in cities may be more susceptible to influenza outbreaks than are their counterparts in rural areas. The occupation of the host must be carefully examined for exposure to pathogens. Historically, one can recall the discovery of the prevalence of lung disease among miners. More recently, researchers have examined the relationship between agricultural pesticide use and disease development among farm workers, as well as between silicate exposure and asbestosis.

The significance of the epidemiologic triad should thus be evident. Equally significant is the interrelationship among the three parts of the triad. For example, occupation is viewed as a characteristic of the host, but where the host works constitutes an environment. Further, the occupation of the host in a particular environment can cause exposure to chemical or mechanical agents. Likewise, socioeconomic status (a host factor) can affect the nutritional state and the ability to obtain adequate and safe housing (an environmental factor). For instance, the media have reported numerous cases of lead poisoning among children who have been exposed to old lead-based paint (an agent) on walls in pre–1950 tenements or on older cribs. Furthermore, disease vectors (agents) including rats, cockroaches, and fleas may also be rampant in substandard conditions. See Figure 11-1 for an illustration of the epidemiologic triad.

Many of the host and environmental factors thus far mentioned constitute distinct areas of scientific study, such as genetics, microbiology, geriatrics, pediatrics, and sociology, to name a few. The task of the epidemiologist is to attempt to examine and integrate pertinent elements from many different disciplines in order to assemble the data needed to analyze a particular disease or condition and trace its etiology (Lilienfeld & Stolley, 1994). The same process may be used by community health nurses in identifying factors related to disease, disability, or injury among their clients.

DECISION MAKING

Lead Poisoning

As a community health nurse, you have determined that several of your youngest clients, who live in a housing project, are exhibiting symptoms of lead poisoning.

- What host factors might predispose the children to this condition?

- How might you determine the agent involved?

- What environmental factors might you suspect that could be related to the condition, and what steps might you advise the parents to take to correct those factors?

It is important to understand the concepts of agent, host, and environment in that they are basic to the science of epidemiology. These three factors and their parts must be considered whenever and wherever the epidemiologist seeks to determine the etiology of a disease, whether the goal is eradication of the disease or the development of preventive measures.

The Natural History of a Disease

One goal of epidemiology is the eradication or prevention of health problems. A logical first step for the epidemiologist, then, is to understand the natural history of the disease in question. The **natural history of a disease** can be defined as the unaltered course that a disease would take without any intervention such as therapy or lifestyle changes. One primary application of epidemiology is to study the natural history of a disease in order to develop therapeutic interventions or prevention strategies. The natural history of a disease can be understood by viewing the concept as a continuum, with exposure to the agent suspected of causing the disease or condition at one end, through the development of signs and symptoms of illness in a progression of severity, to the ultimate outcome of the disease, whether that be disability or death, at the other end (see Figure 11-2).

The most common analytic study design used to determine the natural history of a disease is the cohort study, which will be discussed in detail later in this chapter. Understanding the natural history of disease is of vital importance to epidemiologists and others who seek to discover the etiology of disease, design strategic therapeutic interventions, and develop preventive or screening measures in order to alter the outcome of a particular disease process or condition. Community health nurses also use the concept of the natural history of disease in client education, when informing clients about their diseases or conditions and encouraging behavior or lifestyle modifi-

---

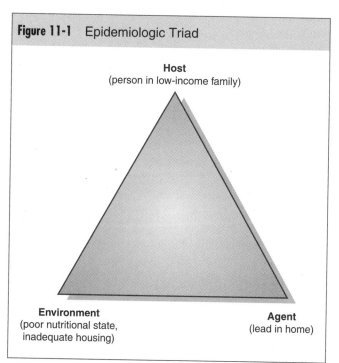

Figure 11-1 Epidemiologic Triad

Host
(person in low-income family)

Environment
(poor nutritional state,
inadequate housing)

Agent
(lead in home)

Figure 11-2 Continuum of Natural History of Disease

Exposure to agent	Development of disease signs and symptoms	Disability or death

cation as a means of altering the course of the disease or condition in question.

Figure 11-3 illustrates the natural history of a disease continuum with incorporation of detection via a screening test in the preclinical stage.

The usefulness of screening tests to detect early disease depends on available and effective treatments at the time of detection. Additionally, the possibility of a **false-negative test** (test that is negative when the individual actually has the disease of interest) and a **false-positive test** (test result that is positive when the individual does not have the disease of interest) should be minimal; that is, the test should have sufficient **sensitivity** (the probability of a positive result for an individual who has the disease) and sufficient **specificity** (the probability of a negative result for an individual who does not have the disease).

Concept of Prevention

Prevention is another key concept to epidemiology. Epidemiologists seek to identify characteristics that cause or predict a disease or condition. This identification of potential risk factors may result in prevention of disease when intervention strategies can be established. Measures that delay the onset of a disease or prevent it altogether are called preventive. The three **levels of prevention** are called primary, secondary, and tertiary.

A taxonomy of the three levels of prevention reflects the continuum of the natural history of a disease. Primary-prevention strategies or interventions foster health promotion and wellness before a disease or symptoms develop (Green, 1990). Secondary-prevention activities target early diagnosis, treatment, and detection of disease to prevent disability. Tertiary-prevention strategies and activities focus on limiting disability once disease develops. Community health prevention strategies include health education for health promotion, public health measures, legal or regulatory sanctions for health protection, and health services for screening and preventive care.

Primary Prevention

Primary prevention typically involves several key strategies: health education, regulatory strategies, and health care services. These strategies are used in many disease-prevention programs. Health-education programs targeting populations at risk for cancer, for example, include antismoking campaigns, fiber-rich diet promotion to reduce colon cancer, and promotion of sunscreen use to prevent harmful sun overexposure. Regulatory strategies that limit carcinogens in the environment and alert the public to potential hazards have been employed in such states as California to promote cancer prevention. Cigarette taxes constitute another example of regulatory strategy, specifically with regard to the primary prevention of lung cancer. Immunization is an example of preventive health care services, constituting an important component in the primary prevention of childhood infectious diseases. Vaccination against hepatitis B to prevent liver cancer is another example of primary preventive health care.

Secondary Prevention

Screening tests constitute a common secondary-prevention strategy to detect disease before symptoms occur or would be detectable by routine diagnosis (Greenberg, Daniels, Flanders, Eley & Boring, III, 1996). Screening tests should provide for early treatment and enhanced outcome. One such example is the Mantoux skin test. This test reliably detects tuberculosis infection in an individual when the health care provider uses proper cutoff points. In addition, the individual with a positive Mantoux skin test may benefit from early chemoprophylaxis with

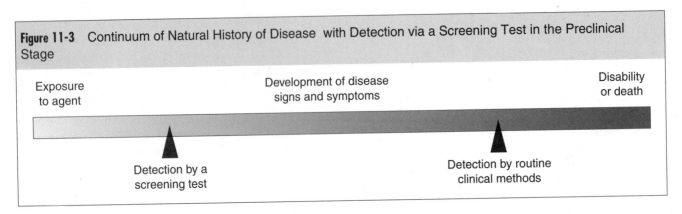

Figure 11-3 Continuum of Natural History of Disease with Detection via a Screening Test in the Preclinical Stage

Exposure to agent	Development of disease signs and symptoms	Disability or death

Detection by a screening test

Detection by routine clinical methods

isoniazid therapy before disease onset. A complete and properly taken course of preventive isoniazid can reduce an individual's lifetime risk of developing active tuberculosis disease by 90%. Secondary-prevention screening programs for tuberculosis infection are used in populations considered at risk of acquiring active disease, such as persons with HIV infection, or groups at risk of recent infection, for example those individuals in institutional settings such as prisons and homeless shelters.

Tertiary Prevention

Tertiary prevention strategies seek to reduce complications and limit disability once disease develops. Tertiary care is the major focus of the health care industry. As the natural history of a disease continuum progresses to disease development, treatment of disease and rehabilitation are the primary activities.

TYPES OF EPIDEMIOLOGIC STUDIES

As mentioned earlier, the purpose of the epidemiologic approach is to study the distribution and determinants of health problems in groups or populations. Epidemiologic methods of study may also be used by nurse researchers. The community health nurse must therefore become familiar with both epidemiologic literature and clinical nursing research in order to integrate both into practice. This section provides an overview of two major approaches to epidemiologic study designs.

Table 11-2 summarizes the types of epidemiologic studies.

Observational Studies

Observational studies are nonexperimental in nature. They primarily describe, compare, and explain disease, disorder, or injury occurrence in a population. There are two general categories of observational studies, descriptive and analytic.

Descriptive Studies

Descriptive epidemiology studies contribute to the investigation and understanding of a health problem by asking the following questions:

Who has the problem (*person*)?

Where does the problem occur (*place*)?

When does the problem occur (*time*)?

These essential features of person, place, and time are the necessary elements of descriptive studies. Data such as sex, age, occupation, ethnicity, marital status, and socioeconomic status may be factors in who gets a particular health problem. Where a person lives or works provides information regarding the place where the disease or injury is occurring. Timing of a disease, such as seasonal occurrence or epidemic outbreak, is important in determining when a disease may occur. For example, descriptive studies were invaluable in initially understanding and identifying the presence of acquired immunodeficiency syndrome (AIDS) among young homosexual males in the United States in the early 1980s. Three types of descriptive studies—correlational studies, cross-sectional surveys, and case reports and case series—are useful in examining the factors of person, place, and time.

A **correlational study** is useful when the community health nurse investigator wants to compare neighborhoods and examine a particular disease in relationship to a potential risk factor. Epidemiologic measures are assessed on a group rather than an individual basis. For example, if a community health nurse notices a number of children with leukemia in the health district and suspects a contributing environmental contaminant in the area, a correlational study could be initiated to compare leukemia rates among children of a health district in a neighboring town. This statistical comparison may or may not confirm higher leukemia rates in the nurse's health district. The information is specific only to the population groups under study in the geographic areas. Correlational studies are used in the initial assessment phase of investigating potential exposures (risk factors) of diseases.

The second type of descriptive study design, the **cross-sectional survey**, also may constitute the initial assessment phase of a more in-depth study. The cross-sectional survey could be used to assess a health problem such as tuberculosis infection among homeless persons, for example. By using a representative group (cross section) of individuals, such as those residing in a particular shelter, to represent the homeless population of a community, a survey using TB skin testing could be performed. This type of study occurs at only one point in time but can be helpful in associating disease prevalence and possible causes.

Case reports and **case series** constitute the third type of descriptive study design. Case reports detail histories of individuals or groups with unusual health problems and are significant in the identification of potential new diseases. For example, some of the first known cases of acquired immunodeficiency syndrome (AIDS) were described in the medical literature as case reports. A case series are compilation of case reports.

Analytic Studies

Analytic studies go beyond describing the occurrence of health problems in a population by comparing groups of individuals in order to study associations and causal relationships. The purpose of **analytic epidemiologic studies** is to search for causes of disease occurrence.

The first type of observational analytic investigation is the **case-control study**. In this look-back study design, also known as a **retrospective study**, groups of individuals are assembled after a disease has occurred. The epidemiologist compares groups with similar characteristics to examine risk factors associated with a disease occurrence. The structure of the case-control study requires that two study groups be assembled by the epidemiologist. One group of individuals who have a specifically defined disease (the cases) is compared with another group of individuals who do not have the disease (the controls). Members of both groups may share certain characteristics such as age and sex. Both groups are then studied using questionnaires, interviews, or testing in order to determine possible exposures or characteristics that may be attributable to the disease under study. Most notable among etiologic associations discovered via the case-control study design are the relationships between viral illness among young children, aspirin use, and with Reye's syndrome and the relationship between toxic shock syndrome and tampon use.

The second type of observational analytic investigation is the **cohort study**, or **prospective study**. In this study design, the epidemiologist assembles a group of individuals who are free of the disease under study (the cohort) and follows the group into the future to determine etiologic factors contributing to disease development. This type of epidemiologic study is one of the most effective methods to show potential causes of a disease. The best-known cohort study in the United States is the Framingham, Massachusetts study, which began in the 1950s. Framingham was chosen as the site for this study because it exhibited a number of characteristics that would allow the investigators to follow the study population for a number of years: a stable population; a wide range of occupations; one hospital, which was utilized by the majority of the population; and annually updated population lists (Hennekens & Buring, 1987). In this study, investigators identified and examined a cohort of 5,127 Framingham men and women, each 30 to 50 years in age and free of coronary heart disease. Data were assembled on demographic characteristics, medical history, cigarette smoking, and several clinical and laboratory parameters. Members of the cohort have been followed and reexamined at regular intervals since the initial information was collected (between 1950 and 1952). Epidemiologists are studying these individuals to determine potential risk and predictive factors contributing to the development of coronary heart disease. Findings from this cohort study have contributed significantly to the understanding of the causal relationship between smoking, high blood pressure, high serum lipids, and heart disease. The study has added significantly to the body of knowledge on cardiovascular diseases. The Framingham Heart Study is considered a classic in the annals of epidemiology, both in describing the natural history of a disease and in determining the etiologic factors in the development of a particular disease.

Another example of an ongoing cohort study is the Nurses' Health Study, which began in 1976. The study uses biannual questionnaires to collect information on reproductive factors, lifestyle practices, and diet in relation to the occurrence of breast cancer, heart disease, and other major illnesses in women (Nurses' Health Study Newsletter, 1996).

Both case-control and cohort studies have limitations in the final analysis of the study results. In the case-control study, the epidemiologist selects individuals who already have a disease, thus, this method is potentially susceptible to selection and observation bias. **Bias** is an error in study design that results in incorrect conclusions regarding the association between potential risk factors and disease occurrence. The cohort study design is less prone to bias because individuals are selected and observed before disease occurrence. Experimental, or intervention, studies greatly reduce the role of bias by randomly assigning individuals to study groups.

Intervention Studies

Intervention studies are experimental in nature and require the epidemiologist to alter the behavior of the individuals participating in the study rather than merely observe the behaviors. Also known as randomized controlled clinical trials, intervention studies can best demonstrate the relationship between cause and effect. The structure of the study design requires a group of individuals (the study population) and a treatment or intervention to be tested. Individuals are randomly assigned to either the experimental (treatment) group or the control (no treatment) group. Members of the experimental group receive the treatment or intervention, and members of the control group receive no intervention. Providing the study is conducted properly, comparison analysis of the two groups following the treatment or intervention may provide epidemiologic evidence of a cause-and-effect relationship. Pharmaceuticals approved for therapeutic use are frequently tested using this study design.

There are two types of intervention studies: prevention trials and therapeutic trials. **Prevention trials** use experimental methodology to test measures or interventions among individuals and groups to prevent disease in a healthy population. Common examples of prevention trials are vaccine field testing and fluoridation of community water supplies to prevent tooth decay. **Therapeutic**

Table 11-2 **Types of Epidemiologic Studies**	
OBSERVATIONAL STUDIES	**INTERVENTION STUDIES**
Descriptive	
Correlational	Prevention trials
Cross-sectional/survey	Therapeutic trials
Case reports and case series	
Analytic	
Case-control study (retrospective)	
Cohort study (prospective)	

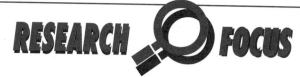

RESEARCH FOCUS

The Long-Term Effects of a Cardiovascular Disease Prevention Trial: The Stanford Five-City Project

STUDY PROBLEM/PURPOSE

This study examined the long-term effects of a community-based health-education intervention trial to reduce the risk of cardiovascular disease. During the last 40 years, epidemiological studies have established that hypertension, cigarette use, obesity, elevated plasma cholesterol, and sedentary lifestyle are related to the pathogenesis of cardiovascular diseases. It is important to conduct community-based education programs as a public health measure.

METHODS

Two treatment cities in California (those who had received a community-based health program) and two control cities were selected to participate in this study. Persons 12–74 years of age who resided in randomly selected households in the four cities were eligible to participate. The initial study (one city) of the intervention trial, with results published in 1990, was designed to test whether a comprehensive program of community organization and health education produced favorable changes in cardiovascular disease risk factors, morbidity, and mortality. This current study (four cities) was conducted as a follow-up, population-based, cross-sectional survey, 3 years following the conclusion of the main health education intervention.

FINDINGS

Blood pressure improvements observed in all cities from baseline to the end of the intervention were maintained during the follow-up in those cities who received the treatment but not in the control cities. Cholesterol levels continued to decline in all cities during follow-up. Smoking rates leveled out or increased slightly in the treatment cities and continued to decline in the control cities but did not yield statistically significant net differences. Both coronary heart disease and all-cause mortality risk scores were maintained or continued to improve in the treatment cities while leveling out or increasing in the control cities.

IMPLICATIONS

These findings suggest that community-based cardiovascular education programs can have sustained effects. However, the modest net differences in risk factors point to the need for new designs and interventions. The use of smaller, more frequent surveys, interventions of shorter duration, longitudinal follow-up of high-risk cohort samples, and evaluation of qualitative parameters at various levels are needed. The Stanford Five-City Project is one of the most comprehensive cardiovascular disease risk reduction studies conducted in the United States and the first to conduct a long-term follow-up of the main intervention effects (the community-based education programs).

SOURCE

From "The Long-Term Effects of a Cardiovascular Disease Prevention Trial: The Stanford Five-City Project" by M.A. Winkleby, C. B. Taylor, D. Jatulis, & S. P. Fortmann, 1996, American Journal of Public Health, 86 *(12), pp. 1773–1779.*

---

trials are usually conducted among individuals who are identified to be at risk of a certain disease or who already have symptoms of the disease being studied. The intervention given to the experimental group may be a drug, behavior change, or surgical intervention, for example, a new medication for hypertension. The control group may receive the current usual care or no intervention. Both the experimental and control groups are followed up for a specified time in order to determine the effects of the intervention.

EPIDEMIOLOGIC MEASUREMENT

As discussed earlier, epidemiology focuses on describing the presence and distribution of a disease or other health-related condition in a population and identifying associations between that disease or health-related condition and possible causative factors. In order to accomplish either of these objectives, the frequency of disease must be measured. Such measurement allows comparison of disease occurrence between groups. Within a given population, groups that exhibit a particular exposure or characteristic can be compared as can groups that either do not exhibit the condition of interest or have not been exposed to the disease of interest. In this way, the epidemiologist may gain information useful in determining disease etiology or developing preventive measures.

Measures of Disease Frequency

Several techniques are used to measure disease frequency. The most basic measure of **disease frequency** is a simple count of those individuals who have the disease of interest. Such a count is of limited use to epidemiologists, however. In order to successfully determine the distribution and probable etiology of disease in a population or geographic area, the epidemiologist must know the size of the population of which affected individuals were a part (e.g., a city) and the time period during which information on the presence of the disease was obtained. Knowing the base population and the time period for data collection permits the comparison of disease frequencies among two or more groups of people or populations. To illustrate this concept, consider the following hypothetical scenario:

> City A reports 56 cases of tuberculosis, while City B reports 35 cases. With only this information, the county public health officer would assume that City A had a larger outbreak of TB and therefore required more financial resources and public health nurses to combat the spread of the disease. However, if City A has a population of 75,000, and City B has a population of 15,000, it can be seen that City B actually has the more severe problem with the disease. If a time element is factored in—for example City A's cases are reported for a period covering one year, and City B's cases occurred during a six-month period—the picture becomes even clearer. Resources should be deployed to City B, where the situation is much more serious.

Prevalence and Incidence Rates

The most commonly used measures of disease frequency are the prevalence rate and incidence rate. The **prevalence rate** is defined as the proportion (percentage) of the population that has the disease or condition at a given time. **Point prevalence** refers to the total number of persons with a disease at a specific point in time. The **incidence rate** is defined as the rate of change from the nondiseased state to the diseased state among persons at risk and reflects new cases of the disease or condition in a specified time period (Hennekens & Buring, 1987). Rates are special forms of proportions that include a time specification. All rates have a numerator and a denominator. The numerator is the number of events (disease incidents) or conditions of interest, and the denominator is the number of people in the population from which the numerator (affected individuals) was derived.

$$\text{prevalence rate } (P) = \frac{\text{number of cases (new and old)}}{\text{size of the population}}\\ \text{at a given point in time}$$

$$\text{incidence rate } (I) = \frac{\text{number of new cases of disease}}{\text{population at risk of becoming}}\\ \text{new cases at the same point in time}$$

Other common measurements of disease frequency with which the student should be familiar are morbidity rate and mortality rates, special types of incidence or prevalence rates. The **morbidity rate** is the incidence of nonfatal cases of disease in the total population at risk during a specified point in time:

$$\text{morbidity rate} = \frac{\text{new nonfatal cases of disease}}{\text{total population at risk}}$$

The **attack rate**, a more specific morbidity rate, expresses the occurrence of a disease among a particular population at risk often due to a specific exposure and is calculated for a limited period of time (Morton, Hebel, & McCarter, 1996).

$$\text{attack rate} = \frac{\text{number of people ill in the time period}}{\text{total number of people at risk}}\\ \text{in the time period}$$

The usefulness of the attack rate is illustrated by the following situation:

> A number of patrons of a local restaurant presented in local emergency rooms on Mother's Day evening with complaints of nausea, vomiting, abdominal pain, and diarrhea. Investigation by the local health department revealed that all of those who were taken ill had eaten brunch at the restaurant. After interviewing all Mother's Day patrons, it was determined that of those attending the brunch, nearly all became ill (attack rate) following the ingestion of certain food items. The source of the outbreak was traced back to poor refrigeration and lack of stringent sanitary measures among staff preparing those particular foods. Public health measures were instituted to prevent further illness.

The **mortality** (death) **rate** can reflect both incidence and prevalence. The general formula used to calculate mortality is:

$$\text{mortality rate} = \frac{\text{number of deaths from a disease}}{\text{total population}}\\ \text{(or all causes)}$$

The **case fatality rate** refers to deaths from a specific disease:

$$\text{case fatality rate} = \frac{\text{number of deaths from a disease}}{\text{number of cases of the disease}}$$

All of these rates are summarized in Figure 11-4.

Vital Statistics

More specific rates are used by scientists, including epidemiologists, when examining incidence or prevalence in special populations. These are major public health rates, also known as vital statistics. **Vital statistics** are the result of systematic registration of vital events such as births,

Figure 11-4 Equations Used in Computing Prevalence, Incidence, Morbidity, and Mortality Rates

$$\text{prevalence rate }(P) = \frac{\text{number of cases (new and old) existing at a given point in time}}{\text{size of the population at a given point in time}}$$

$$\text{incidence rate }(I) = \frac{\text{number of new cases of disease at a given point in time}}{\text{population at risk of becoming new cases at the same point in time}}$$

$$\text{morbidity rate} = \frac{\text{new nonfatal cases of disease}}{\text{total population at risk}}$$

$$\text{attack rate} = \frac{\text{number of people ill in the time period}}{\text{total number of people at risk in the time period}}$$

$$\text{mortality rate} = \frac{\text{number of deaths from a disease (or all causes)}}{\text{total population}}$$

$$\text{case fatality rate} = \frac{\text{number of deaths from a disease}}{\text{number of cases of the disease}}$$

deaths, and health events. The statistical reports generated from the assembled data have many uses. For example, birth and death statistics are used to calculate estimated life expectancy, and health and disease statistics are used to identify changes in leading causes of death over time.

Those rates whose denominators are the total population are as follows:

$$\text{crude birth rate} = \frac{\text{number of live births}}{\text{total mid-year population}}$$

$$\text{crude death rate} = \frac{\text{number of deaths during the year}}{\text{total mid-year population}}$$

$$\text{age-specific death rate} = \frac{\text{number of deaths in a given age group in a year}}{\text{average mid-year population in the age group}}$$

These rates are expressed as a number per 1,000 people. The **cause-specific death rate** is expressed as a number per 100,000 population:

$$\text{cause-specific death rate} = \frac{\text{number of deaths due to a given cause in a year}}{\text{total mid-year population}}$$

Mid-year population, as used in the preceding equations, is an arbitrary but universal population number selected to ensure that calculations are based on the same figure regardless of what agency or person is preparing the information.

Vital statistics of those rates and ratios whose denominators are live births are as follows:

$$\text{infant mortality (death) rate} = \frac{\text{number of infant deaths in one year (under 1 year of age)}}{\text{number of live births in the same year}} \times 1{,}000$$

$$\text{neonatal mortality (death) rate} = \frac{\text{number of newborn deaths (under 28 days of age)}}{\text{number of live births in the same year}} \times 1{,}000$$

$$\text{fetal death ratio} = \frac{\text{number of fetal deaths in one year (20+ weeks)}}{\text{number of live births in the same year}} \times 1{,}000$$

These three equations are expressed as a number per 1,000 live births.

The **maternal mortality rate**, which reflects the deaths of mothers at the time of birth or shortly thereafter, is expressed as a number per 100,000 live births.

$$\text{maternal mortality rate} = \frac{\text{number of maternal deaths in one year (from complications)}}{\text{number of live births in the same year}}$$

A third category of public health rates is one whose denominators are live births plus fetal deaths, as follows:

$$\text{fetal death rate} = \frac{\text{number of fetal deaths in one year}}{\text{number of live births plus fetal deaths in one year}}$$

$$\text{perinatal mortality rate} = \frac{\text{number of fetal deaths (under 7 days)}}{\text{number of live births plus fetal deaths in one year}}$$

These two equations are expressed as a number per 1,000 live births plus fetal deaths. Note that although they sound alike the fetal death *rate* and the fetal death *ratio* are calculated differently.

Sources of data for these measures are many and varied and include birth and death certificates; census figures (for populations); disease registries; the Centers for Disease Control (for notifiable diseases); various national surveys such as the National Health Interview Survey; hospitals (discharge records); insurance providers; exposure or trauma registries; and tumor registries. Also useful to the investigator are employment statistics and air and water quality statistics. The Internet is a newer but valuable source for data on vital statistics.

The measures calculated from information compiled by these various sources allow epidemiologists and public health practitioners to construct a picture of the state of the nation's health. In this way, we can learn which diseases are the leading causes of death in various age groups or in other populations and in the nation as a whole. We can also learn which diseases or conditions are most prevalent in given populations and which are geographically widespread. This information guides scientists (including nurse researchers and investigators), policy makers, and others engaged in research or the development of new treatment modalities. For example, decisions can be made regarding priorities for the allotment of financial and personnel resources and the development of treatment or preventive measures.

The information provided by the various public health measures discussed here also provides a historical record of diseases in the population. For example, according to the U.S. Public Health Service, the two leading causes of death in 1900 were pneumonia/influenza and tuberculosis, whereas heart disease and cancer were the leading causes of death in 1993. Such data provide information about the results of lifestyle changes, treatments developed for disease (including pharmaceuticals), and similar variables. Such information could only be surmised had these vital records not been kept. Figure 11-5 summarizes the formulas used in computing vital statistics.

Measures of Association

Thus, measures of disease frequency are a basis for comparing populations. Such comparisons are valuable to epidemiologists investigating the relationships (associations) between disease agent, host, and environment as discussed earlier in the chapter. In epidemiology, **measures of association** are defined as those statistical measures used to investigate the degree of dependence between two or more events or variables. Events can be classified as statistically associated when they occur more frequently together than could be accounted for by chance alone. Statistical association does not always imply causality, however. For example, when a factor and disease are associated only because both are related to some underlying cause, a noncausal statistical association exists. To illustrate this concept, consider an association found between yellow fingers and lung cancer. In other words, many people who developed lung cancer exhibited the phenomenon of yellow fingers. We can be reasonably certain, however, that yellow stains on the ring and middle fingers do not cause lung cancer. Rather, the underlying cause of these stains is smoking, and many heavy smokers do develop lung cancer. The association between yellow fingers and lung cancer would therefore be labeled noncausal.

Two of the most frequently used measures of association in epidemiology are relative risk and attributable risk. These measures indicate the degree of increased likelihood that one group as compared with another group will develop a disease or condition, or the degree of higher disease frequency in one population as compared with another. The concept of **risk** refers to the probability that a disease or a condition will develop in a given time period.

Relative Risk

Although epidemiologists widely use several relative measures, only the most common are discussed here. Relative measures indicate the likelihood of an exposed group's developing a disease *relative* to those who are not exposed. The rate ratio (*RR*), also called the **relative risk** or the risk ratio, is the ratio between the rates in the exposed and unexposed groups. Cohort studies such as the Framingham Heart Study, discussed previously, are the source of data for relative risk determination.

$$RR = (Ie/Iu)$$

where *Ie* represents the *incidence* rate among the *exposed*, and *Iu* represents the *incidence* rate among the *unexposed*

DECISION MAKING

Teenage Pregnancy and Birth Rates

• What are the pregnancy and birth rates among teenagers in your community? What percentage of infants born to teenage mothers in your community exhibit low birth weight or other neonatal problems?

• What resources exist in your community to advise or assist pregnant teens?

• Where would you look for information on teen pregnancies and births in your community?

Figure 11-5 Equations Used in Computing Vital Statistics

Rates Whose Denominators Are the Total Population

crude birth rate = $\dfrac{\text{number of live births}}{\text{total mid-year population}}$ × 1,000

crude death rate = $\dfrac{\text{number of deaths during the year}}{\text{total mid-year population}}$ × 1,000

age-specific death rate = $\dfrac{\text{number of deaths in a given age group in a year}}{\text{average mid-year population in the age group}}$ × 1,000

cause-specific death rate = $\dfrac{\text{number of deaths due to a given cause in a year}}{\text{total mid-year population}}$ × 100,000

Rates and Ratios Whose Denominators Are Live Births

infant mortality (death) rate = $\dfrac{\text{number of infant deaths in one year (under 1 year of age)}}{\text{number of live births in the same year}}$ × 1,000

neonatal mortality (death) rate = $\dfrac{\text{number of newborn deaths (under 28 days of age)}}{\text{number of live births in the same year}}$ × 1,000

fetal death ratio = $\dfrac{\text{number of fetal deaths in one year (20+ weeks)}}{\text{number of live births in the same year}}$ × 1,000

maternal mortality rate = $\dfrac{\text{number of maternal deaths in one year (from complications)}}{\text{number of live births in the same year}}$ × 100,000

Rates Whose Denominators Are Live Births Plus Fetal Deaths

fetal death rate = $\dfrac{\text{number of fetal deaths in one year}}{\text{number of live births plus fetal deaths in one year}}$ × 1,000

perinatal mortality rate = $\dfrac{\text{number of fetal deaths (under 7 days)}}{\text{number of live births plus fetal deaths in one year}}$ × 1,000

Attributable Risk

Attributable risk provides information about the effect of the exposure or the increased risk of disease in those exposed as compared with those who are unexposed. This measure expresses the number of cases of disease attributable to the exposure of interest. It is useful as a measure of the impact of a particular exposure on public health. Attributable risk is expressed as follows:

$$AR = (Ie - Iu)$$

An allied measure is **attributable risk percentage (AR%)**, which is defined as the proportion of the disease of interest in the population being investigated that could be prevented by eliminating the exposure. This is a measure of the impact of an exposure on public health, assuming that the association is one of cause and effect.

Attributable risk percentage (also called rate difference or risk difference) is expressed by the following formula:

$$AR\% = \frac{Ie - Iu}{Ie}$$

Measures of association are calculated with the aid of a two-by-two table, also called a four-fold table or a contingency table (see Figure 11-6).

The relative risk or risk ratio is also utilized by epidemiologists to judge whether a valid observed association is likely to be causal. A relative risk value of 1.0 indicates that incidence rates of disease in exposed and nonexposed populations are the same and that, therefore, no association exists between the variable, or risk factor, being studied and the development of the disease of interest. A relative risk value greater than 1.0 indicates that a positive association does exist between the exposure to

Figure 11-6 Two-by-Two Table

	(D) Disease	(D̄) No disease	
Exposed (E)	a	b	$a + b$
Unexposed (Ē)	c	d	$c + d$

Using a two-by-two table, relative risk (risk ratio) would be calculated in the following manner:

$$RR = (Ie/Iu) = \frac{a/a+b}{c/c+d} =$$

$$Ie = \frac{\text{those exposed who develop disease}}{\text{those exposed with disease + those exposed with no disease}}$$

$$Iu = \frac{\text{those unexposed who develop disease}}{\text{those unexposed with disease + those unexposed with no disease}}$$

the risk factor being examined and the development of disease. In other words, if an individual or host is exposed to the agent or risk factor, he or she has a greater likelihood of developing the disease under study. Conversely, a relative risk value of less than 1.0 indicates that the individual with that factor is less likely to develop the disease or other event under study. Use of the two-by-two table is illustrated in Figure 11-7.

Figure 11-7 Calculating Relative Risk Using the Two-by-Two Table

Data for 37,840 live births in an urban county for one year, by birth weight

	Outcome at One Year		
	Dead	Alive	Total
≤2,500 g	530 (a)	4,340 (b)	4,870
>2,500 g	333 (c)	32,637 (d)	32,970
	863	36,977	37,840

The relative risk of mortality at one year associated with low birth weight is calculated in the following manner:

$$RR = (Ie/Iu) = \frac{a/a+b}{c/c+d} = \frac{530}{4,870} \text{ divided by } \frac{333}{32,970} = 10.78$$

Stated in words, the relative risk that babies born at 2,500 g or less had a death rate at one year of 10.78 times that of babies born over 2,500 g.

Odds Ratio

The last relative association measure to be discussed here is the exposure odds ratio, which is calculated when incidence rates are unavailable. The **odds ratio (OR)** for a population approximates the relative risk (*RR*) when the specific risk of disease for both the exposed and unexposed groups is very low. The odds ratio is expressed by the following formula:

$$OR = \frac{a/c}{b/d} = \frac{ad}{bc}$$

A two-by-two table can be used to determine this measure.

Information used to calculate the odds ratio is collected via a case-control study, discussed earlier in this chapter. Because the disease status of the two populations being investigated is already known, case-control studies can be conducted with fewer subjects than is possible in cohort studies. The case-control study is particularly useful in the development of knowledge about a particular disease and its possible causative factors and is frequently used to test hypotheses about the etiology of a disease. In the case-control study, the control group must be carefully selected and must be comparable in demographic characteristics to the case group in order for the results to be valid, that is, to have scientific merit. In other words, the control group must, as nearly as possible, mirror the case group except that they do not have the disease or event of interest. Several sources of controls are commonly utilized in the development of a case-control study. These sources include hospitals, the general (but similar) population, or special groups such as friends, relatives, or neighbors of the cases. The analysis of the case-control study involves comparing cases and controls with reference to the frequency of the exposure or characteristic that is being investigated as a possible etiologic, or causative, factor. This comparison is effected by estimating the relative risk as computed by the odds ratio. A case-control study often precedes a cohort study as an important initial attempt in identifying the risk factors for a particular disease or event. Figure 11-8 illustrates the use of a two-by-two table to calculate the odds ratio in a case-control study. Figure 11-9 summarizes the measures of association.

DECISION MAKING

Disease and Risk Factors

- What are the incidence and prevalence of breast cancer in your community?

- Is Lyme disease present in your state?

- If so, identify any risk factors associated with the presence of this tick-borne disease in your community.

Figure 11-8 Calculating Odds Ratio Using the Two-by-Two Table

Researchers reported on a case control study of the relationship between pancreatic cancer and various lifestyle habits, including coffee drinking. Of 902 cases with pancreatic cancer, 347 reported drinking one or more cups of coffee per day. Eighty-eight of the 108 controls reported drinking no coffee per day (Hennekens & Buring, 1987).

	(D) Disease	(D̄) No disease	
Risk factor: coffee drinking	347	20	$a + b$ 367
	a	b	
	c	d	
absent	555	88	$c + d$ 643
			1,010
	$a + c = 902$	$b + d = 108$	

$$OR = \frac{a/c}{b/d} = \frac{ad}{bc} = \frac{347 \times 88}{555 \times 20} = \frac{30{,}536}{11{,}100} = 2.75$$

Stated in words, people who drank one or more cups of coffee per day exhibited odds of having pancreatic cancer 2.75 greater than those of people who drank no coffee.

Figure 11-9 Measures of Association

$$\text{relative risk} = \frac{\text{incidence rate among the exposed } (Ie)}{\text{incidence rate among the unexposed } (Iu)}$$

$$\text{attributable risk} = \text{incidence rate among the exposed } (Ie) - \text{incidence rate among the unexposed } (Iu)$$

$$\text{attributable risk \%} = \frac{Ie - Iu}{Ie}$$

$$\text{odds ratio} = \frac{a/c}{b/d} = \frac{ad}{bc} \text{ (using two-by-two table)}$$

veillance information, then, is key to the public health approach to prevention of diseases and injuries.

As practitioners, educators, and health planners, community health nurses must have fundamental knowledge of and access to population-based disease and health-status surveillance data. Such data may be obtained from a variety of sources such as government agencies or may be directly collected by the community health nurse who conducted, for example, a neighborhood needs assessment. State and local public health jurisdictions collect and analyze the immunization rates of school-aged children in most communities. Audits of immunization records may reveal demographic features of the children. This information may, in turn, lead to the identification of barriers to vaccination or of poor access to health care.

Computerized health information systems and registries facilitate the use of medical information in a timely manner. Governmental agencies also publish data on the Internet. Common sources of routinely collected data in the United States include the following:

Centers for Disease Control and Prevention (CDC)

National Center for Health Statistics (NCHS)

Health Care Financing Administration (HCFA)

Bureau of the Census

Agency for Health Care Planning and Research (AHCPR)

National Institutes of Health (NIH)

USING THE EPIDEMIOLOGIC APPROACH IN COMMUNITY HEALTH NURSING

Disease and Health Status Surveillance

Epidemiologic measurement and analysis allow community health nursing researchers to measure health status and disease occurrence in populations. Health-status indicators are used to provide a snapshot of the major diseases, disabilities, and injuries in a community for use in establishing health priorities and plans and evaluating programs. **Surveillance** of disease occurrence yields epidemiologic intelligence data by providing a systematic count of disease frequency. These data, in turn, can be used to estimate the magnitude of health problems in the community, detect epidemics, understand the natural history of a disease, or detect potential emerging infectious disease threats (Teutsch & Churchill, 1994). Timely sur-

The Search for Etiology

The community health nurse is an instrumental link in the search for and detection of potential health problems or hazards in a health district. Using the epidemiologic approach, the community health nurse can identify connections between community demographics or environmental characteristics and disease occurrence. In a given health district, for example, children with elevated serum lead levels may be treated and returned to the same lead-contaminated environment unless the community health nurse determines the source of exposure. The community

Perspectives...

Insights of a Community Health Nursing Professor

Epidemiology is a public health science essential to nursing practice. With the increased emphasis on population-focused practice in nursing, a knowledge of the science of epidemiology is critical. The study of the distribution of diseases, accidents, and other health-related conditions and of the factors or determinants of health-related problems is central to community health nursing in particular.

As one of the coordinators of a 1998 regional community health nursing conference which focused on building health caring communities, I had the opportunity to participate in the selection of conference speakers. One of the public health nursing directors in Northern California was a speaker at the conference and was recognized for her leadership. She clearly demonstrated the application of epidemiology in the practice setting and discussed its importance for the future.

The director described the role of public health nurses in her county specific to identifying high risk population groups with designated public health problems. Those groups with a higher inci-

dence and prevalence of selected health-related problems were targeted for public health nursing interventions, with a focus on health promotion and prevention efforts. The public health nurses worked to develop community coalitions comprised of various community representatives to further examine the nature of the health problems, propose interventions, and work to reduce the incidence and prevalence of them. The coalition partnership model was an effective approach in community building efforts.

Building healthy communities requires knowledge of epidemiological methods in order to understand those population groups that require targeted attention and intervention. As community health nurses, we can play a vital role in coalition building in order to enhance community health and reduce the incidence and prevalence of health-related problems. Working together with other health professionals and community members to build healthier communities is central to community health nursing practice.

—*Sue A. Thomas, RN, EdD*

health nurse would use the epidemiologic approach and knowledge of abatement resources in order to eradicate the lead source.

Health Planning and Program Evaluation—PRECEDE–PROCEED Model

Community health nurses are frequently involved in planning and implementing new health programs or are asked to identify the health needs of their communities. For example, legislation may mandate that local services be implemented for an identified vulnerable population such as pregnant teens or homeless youth. Changes in national immigration policy may result in an influx of refugees requiring specialized health screening. The PRECEDE–PROCEED model uses deductive reasoning in applying an epidemiologic approach to community health planning. Developed by Green and Kreuter (1991), the **PRECEDE–**

PROCEED model is a health-promotion planning framework consisting of two components: a diagnostic component called PRECEDE and a developmental component called PROCEED. PRECEDE was conceptualized by the authors as an acronym for *p*redisposing, *r*einforcing, and *e*nabling *c*onstructs in *e*ducational *d*iagnosis and *e*valuation. PROCEED is an acronym for *p*olicy, *r*egulatory, and *o*rganizational *c*onstructs in *e*ducational and *e*nvironmental *d*evelopment. The model can be used at the primary (hygiene- and health-enhancement), secondary (early-detection), or tertiary (therapeutic) stage of prevention or treatment and may be viewed as an intervention whose purpose is to "short-circuit illness or enhance quality of life through change or development of health-related behavior and conditions of living" (Green & Kreuter, 1991, p. 22). Green and Kreuter believe that the PRECEDE framework takes into account the multiple factors that shape health status, thereby assisting the user in developing a subset of those factors as targets for intervention and in generating objectives and evaluation criteria.

PRECEDE–PROCEED includes a series of phases in the planning, implementation, and evaluation process. Six phases of the model are considered basic; phases seven, eight, and nine are seen as extensions, depending on the evaluation needs of the health planners. The phases defined by Green and Kreuter (1991) are presented in an abridged format here. The following scenario provides examples of how PRECEDE–PROCEED may be used.

The number of pregnancies among noncaucasian adolescents is of concern in a particular community. Community health nurses at a teen clinic have been directed to create and implement a program to decrease pregnancies among the target population (noncaucasian teens).

Phase 1. Assessment of needs or problems of the target population. The population concerned should be involved in the process.

A questionnaire is prepared to ask young women about their level of sexual activity, use of contraceptives, use of condoms as protection against sexually transmitted diseases (STDs), presence of

support systems, educational and life goals, feelings about themselves (self-esteem), and other pertinent issues. Other medical or psychosocial staff are asked for their assessment of problems pertaining to their clients.

Phase 2. Identification of the specific health goals or problems that may contribute to the needs or problems identified in Phase 1. Health problems are ranked, and the problem most deserving of scarce resources is targeted.

Among the problems identified in Phase 1, those identified most often were low self-esteem, inconsistent contraceptive use, and sexual partners who disliked using protection. These and other identified needs or problems are ranked and resources are allotted to those problems that can be addressed in the clinic setting.

Phase 3. Identification of specific health-related behavioral and environmental factors (risk factors) that are linked to the targeted problem.

Identified behavioral risk factors are inconsistent contraception use on the part of the young women

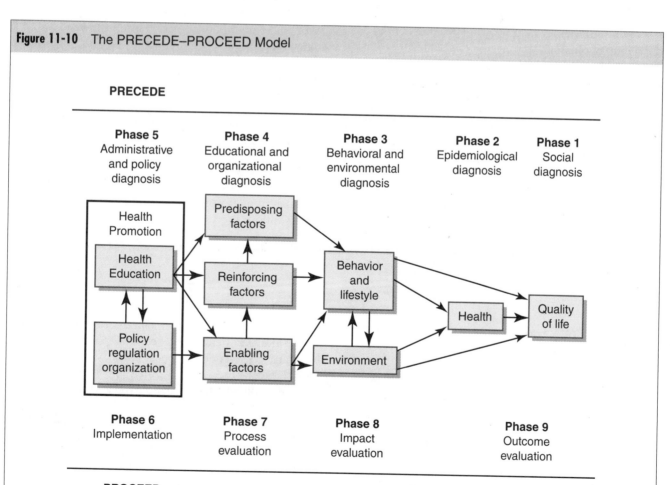

Figure 11-10 The PRECEDE–PROCEED Model

From Health Promotion Planning: An Educational and Environmental Approach *by L. Green and M. Kreuter, 1991, Mountain View, CA: Mayfield Publishing Company. Reprinted by permission of the publisher. Copyright 1991 by Mayfield Publishing Company.*

COMMUNITY NURSING VIEW

One day during the winter of 1981, seven Laotion refugees, who recently came to the United States, ate mushrooms from the same batch, picked at a local park that same day. The next day six of the seven were admitted to a small community hospital with symptoms of nausea, vomiting, diarrhea, dehydration, and elevated liver enzyme tests. Although the onset time of the symptoms varied within the group, most experienced gastrointestinal distress within eight hours. Three of the seven individuals were monitored for liver, kidney, and circulatory complications for 24 hours in the intensive care unit. All seven individuals were discharged without complications within seven days.

Samplings of the remaining mushrooms collected by the hospitalized group were sent to a local university for identification. These mushrooms were identified as belonging to a poisonous genus, *Amanita*.

With help from a Laotian-speaking community outreach worker, the community health nurse interviewed several members of the group. These individuals stated that foraging of wild mushrooms was customary in their homeland and that they therefore continued to forage mushrooms following their arrival in the United States. They further reported that in Laos, a simple boiling method was used to determine whether mushrooms were poisonous or harmless. In Laos, when poisonous mushrooms are boiled with rice, they turn the rice red. Because the locally

gathered batch did not turn the rice red, the mushrooms were ingested. The community health nurse determined that several steps needed to be taken to prevent further poisoning from wild mushrooms. The nurse knew that foraging wild mushrooms was not unique to Laotians or Southeast Asian groups.

Nursing Considerations

ASSESSMENT
• What data including cultural factors would the nurse need to collect to assess the problem of mushroom poisoning?

DIAGNOSIS
• What diagnosis might be made given the data included in the case scenario?

OUTCOME IDENTIFICATION
• What outcomes might be formulated specific to a community approach to mushroom poisoning?

PLANNING/INTERVENTIONS
• What community notification and educational strategy might the nurse develop and implement to deal with the problem of mushroom poisoning?

EVALUATION
• How would the community health nurse evaluate the effectiveness of the community intervention?

---

and dislike of condoms by their partners. Environmental factors include lack of familial support for educational goals and the acceptance of sexual activity and child bearing as a norm by the peer group.

Phase 4. Classification of factors that have direct impact on the target behavior and environment into one of three categories: predisposing factors (knowledge, attitudes, beliefs, values, and perceptions that facilitate or hinder motivation for change), enabling factors (skills, resources, or barriers that help or hinder desired behavioral or environmental changes), and reinforcing factors (rewards and feedback received by the learner following adoption of the behavior).

Predisposing factors may include knowledge about reproductive health and contraception, attitudes toward contraception versus child bearing on the part of both the young women and their partners, and the value system of the peer group, among others. Identified enabling factors might be barriers to contraception, as outlined for predisposing factors. Identified positive enabling factors might include a program designed to assist in behavior change, specifically, a counselor-facilitated young women's support group where contraceptive issues are discussed, the positive aspects of postponing child bearing are set forth, and self-esteem issues are addressed. Reinforcing factors might be the support for contraception use among the young women in the group, increase in self-esteem fostered by the support group, and the achievement of educational goals such as high-school graduation.

Phase 5. Assessment of organizational and administrative capabilities and resources for the development and implementation of a program.

The clinic determines which personnel are available to create and administer the questionnaire, tabulate and analyze completed questionnaires, facilitate the support group, provide contraceptive and STD education, provide educational and self-esteem counseling, and evaluate the program's achievements.

Phase 6. Implementation of the program.

The program is implemented.

Phase 7. Evaluation of the process, which includes examining the program implemented by determining whether the program has met the requirements outlined in each of the previous steps.

An evaluation is performed to determine whether the program met the requirements outlined in the previous steps. Were questionnaires, support groups, and one-on-one interventions or other program components well designed to elicit the information needed and to provide the support needed for goal attainment?

Phase 8. Impact evaluation. Examined are the goals of the implemented program and whether the actions implemented affected the problem being addressed by the model.

An evaluation is performed to determine whether the support group, contraceptive education, and educational and self-esteem counseling components of the program improved low self-esteem, changed contraceptive behavior, increased the frequency of young women remaining in school, or improved other aspects of the clients' lives.

Phase 9. Outcome evaluation. The results of the implemented program are examined to determine whether the program accomplished the goals for which it was designed.

An evaluation is performed to determine whether the program accomplished its goal of decreasing pregnancies among noncaucasian adolescents utilizing this clinic.

The uniqueness of the PRECEDE–PROCEED framework allows the community health nurse to determine population needs prior to a program's implementation. Because evaluation methods are established in the planning phase, the achievement of program objectives can be measured throughout the program's phases. The model also was specifically developed with the community rather than the individual in mind, making it particularly useful to community health nurses. See Figure 11-10 for an illustration of the PRECEDE–PROCEED Model.

Key Concepts

- Epidemiology is an applied, population-based science embracing the related community health sciences of ecology and demography and focusing on the distribution and determinants of diseases or conditions.

- A basic understanding of the epidemiologic approach provides the community health nurse with necessary language and methodology to understand, describe, and analyze health problems of communities.

- Epidemiology methods are used to investigate the natural history of a disease, to search for disease causes (etiology) or risk factors, to conduct disease surveillance, and to test new treatments.

- Concepts basic to the epidemiologic approach are that health problems in a population do not occur randomly; that causes are interactions between agent, host, and the surrounding environment; and that the natural history of a health condition provides fundamental information on how to intervene or prevent that condition from occurring.

- Observational or nonexperimental epidemiologic study designs are used when little is known about a disease, when a disease occurrence is rare, and to make associations or comparisons between those with and those without a disease. Intervention studies or experimental methods are used to compare therapeutic or preventive treatments.

- Epidemiologic measurements typically encountered by the community health nurse are measures of disease frequency expressed as rates and measures of association (ratios and percentages).

- The epidemiologic approach is particularly useful to the community health nurse because the focus is population-based and the approach provides tools to collect, describe, analyze, and evaluate information about a community.

Assessing the Community

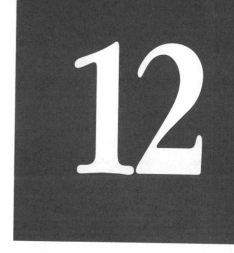

Andrea Wass, RN, BA, MHlth Sc, DRM, MRCNA

12

KEY TERMS

community
community assessment
community capacity
community competence
community of interest
community participation
comparative need
expressed need
felt need
normative need
population
project team
steering committee
windshield survey

A healthy city is one that is continually creating and improving those physical and social environments—expanding those community resources which enable people to mutually support each other in performing all the functions of life and in developing to their maximum potential.

—*Hancock & Duhl, 1985, p. 29*

COMPETENCIES

Upon completion of this chapter, the reader should be able to:

- Describe the various ways that communities are defined.
- Discuss the influence of values on need and explain the various types of need.
- Describe in detail the participation of community members in community assessment.
- Outline the steps in conducting a community assessment.
- Discuss the sources of information about communities.
- Explain the various tools used in community assessment.
- Discuss ways to determine appropriate responses to an identified need.
- Outline the process of setting priorities for action.

In Chapter 1, a number of definitions of community health nursing and the scope of community health nursing practice were presented. A common theme, however, pervaded all these definitions: The focus of community health nursing is the promotion and maintenance of health of whole populations or communities. This responsibility is ongoing, underpinning the daily practice of community health nurses. If they are to effectively promote the health of the communities they serve, community health nurses must have the knowledge and skills to effectively assess community needs and resources. This chapter explores some key issues in community assessment, including the importance of community participation in community assessment, the stages of the community assessment process, and a number of tools and methods useful in the collection of information required for community assessment.

A POPULATION OR COMMUNITY FOCUS

Since the development of Health for All by the Year 2000, countries around the world have been attempting to implement the principles outlined in the Alma-Ata Declaration (World Health Organization [WHO], 1978) and the Ottawa Charter for Health Promotion (WHO, 1986). National policies have been established to implement Health for All in many countries, and international and national health professional associations have committed themselves to the principles of social justice, equity, and community participation.

Through the International Congress of Nurses and various national nursing and public health associations, community health nurses have made a formal commitment to improve the health of the world population. This commitment, like the declarations from which it arose, is based on the recognition that health is determined largely by the social, economic, and political environments in which people live and that effective solutions to health problems must therefore address social, economic, and political issues.

Community assessment is an extremely important component of community health nursing practice. Without adequate assessment, nurses may identify a problem and a corresponding solution before having explored the situation in sufficient depth to fully understand it (Rorden & McLennan, 1992). Comprehensive community assessment not only identifies problems but also addresses the nature of those health problems. Because of the primary role that health assessment plays in promoting the health of communities, community assessment has been identified as one of the three core functions of public health (Institute of Medicine, 1988).

Community assessment is not achieved simply by assessing the health of individuals within a community. Community health nurses must also assess the health of the community itself; identify the characteristics, resources, and needs of the community; and work with community members on those issues that arise, addressing not only individual behavior but also applicable environmental variables. Working to change individual behavior when the environment in which those individuals live has a greater bearing on health results in "blaming the victim" (Ryan, 1976).

Focusing on the community as a whole requires a population focus and the recognition of the community as client (Anderson & McFarlane, 1988; Kuehnert 1995). In order to understand the full implications of such an approach, we must first consider the meaning of the terms *community* and *healthy community* and how need is conceptualized.

DEFINING THE COMMUNITY

The term **community** has been used in a myriad of ways, ranging from the very specific to the quite broad and general. In 1955, Hillery identified 94 different definitions of the term (Rissel, 1996); many more have been developed since. Some authors suggest that the result has been a confusing array of definitions (Rorden & McLennan, 1992). Given its central place in the discussion and analysis of communal life, however, *community* as a term cannot be avoided. An examination of the term and of the common dimensions among its various definitions constitutes an important preface to a discussion of community assessment.

Many of the broader definitions of the term refer to *community* as simply a large group of people or "community as population" (Hawe, 1994, p. 200). **Population** has in turn been defined as "an aggregate of individuals with similar or the same characteristics" (Wadsworth, 1988). According to these definitions, then, communities are little more than large numbers of individuals.

Such definitions have some similarities to geographic definitions of community, wherein communities are seen as groups of people living in particular places, with locality central to their definition as communities. Definitions of community as populations and geographic areas are those that have generally been used by health planners in their assessment and planning work (Rissel, 1996).

The Health for All by the Year 2000 movement strengthened the commitment on the part of community health nurses and other health professionals to communities, requiring a more dynamic definition of community. One definition that has emerged in response to this movement is "a 'living' organism with interactive linkages among families, friends, organizations, and neighborhoods" has evolved among some health professionals (Eng, Salmon, & Mullan, 1992, p. 1).

Sociologists have long seen community as more than a large collection of individuals. Dynamic definitions of communities emphasize that communities are social systems bound together by either shared values or shared interests (Hawe, 1994). Wadsworth's (1988) definition of a community as an interacting group of people with shared needs and interests captures this idea. In such definitions, participation in the life of the community and identification as a member of the community are important and result in a sense of belonging. This sense of belonging is important in fostering a sense of connectedness in the community (Daly & Cobb, 1989).

Definitions of community are further complicated by the value-laden nature of the term itself. For example, the notion of *community* has been romanticized (Labonte, 1989), with communities often being conceived as close-knit groups of people among whom little, if any, conflict or harm occurs. The reality is that communities may be divided by opposing values and may reflect racism, sexism, ageism, homophobia, or some other catalyst of divisiveness among community members (Minkler, 1994). Similarly, community members may share an interest in a particular issue but may at the same time hold divergent beliefs and values regarding other aspects of their common life. That is, elements of consensus and conflict may exist side by side.

Bryson and Mowbray, in a now classic Australian article (1981), suggest that, because of the positive light that it seems to imbue, the term *community* has also become a "spray-on solution" to difficult issues. Community programs may be seen in a positive light simply because they are described as such, although the reality may be quite different. For example, much deinstitutionalization of people with serious mental illness has occurred under the guise of community programming but without the necessary resource support to be effective (Bryson & Mowbray, 1981). Similarly, although "community care" may sound like an inherently good thing, it may in reality mean care provided by unrecognized and unpaid caregivers, usually women who provide the care sometimes at the expense of their own health.

Because community health nurses typically work in particular geographic areas, it is reasonable to expect that the majority of communities or populations with whom community health nurses work will be geographically based. Community health nurses may also work with communities having shared interests and a common sense of belonging as well as with **communities of interest**, groups of people who share beliefs, values, or interests in a particular issue (Clark, 1973) but whose membership may or may not be restricted to the particular geographic area.

Because communities are not homogeneous but, experience varying degrees of consensus and conflict, community health nurses may also find themselves working with a number of communities of interest having dissimilar—or even conflicting—needs. For example, one group of people may be working to preserve parkland within a community, while another group may be urging the development of this land for public housing for low-income earners. Community health nurses may also find themselves working with a community whose values are in opposition to those of community health nursing, for example, a group creating racial disharmony. Minkler (1994) warns us that

> while we do need to work closely with communities, to respect their capacities and rights to self-determination, we must at the same time strive to live up to our own ethical standards and those of our profession in not letting blind faith in the community prevent us from seeing and acting on the paramount need for social justice (p. 529).

Similarly, community health nurses may find themselves working with populations or groups who may or may not recognize a sense of common purpose or belonging. For example, a number of elderly people may be living alone and experiencing social isolation within a particular community. These people may seem to the community health nurse to be a community of interest, but they may have no awareness of their shared experiences or needs. Just as the complexity in defining community is reflected in community health nursing practice, so is it reflected in the community assessment process.

DEFINING HEALTHY COMMUNITY

The goal of community health nursing practice—and, hence, the ultimate goal of community assessment—is to promote community health. This raises the questions, "What is a healthy community?" and "How will we know when we've attained one?"

Unfortunately, most definitions of health focus solely on individuals, a legacy of the power of the medical model. Given what is known about the influence of the

> ## ⚬ REFLECTIVE THINKING ⚬
>
> ### *Communities and Communities of Interest*
>
> Consider an area where you plan to conduct a community assessment.
>
> • To what communities and communities of interest do members of this area belong?
>
> • Can you identify areas of conflict between any of the communities and communities of interest that you have identified?
>
> • Consider what steps you could take to deal with conflict between competing communities of interest.
>
> • What values would guide your decisions?

social, economic, and political environments on individual health, being able to define a healthy community may be an important first step in making a significant difference in the population's health.

The World Health Organization's (WHO) definition of health as a positive concept, rather than as the absence of disease, is a useful point from which to begin consideration of a healthy community. Although the WHO was referring to the health of individuals in its definition, the point that health is much more than the absence of disease is equally relevant to communities. Unfortunately, current population health indices—mortality and morbidity data—focus on disease. Other more positive indicators are needed in order to develop a vision of a healthy community. In response to this need, Brown (1985) has called for an "epidemiology of health". In fact, health professionals attempting to examine healthy community indicators as part of recent WHO Healthy City projects have lamented the lack of positive health concepts at the community level (Hayes & Willms, 1990).

One approach to developing a definition of community health is to consider three dimensions of community health: status, structure, and process (Goeppinger & Shuster, 1988). These three dimensions may point the way to a broad definition of a healthy community, though care must be taken to ensure that a positive concept of community health is developed.

• The status dimension of community health refers to the information available about a community from outcome measures, such as morbidity and mortality data, life expectancy, crime rates, and education levels.
• Structure refers to the composition of the community itself, in terms of the socioeconomic, age, gender, and ethnic distribution of the population, as well as the types of health and social services available in the community.
• Process refers to the manner whereby the community operates and its effectiveness in functioning as a whole to solve problems that arise.

The first two of these dimensions—status and structure—have traditionally been recognized as important.

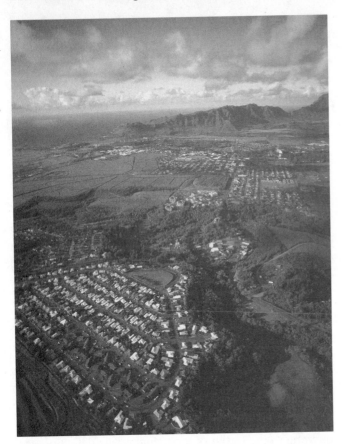

Community health nurses tend to work within geographic boundaries with either the entire community or particular communities of interest. Photo courtesy of Douglas Peebles/Corbis.

The third—process—has been largely ignored until recently, though it offers a broad scope in examining the health of a community.

Community competence and **community capacity**, two concepts that have emerged in recent years, describe the process dimension of a healthy community. These two related concepts are particularly important with regard to their focus on capability rather than deficiency. Cottrell defined a competent community as one in which members of the community:

(1) collaborate effectively in identifying the problems and needs of the community; (2) achieve a working consensus on goals and priorities; (3) agree on ways and means to implement the agreed-upon goals; and (4) collaborate effectively in the required actions (Goeppinger & Baglioni, 1985, p. 508).

Building on the notion of community competence, community capacity has been defined as the strengths, resources, and problem-solving abilities of a community (Robertson & Minkler, 1994).

Progress has been made in developing the concept of a healthy community. It is possible, however, that a concrete definition will never be found. Indeed, Hayes and Willms (1990) suggest that definitions of a healthy community may vary from one community to another and that, on the basis of its own culture and values, each community should be afforded the opportunity to establish its own vision of a healthy community.

At the same time, the health of individual communities should not be considered outside the context of the health of other communities. With major disparities between groups both within and among countries, improving the health of one community at the expense of others threatens the values of social justice and equity, which form the basis of community health nursing practice and constitute part of the definition of a healthy community.

DEFINING NEED

Determining need is primary to community assessment, however, a community assessment also includes a focus on community assets or strengths. Because the concept of need is not value free, determining need is not a simple process. Which issues are identified as needs depends very much on the perspective and values of the person or people identifying them. Rather than deny the value-laden nature of needs assessment, it is important to acknowledge and make explicit the values that should be driving the process. In community health nursing practice, these values include social justice, equity, and the importance of meaningful community participation.

Types of Need

Bradshaw (1972) is one author who recognized the value-laden nature of need assessment, and his framework for examining need takes this nature into account. Bradshaw's taxonomy of need outlines four different types of need based on whether need is identified on the basis of community-member opinion, professional opinion, or precedent. These four types of need are felt need, expressed need, normative need, and comparative need.

Felt Need

Felt need is described as that which people say they need. For example, community members may tell staff at a community health center that they need more antenatal care services within the area. Felt need is important because it reflects that which the people themselves identify as their problems. By itself, however, felt need is unlikely to be comprehensive for a number of reasons. First, people may say that they need only those things that they believe are within the realm of possibility for them; they may not be able to identify those needs of which they are unaware, or those needs that they believe will not be met. Second, people may identify only those needs that they believe the person who is conducting the needs assessment wants to hear. They may not, for example, describe anything other than medical needs to a community health nurse if they do not understand the broad population-level role of the nurse and, instead, believe that the nurse's role is primarily the provision of clinical care. Third, felt need may be easily influenced by opinion leaders and the mass media, and people may not always have opportunities for informed decision making. This can particularly be the case in health care delivery, where the medical model and the provision of acute care services dominate public debate. Fourth, as with the other types of need discussed further, it cannot be assumed that the felt need of a few community members reflects the perspective of the whole community, or even of a significant proportion of the community. Care must therefore be taken in community assessment to ascertain the views of a representative sample of the community before coming to conclusions about a community's felt need. Despite these shortcomings, however, felt need is extremely important because it is determined by community members.

Expressed Need

Expressed need is described as felt need turned into action, demonstrated by such things as the number of names on a waiting list. Although expressed need is somewhat more concrete than felt need, it remains problematic because people can sign up only for those services that already exist. Demand for a service may occur simply because the service represents the only solution currently offered for a particular problem. For example, long waiting lists to see obstetricians may not necessarily indicate a shortage of obstetricians in the area. Rather, lack of other services such as midwifery may be the problem, or community members may be highly concerned regarding the effects of environmental pollution on the developing fetus, causing many people to visit existing services for additional checkups. Thus, although these problems may manifest as long obstetric waiting lists, more obstetricians may not be the best solution. Also, people tend to sign up on more than one waiting list. For example, people waiting for a nursing home placement may sign up on the waiting list of every nursing home in the area, although they will eventually accept only one place. Thus, adding together the numbers of names on waiting lists may yield an inaccurate picture of need.

Normative Need

Normative need is need determined by experts on the basis of professional analysis. For example, dietitians may determine the recommended daily allowance of protein or fat. Although normative need is the type of need most often regarded as objective and unbiased, it is not without its problems. Professional judgment is based on values in the same way as is felt need, a fact reflected in the way that professional judgment changes over time. Changing beliefs about acceptable cholesterol levels constitute just one example (Becker, 1986). Professional judgment is also often influenced by political agendas, which

DECISION MAKING

Needs

A local community group of nonsmokers has asked that a smoking-cessation class be added to services already offered at a local clinic. They state that a neighboring community clinic offers one such class.

• Which type of need is expressed in their initial request to you?

• Given this type of need, what must you consider before making any decision regarding the request?

may make professionals more or less willing or able to publicly present their opinions.

Comparative Need

Comparative need is need determined by comparing the resources or services of one group or area with those of another similar group or area. For example, a given area may be designated as needing more public housing because it has less than do other areas of a similar size and demography. The main shortcomings of this type of need are related to the assumptions on which it is based: that similarity exists between the areas and that the response to the need in the area of comparison was the most appropriate response to the problem, neither of which may be true.

As the preceding discussion illustrates, there are strengths and weaknesses inherent in each of the types of need outlined by Bradshaw (1972): No one type presents a complete picture. When considered together, however, the various types of need provide a much more comprehensive picture than that provided by assessing need via only one method. The responsibility of community health nurses lies in critically examining the types of need present in any situation and ensuring that both professionals' and community members' perspectives are included in the process of identifying need.

REFLECTIVE THINKING

What Type of Need?

• Identify an issue that has been described as a need in your local area.

• Which types of need are present: felt need, expressed need, normative need, and/or comparative need?

COMMUNITY PARTICIPATION IN COMMUNITY ASSESSMENT

The WHO, through its Health for All by the Year 2000 program, has identified the importance of active **community participation** at all stages in the assessment, planning, delivery, and evaluation of health services. This sentiment has been echoed at the national level by the American Public Health Association (1991). Attainment of effective community participation is by no means a simple process, however. As is the case with the concept of community, *community participation* must be defined and those kinds of participation likely to be meaningful and effective identified.

Arnstein (1971) characterizes the romantic manner in which participation is often regarded, pointing out that "the idea of citizen participation is a little like eating spinach: no one is against it in principle because it is good for you" (p. 71). Health professionals, including nurses, have been accused of often allowing only limited, passive participation, for example, by implementing plans already developed by professionals (Goeppinger & Shuster, 1988; Chalmers & Kristajanson, 1989). Effective participation must be active and meaningful to participants if it is to achieve its goals of empowerment and self-reliance. The community health nurse must critically review participation processes to ensure that they facilitate meaningful participation of community members in the community assessment process, as opposed to merely co-opting community members to the ideas of professionals.

In her now classic work, Arnstein (1971) describes eight rungs on a ladder of citizen participation (see Figure 12-1). These rungs of participation range from manipulation and therapy (which is described as nonparticipation), through informing, consultation, and placation (which is identified as degrees of tokenism), to partnership, delegated power, and citizen control (which is identified as degrees of citizen power). Arnstein argues that true participation occurs only when the relationship between health professionals and citizens is one of either partnership, delegated power, or citizen control. Arnstein's critical evaluation of participation provides a useful framework for reviewing and planning participation processes.

If they are to take seriously the commitment to community participation established as part of Health for All by the Year 2000, community health nurses must ensure that community members have opportunities to effectively participate in the decision-making processes associated with the assessment, planning, implementation, and evaluation of health programs. Merely consulting with community members about their opinions is not sufficient. Effective participation requires a true partnership between community health nurses and community members (Wass, 1995; Courtney, Ballard, Fauer, Gariota, & Holland, 1996). The community health nurse plays an important role in supporting and empowering community members, in identifying their problems and needs, setting

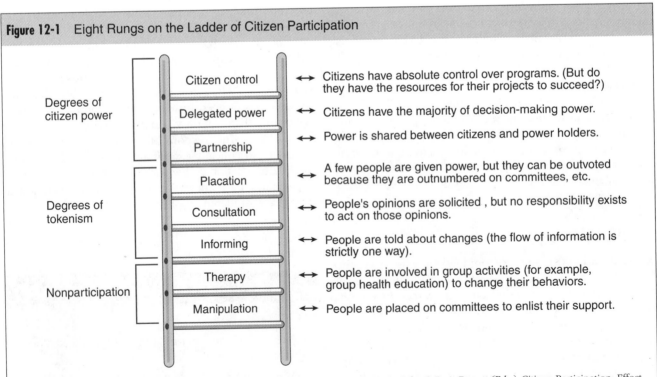

Figure 12-1   Eight Rungs on the Ladder of Citizen Participation

Degrees of citizen power
- Citizen control ↔ Citizens have absolute control over programs. (But do they have the resources for their projects to succeed?)
- Delegated power ↔ Citizens have the majority of decision-making power.
- Partnership ↔ Power is shared between citizens and power holders.

Degrees of tokenism
- Placation ↔ A few people are given power, but they can be outvoted because they are outnumbered on committees, etc.
- Consultation ↔ People's opinions are solicited , but no responsibility exists to act on those opinions.
- Informing ↔ People are told about changes (the flow of information is strictly one way).

Nonparticipation
- Therapy ↔ People are involved in group activities (for example, group health education) to change their behaviors.
- Manipulation ↔ People are placed on committees to enlist their support.

From Eight Rungs on the Ladder of Citizen Participation by S. Arnstein, 1971. In E. S. Cahn & B. A. Passett (Eds.), Citizen Participation: Effecting Community Change (p. 70). New York: Praeger Publishers. Copyright 1971 Praeger Publishers. From Promoting Health: The Primary Care Approach by A. Wass, 1994, Sydney, Australia: Harcourt Brace and Company. Used with permission.

their priorities for action, and in proposing solutions that require community members to assume active leadership roles (Courtney et al., 1996).

Developing such a partnership with community members requires recognizing the particular expertise that community members have with regard to their lives and experiences. This expertise is complementary to that of community health nurses and other health professionals; such combined expertise is much broader than that of health professionals who attempt to solve health problems alone. Recognition is, in fact, growing regarding the importance of participatory research and of health professionals and community members working alongside each other on issues of mutual concern (Kelly, 1988; Oakley, 1989; Matrice & Brown 1990; McTaggart, 1991; Flynn, Ray, & Rider, 1994; Rains & Ray, 1995).

Community members also may gain from being involved in the decision-making process, and the skills they develop may have a positive influence on community and individual well-being long after a particular community assessment has been completed. That is, via their active involvement, community members may further develop skills in such areas as communication, working in groups, negotiation, dealing with the mass media, organization, and submission writing (Wass, 1994), thereby increasing their sense of self-reliance and efficacy. Community participation in community assessment may in and of itself, then, add to the resources and competence of the community (Eng et al., 1992), increasing community capacity (Kang, 1995) and, therefore, the community's ability to respond to future issues that may arise. There is also growing evidence that the resulting empowerment may itself have direct positive effects on health (Wallerstein, 1992).

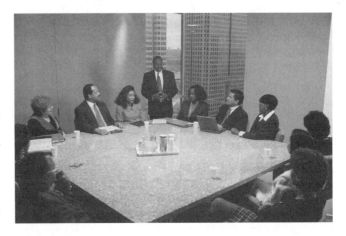

Effective participation requires a true partnership between health care professionals and community members. *Photo courtesy of PhotoDisc.*

APPROACHES TO COMMUNITY ASSESSMENT AND PROGRAM DEVELOPMENT

As mentioned in the previous section, building relationships within the community is a critical part of the community assessment process. The consensus process encourages the involvement of community leaders in developing goals, outcome and process objectives, and plans to meet the objectives. A number of models have been developed and effectively used to develop an effective partnership with community members and to facilitate community participation. These models include the Assessment Protocol for Excellence in Public Health, the Planned Approach to Community Health, and Healthy Cities (Katz & Kreuter, 1997).

The Assessment Protocol for Excellence in Public Health (APEX/PH) was developed in the United States and designed to facilitate the process of improving public health. The APEX/PH model provides a process for local health departments to assess their capacity to build stronger partnerships with their communities, involve community representatives in identifying their health problems and priorities, and develop a community plan for improving the ability of the health department to meet community health needs identified in the assessment process.

The Planned Approach to Community Health (PATCH) was developed by the Centers for Disease Control and Prevention (CDC) in the United States as a means to plan, deliver, and assess the progress of community-based health-promotion programs. The PATCH program is basically a system—a working partnership among the CDC, state health agencies, and the community. There are five general phases in the process (Kreuter, 1984): (1) mobilizing the community by establishing a core of representatives at the local level, (2) collecting and organizing data reflecting local community opinion and health-related

---

◎ REFLECTIVE THINKING ◎

Arnstein's Ladder of Citizen Participation

Consider some times when you were asked to participate in decision making.

• Where on Arnstein's ladder of citizen participation would you place your opportunities to participate?

• Did your participation take the form of effective participation, tokenism, or nonparticipation?

Now consider opportunities for community participation in the practice of health professionals with which you are familiar.

• Where on Arnstein's ladder of citizen participation would you place these activities?

• How would you, as a community health nurse, respond to these situations to increase the effective participation of community members?

variables, (3) choosing health priorities, (4) designing interventions, and (5) evaluating results.

The Healthy Cities model, a demonstration project developed initially in the European office of the WHO, is a model that emerged from the Alma-Ata Declaration and the Health for All strategy. Two key principles of the Health for All by the Year 2000 initiative—multisectoral collaboration and public participation—constitute a central focus of the Healthy Cities model. Although originating in Europe, the Healthy Cities model has been applied in cities and communities throughout the world.

As discussed in Chapters 1 and 30, the Healthy Cities model focuses on the need to reorient medical services and health care systems toward primary health care. The model emphasizes the importance of public involvement in the creation of partnerships between the public, private, and voluntary sectors. The concept of health promotion is central to this model.

THE COMMUNITY ASSESSMENT PROCESS

Having examined some of the main concepts relevant to community assessment, we can now review the community assessment process itself. A number of terms are used to describe this process, including community assessment, community profiling, and community analysis. These terms may also be defined in varying ways. This chapter uses the term **community assessment,** defined as the process of critically examining the characteristics, resources, assets, and needs of a community, in collaboration with that community, in order to develop strategies to improve the health and quality of life of the community (Hawtin, Hughes, & Percy-Smith, 1994).

Community assessment is not an end in itself, but the beginning of a process that addresses the community's needs and makes a difference in people's health (Rorden & McLennan, 1992). Unfortunately, community assessments are often conducted at the expense of other parts of the process.

Community assessments are more likely to be useful when they are conducted for positive reasons, such as to:

- Review existing practices in order to bring about refinement and change
- Provide information for policy formulation, funding allocation, and planning of new initiatives
- Prevent costly mistakes resulting in inappropriate or underutilized programs and services
- Challenge accepted beliefs and practices
- Encourage lateral thinking and provide people with an opportunity to challenge long-accepted ideas with new information (Baum, 1992)

It is important that all participants in the community assessment have a common understanding of its purposes. Otherwise, people may be inadvertently working toward different—or even conflicting—goals, which could significantly hinder the project (Southern Community Health Research Unit [SCHRU], 1991).

Identification of Available Resources

Early in the process, it is necessary to ascertain the time and money available to conduct the community assessment. In this way, the size of the project can be made to correspond to the available resources. The skills and time required of the team involved in the assessment must also be established. Proper review of resources will also help ensure that adequate resources are allocated to address the issues identified in the community assessment. There is little point in expending resources to complete a community assessment if there are neither sufficient resources nor commitment to respond to the needs that arise (Rissel, 1991).

If other community agencies are interested in the community assessment, they may be willing to contribute some resources to the project, particularly if their needs are also addressed. This could constitute a very efficient use of both agency and community resources.

Establishment of Project Team and Steering Committee

Having established why and with what resources the assessment is being conducted, it is then important to establish the project team and steering committee. Community assessments are rarely completed by a single person; rather, they are best conducted by a group of people with complementary skills.

The **project team** is the group of people who will conduct the community assessment. The team must include a number of people with varying expertise, such that, together, the team has a broad range of skills. It may be made up of outside experts employed specifically for the assessment or employees of local agencies allocated to the project.

The **steering committee** is a group of people from outside the project team who oversee the project, providing outside advice and ensuring that the project achieves its goals. The steering committee typically comprises members of three groups: community health professionals from the area in question, representatives from other organizations that are able to respond to the findings of the community assessment, and representative community members (SCHRU, 1991).

The steering committee is a valuable source of expertise, direction, and support for those conducting the community assessment. This committee also ensures a link between community and project team (necessary if the assessment is to include a community perspective) and plays an important role in formulating recommendations for action on the basis of the community assessment. The steering committee should be of manageable size to facilitate problem solving and decision making; between six and twelve people is usually considered workable (SCHRU, 1991).

The steering committee takes on particular importance when the project team is composed of people who are outsiders. If an outside body is commissioned to perform as the project team on a community assessment, the lack of insider knowledge on the part of team members may cause them to miss or misinterpret important information about the community's history or values. They will also be unaware of any contentious issues about which community members are not speaking. Having community insiders on the steering committee helps compensate for such difficulties (see Figure 12-2).

Development of Research Plan and Time Frame

Developing a plan for the entire community assessment process at the beginning will enable the team to keep more or less on schedule. Changing circumstances may, however, require some flexibility in the plan. Outlining a

clear time frame at this point will also ensure that all members of the project team and steering committee are aware of the time commitment expected of them (SCHRU, 1991).

Collection and Analysis of Information Already Available

Regardless of the number of potential new resources available for the assessment, it is advisable not to reinvent the wheel. Nor can one ignore that which has already been learned about the particular issues being addressed. It is thus wise to collect information that is already available. A literature review to identify ways whereby similar issues have been dealt with elsewhere is invaluable. It is also important to identify the information about the area that is available from secondary sources, information previously collected by local, state, and federal governmental bodies. Such information may take the form of epidemiologic and demographic data about the area, policy documents developed at the national or state level, and the like. These are discussed in more detail later.

Any community assessments previously conducted in the area should also be examined. Some such assessments may have examined one particular group of the community rather than the community as a whole. Analysis of the information obtained from the various sources will help the team identify the need for further information.

Completion of Community Research

Having developed an overview of the characteristics of the community and having examined any previously col-

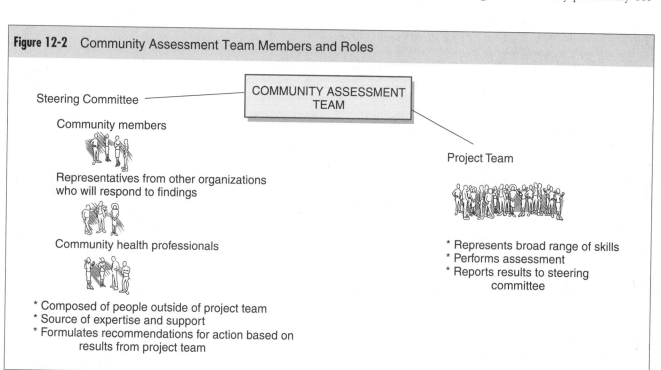

Figure 12-2   Community Assessment Team Members and Roles

Steering Committee — COMMUNITY ASSESSMENT TEAM

Community members

Representatives from other organizations who will respond to findings

Community health professionals

* Composed of people outside of project team
* Source of expertise and support
* Formulates recommendations for action based on results from project team

Project Team

* Represents broad range of skills
* Performs assessment
* Reports results to steering committee

lected information about the community's needs, to plan ways to collect additional data that are needed. Such data are likely to include needs identified by local community members and other health and social welfare personnel, as well as information related to community history and values. Techniques such as surveys, interviews, and group discussions are particularly useful in data collection. The various methods are discussed in further detail later in this chapter.

Analysis of Results

Once the data collection process is complete, analysis of the results is the next step. This is a crucial stage of the process and includes analysis of both community resources and needs. In needs analysis, it is important to express the need as a problem, rather than a potential solution to the problem. For example, it might be said that there is a need for more dentists in a community. This, however, describes a solution to the problem rather than the problem itself. The problem may be better described as long waiting lists to see dentists. More dentists in the community might then be identified as one of a number of potential solutions to the problem. Making explicit this difference between problems (needs) and solutions may alert the project team and steering committee to a number of possible causes and solutions to each need identified. During the analysis of results, it is important to be mindful of the original purpose of the assessment and to link the analysis back to that purpose.

Another important aspect of the analysis process is to look beyond the immediate issue identified to any underlying problems. Time should be spent critically analyzing any underlying causes of each problem. Analyzing the data in this way increases the likelihood of identifying, and, later, addressing the root causes of issues affecting the health of the community. It may also facilitate the identification of a common basis for a number of seemingly unrelated issues and, thus, a comprehensive response. For example, in exploring the issues facing the Fitzroy Community Health Centre in Melbourne, Australia, staff identified poverty as the underlying cause of a number of these issues (McBride, 1988). Having done so, they were then in a position to identify strategies to address this problem directly, rather than by continuing to react separately to multiple results of poverty.

Reporting Back to the Community

Reporting the findings of the community assessment to members of the community is a vital part of the community assessment process. Community members "own" the information collected in a needs survey as much as do the team members involved in collecting it. Effort should thus be made to ensure that the information collected is returned to the community (SCHRU, 1991).

Reporting back to the community is much more than a formality; doing so provides an opportunity for verification of the findings and identification of any potential problem areas prior to final publication (Barton, Smith, Brown, & Supples, 1993). For these reasons, it is recommended that a penultimate draft be presented to the community for response, rather than simply presenting the final report as a *fait accompli* (Russell, Gregory, Wotton, Mordoch, & Counts, 1996). Any important omissions or areas of contention can then be identified and acted on.

Results can be presented in both verbal and written forms. A combination of approaches is most likely to ensure effective dissemination of the results. Reports must be written clearly to ensure accessibility to a wide range of community members. Some examples of ways to report the findings of the assessment to the community are as follows:

- A brief, widely distributed, user-friendly report
- Public meetings
- Press releases
- Displays in well-frequented areas such as shopping centers
- Presentations to local government and community groups

In addition to fulfilling the moral obligations of the project team, reporting back to the community enables other agencies to act on needs identified and allows community members to lobby for further action if the issues identified so warrant. Conclusions and recommendations from the community assessment direct both the community and health agencies toward appropriate action (SCHRU, 1991).

Setting Priorities for Action

Once the needs assessment is complete and the issues requiring attention are identified, identification of priorities for action is the next important step. This is a point at which the differing values of steering committee members may become apparent, and the perspectives of community members on the steering committee become particularly important (Kang, 1995).

Ruffing-Rahal (1987) identifies consistent contrasts between priorities identified by community members and those identified by health professionals. The danger lies in deciding whose priorities take precedence. Labonte (1994) highlights a PATCH project wherein community members' priorities were ignored because they did not match those identified by a risk factor survey. This is a point at which the full implications of a partnership approach become apparent.

Determining priorities for action is a complex process that must begin with a confirmation of those values that will guide the process. Decision making may be guided by the principles of social justice and equity, which drive primary health care and the new public health movement, as well as by the values implicit in an agency's mission statement and philosophy. A series of questions, such as those listed, may help guide decision making.

- What types of need are present? Do community members consider these to be needs?
- How many people are affected?
- What will be the consequences if these needs are not met?
- Are there critical needs that should be met before other needs are addressed?
- Is it possible to address these needs?
- Do the needs coincide with governmental policies or the department's mission statement?
- Are resources (funds, staff) available? (Wass, 1994, based on Gilmore, Campbell, and Becker, 1989)

The process for determining priorities must also ensure that everyone has an equal opportunity to participate and to influence any decisions. Group rules that recognize everyone's right to speak are important, as are voting processes that allow everyone an equal vote. One process that has been used quite successfully is the nominal group process. This process is discussed in the section on community assessment tools.

Determination of Responses to the Needs Identified

Once the community needs have been identified, it is necessary to determine ways to best address those needs. Once again, it is important that community members be actively involved in this process. This is a point at which the contributions of community members may be vital, because understanding the issues from their perspective may highlight particular approaches that are either likely or unlikely to be successful. As is true at earlier stages of the community assessment, one of the first steps in this process is to ensure clarity regarding actual needs so that appropriate responses to those needs may be generated.

The Ottawa Charter for Health Promotion (WHO, 1986) provides a useful framework around which responses to needs can be identified. The five levels of action listed by this charter identify a broad range of activities at both the environmental and the individual levels, serving as another reminder that change at the individual level may not necessarily be the most appropriate response to identified needs. A comprehensive response is likely to include action on a number of these five levels, listed in Figure 12-3.

Discussion and idea-generating processes are important at this stage to enable the group to identify a range of innovative and comprehensive responses to the identified needs. One such process is brainstorming. The brainstorming process can prove quite useful for a committee or group trying to decide ways to best address identified problems. The value of the brainstorming process lies in the fact that it provides a forum wherein creativity is

---

Figure 12-3   The Ottawa Charter for Health Promotion's Five Levels of Action

- Build healthy public policy.
- Create supportive environments.
- Strengthen community action.
- Develop personal skills.
- Reorient the health system.

From Ottawa Charter for Health Promotion *by World Health Organization, Health and Welfare Canada, Canadian Public Health Association, 1986, Copenhagen, Denmark: FADL Publishers. Copyright 1986 by WHO.*

---

encouraged and judgment of ideas is suspended, enabling the development of hitherto unthought of solutions. Brainstorming has been used successfully in a variety of scenarios and may be a valuable tool in developing creative ideas. The steps of brainstorming are listed in Figure 12-4.

Planning and Implementation

Once a strategy or set of strategies to address identified problems has been developed, the next step is to plan the ways that these strategies will be implemented. This does not mean that the assessment phase is entirely over; rather, the process must remain flexible and sensitive to changing circumstances and the needs of the community throughout the planning and implementing phases. Certainly, though, a large component of the assessment phase is over, and attention can be focused more fully on the very different set of skills required in effective plan-

---

Figure 12-4   The Steps of Brainstorming

1. Present the issue to the group.
2. Invite the group to suggest solutions to the issue.
3. Encourage group members to be creative and to not judge the value of an idea before suggesting it.
4. Write down all suggestions without comment or criticism.
5. Continue the process until all ideas are exhausted.
6. When no more suggestions are forthcoming, analyze the responses.

If the brainstorming process is used to identify appropriate responses to a health issue, the next step involves discussing each suggestion to identify its merits and shortcomings. Suggestions may then be scaled according to their usefulness.

Adapted from Promoting Health: A Practical Guide *by L. Ewles and I. Simnett, 1992, London: Scutari Press. Copyright 1996 by Bailliere Tindall, London.*

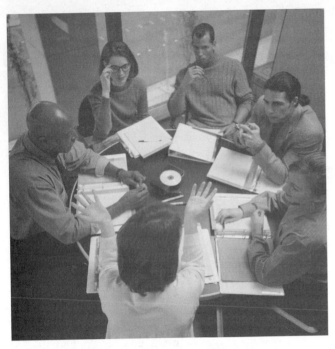

Creative ideas often stem from brainstorming. Present an issue to a group of classmates and then have a group brainstorming session to suggest solutions. Photo courtesy of PhotoDisc.

ning, implementation, and evaluation (examined in the Chapter 13).

FRAMEWORKS FOR DOCUMENTING A COMMUNITY ASSESSMENT

A number of authors have developed frameworks around which information for a community assessment can be organized and documented (including De Bella, Martin, & Siddall, 1986; Henderson & Thomas, 1987; Anderson & McFarlane, 1988; Stoner, Magilvy, & Schultz, 1992; and Russell et al., 1996). Other authors resist the use of a framework on the grounds that themes should be allowed to emerge from the data rather than being imposed (Barton et al., 1993). A number of themes are common across certain community assessment frameworks. These themes fall into broad categories such as history, culture, politics, education, employment, economics, environment, organizations, power and leadership, communication, population, health status, health services, and social services.

An examination of the various available frameworks is desirable. The use of a framework assists in the assessment process. Although most frameworks have been developed for use with geographic communities, these frameworks are generally just as useful for other forms of communities, including communities of interest.

An example of a framework is one developed by Anderson and McFarlane (1988). This framework includes information about the place (e.g., history, boundaries, topography, climate, housing, and physical environment),

the people (e.g., demographics, vital statistics, morbidity and mortality, households by type of families, values, beliefs, religion), the social system (e.g., safety and transportation, politics and government, communication, religious organizations, education), and the health and social services (e.g., hospitals, rehabilitation facilities, extended care, home health agencies, respite care services, ambulatory clinic services, public health and social services, and voluntary organizations).

COMMUNITY ASSESSMENT TOOLS

There are a number of valuable tools for use in collecting the information required in a community assessment. The kind of information obtainable through these tools varies considerably. Some tools facilitate the collection of quantitative data, whereas others provide qualitative data. It is important to note that no one method is likely to provide the full range of information needed in a community assessment. Rather, the kind of information provided by these methods is likely to be complementary; thus, use of multiple methods is warranted. As a general rule, quantitative methods facilitate a description of the extent of social phenomena, whereas qualitative methods facilitate the exploration of the underlying rationale of attitudes and behaviors (Chu, 1994). If the community assessment is to move beyond describing an area to *understanding* that area and its related issues of concern, some in-depth, qualitative methods must be used. In this way, the issues raised and their contributing factors can be explored (Baum, 1995). Regardless of the tools ultimately chosen, it is important to have people with expertise in the available assessment methods on either the project team or the steering committee.

The following summary of the various tools and methods constitutes an introduction to this topic. Some of the methods involve the analysis of information already collected, whereas others involve the collection of new information. Examination of information already collected is referred to as secondary data analysis. Applicable data include epidemiologic and demographic information, national or regional policy documents, and previously conducted needs surveys. Methods that involve the collection of new information, or primary data, include participant observation, surveys, key-informant interviews, group techniques, and community forums. Figure 12-5 illustrates the various tools used in community assessment.

Demographic and Epidemiologic Data

Demographic and epidemiologic data can provide a great deal of useful information about a community. Demographic information includes the age, gender, and ethnicity compositions of the community. Other social and

Perspectives...

Insights of a Community Health Nursing Professor

The keystone of community health nursing practice is the focus on the community as a whole. Caring for the community is central therefore to the mission of community health practice. This caring mission requires the ability of nurses to assess the health of the community. Community health nurses must be able to identify factors within a community that enhance health and those that predispose to poor health. The identification of high-risk population groups within the community and the available, acceptable, and accessible health care resources are critical factors to assess.

Assessing the health of a community is a complex process that requires flexibility, collaboration, commitment, effective communication skills, diagnostic reasoning ability, and the ability to think critically. We must provide opportunities for students to participate in the community assessment process—to experience its complexity and ambiguity. One of the major themes I teach students is the importance of focusing on community strengths as well as health problems and issues. In addition, I also focus on the complexity of the process and the collaborative efforts required. The importance of assessing the health of a community is difficult for some students to grasp, particularly when their major focus has been the care of individuals in different contexts. The shift to community as the context for practice requires a shift in the mind-set of students.

Because the community is where the action is in relation to innovative and evolving health programs and services, I think it is the most effective place to bring about improvement in the health of the people. One of my former students, for example, identified the need to improve health care services for the homeless and near-homeless in her county. As a result of her participation in the community assessment process, she identified that there was a need to begin a nursing center to serve the homeless and near homeless. She worked to create the center with community participation, and is now the program director of the center. The center today serves many homeless and near-homeless persons who feel respected and treated with caring and compassion. The nursing center is a part of an interfaith council organization whose mission is to serve this population group. Because of its contribution to the community, the nursing center has been highlighted in the news media as a respected community contribution.

—*Sue A. Thomas, RN, EdD*

economic indicators, such as employment levels, levels of home ownership, and population rates, are also valuable. Epidemiologic data identify the rates of morbidity and mortality in the population, for identification of leading causes of death and diseases within population subgroups and local communities. In addition, epidemiologic information now includes data related to injuries (Murray & Lopez, 1996).

In the 1980s there was growing recognition of the limitations of epidemiologic data, particularly since the major indicators used to assess population health status were mortality indices (Brown, 1985). Rather than describing the health of the population, epidemiologic data focused on mortality data. Given the WHO's definition of health as being more than the absence of disease, this has been a shortcoming. Billings and Cowley (1995) further point out that mortality data can be misleading. This is particularly true when rates are relatively low, because the rates say nothing about the state of the majority of the population who remain alive (Patrick, 1986). Morbidity data have also been criticized because it cannot be assumed that incidence rates equate with need for services (Stalker, 1993; Billings & Cowley, 1995).

In addition to the above statistical limitations, there are others as well, ones that reduce their practical value to policymakers (Murray & Lopez, 1996). First, even the mortality data may be fragmented and partial, even not available in some countries. Second, estimates of the numbers killed or affected by certain conditions or diseases may be exaggerated beyond their demographically plausible limits. Third, traditional health statistics do not provide policymakers with sufficient indicators to compare the relative cost-effectiveness of different interventions. Because of these problems with the use of traditional population health status indices, primarily mortality rates, the WHO, the World Bank, and the Harvard School of Public Health

Figure 12-5 Community Assessment Tools

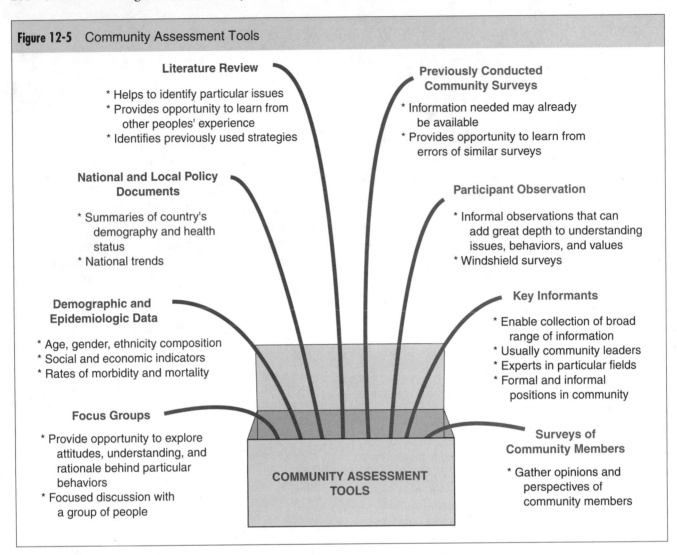

Literature Review

* Helps to identify particular issues
* Provides opportunity to learn from other peoples' experience
* Identifies previously used strategies

Previously Conducted Community Surveys

* Information needed may already be available
* Provides opportunity to learn from errors of similar surveys

National and Local Policy Documents

* Summaries of country's demography and health status
* National trends

Participant Observation

* Informal observations that can add great depth to understanding issues, behaviors, and values
* Windshield surveys

Demographic and Epidemiologic Data

* Age, gender, ethnicity composition
* Social and economic indicators
* Rates of morbidity and mortality

Key Informants

* Enable collection of broad range of information
* Usually community leaders
* Experts in particular fields
* Formal and informal positions in community

Focus Groups

* Provide opportunity to explore attitudes, understanding, and rationale behind particular behaviors
* Focused discussion with a group of people

COMMUNITY ASSESSMENT TOOLS

Surveys of Community Members

* Gather opinions and perspectives of community members

worked to address these problems with their landmark study, *The Global Burden of Disease and Injury*, Further discussion of this study is included in Chapter 29.

Additional concerns about epidemiologic data have also emerged in conjunction with the growing awareness of environmental health issues. Epidemiologic data that focus on those health problems involving a simple cause-and-effect relationship and no delay in the onset of symptoms may be of limited use (Auer, 1988; Brennan, 1992). There are many situations in which long time frames and complex interrelationships result in the suffering of many people before epidemiologic evidence of the problems is identified (Wass, 1994). Even given all of the various shortcomings, however, epidemiologic data, used and recommended for use in the *Global Burden of Disease and Injury* study, remain a key source of information for community assessment purposes.

Barton et al. (1993) warn that secondary data such as demographic and epidemiologic information is often not available for the exact area being assessed. In fact, community boundaries rarely correspond to census tracts. In such situations, inferences may need to be drawn about the community in question on the basis of information

gathered for larger statistical areas. Local information gathered via discussion with local key informants can then be used to determine whether the issues reflected in the broader data are true for the local community (Barton et al., 1993).

Because it constitutes part of the public record, demographic and epidemiologic information should be relatively easy to access in industrialized nations. In addition to being available directly from the governmental bodies that collect it, this information also may be obtained from the regional health department or public health offices. This may not be the case, however, in the developing nations of the world, where information may be difficult to obtain.

National and Local Policy Documents

National policy or strategy documents, such as *Healthy People 2000* in the United States (U.S. Department of Health and Human Services, 1991), *Achieving Health for All: A Framework for Health Promotion* in Canada (Epp, 1986), and *Health for All Australians* in Australia (Health

Targets and Implementation Committee, 1988), may provide useful summaries of a country's demography and evidence of health problems. As national documents, they may also contribute to the decision to address a particular health issue. It must be remembered, however, that these documents are political in nature and that issues may therefore be exaggerated or downplayed depending on current political agendas. Also, as political documents, the extent to which they reflect felt need depends on the extent to which meaningful participation processes were incorporated into the policy-making process. If such participation processes are largely nonexistent, the documents are likely to reflect only normative or comparative needs.

The other important point to note about national documents is that they reflect national trends, which may or may not accurately reflect the local picture. Different localities clearly have different needs; and if local needs do not reflect national needs, national policy documents may be of limited use.

Literature Review

Reviewing current literature can help identify the particular issues facing people in certain situations and can highlight typical or potential needs (McKenzie & Jurs, 1993). A literature review may afford the project team insight garnered from the work of others. In this way, the team can build on, rather than unnecessarily repeat, previous work.

A literature review will also uncover strategies used by others in addressing particular needs. Such information proves very useful when it comes time to plan appropriate responses to the needs identified in the assessment process.

Previously Conducted Community Surveys

Any previously conducted community surveys constitute useful sources of information about a community for three central reasons. First, the local information needed may have already been collected by others, minimizing duplication of effort and the unnecessary use of resources. Second, through either critical examination of any corresponding reports or discussion with those who conducted previous surveys, it is possible to learn from any errors made in those surveys. Third, all necessary information may already be available, and no further community research may be needed, although this is seldom the case.

Participant Observation

Community health nurses are in an excellent position to learn about community beliefs, values, and issues through observation, having many opportunities to observe and listen to people during the daily interactions of community health nursing practice. Such opportunities occur both when working directly with individual clients and groups and when living and moving among the community. This process of observation can be cultivated by taking every opportunity to listen and to take notice of occurrences (Twelvetrees, 1987). For those community health nurses who are not members of the communities with which they work, this may require making a conscious effort to participate in some of the everyday activities of the community: for example, attending local shows, walking through the various parts of the community, or shopping as the locals do. This type of informal observation can greatly enhance understanding of issues, behaviors, and values in a community and becomes particularly important when working with people who are unable or unwilling to articulate their views (Bowling, 1992).

Developing networks with a wide range of individuals and groups as part of daily practice can also help increase awareness of emerging health concerns (Peckham & Spanton, 1994). Indeed, Eng et al. (1992) urge health care professionals to be active members of their communities, while being careful not to take over from community members in local leadership roles.

The term **windshield survey** describes the process of observing a community by driving a car or riding public transportation through that community. Windshield surveys enable the observation of such things as housing quality, recreation facilities, the movement of people throughout the area at varying times of the day, areas of congregation in the streets, and the atmosphere of different areas of town (Shuster & Goeppinger, 1996). All such observations contribute to understanding the area and what it is like to live there.

Key Informants

Interviewing key informants is one relatively efficient way to collect a broad range of information about a community. Key informants are people who, by virtue of their positions in the community as community leaders or experts in a particular field, are able to identify problems and issues affecting that community. Key informants may hold formal or informal positions in the community; it is important to include both types of key informants because their perspectives may vary greatly. For example, the viewpoint of the mayor may differ substantially from that of the leader of a local self-help group. At the same time, however, the perspectives of key informants may differ from that of the general community. Thus, interviewing key informants is never assumed to be equivalent to interviewing community members not in leadership positions.

There are three main groups of key informants:

1. People who are in key positions in the community because of their professions, such as health professionals, social workers, and police

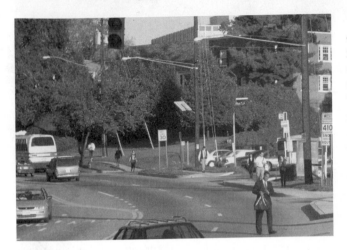

From the car, the nurse can observe communities in action. Photo courtesy of Paul A. Souders/Corbis.

2. People who are leaders within the community, such as leaders of self-help groups or volunteer organizations and counselors

3. People who are centrally placed because of their social roles in the community, such as corner shopkeepers or postal workers (Ong, Humphris, Annett, & Rifkin, 1991)

Because they typically have lived in the area for some time, key informants may be able to tell you a great deal about the community, including the historical and cultural base, the major problems, and the experience of living there. There are some important points to note, however, about the use of key informants. First, key informants must be chosen carefully to ensure that those chosen have a good understanding of the community and that their perspective is likely to be a representative one. Second, key informants should not be used in isolation at the expense of talking to the actual people affected by the issue or problem at hand (Gilmore, Campbell, & Becker, 1989). Doing so introduces the risks that assumptions about community members will be accepted as fact and that vested interests will unduly influence the results.

Because they facilitate exploration and discussion of issues as they arise, semi-structured interviews are commonly used in ascertaining the views of key informants. Although it is possible to use a survey approach with key informants, doing so is unlikely to yield the same depth of material.

Surveys of Community Members

If a community assessment is to take account of felt need, soliciting the opinions and perspectives of community members is vital. Surveys may be used both to ask residents about unmet needs and to evaluate existing services. Surveys may also be used to collect direct information about people's health experiences, attitudes, and behaviors.

A number of different survey methods may be used in community assessment, the most common being face-to-face interviews, telephone surveys, and self-administered questionnaires (Hawe, Degeling, & Hall, 1990). These three forms of information collection are compared in Table 12-1. Which one is used depends on the type of information that must be collected. Information regarding issues that can be clearly and simply expressed may be obtained via a self-administered questionnaire, whereas information regarding issues that require substantial thought and exploration might be best obtained via interviews (Hawe et al., 1990). Similarly, it may be possible to examine some issues via the use of a set of structured questions, whereas a less structured approach in the form of either semi-structured or unstructured interviews may be more suitable for exploring other issues.

The type of information sought is not the only variable to be considered, however. Cultural differences may play an important part. For example, interviews may be the most appropriate method when working with members of an ethnic group having a strong oral culture. Similarly, asking direct questions may be considered rude in some cultures. In such a circumstance, a general discussion may be more appropriate, even if the issues of concern seem straightforward to the professionals involved in the community assessment.

If survey findings are to be generalized to the community, the sample chosen for the survey must be randomly selected to ensure representation of the population in question. Furthermore, the data collection instrument must be valid and reliable (McKenzie & Jurs, 1993). Involving people with expertise in the development of the survey instrument and survey plan is vital.

The Nottingham Health Profile, used in both Britain and Australia, represents a useful example of a questionnaire for collecting information on health experiences and perceived health status. Such information complements information received from analysis of service use and is of particular value because of the likely correlation between perceived health status, health attitudes, and health behavior. The fact that such self-reported information may be more valuable than morbidity and mortality figures in predicting service use means that this profile could be invaluable in community assessments (Baum & Cooke, 1989). Furthermore, because it retains a social health perspective and can be used to demonstrate the influence of socioeconomic status on health, the Nottingham profile, unlike many other behavioral surveys, precludes the risk of blaming the victim.

Focus Groups

When groups of people hold discussions regarding a specific area of interest to the community assessment, the groups are known as focus groups. Focus groups provide opportunities to explore attitudes, understandings, and the rationales behind particular behaviors or attitudes among groups of people (Hawe et al., 1990) and can be

Table 12-1   A Comparison of Three Models of Data Collection

	SELF-ADMINISTERED QUESTIONNAIRES	TELEPHONE SURVEYS	FACE-TO-FACE INTERVIEWS
Cost	Cheapest method per respondent	Low to medium cost per respondent	Most expensive method per respondent
Coverage	Can reach a widely scattered sample	Can reach a widely scattered sample, but only those with phones	Depends on personal contact
Response rate	Lowest, especially with groups of low socioeconomic status	Medium response rate	Highest response rate
Standardization	Standardized	Standardization depends on the interviewer	Standardization depends on the interviewer
Privacy for asking sensitive questions	Good, least likely to cause embarrassment	Some "anonymity" for giving replies	May be difficult
Probing	Does not permit clarification; misunderstanding will go undetected	Allows for probing, reduces misunderstanding and missing answers	Allows for probing, reduces misunderstanding and missing answers
Literacy	Requires literacy	Not restricted by literacy, but language skills important	Not restricted by literacy, but language skills still important
Observation	No observation possible	Listening to respondent	Listening to and watching respondent

From Evaluating Health Promotion by P. Hawe, D. Degeling, & J. Hall, 1990, Sydney, Australia: MacLennan & Petty. Copyright 1990 by MacLennan and Petty, Sydney. Reprinted with permission.

of value in developing a greater understanding of the needs of groups who may have been largely neglected by the health system (Stevens, 1996). They also provide researchers with opportunities to listen to a group of people explore an issue of concern.

A typical focus group is limited in number to eight to twelve people to facilitate in-depth discussion and participation by all group members (McKenzie & Jurs, 1993). Focus groups are conducted in an informal atmosphere. The researcher acts as facilitator, guiding the group through a semi-structured interview schedule related to the topic of interest. Because focus groups are designed to uncover the range of opinions and feelings on various aspects of the topic, the questions used are open-ended, and freedom of expression is encouraged (Murphy, Cockburn, & Murphy, 1992). The facilitator remains relatively unobtrusive and does not disrupt the flow of discussion, thereby enabling group participants to explore the issues and respond to each other's comments without external judgment (Hawe et al., 1990; Stevens, 1996). Focus group discussions are taped so that they can be analyzed after the event (Murphy et al., 1992).

Within the relative safety of such a group, participants may feel comfortable expressing views that they may not be willing to share individually. Also, group members are able to build on each other's comments and come to conclusions that they may not have considered outside of the group context (Stevens, 1996). For these reasons, focus groups can be of great value in community assessment.

Focus groups are most effective when group members are relatively homogeneous. People invited to participate in a focus group may share certain characteristics such as age group, gender, cultural background, education, or socioeconomic status (Stevens, 1996). Within the boundaries of their shared characteristics, however, people may be chosen to reflect a variety of different attitudes toward the topic at hand in order to facilitate discussion and identify important issues. If the people in a focus group were to be too similar, there might be little for them to discuss; conversely, if focus group members were to not share certain assumptions or history, productive discussion may be impossible (Hawe et al., 1990).

Focus groups may be useful at various points during the community assessment process—from exploring the rationale behind a particular high-risk behavior to developing action plans to address community problems from the perspective of those people affected by the problems. For example, a group of young people might be invited together to discuss the issues of mental health or youth unemployment. Through a discussion of the youths' experiences, researchers might reap a deeper understanding of the underlying dynamics of these experiences. The focus group might then be asked to explore possible solutions to the identified problems. Brainstorming, discussed earlier, may be a valuable technique in such a situation.

Focus groups constitute a very useful way of exploring in some depth the perspectives of people who may not normally have a voice but whose inclusion in the assessment process is important. It is important to note, however, that although focus group participants are chosen because they are typical of their particular subgroup, they are not a representative sample. This means that the outcomes of focus groups cannot be generalized to the entire community (McKenzie & Jurs, 1993).

Community Forum

A public meeting or series of public meetings can provide a valuable opportunity to assess the range of public opinion on an issue or to identify a number of possible solutions to an issue. Unlike a focus group, a community forum can be conducted with a large number of people. In fact, community forums are advertised widely to encourage maximum community participation. Because some people are more likely to be able to attend or to publicly express their view, however, a community forum is unlikely to be representative of a community. The purpose of the community forum should be made clear beforehand and again at the outset of the forum so that participants do not expect that issues discussed will necessarily be acted on by health professionals in the manners identified at the forum. This is particularly important because certain people or groups may attempt to dominate discussion, potentially leaving less articulate people concerned that their views will not be considered. If well advertised beforehand and used for the purposes of information sharing and information gathering, a community

DECISION MAKING

Planning an Elder Center

A group of elder adults (ages 65 and over) says that their community needs a center where the elder members of the community can meet and socialize. It is determined that a needs assessment will be done.

• Outline a plan to begin a needs assessment process that you would recommend to the steering committee and project team.

• Include a list of the tools that could be used to identify who would be members of your project team and your steering committee. Incorporate the stages of the community assessment process.

forum can be a valuable tool in the community assessment process (Cooney, 1994).

A community forum should be facilitated by one or several people, depending on the size of the group. In addition, someone should take specific responsibility for recording the proceedings of the forum. As taping of large groups is not always successful, taking notes during the forum is recommended.

Nominal Group Process

Nominal group process is a technique that can be used in small-group settings to identify issues or rank priorities. It was designed to overcome the problem of some group

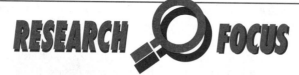

From GENESIS to ACTION—Development and Refinement of a Community Assessment Method

STUDY PROBLEM/PURPOSE

To explore the relevance and accuracy of information gathered during a community assessment using the GENESIS (General Ethnographic and Nursing Evaluation Studies in the State) model.

METHODS

GENESIS, originally created by nursing faculty from the University of Colorado Health Sciences Center School of Nursing, is based on the acceptance of the inextricable relationship between the health of the community and the socioeconomic en-

vironment and values of the community, as well as the importance of the community's felt needs (Stoner, Magilvy & Schultz, 1992). The community assessments are conducted at the request of local community groups or organizations. Assessment consists of two main components: (1) collection and analysis of secondary (epidemiologic and demographic) data and (2) a series of interviews with key informants and primary informants conducted during short but intensive visits to the community. Data are then analyzed, beginning with major themes known to influence health, including environment, recreation, economics, politics, religion, housing, social support, education, and health care services. Other themes

Continued

Continued

that may emerge depending on each local situation include lifestyle, food, families, and employment. Strengths and weaknesses are identified, and recommendations are made for further action. A draft is then presented, first to the community group that commissioned the assessment and then to the broader community. To provide an opportunity for verification of the findings before final publication, copies are also given to the key informants who contributed to the process.

FINDINGS

In reviewing their experience with the GENESIS Model, Barton et al. (1993) make a number of recommendations about methodological issues in the areas of data generation, data analysis, the conceptual framework, dissemination of findings, rigor, and group process. Two potential problem areas in the GENESIS model were identified. First, the research team consists of outsiders. It is thus possible that their interpretations may be incomplete. Outsiders may not, for example, be able to interpret all that they see or hear in the same way that an insider might. Furthermore, they may miss nuances of the community life. Second, GENESIS projects rely on key informant and primary informant interviews to gain a qualitative understanding of life in the community. The perspectives of key informants, while valuable, are unlikely to be representative of the community, solely by virtue of the positions held by the key informants. The primary informant interviews compensate for this shortcoming to some extent, but primary informants also do not constitute a representative sample of community members.

IMPLICATIONS

It is imperative to have insiders and outsiders as members of the project team and the steering committee. A more comprehensive examination of the perspectives of community members would strengthen the research design and increase the confidence of those using the community assessment results to initiate action in the area.

SOURCE

From "Community Analysis in Community Health Nursing Practice: The GENESIS Model," by M. H. Stoner, J. K. Magilvy, & P. R. Schultz, 1992, Public Health Nursing, 9 *(4), pp. 223–227. Copyright 1992 by Public Health Nursing.*

ACTION: Application and Extension of the GENESIS Community Analysis Model

STUDY PROBLEM/PURPOSE

To explore the relevance and accuracy of information gathered during a community assessment using ACTION (Assessing Communities Together in the Identification of Needs).

METHODS

Because the communities being assessed were part of a larger city in which the university was located and much intermingling between communities therefore occurred, the ACTION project team consisted of a mixture of community outsiders and insiders. This brought a mix of perspectives to the project. The ACTION project strengthened its research design in order to ensure adequate representation of the large community. A mail survey of a random sample of community members was conducted, as were telephone surveys of another random sample. Drop-off surveys were also made available at a number of key locations. Finally, in addition to the original key informant interviews of GENESIS, a series of focus groups was conducted.

FINDINGS

The fact that the ACTION project was a more complex research process conducted on a larger community required greater immersion of the research team in the community. The ACTION team was involved intermittently with the community over a five-month period, compared with the five-day period used in many GENESIS projects. Although the extra time involved created some difficulties for the research team, the result was deepened understanding of local issues. The large size of the project also created some difficulty with regard to managing the data generated, resulting in the team's being broken up into several small groups, each with specific responsibility for certain areas. This left only one person with an overall picture of the project, a major difficulty in community assessments involving large communities.

IMPLICATIONS

As a result of their experience, the research team made a number of recommendations for future urban community analysis projects, including more regular meetings of the whole research team, greater attention to group process, the inclusion of some people with specific responsibility for community mobilization and monitoring community involvement throughout the project, and employing a data manager to deal with the large volumes of information generated.

SOURCE

From "ACTION: Application and Extension of the GENESIS Community Analysis Model" by C. K. Russell, D. M. Gregory, D. Wotton, E. Mardoch, & M. M. Counts, 1996, Public Health Nursing, 13 *(3), pp. 187–194. Copyright 1996 by Public Health Nursing.*

COMMUNITY

NURSING VIEW

A community health nurse working in a low-income urban area has been asked to participate on a steering committee working to develop an afterschool program for approximately 200 students whose parents are unable to pick them up until 5:30 P.M. The school day ends at 2:50 P.M. The goal of the program is to keep "latch key" children off the streets and out of trouble.

Several months earlier, an accidental shooting occurred in the home of one of the children who attended this school. The incident occurred when two 12-year-old boys were home alone playing with a rifle. One of the boys accidentally shot and severely injured the other. Since this incident, latch key children have been the focus of articles in the local newspaper.

The idea for the program came from the mayor of the city. If successful, the program will be a model for other schools in the region. The steering committee has been meeting for several months, holding three meetings to date. The only nurses on the committee will be the community health nurse and a school nurse.

Nursing Considerations

ASSESSMENT
• Who else might be on the steering committee? Why?
• Who might be on the project team? Why?
• What questions should be asked about the type of data to be collected?
• What type of data should be collected?
• Which needs assessment tools might be used to collect the data?
• What questions must be answered to ensure appropriate planning?

DIAGNOSIS
• What nursing diagnosis might be formulated specific to the accident?

OUTCOME IDENTIFICATION
• The goal of the program is to keep the children off the streets. What other positive outcomes could be realized if this program is successful?
• What is the benefit to the community?
• What is the benefit to the children and the families?

PLANNING/INTERVENTIONS
• Who should be involved in the planning with regard to the where, when, who, and how of program development?
• What factors should be considered when planning this program?
• How would costs play a part in the planning?
• Given that this is a low-income urban community, who might cover the costs of this program?
• Where could the steering committee look for funds?

EVALUATION
• If the program is shown to have low enrollment, what might be the sources of the problem? How might these sources be identified?
• What might be suggested as the next course of action if the program were to be deemed unsuccessful?
• What might be suggested if the program were to be deemed successful?
• What process could this steering committee use to select its evaluation methods?
• What indicators could the steering committee use to evaluate program effectiveness?
• What process might the steering committee use to evaluate its own effectiveness in program planning and development?

members' dominating the discussion and, thus, preventing quieter members from voicing their perspectives. There are a number of steps in the nominal group process.

First, the question at hand is presented to the group members. This question might be related to problems that they see in the local community or to solutions to particular problems already identified. Group members are asked to work individually on this question for approximately 10 to 15 minutes.

Next, using a round-robin technique so that all group members participate equally, group members are each asked to contribute an answer. This process is continued until all responses are listed on a board; no critiquing or discussion is allowed. Each response is then allocated a number. The meaning of each response is then clarified with the group, allowing participants to explain their rationale when necessary.

Participants are next asked to "vote" on the priority of the identified problems or issues. Each participant is asked to rank, say, the top five issues or responses. Participants allocate from five points (for the issue to which they assign the highest priority) down to one point (for the issue to which they assign the lowest priority). Finally, points allocated by all participants are collected and collated. The problem or issue with the largest number of points is accorded top priority, and so forth, down to those issues with no points being accorded the lowest priority (Van de Ven & Delbecq, 1972; Green & Kreuter, 1991).

In this way, nominal group process allows everyone to vote anonymously and equally. Findings are therefore much more likely to be representative of the group than are the findings of a focus group or community forum, where particular individuals may dominate. For these reasons, nominal group process can be useful in setting priorities.

Key Concepts

- Three dimensions that are important to consider when defining community health are status, structure, and process.
- The population focus of community health nursing requires an understanding of the purpose and process of comprehensive community assessment.

- Community assessment is part of a complex process of identifying and responding to problems, needs, and issues affecting populations.
- The different types of needs that must be considered when conducting a needs assessment include felt need, expressed need, normative need, and comparative need.
- Comprehensive community assessment considers the needs of a community, its assets, and the resources available to perform the assessment.
- Community members and health professionals bring different, but complementary, perspectives to the identification of community health needs and assets. Thus, community members must be involved in the identification of health needs and assets, as well as the planning of programs to address those needs.
- The purpose of the assessment must be clearly defined and the available resources for conducting the assessment identified to ensure that adequate resources are allocated to complete the assessment.
- A research plan and time frame must be developed and agreed on by the project team and the steering committee members.
- A community assessment should include the collection and analysis of data currently available in addition to the collection and analysis of new data.
- A variety of information sources and methods of obtaining data are available to and valuable in community assessment, including: demographic and epidemiologic data, national and local policy documents, previously conducted surveys, literature reviews, participant observation, windshield surveys, key informants, surveys of community members, focus groups, community forums, and the nominal group process.
- The results of the community assessment must be communicated to the community either orally, in written form, or in both ways.
- The plan to address the identified needs must be developed with input from community members.
- Community assessment is the beginning of a process to respond to community health problems and needs; it is not an end in itself.

Program Planning, Implementation, and Evaluation

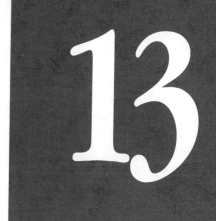

13

Clare Budgen, RN, BSN, MSN, PhD
Gail Cameron, RN, BSN, MN

 KEY TERMS

community organization
cost analysis of health
  programs
formative program
  evaluation
Health for All
health promotion
impact evaluation
outcome evaluation
primary health care
process program
  evaluation
program
program evaluation
program implementation
program planning
programming
programming models
summative program
  evaluation

Go to the people
Live among them
Start with what they know
Build on what they have
But of the best leaders
When their task is accomplished
Their work is done
The people all remark
We have done it ourselves

—*Author unknown*

COMPETENCIES

Upon completion of this chapter, the reader should be able to:

- Discuss ways that the Health for All movement, with its strategies of primary health care and health promotion, is changing community nurses' work with programs and people.
- Describe the ways that societal trends, health care reform, and a broad definition of health affect programs.
- Examine program issues through the different lenses of caring, phenomenological, feminist, and critical social theories.
- Identify the ways that multilevel change theories may be used to guide programming.
- Differentiate among types of community organizing: community development, social planning, and social action.
- Understand the programming processes of planning, implementation, and evaluation.
- Critique programming models for their usefulness in various community situations.

The **Health for All** movement, initiated by the World Health Organization (WHO), has captured the imagination of people around the world (WHO, 1978, 1981). Many countries have responded to this visionary goal with public policy changes and nation-wide health programs. For example, the United States passed federal legislation to support health planning and created a national program, Healthy People 2000 (U.S. Department of Health & Human Services [USDHHS], 1992). Canada, striving to strengthen its national system of health care, has designed numerous programs based on Achieving Health for All: A Framework for Health Promotion (Epp, 1986) and the Ottawa Charter (WHO, 1986) (see also Chapter 1).

Ideas foundational to the Health for All movement are that all people must be included equitably in health endeavors and that all sectors of society must put health on their agendas and be held accountable for the health consequences of their decisions. The underlying belief is that the global population and all aspects of global development benefit from equity in health (Waring, 1996). Social activism and social justice, rather than market justice, are thus integral to the Health for All movement and, therefore, must be integral to programs designed to further the Health for All goal.

The WHO strategies to achieve Health for All are primary health care and health promotion. **Primary health care** is defined as:

> Essential health care based on practical, scientifically sound and socially acceptable methods and technology made universally accessible to individuals and families in the community through their full participation and at a cost that the community and country can afford to maintain at every stage of their development in the spirit of self reliance and self determination (WHO, 1978, p. 21).

This definition is rich with ideas to guide nurses' work in community health programming.

Health promotion is defined as the process of enabling individuals and communities to increase their control over and improve their health (WHO, 1986). Health promotion requires not only individual change but also societal and system change (Green & Raeburn, 1990). Many community health programs have emphasized individual change; fewer efforts have targeted societal and system change. Inherent in primary health care and health promotion is the belief that individuals, communities, and countries have the ability, right, and shared responsibility to take care of their health and the health of others. Health care systems and practitioners act as resources, not central actors. Health care is only one, and not the main, contributor to health (Ritchie, 1997). Although progress has been made, much work remains for these ideas to be fully incorporated into community health programs.

Community nurses use programs to improve the health of communities. *Community* is broadly defined in this chapter as any group of people sharing an interest. An interest might be a geographic location, social network, or characteristic such as age, gender, race, disease, or health issue. The Health for All movement, with its accompanying strategies of primary health care and health promotion, challenges nurses to reconsider their use of programs. Use of primary health care and health-promotion principles in combination with principles of programming means that health programs must be thoughtfully planned, implemented, and evaluated to ensure that, from the viewpoint of the community, priority health issues are dealt with effectively and resources are well used.

In the past decade, one of the biggest challenges and most frequent omissions in health programming has been the full participation of the community. Most health care practitioners (and associated bureaucracies) are not familiar with a partnership model of care and are loathe to give up control. Also, the "health care provider/system as expert" model has predominated to such an extent that many community members are not experienced at gaining control and making decisions in partnership with health care practitioners. Indeed, this can be an overwhelming task, as practitioners frequently learn when they find themselves in the role of client.

Community health nurses have derived basic programming principles from a variety of sources including business, education, and social science theory. The term *program* has various meanings. **Program** is most simply defined as a collection of activities designed to produce particular results (Dignan & Carr, 1992). For community health programs, because the ultimate desired result or outcome is improved health of the community, the substance of programs is health or health related (e.g., environmental determinants of health). The term **programming** is used to encompass the whole sequence of processes that when performed together produce the program and the desired results. Thus, programming is process oriented. Community health nurses most often have conceptualized programming similarly to the nursing process: that is, as assessment, planning, implementation, and evaluation. These terms are in fact used extensively in programming work across disciplines.

A word of caution is needed here. When programs are based on primary health care and health-promotion principles, nurses work to enable communities to increase their control over and improve their health. In the past, however, assessment, planning, implementation, and evaluation activities frequently have not involved adequate community partnership. There is thus value in considering other ways of thinking about programming to ensure that conceptual space is created for processes that truly enable the community (i.e., that give opportunity for control). Lindsey and Hartrick (1996) recommend that nurses use a framework based on the work of Friere (1970/1993) that comprises active listening, participatory dialogue, theme/pattern recognition, envisioning action, action, and reflection on action. Similar ideas and language are beginning to appear in the literature of other disciplines as theorists work on the issue of ways to best effect change through programs (McKenzie & Smeltzer, 1997). Regardless of the programming framework used, knowledge of a variety of frameworks is helpful because community nurses work with people from different programming backgrounds.

Successful programming does not take place in isolation from the situation or setting within which it occurs. In this chapter, health programming is considered in the context of health care reform and societal trends. Also, primary health care and health promotion are examined more closely in relation to a broad definition of health and the practicalities of programming. Some of the theories, models, and "how to's" of program planning, implementation, and evaluation are explored. Because change is inherent in programming, the use of change theories is also discussed. For example, community organization is presented as a multifaceted theoretical approach to community change. The intent of this chapter is to provide nurses with background enough to reasonably begin the work of community health programming.

HEALTH PROGRAMMING IN CONTEXT

Thoughtful consideration of the context within which a health program will be developed and implemented contributes directly to program success. Local contexts are nested with regional, national, and international contexts. Although contexts vary considerably, important factors and trends relevant to health usually can be identified if the nurse is open minded, observant, and questioning.

Health Care Reform and Societal Trends

Health care reform issues and societal trends are macro-level contextual factors that must be considered in programming. Societal trends include increasing global interconnection, environmental degradation, and changing demographics and health issues; the response has been the restructuring of health care organizations. Organizations generally are under strong pressure to change in order to survive in rapidly changing local and global environments. Hammer and Champy (1994) recommend that, in order to remain competitive and profitable, organizations undergo reengineering, defined as a "fundamental redesign of business process to achieve dramatic improvements in critical, contemporary measures of improvement, such as cost, quality, service and speed" (p. 32). Hammer and Chamby argue that the basic idea of "doing more with less" requires a shift in focus to a process orientation, rule breaking, better team building, and the creative use of information technology.

Health care systems, under pressure "to do more with less" or "to do better with the same," are using industrial business models such as Hammer and Champy's (1994) to guide reform. Of greatest concern in health care are appropriateness of care, quality, accessibility, and costs. Business theories can provide useful ideas for the administration of health care. Nurses must be aware, however, that business theories generally are based on market justice principles that may conflict with a social justice orientation and cause programmers to be "insufficiently appreciative of the human dimension" (Hammer, as cited in Pratt, 1997, p. 81).

The values underlying reform approaches and program decisions must be openly examined so that profit or short-term cost savings do not take precedence over people and long-term costs. For example, in the health maintenance organization initiative in the United States, *prevention for profit* has many times taken precedence over *prevention*

to improve the health of the population; the original goal of increasing access to prevention services has been overshadowed by excessive profit taking. To achieve the Health for All goal, programmers must consider health program appropriateness, accessibility, and quality of outcomes for communities in relation to human and material costs for both the short and the long term. Nurses working in community programming are well positioned to participate in reform; to anticipate and observe the impact of various strategies; to ask and to assist communities to ask critical questions; and, through the inclusion of political-action strategies in programs, to influence the direction of system changes and resource use. In the past, nurses might not have considered this sociopolitical type of work as part of programming; but nurses are accountable to the public, and if health care system issues are a priority for the community, their inclusion in programming is appropriate (White, 1995) (see also Chapters 4 and 30).

Health problems also are changing. Epidemiologic data in the United States and Canada reveal high mortality and morbidity related to chronic disease (e.g., cardiovascular disease, cancer, HIV/AIDS, diabetes), substance misuse/abuse, accidents, violence, physical and mental abuse, suicide, homelessness, occupational and environmental hazards, inadequate nutrition and activity, and teenage pregnancy. To a large extent, these conditions are preventable. Needed are effective prevention programs at the societal, community, and individual levels (see Figure 13-1). Research on prevention programs has increased significantly in the past decade. Studies rich in information about the content and effectiveness of different programs can be found via health care database searches. Appropriate allocation of health care resources to prevention

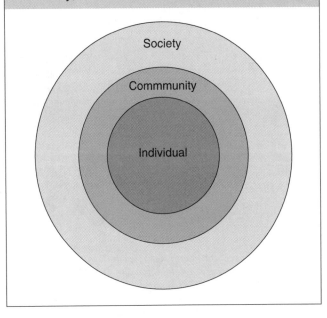

Figure 13-1 To improve health care, effective prevention programs are necessary on societal, community, and individual levels.

programs, in comparison with treatment services, has not yet occurred in most countries. Nurses involved in programming may need to search for resources to support preventive programs. National coalitions and associations are sources of support for prevention program information, funding, and other resources (see Appendix B).

Dramatically changing technologies have created an unprecedented flow of information and a multitude of new health programs. Technologies have "done wonders" but have also engendered ethical, legal, social, and economic dilemmas, as well as iatragenic health effects (Vail & Shetowsky, 1997). Nurses should anticipate encountering these dilemmas and effects in their work in programming. Careful programming in partnership with communities helps ensure that the technologies used are acceptable, appropriate, and affordable.

Demographic data in the United States and Canada indicate an increasing proportion of elderly people, increasing cultural and racial diversity, increasing poverty (and wealth), and changes in the profile of families and communities (Creese, 1994; Porter-O'Grady, 1994) (see also Chapter 29). Increasing global population, political problems, and wars put pressure on countries to accept immigrants and to share resources. Equitable creation and distribution of resources is a challenge for all levels of government and for nurses involved in programming. Distribution of wealth in countries is strongly correlated with health; where there are wide gaps between rich and poor, health is negatively affected. Racial, socioeconomic, and other prejudices are impediments to equity that nurses must be prepared to counteract or circumvent. Smith (1997) encourages community health nurses to mobilize resources through the development of both local and global partnerships rather than focusing on scarcity of resources. Resources can be created, used, counted, and distributed in many different ways.

Societal trends are significant to health programming because they are linked with the health of communities and with the types of programs that would be most helpful. Certain groups are at greater risk, and the health-related circumstances of these groups need careful consideration for the benefit of the whole community. Also, programs must be designed differently for different subpopulations or aggregates within communities. Nurses who consider the ways that health care system changes and societal trends are affecting communities and subpopulations can use this knowledge to avoid pitfalls, realize opportunities, and improve programming success. Opportunities for nurses to make positive contributions through programming have never been greater.

Health Broadly Defined

With regard to health programming, the term *health* must be defined. Current major health problems in Canada and the United States are the result of a multitude of determinants; many of these determinants are socially constructed and can therefore be changed (Lalonde, 1974; USDHHS, 1992; Frank, 1995). Of importance to programming is expansion of definitions of health beyond the absence of disease and disability so that health is viewed as a resource for living (WHO, 1986). Contemporary definitions link health closely with the social and economic environment and to the ways society and its institutions operate.

To act consistently with a definition of health that incorporates social as well as physical determinants, nurses involved in health programming must cast their sights broadly to ensure that all critical factors influencing the health of a given community are taken into consideration. For example, a community plagued by violence

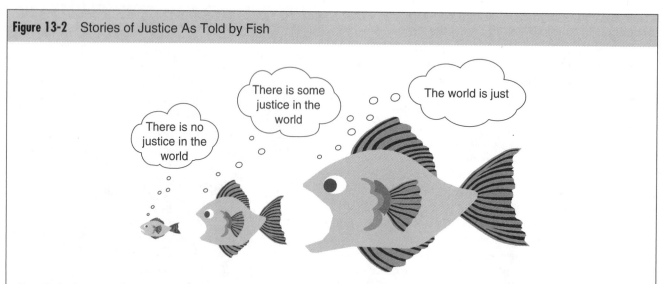

Figure 13-2   Stories of Justice As Told by Fish

From Basic Concepts of International Health *(Reading Module, p. 13) by K. Wolton, H. Amit, S. Kalma, L. Hillman, D. Hillman, & N. Cosway, January 1995 , Ottawa, Canada: Canadian University Consortium for Health in Development. Copyright 1995 by Canadian Society for International Health. Reprinted by permission of Canadian Society for International Health.*

may benefit from a program that includes initiatives to improve employment, housing, neighborhood support, and recreation in combination with initiatives directed toward assisting those who are attacked, at risk, or perpetrators (Stokols, 1992). Nurses involved in programming have many opportunities to promote the use of a broad definition of health.

Medical, Behavioral, and Socioenvironmental Approaches to Health Programs

In health programming work, nurses will encounter three common approaches to health: medical, behavioral, and socioenvironmental (Labonte, 1993). Health and health problems are defined differently within each, and each is associated with different types of programming. The medical approach focuses on disease and disability. Health programs using this approach tend to be practitioner managed and focus on detection, treatment, and reduction of risk factors. In preventive practice (public health in the United States and Canada), although the program is delivered to the individual, the intent is improvement in the population's health (e.g., hearing and vision screening of young children and immunization programs). A high percentage of the population must therefore be reached. The irradication of smallpox through massive immunization programs is an example of the successful application of the medical approach in the global population.

In the behavioral approach, health is defined as physical functional ability and healthy lifestyle behavior. Behavioral programs thus focus on the reduction of risky behavior and the promotion of healthy lifestyles. Such programs may be supported by public policy such as "no smoking" and seat belt legislation. Again, the underlying intent is to improve the health of the population. With the behavioral approach, practitioners and communities may negotiate strategies to improve health behavior.

The socioenvironmental approach encompasses social wellness, being connected to others, having a meaningful life, and being in control. Socioenvironmental programs are intended to improve social and environmental conditions that support health and to reduce both psychosocial risk factors (e.g., isolation, low self-esteem, and low perceived power) and socioenvironmental risk conditions (e.g., poverty, dangerous environments, consumerism, and inadequate education). With this approach, communities are likely to determine the issues, goals, and strategies; practitioners then assist communities to plan and implement programs. Examples are family caregivers, support networks, and media watch programs to detect and change media messages that are hazardous to health. The socioenvironmental approach is receiving renewed attention in nurses' programming work.

Each of the three approaches has appropriate and inappropriate applications; a collaborative rather than competitive view is helpful overall. Community health nurses may want to use a single approach or a combination of approaches within a given program, depending on the situation. Familiarity with each approach and a critical view regarding the most appropriate approaches for given situations are strengths nurses can develop and bring to community health programming. Health care practitioners tend to use the single approach with which they are most familiar; community health nurses who understand all three approaches can work effectively with a wide variety of others and, in some cases, help diverse groups work more effectively together.

Ecological Approaches to Health Programs

Of particular interest to community health nurses is a fourth approach to health. Ecological approaches are wholistic and encompass aspects of the previous three approaches. These models of health are based on ecosystem theory; thus all biological, behavioral, and socioenvironmental factors are viewed as interconnected. The Mandala of Health (Hancock, 1993) (see also Chapter 1) is an ecological model as are two additional ecological models put forward by Hancock. The Human Development Model emphasizes connections between health and environmental and economic well-being, with a particular focus on the principles of equity and sustainability. The Health and Community Ecosystem Model uses equity and sustainability principles at the community level, introducing issues such as viability, conviviality, adequate prosperity, and livability (see Figure 13-3). This latter model originated from Healthy Cities/Communities program work within the Health for All movement. Methods for evaluating results of these ecological models are under development. Hancock sees ecology as a critical science because it promotes an equalization of power relationships among societal sectors. Ecological health models are especially relevant for nurses working toward the goal of Health for All. For example, an immunization or infant-rehydration program may save the lives of children, but unless those children have enough to eat, death and disability are simply delayed. Ecological models invite the practitioner to look holistically at the situation, enabling more effective programming.

Programming Upstream

Regardless of the health approach favored, consensus is growing that health programs must focus more "upstream," meaning taking into consideration the societal context that manufactures health or health problems (Butterfield, 1990; Steingraber, 1997). The community health nurse might, for example, examine demographic and epidemiologic data about smoking and raise questions regarding the reasons that smoking predominated among the more established and affluent male members of society until its health hazards were recognized. Other questions that might be raised include why it now predominates among those with fewer social and economic

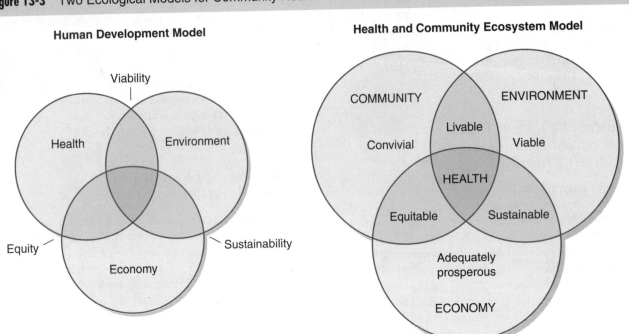

Figure 13-3   Two Ecological Models for Community Health

From "Health, Human Development & the Community Ecosystem: Three Ecological Models" by T. Hancock, 1993, Health Promotion International, *8(1), pp. 43, 44. Copyright 1993 by Oxford University Press. Used with permission.*

resources, including young people, particularly young females (Evans & Stoddart, 1990; Provincial Health Officer, 1996). In a community where increasing numbers of young people are starting to smoke, an upstream approach would guide the nurse to consider the context within which individual smoking behavior is created and maintained. A smoking-prevention program in the local community might include working with young people and other groups to assist them in critiquing market and social forces, lobbying local merchants to reduce marketing of tobacco to young people, and developing environments for young people that promote nonsmoking. Further upstream, the program might include sharing of information from regional, national, and international antismoking groups to give interested community members the opportunity to gain skills at coalition building to further curtail tobacco marketing, use, and production.

In the United States, where in 1997 tobacco companies agreed to pay substantial funds to governments for tobacco-related health costs, a community smoking-prevention program might also involve lobbying governments to influence the ways that these funds will be spent in an effort to ensure that a substantial portion is directed upstream and toward the protection and strengthening of youth. "Downstream" approaches, which focus on prevention at the individual level, might involve programs for developing personal efficacy around not smoking for young people at risk and for helping those who smoke to quit. The furthest downstream work would not occur until tobacco-related health problems were identified.

PRIMARY HEALTH CARE PRINCIPLES FOR PROGRAMS

As a component of an integrated health system, primary health care focuses on the main health issues of a community as defined by that community. This does not mean, however, that practitioners never bring issues to a community (e.g., new immunization programs). Primary health care, done well, may look different in different regions or countries. Primary health care encompasses a broad range of health strategies; primary are health pro-

DECISION MAKING

Which Health Approach to Use?

In the region where you work, several cases of active tuberculosis and two deaths from untreated tuberculosis have been identified. Neighborhoods in the region are diverse (e.g., some very poor, others affluent). You have been asked to help plan new programs to deal with the problem.

• What do the various health approaches offer in this situation?

• Which approach(es) would you recommend using? Why?

motion, prevention, rehabilitation, and supportive services. Curative services are an essential but not dominant component. This comprehensive, non-discipline-specific model should not be confused with selective primary care models such as primary nursing and primary care medicine (Registered Nurses Association of British Columbia, 1994). Enactment of Health for All/primary health care principles in community health programs means:

- Essential programs with increased health promotion and illness and injury prevention
- Full community participation throughout the programming process, including defining issues and making decisions about actions
- Use of socially acceptable, appropriate, and affordable methods and technology
- Universal, equitable access to programs close to where people live, work, play, and study
- Collaboration among all sectors (community, health, environment, social, political, economic, business, education, religion, private and public organizations, government) (WHO, 1986; Stewart, 1995)

On the basis of primary health care principles, nurses involved in community programming must be prepared to work with a wide cross section of people in ways that support meaningful participation (Clarke, Beddome, & Whyte, 1993). Knowledge and skills are useful in the areas of:

- Forming a working relationship with a community
- Building intersectoral relationships
- Negotiation
- Conflict management/conflict resolution
- Advocacy
- Consensus building
- Coalition building
- Written and verbal communication
- Group facilitation
- Networking
- Committee work
- Resource finding
- Lobbying
- Teaching/learning
- Social marketing
- Use of media
- Proposal and report writing
- Political action
- Budgeting

The reader is referred to the extensive multidisciplinary literature available on these topics (nursing, social work, political science, community psychology, business, and education).

Participation does not mean that community members are expected to carry out work that is in the practitioners' areas of expertise and responsibility; rather, it means being fully informed, making decisions, and being adequately supported. The views of community members must always be given priority consideration in programming. Further, the views of those external to the community must be considered in relation to the views of those

DECISION MAKING

Is Primary Health Care Achievable?

In the region where you work, families with members experiencing cancer must travel for treatment to a city 250 miles away. Costs to families are high in terms of both dollars and disruption to work, school, and support networks.

- Using primary health care principles, what possibilities do you see for improving this situation?

in the community. Programming is a mutual process. This is not to idealize the notion of community. However, programming will not be helpful if nurses do not ground their work in the community.

Health-Promotion Programs

Health promotion, health protection, and disease prevention, although closely related and sometimes overlapping in the realm of application in programs, can be differentiated theoretically (see Chapter 9). Prevention programs are geared toward eliminating the negative, that is "to prevent the occurrence of specific diseases and disorders" (Stoto, Behrens, & Rosemont, 1990, p. 6), rather than enhancing the positive (e.g., well-being) (Stachtchenko & Jenicek, 1990). *Health protection,* a term used primarily in the United States, implies changing the physical and social environment to improve health; changes in legislation and regulation are components. In Canada, the term *health protection* is not widely used; instead, prevention and health promotion are understood to include environmental change.

Health promotion is framed positively; thus, health-promotion programs are aimed at maintaining and enhancing health and well-being. Health promotion has especially captured the interest of (over)developed countries (Pederson, O'Neill, & Rootman, 1994). Conceptualized as occurring in any situation that enables people to take control of and improve their health, health promotion has been defined by some practitioners as a way of "being" rather than of "doing." When guided by the WHO definition, health-promotion programs and health-promoting practices have a distinctly political and socially critical dimension. Those other than health care practitioners or institutions are viewed as the active agents (Stokols, 1992). The politics of enabling others to increase control implies that the "others" will experience an increase in power to act on their own behalf. The status quo is challenged when power is directed toward changing inequities that negatively affect health.

Theorists and activists in health promotion caution about professional practitioners' inclination to take over processes intended to strengthen others; governments and organizations tend to do the same (Grace, 1991; Baum & Sanders, 1995). It is tempting to take over control when one believes one knows that which is best in a given situation. The result is another form of "power over," implying social control and maintenance of inequities, rather than the intended "power with," implying social change and transformation to a more equitable state. Social control has contributed to community health. Given the current health care context and broader definition of health, however, it is clear that social control has been overused and social change neglected. Eng, Salmon, and Mullan (1992) have identified different models of intervention for social change and social control (see Table 13-1). Social change is required if the Health for All goal is to be reached (Maglacas, 1988; American Nurses Association, 1991; Porter-O'Grady, 1994).

EMPOWERMENT AND PARTNERSHIP

Central to health promotion are the concepts of empowerment and partnership. The concept of empowerment has multiple meanings and, as both a process and an outcome, is not straightforward to enact in practice (Wallerstein, 1992; Rissel, 1994; Robertson & Minkler, 1994; Skelton, 1994. Empowerment can be simply defined as taking power. Most appealing is the notion that power can be created through transformative interactions among people: the power of possibility, the power of affirmation, the power of new ideas, and the power of self-created knowledge (Friere, 1970/1993; Chinn, 1995). Rissel (1994) argues that this win–win form of empowerment occurs only in the psychological realm and that when material resources are involved, empowerment means win–lose, hence the struggle to maintain the status quo by those who benefit materially from it. Others see this win–lose conceptualization as learned, unhealthy for communities, and subject to change (McKnight & Kretzmann, 1992).

In health care, the implications are that empowered individuals and communities will make positive use of the power they gain; that is, they will be able to think critically, act in their own best interests, create more equitable access to resources, develop their own resourcefulness, work well with others, and respect their own and others' diversity. Obviously, certain values, knowledge, and skills are components. A further implication is that empowerment is associated with improved health and a reduced need for health care services (Frank, 1995). Community empowerment is associated with the concept of community competence, the ability of the community to function effectively as a unit of problem solving (Ross, 1955, as cited in Minkler, 1990, p. 268). These idealized views of empowerment have been tested and critiqued as practitioners have attempted to shape their practices in ways that support others' empowerment. Labonte (1993) derived from his varied community practice an empowerment pathway from personal care (individual development), to small-group development (mutual support), to community organizing (around issues), to coalition building/advocacy, to collective social and political action.

Concern has been expressed that empowerment and health-promotion theory may be used by some as insincere rhetoric to disguise a shifting of the burden, as opposed to the profit, of health care to someone else (e.g., from government to citizens or from health care practitioners to families) (Grace, 1991; Labonte, 1994). Bringing the idea of empowerment into health programming suggests that nurses must tend to their own empowerment as well as to the empowerment of others. Nurses have been observed at some times to be the recipients of disempowering behavior, at other times, the perpetrators (Roberts, 1983). Although this is not surprising in a world where disempowering acts are prevalent, it does not need to continue. Nurses have been challenged to value their knowledge and closeness with people and to use their considerable strengths to address health problems, health determinants, and the inequities and power imbalances that negatively affect health (Mahler, 1985; Moccia, 1990). This challenge can be met, at least partially, through the thoughtful planning, implementation, and evaluation of community health programs

Empowerment, partnership, and participation are fundamentally linked. It seems reasonable that, to support empowerment, community health nurses must work more

Table 13-1 Comparison of Social Change and Social Control Models of Intervention	
SOCIAL CHANGE	**SOCIAL CONTROL**
• Social analysis	• Epidemiologic/demographic analysis
• Focus on strengths	• Focus on weaknesses
• Goal is health outcome and increased community competence	• Goal is health outcome
• Organized around human categories	• Organized around disease
• Asks "What are people's motives?"	• Asks "How can we motivate people?"

From "Community Empowerment: The Critical Base for Primary Care" by E. Eng, M. E. Salmon, & F. Mullan, 1992, Family Community Health, 15(1), p. 5. Copyright 1992 by Aspen Publishers, Inc. Reprinted with permission.

in equal partnership "with" others rather than "doing things to" or "for" others. In the familiar "doing to/for" style, the nurse as "expert" may simply decide that which must be done and do it, or the nurse may act under the direction of another "expert" such as an organization. In the partnership style, the nurse is a collaborator in achieving improved health, a co-learner/teacher, co-decision maker, and facilitator. Nurses and others alike contribute their knowledge and skills. Partnership implies shared responsibilities, decision making, commitment to outcomes, and benefits. Practitioners have expertise in health care; clients have expertise in their own lives (including their health) and in their own communities.

This partnership style is applicable to all nursing relationships: that is, with individuals, communities, colleagues, other practitioners, agencies, and government. Skelton (1994) argues that partnerships create participation and empowerment. In situations where health programming is actually taking place, the partnership and "doing for" styles are not mutually exclusive. To support empowerment and participation, nurses must work fundamentally from the place of partnership and shift to a more "doing for" style only as temporarily needed, for example, in crisis or emergency situations when quick action is required, such as during a sudden outbreak of a communicable disease.

THEORETICAL LENSES

Theory-based programming enables community nurses to use already developed ideas to guide and strengthen their work. The adage about not needing to "reinvent the wheel" applies here, as do the ideas about "improving the wheel" through testing and altering the wheel to suit different situations. Theories provide nurses with different lenses through which to see situations; each lens provides a different view and different understandings. According to McKenzie and Smeltzer (1997), theories are the backbone of the processes of programming and models are representations of these processes. Bateson (1990) speaks about the value of improvisation and reflection as one lives, works, participates, and observes. As theories are the science of programming, improvisation and reflection are the art.

Meta-Theories

If you have come to help me, you are wasting your time. But if you have come because your liberation is bound with mine, then let us begin. (Lily Walker, an Australian aboriginal woman, as cited in Labonte, 1993, p. 35)

Meta-theories provide broad descriptions and explanations of general happenings in the world. Of particular interest in nursing at this time are caring, phenomenological, feminist, and critical social theories. Phenomeno-

logical, feminist, and critical social theories are helping nurses understand and transform the underlying ideas and responses that support the social construction of inequities.

Caring

Caring has been defined as the moral imperative to act ethically and justly and the motivating power underlying all nursing realities and possibilities (Hills et al., 1994) (see also Chapter 1). Bateson (1990) defines caring as "a quality of attention, a total commitment to looking and listening" (p. 158) and care or caretaking as action that "at its best . . . creates freedom" and enables the cared for and caretaker to thrive (p. 156). Bateson contends that these principles apply equally to the care of humans and the care of the earth.

From these definitions, caring is understood as the attitude and activity of nursing and is inherent in every nurse–client interaction, including programming. Community health nurses are commissioned to provide care (programs) in ways that maintain dignity and respect, knowing that the ways will vary for different people (Canadian Nurses Association, 1997). Watson (1988) emphasizes mutual, reciprocal, and interactive experiences directed toward the preservation of humanity. Within these mutual, reciprocal, and interactive experiences, nurses and clients make choices about that which is needed from each. These ideas are consistent with empowerment and partnership. For example, in programming, depending on what is jointly decided, nurses may take direct action on behalf of clients or may act to support action by clients themselves.

Phenomenological Theory

Inequities, a main focus of Health for All programming, are associated with the categorizing of and responses to differences. Use of phenomenological theory enables nurses to appreciate the lived experiences of others, within the context of such things as culture, time, and place. It is the meaning of people's lives as lived by them (Leonard, 1991). For example, people who are living in poverty may experience their lives as a daily struggle to satisfy basic needs (food from foodbanks), relieve stress (a cigarette butt to smoke), or avoid hazards in the environment (gangs, thieves, police).

Phenomenology provides community health nurses a lens through which to understand the world from the viewpoint of clients. The nurse asks clients to speak of their experiences, listens carefully, and avoids translating the story into nurse language or jumping in with interpretations. The nurse may learn that the idea of impoverishment as avoidable may not be part of the lived experience of poverty. From this place of understanding, meaningful work with clients can begin. Thus, that which is sometimes called "the apathy of the poor" can be reconceptualized into the need to create possibilities.

The experience of being listened to and understood is

a powerful one that validates and strengthens clients (Attridge et al., 1997). Most practitioners would say they routinely work this way, but clients would disagree. Although it is challenging to work in this way when pressures of busy schedules and agency policies impinge, doing so is essential. Using phenomenological theory in programming can help the nurse understand the experiences of the different people who compose a community and a programming team. Effective action is based on understanding (Covey, Merrill, & Merrill, 1997).

Feminist Theory

Feminist theories provide a lens through which socially constructed inequities based on gender can be seen and challenged (Bent, 1993). For example, when poverty is examined as a gendered situation, research reveals that poverty is not equally distributed among males and females and that the causal patterns as well as the impacts and the responses of others such as social organizations are different. Gendered beliefs are embedded in the operation of social, educational (including family), political, and legal institutions around the world. Some gendered practices are harmful to a particular gender, such as the practice in some countries of males' eating before females, leaving females inadequately nourished and at risk, especially during childbearing.

Bateson (1990) points out that certain gendered knowledge is health promoting and may be helpful to the other gender. For example, women's greater experience with balancing multiple commitments and handling discontinuities and diversities (as a result of their family and work roles) makes them a source of knowledge about interdependence and flexibility. Often, there is value in critical examination from the perspective of each gender.

> Many women raised in male dominated cultures have to struggle against the impulse to sacrifice their health for the health of the other. But many men raised in the same traditions have to struggle against pervasive imageries in which their own health or growth is a victory achieved at the expense of the other (p. 240).

Programming based on gender-sensitive research can take into account the different experiences of males and females, and more helpful programs can be designed (Van Norstrand, 1993). Feminism challenges community health nurses, first, to question the influence of gender in a given situation (in combination with other categorizations such as culture, age, size, sexual orientation, ability, and the like); second, to determine whether the influence is benefiting or harming the health of the various people involved; and, third, to support beneficial influences and reduce influences embodying harmful inequities.

Critical Social Theory

Critical social theory is a lens that focuses on the transformation of existing social orders with the intent of promoting greater freedom, equality, and social justice. Social orders determine: the distribution of wealth and work, including that work which does not count (e.g., housework); access to resources such as education, health care, and law enforcement; and media images about various groups including religious, ethnic, family, age, and the like (Habermas, as cited in Stevens, 1989). There is no one critical social theory. Rather, from systematic social critique by those who are in oppressed positions, critical theories are developed relevant to the specific position (e.g., from experience with racism, poverty, environmental destruction, homophobia, or gender bias) (Kendall, 1992).

The domination and privileges of one group over another often are assumed to be natural or "just the way it is." For example, the work of one health care discipline may be taken for granted to be more important than the work of another; the existence of poverty may be viewed as a natural phenomenon or the result of an inadequate work ethic; the superior socioeconomic status of one race or class over another may be assumed to be the result of natural superiority; and the protest that industry cannot switch to environmentally safe production methods without shattering the local, national, or global economy may be viewed as a basic truth. Historical and cultural comparisons can help uncover the roots and development of dominant social constructions.

Use of a critical social theory lens invites the nurse to ask questions:

- *To expose existing social formations*: Whose voice is heard? Not heard? Is my voice heard? What is frustrating or contradictory in my position?
- *To raise questions about those interests that are served and not served by these social formations:* Who benefits? Who does not benefit?
- *To explore the way social formations are produced and reproduced:* What is actually taught in families? In schools? In health care agencies?
- *To create images of new possibilities:* What would "better" look like?
- *To identify actions through which transformation can be achieved*: What must happen to create "better"? (Bassett-Smith, 1997)

Dialogue (mutual interaction) and consciousness raising are part of critical theorizing. The social critique does not end at the point of blaming the oppressor or the oppressed but at the place of challenging and changing the rules that support the undesirable imbalance in power. Use of critical social theory is an optimistic act that enables nurses and communities to see the established order of society as only one way the world can be constructed and to appreciate and use the power they have to transform their worlds for the better (Hagedorn, 1995; Bassett-Smith, 1997).

Caring, phenomenological, feminist, and critical social theories can assist community health nurses to achieve Health for All goals in their programming work. These theories offer explanations about how meaningful connections can be made with people having diverse characteristics, how people experience the world, and how people hold different truths and ideas about that which is desirable and that which is possible. Further, use of these theories can raise awareness about barriers to health and can facilitate health-promoting action.

Change Theories

Other theories useful in programming are change theories. Programs always have some level of change as a goal: individual, family, group, organization, community, societal. Programs often are directed at more than one level of change. For example, a program aimed at assisting teenage mothers and fathers may include change at the individual level to increase the mothers' and fathers' interpersonal and parenting knowledge and skills; change at the family and group levels to build mutual support and problem solving; and change at the organizational, community, and societal levels to provide employment and housing that enables teenage parents to care for their chil-

dren while completing school, participating in neighborhood support networks, and working for pay via flexible arrangements with employers and social agencies. Societal change is connected to public policy and politics (see Chapter 31). Change theories are interspersed throughout this text. Of particular interest in this chapter are change that is emancipatory or empowering and change at the community level.

Transtheoretical and Relapse-Prevention Models of Change

The nurse will encounter many programs aimed toward individual change, often as components of larger community change programs. Social learning and cognitive theories inform the transtheoretical (Prochaska, Redding, Harlow, Rossi, & Velicer, 1994) and relapse-prevention (Marlatt & Gordan, 1985) models of individual change (see Figures 13-4 and 13-5). Learning is viewed as occurring when individuals interact with others, and challenges arise when individuals work to change behavior patterns that have been constructed and maintained through social interaction.

In the transtheoretical change model, the individual moves from not thinking about change in the near future, to seriously thinking about change (in the next six months), to actively planning changes, to overtly making changes and taking steps to maintain changes and avoid relapse (McKenzie & Smeltzer, 1997). Relapse is common, but the opportunity is there for another change effort, hence the spiral diagram. Individuals can identify where they are at in the model, and strategies to assist them can be designed accordingly.

According to the relapse-prevention model because relapse is common in health behavior change, the programmer needs to prepare individuals for the possibility of relapse and teach them how to avoid relapse and, in

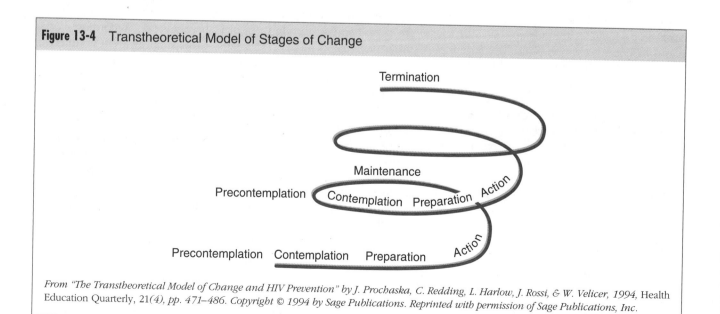

Figure 13-4 Transtheoretical Model of Stages of Change

From "The Transtheoretical Model of Change and HIV Prevention" by J. Prochaska, C. Redding, L. Harlow, J. Rossi, & W. Velicer, 1994, Health Education Quarterly, 21(4), pp. 471–486. Copyright © 1994 by Sage Publications. Reprinted with permission of Sage Publications, Inc.

Figure 13-5   Relapse-Prevention Model

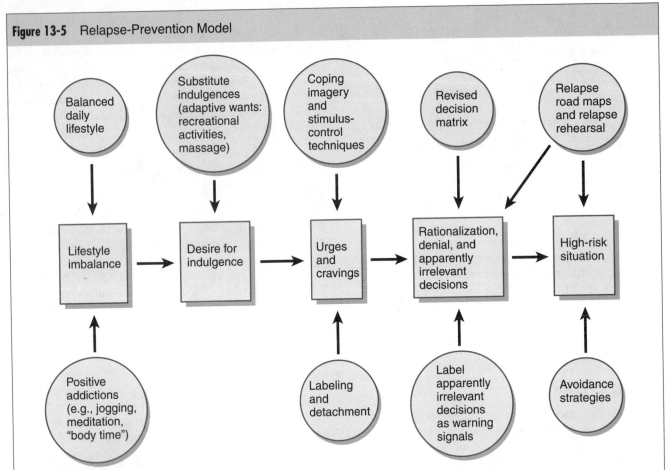

From: "Relapse Prevention: Theoretical Rationale and Overview of the Model" by G. Marlatt, 1985. In G. Marlatt & J. Gordon (Eds.), Relapse Prevention (p. 61), New York: Guilford Press. Copyright 1985 by Guilford Press. Reprinted by permission of Guilford Publications, Inc.

case of relapse, how to get back on track without guilt or giving up. Possible global self-control strategies are identified in the circles of the model, in correspondence with specific experiences of the individual, identified in rectangles. Use of the model is intended to improve personal knowledge and skills so that individuals are prepared to cope well with typical experiences as they try to develop healthier behaviors. Therefore global strategies need to be translated into specific strategies for individuals. Role playing, relaxation and imaging techniques, contracts and reminder cards have been used to help individuals develop personally relevant self-control strategies. Those individuals who have made changes are often very helpful in assisting others to change (ripple effect).

The transtheoretical and relapse-prevention models both involve critical awareness and skill building at each stage and are cyclical. Individuals may move through the stages several times before their lifestyle patterns are as they want them to be. The use of these theories can be empowering when a program incorporates a critique of societal influences along with the strengthening of individual competence as long as individuals are neither pressured nor blamed.

Diffusion Theory

Diffusion theory provides a useful lens through which to view group, organizational, and population change. The theory explains the way that information and change spread through populations unevenly. According to diffusion theory, systematic processes (awareness, interest, trial, and adoption) are engaged in sequentially by different segments of the population (Rogers, 1983, as cited in Dignan, Tillgren, & Michieulutte, 1994). Change is seen as progressing in an approximately normal bell-shaped curve from innovators (risk takers), to early adopters (respected opinion leaders), to early majority adopters (deliberators), to late majority adopters (responders to the norm), to laggards (marginalized people or cynics). Diffusion processes are enhanced when people are aware of the advantages of the change, are provided opportunities to explore the compatibility of new and current practices, are supported in adopting change, and are offered opportunities for trial and modification (Parcel, Perry, & Taylor, 1990).

Implications for programmers are that different approaches must be used to reach (i.e., establish meaning for) different segments of the population at different times. For example, according to the theory, innovators respond best to cognitive approaches, early majority adopters to motivational approaches, late majority adopters and laggards to reducing perceived barriers. The approaches must be timed so that each of the various segments in the population are introduced at the right time to that which is most meaningful to them. Diffusion theory can be used to guide programming aimed at multiple levels of change (e.g., adoption of healthier eating habits by high-school students, or a "healthier eating" program in a school food service, or of a Heart Smart nutritional program in restaurants across a region). Use of diffusion theory is compatible with Health for All programs when the focus is on social change as opposed to control.

Freire's Theory of Freeing

To support emancipatory change and empowerment, Freire (1970/1993), a Brazilian educator, developed a methodology of problem-posing dialogue (termed by some a theory of "freeing") intended to help people uncover the root causes of problems, see possibilities for transformative actions, and act to change social inequities rather than adapting. Practitioners around the world have found Friere's methods highly effective for helping people who are stuck in complex, disadvantaged, and marginalized situations become effective in improving their health and health-related situations. The underpinnings of critical social theory are apparent in Friere's use of "conscientisation, that is, bringing to awareness hidden power relationships and overcoming the culture of silence that accompanies oppression.

Rather than telling people what they ought to do or think, Friere invites people to engage in an egalitarian conversation (dialogue) to identify and pose questions about issues. Communities work from their own values, experiences, and definitions of situations, and practitioners work to support the process. Friere's approach may be represented as:

1. Listening to understand community issues and themes:

   • Community identifies issues; practitioners ask: "What is important to you?"
   • Practitioners learn/use the community language to depict that which is important.
2. Problem-posing dialogue:

   • The community selects codes (physical representations of the issue—stories, pictures, songs, role plays—that place the issue in social context).
   • Question posing moves from personal to social analysis; practitioners ask:
   "What do you see and feel? What is happening here?"
   "What experiences have you had with this?"
   "What are the many parts of this problem?"
   "Why does this problem exist?"
   "Can you imagine a better situation? What does it look like?"
   "What actions would create a better situation?"
3. Action and reflection:

   • Community tests out their ideas for action in the world.
   • Community reflects on their action.
   • Action and reflection become a deepening spiral over time as the community works to change complex, embedded problems. (Wallerstein & Bernstein, 1988; Bassett-Smith, 1997; Verhey, 1997)

Community Organization

Community organization, a muiltifaceted theoretical approach to promoting change at the community level, incorporates many of the concepts of interest to nurses. Community organizing has a long history, originating in situations where adverse social conditions prompted the formation of coalitions to create systemwide change. Lillian Wald's work in the late 1800s with the settlement house population of New York constitutes one example of the way that community nurses can use community organization to dramatically improve the health of a community.

Community organization, a term coined by social workers, represents a collection of principles and methods for influencing change (Drevdahl, 1995). Rothman and Tropman (1987, as cited in Minkler, 1990) developed

DECISION MAKING

Top-Down and Grassroots Processes

You work for an agency that offers a program for teen mothers. You have been given an educational plan with corresponding videos and handouts covering topics such as baby development, feeding, crying, birth control, and the like. At the first meeting of the program, you ask the mothers about their interests and issues. Your focus is on ensuring that everyone gets to speak and be understood. The teens talk about always being "on call" and having no social life. They also speak of being worried about money and whether they will ever get off social assistance. After the meeting, you realized that you had not covered the educational plan.

• Using Friere's ideas, how might you continue to facilitate the process in the meetings so that the teens' priorities guide the group?

• How might you support the development of their competence?

• How will you explain your choices to your employer/supervisor?

a classic typology of three models of community organization: locality development (commonly called community development), social planning, and social action. Incorporated, in varying degrees, are the concepts of participation (people working together), relevance (starting where people are), and empowerment (increasing community choice and competence). Each model is associated with different change strategies and roles for health care practitioners (see Table 13-2).

Social planning is the most "top-down" of the models. In this model, much of the planning work is carried out by practitioners. Issues may be identified by the practitioner rather than (or, sometimes, in addition to) the community. The process is one of rational problem solving based on empirical data and expert technical assistance. Social planning is a familiar model in public health programs based on a population-focused, epidemiologic problem-solving approach. Many programs offered by community nurses, are based on a social planning model. For example, in well baby programs topics and activities may be largely predetermined by practitioners, who gather and analyze data about the baby and parenting and design interventions accordingly. The process whereby community nurses advocate for babies (child protection) while maintaining caring, empowering relationships with parents (parenting support) has been described as a "figurative dance" and "exquisitely complex" (Zerwekh, 1992, pp. 102, 104) .

Community development and social action models are more grassroots, or "bottom up"; in other words, the community identifies the issues, is fully involved in decision making throughout all processes, and most often determines the processes. Practitioners may teach community people needed skills so that they can act on their own behalf. Community development is intended to bring people together to solve community problems and build community competence, consensus, and a sense of community. Social action is the most political of the models, with the intent of action being inequity correction, institutional change, and power redistribution. In using community organization, Drevdahl (1995) cautions:

> When professionals initiate a program they may think, "How can I get you (the community members) to participate in what I want to achieve?" This reasoning is antithetical to community organization tenets when the objective is to examine relationships of power and create opportunities for community change (p. 16).

Community nurses are exploring the potential of community organization models and meeting with impressive successes (English, 1995) as well as some frustrations (Chalmers & Bramadat, 1996). Employing agencies and program funders sometimes want greater up-front specification of program goals, timelines, and quantifiable results than is possible with minimally pre-structured models of programming, such as community development and social action. Also, the targets for change under the social action model may be either the agency (or government) that employs the nurse or powerful organizations in the community (e.g., a factory polluting or a gang terrorizing a neighborhood). These situations create conflict and in some cases result in sanctions against involvement. Other confounding factors may arise from the need for confidentiality versus the open information sharing inherent in participatory processes, and from the nurse's personal desire for control or discomfort with conflict. Despite these challenges, community organizing "shows promise as an important mechanism to promote community health" (Chalmers & Bramadat, 1996, p. 725).

In programming practice, community organization models often are blended to address the multiple factors influencing the health of a community. Of importance is

Table 13-2 Community Organization Models

	COMMUNITY DEVELOPMENT	SOCIAL PLANNING	SOCIAL ACTION
Categories of community action	Self-help; community capacity and integration (process goals)	Problem solving with regard to substantive community problems (task goals)	Shifting of power relationships and resources; basic institutional change (task or process goals)
Practitioner roles	Enabler, catalyst, facilitator, teacher	Fact gatherer and analyst, program implementer	Activist, advocate, negotiator
Change strategies	Building community connection and caretaking	Planned change, social marketing, health education	Political action, lobbying, confrontation
Primary definer of issues and actions	Community (practitioner input)	Practitioner (community input)	Community (practitioner input)

From "Models of Community Organization & Macro Practice: Their Mixing and Phasing" by J. Rothman & J. Tropman as cited in "Improving Health through Community Organization" by M. Minkler, 1990. In K. Glanz, F. M. Lewis, & B. K. Rimer (Eds.), Health Behavior and Health Education *(pp. 264–265), San Francisco: Jossey Bass. Copyright 1987 by Itasca County Historical Society. Adapted by permission of the publisher, F. E. Peacock Publishers Inc., Itasca, Illinois.*

that nurses use these models, as well as other models and theories, on the basis of thoughtful judgment regarding that which would be most helpful to the community. Although nurses may feel passionately about a particular model or theory, being dogmatic is not useful.

Community Organization in Action: Planned Approaches to Community Health (PATCH) and Healthy Cities/Communities

Two examples of community organizing associated with the Health for All movement are the Planned Approach to Community Health (PATCH) and Healthy Cities/Communities programs. The PATCH programs are sponsored by the Centers for Disease Control and Prevention (CDC) in the United States to promote partnerships among the CDC, local communities, and state and local health agencies to plan, implement, and maintain local health-promotion programs (Goodman, Steckler, Hoover, & Schwartz, 1993). The PATCH programs use a social planning approach that incorporates some features of community development. Communities develop advisory committees with representatives from agencies and the public. The CDC provides training and technical assistance so that the advisory committee can conduct structured interviews with identified community leaders and assess needs using an established behavioral risk survey oriented to major chronic diseases. The committee collects and analyzes data, designates priority health issues, and designs and implements interventions to improve health in these areas.

Many PATCH programs have been implemented and evaluated throughout the United States. Results from an evaluation of 27 programs (Steckler, Orville, Eng, & Dawson, 1992) were that awareness of health issues increased; programs were implemented that otherwise would not have been; communication between agencies and the CDC improved; participants wanted more information sharing with other PATCH programs; and agency participants reported improvements in their skills, whereas public participants reported becoming more informed about their communities. Not surprising, but of concern, was the additional finding that the risk survey was too complex for the community partners to deal with, and it directed attention to predetermined health problems, which were not necessarily of primary interest to the community. The evaluators further concluded that funding and technical support were insufficient throughout to fully support program goals. Overall, participants expressed enthusiasm for PATCH but noted difficulty in maintaining the considerable commitment required.

Commenting on these PATCH evaluations, Green and Kreuter (1993) suggest that future technical tasks be done by professionals. Tensions such as those that arose around the use of the predetermined risk survey are common with social planning approaches. Local people are most keen to participate when issues have personal meaning for them (community development), whereas health professionals may be assigned responsibility for preventing and controlling the most prevalent population health problems as determined by epidemiologic data (social planning). Green and Krueter question, "Is it necessary for us to create an integrated model that intertwines these two divergent approaches through all aspects of the planning and implementation process?" (p. 221). One might further ask, "Is this possible?"

In operation worldwide are WHO-inspired Healthy Cities/Communities programs (Baum, 1993; Flynn, Ray, & Rider, 1994; Ouellet, Durand, & Forget, 1994). These programs are based on community development and social action models. Related successes have been credited to the wide general appeal of the concept and the use of strategies that promote intersectoral collaboration, local participation, shared vision, and community ownership. Program foci and processes are determined by the participants.

The Healthy Cities/Communities initiative has stimulated a diverse range of programs that are meaningful to specific communities and "potentially effective in addressing risk conditions that predetermine the risk factors for disease" (e.g., making public parks safer, refitting a town water system, and the like) (Higgins & Green, 1994, p. 318). Difficulties arise when funders from the health sector want to see measurable reductions in disease risk factors (which the programs are not immediately geared toward) and measurable improvements in health (although tools for measuring "broadly defined" health are not well developed). Funders from sectors other than health have other interests that must be addressed. Programmers may not be able to bridge the gap between that which the program can realistically affect and that which funders recognize as worthy. As a result of such difficulties, the federal Healthy Communities program in Canada lost its funding in 1991 (Manson-Singer, 1994).

Another challenge for Healthy Cities/Communities programs is that social action naturally gives rise to conflict between competing interests of the powerful and less powerful (e.g., developers' wanting land rezoned for building versus parents' wanting a park for youth recreation). In addition, local issues often are affected by external forces such as national policies or multinational corporations (Higgins & Green, 1994). Because the vision of Healthy Cities/Communities programs has public appeal, those who do not want a particular change may stall and use diversionary tactics rather than being open about the conflict and thus risking political fallout. Skillful negotiation, early conflict recognition, and open conflict management have proved essential in most community organizing efforts (Flick, Reese, Rogers, Fletcher, & Sonn, 1994; Bless, Murphy, & Vinson, 1995). Sustaining Healthy Cities/Community programs takes considerable energy and political savvy; nevertheless, the concept continues to inspire commitment. The Canadian Forum on Health (Ritchie, 1997) and the Healthy People 2000 Midcourse Review (USDHHS, 1995) document the gains made through community social action and Healthy Cities/Communities programs and continue to recommend community action as a national health strategy.

PROGRAMMING THEORIES AND PRACTICALITIES

With context appreciation and an array of potentially helpful theories providing the background, the nurse is well prepared to bring programming into the foreground. Nurses may use their knowledge of context and theories to assist with both the substantive content and organizational process requirements of programming (i.e., the focus of the program and the way the program will operate). (See Figure 13-6.). Community health programs vary from being relatively simple and narrowly focused, such as a heart health program for local firefighters, to being highly complex and broadly focused, such as a Healthy Cities program. When a program is broadly focused and comprises many different components, the term *project* rather than *program* may be used; however, basic programming ideas continue to be applicable.

The language appropriate for nurses to use in programming varies depending on the participants. When a nurse is submitting a proposal to get funding support for a program from a level of government, the language used will be different from that used by a nurse working with a group of laypeople to create an action plan that everyone can follow. The nurse must therefore be "multilingual" within English (or other languages). Adjustment of language to suit the situation and participants supports primary health care and health-promotion principles and enables participation throughout programming by all stakeholders (those who are likely to be affected by the program in some way). Stakeholder participation and partnership increase the likelihood that the program will cre-

ate the desired health outcomes, including increased community competence.

Decisions about participation should be based on the community situation, the theories being used, and stakeholder preferences. To support partnership throughout the processes, planning and advisory groups of some type with representatives from all stakeholder groups may be formed, or the style may be more loosely structured (Bracht, 1990). Organizational support structures and styles of operating often change during programming to facilitate progress toward the desired results and, also, because participation may change over time.

Programming processes of planning, implementation, and evaluation are most easily described in a linear sequential format. In practice, however, these processes overlap and must be revisited often during the time span of a program. Community assessment, sometimes called community analysis, may be viewed as either a part of planning or a separate process occurring prior to planning. Evaluation, in particular, must be integrated throughout. To be done well, the processes of planning, implementation, and evaluation, like most things, require practice, particularly given the constantly changing nature of people, settings, and resources (McKenzie & Smeltzer, 1997). Nurses should anticipate ambiguity and remember that reflection and improvisation will contribute to clarity and direction.

Programming Models

Programming models are representations of approaches to programming that offer explanations of the processes involved. To provide guidance throughout programming processes, communities and nurses together may either create their own model or choose to use an already tested programming or planning model. Sometimes a model is recommended by a funding agency. Numerous choices are available in the literature. Because all models are based on values and assumptions, the nurse should ensure that the chosen model is either consistent with Health for All ideas or can be adequately adapted. Several models are described next: Two are designed to guide process decisions; two focus on decision making about program activities or content; and one focuses on both process and content. Following these descriptions is a section on some practicalities of programming.

Healthy Communities: The Process

Grassroots community development is the focus of the Healthy Communities: The Process model (British Columbia Ministry of Health, 1989). This model is useful when diverse community people come together to work on health issues; a brief manual is written in language intended to be discernable to people lacking community organizing experience. The phases of the model are entry, needs assessment, planning, doing, and renewal. The circular movement through the phases and the main tasks to

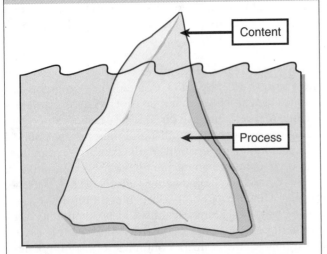

Figure 13-6 The Process–Content Iceberg

Content

Process

From Basic Concepts of International Health *(Reading Module, p. 13) by K. Wolton, H. Amit, S. Kalma, L. Hillman, D. Hillman, & N. Cosway, January 1995, Ottawa, Canada: Canadian University Consortium for Health in Development. Copyright 1995 by Canadian Society for International Health. Reprinted by permission of Canadian Society for International Health.*

be accomplished during each phase are depicted in Figure 13-7. Near the completion of each phase, a pause is recommended so that the community group can reflect on "Did we get the job done? Where are we now? What worked? What didn't and why? What next?" (p. 11).

Health Promotion at the Community Level

Bracht and Kingsbury's (1990) model for health promotion at the community level is well grounded in community organization theory (see Table 13-3). Although this model is similar to Healthy Communities: The Process, the language is intended for practitioners. The model has effectively guided extensive as well as small community programs. The five phases of the model are community analysis, design initiation, implementation, maintenance/consolidation, and dissemination/reassessment (see Figure 13-8).

Population Health-Promotion Model

The broad planning model referred to as Population Health Promotion combines the main ideas that have emerged from health-promotion and population-health theory and practice over the past two decades (Hamilton

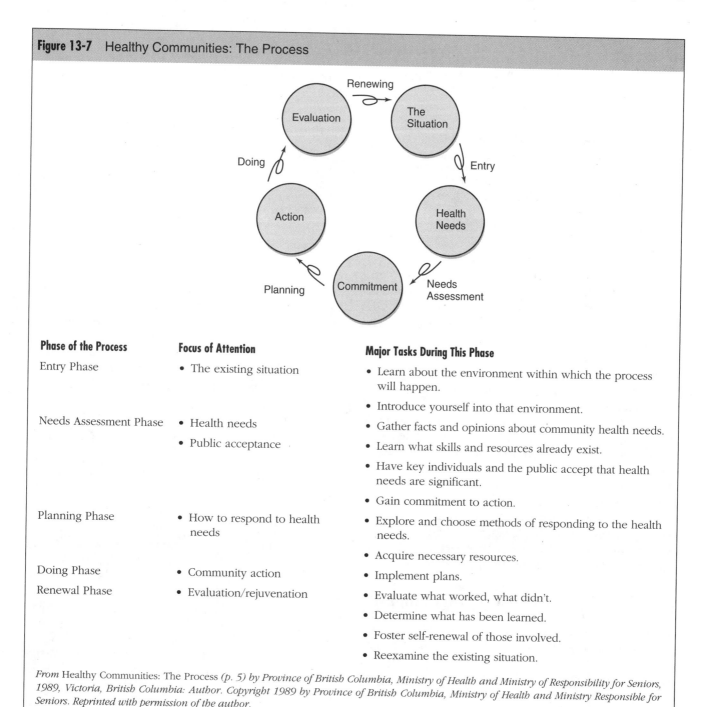

Figure 13-7 Healthy Communities: The Process

Phase of the Process	Focus of Attention	Major Tasks During This Phase
Entry Phase	• The existing situation	• Learn about the environment within which the process will happen.
		• Introduce yourself into that environment.
Needs Assessment Phase	• Health needs	• Gather facts and opinions about community health needs.
	• Public acceptance	• Learn what skills and resources already exist.
		• Have key individuals and the public accept that health needs are significant.
		• Gain commitment to action.
Planning Phase	• How to respond to health needs	• Explore and choose methods of responding to the health needs.
		• Acquire necessary resources.
Doing Phase	• Community action	• Implement plans.
Renewal Phase	• Evaluation/rejuvenation	• Evaluate what worked, what didn't.
		• Determine what has been learned.
		• Foster self-renewal of those involved.
		• Reexamine the existing situation.

From Healthy Communities: The Process *(p. 5) by Province of British Columbia, Ministry of Health and Ministry of Responsibility for Seniors, 1989, Victoria, British Columbia: Author. Copyright 1989 by Province of British Columbia, Ministry of Health and Ministry Responsible for Seniors. Reprinted with permission of the author.*

Table 13-3 Guiding Principles for Health-Promotion Organizing

- Planning must be based on a historical understanding of the community. Conditions that inhibit or facilitate interventions must be assessed.

- Because the issue or problem is usually one of multiple (rather than single) causality, a comprehensive effort using multiple interventions is required.

- It is important to focus on community context and to work primarily through existing structures and values.

- Active community participation, not mere token representation, is desired.

- For the project to be effective, intersectoral components of the community must work together to address the problem in a comprehensive effort.

- The focus must be on both long-term and short-term problem solving if the change is to endure beyond the project's demonstration period.

- Finally, and most important, the community must share responsibility for the problem and for its solution.

From "Community Organization Principles in Health Promotion: A Five Stage Model" by N. Bracht & L. Kingsbury, 1990. In N. Bracht (Ed.), Health Promotion at the Community Level (p. 74), Newbury Park, CA: Sage. Copyright © 1990 by Sage Publications. Reprinted by permission of Sage Publications, Inc.

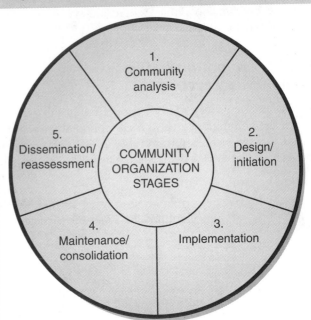

Figure 13-8 Model of Community Organization Stages

From "Community Organization Principles in Health Promotion: A Five Stage Model" by N. Bracht & L. Kingsbury, 1990. In N. Bracht (Ed.), Health Promotion at the Community Level (p. 74), Newbury Park, CA: Sage. Copyright © 1990, Sage Publications. Reprinted by permission of Sage Publications, Inc.

& Bhatti, 1996) (see Figure 13-9). The model guides program content decisions; that is, it answers the questions "On what should we take action?" "How should we take action?" and "With whom should we act?" (p. 6). The model is new and, therefore, has not been extensively tested; it is appealing, however, because of its integration of Health for All concepts and strategies. Depicted in the cubic-style model are health determinants, health-promotion strategies, and levels at which action can be taken (Epp, 1986; WHO, 1986). A short manual gives multiple examples of ways the model can be used to create a program, starting from a health determinant, health concern, specific population, or at-risk group (see Figure 13-10). Some community health providers have redesigned the Population Health-Promotion Model by converting the cube into a North American native medicine wheel style (nesting circles) and adding gender and culture as health determinants (Health & Community Services, 1998.) Manuals and a colorful mobile model are available.

Diagrammatic Models for Programming

If a program is defined as a collection of activities designed to produce particular results, it is reasonable that diagramming that which is envisioned would be helpful to those involved. Diagrammatic models show via graphic designs how program components are related to produce desired results. The exercise of creating the diagrams (sometimes called maps) brings people together to think through on paper the relationships among goals, program activities, and predicted outcomes. The values, assumptions, and hypotheses shaping the program can thus be made more visible. Choices can then be made about those things that should and should not be included (program content). Examples of diagramming approaches are modeling (Budgen, 1987) and logic charts (Wong-Reiger & David, 1995).

Modeling, based on systems theory, was originally developed for educational programs (Borich & Jemelka, 1982). A series of sketches are used to diagram inputs (basic requirements for the program to work), activities (events intended to produce change), modifiers (factors that affect program activities and, thus, influence outcomes for better or worse), and outcomes (the changes following from program activities) (see Figure 13-11). In accordance with force field analysis theory, modifiers may be conceptualized as restraining and driving forces, respectively hindering and helping a particular change (Brager & Halloway, 1978, cited in Bracht, 1990, p. 75).

Program logic charts are another way to show the relationships between program activities and outcomes. Wong-Reiger and David (1995) suggest working backward, from the long-term desired outcomes, to intermediate outcomes that indicate progress, to program activities (see Figure 13-12).

Outcomes produced by the program should be related directly to the situation (i.e., the issues, values, needs, or goals) that gave rise to the program. When predicting outcomes, the programmer must carefully consider the

Figure 13-9   Population Health-Promotion Model

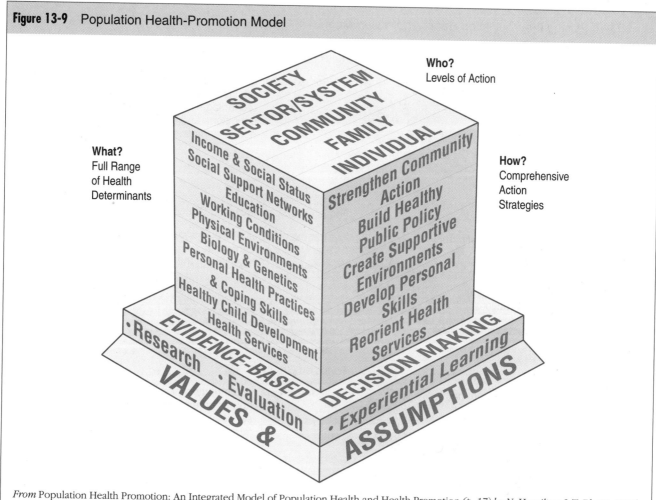

From Population Health Promotion: An Integrated Model of Population Health and Health Promotion (p. 17) by N. Hamilton & T. Bhatti, 1996, Ottawa, Canada: Health Promotion Development Division. Copyright 1996 by Health Promotion Development Division, Health Canada, Ottawa, Canada. Reprinted with permission of Health Canada.

strength of program activities; it is tempting for the novice to expect too much from small programs (e.g., to prevent teen smoking via a two-hour educational program). After program components have been identified, the relationships among them are mapped; in instances where relationships are not sound, changes in components are made. Also, gaps or extensive overlaps between desired outcomes and activities are eliminated.

Use of diagrammatic models can expedite understanding of the program by funders and others. The language can be adjusted to suit the audience. Several diagrams may be drawn for a program, starting with general program components and moving to greater specificity as needed. For example, a program for people experiencing family violence might include components of education and support for women, children, and men; coalition work with community groups and agencies to increase shelter facilities; and collaboration with police to ensure protection. The overall program as well as each of the components may be diagrammed. Funders may appreciate diagrams at the most general level; practitioners and others may prefer more specific diagrams.

Although the primary intent of diagrammatic models is

to make clear the connections between values, goals, program activities, and outcomes, other relevant program dimensions may be included for practical purposes. For example, specific resource requirements may be noted (e.g., 20 hours of nursing, space for group meetings, 60 handouts), and the power, or "dose," of activities may be shown (e.g., two-hour support group once a week for six weeks). Program costs are then easy to estimate, and, if the evaluation shows that the outcomes are positive but not to the extent desired, a power increase may be recommended (e.g., extending the support group to 12 weeks or making it ongoing).

Logic charts, program models, and other diagrams such as conceptual maps may be created in many forms for planning purposes, updated later as programming progresses, and used finally to guide evaluation. Cartoonlike sketches are sometimes helpful in depicting the human experiences represented within the diagrams. Of importance is not the form of the diagrams per se, but that the diagrams visually depict that which is planned, is happening, or has happened. Constructing diagrams in conjunction with community participants promotes clarity, shared vision, and ownership.

Figure 13-10 Using the Population Health-Promotion Model

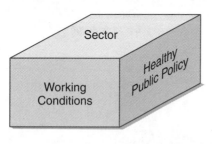

Focus on the Determinants of Health

For example, industry can examine the effects of emerging technologies on working conditions and can adopt health-enhancing options.

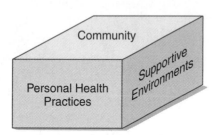

Focus on a Specific Health Concern

For example, schools and workplaces can make nutritious foods available in their cafeterias.

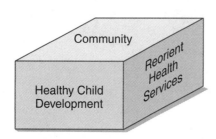

Focus on Group at Risk

For example, community clinics can make appropriate primary care services accessible to young families.

From Population Health Promotion: An Integrated Model of Population Health and Health Promotion *(p. 17) by N. Hamilton & T. Bhatti, 1996, Ottawa, Canada: Health Promotion Development Division. Copyright 1996 by Health Promotion Development Division, Health Canada, Ottawa, Canada. Reprinted with permission of Health Canada.*

Figure 13-11 Modeling: A Group Support Program

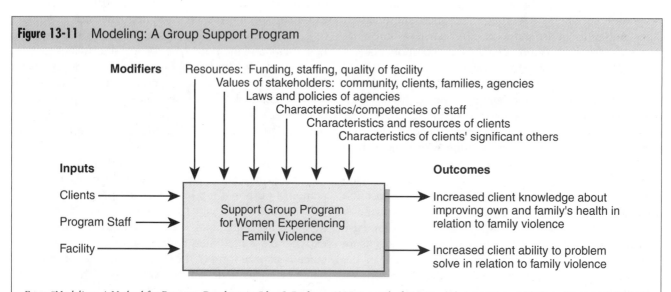

From "Modeling: A Method for Program Development" by C. Budgen, 1987, Journal of Nursing Administration, *17(12), p. 22. Copyright 1987 by Lippencott-Raven. Adapted by permission of Lippincott-Raven Publishers.*

Figure 13-12   Logic Model for Public Awareness Program

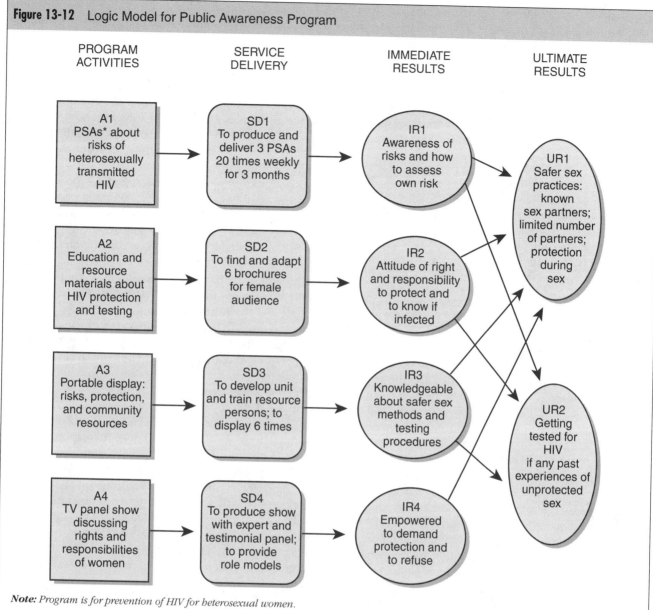

Note: Program is for prevention of HIV for heterosexual women.

*PSA means public service announcement.

From "Using Program Logic Models to Plan and Evaluate Education and Prevention Programs" by D. Wong-Rieger & L. David, 1995. In A. Love (Ed.), Evaluation Methods Sourcebook II (p. 122), Ottawa, Canada: Canadian Evaluation Society. Copyright 1995 by Canadian Evaluation Society. Adapted by permission of Canadian Evaluation Society.

PRECEDE–PROCEED

The PRECEDE–PROCEED model (Green & Kreuter, 1991) is a comprehensive social planning framework that has been used in a myriad of ways to guide the planning, implementation, and evaluation of numerous large and small health programs (see Chapter 11). Social, behavioral, epidemiologic, educational, organizational, policy, and administrative dimensions are analyzed; diagnoses are made; and multilevel strategies are designed to improve health status and quality of life. Subjective quality of life is placed ahead of objective health status. The

long-term use of the model has permitted refinement. For example, PATCH programs were based on PRECEDE, and the results led to the development of PROCEED.

Program Planning

Whether a specific programming model or a more ad hoc approach is used, the nurse will benefit from additional organizational skills and knowledge about ways to actualize programs. The subsequent several sections focus on the practicalities of planning, implementation, and evaluation, with Health for All theory providing an underlay.

Program planning is the process of identifying the situation, deciding on a more desirable situation, and designing actions to create the desirable situation. The nurse who is new to programming may be impatient to proceed to the "action" and do something about that which from the nurse's point of view is an obvious health problem or issue. But planning is action and

should not be considered simply as a prelude to . . . action, although it does play a vital role in this respect. Not only does it have its own (intervention) implications, it is a process that continues through all action phases, making a total programme more purposeful, giving it a greater direction, increasing its amenability to control, and yielding a clearer vision of its effectiveness (Steuart, 1959/1993, p. S22).

An analogy can be made between planning a health program and creating an architectural design for a building. The more carefully the architects consult with the people for whom the building is being constructed, the greater the likelihood that the building will be satisfactory to those people. The more clearly specified the vision of that which is wanted, the more likely the vision's realization. Although it is impossible to anticipate and plan ahead for everything, the more thoroughly the components are detailed, and possible pitfalls are anticipated, the greater the chance that the actual building process will proceed smoothly and the building will meet the needs of the clients. Also, the more the architects attend to the physical and social environments where the building is to be located, the more likely the building to be compatible with the environment, appreciated by the neighbors, and viewed as an overall positive addition to the neighborhood. It is much the same with program planning.

To carry the analogy a bit further, if a social planning approach were to be used, the architects might bring one or several building plans for consideration, oversee the project, and provide expert assistance; the people for whom the building is being constructed might, in turn, suggest alterations and provide information about preferred choices throughout. In a community development approach, the architects might work to assist the people to plan and build the building themselves and provide assistance as needed and as negotiated. In a social action approach, the architects might join with the people in lobbying to get resources and to change zoning in a neighborhood so that the desired and needed building can be constructed in the location where it is most needed.

Community Analysis

What is the situation?

Planning basically consists of identifying the situation, deciding on a more desirable situation, and designing actions to create the desirable situation. In nursing language, this translates to assessment, issue identification

(diagnosis), clarification of goals, and creation of actions or intervention strategies to achieve the goals. Again, it is important to remember that in actual situations, these processes are intertwined; and depending on the situation, the community and nurse may start with an issue, goal, idea for action, or assessment and work in a circular fashion to complete the picture. For example, a community group may ask the nurse for assistance to decrease violence (goal), implement a heart health program (action), or assess the community in order to establish health-planning priorities.

Community analysis or assessment for programming purposes may thus be done in a comprehensive, largely "up front" way or in more targeted or ongoing ways as people come together to plan and more information is needed. Assessment frameworks are developed from particular perspectives. Assessment consistent with Health for All strategies focuses on community competence as much as (or more than) needs. And, of course, the community and the nurse work in partnership to determine ways and times to best accomplish assessments. McKnight and Kretzmann (1992) describe ways to map community capacity so that communities can be built "from the inside out," thereby increasing community competence rather than community dependence on outside services.

In the United States, the Assessment Protocol for Excellence in Public Health (APEX/PH) tool was developed by local health departments in response to the recommendation that all departments regularly and systematically evaluate community needs (McKenzie & Smeltzer, 1997). Currently, an environmental addendum is being piloted. The APEX/PH tool has been used extensively to collect communitywide data that can provide valuable information for community health programs. Similar data sources are available in many countries. Chapter 12 includes a comprehensive discussion of community assessment.

Identifying Issues

What is important?

Whose views have been heard?

Whose views have not been heard?

What issue is most important at this time?

What are the parts of the issue?

Why does the issue exist?

Issues of interest or concern must be identified. Friere's problem-posing dialogue can be helpful for doing so, especially if the participants are struggling to identify the determinants of an issue. When a more desirable situation is envisioned, action plans (community development and social action language) or intervention strategies (social planning language) can then be developed to change the current situation.

Planning should not proceed unless there is strong consensus within the community that the issue in question is a priority. Because communities often are not homogeneous, achieving a shared view may take time. Nurses sometimes are sent to a community to address an issue or problem that has been identified outside the community; for example, a nurse working for a public health service may be asked to develop an immunization program or a wellness program for teens. Dialogue around any such issue must occur to foster community ownership of the issue and the solutions. Often, a nurse or agency issue is intertwined with an issue of priority to the community. After the community connects with an issue, the community and nurse can proceed to work together. If the community does not connect with an externally identified issue, the nurse must either drop or delay that issue and instead address the priorities of the community. Why should the community become involved with something that is not important to them?

Information-generating strategies that nurses can use in assisting a community to clarify and rank issues include community forums, focus groups, nominal group processes, Delphi techniques, key informant interviews, and surveys (Dignan & Carr, 1992; McKenzie & Smeltzer, 1997) (see also Chapter 12). These strategies also can be used to uncover community views on program goals and preferred actions to achieve those goals. There is no one right way to use these strategies. For example, nominal group process can be particularly helpful when consensus decisions must be made at a community meeting by people who have varying levels of skill at expressing themselves in groups. One way of using nominal group process is to ask the group to brainstorm by having each person contribute an idea (possibly in round robin style) until everyone has exhausted all their ideas. During brainstorming, the group is encouraged not to censor any ideas but, rather, to bring forward as many ideas as possible. All ideas are written down (e.g., on chalkboards or large paper fastened to the wall). After brainstorming, time is taken for people to clarify (but not debate) the proposed ideas. Everyone is then invited to vote for the ideas that they think are priorities (or best action strategies). Voting can be achieved by giving everyone a marker or a predetermined number of stickers and asking them to mark ideas as they walk around the room during a refreshment break. The priority ideas are then discussed, and plans are developed. Remaining ideas are recorded for possible consideration another time.

The Delphi technique is a multistep survey method that is useful for identifying issues of importance and achieving consensus when it is not practical for people to meet face to face. Advantages are that input is obtained via regular or electronic mail and everyone is given equal chances for input without undue influence from other participants. A limitation is that participants must be comfortable with reading and writing and prompt about returning mail. Participants receive initial questions, data are analyzed, results (issues identified and rankings) and any new questions arising are returned to participants for further comment, and so on, until adequate information and consensus are obtained (Green & Kreuter, 1991). Sometimes a planning group generates the first list of issues; other times, one or two broad questions are asked: for example, What are the most important health issues in your community? and Why do these issues exist? Following the Delphi, program planning proceeds around the top ranked issues. By regular mail approximately 45 days are required for three survey rounds; occasionally more rounds are needed (Dignan & Carr, 1992; see Clark, Beddome, & Whyte, 1993, for an example).

The people who are hardest to reach are sometimes neglected in the planning phase These people, who often do not come to events such as community forums, may be the most marginalized or at risk—and may be the people whom the program is most intended to benefit. Bracht (1990) argues that it is the practitioner who finds it "hard to hear" rather than the client who is "hard to reach" (p. 256). Whatever must be done to make early, meaningful connections with these people should be done. Much time has been wasted planning programs for people who have not participated in the process, with program failure a common result. Skelton (1994) speaks of empowerment in terms of the power of voice and exit: that is, being heard and leaving or not participating. From this point of view, nonparticipation may be seen as positive for the participants and as requiring a change in the nurse's approach. If the planning phase is not appropriately welcoming for people, why should they later be receptive to intervention strategies?

A method of fostering participation (and voice) among seniors was incorporated in one community development project, in which one of the authors (Cameron) participated. A steering committee with a balance of seniors and practitioners was formed. Community forums were held in settings frequented by seniors. Those who came to community forums were invited to join a networking process whereby they designed questions, practiced interviewing, and then went into the community to interview other seniors. Through snowball sampling, interviewees suggested additional names of people who had not participated (for example, housebound seniors). The interviewers were paid as research assistants from a government grant. Opportunities for empowerment and increased community competence among seniors are apparent in this method, and, not surprisingly, meaningful information was gained about seniors' views and wishes (goals).

Clarifying Goals

What would be a more desirable situation?
What do we want to happen?

Communities sometimes express their goals broadly. For example, the community may want children to grow up healthier. In this case, further exploration is required to identify factors that are influencing the situation (e.g., poor food or a lack of safe places to play and learn). Sometimes called targeted assessment, this more specific exploration ensures that action strategies can be sensitively designed to achieve desired results. Action strategies are different depending on the determinants. More specific and detailed subgoals (termed objectives in social planning language) can provide better direction for the action plan (e.g., to provide adequate daily nutrition for all children). Although familiarity with this more formal programming language is a necessity, the nurse must not use such language in a way that obscures meaning for those involved. Program goals and objectives become the intended results (see the discussion on diagrammatic models).

Program subgoals, or objectives, may be devised for all factors that influence an issue, thereby interconnecting the subgoals with the achievement of the overall goals. Priorities can then be established relative to importance and resource availability. In doing so, it is helpful to consider both significance and likelihood of achieving success. The first objective may be to identify and mobilize resources. When possible, objectives are phrased to specify the desired results, those persons being targeted, and the time frame. Early in programming, striving for this degree of specificity may not be helpful, for example, in community development programs. After goals and objectives are established to the degree of specificity appropriate, alternative strategies for achieving them are considered and, finally, actions are selected for implementation.

For U.S. nurses, the national goals and objectives outlined in the Healthy People 2000 document (Stoto, Behrens, & Rosemont, 1990) and the Healthy Communities 2000: Model Standards (American Public Health Association, 1991) are very helpful, because they target specific priority needs of the U.S. population, as identified by a cross section of practitioners and interested citizens. For example, in the area of nutrition, Healthy People 2000 has an objective to "reduce iron deficiency to less than 3 percent among children aged 1 through 4" (USDHHS, 1992, p. 94). In a community development process, the community might evaluate how well they meet national or state objectives, decide the significance of the objectives for them, and use gaps as starting points for action. Communities also could be encouraged to think about health care in a different way via introduction to the primary health care model. The *Midcourse Review* of Healthy People 2000 (USDHHS, 1995) describes many programs across the United States that are helping the country move toward Health for All goals. Nurses in other countries also may find the Healthy People 2000 documents useful because of their comprehensiveness and specificity.

Keeping information organized is an important part of programming. A chart with columns or a diagrammatic model can be used to keep track of goals, objectives, corresponding actions, and desired outcomes. The formality of the documentation will vary depending on the complexity of the program and those who will be using the chart. For example, handwritten lists or diagrams using lay terms may be appropriate for one program (e.g., a community development program for homeless children who live on the streets), whereas typewritten documents using practitioner/bureaucratic language may be appropriate for another program (e.g., a citywide program for sexually transmitted disease prevention).

Designing Actions

What should be done to create the more desirable situation?

What resources are needed, and where can they be obtained?

Who can do what?

Many choices confront nurses and communities as they decide which actions or intervention strategies will be used to achieve the desired results. Programs may include, for example, health education, environmental change, health assessment, immunization, risk screening, illness management, political action, regulatory activities, advocacy, and the like. Each of the change theories and programming models is associated with (but not limited to) particular action strategies. For example, health education and social marketing (e.g., public awareness campaigns) are associated with social planning; these strategies are used in nationwide school and media initiatives in the United States and Canada to stop drinking and driving. Social action commonly uses lobbying strategies such as letter writing and telephone campaigns to change policy, laws, and regulations. Community development uses strategies such as community forums where critical dialogue is supported.

Questions regarding appropriate strategies must be considered simultaneously with questions about resources, including people and time. This tends to be an iterative (back and forth) process involving consideration of those strategies that would likely achieve the desired results, the resources that would be required, and the likelihood of getting those resources. Adjustments are made until all three aspects are in reasonable accord. The use of diagrammatic models can be helpful in this process.

Many kinds of action strategies can be created, and imagination is an essential ingredient. Actions may be targeted to change any relevant health determinants. When nurses and their community partners find themselves at a loss to answer the question "What can be done to improve this situation?" use of the theories discussed earlier may generate possibilities. Community pressures and problems—and the efforts to improve them—are seldom unique to any one setting. Valuable ideas may be garnered by investigating the approaches being used elsewhere. Programs addressing most issues of community concern will have been previously developed, and ideas can be adapted to suit the community in question. Searching the literature is one strategy for making such connections; networking via word of mouth, the Internet, and the telephone are other strategies.

Resources, Budgets, and Feasibility

Resources should be sought both within and outside the community. Capacities within the community may be thought of as resources and, to promote community self-reliance, should be considered before looking for resources outside the community (McKnight and Kretzmann, 1992). For example, a community kitchen program to help teen parents may be well served by having experienced older people or students from a cooking school take turns teaching, rather than bringing in outside assistance. Possible sources of support both within and outside of the community include businesses, social and professional clubs, volunteers, community institutions, and agencies such as churches, schools, colleges, hospitals, and mental health and social services. People will create and mobilize resources and take on a multitude of tasks to achieve goals that are meaningful to them. And, of course, the skills and time the nurse will commit to the program must be counted. Programs involving volunteers of all sorts are becoming popular as a way to contain costs and, hopefully, support community empowerment (Hutchison & Quartaro, 1995). This is an example where the art of programming is important. To help justify the use of their valuable energy toward a given program, volunteers must benefit from their involvement in some way. The community health nurse can ask volunteers to think about those things that they would find beneficial.

To be feasible, a program must have adequate resources. Resource needs can be determined by noting the resources required next to each action strategy. Expenses can then be listed next to the resources, and a budget can be prepared. A budget lists expenses (costs for the resources required) and expected income (available funds or donations) and specifies sources. Resource documents must be updated on an ongoing basis; the complexity of such documentation varies with the nature of the program. Resource documents guide the distribution and tracking of

program resources and are also useful when applying for resources (e.g., for funding from an agency) and when compiling program reports (see Figure 13-13).

Managing Tasks and Time

Program planning must be linked with time estimates and task specification. Preliminary time frames are developed on the basis of any fixed time requirements. For example, if students are involved, note when the students must have their work completed; if elders need immunizations prior to flu season, note when the immunizations should be finished; or if an agency has provided funding for a project, note when a final report is expected. From fixed time requirements, the nurse and community can work backward to the present; if there are no time requirements, working forward from the present is possible.

Time and task management tools may be used during all phases of programming and are especially helpful when a number of people are working on different aspects of the program. All tools can be modified, for example in terms of the language used. A simple tool can be created by expanding diagrammatic models or the previously described chart that lists goals, objectives, and action strategies. Timelines indicate tasks or activities that must be done and by whom and when. Making an optimistic and an alternative timeline (if things take longer) may be wise. As with all aspects of programming, flexibility is needed in combination with goal directedness.

A commonly used time and task management tool is a Gantt chart, which has the tasks to be completed listed on the vertical axis and the time periods (days, weeks,

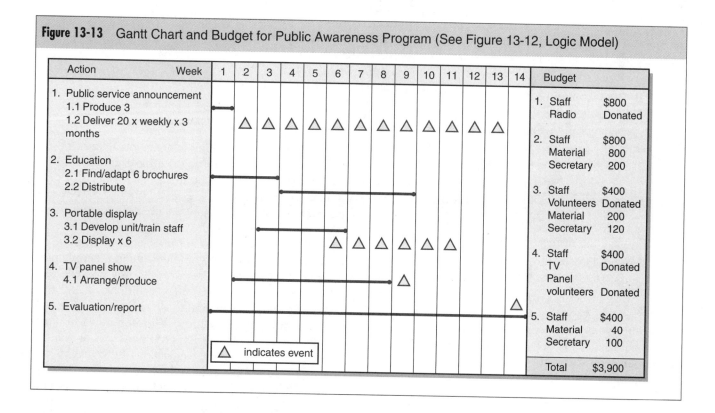

Figure 13-13 Gantt Chart and Budget for Public Awareness Program (See Figure 13-12, Logic Model)

months) marked on the horizontal axis (Hale, Arnold, & Travis, 1994). Dots indicate the start and completion points for each task, and the connecting line provides a visual indicator of the time period estimated (see Figure 13-13).

Grant Writing

To get adequate resources for a program, nurses may need to submit a proposal to an agency or foundation that grants funds for health programs. Sometimes nurses submit proposals to their own employing agency. A grant proposal is simply a written request for money (and occasionally for other resources). Writing a grant proposal is a systematic, step-by-step process (McKenzie and Smeltzer, 1997, p. 178):

- Locate grant money.
- Find out how to apply for it.
- Write a request.

A source must be found that grants funds for the kind of program the nurse is undertaking. For example, a community service group, such as Kiwanis, may focus on helping children and be willing to fund a program to improve youth health in a community, or a cancer society will fund a smoking-prevention program. Local, state or provincial, and national sources may also have funds available (see Appendix B for an inventory of U.S., Canadian, and other national sources). Also, funding agencies may send out requests for proposals; nurses need to watch for these and be prepared to work in a short time frame.

After a potential funding source is located, it is a good idea to contact the funding agency to discuss whether the nurse's program idea "fits well" with agency interests and to clarify what should be included in the proposal (questions to be answered, deadlines for submissions, and format). Although guidelines vary among agencies, particularly in the amount of detail required, certain questions usually must be answered:

1. What do you want to do, how much will it cost, and how much time will it take?
2. How is the proposed project related to the sponsor's interests?
3. What has already been done in the area of the project?
4. What will be gained if this project is carried out?
5. How do you plan to do it?
6. How will the results be evaluated?
7. Why should you, rather than someone else, conduct this project?

(McKenzie and Smeltzer, 1997, p. 179)

In writing the grant proposal, the wise nurse follows agency guidelines precisely, uses language familiar to the agency, and makes use of any work already completed (for example a Gantt chart developed with a community). Accuracy, clarity and appearance (grammar and spelling)

are important because the reviewer must make a judgment based on what is visible, and competition for funds usually is keen (similar to a job application). Helpful strategies for improving the quality of a proposal are to ask others (respected colleagues or persons familiar with the agency) to critique the proposal prior to submission and to review a proposal that was previously funded by the agency.

Documenting Programs

Record keeping should be accurate and designed specifically to support programming processes and program activities. Program documentation is comparable to record keeping for individual clients in agencies, although community participants may maintain the records themselves, and records may be kept open to all participants. Record keeping can serve to promote participation. Both quantitative data (objective measures such as dates of meetings and numbers of participants) and qualitative data (verbal descriptions, journals, pictures, and case stories) can be used to document processes and program activities. Keeping a simple journal can assist the nurse in tracking actions and the nurse's reflections on processes and events. Documentation can save time and prevent conflict by designating previous decisions, meeting attendees, and discussions among attendees. Documentation is also a rich source of data for program evaluation because it serves as a record of those things that actually occurred. Accuracy and usefulness are improved when documents are compiled promptly.

Program Implementation

Program implementation is the process of putting the program plan into action. Some questions to consider are:

How can we ensure that we do "good" and "no harm"?

How can we keep things on track?

How can we deal with the unexpected?

Ethics

Of special interest during implementation are ethical considerations and follow-through. Ethical codes apply in programming just as they do in all other aspects of nursing practice (Canadian Nurses Association, 1997). Nurses must ensure that activities are adjusted if anyone is experiencing negative effects (the ethical principle of doing no harm). Principles related to informed consent must be adhered to before and during implementation. People must understand the program, its purposes, any possible risks and benefits, and that they may withdraw at any time without difficulty. People must also understand confidentiality and negligence (failure of a person to act in a reasonable manner given the accepted standards of conduct for persons with the same qualifications and background). Safety issues must be considered throughout; for example, people who work in high-crime neighborhoods must take precautions such as traveling in pairs and during daylight hours, and meetings must be held in locations offering safe and easy access.

Follow-Through

The implementation of a program may be time limited (e.g., a six-week healthy lifestyles program or a six-month letter-writing campaign) or may occur over a long period and in a more intermittent manner (e.g., a community development project that takes place over a period of many months). Structured social planning or social action interventions may be piloted, phased in over time, or implemented in totality (McKenzie & Smeltzer, 1997). Tasks, time, and resources must be carefully monitored during implementation (e.g., staying within budget).

Just as they did in earlier processes, the concepts of partnership and participation apply during the implementation process (e.g., getting people together regularly to refresh their sense of purpose and humor). All involved should be invited to use their observation skills to ensure that actions are implemented as planned or adjusted as necessary to keep the actions moving toward the desired result. With community work, the follow-through process is sometimes like trying to keep an eye on a ball when the ball is moving in an unpredictable pattern and the playing field is full of hills and gullies. Continue to listen, negotiate, and deal promptly with conflicts. If the program must continue after the nurse's involvement has ceased, community follow-through and its long-term implications should be incorporated into planning to ensure program continuity after the nurse leaves (Bracht et al., 1994).

Program Evaluation

Was the program carried out as planned?

What has changed as a result of the program?

Were the results worth the effort?

What is the situation now?

DECISION MAKING

Disaster Planning: What Applies?

You have been invited to join a committee to design a disaster plan for a small town.

- Drawing on your community health programming knowledge, what ideas, principles, and processes do you think might prove useful in this different programming context?

- What ideas would likely not prove useful or would need modification?

Program evaluation is a process of inquiry to assess the performance of a program (Dignan & Carr, 1992, p. 143). Health care programs commonly are evaluated in terms of three dimensions: the extent to which the issues that gave rise to the program were addressed (responsiveness), the extent to which the desired outcomes were achieved (effectiveness), and whether as much as possible was achieved with the least expenditure of resources (efficiency) (Mullett, 1995). Evaluation of these dimensions is not always straightforward.

A systematic sequence of activities is performed to complete an evaluation: choosing questions to be answered, creating an evaluation plan or design, deciding the kinds of data needed to answer the questions and ways of obtaining these data, collecting and analyzing the data, and interpreting the results. Dignan and Carr (1992) emphasize that no set of fixed rules applies; rather, evaluation approaches must be flexible to permit answering of the most important questions. Nurses must remember that different questions are important to different stakeholder groups. Use of basic research principles (including ethics) will ensure both rigor and relevance. Method selection from quantitative (empirical analytic), qualitative (interpretive), and participatory action (critical) research traditions facilitates appropriate evaluation of any program. The selection of specific methods should be based on the nature of the evaluation questions.

The extent of evaluation possible is largely determined by resource availability. Resource considerations must include appropriate expertise to design and conduct the evaluation. If people working directly with the program do not have the necessary expertise, they should find an external consultant who does. University faculty and private consultants usually can be found. Practitioners and community people are sometimes reluctant to designate resources for evaluation, preferring instead to see the resources used to enhance the program. In response, the nurse–programmer might ask the question "Why would you want to do more until you know the effectiveness of what you are already doing?"

Evaluation Types

Evaluation may be formative, occurring throughout all programming processes, or summative, occurring at an end point. **Formative program evaluation** provides information to those planning and implementing the program "along the way" and permits improvements to the program while activities are in progress. **Summative program evaluation** provides retrospective information about the performance of the program up to the point when the evaluation was completed. Summative evaluation is more likely to be used to make decisions about whether the program should continue, and if so, with what changes. According to Pirie (1990), it is important to inform program stakeholders that evaluation results are not the only factor in such decisions; for example, budget cuts and political pressures may result in the termination of a successful program.

Evaluation is also sometimes conceptualized in terms of process, structure, impact, and outcomes. *Process* is the term used to describe all the activities undertaken to produce change. **Process program evaluation** is the assessment of the extent to which the program activities as carried out corresponded to the activities as planned. If that which happened is different from that which was planned, the evaluator will want to know the reasons so that implementation issues can be understood. *Structure* (or inputs) is the term used for all the resources required to support the program process. Data about structures are used to help determine costs. Process and structural evaluations provide an essential underlay for outcome evaluation because the interpretation of program outcomes rests on an understanding of the program as it was actualized. The program could erroneously be judged as unsuccessful when, in fact, it was not fully implemented.

Impact evaluation (a form of outcome evaluation) is the determination of the immediate effects of the program and whether those effects were the effects intended (e.g., teen mothers' gaining knowledge about child care and self-care). **Outcome evaluation** is the assessment of long-term change and whether that change was the result intended (e.g., healthier teen mothers and their children). Outcome evaluation requires resources for longitudinal tracking. Sensitive indicators of impacts and outcomes are selected on the basis of the following questions:

What changes are reasonable to expect?

What would indicate that the program resulted in changes?

What would permit discovery of unexpected changes?

Indicators might be, for example, safety, behavior, quality of life, health-related policies, participation, individual health status, population health status, use of resources, and the like. Satisfaction of stakeholders may or may not be a good indicator of program success (e.g., parents of teens may not be satisfied about condom machines in school washrooms, but the program may help prevent disease and unwanted pregnancy).

Evaluation As Comparison

Evaluation is a process ultimately intended to determine the worth of something, presumably in comparison with some norm or standard of "goodness." In program evaluation, comparison may be made with:

- A similar program (e.g., comparing one nursing center with another);
- A different program (e.g., comparing weight gains of infants going home on an early maternity discharge program with weight gains of infants who are kept longer in the hospital);
- Established norms (e.g., comparing condom use by local teens with condom use by teens as reflected in national data);
- A preprogram assessment (e.g., nutritional patterns of college students before and after the lowering of cafeteria prices for healthy foods);
- The same program over time (e.g., historical record keeping with documentation of activities and changes over time; periodic inventories that permit comparison with previous performance (Green & Kreuter, 1991).

In instances where some control is possible and resources permit, time series, quasi-experimental, and experimental designs may be used. Comparisons can be difficult with new innovative programs and with programs in uncontrolled natural community settings. Creativity is helpful (e.g., the nurse may consider that which would likely have happened to the people or in the community if the program had not been implemented and provide evidence to substantiate the answer).

DECISION MAKING

Sensitive Indicators

You are a resource person for a self-help support group for people experiencing chronic pain. Group members are helping each other manage pain by sharing ideas and encouragement. At the group's request, you have invited different health care practitioners (e.g., Therapeutic Touch, massage, medical, physiotherapy) to share their approaches. Group members also are working to change the regional government's compensation policy, which restricts benefits for persons who experience chronic pain following on-the-job injuries.

- What indicators might be sensitive to and reflect changes resulting from the group activities?

Data Sources and Collection Methods

After evaluation questions have been determined, the type of evaluation needed, the approach or design to be used, data sources, and collection methods can be selected. Data already collected for purposes related to assessment, planning, and implementation should be used for evaluation whenever possible. For example, assessment data may have been gathered about the community health status during program planning; after program implementation, these same kinds of data may be gathered and a before-and-after comparison performed.

Data sources usually are people and documents; collection methods include interviews, focus groups, observations, standardized tools, and tools created specifically for the program. As appreciation increases for clients' rights, abilities, and responsibilities, the subjective perspectives of program participants are becoming more valued by programmers and funders. All program documentation has potential for use in evaluation (e.g., records of meetings and group sessions, letters, media coverage, pictures). Nurses are encouraged to use innovative as well as traditional data sources and collection methods.

Evaluation Models

As much as is possible, evaluations must be designed to answer questions pertinent to each of the stakeholder groups, possibly including practitioners, various groups of community people, agencies, and funding bodies. Each group will likely be interested in different aspects of the evaluation; dissemination of findings to these groups may therefore require the preparation of separate reports and recommendations. Funders generally want quantified information derived from measurements of risk-factor reduction or improvements in health. In some situations, providing such information is not feasible; in other instances, that which is important to health cannot be quantifiably measured. Because funders deal primarily in these terms, however, the nurse must find a way to translate the effects of the program into terms meaningful to funders (or others).

Numerous models for program evaluation exist. Diagrammatic models developed earlier in the process may be used to guide evaluation. Two evaluation frameworks that are especially useful in the current health care context are those of Pirie and Mullett. Pirie (1990) designed a series of questions to ensure that evaluation information would be directly useful "to people and their programs" (p. 201). The questions as outlined below have been altered to reflect a partnership, health-promoting style of relating.

- *Questions for the planning stage:*
  Why should this program be developed?
  Are the resources appropriate?

- *Questions for the program implementation stage:*
  Is the program being implemented as planned?
  Is the program reaching the people/organizations intended?
  Who is the program failing to reach and why?
  What are participants' views about the program?
  Are participants satisfied with their experience?

- *Questions about program outcomes:*
  What, if anything, is changing as a result of the program?
  Is the program having the effects it was designed to have?

On the basis of these general questions, nurses and their community partners can design specific evaluation questions relevant to their programs. This framework can be used to guide formative or summative evaluation by altering the tense of questions.

A framework developed by Mullett (1995) for British Columbia's health care reform effort is intended to be a user-friendly evaluation guide for a broad range of health programs and stakeholders (see Figure 13-14). This framework can be readily adapted. In particular, the "How to

DECISION MAKING

Evaluation

A community agency funding a public awareness program for HIV prevention in heterosexual women has asked you for advice about the evaluation (see Figures 13-12 and 13-13 for program activities, desired results, evaluation budget, and timeline).

- Given the limited evaluation budget and short timeline, which types of evaluation would you recommend?

- What comparisons might be made?

- What data sources and collection methods might be used?

Evaluate" examples are primarily geared toward social planning and must be significantly modified to be appropriate for community development, social action, and small programs.

Cost Analysis

In this era of health care reform and associated concerns regarding cost control, evaluation is linked with accountability to the public to ensure that health improvements are worth the funds spent. **Cost analysis of health programs** is the evaluation of the costs of a program in relation to health outcomes. There are many ways to examine cost: for example, cost effectiveness (comparison with another program, cost per effect achieved), cost benefit (comparison of dollar benefit of different programs with costs of those programs), and cost utility (amount of improvement in quality of life per dollar spent) (Vail, 1995; McKenzie & Smeltzer, 1997). Because all that is important to health is not readily measurable or easily converted into monetary terms (e.g., community competence, environmental change, quality of life, adding life to years), new approaches to cost analysis are needed. Values and needs that gave rise to a program, short- and long-term health outcomes, and human and material costs must be considered. The use of a case study is often helpful to illustrate the human dimension along with material costs (Vail, 1997). With large programs, community health nurses are advised to seek the assistance of a consultant; with small programs, nurses can analyze the resource and budget information in combination with the process, structure, and outcome evaluation data.

Cost analysis is sometimes simple; at other times, it is complex. For example, the cost analysis for a home intravenous drug therapy program may simply compare the costs of home care with the costs of hospital care. In contrast, the cost analysis for a community cardiovascular disease–prevention program may require 20 years of

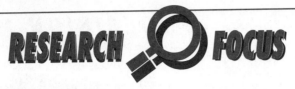

Effectiveness of Community-Directed Diabetes Prevention and Control in a Rural Aboriginal Population

STUDY PROBLEM/PURPOSE

The increasing prevalence of non–insulin-dependent diabetes mellitus (NIDDM) in native Canadian populations is having profoundly negative health impacts. The strongest risk factors for NIDDM are lifestyle related, including obesity, physical inactivity, and inappropriate diet. Lifestyle is shaped by the cultural, health, social, educational, and economic environment of the community. In response to the problem, a community-based diabetes prevention and control project of 24 months duration was initiated. General aims of the project were to modify risk factors, encourage meaningful community participation, develop culturally relevant interventions, and enable the community to assume responsibility upon completion of the project. The project was federally funded (NHRDP-Canada).

METHODS

The study combined community development, participatory action research approaches, and quasi-experimental design. An intervention community and two control communities were chosen so that comparisons could be made. Sites were semirural Okanagan First Nations communities. The intervention community had a population of 707, high-risk cohort n=62; the two control communities, 659 total population, high-risk cohort n=43. The research team included six native tribe members from the study community, one native nurse, a diabetes nurse specialist, two nursing faculty members, and a doctoral student. An advisory team of eight community members worked with the research team. Nursing students worked as research assistants.

A seven-month pre-intervention included training of workers and interaction with the communities to achieve mutual understanding of the situation. Measurements of physiological, anthropometric, and behavioral variables among established diabetics and persons at familial risk were taken prior to and at two points after the eight-month intervention. Program implementation consisted of socioenvironmental and behavioral interventions designed by the community and research team together. Interventions stressed individual and community strengths and capabilities to deal with diabetes. Interventions comprised numerous communitywide, group, and individual activities combining exercise, education, nutrition, smoking-

cessation, and social interaction activities. An array of people with special knowledge and skills participated in health activities (e.g., community members of all ages, tribal council, media, diabetic/heart/cancer associations, grocery stores, health practitioners, etc.). Over the duration of the study, quantitative and qualitative data were collected via minimally structured interviews, lifestyle surveys, blood tests, blood pressure readings, anthropometric measures, and observation.

FINDINGS

Prior to the interventions the communities had limited knowledge about healthy lifestyles and diabetes. This was also true of those members with diabetes. Following the interventions knowledge increased; health-promoting activities were designed and people participated; outside resource people were invited into the community for the first time; the tribal council hired a full-time recreation coordinator; and several activities have continued after the project. One continuing activity is a walking event in remembrance of a beloved native research team member who was killed near the end of the study; the walk has been held every six months (three times). Approximately 200 people (20% of community) have participated each time.

Community members reported that they are developing a sense of community cohesiveness and of possibilities and that internal community conflict is decreasing. These data were provided during open interviews, rather than via questionnaires. Although efforts were made to adapt the questionnaires to the cultural perspective of the community, participants reported "hating" filling out the questionnaires. Among high-risk cohorts, although individuals reported that their lives were "getting better" and that they were hopeful for the future, individual behavior and physiological status did not improve.

IMPLICATIONS

The project was not successful in reducing risk factors in the high-risk cohort. The project was successful at helping the community increase competence, mobilize resources, and begin to change their social and political environments in directions supportive of healthy lifestyles. The change theories on which the study was based suggest that environmental and lifestyle changes take considerable time, especially with populations who have been severely marginalized. The project likely was too short. Also, interventions must be powerful enough to create the
Continued

Continued

desired changes. Because the interventions were largely carried out by community people who were themselves learning about diabetes and modification of environments and lifestyles, the interventions may not have been strong enough. The researchers concluded that replication of the study over a longer period and with increased intervention strength and measurement tools more appropriate to the people and the community is warranted.

SOURCE

From Aboriginal Community-Directed Diabetes Prevention and Control: The Okanagan Diabetes Project *(project report for the National Health Research and Development Program, Ottawa, Canada) by M. Daniels and D. Gamble, 1996, Ontario, Canada: National Health Research and Development Program; and* Effectiveness of Community-Directed Diabetes Prevention and Control in a Rural Aboriginal Population *(Doctoral dissertation, University of British Columbia, Vancouver, British Columbia) by M. Daniel, 1997, University of British Columbia.*

Figure 13-14   Program Performance Evaluation Framework

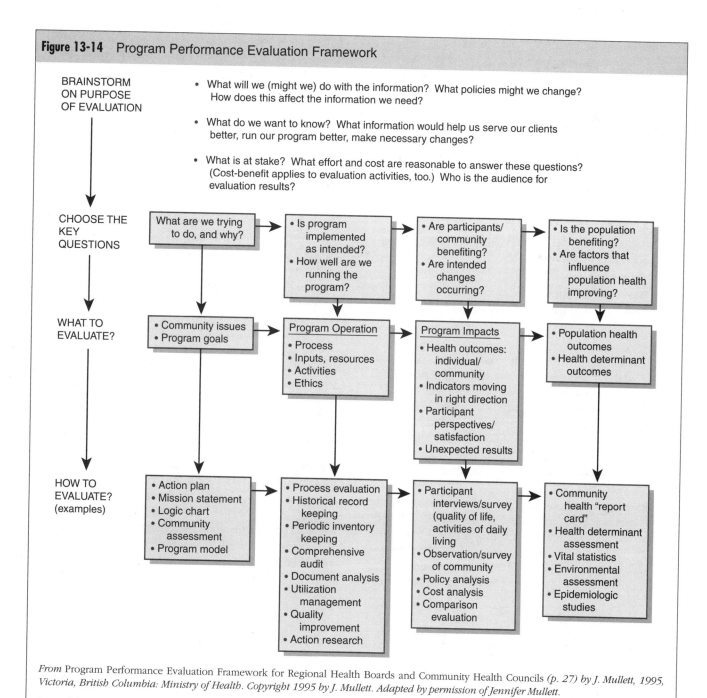

From Program Performance Evaluation Framework for Regional Health Boards and Community Health Councils *(p. 27) by J. Mullett, 1995, Victoria, British Columbia: Ministry of Health. Copyright 1995 by J. Mullett. Adapted by permission of Jennifer Mullett.*

Perspectives...

Insights of Student Nurses

Based on the observation that pregnant women often were not well prepared for hospital delivery or for early discharge, our plan was to develop an antenatal clinic. In a BSN health-promotion course, we learned the importance of clients' identifying their own needs and of the input of other health care providers. We therefore conducted interviews and a survey of clients, public health nurses, hospital maternity nurses, and physicians. Results revealed that there were already a number of programs in place. Our question then became, "Why aren't clients using them?" Further investigation indicated the need for integration of hospital and community resources and for consistent information for clients, especially about breastfeeding. We thus changed our plan to focus on the following:

- Improve continuity of care (reduce the need for multiple visits)
- Identify at-risk clients early (those with particular needs)
- Increase access to prenatal classes and other educational opportunities
- Streamline hospital admission
- Decrease the amount of paperwork
- Provide consistent breastfeeding information postpartum

We developed a working committee that included a public health nurse who works with pregnant teens, the planned maternity care coordinator (who liaises between hospital and public health nurses), a family physician, an obstetrical nurse (who also was pregnant), an obstetrical unit clerk, and the obstetrical and pediatric clinical coordinators. We also obtained additional input from clients, midwives, obstetrical nurses, obstetricians, and the college prenatal educator.

Many viewpoints were presented, and it was challenging to obtain consensus on the way to achieve the client's needs while meeting regional, community, and hospital philosophies and fiscal responsibilities. As discussions and meetings were held, actions were gradually agreed on, and progress was made.

- Approval was given by administration for a preadmission clinic for clients at 28 to 30 weeks of gestation. The focus is client-identified educational needs, risk identification and referral, completion of hospital forms, admission and discharge planning, and a tour of the obstetrical unit.
- To improve prenatal education, support for clients to attend prenatal classes is offered at the clinic (e.g., funding), as will information about prenatal videos available at the public library and video stores.
- To streamline information and reduce paperwork, care mapping has been developed with the help of interested hospital nurses and implemented. The form replaced three other forms, and the information obtained is faxed to public health nurses to improve continuity of postpartum follow-up.
- A breastfeeding workshop was held for public health nurses, hospital nurses, and lactation consultants. Nurses were encouraged to identify their learning needs, and client feedback about inconsistencies in teaching was incorporated. Nurses were given paid time from work to attend.

Implementation of the preadmission clinic is the joint responsibility of hospital and public health nurses. Depending on client demand, a clinic will be held one afternoon per week and one Saturday per month. Public health nurses, hospital nurses, and prenatal educators interested in working at the clinic are mentored by the obstetrical coordinator.

Evaluation of the clinic will include surveys of clients, nurses, and physicians to obtain quantitative and qualitative information about their positive and negative experiences. For comparison purposes, length of stay statistics were gathered prior to and following the implementation of the clinic.

During the year-long programming process to streamline and improve maternity care, we learned the importance of letting go of our own ideas. Obtaining input from all involved shaped and helped with the acceptance of change. In acknowledging and respecting diverse views and working together, we were able to achieve the consensus necessary to make the program a reality. Support and encouragement for each other as agents of this change are assisting us to maintain the momentum to follow through on the work.

—Maureen Spinks, RN, BSN student
Jean Jacobsen, RN, BSN student
Lisa Porter, RN, BSN student

COMMUNITY NURSING VIEW

A nurse has been asked to develop a program for teens at a local high school. The nurse has been told that: teachers are concerned about "bullying" on the school grounds; parents are worried about conflict among students from different cultural backgrounds; and the school principal would like help to improve support for students with serious medical problems.

Nursing Considerations

PLANNING/IMPLEMENTATION
- Given the preliminary information available about the high school, what overall *approaches to health* might be most helpful for this high-school community?
- What *theories and models* might be useful initially? Later?
- *Who* should be included in the initial work? *What* are the urgent and longer-term issues?
- *How* should the nurse deal with the fact that three issues have been raised?
- How might the nurse and community find out more about the current situation and issues of importance? (*diagnosis)*

- What would be a better situation? (*identification of goals/outcomes*)
- How can the desired situation be created? (*action strategies*)
- What are the resource requirements and availability? (*feasibility*)
- Among the many possible actions that could be undertaken, how would the nurse determine those that are best?
- What *ethical issues* might be anticipated?
- What forms of *documentation* might be useful?

EVALUATION
- What would indicate that programming work was helping the community?
- What *types* of evaluation would be appropriate?
- The nurse will be able to work with the school intensively for a year but then will need to decrease involvement. What might be done to assist the high school to continue on with the program after the nurse's involvement has decreased or ceased?

follow-up. When more immediate information is needed with regard to programs such as the latter, the nurse can make comparisons with other similar programs for which cost analysis has already been performed. With prevention program cost analysis, a bit of a conceptual leap must often be made when comparing the cost of prevention with the cost of disease. For example, a campus health program (along with other factors, no doubt) was associated with a 30% reported increase in condom use by students (Budgen & Bates, 1996). Condoms are highly effective (but not foolproof) in reducing the transmission of sexually transmitted disease. Cost estimates in the literature indicate that health care for one person with HIV/AIDS dramatically exceeded the annual costs of the health program. The conclusion was thus drawn that the program was worth the cost.

Cost analysis, like other components of programming, becomes easier with practice. The community health nurse who adds the skills of cost analysis to program planning, implementation, and evaluation will be well equipped to make a significant contribution to the Health for All initiative.

Health for All goals can be achieved through programs when nurses understand the context, use theory thoughtfully, and work with communities in partnership (see Figure 13-15). See Table 13-4 for a review of questions to

ask in relation to program planning, implementation, and evaluation. The community health nurse can be a significant force in the Health for All initiative.

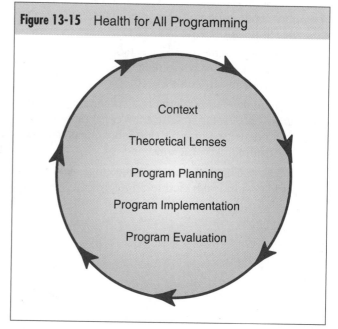

Figure 13-15 Health for All Programming

Context

Theoretical Lenses

Program Planning

Program Implementation

Program Evaluation

Table 13-4 Program Planning, Implementation, and Evaluation: Questions to Ask		
PROGRAM PLANNING	**PROGRAM IMPLEMENTATION**	**PROGRAM EVALUATION**
Analyzing the Community		
What is the situation?	How can we ensure we do "good" and "no harm"?	Was the program carried out as planned?
Identifying Issues	How can we keep things on track?	What has changed as a result of the program?
What is important?	How can we deal with the unexpected?	Were the results worth the effort?
Whose views have been heard?		What is the situation now?
Whose views have not been heard?		
What issue is most important at this time?		
What are the parts of the issue?		
Why does the issue exist?		
Clarifying Goals		
What would be a more desirable situation?		
What do we want to happen?		
Designing Actions		
What should be done to create the more desirable situation?		
What resources are needed, and where can they be obtained?		
Who can do what?		

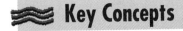 **Key Concepts**

- The WHO's primary health care and health-promotion strategies are of special interest to nurses as they create programs that contribute to the goal of Health for All.
- Dramatic, multilevel change (societal, community, individual, and environmental) is required for the achievement of Health for All.
- Community empowerment, community competence, partnership, intersectoral collaboration, and a broad definition of health are fundamental concepts in Health for All programs.
- Successful health programs take into account the societal and health care reform context.

- Community health nurses use caring, phenomenological, feminist, critical social, and multilevel change theories to assist their work with people and programs.
- Community organization, a multilevel change theory comprising community development, social planning, and political action, provides useful guidance for many Health for All programs.
- Health programming work includes the processes of planning, implementing, and evaluating programs for the purpose of improving health.
- The science of programming is the theoretical knowledge that community nurses use; the art is the way nurses work with communities.

The Varied Roles of Community Health Nursing

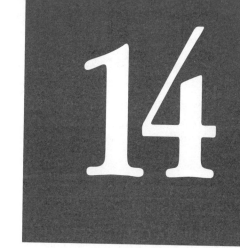

14

Susanne F. Wilkey, RN, MS
Susan S. Gardner, RN, ANP, MS

. . . Your behavior influences others through a ripple effect. A ripple effect works because everyone influences everyone else. Powerful people are powerful influences.
If your life works, you influence your family.
If your family works, your family influences the community.
If your community works, your community influences the nation.
If your nation works, your nation influences the world.
If your world works, the ripple effect spreads throughout the cosmos.
. . . All growth spreads outward from a fertile and potent nucleus. You are a nucleus.

—Heider, 1985, p. 107

COMPETENCIES

Upon completion of this chapter, the reader should be able to:

- Discuss possible effects on the nurse when making a role transition from an acute care practice to community-based practice.
- Compare and contrast the roles of community health nurse generalist and community health nurse specialist.
- Compare and contrast the multiple role functions (clinician, advocate, collaborator, consultant, counselor, educator, researcher) of the community health nurse.
- Analyze the significance of nurse actions in the role of case manager for the client maneuvering through a complex health care system.
- Describe the similarities and differences between home health nursing and community health nursing.
- Discuss the role of the nurse in a public health setting.
- Recount the role of the nurse in providing hospice services to dying clients and their families.
- Describe the role of the school nurse in meeting the broad health needs of students, staff, families, and the community for whom he or she is responsible.
- From administrative/management, nurse, and worker perspectives, the role of the occupational health nurse in implementing cost-effective programs.
- Chronicle the challenges in providing quality nursing services to clients in a correctional setting.
- Compare and contrast the differing standards of nursing practice as outlined by the American Nurses Association (ANA), the American Association of Occupational Health Nurses (AAOHN), and the National Association of School Nurses (NASN).
- Review the recommendations outlined by the ANA, the National League for Nursing (NLN), and the National Institute of Nursing Research (NINR) for meeting challenges confronting nursing practice in the United States.

KEY TERMS *(Continued)*

role socialization
role taking
role transition

school nursing
self-care
self-determination

teaching
toxicology

As health care continues to evolve and change, delivery systems and practice settings must also change. Consistent in all discussions of such transition is the recognition that delivery of health care services will shift to community settings. The health needs of society and consumer demand will bring about community-based and community-focused services. Nursing assessment and intervention will address the needs of **aggregates** (groups of people with similar needs) as well as individuals. To fulfill these expectations, the nurse must be prepared to practice autonomously in a variety of settings while enacting many functional roles.

ROLE TRANSITION

Nursing roles are ever changing. The **roles**, or sets of expectations associated with given positions, of all health care professionals are continuously redefined and realigned in response to changing knowledge, technology, cost, and consumer need. Roles exist and evolve in order to meet societal demands (Rubin, 1988). As health care delivery systems change, the practice of nursing continues to shift from acute care, institution-based settings to community settings. For many nurses, the transition from an acute care focus to a community focus is challenging.

To enact a role, the nurse must have a clear idea of the expected behaviors associated with that role. **Role socialization** is the process by which persons acquire knowledge, skills, and attitudes that enable them to fulfill assigned roles. Transitions into new roles require mastering and incorporating new knowledge and expectations (**role clarification**). This requires the nurse to change both overt behavior (**role taking**) as well as the inner definition of self so that the new roles are both internally and externally validated (Rubin, 1988; Clarke & Strauss, 1992).

Role stress and strain can result from deficient role socialization and may manifest in a number of ways. **Role ambiguity** results from vague, ill-defined, or unclear norms. There may be disagreement or lack of clarity about role expectations. **Role conflict** occurs when existing role expectations are contradictory or incompatible. **Role incongruity** develops when role expectations are not in agreement with self-perception, disposition, attitudes, and values. **Role overload** manifests when the nurse is confronted with excessive demands; although able to perform each role demand, the nurse is unable to carry out all of them in the available time. **Role incompetence** is felt when the nurse's resources are inadequate to meet the demands of the job, whereas **role overqualification** occurs when the nurse's resources are in excess of those necessary for the job (Hardy & Conway, 1978).

A structured program to assist the new community health nurse in acquiring the knowledge and skills necessary to fulfill a new role eases **role transition** and fosters role socialization. When transitioning to a new role, a nurse must learn new role behaviors, review previously learned material, and mediate any conflicts between the different role expectations. The nurse must internalize the values of the new role, adopt the appropriate behaviors, and identify significant role models. Role socialization is enhanced by observation of others in the role (**role modeling**), internal preparation and overt practice of new role behaviors (**role rehearsal**), and participation in planned group activities with others involved in role transition (i.e., a **reference group**) (Rubin, 1988; Clarke & Strauss, 1992). The nurse manager along with other health care professionals, the **multidisciplinary team**, are critical factors in the success of the nurse's development in a new role. The new community health nurse must recognize the broader scope of practice, embrace the autonomous nature of the practice, and communicate needs to those who may be of help during the role transition.

MAJOR ROLE FUNCTIONS

The community health nurse must be capable of performing multiple role functions regardless of the setting of employment. These role functions include:

- Clinician
- Advocate
- Collaborator
- Consultant
- Counselor
- Educator
- Researcher
- Case manager (see Figure 14-1)

The nurse who implements these roles demonstrates a caring and comprehensive client-centered nursing practice.

Clinician

Community health nursing differs from most traditional nursing roles in its focus on the community as client. Personal health services focus on individuals and may

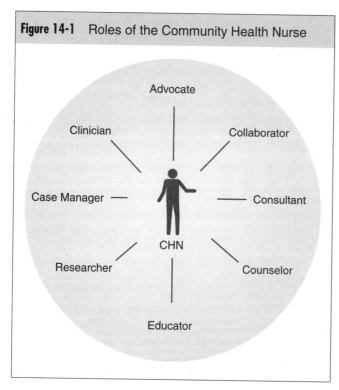

Figure 14-1   Roles of the Community Health Nurse

Advocate
Collaborator
Clinician
Consultant
Case Manager
CHN
Consultant
Researcher
Counselor
Educator

Figure 14-2   Standards of Community Health Nursing Practice

Standard I. Theory: The nurse applies theoretical concepts as a basis for decisions in practice.

Standard II. Data Collection: The nurse systematically collects data that are comprehensive and accurate.

Standard III. Diagnosis: The nurse analyzes data collected about the community, family, and individual to determine diagnoses.

Standard IV. Planning: At each level of prevention, the nurse develops plans that specify nursing actions unique to client needs.

Standard V. Intervention: The nurse, guided by the plan, intervenes to promote, maintain, or restore health, to prevent illness, and to effect rehabilitation.

Standard VI. Evaluation: The nurse evaluates responses of the community, family, and individual to interventions in order to determine progress toward goal achievement and to revise the database, diagnosis, and plan.

Standard VII. Quality Assurance and Professional Development: The nurse participates in peer review and other means of evaluation to ensure quality of nursing practice. The nurse assumes responsibility for professional development and contributes to the professional growth of others.

Standard VIII. Interdisciplinary Collaboration: The nurse collaborates with other health care providers, professionals, and community representatives in assessing, planning, implementing, and evaluating programs for community health.

Standard IX. Research: The nurse contributes to theory and practice in community health nursing through research.

Adapted from Standards of Community Health Nursing Practice, *by American Nurses Association, 1986, Kansas City, MO: Author. Copyright 1986 by American Nurses Publishing, American Nurses Foundation/American Nurses Association. Used with permission.*

include services to help individuals maintain health, recover from illness, or adapt to long-term disabilities. Public health, however, addresses the health of individuals within the broader context of the community. Although community health nursing practice may include nursing care of individuals, families, and groups, the primary responsibility is to the health of the community as a whole (Williams, 1992). Community health nursing promotes the health of the public. The services and programs emphasize health promotion and maintenance and the prevention of disease. The aim of illness prevention and risk reduction is the promotion of optimal health of the total community. Although community health activities may change over time, the goals remain those of reducing disease, discomfort, disability, and premature death (American Nurses Association [ANA], 1986a; Laffrey & Page, 1989; Riner, 1989). Refer to Figure 14-2 for further elaboration of expectations for community health nurses.

Most nurses with a background in acute care do not have experience with a broad, community-based practice perspective. Associate degree and diploma programs in nursing generally do not provide a theoretical background for community health nursing practice. Yet, recent surveys have indicated that during the next 10 years, the majority of nurses will find employment opportunities in the community rather than in acute care facilities. This transition and relocation of the acute care work force to community and public health delivery systems will present many challenges. Current surveys indicate that less than 50% of the nurses now employed in community health have the minimum recommended educational preparation of a baccalaureate degree in nursing. This shortage of adequately prepared community health nurses is likely to continue in the foreseeable future (Mason Knight, Toughil, DeMaio,

Beck, & Christopher, 1992; Association of Community Health Nursing Educators, 1993)

The American Nurses Association (ANA) and the Association of Community Health Nursing Educators (ACHNE) recommend that two levels of community health nurses form the core personnel for community health nursing practice: the **community health nurse generalist**, educated at the baccalaureate level, and the **community health nurse specialist**, prepared at the master's or doctoral level. In this model, the focus of baccalaureate-prepared nurses is clinical practice with individuals and families within a community context. The focus of master's-prepared nurses is the health needs of the community, whereas the doctorally prepared nurses focus on health policy and research. This staff might be assisted by clinical nurse specialists from other nursing fields, nurse practitioners, nursing care associates, and ancillary nursing personnel. Community health nurses also work with and collaborate with other members of a multidisciplinary team (ANA, 1986a; Laffrey & Page, 1989; ACHNE, 1993).

Community Health Nurse Generalist

The community health nurse generalist functions in the broadest practice role. This role combines nursing, epidemiology, case management, and resource coordination. The generalist provides care in a wide variety of settings to individuals, families, and groups while maintaining an understanding of the values and concepts of population-based practice. The community health nurse generalist participates with the specialist in communitywide assessments, and in the planning, implementation, and evaluation of programs and services (ANA, 1986a; Laffrey & Page, 1989; Riner, 1989).

Community Health Nurse Specialist

The community health nurse specialist may perform all of the functions of the generalist. In addition, the nurse specialist brings expertise in working with families and groups, in formulating health policy, and in assessing communities and has proficiency in carrying out all phases of population-focused programs. The specialist has skills in epidemiology, **demography** (the statistical study of populations, including health, disease, births, and deaths), **biometrics** (the application of statistical methods to biological facts), community development, and management. The community health nurse specialist engages in research, theory development and testing, and health policy development (ANA, 1986a).

Graduate programs to prepare community health nurse specialists may prepare nurses as **clinical nurse specialists** (CNS) or **nurse practitioners** (NP). Much debate has centered on the similarities and differences in these two roles. Both roles originated in the mid-1960s to meet perceived health care needs. The CNS role was proposed by nurse educators in response to a need to improve client care. The CNS role was envisioned as an avenue for advancement for the talented nurse who wished to remain in direct contact with clients. The CNS would provide expert physical, social, and psychological support to clients; educate clients and families in the management of health problems; consult with nursing staff and other disciplines; and conduct research related to nursing practice outcomes (Elder & Bullough, 1990).

The CNS is described as an expert practitioner with graduate preparation in a nursing specialty. Subroles of practice include clinical practitioner, educator, researcher, and consultant. According to Brunk (1992), "the CNS is capable of planning, implementing, and delivering quality care to complex patients; planning and implementing educational programs for staff and patients; using research findings in the clinical setting as well as conducting clinical studies; and serving as a change agent to promote quality care" (p. 2). The community health CNS would fulfill all of the roles of the community health nurse generalist plus be involved in conducting community assessments, assess-

ing for populations at risk, and developing and implementing population-focused programs (ANA, 1986a; Selleck, Sirles, & Sloan, 1992).

The nurse practitioner (NP) movement evolved in response to a perceived shortage of physicians, particularly generalists willing to meet the needs of underserved populations. This new role was not supported by all nurses. Health professionals of the 1960s divided health care workers into those who cured illness and those who gave care. Nursing was seen as a caring profession, and, whereas clinical nurse specialists were applauded for expanding that role, nurse practitioners were categorized as suspect because their role included both caring and curing. Some experts felt the NP role was a step backward because it threatened the independence of the nursing profession (Elder & Bullough, 1990).

Many community health nurses have pursued additional education to assume the role of advanced practice nurse practitioners providing primary care services. Nurse practitioners are prepared to provide a full range of primary health care services. They engage in independent decision making and provide health care to individuals, families, and groups throughout the life span. Nurse practitioners are skilled in assessment and intervention. In many states, their practice includes prescriptive privileges and other treatments commonly viewed as within the domain of medical practice. Nurse practitioners maintain a strong nursing focus by providing anticipatory guidance and counseling about health maintenance and disease prevention. The NP diagnoses actual and potential health problems and, with the client, plans appropriate treatment. Nurse practitioners operate under protocols and consult with and refer to other disciplines (Riner, 1989; Jones & Clark, 1990; Selleck et al., 1992).

Despite the differences, there are many similarities in the components of the NP and CNS roles. Teaching and counseling individuals, families, and groups are major responsibilities for both groups. Although the tasks of conducting physical examinations, ordering laboratory tests, and prescribing medications are commonly associated with the NP role, a significant number of clinical nurse specialists also carry out these activities depending on their legal authority and scope of licensure. Clinical nurse specialists are more likely to be expected to teach staff and run support groups, but many nurse practitioners also perform these functions. Although differences remain in terminology and description of practices, there are many overlapping functions in the two roles, and some nurse educators see further merging of the roles in the future (Elder & Bullough, 1990).

The need for community health nurses prepared at the generalist and specialist levels will increase in the future. To truly function in the clinician role, the nurse must remember that community health nursing is not defined merely by the setting. Community health nursing practice is characterized by its focus on aggregates, the community, and high-risk populations. The beginning community health nurse may face the dilemma of "not seeing the forest for the trees" (individuals versus aggregates). Most baccalaureate nursing programs still devote the majority of their time to care focused on sick individuals. In community health, such graduates must expand their thinking from individuals to families, high-risk groups, and the entire community. Concurrently, emphasis must shift from treatment of acute illness to the prevention of illness and promotion and maintenance of health. Community health nurses who do not focus care on the total community are not fulfilling the potential of the role in promoting the health of the community (Laffrey & Page, 1989).

The present trend in community health nursing is to bring about the need for more graduate-prepared clinical specialists. Populations most in need of graduate-prepared community health nurses include elders, the homeless, adolescents, the unemployed, and other populations at risk. Health conditions needing specialist services include at-risk pregnancies and low birth weight; HIV and AIDS; Alzheimer's and other chronic diseases of elders; and stress-related injuries and illness. Community health nurses are being employed throughout the community, in health departments, schools, industries, home health, hospice, and multiple other settings. Current health care changes hold many possibilities and exciting opportunities for community health nursing as the health care system rediscovers the importance and cost-effectiveness of prevention, and caregivers again teach people ways to be in control of their own health via healthy lifestyles. The objectives of the Healthy People 2000 initiative serve to outline the numerous ways that the nurse may influence the health of communities (see Appendix A). Nurses have a great opportunity to be key players in addressing many of the health care problems facing society in the immediate future (Riportella-Muller, Selby, Salmon, Quade, & Legault, 1991; Selleck et al., 1992). The development of the national health objectives for Healthy People 2010 is currently in progress. Public involvement in this process will continue into 1999 and Healthy People 2010 will be released in January, 2000 (Office of Disease Prevention and Health Promotion, 1998). Nurses also have the opportunity to contribute to this major national effort.

Advocate

The community health nurse acts as **advocate** for the individual, group, or community client. Advocacy is the act of speaking or acting for an individual or group of individuals who may be unable to speak for themselves. In the health care system or larger social system, clients may be unable to speak for themselves for multiple reasons. These reasons may include lack of knowledge; difficulty or inability to articulate needs or ideas; perceived lack of power; fear; and physical or mental disability. Because of close and frequent contact with the client, the nurse is often the best health professional to promote the needs and desires of the client within the realm of a complicated and potentially cumbersome system.

Concepts of Advocacy

Client advocacy is essential to the nurse–client relationship (Bandman & Bandman, 1995; Klainberg, Holzemer, Leonard & Arnold, 1998). A professional responsibility for all nurses, advocacy is especially important for the community health nurse, who has a broad exposure to social situations, is closely tied to the family and community, and has a philosophical basis for advocating for the group (Kosik, 1972). Public health philosophy supports the appropriate use of social programs, fosters decision making within the family or community network, and promotes **self-care** (health care performed by the client) and **self-determination** (the right to make one's own choices) by the individual or group.

Advocacy has been described as encompassing both simplest and complex actions. Kohnke (1980) suggests that advocacy is perhaps simplest when it involves actions of loving and caring for others. This premise of caring is supported by Mayeroff (1971), who in his classic reference describes caring actions that may precisely apply to the role of the nurse advocate:

> When I care for an adult, . . . I try to avoid making decisions for him. I help him make his own decisions by providing information, suggesting alternatives and pointing out possible consequences, but all along I realize that they are his decisions to make and not my own. If I made his decisions for him, I would be condescending to him and treating him as a child; and by denying his need to take responsibility for his own life, I would be denying him as a person (p. 34).

To advocate for the client is to care for that individual. To care for the individual is to help the client develop full potential. The nurse as advocate is dedicated to supporting this process.

Kohnke (1980) describes advocacy as complex because it demands that the nurse be knowledgeable about the health care system, the law, and the unique characteristics of the client. The advocate must know ways to use the system to achieve the desired outcomes while still promoting client self-determination. Advocacy is essential for the provision of ethical health interventions.

As an advocate, the nurse informs the client of available services, supports the client's requests, and assists with the receiving process. Being a true advocate requires a willingness on the part of the nurse to fully invest in the client–nurse relationship. Advocacy is time consuming and demands a client-focused approach. The nurse must in one sense be a risk-taker, being willing to intervene on behalf of the client to ensure that the system does not prevent access to necessary services to which the client is entitled.

Characteristics of an Advocate

The National Society of Patient Representatives, as cited by Robinson (1985), identifies multiple characteristics desired in an advocate. Included in this list are the abilities to relate to clients and staff, to cope with pressure, and to manage stress. Desirable personal attributes include self-motivation, objectivity, empathy, tact, flexibility, tenacity, and a sense of humor. Leadership skills such as risk-taking, vision, confidence, assertiveness, accountability, the ability to articulate ideas and resolve conflict, and the appropriate use of power are also essential for the nurse-advocate (Robinson, 1985; Marquis & Huston, 1992). A genuine concern and regard for the client as a total person is the foundation on which the advocate builds all other skills and attributes. The advocate values the humane and just treatment of others, including equality, respect, and dignity (Kosik, 1972).

As an advocate, the nurse supports the client's right to make decisions freely and without persuasion. Nursing actions include supporting the client so that the client can make the best possible decisions regarding health (Kohnke, 1980). With the client, the nurse evaluates the validity of the client's choice. This process affirms whether the client's choices are consistent with personal desires. **Affirming** is an important process that allows the client to review the motives behind his or her choices. Via this process, the client may identify areas requiring further information, support, or time (Cary, 1996).

Client decisions may conflict with the desires of the nurse. The nurse must be on guard not to persuade the client. It is essential that the advocate examine personal attitudes, knowledge, and responses to client choices. The nurse as advocate must be sensitive to possible conflicts of interest. The advocate must maintain an accurate awareness of self while managing interactions for the client, thus allowing the client to freely choose a direction (Robinson, 1985; Cary, 1996).

Goals of Advocacy

The goal of client advocacy is twofold: client independence and system improvement. In making the client more independent, the nurse encourages the client to be an active participant in individual health care. The client must remain at the center of the care process and feel supported in decisions. To this end, the nurse expands the client's understanding of those services that can be expected from the system, the reasons those services are needed, and the ways that those services might be obtained. In all actions of advocacy, the nurse fosters both client and system acceptance of client participation. The system must support active participation by clients and social groups in health care decisions that affect them. Active decision making ensures the client's progress toward self-care, the desired outcome of advocacy interventions (Kosik, 1972).

The second goal of advocacy is to improve the system to make it more sensitive and relevant to the needs of the individual or group (Kosik, 1972). The community health nurse "uses tools of public health policy development and advocacy for needed policy changes to improve the health of communities" (Kuehnert, 1991, p. 5). This is accomplished by implementing such actions as assessing client/community needs, planning appropriate programs, developing policies, implementing change, evaluating outcomes, and remaining committed to the process until change is accepted.

Advocacy Interventions

Advocacy interventions are implemented on multiple levels. Advocacy occurs with individuals, families, communities, and social systems (Kuehnert, 1991; Murphy, 1992; Wagner & Menke, 1992). The community health nurse is active at each of these levels during the course of professional practice. At times, the focus may be on one level more than on another. The needs of different clients, groups, or social situations require varied time and energy commitments from the advocate. The nurse must be sensitive to difficulties the client may encounter and must develop the ability to identify potential barriers to the well-being of the client at each level.

For example, an unmarried teen mother may not be able to negotiate the health system to apply for Medicaid coverage, thereby restricting access to health care for herself and her infant. The community health nurse can advocate for the teen mother by implementing interventions that reduce barriers to the services.

Some advocacy changes may be possible only at the community level. Larger social issues, for example, may be addressed at the level of public policy development. Such larger social issues may include, but are not limited to, poverty, homelessness, unemployment, gender issues, violence, and illiteracy. The nurse advocating at the pub-

DECISION MAKING

Client Advocacy

Nurses often interact with clients whose values and beliefs differ from their own. It is important to identify ways that your own values and beliefs affect your interactions with clients. How might you respond to the following situations?

• Your belief system supports abstinence as the only acceptable contraceptive practice. You are a school nurse and are approached by a teenaged girl who is sexually active and desires information and access to condoms and the birth control pill.

• You believe that people must have their basic safety and security needs satisfied in order to progress to independence. You are the case manager for several families whose income is significantly below the poverty level. The families live in substandard housing, and their apartments are vermin infested. How might you advocate for these families? To what community groups would you address your concerns?

lic policy level needs expertise in skills of problem solving, negotiation, conflict resolution, and change processes (Kuehnert, 1991; Spradley & Allender, 1996). The political arena provides access to the legislative system, an established vehicle for social progress. Involvement in the political process challenges all of the abilities of the nurse in the advocate role.

An example would be a community health nurse who sits on the board of directors of a women's crisis shelter. In this example, the nurse is aware that recent legislation and new state guidelines mandate that an increase in shelter services be provided. However, no increase in state funding has been appropriated to support the newly mandated services. The community health nurse takes the problem to the county commission to petition for county funding as a yearly budget item. Such funding would ensure a state source of income for the women's shelter, allow for an increase in services to cover the state mandate, and generate local commitment to women's needs in the county.

Consumers of health care demand that they be participants in the decisions affecting their health care at both the individual and group levels (Bramlett, Gueldner, & Sowell, 1990). It is the responsibility of the advocate to foster this participation. As the consumer becomes more involved, the advocate must become better prepared in order to impart the necessary knowledge and power to the consumer. The nurse must develop expertise in political processes, client-focused care, community and social issues, and the acquisition of health care resources in order to empower the client in self-management.

Collaborator

To **collaborate** means to work with others toward a common goal. It is a process of joint decision making in an atmosphere of mutual respect and cooperation. Collaboration should always be the mode of interaction between the community health nurse and the client and is an equally important nursing role when the nurse functions as part of a team. Whether collaborating with an individual, a family, or an agency or as part of a team, the community health nurse is involved in joint decision making regarding the most appropriate action to be taken to resolve problems (Spradley & Dorsey, 1992; Clark, 1996).

Concepts of Collaboration

Nurses in all settings work as members of a team. In acute care settings, team members are generally other health care professionals. In community health settings, the nurse is part of a truly multidisciplinary team that includes not only other health care workers but also members from community organizations, social service agencies, judicial systems, political entities, schools, religious organizations, volunteer networks, and other non–health-related profes-

sions. The complex demands of clients and populations in many community health settings require a multidisciplinary approach in order to promote optimal outcomes. All members of this multidisciplinary team work together to bring about optimal health and well-being for the client, whether that client be an individual, family, group, or community (ANA, 1987; Proctor, Lordi, & Zaiger, 1993). As described in the ANA's *Standards for Community Health Nursing* (1986a), "community health nursing practice requires planning and sharing with others in the community to promote health for the community, family, and individual. Through the collaborative process, the special abilities of others are used to communicate, plan, solve problems, and evaluate services" (p. 14).

Successful collaboration requires that the multidisciplinary team develop a common purpose, communicate to effectively coordinate efforts, and recognize the unique and complementary skills possessed by each team member (Brunk, 1992). Each team member brings special abilities and expertise to the collaborative process. With strong support and active participation of all members, "the team communicates, plans, anticipates and solves problems, and evaluates services" (ANA, 1987, p. 4).

Although they do share some similarities, collaboration and coordination are inherently different. **Coordination** is the efficient management of services without gaps or overlaps. The nurse as coordinator may or may not consult with others in carrying out that which is essentially a management function. Collaboration, on the other hand, involves joint decision making between two or more people (Clark, 1996).

Characteristics of a Collaborator

Effective collaboration requires skills in communication and problem solving. The nurse must be able to communicate effectively with the client, family, group, or team. With other team members, the nurse shares client needs and possible interventions to bring about the resolution of problems. With the client, the nurse engages in joint problem solving to identify needs and evaluate alternative solutions. Together, all members of the team, including the client, select an appropriate alternative. Collaboration continues as solutions are implemented and evaluated. Collaboration does not work when each team member designs and provides a program from a particular area of expertise and then "coordinates" by informing others of the plan. To be successful, collaboration must be a joint effort on the part of the client and all team members to identify mutual goals and acceptable means for meeting those goals (Clark, 1996).

The community health nurse as team member must develop assertive communication skills and be able to describe the nurse's unique contribution to the health team as an equal partner. The nurse as collaborator works with individuals from other disciplines, service providers, political entities, and community agencies to establish effective networks to expedite client services. This networking may require continual redefinition and development. Political astuteness and maturity on the part of the nurse will assist in overcoming the turf issues, financial constraints, and competition that combine to make collaboration a complex and involved process. Although collaboration is a relatively new role for nurses, they must actively promote the collaborative process to secure the delivery of high-quality services to the client. Collaboration succeeds when there are feelings of mutual respect and collegiality among all members of the team (ANA, 1986b; Kenyon, Smith, Hefty, Bell, McNeil, & Martans; 1990; Clark, 1996).

Consultant

Every community health nurse is a **consultant**. Each time a nurse gives information or assists a client in choosing between alternative actions, the nurse is using consulting skills. Consultants help clients understand their problems and assist them in making wise decisions. Consultants are catalysts, persons who bring about change or changes. From a perspective of expertise, the nurse consultant promotes decision making and change by providing information and alternatives. Consultation as a skill is part of almost every professional activity that involves problem solving. The nurse also acts as consultant when helping a client improve specific skills or make more effective plans (Lange, 1987; Schneider, 1992; Hazelton, Boyum, & Frost, 1993).

Components of Consultation

The consultant has traditionally been viewed as an expert, or someone with specialized skills and knowledge who is able to propose solutions for identified problems. The consultant is expected to be a resource, someone who can provide information that will assist the client to make decisions based on alternatives. The consultant may be viewed as a change agent who uses process consultation

Figure 14-3 Types of Clients Encountered in Nursing Consultation

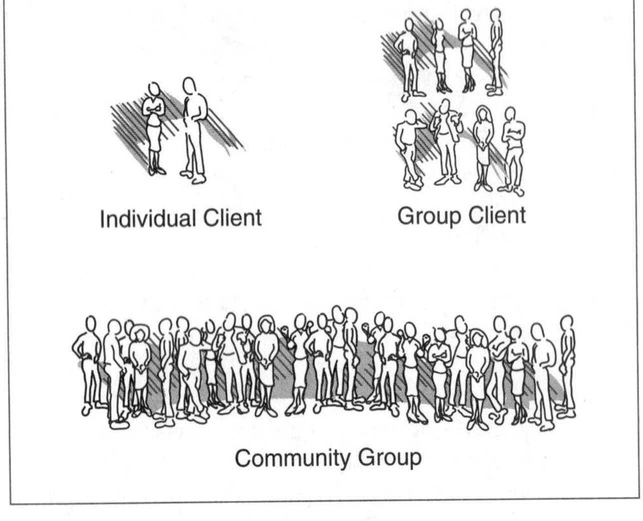

Individual Client

Group Client

Community Group

to bring about change in a given situation. In process consultation, the consultant helps the client perceive, understand, and act on events that occur in the client's environment. A consultant can be seen as a trained teacher and an expert in a particular specialty. The successful consultant must be able to motivate others and be able to get things done even when not in direct charge of the people concerned (Lange, 1987; Wright, Johnson, & Purdy, 1991; Brunk, 1992).

In nursing consultation, there are generally three types of clients: the individual client, the group client, and the community or secondary group (see Figure 14-3). The individual client may be a patient, family member, fellow nurse, or other professional. The group client is usually a small cohesive unit or primary group of 10 or fewer people. Examples of such groups include families, unit staff nurses, or other nurse groups. The community or secondary group is a larger, more diverse and complex social system. This community group is more impersonal; examples include community organizations, large health care agencies, schools, governmental agencies, and foundations (Lange, 1987).

The nurse consultant fulfills multiple roles. In addition to specific consulting duties, the nurse will likely be expected to fill one or more of the following roles: leader, expert, coordinator, resource person, clinical specialist, teacher, and researcher. As leader, the nurse consultant assists and directs others toward a desired goal. The quality of leadership is key in determining the success or failure of a consultant. In a consulting arrangement, the nurse must develop informal power based on interpersonal relationships and expert knowledge. As expert, the nurse has unique skills to bring to a particular problem. The client must believe that the consultant has pertinent information, skill, or ability that can help. As coordinator, the nurse plans, organizes, supports, energizes, and inspires. The nurse is able to manage conflict and to synchronize events to produce minimum conflict and maximum collaboration. As resource person, the nurse consultant brings knowledge and assistance in the wise use of resources. The nurse provides information about resources so the client can make informed choices from a variety of alternatives. As clinical specialist, the nurse consultant provides a unique service by bringing specialized knowledge, skill, and experience to the situation. As teacher, the consultant helps the client actively learn new information, skills, and abilities. As researcher, the nurse consultant is involved in fact-finding. This is a key function of the consultant, whether in developing a database, assessing and diagnosing client problems, or producing a formal research proposal. The consultant is researching, whether by simply listening or by conducting a complex formal survey (Lange, 1987).

Many nurses may initially be uncomfortable functioning in the role of consultant because it differs from the traditional role of "doing for" the client and, instead, consists of helping others gain the expertise and ability to do for themselves. A consultant remains relatively distant from the problem at hand, giving advice but not personally investing in the outcome. Indeed, a consultant must be willing to stand by without directly controlling anything. Although there to influence and give advice, the consultant generally does not have the authority or position power to implement change. The optimal relationship is one in which the consultant shares knowledge and expertise in a collaborative relationship. The client allows the consultant to take the lead in exploring a problem, and the consultant respects the client's right to make the final decision. It may be a challenge for the consultant to balance the supportive role with the objectivity and distance that must be maintained for credibility to be enhanced (Butler, 1986; Lange, 1987; Wright et al., 1991).

Counselor

Counseling at its most basic level is the process of helping clients choose appropriate solutions to their problems. Counseling is not telling people what to do; instead, it is the process of assisting them to use problem-solving processes to decide on the course of action most appropriate for them. The counselor's role is to listen objectively, clarify, provide feedback and information, and guide the client through a problem-solving process (Thompson, 1989; Igoe & Speer, 1996; Clark, 1996).

Clients generally seek counseling when they are unable to make decisions about health or personal concerns. Counseling involves exploration of feelings and attitudes on the part of the client and is directed toward helping the client develop self-understanding. Counseling requires trust, empathy, respect, confidentiality, and good communication skills on the part of the nurse. Good listening skills and the ability to clarify and ask open-ended questions in a nonjudgmental way will assist the client in arriving at appropriate solutions to individual problems (Lange, 1987; Thompson, 1989; Igoe & Speer, 1996; Balzar-Riley, 1996).

Counseling may be confused with either educating or consulting. As educator, the nurse is presenting information and facts but is not necessarily seeking to assist in problem solving or decision making. The goal of both consulting and counseling is decisive action. But, whereas counseling involves the exploration of feelings and attitudes directed toward assisting the client to understand him- or herself more openly and honestly, consulting is a mutually planned, purposive process whereby client and consultant set goals and objectives to meet identified needs and then put in place processes and practices to meet those needs. The consultant is not necessarily concerned with subjective understanding on the part of the client. The nurse works with the client to achieve preset goals in an efficient way so that the tasks at hand can be accomplished. Counseling may be a skill used in the consulting process to create a climate within which to explore solutions to problems, or it may follow education to assist the client in making decisions based on the information given (Lange, 1987; Clark, 1996). Regardless of the context, counseling remains an important component of community health nursing. Table 14-1 illustrates the differences between education, counseling, and consulting. For more detailed information on counseling, refer to Chapter 8.

Educator

Community health nursing has embraced the responsibility of educating individuals, families, and communities since the days of the Henry Street Settlement. Health teaching is considered one of the major functions of the community nurse and is deemed an essential nursing responsibility regardless of the setting where the nurse is employed (Lee, 1992; Babcock & Miller, 1994; Balzar-Riley, 1996). Teaching is a necessary role function for the promotion of health and welfare of individuals and societies. Teaching is one of the avenues via which the nurse enables the client to make informed decisions regarding personal, family, or community health practices and lifestyle choices. Although teaching the individual is considered important, the majority of teaching implemented by the community health nurse is directed toward aggregates rather than the individual (Lee, 1992; DeBella, 1993), and focuses on health promotion, health maintenance, and disease prevention.

An understanding of the teaching–learning process is especially vital to the community health nurse. The nurse is expected to teach individuals, families, and communities on a wide range of topics, in various settings, and

Table 14-1   Comparison of Educating, Counseling, and Consulting

EDUCATION GOAL	COUNSELING GOAL	CONSULTING GOAL
Present facts No decisive action taken	Decisive action	Decisive action
Example	**Example**	**Example**
Present dangers of smoking Present cessation techniques	Explore methods of cessation and help client decide best course of action	Set goals and objectives to stop smoking (obtain nicotine gum; begin program within two days of obtaining nicotine gum; complete prescribed regimen; monitor adherence to regimen; monitor nonsmoking for a period after regimen has been completed)

under different circumstances. Because it is grounded in theory and concepts from professional education teaching is one of the most technical and difficult roles in nursing (Van Hoozer et al., 1987). See Chapter 8 for further discussion of teaching and learning.

Teaching is defined as the process of providing a person or group of persons with the knowledge and skills necessary to make appropriate choices and decisions. To educate or teach others is to provide them with the skills to adapt to their circumstances (Clark, 1996; Murray & Zentner, 1997). Teaching includes the ability to identify learning needs of populations at risk and to plan and implement teaching strategies that will lead to adaptation (Kenyon et al., 1990). **Learning** (the gaining of knowledge, understanding, or skill) is considered a lifelong rather than a short-term process. Therefore, strategies for continued learning must be encouraged and reinforced in the learner (Murray & Zentner, 1997).

Goals of Client Education

The goal of the nurse as educator is to ensure optimal learning by the client in order to encourage improved health behaviors. Teaching includes developing activities that provide the client with new information and with opportunities to practice new skills. Ideally, the client will embrace this information, develop skills, and implement improved behaviors that lead to the highest level of wellness possible (DeBella, 1993; Babcock & Miller, 1994). It is the challenge of the nurse–educator to identify the specific needs of the individual or group, to implement an appropriate plan for learning, and to evaluate outcomes in order to modify or repeat content and practice and to reinforce positive changes.

Characteristics of a Nurse–Educator

It is important that the nurse–educator view the client as a responsible, thinking individual who has the right to make choices regarding individual health behavior (Babcock & Miller, 1994). With this perspective, the nurse–educator will include the learner in the planning process and will advocate for the learner until the individual can take responsibility. The attitudes, behaviors, and style of the teacher affect learning outcomes (Rankin & Stallings, 1996).

In order to foster success in the learner, the professional nurse–educator must keep several important concepts in mind and must continuously evaluate him- or herself with respect to these concepts. By doing so, the nurse will develop further skill in interpreting the needs of the learners and in adapting the teaching process to best meet those needs. Figure 14-4 lists several concepts identified by Van Hoozer et al. (1987) as being critical to maximizing teaching effectiveness.

The role of nurse–educator is challenging, yet offers significant rewards. Community health nursing affords boundless opportunities to teach in any setting with any number of individuals. This teaching–learning exchange is

Figure 14-4   Critical Concepts in Maximizing Teaching Effectiveness

The nurse–teacher will:

- Diagnose learning needs and problems.
- Assess learner characteristics and readiness to learn.
- Consider learning theory, forces that affect learning, and learning principles in shaping the learning experiences.
- Realize that learner participation promotes achievement.
- Analyze content and tasks.
- Employ teaching strategies based on the characteristics of the learner, the learning environment, and the expected outcomes.
- Identify, select, and design teaching actions.
- Foster teacher–learner relationship.
- Be attentive to common group needs while remaining sensitive to individual needs.
- Recognize that the behaviors, attitudes, and style of the teacher affect achievement of the learner.
- Create an optimal learning environment.
- Validate, implement, and evaluate teaching process and learning outcomes

Adapted from The Teaching Process: Theory and Practice in Nursing *by M. L. Van Hoozer, B. D. Bratton, P. M. Ostmoe, D. Weinholtz, M. J. Craft, C. L. Gjerde, & M. A. Albanese, 1987, Norwalk, CT: Appleton-Century-Croft. Copyright 1987 by Appleton-Century-Croft.*

vital in developing an informed client who is capable of making health-promoting changes in self, family, and the community. An in-depth discussion of the education process, including teaching methodologies and learning theories, is presented in Chapter 8.

Researcher

The community health nurse participates in the research process at multiple levels. The nurse may be involved in activities such as identifying problem areas; collecting, analyzing, and interpreting data; applying findings; and evaluating, designing, and conducting research. All research efforts are designed to provide a specialized, scientific knowledge base for nursing practice. This foundation enables the nursing profession to anticipate potential health problems of society and to remain accountable for care interventions. This ability, in turn, ensures that nursing interventions remain current and relevant to society's needs. At a minimum, the community health nurse is expected to read current research and apply the findings to practice as a consistent part of professional actions (LoBiondo-Wood & Haber, 1994).

Goals of Nursing Research

As researcher, the nurse seeks to discover, investigate, understand, explain, and predict phenomena. The research process comprises specific actions to collect data and synthesize information. The steps of the scientific research process are as follows:

1. Identify the question.
2. Review related literature.
3. Select a conceptual framework or model.
4. Select a research design and methodology.
5. Collect and analyze data.
6. Interpret and discuss results.
7. Identify implications for practice.
8. Communicate findings to others.

These steps ensure that the research process as well as the findings can be reviewed, evaluated, and critiqued by other investigators (LoBiondo-Wood & Haber, 1994).

To manage future health concerns, the researcher will be challenged to answer research questions on issues related to HIV/AIDS, infectious disease, chronic physical and emotional conditions, and injury prevention. Social issues including escalating health care costs, disability related to aging, social violence, poor pregnancy outcomes, poverty, homelessness, substance abuse, and other such community-level concerns must also be studied thoroughly (Laffrey & Page, 1989; Shelov, 1994). Other broad areas for nursing research as outlined by the National Institute of Nursing Research (NINR) are discussed later in this chapter. Participation in research at the community level can range from collecting data to chart auditing and participating in small pilot studies to creating and managing large longitudinal studies. There is a place for community health nurses at all levels and in all settings to be involved in ongoing research.

Characteristics of a Nurse–Researcher

The researcher embodies several characteristics. Among these are a spirit of inquiry, energy, drive, creativity, and perseverance. The investigator must be open minded, analytical, detail oriented, and able to communicate findings. Even if not involved in the full research process, the nurse must actualize these characteristics in order to critically review and analyze the research of others before applying findings to practice (Spradley, 1990; Shelov, 1994).

To develop new strategies and new tools to meet the changing needs of clients and health care delivery systems, the researcher must prepare to meet research challenges. Shelov (1994) outlines several necessary components for meeting future needs:

- The community health researcher must gather good data. Data must be reliable, valid, reproducible, objective, and sufficiently flexible for application over time.
- The researcher must carefully identify the needs of populations. High-risk population groups must be targeted so that specific and relevant strategies can be developed and implemented. The population group must be involved in the processes of decision making and program and/or policy development in order to increase group interest and commitment to behavior changes.
- The researcher must measure and analyze the outcomes of the specific interventions. Accurate evaluation provides information necessary to modify or restructure future interventions.
- The researcher must accept that technology cannot answer all social and health problems. The greatest research challenges lie in the psyche, behavior, motivations, values, and needs of individuals and populations. These phenomena may be the most difficult to assess through the scientific process as it is now designed.

Research-based solutions to current and future health issues are necessary to enable society to work toward a healthier future. Critical-thinking skills, creativity, flexibility, and tenacity are essential to ensure the success of research-based decision making and practice in community health nursing. The research role of the community health nurse is an essential component in the identification, analysis, and application of strategies that lead to positive health outcomes and promote the self-care of populations.

DECISION MAKING

Nursing Research

Research in community health practice is challenging. The variables can be difficult to identify and measure. Consider ways that you might structure your research to answer the following.

- How might you measure the "health" or "wellness" of your community?

- You have decided to implement a teaching project on stress management to a group of well elders. What criteria might you use to measure the effectiveness of your nursing interventions?

- You are a new occupational health nurse at a local plastics factory. What questions might you ask the employees to better understand their need for and interest in health-promotion topics?

Case Manager

Coordination of care is difficult in a health care system with many differing public and private programs, services, agencies, and institutions. Because of its complexities, the system frequently breaks down, creating fragmentation of care for the client. Obvious gaps in services, duplication of resources, and difficulty in accessing care are among the manifestations of this breakdown, some of which contribute to escalating health care costs. Furthermore, concerns regarding the quality of services rendered are ever-present. One response to the problems of our health care system is **case management**. Case management is the application of strategies for coordinating and allocating services for individuals who cannot manage their own care or who cannot negotiate the health care system (Redford, 1992). Case management is also a framework used by managed care programs to control access and use of health care services by enrollees.

Case management programs are becoming increasingly common and have been implemented in every conceivable public and private setting throughout the United States. Case management is seen as an effective method of delivering services to individuals needing assistance maneuvering through the health care system and is especially effective for those with long-term care needs. Those who are physically and emotionally disabled, frail and elderly, chronically ill, nursing home residents, or members of high-risk groups—those who require multiple services and who are involved in the system over a long period of time—are excellent candidates for case managed services (Molloy, 1994).

Rogers, Riordan, and Swindle (1991) define a case manager as "a single health care professional—whether social worker, physician, or nurse—who oversees, manages, and accounts for the total health care of a client or given caseload over time" (p. 30). Case managers expedite the implementation of a comprehensive service plan, attain services to meet treatment goals, and monitor the effectiveness of interventions (Epstein, Nelson, Polsgrove, Coutinho, Cumblad, & Quinn, 1993). The community health nurse is in an excellent position to function in the role of case manager because of long-term commitment to the client, a focus on considering the wide range of client needs and matching the client to needed services, experience with the referral network, and professional skills in comprehensive assessment and care planning, implementation, and evaluation (Kane, 1990; Wagner & Menke, 1992).

Concepts in Case Management

Multiple concepts are inherent in case management. Kane quotes the *Encyclopedia of Aging* definition of case management as "a service function directed at coordinating existing resources to assure appropriate and continuing care on a case-by-case basis " (1990, p. 2). Case management requires focused and skilled assessment in the planning of services. The process is built on comprehensive functional assessment, identifies measurable outcomes, and incorporates collaboration and networking for the allocation of health services (Kane, 1990).

Case management is further identified as a process that coordinates services by implementing an individual service plan developed in response to client needs and problems (White et al., 1989). This plan addresses the gap between complex client needs, services offered by providers, and increasingly limited health care resources. The overriding goals of case management are to minimize fragmentation of services and maximize individualization of care (Strong, 1992).

Managed Care and Case Management

The definition and role of the nurse as case manager are fluid in today's health care system and will continue to evolve. The advent of managed care will affect the community nurse in functional roles and practice settings. Because Medicaid and Medicare populations in the United States are rapidly being moved into mandated managed care programs, implications for the role of community nurses in health departments, clinics, home health agencies, and other organizations using managed care frameworks are profound. Because they are likely to lose the safety net funding they have received for providing primary care services to Medicaid clients, public health departments will undoubtedly see changes. There is a concern that the growth of managed care will lead to closure of home health agencies because authorization of services will be denied or severely restricted. This presents a dilemma as the population in need of home health services will continue to grow. Nurses employed in managed care organizations will be challenged to incorporate community nursing principles into their practice as they become responsible for applying population-based care to system enrollees in a cost-effective manner. Case management functions may potentiate nurses' becoming administrators of client care rather than being caregivers (Rheaume, Frisch, Smith, & Kennedy, 1994). This shift from a primary care focus will have ramifications for nursing practice, such as increased need for task delegation, increased use of unlicensed assistive personnel, and a blurring of practice boundaries and authority lines.

Functions in Case Management

Case management comprises six major functions that must be present in all case management models. These functions are: case finding, assessment, care planning, implementation, monitoring, and reassessment and evaluation (Kane, 1990).

Case finding: Case finding is the identification of those individuals from a population who will benefit from case management services. Case finding was founded on the philosophy that not all individuals require case management. Only those individuals who were unable to function at the level necessary to effectively care for themselves or manage independently were considered for case management (Kane, 1990; Redford, 1992). Appropriate cases were identified through the screening of applicants, information and referral networks, or brief assessments of key dimensions that showed need or eligibility. Case finding has evolved to now include many or all of the enrollees in health maintenance organizations (HMOs) or other managed care programs. Such programs manage enrollees to the degree necessary to reduce costs while striving to ensure access to quality care. Enrollees may be grouped with other individuals with similar health needs and be assigned to specific case managers in order to more effectively track concerns and facilitate services.

Assessment: Assessment means a full-scale, multidimensional, standardized, functional assessment of the client's needs and resources. Assessed are a comprehensive range of dimensions, including functional abilities, physical health, emotional well-being, social function, environment, current service involvement, and family support. The information obtained from the assessment process provides the case manager with practical and measurable data from which problems are identified and service plans are developed, implemented, and evaluated (Kane, 1990; Redford, 1992).

Care planning: Care planning is the core function of the case management process. The case manager takes the data identified via the assessment and, with the client, develops a service plan. This plan incorporates client preferences; specifies the type, amount, and source of services; identifies family roles and responsibilities; and specifies the nature and intensity of the case manager's role (Kane, 1990). According to Schneider (1992), service planning commits the agency to the client for a specified period of time, makes claim to identified resources, and establishes client and provider expectations. Regardless of the format, the service plan incorporates seven basic elements, as identified in Figure 14-5.

Service planning requires the case manager to have a broad knowledge base, abilities in the analysis and synthesis of information, and skills in client teaching, counseling, and service negotiation. The case manager must be aware of the availability, limitations, and accessibility of service alternatives and must be skilled in the effective integration of these services (Redford, 1992).

The use of standardized care plans and critical pathway tools is increasing in the community setting. The data derived from these processes allow agency nurses to better track clients by monitoring their signs and symptoms and contrasting and comparing variances to expected health responses. Tracking client health in this manner allows the nurse to anticipate potential problems and respond quickly to actual problems to minimize untoward health responses. The use of computers to track and compile the data collected from these tools is helpful to the nurse in providing high-quality care.

Implementation: Implementation is when the service plan is enacted. It is challenging to arrange services that adequately and effectively meet the needs and preferences of the client while also keeping costs to a minimum. Costs of services must be factored into deci-

Figure 14-5 Elements of Service Planning in Case Management

- A comprehensive problem list
- A desired outcome for each problem being addressed
- A determination of the type of help needed to achieve each desired outcome
- A list of the services and providers that will be supplying the type of help listed
- An indication of the amount of each service to be provided
- A calculation of the costs of providing the listed services for a specific period of time and an indication of the sources of payment
- An indication of agreement by the client and, when appropriate, informal caregiver

Adapted from Care Planning in the Aging Network by B. Schneider, 1992. In R. Kane, K. Urv-Wong, & C. King (Eds.), Concepts in Case Management (pp. 3–27), Minneapolis: University of Minnesota Long-Term Care DECISIONS Resource Center. Copyright 1992 by University of Minnesota.

sions regarding the best service alternatives. Both formal and informal, traditional and nontraditional networks and resources are used to enact the service plan (Redford, 1992).

Monitoring: Monitoring is the function that provides information regarding the appropriateness, adequacy, and effectiveness of the service plan. The case manager monitors the well-being of the client in response to the service plan. Changes in the condition or circumstances of the client are noted. The services received are also evaluated. Services are monitored for timeliness, appropriateness, amount, duration, and effects. Monitoring service providers is important. Each provider is evaluated against specified performance standards. The overall purpose of the monitoring function is to ensure that the service plan is assisting the progress desired for the client. Monitoring requires knowledge of the services requested, an understanding of specific performance standards, attention to service goals, and responsible documentation. Modifications are made to the service plan as necessary (Kane, 1990; Redford, 1992).

Reassessment and evaluation: Reassessment and evaluation is a formal process that occurs at regularly scheduled intervals. Evaluation also occurs at times of client hospitalization, nursing home admission, illness, family crisis, or other precipitous, triggering events. This function provides for the assessment and evaluation of the total service plan and/or the entire case management process. Data are used to evaluate the effectiveness of the service plan in meeting the identified client goals and outcome objectives. This function provides information regarding the effectiveness of case management as a service-coordinating strategy.

The information collected may be used in research investigations targeting client outcomes following case management interventions (Kane, 1990; Redford, 1992).

Characteristics of a Case Manager

The case manager must have a high level of professional competence, including in-depth clinical knowledge, an understanding of the service system, and experience with cost-containment strategies. The case manager needs skills in negotiation, collaboration, and conflict resolution in order to broker for services. An appropriate educational background is necessary to better prepare nurses in these areas. An integration of case management content in baccalaureate and master's nursing programs is essential for professional preparation. Continuing-education programs are necessary for nurses who must incorporate case management skills into their careers. Opportunities for nurses as case managers will continue to expand in the future (Redford, 1992).

An example of a planned case management program is the Registered Nurse Specialist Program at the University of Miami. This program develops nurse case managers for chronically ill children through a formal, continuing-education program. It was implemented to reduce the fragmentation of services for children and families needing long-term interventions. The goals of the program are to:

- Promote integration of services.
- Reduce unnecessary health care expenditures.
- Promote the integrity of the family unit and the family's ability to access health services.
- Empower family members to better manage their children's care.

This unique nursing program has improved health care delivery, has met an urgent statewide need for children and families who meet eligibility, and has expanded the role of the nurse as case manager (Urbano, von-Windeguth, Siderits, Parker, & Studenic-Lewis, 1991).

The increasing demand for well-managed and coordinated client services requires a pool of highly qualified and well-educated professionals. Case management is a logical path for community health nurses because of their educational preparation and community experience. Continuing-education programs that update knowledge, skills, and experiences in case management strategies will enhance the nurse's proficiency as a case manager. Legal, ethical, and social obligations must be well understood by the nurse and incorporated into the service delivery plan. As case manager, the nurse, along with other community service providers, is challenged to develop and refine management systems that promote client well-being, that are fair to all (clients, case managers, and service providers), and that cost no more than necessary (Kane, 1990). Table 14-2 presents examples of the roles of community health nurses.

PRACTICE SETTINGS FOR COMMUNITY HEALTH NURSING

Community health nurses provide care to aggregates in multiple settings. Some nurses function as home health or hospice nurses, for example. In each of these capacities, the nurse delivers care in a variety of locations, but generally in the client's home. The nurse's caseload is an aggregate assembled because of individual disability, diagnosis, or need. Other nurses practice in stationary community settings such as public health departments, neighborhood schools, industrial or business environments, or correctional facilities. Such caseloads are composed of groups of people within these settings who need interventions for actual or potential health needs. Regard-

Table 14-2 The Various Roles of the Community Health Nurse

ROLE	EXAMPLE
Clinician	Provide information to a group of teenagers regarding safe-sex practices. Plan, implement, and evaluate a program to decrease drug use by adolescents.
Advocate	Speak for the needs of the homeless
Collaborator	Work with a parent, teacher, principal, physician, and social worker to develop a plan to facilitate the successful integration of a child with a disability into a public school setting.
Consultant	Provide assistance to a program coordinator to develop a client satisfaction questionnaire.
Counselor	Assist adult children to explore their feelings about nursing home placement for a parent and discuss other options available to them.
Educator	Teach a prenatal class on nutrition and healthy habits.
Case manager	Coordinate support services for an elderly woman and her husband, who has Alzheimer's disease. Explain Alzheimer's respite services, support groups, nursing home and long-term care facilities. Assist with insurance issues. Assist the woman to obtain transportation as she no longer drives.

less of the location or setting, the community health nurse provides a comprehensive health program for individuals, families, groups, and communities. In each setting, with all clients, the nurse provides services that emphasize caring, compassion, respect, and dignity.

Public Health Nursing

Previous generations of public health nurses identified the need for community-based programs whereby people who were at risk were connected with community services such as those provided by health departments. Public health nurses were at the forefront of many policy reforms that helped bring family planning, workplace safety, and maternal and child health services to people in need.

Since the inception of public health nursing, public health nurses have made a unique contribution to the health care system. Beginning with Lillian Wald, visiting families in their homes has been central to public health nursing practice, thereby providing nurses with the opportunity to see firsthand the difficulties that individuals and families experience in their homes and communities. In addition to the home-based interventions, public health nurses work in other community-based services such as nursing centers, screening programs, and health education outreach efforts (Rector, 1997).

Today, they continue to contribute significantly to the health of the community. As discussed in Chapter 1, public health nursing, as defined by the American Public Health Association, Public Health Nursing Section (1996), is "the practice of promoting and protecting the health of populations using knowledge from nursing, social, and public health sciences" (p. 1). The primary focus of public health nursing is to promote health and prevent disease for population groups. Public health nurses may provide care to individuals and families within a population group; however, the focus is on the population, with an emphasis on identifying individuals who may not request care but who have health problems that put them and others in the community at risk.

Role Functions of the Public Health Nurse

Public health nurses work in the neighborhoods and homes of some the most vulnerable people (Zerwekh, 1993). Their practice includes the assessment and identification of populations who are at risk or high risk for disease, threat of disease, poor recovery, and injury. These populations include the aging population, whose numbers will increase significantly in the near future, children and adults with chronic illness and disabilities, impoverished women and children, homeless and near-homeless persons, families who are dealing with violence in their homes and neighborhoods, those with substance abuse problems, and people threatened by the return of acute and chronic communicable diseases.

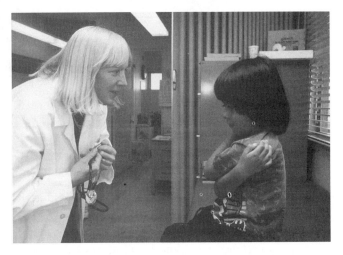

A few of the many places community health nurses can be found working and caring for clients are schools, correctional facilities, and places of business.

Public health nurses are involved in the interdisciplinary activities associated with the core public health functions of assessment, assurance, and policy development. Public health nurses translate knowledge from the health and social sciences to individuals, families, and population groups through advocacy, targeted interventions, and program development. Public health nurses work to ensure that services are available and accessible. They function as health educators and care managers, working with and through relevant community leaders, interest groups, employers, families, and individuals, and they are involved in social and political actions, all to improve health care access and availability (American Public Health Association, 1996).

Public health nurses practice in community-based health agencies, particularly health departments in counties throughout the United States. In health departments, public health nurses contribute to the surveillance and monitoring of disease trends within the community. Emerging patterns of diseases that may threaten the public's health are identified, and interventions are planned, implemented, and coordinated. Public health nurses also contribute to the monitoring of environmentally caused illnesses, immunization levels, lead poisoning incidence, infant mortality rates, and communicable disease occurrence in order to identify problems that threaten the public's health. Public health nurses also function in other community-based agencies with varying degrees of public health focus.

Home Health Nursing

Home health nursing is a rapidly expanding and dynamic specialty in health care delivery. Burbach and Brown (1988) cite Warhola's definition of home health nursing as a "component of comprehensive health care whereby health services are provided to individuals and

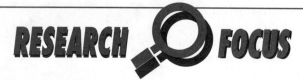

Perceptions of Public Health Nursing: Views from the Field

STUDY PROBLEM/PURPOSE

The purpose of this study was to gather information about the experiences and perspectives of practicing public health nurses. System changes affecting public health nursing may potentially lead to role conflict, role ambiguity, and role overload, resulting in role stress and strain, and may influence the provision of care. An understanding of what public health nurses do and how they feel about that which they do can be used to support public health nurses during times of restructuring and shifting demands.

METHODS

A descriptive, qualitative research design was used with 28 female public health staff nurses from six health units serving urban and rural populations in Alberta, Canada. Participants' length of experience in public health nursing ranged from 8 months to 24 years, with a mean of 12 years.

FINDINGS

Four main themes were inductively derived from interviews regarding nurses' feelings about their work. These nurses perceived their work as valuable, worthwhile, enjoyable, demanding, and not well understood by others.

IMPLICATIONS

These findings can be used to provide support for nurses in times of uncertainty and to design strategies that will ensure nurses' optimal contribution to enhancing health in communities. Workloads that provide variety and autonomy, resources that provide necessary services, marketing that encourages community support, and networking that educates professionals and the public alike in the role of the public health nurse are some of the many methods available to sustain these nurses.

SOURCE

From "Perceptions of Public Health Nursing: Views from the Field" by L. Reutter & J. Ford, 1996, Journal of Advanced Nursing, 24, *pp. 7–15.*

families in their places of residence for the purpose of promoting, maintaining, or restoring health" (p. 119).

Lyon and Stephany (1993) state that the primary purpose of home health services is to allow clients to remain in their homes to receive health care services that would otherwise be offered only in health care institutions. The home health nurse provides skilled nursing interventions to clients who have acute or intermittent medical conditions or who are terminal. The client must be under the supervision of a physician who writes orders and monitors medical responses (Snow, Giduz, McConnell, Sanchez, & Wildman, 1988). The nurse implements these medical orders as a part of the overall nursing care plan.

Home health nursing is delivered through a variety of agencies and organizations. Home health services have traditionally been provided through visiting nurses' associations and community health agencies. As demand for services increases and opportunities for business emerge, however, hospitals are expanding their services into the home health field, and other private organizations are entering the arena. The inclusion of private, for-profit businesses in home health has affected the delivery of care by community, nonprofit health care agencies. This highly competitive market has made it difficult for many community agencies with limited resources to survive (ANA, 1986b; Spradley & Dorsey, 1992).

Home Health Links to Community Health Nursing

Home health nursing's historical link to community health agencies has forged multiple similarities between these specialties. (See Chapter 2 for further discussion of the history of community health nursing.) Social and cultural changes and economic and business trends, however, have led to the development of some significant differences. Burbach and Brown (1988) identify similarities (Figure 14-6) and differences (Table 14-3) between home health nursing and community health. It is important to distinguish between the two areas in order to understand performance expectations, to appreciate the common historical origins, and to identify present dichotomies. By clearly distinguishing between the two, one can acknowledge, appreciate, and evaluate the integrity and uniqueness of each specialty. It is also important to recognize the commonalities between the two areas to foster the sharing of information that supports the practice of each. It is vital that the home health nurse have knowledge of broad community health practices and have the skills to provide a community/family focus. Likewise, in order to enhance community support of clients who require home health services and the nurses who provide those services, the community health nurse must be aware of the needs of this aggregate.

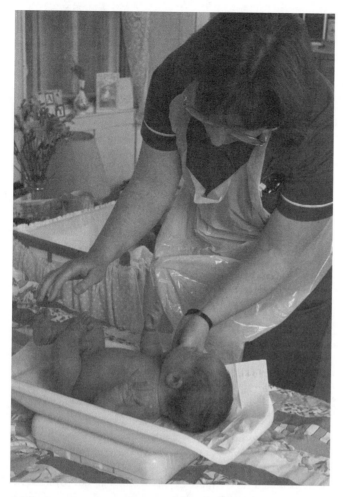

With the assistance of the community health nurse, clients are able to stay at home to receive health care services. *Photo courtesy of Jennie Woodcock; Reflections Photolibrary/Corbis.*

Figure 14-6   Similarities between Community Health Nursing and Home Health Nursing

Setting: Nursing care is provided to clients in places of residence or in their community environments.

Independent Nature of Practice: Nurses practice independently outside institutions. Community and homes are less controlled environments.

Control and Environment: Client is active participant in care decisions. Control is shifted to client. Environment empowers client.

Family-Centered Care: The family is considered as a unit of care. Family members contribute significantly to client care.

Organization and Provision of Services: Community and home health services may be offered by the same institution. Multiple combinations of agency structure exist.

Broad Goals: Community and home health services strive to promote, maintain, and restore health in the community.

Adapted from "Community Health and Home Health Nursing: Keeping the Concepts Clear" by C.A. Burbach, & B. E. Brown, 1988, Nursing and Health Care, 9, pp. 97–100. Copyright 1988 by National League for Nursing.

A comprehensive program of care for the home health client requires multidisciplinary expertise over a wide range of services. The home health nurse must be well informed and skilled in the various community health role functions in order to ensure the delivery of comprehensive and effective care to the client and family. The *Standards of Home Health Nursing Practice* (ANA, 1986b) identify specific nurse responsibilities and actions for quality client care (see Figure 14-7).

Role Functions of the Home Health Nurse

The functions of home health nurse as clinician, educator, and collaborator merit special mention. As clinician, the nurse works with clients throughout the life span as well

---

Table 14-3   Differences between Community Health Nursing and Home Health Nursing

	COMMUNITY HEALTH NURSING	HOME HEALTH NURSING
Focus of Interventions	Population	Individual/family
Caseload Acquisition	Case finding in community at large	Referral by agency or physician
Interventions	Continuous	Episodic
Orientation	Wellness	Illness
	Primary prevention	Secondary prevention
		Rehabilitation
		Tertiary prevention
Entry into Services	Risk potential/social diagnosis	Medical diagnosis

Adapted from "Community Health and Home Health Nursing: Keeping the Concepts Clear," by C. A. Burbach, & B. E. Brown, 1988, Nursing and Health Care, 9, pp. 97–100. Copyright 1988 by National League For Nursing.

Figure 14-7 Standards of Home Health Nursing Practice

Standard I. Organization of Home Health Services: All home health services are planned, organized, and directed by a master's-prepared professional nurse with experience in community health and administration.

Standard II. Theory: The nurse applies theoretical concepts as a basis for decisions in practice.

Standard III. Data Collection: The nurse continuously collects and records data that are comprehensive, accurate, and systematic.

Standard IV. Diagnosis: The nurse uses health assessment data to determine nursing diagnoses.

Standard V. Planning: The nurse develops care plans that establish goals. The care plan is based on nursing diagnoses and incorporates therapeutic, preventive, and rehabilitative nursing actions.

Standard VI. Intervention: The nurse, guided by the care plan, intervenes to provide comfort; to restore, improve, and promote health; to prevent complications and sequelae of illness; and to effect rehabilitation.

Standard VII. Evaluation: The nurse continually evaluates the client's and family's responses to interventions in order to determine progress toward goal attainment and to revise the database, nursing diagnoses, and plan of care.

Standard VIII. Continuity of Care: The nurse is responsible for the client's appropriate and uninterrupted care along the health care continuum and therefore uses discharge planning, case management, and coordination of community resources.

Standard IX. Interdisciplinary Collaboration: The nurse initiates and maintains a liaison relationship with all appropriate health care providers to ensure that all efforts effectively complement one another.

Standard X. Professional Development: The nurse assumes responsibility for professional development and contributes to the professional growth of others.

Standard XI. Research: The nurse participates in research activities that contribute to the profession's continuing development of knowledge of home health care.

Standard XII. Ethics: The nurse uses the code for nurses established by the American Nurses Association as a guide for ethical decision making in practice.

Adapted from Standards of Home Health Nursing Practice *by American Nurses Association, 1986, Kansas City, MO: Author. Copyright 1986 by American Nurses Association. Used with permission.*

obtained from continuous physical and functional assessment and evaluation of client response to interventions.

As clinician, the nurse is confronted with advancements in health-related technology. Improvements in home intravenous therapy, pain management techniques, portable ventilator management, total parenteral nutrition, computer-assisted documentation, and other intervention tools increase the nurse's need for continuing education. This education may be formal or informal but must be supported by nursing management to guarantee the delivery of up-to-date, skilled nursing interventions.

As educator, the nurse provides information to promote health for the client and family. The nurse is responsible for implementing teaching/learning strategies to assist the client in adapting to personal circumstances. The nurse and client, in partnership, identify needs, set goals, and develop and implement an educational plan. Interactions characterized by caring and compassion throughout the teaching/learning exchange support the development of trust between the nurse and client.

The nurse collaborates with the multidisciplinary team to create a plan that optimizes client response. This collaboration is required in home health nursing in order to ensure continuity of care. Although members may vary, the team frequently includes a nurse, physician, physical therapist, occupational therapist, speech pathologist, social worker, homemaker/home health aide, and clergy member (Stanhope, 1996). Regardless of the composition of the team, it is important to remember that the delivery of comprehensive, skilled nursing care is and will continue to be the predominant component of home health services (ANA, 1986b). The home health nurse is responsible for the management and coordination of care. As such, the nurse coordinates client access to multiple community resources. The home health nurse must therefore have a working knowledge of broad community health concepts.

The population in need of home health nursing services continues to grow and will do so in the future. As it does there will be increased competition for clients as well as for qualified personnel. Increasingly, health services are being provided by private organizations. Services are expected to expand to include wellness and health-promotion activities and high-technology interventions. In order to meet this broad scope of services and to implement the professional standards set forth for home health nursing, registered nurses holding a minimum of a baccalaureate degree in nursing—and whose competencies and skills therefore parallel practice expectations—will be sought after (Lyon & Stephany, 1993). Specialization via master's preparation and professional certification are endorsed by professional nursing as means to better prepare the nurse to assist clients and families, enact social policy, and conduct research (ANA, 1986b).

Hospice Care

Hospice care is a coordinated program of **palliative** services (which alleviate pain or other symptoms without

as along the wellness–illness continuum. The nurse must be creative and adaptable when providing interventions in light of limited resources, in restricted environments, and in practice isolation. The home health nurse is the practitioner who provides critical information regarding client status to the multidisciplinary team. This information is curing) delivered to terminally ill clients and their families. Interventions provide for the physical, psychological, social, and spiritual care of dying persons and their families (Spector, 1984; ANA, 1987; Murray and Zenter, 1997). Hospice emphasizes the caring and comfort aspect of care over the curing aspect via interventions to alleviate symptoms and control pain in the client and provide support and instruction to the family and significant others (Samarel, 1989; Lyon & Stephany, 1993). Caring and comfort interventions include actions that preserve the humanity and protect the dignity of dying clients and their loved ones. Such interventions take place in a variety of settings, depending on the availability and accessibility of services. To support the restoration of health to the survivors, bereavement interventions continue for loved ones after the death of the client. Figure 14-8 lists philosophical foundations essential to hospice care.

Clients are eligible to receive hospice care when it is certified by a physician that the client has fewer than six months to live and when the client is willing to receive palliative, as opposed to curative, care (Schultz, 1984; Snow et al., 1988). Clients are best served by a comprehensive hospice program that "provides centrally coordinated home care, inpatient, acute, and respite care, and bereavement services for the family and others deeply affected by the death of a client" (ANA, 1987, p. 17). Such a program is guided by a multidisciplinary team of professionals who coordinate skilled care through a holistic, dynamic, individualized plan of care that prescribes interventions to attain expected client and family outcomes (Hospice Nurses Association [HNA], 1995). The client and family are integrated into the team and define their rights and responsibilities regarding pain and symptom control, comfort interventions, home emergencies, and identification and use of available resources (ANA, 1987).

Standards of hospice practice define the basis of responsibility and accountability of the nurse providing hospice services. Current standards are designed to "promote and enhance the quality of hospice clinical practice and to define the nature and scope of hospice nursing practice" (HNA, 1995, p. 2). Refer to Figure 14-9 for practice standards.

Figure 14-8 Philosophical Foundations of Hospice Care

- Hospice offers comfort and support, rather than seeking to cure.
- Hospice considers the client and the family as the basic unit of care.
- Hospice provides care in institutional, home, and community settings.
- Hospice continues bereavement care to the survivors following the client's death.

Adapted from What Makes Hospice Unique? by R. Spector, 1984. In S. Schraff (Ed.), Hospice: The Nursing Perspective (pp. 1–15), New York: National League for Nursing. Copyright 1984 by National League for Nursing. Used with permission.

Figure 14-9 Standards of Hospice Nursing Practice and Professional Performance

Standards of Hospice Nursing Practice

Standard I. Assessment: The hospice nurse collects client and family data.

Standard II. Diagnosis: The hospice nurse analyzes the assessment data in determining diagnosis.

Standard III. Outcome Identification: The hospice nurse identifies expected outcomes individualized to the client and family.

Standard IV. Planning: The hospice nurse develops a nursing plan of care that prescribes interventions to attain expected outcomes.

Standard V. Implementation: The hospice nurse implements the interventions identified in the plan of care.

Standard VI. Evaluation: The hospice nurse evaluates the client's and family's progress toward attainment of outcomes.

Standards of Professional Performance

Standard I. Quality of Care: The hospice nurse systematically evaluates the quality and effectiveness of nursing practice.

Standard II. Performance Appraisal: The hospice nurse evaluates his or her own nursing practice in relation to professional practice standards and relevant standards and regulations.

Standard III. Education: The hospice nurse acquires and maintains current knowledge in hospice nursing practice.

Standard IV. Collegiality: The hospice nurse contributes to the professional development of peers, colleagues, and others.

Standard V. Ethics: The hospice nurse's decisions and actions on behalf of client and family are determined in an ethical manner.

Standard VI. Collaboration: The hospice nurse collaborates with the client and family, other members of the interdisciplinary team, and other health care providers in providing client and family care.

Standard VII. Research: The hospice nurse uses research findings in practice.

Standard VIII. Resource Utilization: The hospice nurse considers factors related to safety, effectiveness, and cost in planning and delivering client and family care.

Adapted from Standards of Hospice Nursing Practice and Professional Performance by Hospice Nurses Association, 1995, Pittsburgh: Author. Copyright 1995 by Hospice Nurses Publishing. Used with permission.

The importance of the multidisciplinary team is addressed in the standards. The HNA (1995) describes hospice practice as conducted within an "affiliative matrix" (p. 2). In such a matrix, the development and maintenance of collaborative relationships within the hospice team are critical. Role blending occurs as the nurse functions as case manager, coordinator of the plan of care, advocate, and educator. Because of the associated clinical expertise and close contact with the client and family, nursing care is recognized as the cornerstone of hospice services (ANA, 1987).

Dimensions of Hospice Care

Healing is an essential concept of caring and underlies hospice philosophy. Healing may be analyzed across physical, psychosocial, and spiritual dimensions (Spector, 1984). Interventions related to the physical dimension are geared toward supporting restoration to maximum wholeness. In this dimension, the client is assessed for physiological responses to his or her disease process. Interventions related to the physical dimension include pain relief, symptom control, maintenance of skin integrity, energy conservation, and nutrition management. Modalities that enhance client control of these responses may include autogenic training, relaxation techniques, biofeedback, self-hypnosis, and/or Therapeutic Touch (Keegan, 1994).

The psychosocial dimension refers to the emotional, psychological, and social health of the client and family despite loss and grief (Spector, 1984). Related interventions are geared toward optimizing this dimension and include supporting a sense of power and control in the client and family, promoting positive self-concept, alleviating feelings of loneliness and isolation, and fostering the communication of feelings and needs. The hospice nurse strives to assist with the peaceful acceptance of inevitable death by fostering communication and encouraging the life-review process. Interventions that promote client control over his or her life may reduce anxiety and generate feelings of harmony for the client and the family (Keegan, 1994).

The spiritual dimension refers to the spiritual, religious, and relationship needs of the client and family (Spector, 1984). With hospice care, spiritual interventions support the client and family to come to terms with death. Assessment of the spiritual needs of the client and family is the responsibility of the hospice nurse. Interventions include recognizing the spiritual needs of the dying person, assisting the client in meeting those needs, and enhancing a sense of wholeness and closure. The importance of the spiritual dimension in working with the dying cannot be overemphasized. Igou states, "The essence of hospice seems to be found in the spiritual dimension" (p. 160). It is critical that the caregiver assure hospice clients that they will be well cared for, surrounded by those they love, and treated with love and respect in their efforts to arrive at spiritual peace (Igou, 1984).

Types of Hospice Programs

Hospice programs vary in organizational structure and service delivery. Community needs, leadership, funding sources, political influences, and available resources for health care, spiritual care, and social services affect the availability and structure of hospice care. Hospice programs may be owned and operated by public agencies, hospitals, home health agencies, extended care facilities, or other independent organizations. As with home health services, hospice organizations may be financially structured as nonprofit or for-profit. They may serve clients in their homes or in inpatient facilities, be freestanding or part of a larger institution (Spradley & Allender, 1996). Regardless of the organizational structure, a hospice program must meet strict criteria to become Medicare certified and receive reimbursement for services rendered (Schultz, 1984).

Hospice programs employ registered nurses as either full-time hospice nurses or home health, hospital, or community staff nurses with varying hospice caseloads. Trained volunteers are critical members of the hospice team and constitute a significant source of support for the client and family (ANA, 1987). Also provided by hospice programs are physician services, various therapy services, spiritual and bereavement counseling, home health aide services, homemaker services, medical supplies, short-term inpatient care, and other specialized care providers as necessary to achieve the outcomes of the plan of care (Schultz, 1984; HNA, 1995).

Role Functions of the Hospice Nurse

A high level of professional competence is required to function effectively as a hospice nurse (ANA, 1987). The hospice nurse must be skilled in all of the functional roles required of the nurse in the community setting and also have a strong background in acute care. Three role functions deserve specific discussion with regard to hospice care. As educator, the hospice nurse supports client and family decision making by providing information specific to the client's situation across the physical, psychosocial, and spiritual dimensions. As consultant, the nurse provides expert knowledge combined with an understanding of the client's needs and strengths to empower the client to make decisions about the dying process. The other members of the multidisciplinary team rely on the nurse's accurate and comprehensive judgment in order to make appropriate decisions regarding care (Spradley & Allender, 1996). As advocate, the hospice nurse upholds the desires of the client. In the dying process, clients often become too weak and disadvantaged to defend their wishes. The hospice nurse must practice with a heightened sense of ethics in considering the client's decisions (ANA, 1987; HNA, 1995).

The nurse is responsible for coordinating the services provided to the dying client and grieving family members (Gurfolino and Dumas, 1994). Close and frequent interaction with dying clients and their distressed families may deplete the nurse's physical and emotional reserves. The

╭───╮
🌀 **REFLECTIVE THINKING** 🌀

Hospice Care

- How might you provide spiritual support to those with values that differ from your own?

- In what ways do you manage your needs when you are experiencing loss?

- How has your ability to communicate been affected when you are grieving?
╰───╯

nurse must therefore carefully balance the needs of the client and family with personal limitations. The hospice nurse requires administrative and peer support in order to manage personal needs as they arise. Appropriate interaction with and utilization of all members of the multidisciplinary team will strengthen the support network for the hospice nurse as well as for the client and family.

Hospice nursing involves the delivery of holistic, sympathetic, empathetic, personal care to dying individuals and their families during a critical phase of family life (Spector, 1984). The provision of such comprehensive client/family care and the autonomous professional practice characteristic of hospice nursing afford the nurse numerous opportunities to develop clinical and leadership skills. The hospice movement is expected to grow rapidly as individuals and families continue to seek a comfortable and humane death with caring professionals who will assist and guide the process without controlling it.

School Nursing

School nursing is a branch of community health nursing that seeks to identify or prevent school health problems and intervenes to remedy or reduce these problems. The school nurse is a licensed, professional nurse; licensure or certification is preferably through an appropriate association (Proctor et al., 1993). The nurse implements primary, secondary, and tertiary prevention strategies to promote optimum wellness in the school-aged client. Prevention interventions target students who have potential health concerns, acute or chronic diseases, handicapping conditions (speech, hearing, visual, and orthopedic impairments), emotional or family problems, mental retardation, or learning disabilities. Other health-related issues that demand attention include accident awareness, tobacco use, chemical abuse, sexual activity, pregnancy, and various types of violence. The school nurse should be familiar with the year 2000 national health objectives in order to provide appropriate screening, monitoring, and services that will support meeting these objectives. The school nurse contributes directly to the students' education by implementing prevention strategies that promote the physical, emotional, and social health of students so they are prepared to learn (Zanga & Oda, 1987; Farnsworth & Gutterres, 1989; Proctor et al., 1993).

School Nursing Service Populations

School nursing takes place in both public and private schools with enrollments ranging from several students to several thousand students. Services are delivered to students and staff across the health care continuum. Nurse competencies must therefore run the spectrum from pediatric and adolescent to general adult health care. Because the school community is a microcosm of our society, a functioning knowledge of public health concepts and occupational health principles is vital to the school nurse. School nursing is considered "community-based and community-focused, with the school community at the center of interest and the recipient of nursing services" (Proctor et al., 1993, p. 11).

School health services have expanded in recent years due to the inclusion of programs for disabled and disadvantaged students, the relatively new phenomenon of children with acute or chronic health problems attending school, the increased numbers and types of communicable diseases, and the incorporation of students in need of specialized treatments. Contemporary school services may also include wellness programs for students and staff. The challenge of keeping students and staff healthy enough to attend school and be in condition for optimal teaching and learning will continue. As such challenges continue and grow, so too will the responsibilities of and opportunities for the school nurse (Farnsworth & Gutterres, 1989; Thurber, Berry, & Cameron, 1991; Proctor et al., 1993).

As a specialty practice, school nursing has identifiable and measurable standards of practice. Because the school nurse most often works in isolation and is generally evaluated by nonnurse administrators, these standards are an essential foundation of practice. Both the administrator and the nurse must have an in-depth understanding of these standards and be committed to applying them (Proctor et al., 1993). A summary of these standards is provided in Figure 14-10.

Role Functions of the School Nurse

The National Association of School Nurses (NASN) outlines three overlapping roles for the school nurse: the generalist clinician role, the primary care role, and the management role. The nurse in the generalist clinician role provides health services, counseling, and health education to students and families. These services are integrated into the school as an important part of the total educational program. This nurse is usually employed by the school, by the school district, or by a local governmental agency such as the health department (Proctor et al., 1993).

The generalist clinician is located in the school and provides services during school hours. The nurse is incorporated into the daily functions of the school community. Students, families, faculty, and staff recognize the nurse as being an available professional resource for health concerns. In this role, the nurse is able to identify students, families, and staff at risk (case finding), develop and implement appropriate interventions for identified health needs,

Figure 14-10   Standards of School Nursing Practice

Role Concept I: Provider of Client Care

NASN Standard 1. Clinical Knowledge: The school nurse utilizes a distinct knowledge base for decision making in nursing practice.

NASN Standard 2. Nursing Process: The school nurse uses a systematic approach to problem solving in nursing practice.

NASN Standard 3. Clients with Special Health Needs: The school nurse contributes to the education of the client with special health needs by assessing the client, planning and providing appropriate nursing care, and evaluating the identified outcomes of care.

Role Concept II: Communicator

NASN Standard 4. Communication: The school nurse uses effective written, verbal, and nonverbal communication skills.

Role Concept III: Planner and Coordinator of Client Care

NASN Standard 5. Program Management: The school nurse establishes and maintains a comprehensive school health program.

NASN Standard 6. Collaboration within the School System: The school nurse collaborates with other school professionals, parents, and caregivers to meet the health, developmental, and educational needs of clients.

NASN Standard 7. Collaboration with Community Health Systems: The school nurse collaborates with members of the community in the delivery of health and social services, and utilizes knowledge of community health systems and resources to function as a school–community liaison.

Role Concept IV: Client Teacher

NASN Standard 8. Health Education: The school nurse assists students, families, and the school community to achieve optimal levels of wellness through appropriately designed and delivered health education.

Role Concept V: Investigator

NASN Standard 9. Research: The school nurse contributes to nursing and school health through innovations in practice and participation in research or research-related activities.

Role Concept VI: Role within the Discipline of Nursing

NASN Standard 10. Professional Development: The school nurse identifies, delineates, and clarifies the nursing role; promotes quality of care; pursues continued professional enhancement; and demonstrates professional conduct.

Adapted from School Nursing Practice: Roles and Standards *by S. T. Proctor, S. L. Lordi, & D. S. Zaiger, 1993, Scarborough, ME: National Association of School Nurses. Copyright 1993 by National Association of School Nurses. Used with permission.*

Figure 14-11   Examples of Items to Monitor in the School-Age Client

Physical health

Emotional health

Health habits (smoking, eating, drug abuse, sexual activity)

Pregnancy

Potential abuse (sexual, emotional, verbal, physical)

Chronic absenteeism

Failing grades

Medicine intake and reactions

Interaction with peers, teachers, and other authority figures

Safety issues

Social concerns (home environment, homelessness, poverty, domestic violence)

and formulate appropriate policies and programs to resolve actual and potential problems (Proctor et al., 1993).

The primary care role is carried out by nurse practitioners who practice under physician-approved protocols and standardized procedures. The school nurse practitioner diagnoses and treats health problems and coordinates care with other health professionals. Management of minor acute and chronic illnesses, health education, and environmental health support are provided (Igoe & Giordano, 1992). Annual health assessment for the well child/adolescent and developmental assessment are included within this primary care role (Zanga & Oda, 1987). Many of these practitioners have implemented school-based clinics; school-linked services; and collaborative, community-based services. School-based clinics are offered near the families who need them and furnish an

DECISION MAKING

School Nursing

As the nurse in an elementary school, you have witnessed an increasing number of students with complex physical and emotional problems being mainstreamed into the classroom. At the same time, money, resources, and services are dwindling.

• What school and community resources might you approach for assistance in meeting the needs of these students?

• As the school nurse, how would you influence the health of aggregates faced with decisions regarding gang membership? Violence? Drug and alcohol use? Cigarette use? Teen pregnancy?

Figure 14-12   Management Functions of the School Nurse

- Development, coordination, and evaluation of school health programs

- Development and implementation of school health policy and procedure

- Case management of students and families with special health needs

- Acquisition and management of funds for implementation of health services

- Supervision and evaluation of other professional and support personnel

Adapted from School Nursing Practice: Roles and Standards *by S. T. Proctor, S. L. Lordi, & D. S. Zaiger, 1993, Scarborough, ME: National Association of School Nurses. Copyright 1993 by National Association of School Nurses.*

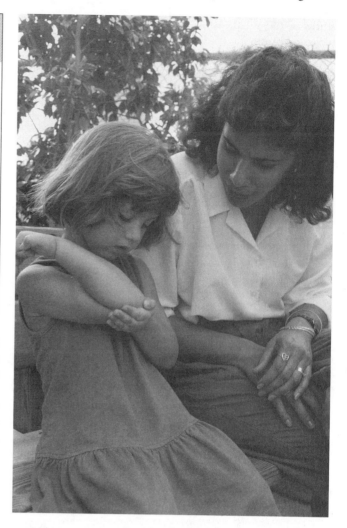

The school nurse treats injuries as well as offering counseling, screening, and other services.

accessible location for persons seeking professional health care (Feroli, Hobson, Miola, Scott, & Waterfield, 1992; Igoe & Giordano, 1992; Proctor et al., 1993). Figure 14-11 offers examples of items to monitor in the school-age client.

As manager, the school nurse is responsible for a variety of actions defined by the NASN and outlined in Figure 14-12. The management role includes program planning for the provision of comprehensive services to clients in the school community. Effective management strategies ensure a continuum of care from the student's home, to community health provider, to school, and back to home (Zanga & Oda, 1987).

Because the school nurse may coordinate programs on several campuses, carry a large and active caseload, and supervise other school nurses, volunteers, or health aides, management and leadership skills are crucial. The school nurse is in a position to influence health policy formation, to obtain political and parental support for program development, and to secure maximum participation from the community (Zanga & Oda, 1987; Proctor et al., 1993).

An essential management function of the school nurse is to conduct research. The NASN's Standard 9 addresses the need for school nurses to participate in research or research-related activities to further the knowledge base for school-based health outcomes. Many studies conducted on the school-aged population have been done by professionals other than school nurses. The NASN challenges nurses within the specialty to conduct studies and promote research-based practice (Proctor et al., 1993). Data collection and documentation of school health efforts, interventions, and outcomes are beneficial to the development of effective programs. Such information is crucial to the formation of district and/or governmental health policy and to the delineation of the scope of school nursing practice (Zanga & Oda, 1987; Thurber et al., 1991).

The school nurse of today is a valuable resource for students, families, and staff who are continually confronted with a multitude of physical, mental, social, and behavioral issues. The nurse is a competent case finder, clinician, educator, manager, collaborator, and researcher and is available as a health resource for the community served. As the center of school health services, the school nurse supports the education process by promoting the overall health of students and staff.

Occupational Health Nursing

According to the American Association of Occupational Health Nurses (AAOHN), **occupational health nursing** is a specialty practice providing health care services to workers and worker populations (AAOHN, 1994). This practice is an extension of community health nursing and focuses on the promotion, protection, and restoration of workers' health within the context of a safe and healthy work environment. Occupational nursing is a synthesis and application of principles from nursing, medicine, **environmental health** (the study and prevention of environmental problems), **toxicology** (the study of poisons), and epidemiology. It incorporates concepts from safety, **industrial hygiene** (the study of the workplace environment and its relationship to impaired health of workers or community citizens), and **ergonomics** (the study of the relationship between individuals and their work environment) and adopts principles from the social and behavioral sciences. A rapidly changing and evolving practice setting, occupational health is dynamic and fluctuates in response to changing health care, business, economic, political, ecological, social, and cultural demands (Barlow, 1992; AAOHN, 1994).

Goals of Occupational Health Nursing

The occupational health nurse, often the only health care professional in the industrial setting, holds a key position working with management to develop strategies to improve the health of workers. The work of the occupational health nurse benefits the corporation by giving rise to a healthy, involved, and productive work force (Miller, 1989; Cookfair, 1996).

The workplace provides an ideal community for the implementation of health-promotion, health-protection, and health-restoration strategies. Individuals come together in the workplace, representing a cross section of the societal picture of physical, behavioral, cultural, and emotional variables. The workplace environment changes as society transforms. Work-force demographics mirror these societal transformations. The work force is increasing in age, diversity, educational level, skill, and desire to influence changes in work environment (Barlow, 1992; Haag & Glazner, 1992; Travers & McDougall, 1997). The health and wellness issues that emerge in conjunction with changing demographics are the domain of the occupational health nurse.

Role Responsibilities of the Occupational Health Nurse

The occupational health nurse has multiple clinical, educational, and administrative responsibilities. Clinical responsibilities include pre-placement assessment, annual physical examination, diagnosis and treatment of acute minor illnesses, emergent care, and counseling. Educational obligations consist of identifying teaching/learning needs, developing programs, and evaluating learning outcomes. Administrative duties include performing referral and follow-up, monitoring the worksite, implementing corporate and governmental regulations, communicating worker health needs to corporate management, and various other administrative tasks (Atherton & LeGendre, 1985; Cookfair, 1996). Nursing interventions may be geared toward the individual worker, a group of workers on the same unit, or a population of workers with similar actual or potential needs. Standards for clinical and professional performance are determined by the AAOHN and are outlined in Figure 14-13.

Traditionally, the occupational health nurse has delivered direct care on a one-on-one basis. In this individual orientation, the occupational health nurse is usually located in an office, and the worker approaches the nurse for assistance. Interventions include direct services such as individual assessment, one-on-one counseling, treatment of illness and injury, worker compensation case management, or individual crisis management (Maciag, 1993).

Although individual interventions are important, occupational health nurses must consider alternative ways of providing health services with limited resources. Individual interventions are narrowly focused and expensive in terms of time and resource allocation (Miller, 1989). With the rising cost of providing individual health care interventions, the occupational health nurse must meet the challenges of containing costs, ensuring quality programming, and targeting services via planning, research, and policy development (Barlow, 1992). A section of the Healthy People 2000 objectives addresses occupational safety and health challenges. The related objectives guide actions for occupational health services. It is the nurse's responsibility to implement cost-effective interventions to achieve these objectives. Refer to Appendix A for a review of these objectives (Hart & Moore, 1992).

The occupational health nurse plays a big role in maintaining the health and safety of employees by assessing the worksite for hazards and potential hazards and reducing risks that could lead to a disaster situation. The nurse assists in developing written disaster plans appropriate to risks inherent in the worksite. The nurse must be versed in disaster prevention and planning and must be skilled in communicating with company administration, community resources, and at-risk workers. Disaster plans are designed to prevent or minimize injury and death of workers and nearby residents. Additional priorities for planning include development of an effective triage system, interface with community resources (fire, police, emergency, hospital and public health departments), minimizing property damage, and facilitating resumption of business activity (Ossler, 1992). Although the nurse is rarely solely responsible for planning and implementing the disaster plan, as a member of the team, the occupational health nurse may function as clinician.

Future occupational health nurses will need broad business skills. The nurse analyzes trends, develops programs, contains costs, identifies problems, and proposes solutions to health-related issues. Occupational health services, like other corporate functional areas, exist solely to support the overall goals of the corporation. In addition to the health and welfare of the workers, the corporation is critically concerned about profits, losses, productivity, and future economic health. The occupational health nurse must be committed to supporting the goals of the organization. The nurse attends to the health of workers, realizing that a sick, less-productive work force is expensive to the economic health of the organization (Hart & Moore, 1992).

The occupational health nurse is responsible for proposing well-planned and cost-effective health programs to corporate management. Expert skills in data collection, data analysis, and program planning, combined with abilities in persuasive communication, are essential for obtaining corporate support and resources for service needs (Maciag, 1993). The nurse must be familiar with the current and future goals of the corporation to be suc-

Figure 14-13 Standards of Occupational Health Nursing Practice

Standards of Clinical Nursing Practice

Standard I. Assessment: The occupational health nurse systematically assesses the health status of the client.

Standard II. Diagnosis: The occupational health nurse analyzes data collected to formulate a nursing diagnosis.

Standard III. Outcome Identification: The occupational health nurse identifies expected outcomes specific to the client.

Standard IV. Planning: The occupational health nurse develops a plan of care that is comprehensive and formulates interventions for each level of prevention and for therapeutic modalities to achieve expected outcomes.

Standard V. Implementation: The occupational health nurse implements interventions to promote health, prevent illness and injury, and facilitate rehabilitation, guided by the plan of care.

Standard VI. Evaluation: The occupational health nurse systematically and continuously evaluates the client's responses to interventions and evaluates progress toward the achievement of expected outcomes.

Professional Practice Standards

Standard I. Professional Development/Evaluation: The occupational health nurse assumes responsibility for professional development and continuing education and evaluates personal professional performance in relation to practice standards.

Standard II. Quality Improvement/Quality Assurance: The occupational health nurse monitors and evaluates the quality and effectiveness of occupational health practice.

Standard III. Collaboration: The occupational health nurse collaborates with employees, management, other health care providers, professionals, and community representatives in assessing, planning, implementing, and evaluating care and occupational health services.

Standard IV. Research: The occupational health nurse contributes to the scientific base in occupational health nursing through research, as appropriate, and uses research findings in practice.

Standard V. Ethics: The occupational health nurse uses an ethical framework as a guide for decision making in practice.

Standard VI. Resource Management: The occupational health nurse collaborates with management to provide resources that support an occupational health program that meets the needs of the worker population.

Adapted from Standards of Occupational Health Nursing Practice *by American Association of Occupational Health Nurses, 1994, Atlanta: Author. Copyright 1994 by American Association of Occupational Health Nurses, Inc. Used with permission.*

cessful in providing services that complement and support these objectives (Miller, 1989). Adaptability and flexibility are skills required for the nurse to meet these responsibilities.

The occupational health nurse influences worker health behavior in numerous ways and may be a catalyst for voluntary personal behavioral change on the part of the worker. The nurse may implement strategies such as simple awareness-promoting interventions (e.g., posters, lectures, or demonstrations), information contests, or worksite health and nutrition fairs to educate the work force about healthy lifestyles and behaviors (Dalle Molle & Allan, 1989).

More stringent measures that affect worker behavior are by-products of mandatory governmental regulation. Many environmental interventions are the result of governmental policy. The Occupational Safety and Health Administration (OSHA) and the National Institute of Occupational Safety and Health (NIOSH) are federal agencies involved in developing regulations related to occupational health and safety. The Occupational Safety and Health Administration is part of the U.S. Department of Labor. It enforces occupational regulations at the federal, regional, and state levels. The National Institute of Occupational Safety and Health is a division of the Centers for Disease Control and Prevention, a part of the U.S. Public Health Service. The National Institute of Occupational Safety and Health is a data-collection center that makes recommendations regarding occupational hazards. The increase in regulations to ensure safe work practices, smoke-free environments, and employee-exposure control necessitates that the occupational health nurse be well-informed regarding current regulations and be able to understand and apply OSHA and NIOSH regulations (Ossler, 1992). The nurse should be skilled in educating the work force regarding all regulations and be supportive of efforts to comply with them. Figure 14-14 lists items of which the occupational health nurse should be cognizant.

Employee Assistance Programs

Large companies with sufficient resources may finance long-term, in-depth programs designed to affect worker behaviors, beliefs, and attitudes in an effort to improve morale and productivity and reduce health risks and absenteeism (Dalle Molle & Allan, 1989). One example is the **employee assistance program (EAP)**.

Employee assistance programs may take the form of counseling, chemical rehabilitation, stress management training, or other similar initiatives considered helpful in supporting workers' attempts at maintaining or restoring productivity. The occupational health nurse's involvement in an EAP may be at the referral level, or the nurse may function as coordinator or counselor. Occupational health is currently seeing growth in employee assistance programs. Such programs benefit workers by supporting them in regaining or maintaining productivity and benefit corporations by creating a human-oriented, supportive

Figure 14-14 Examples of Potential Agents That the Occupational Health Nurse Needs to Monitor

Exposure to:

- Pesticides
- Allergens
- Asbestos
- Wood dust
- Cement dust
- Metal dust
- Lead
- Noise
- Repetitive motion problems
- Safety violations

REFLECTIVE THINKING

Occupational Health Nursing

- To what degree should the occupational health nurse be involved in employee assistance programs?
- What about confidentiality? If an employee were considered unstable and a risk to fellow employees, would you report this finding to appropriate management/authorities?

environment for their workers and by sustaining a productive work force (Thompson, 1989).

Role of the Occupational Health Nurse

Multiple factors will determine the role functions, scope of practice, and contributions of the occupational health nurse in the future. Among these factors are the ways that occupational health nurses execute the scope of occupational health practice; are viewed by other nurses and professionals in related fields; perceive themselves in the professional role; organize as a professional group; involve themselves in corporate and/or governmental affairs; and generate scholarly research. The role of the occupational health nurse will also be affected by the types of injuries, illnesses, and issues encountered by the worker of the future (Barlow, 1992). Occupational health nursing is creating a solid and unique framework for practice by fostering research. In a rapidly changing and increasingly complex work environment, research is a vital component for the delivery of appropriate, quality services. Rogers (1989) states that occupational health nursing is a scientific, applied discipline that "has an obligation to seek opportunities to expand the frontiers of occupational health nursing knowledge and to be discontent with the status quo" (p. 497).

The role of the occupational health nurse is diversified and complex. The occupational health nurse is in a position to coordinate a holistic approach in the delivery of health services in the work environmental (American Association of Occupational Health Nurses, 1994). The nurses in the occupational health setting must embody new ways of thinking, demonstrate political astuteness and expertise in communication, demonstrate flexibility and the ability to deal with ambiguity, as well as possess a knowledge of economics and health care delivery. Population-based practice that focuses on outcomes measurement, quality assurance, and advocacy will continue to be imperatives for practice in the 21st century.

Research in Occupational Health Nursing

Occupational health nurses are invited to create opportunities for participating in and conducting research to contribute to the growing body of knowledge (Rogers, 1989). Occupational nursing research priorities have been identified and targeted; with the AAOHN Board categorizing 12 research priorities into 3 broad areas. The first area of research is related to the effectiveness of occupational health nursing interventions in the following areas:

- Primary health care delivery at the worksite
- Health-promoting nursing interventions
- Programs on employee productivity and morale
- Ergonomic strategies to reduce worker injury and/or illness

The second broad area of research targets the strategies for dealing with occupational health issues, including the following:

- Methods for handling complex ethical issues related to workers' health
- Strategies for minimizing work-related health outcomes
- Mechanisms to ensure quality and cost effectiveness of programs
- Factors that influence worker rehabilitation and return to work

The final area of research is related to identifying hazards and reducing risks at the worksite. Areas of interest include the following:

- Occupational hazards of health care workers
- Factors that contribute to behavioral changes and self-care
- Factors that contribute to sustained risk-reduction behavior related to lifestyle choices (Rogers, 1989).

Correctional Health Nursing

Correctional health nursing is a branch of professional nursing that provides nursing services to clients in correctional facilities. Facilities in which individuals are incarcerated include prisons, jails, youth detention/correction centers, adult probation/parole divisions, and other similar restricted settings. Individuals who are perceived to be threats or to owe debts to society are retained in correctional facilities to maintain the public order. Individuals incarcerated in such environments vary from juveniles to aged adults and include both women and men (Moritz, 1982; ANA, 1995).

Challenges in Correctional Nursing

The correctional health nurse functions in a non–health care setting governed by an overriding attention to individual safety and institutional security. The nurse works with men, women, and youth for whom society has little regard and minimal interest in spending scarce public resources on personal health needs. The inmate/client usually does not have a choice regarding the services provided or the practitioner providing those services (Moritz, 1982; ANA, 1985). Furthermore, the health services provided may be inadequate because of poor resources, outdated equipment, difficulty in accessing the client for assessment and treatment, lack of health or security personnel, or limited opportunity to involve support services and networks (Little, 1981; Peternelj-Taylor & Hufft, 1997). These factors combine to create a stressful, complex, and challenging work setting that demands the nurse be competent in multiple areas.

Scope of Nursing Services in Correctional Settings

Nursing services provided to inmates range from brief ambulatory or emergent care to comprehensive health programs. Clients range from the healthy to the acutely or chronically ill and include individuals who are mentally ill and/or developmentally or physically challenged. Nursing responsibilities to incarcerated clients include health education, suicide prevention, communicable disease control, alcohol and drug rehabilitation, somatic therapy, psychosocial counseling, emergency care, and environmental health. The nurse must be educationally and experientially prepared to provide and/or coordinate comprehensive services for clients needing interventions in these areas (ANA, 1985). As the number of women inmates increases, women's health issues will move to the forefront. Incarcerated women will need obstetric, gynecological, and parenting services and support. The correctional health nurse is committed to the provision of care to all individuals regardless of the nature of their crimes or the duration of their incarcerations (Moritz, 1982; ANA, 1995).

The scope and standards for practice in a correctional facility as outlined by the American Nurses Association have been adopted by the American Correctional Health Services Association, an organization open to all correctional health care professionals. The *Scope and Standards of Nursing Practice in Correctional Facilities* (see Figure 14-15) guides professional practice and performance for the correctional health nurse (ANA, 1995). The standards recognize the right of all people to have access to ade-

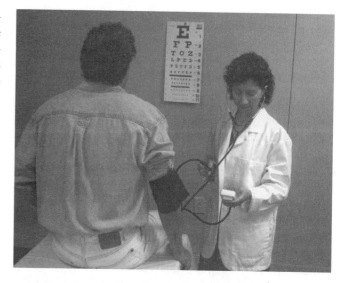

Working in a correctional facility offers many challenges to the nurse; however, rewards can be found in opportunities to function as a group leader, innovator, teacher, planner, and caregiver.

quate health care and are based on principles "that ensure that the incarcerated have access to nursing services; that health care not be compromised by detention or incarceration; that health care be provided in an atmosphere which fosters dignity and reinforces the worth of both the individual and the health professional; and that health services be the direct function of health professionals" (Moritz, 1982, p. 254).

Case finding is particularly important in the correctional setting. The nurse must be able to assess individuals who, among other things, are at risk for suicide, communicable disease, and alcohol and drug problems. Suicide is a significant cause of death for incarcerated youth. Potential for suicide is especially high for juveniles housed in adult facilities. Identification of at-risk individuals is critical for providing effective interventions to reduce suicidal tendencies and behaviors (ANA, 1985; Peternelj-Taylor & Hufft, 1997).

Crowded facilities, poor hygiene, and sexual activity may contribute to the transmission of communicable disease. Health education coupled with epidemiologic strategies is necessary to reduce new disease cases and lessen the effects of current cases. Chemical abuse is another serious problem for many inmates before, during, and after incarceration. In order to effect change, the nurse must therefore be competent in the areas of case finding, treatment programs and detoxification regimes, individual and group counseling, health education, and client referral (ANA, 1985).

Individuals in correctional facilities are isolated from family and other social support systems. This separation can result in significant distress to the individual and the family. Clients and/or family may be sullen, angry, or scared and may therefore be unwilling or unable to communicate needs. Manipulative behaviors and "game-playing" are frequent patterns displayed by inmates. These issues demand skilled communication from the nurse in

Figure 14-15 Standards of Nursing Practice in Correctional Facilities

Standards of Care

Standard I. Assessment: The nurse collects client health data.

Standard II. Diagnosis: The nurse analyzes the assessment data in determining diagnoses.

Standard III. Outcome Identification: The nurse identifies expected outcomes individualized to the client.

Standard IV. Planning: The nurse develops a care plan that prescribes interventions to attain expected outcomes.

Standard V. Implementation: The nurse implements the interventions identified in the care plan.

Standard VI. Evaluation: The nurse evaluates the client's progress toward attainment of outcomes.

Standards of Professional Performance

Standard I. Quality of Care: The nurse systematically evaluates the quality and effectiveness of nursing practice.

Standard II. Performance Appraisal: The nurse evaluates his or her own nursing practice in relation to professional practice standards and relevant statutes and regulations.

Standard III. Education: The nurse acquires and maintains current knowledge in nursing practice.

Standard IV. Collegiality: The nurse contributes to the professional development of peers, colleagues, and others.

Standard V. Ethics: The nurse's decisions and actions on behalf of clients are determined in an ethical manner.

Standard VI. Collaboration: The nurse collaborates with the client, significant others, other criminal justice system personnel, and health care providers in providing client care.

Standard VII. Research: The nurse uses research findings in practice.

Standard VIII. Resource Utilization: The nurse considers factors related to safety, effectiveness, and cost in planning and delivering client care.

Adapted from Scope and Standards of Nursing Practice in Correctional Facilities *by American Nurses' Association, 1995, Washington, DC: Author. Copyright 1995 by American Nurses Publishing. Used with permission.*

Under no circumstances should the nurse participate in activities linked to security or inmate correction. The nurse does not participate, either directly or indirectly, in surveillance, strip searches, disciplinary decisions, or health-threatening actions such as lethal injections. Rather, the nurse implements all aspects of the nursing process to promote, maintain, or restore the health of the client (ANA, 1995). Figure 14-16 lists several health-related concerns that the correctional health nurse must monitor in the inmate.

Attention to safety is particularly important for the nurse working in a correctional setting. It is imperative that the nurse retain a deep respect for the nature of the environment and be committed to security protocol. The nurse is held to all security regulations that apply to other facility personnel and must maintain a balance between the risks inherent in a controlled environment and the delivery of quality care (ANA, 1995). This balance challenges the nurse's ability to provide nondiscriminatory, nonprejudicial services to inmates within a setting characterized by opposing philosophical orientations: Whereas corrections officers focus on security for both the setting and the inmates and staff, inmates focus on personal survival and hopes for freedom, and nurses and health care staff focus on the health and well-being of the inmates whom they serve. Given these differing orientations and foci, the potential for conflict is great (Moritz, 1982; Ogle, 1990; Peternelj-Taylor & Hufft, 1997).

Communication strategies that foster rapport and open exchange with correctional personnel (e. g., guards, counselors, and administrators) are critical in order to continue appropriate interventions without breaching safety and security protocol (Little, 1981; ANA, 1985; Ogle, 1990; Peternelj-Taylor & Hufft, 1997). Educating each group about the functions and expanded services that can be provided by the nurse will promote the acceptance of the nurse as a capable and valuable member of the facility. In return, the nurse must respect the responsibilities and actions of members of the other groups and function within the standards and scope of practice. Communication efforts that further understanding among groups will lead to collaboration, mutual assistance, and coordination of actions to ensure positive outcomes (Chaisson, 1981; Little, 1981; Moritz, 1982; Peternelj-Taylor & Hufft, 1997).

attempting to build rapport and develop a therapeutic relationship with clients. To be successful, the nurse must know ways to respond to and manage these patterns (Ogle, 1990; Peternelj-Taylor & Hufft, 1997). It is important for the nurse to include family and significant others in the plan of care as much as possible. A solid background in communication theory, family theory, and group work is essential to the success of interventions (ANA, 1985).

The scope of practice for the nurse in a correctional setting is limited strictly to the delivery of nursing services.

Figure 14-16 Examples of Problems the Correctional Health Nurse Needs to Monitor

- Depression
- Communicable diseases
- Rape
- Signs of trauma
- Substance abuse
- Chronic and acute illnesses
- Pregnancy

REFLECTIVE THINKING

Treating Clients Incarcerated in a Correctional Facility

How do you feel about providing health care to an individual who has committed murder? A client who has been convicted of sexually abusing a child? A client convicted of selling drugs?

Ideally, the nurse in the correctional setting should receive specific orientation, inservice education, and continuing education to support practice in this specialty (Niskala, 1986). The nurse should be minimally prepared with a baccalaureate degree in nursing. Nurse specialists and nurse practitioners with masters preparation are frequently employed in correctional facilities. These nurses function in broad clinical and administrative roles. They participate in and conduct research to further the foundation of correctional health nursing practice (ANA, 1985).

Many issues combine to make nursing in the correctional setting a challenge (Little, 1981). The nurse practicing in the correctional setting is often the only health care provider in the facility, a setting that is focused on security needs rather than health needs and that allocates few resources to adequately support nursing interventions. The nurse may have few role models and may receive little or no feedback regarding interventions or practice competency. Furthermore, the nurse has little control in the decision-making processes related to inmate health needs and treatment options. Also, educational programs to obtain training in correctional health practice may be unavailable. Finally, the nurse may perceive a lack of support and feel isolated and misunderstood by peers.

Correctional health nursing also offers many potential rewards, however. Such rewards include opportunities to function as group leader, innovator, teacher, planner, caregiver, counselor, coordinator, and researcher. Furthermore, the opportunity for personal growth via identifying values, studying human behaviors, and contributing to the health and well-being of those who otherwise may not receive such care can generate a sense of personal satisfaction (Bridges, 1981; Peternelj-Taylor & Hufft, 1997). Nursing practice in the correctional setting is, and will continue to be, exciting, stimulating, challenging, and potentially rewarding and enjoyable work.

Parish Nursing

Parish nursing is a relatively new adaptation of the older religion-based nursing models of health care delivery. This congregation-based approach to health care delivery was revived during the mid-1980s by Reverend Granger Westberg to better employ the faith and support network of congregations to meet the health-promotion and disease-prevention needs of members. Grouping individuals by congregation or religious affiliation provides a means of identifying populations by value orientation, spiritual direction, and community and cultural associations. Reverend Westberg considered spiritually motivated registered nurses as ideal practitioners to provide the link between health sciences and human needs (Westberg, 1990; Schank, Weis, & Matheus, 1996).

Description of Parish Nursing

A parish nurse is a registered nurse who provides holistic nursing services to the members of a faith congregation as a part of the ministerial team. The nurse promotes the health of parishioners and their families by integrating theological, psychological, sociological, and physiological perspectives of health and healing with the beliefs and culture of the congregation (Ryan, 1990). Principles of holistic health and human caring are employed. These nurses work with other practitioners and health care agencies and with the ministerial team to enhance the quality of life for all members of the congregation (Schank, Weis, & Matheus, 1996). Parish nurses do not provide hands-on, invasive treatments; rather, they provide a framework to move individuals and families toward better health states (Solari-Twadell & Westberg, 1991).

Because the parish nurse functions independently and must be proficient in accessing community resources, it is recommended that entry-level parish nurses have baccalaureate degrees and three to five years of nursing experience. Additionally, the parish nurse must be spiritually

DECISION MAKING

Correctional Nursing

All clients, including those who are incarcerated, have basic rights that must be upheld. They have the right to individualized care; the right to act according to their own values, beliefs, and cultural practices; and the right to know about and participate in personal health care decisions (Faris, 1995).

• How might you preserve individual cultural practices of incarcerated individuals?

• What could you do to encourage clients who may lack fundamental interpersonal and social communication skills to participate in their personal health care decisions?

• Examine your personal values regarding the right to live in a safe, free society and your right to be treated with dignity.

• How would you assist imprisoned clients to improve their health and quality of life if their values and their behaviors toward others in society were in conflict with your own?

mature and have the confidence and experience to fulfill multiple roles. Participation in a parish nursing educational program is considered essential for successful practice (Schank, Weis, & Matheus, 1996). Information about such programs in the United States can be obtained through the National Parish Nurse Resource Center.

The Congregation As a Community Setting

Religious congregations are considered effective settings for addressing the health needs of a population for a variety of reasons. First, religious organizations and congregations are found in virtually every community in every culture. Second, faith congregations have long histories of serving their communities through social activities and educational programming. Third, religions focus on problems of the human spirit, problems that often are related to the development of and/or response to illness. Fourth, religious communities are rich in traditions of service, support, and volunteerism in humanitarian efforts. Fifth, religions can provide a model of cooperation between science, medicine, and faith communities to better serve populations (Westberg, 1990). Nurses working closely with parishioners can facilitate this desirable cooperation. Finally, faith congregations are one of the few institutions that interact with individuals and families from birth through death (Solari-Twadell & Westberg, 1991). This relationship allows the parish nurse to effectively use a lifespan approach when managing client and family health needs.

Role Functions of the Parish Nurse

The role of the parish nurse incorporates "whole-person ways of ministering to people who are hurting" (Westberg, 1990, p. 38). Parish nurses can integrate caring principles into practice by focusing on the beliefs and values of the individual and can effectively combine the strengths of humanities and science, medicine and religion, doctors and clergy, and spirituality and health to better client outcomes (Holst, 1987; Westberg, 1990).

Several functional roles are paramount to the practice of parish nursing. These include counselor, collaborator, case manager, manager, educator, and advocate (Holst, 1987; Boss & Corbett, 1990; Miskelly, 1995). As counselor, the parish nurse discusses individual health concerns, refers clients for health interventions, and makes home, hospital, and nursing home visits (Holst, 1987; Westberg, 1990). In this role, the nurse may empower clients to better express themselves to both health professionals and other members of the ministerial team (Westberg, 1990). As collaborator, the parish nurse serves as a liaison to multiple community resources and services. The nurse may also function as a case manager, assisting clients in navigating the complex health care system (Schank, Weis, & Matheus, 1996). As manager, the nurse organizes support groups within the congregation

and recruits, trains, and supervises volunteers to extend resources throughout the parish community (Holst, 1987; Westberg, 1990). As educator, the parish nurse promotes health through various teaching modalities. The nurse provides seminars, conferences, classes, and other educational activities to raise the health consciousness of the parish community and to "foster an understanding of the relationship between lifestyle, personal habits, attitudes, faith, and well-being" (Holst, 1987, p. 15). The nurse strives to enable individuals to become more active partners in the management of their personal health resources. A nurse working with a congregation can reinforce and validate religion's ancient and contemporary concerns about personal hygiene, health, and well-being (Holst, 1987). As advocate, the nurse attends to the needs of the underserved members of the congregation and focuses on gaining access to needed services (Schank, Weis, & Matheus, 1996).

Models of Parish Nursing Practice

Most parish nursing practice is described as one of four differing models: the institutional/paid model, the congregational/paid model, the institutional/volunteer model, and the congregational/volunteer model. In the institutional/paid model, the nurse is employed by a local hospital, community agency, or long-term care facility that contracts with one or more congregations for nursing services. The employing agency provides the salary, benefits, institutional support, and supervision to the nurse. In the congregational/paid model, the congregation employs the nurse directly, providing salary, benefits, and supervision through the congregation and the ministerial team. In the institutional/volunteer model, the agency and the congregation have a contractual relationship for services and support, and the nurse volunteers his or her time when rendering needed services. The contract, when the services are volunteered, outlines actions and expectations of involved parties to ensure a well-communicated and well-structured program of services. The congregational/volunteer model differs from this in that the contractual relationship is between the nurse–volunteer and the congregation (Solari-Twadell, 1990; Miskelly, 1995). Models will continue to develop or be modified as the role of the parish nurse is shaped and refined.

Future Development

Parish nursing is a developing specialty area in community health nursing that is making a significant contribution to the advancement of the health of faith communities. Parish nurses enjoy the unique opportunity of discovering the ways that deep spiritual beliefs and religious values affect health by working with individuals and families of faith communities. This increased awareness of beliefs and values in the faith community in turn allows the nurse to effectively support parishioners in improving their health practices. Understanding a faith tradition, using the

Perspectives...

Insights of a Community Health Nursing Professor

Nurses who practice in community settings must have a different skill set from nurses who practice in structured settings such as hospitals or skilled nursing facilities. Community health nurses have to be more independent, more creative, and able to apply knowledge from a broad range of disciplines. We must be flexible to work effectively with a wide variety of clients and staff from other disciplines. We must have excellent communication skills and a sound theoretical grounding in systems theory, family theory, and epidemiology in addition to a broad generalist knowledge in nursing. I like to focus on three main themes—tolerance of ambiguity, management of complexity, and appreciation of context—to guide the thinking of nursing students in developing practice skills appropriate for community health nursing.

I tell students at the beginning of my rotation that one of the most important attributes of a community health nurse is a tolerance of ambiguity. When we enter the world controlled by the client, as in a home visit, we frequently enter uncharted territory. My major challenge, in teaching community health to BSN students, has been to convince students to "unlearn" the task orientation so carefully cultivated in the hospital settings, while retaining the skill sets needed to provide care to clients. Nursing students frequently measure "nursing worth" by the number of concrete psychomotor skills, such as injection and IV insertion, that they have mastered and may not consider therapeutic communication, for example, as a skill to be mastered. They are anxious to "do to" rather than "be with." They want to see patients, rather than clients. They are used to specific direction, in the form of procedures, policies, and definite time schedules for the completion of tasks. Lacking the protocols that closely define nursing activities in the hospital setting, they frequently assume that nothing important is being offered in this particular clinical rotation. They are uncomfortable with ambiguity and unable to operate independently without "permission." It is my responsibility to teach students how to function in a world where the details may not be neatly compiled in a patient record, complete with medical diagnosis and treatment plans. They must develop a tolerance for ambiguity.

The complexity of clinical decisions made with clients and vulnerable populations in unstructured environments requires a level of clinical decision making different from that of the hospital or clinic nurse. Nursing practice has dependent functions and independent functions. Community health nurses frequently provide those independent nursing functions that are not dependent on physician's orders. They must decide which nursing interventions are most appropriate, based on an assessment of the client, family, environment, and availability of resources. Many of my clinical teaching strategies revolve around managing the tension between the challenge and the frustration for a student with novice skills who is faced with complex situations. Rarely will the community health nursing student work with clients in need of a simple intervention. Most of our clients have multiple needs and lack resources to meet those needs. If students feel they are unable to "make a difference" for those clients, they may lose motivation in the course. In order to prepare students for these situations, I use case studies and small group work to critically examine problems in a wide variety of clients and situations. I can then guide students through simulated problem-solving scenarios based on the realities that they will encounter in the field.

The context of hospital nursing practice can easily become the hospital. Personnel, clients, and visitors operate within the context of the hospital. Consequently, we begin to view our interactions with clients and family through a unidimensional lens. This helps the hospital nurse to become "more efficient" and increases productivity in accomplishing hospital tasks. Nursing in the community cannot be unidimensional. We must understand the context within which the particular client and family relate to each other and to the larger community. An ability to appreciate contextual variations and design nursing interventions accordingly is a skill necessary in expert community health practice.

Understanding tolerance of ambiguity, management of complexity, and appreciation of context can bring a depth and richness to nursing practice in the community. Nurses, whether they are novice or expert, who can think in multidimensional ways using these concepts are needed in community-based settings.

—*Marjorie Barter, EdD, RN*
Associate Professor, University of San Francisco

health ministry, employing the support community, and providing opportunities for service and spiritual growth combine to make parish nursing fascinating, stimulating, and meaningful.

FUTURE DIRECTIONS

The future holds exciting and challenging opportunities for community health nursing. Proposed health care reforms will alter the education and practice of all nurses. Consistent in all discussions of health care reform is the recognition that delivery of health care services will continue to move into community settings. The practice of nursing will become more community based, population focused, and prevention oriented. Community health and community health nurses as we know them today may not fit all the needs of a new system. Education and practice must work together to develop the training and the delivery systems appropriate to the future (National League for Nursing, 1993).

In the United States, nursing's professional organizations have taken a proactive stance in the ongoing debate surrounding health care reform and the need for new delivery systems. Of particular significance to the field of community health nursing are positions taken by three professional nursing organizations: the American Nurses Association (ANA), the National League for Nursing (NLN), and the National Institute of Nursing Research (NINR).

The ANA (1991) proposed and widely disseminated *Nursing's Agenda for Health Care Reform*, a call for a restructured health care system that places consumers and their health at the center of health care delivery. This document proposes that services be delivered in "familiar, convenient sites, such as schools, workplaces, and homes" and calls "for a shift from the predominant focus on illness and cure to an orientation toward wellness and care" (ANA, 1991, p. 2). Those components of this plan that are relevant to community health call for a restructured health care system that simplifies consumer access to services through community-based delivery sites. Self-responsibility would be fostered through increased consumer responsibility for personal health and self-care. Nurses would assist the consumer in making informed decisions about services. Cost-effective providers in multiple settings would promote the efficient use of health care services. Case management would be featured for those clients with chronic, complex needs, thus reducing the current fragmentation of services. Case managers consult, advocate, and collaborate with consumers to assist them in making the best decisions about their health. Thus, nursing's plan for health care reform would transform a system that focuses on the treatment of illness at ever-spiraling costs to one that emphasizes primary health care services and the promotion, restoration, and maintenance of health. Consumers would take more responsibility and an active role in decisions about health care as new partnerships between consumers and providers developed. Health care would become a vital part of individual and community life (ANA, 1991).

The National League for Nursing (NLN) is just one of the many nursing organizations that have gone on record in support of the ANA agenda for reform. The NLN recognizes that education programs must be redirected and reformed to adequately prepare nurses to deliver care in a consumer-driven, community-based system of primary care providers. Successfully implementing nursing's suggested approach to health care delivery requires the following:

- Significant increases in nurses prepared to deliver primary health care as advanced nurse practitioners
- Preparation for all nurses, regardless of educational background or practice setting, to function in a community-based, community-focused health care system
- Increased numbers and utilization of community nursing centers as clinical sites for nursing students
- More faculty prepared to teach in a health care delivery system that is community based
- Further nursing research in the areas of health promotion and disease prevention at the aggregate and community levels
- Recruitment and retention of nurse clinicians, faculty, administrators, and researchers representative of diverse ethnic, racial, and cultural backgrounds (NLN, 1993)

The NLN recognizes that the nurses needed for the proposed system differ both in profile and number from those currently practicing. Nurse educators must be willing to modify or redesign curricula with the proposed reforms in mind. Graduates of all programs must be prepared to deliver culturally appropriate care to diverse populations. Educational experiences must be planned not just at hospitals but also at sites accessible to the population, such as homes, schools, worksites, ambulatory clinics, long-term care facilities, shelters, and community agencies. Nursing programs across the country are likely to become very dissimilar as they respond to unique settings and population needs. Educational programs must incorporate a macro focus on aggregates and populations rather than maintaining a strictly micro focus on individuals. The need to promote increased consumer accountability, authority, and responsibility must be emphasized in nursing education. To accomplish these goals, nursing education must shift its focus from content to process. Successful nurses of the future will be skilled in critical thinking, collaboration, and shared decision making. They will be able to function from a social/epidemiologic viewpoint and will be able to provide analyses and interventions at the system and aggregate levels. A full implementation of the proposed educational and delivery reforms will shift nursing's focus on the community from the philosophical to the real for the majority of nurses in the future (NLN, 1993).

The NINR, a division of the U.S. National Institutes of Health (NIH), also recognizes the changing focus of nursing practice. The National Nursing Research Agenda (NNRA) originated in 1987 to deepen the knowledge base

COMMUNITY NURSING VIEW

After one month of orientation that included observation of home visits, a new public health nurse working for the health department is excited at the prospect of performing independent home visits. This is her first day doing so.

The nurse's first client today is Sophia, an 18-year-old who has a 2-month-old daughter. Sophia is being followed through the teen parenting program. The program services include assessment for growth and development of the baby; nutritional status of the mother and infant; mother–child relationship; family support system; education regarding parenting, birth control, and nutrition; referrals to support groups; community resources; and educational and child care opportunities.

Sophia recently enrolled in the program, and this is her first experience with a public health nurse. The nurse phoned Sophia prior to the home visit and reviewed her role and the program services. When the nurse arrives at the door, Sophia is sitting on the back porch drinking tea and smoking cigarettes. The baby is lying in a playpen nearby. Sophia tells the nurse that she has been looking forward to the visit. "My friend had a nurse visit her too, and she really thought it was cool. I have been waiting to talk with you about my boyfriend and what I should do—he's a pain, and I'm really upset. He isn't helping me out with the baby. I've asked him and he doesn't want to do anything. What can I do?"

Nursing Considerations

ASSESSMENT
- How might the nurse establish rapport with Sophia?
- What data should be collected regarding Sophia's request for the nurse to help her with the issue regarding her boyfriend?
- What additional data should be collected on this first home visit?

DIAGNOSIS
- What initial diagnoses might be formulated?

OUTCOME IDENTIFICATION
- What initial outcomes would be formulated specific to Sophia's anxiety related to her boyfriend?
- How should the nurse intervene following Sophia's statements about feeling upset?

PLANNING/INTERVENTIONS
- What critical factors should the nurse include in the planning process?
- What would the initial plans be for working with Sophia?

EVALUATION
- How would you evaluate the outcome of the nurse's interaction with Sophia?
- What would you include in the evaluation?

for nursing practice. In 1988, the NNRA set the first series of nursing research priorities, which were implemented through 1992. In 1992, the second Conference on Nursing Research Priorities (CORP 2) resulted in five research priorities that were to guide research funding from 1995 through 1999. All of these research priorities emphasize the increasing importance of community-based, community-focused nursing care. The priorities for 1995–1999 are as follows:

- *Community-Based Nursing Models* (1995): Development and testing of community-based nursing models in rural and underserved populations.
- *Effectiveness of Nursing Interventions in HIV/AIDS* (1996): Assessment of biobehavioral nursing interventions that are effective in alleviating the effects of illness in persons infected with HIV/AIDS and that foster health-promoting behaviors in individuals at risk for infection. Women and individuals of different cultural backgrounds constitute the focus of the research priority.
- *Cognitive Impairment* (1997): Development and testing of approaches to remediate cognitive impairment.
- *Living with Chronic Illness* (1998): Testing of interventions that strengthen the individual's resources in dealing with chronic illness.
- *Biobehavioral Factors Related to Immunocompetence* (1999): Identification and testing of biobehavioral interventions that promote immunocompetence (NINR, 1993).

Each priority area is to be refined by a multidisciplinary Priority Expert Panel, with subsequent implementation of one priority a year. These research priorities will further the nursing knowledge base in the field of community health nursing and community-based care.

Community health nursing will be the core of nursing practice in the future. Many view the prospects for health care reform and changes in the delivery of health care services as a crisis of growing magnitude. Nurses would do well to remember that the Chinese word for *crisis* comprises the characters representing both challenge and opportunity. Nurses are well prepared to meet the challenges of the future and will experience unlimited opportunities to blossom and grow as individuals and professionals.

Key Concepts

- The transition from acute care practice to community-based practice requires the nurse to broaden professional skills and personal perspective and to view the community as client.

- There are multiple clinical roles and preparation levels for the community health nurse. Both generalist and specialist skills are necessary to provide interventions to aggregates with varying needs.

- The community health nurse is an advocate for individuals, families, groups, and communities. The nurse is influential in the development of independence and self-determination (self-care) in the client/community.

- In implementing health-promoting interventions with clients, the community health nurse fulfills multiple functional roles such as collaborating, consulting, and counseling. The nurse implements the educational process to enhance the client's understanding of beneficial lifestyle and behavioral changes and is committed to the implementation of research-based practice. The nurse participates in the research process to varying degrees.

- The community health nurse implements case management strategies to reduce the fragmentation of care that is common for individuals who are unable to negotiate the complexities inherent in the health care system.

- The public health nurse promotes and protects the health of populations, incorporating knowledge from nursing and the social and public health sciences. The public health nurse uses an interdisciplinary approach associated with the core public health functions of assessment, assurance, and policy development.

- The nurse employed in the home health specialty creates a bridge between the acute care institution and community practice. The home health nurse incorporates a multidisciplinary approach to provide skilled interventions to the client and family. When delivering health services in the home environment, the nurse considers the family as the basic unit of care.

- The hospice nurse delivers holistic and personal palliative nursing interventions to dying clients and their families. The nurse provides the client and family with skilled interventions, counseling, and emotional support and is considered the cornerstone of hospice services.

- The school nurse functions as a total health resource for the students, staff, families, and community with whom he or she interacts. The nurse's overriding objective is to promote optimal health in the school population and, in turn, support the educational process.

- The occupational health nurse safeguards the safety and health of workers through the implementation of interventions derived from numerous other disciplines. The nurse synthesizes principles from these multiple disciplines and blends them with objectives outlined by business and industry to promote a healthy and productive work force.

- The nurse practicing in a correctional facility functions as health advocate for incarcerated clients. The nurse ensures that clients have access to quality health services in an atmosphere of dignity and individual worth.

- Standards of community health practice have been outlined by the ANA. These standards have been modified by professional nursing organizations such as AAOHN and NASN for application to specific community-based nursing specialties. The standards address elements essential to the delivery of quality interventions.

- The ANA, NLN, and NINR have outlined recommendations for meeting the challenges of nursing practice in the United States. These recommendations emphasize cooperation between nursing education and clinical delivery systems to prepare nurses for community-based, population-focused, and prevention-oriented practice.

Caring for Individuals and Families in the Community

The focus of Unit V is on those processes that are important to caring for individuals and families in the community including the home visit, the developmental issues needed to be considered, and the understanding of family dynamics.

The Home Visit

Janice E. Hitchcock, RN, DNSc

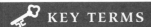

KEY TERMS

caregiver
contacting phase
contract
entry phase
family strengths
partnership
termination phase

This is the true nature of home—it is the place of Peace; the shelter, not only from all injury, but from all terror, doubt, and division.

—Ruskin, 1865, p. 606

COMPETENCIES

Upon completion of this chapter, the reader should be able to:

- Recount advantages and disadvantages of the home visit.
- Describe the process and issues of the home visit.
- Relate the dimensions of assessment in the home setting.
- Explain the use of nurse–client contracting to keep the nursing process goal directed and focused.
- Cite the most common interventions used when providing home care to families.
- Explain the community health nurses's focus on health promotion and prevention when working with families in the home.
- Detail issues of termination of the nurse–client relationship.

Nurses make health care visits to the home for many reasons. The emphasis of public health nursing visits is health promotion and disease prevention. Public health nurses carry out communicable disease investigations and monitor many family health concerns such as maternal–child health and geriatric health care needs. Home health care providers focus primarily on care of the sick and, in the case of hospice nursing, the dying (Humphrey & Milone-Nuzzo, 1991). Although nurses who visit families in the home sometimes have different objectives, the process of the home visit remains essentially the same.

THE HOME VISIT

Zerwekh (1992b) notes that the goal of community health nursing remains the same as when the specialty was founded in the 1890s: "to encourage self-help by promoting capacity to make health choices" (p. 90). One of the ways whereby this goal is met is through the provision of health care to families in their homes. Specific activities depend on the needs of the family and on the agency for which the nurse works. Agencies from which nurses make home visits include visiting nurse associations, hospice, public health departments, home health agencies, and school districts. Many hospitals also have home care programs that employ community health nurses to provide follow-up for the hospital's clients.

Advantages

The advantages of home visits over providing care to clients in an agency setting are multiple. When family members can be cared for at home, hospital stays are shortened and overall costs to the family are reduced. From the client's point of view, the client has greater control over the interaction. The nurse is in the client's home and must adhere both to the client's wishes regarding interactions and to the goals of the visit. In many families, for instance, the offer of food or drink to a visitor is a ritual that conveys welcome. A caring way to respond in such a situation is suggested by Wright and Leahey (1994), who recommend a statement such as "Thanks, but maybe we could work first and then have coffee afterward" (p. 151). In this way, work and social boundaries are differentiated without offending the family's sense of hospitality.

Families tend to be more comfortable and, therefore, less anxious in their home environments; thus, they are also more receptive to teaching. Their motivation to learn necessary skills is enhanced because, at home, they have direct experience in the daily management of their health problems. They have identified areas in which they lack knowledge and are inspired to learn how to more effectively care for themselves. Their interest in participating in the health care needs of family members is also increased.

The nurse is able to observe the interplay of factors that influence the client's health status as the process is happening. Specifically, the nurse has more access to infants, children, and other members of family life such as pets, boarders, roommates, and grandparents. The family's social environment and rituals can also be observed (Wright & Leahey, 1994). Through interactions with the family, the nurse comes to understand potential as well as actual health problems and is therefore able to intervene before problems escalate into serious health concerns (Deal, 1993). The nurse can identify environmental resources and hazards that affect the client's health. Because contact with the family usually occurs over a longer time period than that associated with hospital care, the nurse also has an opportunity to assess the client in activities of daily living and to note health changes. While the mandate of the home health nurse is providing care to the ill client rather than to the family as a whole, the broader family assessment is also important because it affects the health of the individual client.

Disadvantages

Although home visiting provides valuable insights into families and offers interventions unavailable in the hospital, there are disadvantages to be considered. Nurses must weigh whether their value systems and styles of practice are compatible with providing nursing services in the home setting. Nurses with a strong need to control a situation or to be perceived as an authority would have difficulty with ever-changing family circumstances and different lifestyles. Kristjanson and Chalmers (1991) suggest several questions that nurses can ask themselves regarding these issues: "Do [I] hold on to power and control? Do [I] like to be the authority and the expert? Can [I] work in a non-judgmental way with different families?" (p. 152).

🌀🌀 REFLECTIVE THINKING 🌀🌀

Advantages and Disadvantages of Home Visiting

Consider your own experiences and expectations of home visiting.

- Do you agree with Table 15-1 regarding the advantages and disadvantages of home visiting?

- For you, do the advantages outweigh the disadvantages, do the disadvantages outweigh the advantages, or do you think they are evenly balanced? Why?

Visiting a client at home takes more time than does an appointment in the hospital or clinic setting. Home visiting also negates working with groups of people having similar concerns. Home visiting assumes a greater likelihood that the interview will be interrupted by things such as children needing attention or a visiting neighbor. The home setting offers no immediate access to emergency equipment or to consultation with other disciplines as is available in a medical setting. Furthermore, the client's home may be situated in a neighborhood that is known to be dangerous. In addition to these aforementioned disadvantages, the family caregiver may consider home care a drawback, as well. Providing care to a family member in the home can be exhausting for the **caregiver**. In the family, the caregiver is usually a spouse, parent, or child. It is thus important to assess caregiver needs and arrange for support as needed. (See Chapter 18 for further discussion of caregiver issues.)

Some clients resent the intrusion of the health worker into their homes and prefer the more formal climate of the health care setting. In appropriate situations, however, the home visit offers a dimension of health care that can be provided in no other setting. See Table 15-1 for a summary of advantages and disadvantages of the home visit.

Home Visit Considerations

Community health nursing is guided by the nursing process just as is nursing care of individuals. Most family nursing involves working with both individuals in the family and the family as a whole: Individual members may have specific health problems and needs that must be addressed, these problems may have an impact on the family, and the family may have a specific impact on the individual and his or her health. Family decisions regarding the needs of an ill family member play a large part in the progression of treatment and recovery.

Phases of the Home Visit

Byrd (1995a, 1995b) developed the concept of home visiting as a process having three phases. The first phase, the **contacting phase**, encompasses the antecedent event (when the nurse becomes aware of an individual or family who is identified as desiring or needing a visit) and the

Table 15-1   Advantages and Disadvantages of Home Visiting

ADVANTAGES	DISADVANTAGES
Costs less than hospitalization.	Nurse's value system and style of practice may not be compatible with providing services in the home.
Affords client greater control over interaction.	More time consuming than care provided in a hospital or clinic setting.
Family more amenable to health education.	No easy access to emergency equipment or consultation.
Nurse can observe factors that influence family health.	Personal safety concerns.
Nurse can observe family interactions.	Cannot work with groups.
Allows for early intervention.	Distractions more difficult to control.
Allows for identification of environmental resources and hazards.	Family resents intrusion into home and/or prefers health care setting.
Allows for assessment of family over longer period of time than is possible during hospitalization.	Potential for caregiver exhaustion.
Facilitates family participation in health care.	
Facilitates family focus and individualized care.	

going-to-see phase (when the nurse journeys to the home and gains information about the neighborhood and the family's place in it). The context of the antecedent event may be a voluntary or required request for service because of illness or the identification of a risk for health problems. The nursing strategies for promoting trust ease movement into the second phase, the **entry phase,** which moves from the going-to-see phase to the seeing phase. During this phase the nurse observes and interacts with the family, learning about them and their life situation and planning interventions with their input. These experiences facilitate the **termination phase**, which encompasses the telling phase. The telling phase emphasizes referral and documentation of the situation. During this phase, interventions are evaluated and plans made with the family for future visits. Although most visits provide interventions that support family life, Byrd (1995a) cautions that "the visit may have had negative consequences such as stigmatizing the family as neglectful or poor" (p. 87). It is important that the nurse consider strategies to minimize these negative outcomes: for instance, by reinforcing **family strengths** (those characteristics that allow a family to manage its life successfully). See Chapter 18 for a more detailed discussion of family strengths.

The first contact with the family is usually via telephone to arrange a time for the home visit. On this initial call, the nurse introduces herself, identifies the purpose of the visit and the agency to which the referral has been made, confirms the client's address, and requests permission to make a home visit at a mutually acceptable time. If the client does not have a telephone, it may be necessary to make an unscheduled visit. After the nurse has met with the family, a neighbor may be identified who can take calls for future contacts. If the family is not home, the nurse should leave a card providing the nurse's name, telephone number, and agency and either asking the client to call to schedule an appointment or indicating a

time when the nurse will return. There will be times when the family is consistently unavailable or has moved. Zerwekh (1992a) asserts that knowing ways to locate disappearing families is a skill that is foundational to all other work with families in the home. "Effective locating requires community networking, persistence, an extensive map collection, the courage to knock on many doors, and the wisdom to 'sniff out violence' and back away as needed from a threatening household or neighborhood" (Zerwekh, 1997, p. 26). A reasonable effort should be made to effect a successful contact.

In many cases, a health provider, rather than the client, seeks the nurse's services. Under such circumstances, the nurse particularly needs effective social skills to convey caring for the family and to clarify the purpose of the visit with the family. It is important to listen to the family's concerns and to work with them. An authoritative approach is likely to result in a passive or rejecting response (Kristjanson & Chalmers, 1991). Zerwekh (1997) notes that trying to take over in the home is a prescription for alienation and disconnection.

Prior to a subsequent visit, it is important to call and reconfirm the appointment. Families are likely to be distracted by other concerns and may therefore forget a scheduled visit. A brief call will remind them of the nurse's visit and provide the opportunity for the nurse to assess the current status of the client. It is important to remember that priorities and clients' needs change (Humphrey & Milone-Nuzzo, 1991).

Safety

When making home visits, the nurse must consider her own safety. Although most home visits do not present a safety risk, some do. Areas of particular concern are those where gangs are known to exist or those having a high proportion of drug users. Review Figure 15-1 for guide-

Figure 15-1   Visitor Safety Issues

Appearance and Communication

1. Wear a name badge and/or uniform that clearly declares your professional affiliation.

2. Be sure that agency staff know your visiting schedule, including the name, the date, and the time of the visit and your expected return.

3. Let clients know in advance the approximate time of your visit. If you need further directions, ask the client for them rather than stopping to ask someone on the way. If possible, call clients just before the home visit so they can watch for you and come out to greet you.

4. Walk slowly around animals so that you do not frighten them. Ask clients to secure menacing pets before the visit. Never run away from a dog.

5. Do not carry a purse. Before leaving for the visit, lock your purse in the trunk of your car or cover it with a blanket. Keep change for a phone in a shoe or pocket.

6. Use a mobile car phone; however, do not leave it in the car during a visit.

7. If you enter the residence during a domestic dispute, leave and call to make another appointment.

When Traveling

By Car

1. Be sure your car is in good working order and has enough gas to get you back to your agency.

2. Provide for the unexpected in winter by keeping a blanket in the car; in the summer, keep a thermos of cool water. It is also prudent to keep a nonperishable snack in the glove compartment.

3. If you have car trouble, do not accept rides from strangers. Turn on emergency flashers and wait for the police, or call for help if you have a mobile car phone.

4. Keep your car locked when parked or driving. If possible, keep windows closed.

5. Stay in your car or leave the area if confronted with a situation that does not feel right.

6. Park in full view of the client's residence. Avoid parking in alleys or deserted side streets. Put a sign in your car that identifies your agency.

7. If safe parking is a question, it may be necessary for your agency to hire a driver to take you to and from the client's residence.

On Foot

1. Keep one arm free and have nursing bag and equipment ready when exiting from the car.

2. Walk directly to the client's residence in a professional, businesslike manner.

3. When passing a group of strangers, cross to the other side of the street, if appropriate.

4. When leaving the client's residence, carry car keys in your hand, holding the pointed ends between your fingers. Doing so renders the keys an effective weapon.

During Visits

1. Use common walkways in buildings; avoid isolated stairs.

2. Always knock on the door before entering a client's residence.

3. If relatives or neighbors become a safety problem, make joint visits, arrange for escort services, schedule visits when they are gone, or close the case.

Other Tips for Safety

Defense Techniques

1. Scream; yell "FIRE!"

2. Kick shins, instep, or groin.

3. Bite, scratch.

4. Blow a whistle attached to your key ring.

5. Use chemical spray.

6. Use your nursing bag as a defense weapon.

Nursing Considerations

1. Visit neighborhoods of questionable safety in the morning.

2. Neighborhoods that are extremely unsafe may be ones that cannot be served.

3. In the event of robbery, never resist.

4. Notify your agency for further instructions in the event of any car trouble, auto accident, or other incident when personal safety is in question.

5. Document:

   a. Any threat to personal safety while on duty.

   b. Any animal or human bites (give paperwork to infection control manager).

6. Seek medical attention as needed.

7. Consult with agency manager about notifying appropriate public officials of personal safety violations.

Adapted from Manual of Home Health Nursing Procedures *by R. Rice, 1995, pp. 303–304, St. Louis: Mosby-Yearbook, Inc.*

DECISION MAKING

Breastfeeding at Home

It is Jean's second day home from the hospital following the delivery of twins. She was in the hospital for only 24 hours and received some instruction about breastfeeding. Her recollection of the information is fuzzy, however, and she's lost the written material given to her by the nurse before Jean left the hospital. Jean still feels exhausted from her labor and delivery, and one twin is not nursing well. Jean is ready to forget the breastfeeding and, instead, use a bottle. The community health nurse from the hospital is scheduled to make a visit today.

• What can the nurse do to help Jean in her dilemma about breastfeeding?

• What anticipatory guidance can the nurse give?

• What other aspects of Jean's life should the nurse assess with regard to caring for the twins?

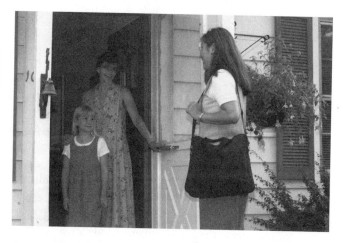

Being perceived with apprehension by the family is commonplace for the nurse conducting an initial home visit. The effective use of social skills to convey caring can ease the family's apprehension.

lines to maximize the personal safety of health care professionals working in the community and home settings.

Fostering Positive Client Response

When preparing for a subsequent visit, review plans from the previous visit and establish priorities with regard to the problems or issues to be addressed. In consultation with the family, develop objectives at primary, secondary, and tertiary prevention levels and relative to the client's readiness to deal with the issues at hand. Detecting the client's readiness to change is an important competency. Zerwekh (1997) cites three dimensions of timing interventions to foster a positive client response. The first is detecting the right time to initiate an approach: for instance, recognizing that a client needs to tell his or her story before considering possible solutions. The second dimension is the persistence of the nurse in visiting so that she or he will be there when the client is ready. If visits are not consistent, the client has no opportunity to develop enough trust to be willing to discuss true concerns. The third dimension is timing interventions on the basis of future problems and possibilities. This aspect of timing anticipates family needs, such as changes in developmental stages, and allows the nurse to discuss these expected changes with the family so that they will be prepared for the changes when they occur.

In consultation with the family, the nurse plans both interventions related to the nursing diagnoses and ways to evaluate the outcome of the interventions. It is important to remember that planned assessments and interventions may have to be postponed because of other family needs that take priority during a particular visit (Byrd, 1995a). Because there is usually a specific health problem to be

addressed, home care interventions may be prescriptive. In all cases, however, the best results will occur when the family is fully involved in the care and is ready to assist as needed.

The Nursing Bag

When making a home visit, the nurse comes equipped with a nursing bag. This bag usually contains equipment for basic assessment (sphygmomanometer, stethoscope, thermometer, etc.), medical asepsis (disinfectant, soap, toilettes, etc.), and waste disposal (plastic bags). During the home visit, universal precautions must be observed. Although the principles are the same in any situation, some special considerations apply when practicing universal precautions in the home environment. Figure 15-2 outlines information about the proper maintenance of the nursing bag, and Figure 15-3 provides information about maintaining universal precautions in the home.

Health Care Team

The community health nurse works as part of a team of health care providers. The family may have a social worker, rehabilitation therapist (e.g., a physical or speech therapist), or a home health nurse or aide. The nurse must participate in the coordination of health care provided by health personnel. This coordination often includes taking steps to resolve "divergent opinions that occur when different disciplines approach common problems" (Zerwekh, 1991, p. 216). At the same time, the nurse works alone in the home and, with the family, makes decisions about care appropriate to the family's ever-changing needs. In addition, the nurse often helps the family to connect with other community resources. To help make these connections, the nurse must develop a network of relationships with all sectors of the community.

Figure 15-2   Bag Technique

1. Maintain the inside of the nursing bag as a clean area.

2. Set the nursing bag on top of fresh newspapers when transporting it in the car.

3. In the client's residence, spread newspapers over cleanest or most convenient work area removed from children and animals. Place the bag on the newspapers.

4. Keep handwashing supplies at the top of the bag. Remove handwashing items and close bag. Go in and out of bag as few times as possible.

5. Take handwashing items to sink area. Use one paper towel on which to place other items. Use a second and third towel for washing and drying hands before and after care has been given.

6. After drying hands, use the paper towel to turn the faucet off.

7. Open nursing bag again and remove items necessary for the visit. If additional equipment or supplies are needed from the bag during the home visit, the handwashing procedure must be repeated.

8. Use soap and water or disinfectant to clean all equipment before returning it to the bag. Contaminated equipment or equipment that cannot be cleaned may be transported to the agency in a sealed plastic bag for disinfection. Never place used needles or dirty equipment or dressings in the nursing bag.

9. Do not expose the bag to extreme temperatures or leave it in the car for long periods.

10. Clean, disinfect, and restock the nursing bag weekly.

Adapted from "Principles of Universal Precautions/Body Substance Isolation" by R. Rice, 1993, Home Healthcare Nurse, 11(4), pp. 55–59. Copyright 1993 by Lippincott-Raven Publishers. Adapted with permission.

Figure 15-3   Use of Universal Precautions in the Home Environment

Items to Carry with You

- Sterile (for procedures that require sterile technique), nonsterile (for procedures that may expose staff to the client's blood or other body substances), and utility gloves (to clean up equipment, the work area, or spills)
- One disinfectant that is tuberculocidal and another disinfectant that is effective against human immunodeficiency virus (HIV)
- A solution of 5.25% sodium hypochlorite (household bleach) diluted with water to 1:10 (mix fresh daily to maintain effectiveness)
- Masks
- Cardiopulmonary resuscitation (CPR) masks
- Goggles
- Moisture-proof aprons/gowns
- Leak-proof specimen containers
- Sharps containers
- Liquid soap, soap toilettes, dry hand disinfectants (alcohol based)

Handwashing

- Wash before and after client contact.
- Wash during client contact if soiled.
- Wash with soap and water immediately after removing gloves (may substitute antiseptic hand cleaner or toilettes but wash hands with soap and water as soon as possible).

Use of Gloves

- Wear before contact with nonintact skin, blood, and body substances.
- Change after each procedure.
- After each use, dispose of sterile and nonsterile latex gloves in a leak-resistant waste receptacle such as a plastic trash bag.
- Disinfect and reuse utility gloves. Dispose of and replace when signs of deterioration are apparent.

Use of Other Protective Equipment As Needed

- Wear disposable gowns or aprons when there is a reasonable expectation of contamination by blood or other body substances. After use, remove and dispose of in a plastic trash bag in the client's residence.

Continued

Figure 15-3   Use of Universal Precautions in the Home Environment *(Continued)*

- Wear a face mask whenever there is a reasonable expectation of aerosolization or splattering of blood or other body substances. After use, remove and dispose of in a plastic trash bag in client's residence.
- Wear a face mask and instruct family members to each wear one when caring for a client who needs respiratory isolation. Paste a homemade "STOP" sign outside the client's room to remind family to put on the mask.
- Wear goggles or safety glasses with side shields when there is a reasonable expectation of aerosolization or splattering of blood or other body substances near the nurses's eyes. Clean with soap and water after each use. Discard in plastic trash bag if cracked or heavily contaminated.
- Use disposable CRP masks if required to provide artificial mouth-to-mouth or mouth-to-stoma ventilation.

Sharp Objects and Needles

- Place in a puncture-proof disposable container. A needle must not be bent, sheared, replaced in the sheath or guard, or removed from the syringe after use. Avoid capping needles unless through the use of a mechanical device or a one-handed technique.
- Store sharp's containers on top of the refrigerator in the residence or some other place out of reach of children.

Specimen Collection

- Place blood or other body substances in a leak-proof container and secure in a puncture-proof container during collection, handling, storage, and transport.
- Label the specimen with client's name and identifying data.
- Handle all specimens in a manner to minimize spillage.
- Place containers on the floor of the car during transport.

Exposure Incident

- Use water to irrigate the eye.
- Use soap and water to wash the exposed body part.
- Contact agency for follow-up instructions.
- Document incident.

Adapted from "Principles of Universal Precautions/Body Substance Isolation" by R. Rice, 1993, Home Healthcare Nurse, *11(4), pp. 55–59. Copyright 1993 by Lippincott-Raven Publishers. Adapted with permission.*

IMPLEMENTATION OF THE NURSING PROCESS IN THE HOME

It is as important to follow the nursing process in the home setting as in any other setting. Assessment incorporates all family members, both as individuals and as a family unit. Family nursing diagnoses are important in developing appropriate plans and interventions, in collaboration with the family. Evaluation is an ongoing component of the nursing process and is crucial to a timely termination.

Assessment

The nurse's assessment of the family begins before the first home visit. It is important that the nurse review the referral information concerning the client. This information provides basic information such as name, age, diagnosis, address, telephone number, insurance coverage, reason for referral, and source of referral. The referral source will vary with each client. A common source is the client's doctor, who recognizes that certain services are needed at home. Because hospital clients are discharged after very short stays, continued teaching and nursing care are often needed after the client returns home.

The first telephone contact is an opportunity to gather data. The nurse should note the client's response to the call. Is the client open to the visit? Does the client remember that a referral had been made? Does the client agree with the reason for the referral or have a different understanding of the reasons that the nurse wants to see him or her? The client's responses and demeanor give the nurse some clues as to the client's perception of the meaning of the home visit.

The purpose of the first home visit is to begin to identify the family's strengths and health needs. It is unreasonable to expect the family assessment to be completed in one visit, or, indeed, in many visits. The first meeting is usually at a time of stress related to the event that precipitated the need for a home visit. The nurse must remember that the family's usual functioning is compromised and that their current behavior may not reflect their usual coping abilities. Objectively assessing families is difficult. It is important to recognize personal bias. The use of assessment tools helps the nurse maintain objectivity. Common assessment tools are interviewing, observation, standard-

Perspectives...

**Insights of a Registered Nurse
Stories into Lessons**

I
How to tell my story
   of the stories
   I've been allowed
   to know?
Each with a heroine/hero
each with myth and magic
each sad and true
each strong and full of wonder
   amazing
   I repeat
amazing the lives
   however ordinary
amazing they would tell me
   a stranger
my entré
   is the assumption they make
   about NURSE
I think, I wonder, I worry
will I live up to this?
At times I know
   I don't,
I count on grace.
Lives seem too important to make mistakes
   Yet I learn the human spirit is
      too sturdy
      to crumble completely.
I take their stories in
   absorbing the life so
      that mine is enhanced.
      I'm a robber
but they seem not diminished
   but grateful somehow
   to have a listener.
It's got to be more than that
What about all those theories?
   What about all the postures/
   and definitions?

II
A ninety-year-old professor
   proud and dignified
   took me in and shared the
history of his life
   mostly the good parts

very few of the bad
   but they were
      there.
The twenty-five year old
   recovered heroin and
   cocaine user
raising a young family
trying in many ways
   beyond herself
to cope with what she had chosen to escape
"It's all still there when
   you come down" she once told me.
Compromising to fit and do the right thing
   in a society that does not
   welcome her
Wanting all the things for her kids
   that others want for theirs,
peacefulness, some joy, a well-received mind
she struggles and her struggles
   make her strong
   a survivor.
A tragic family tale
   of loss and abandonment
   of fear and flight
   of survival
remembered by a child who at seven
   left the only world she
      ever knew
a quiet life on a village farm
   in Cambodia.
Two children for each parent
   to carry
   and one hidden in a womb
   yet to be discovered
But two left behind
   who would surely die
The inconsolable loss sustained
   in an effort that more
   might survive.
The tears in her eyes
   as this
   now eighteen-year-old
   remembers
She rubs her pregnant belly
   just now understanding
   the proportions
   of her mother's loss.

Continued

Continued

Take it from Helen,
    Life is Hell.
she will engage me and then set
    me to anger and bring me back
        again to an enormous
        attraction.
She could be my aunt Mary
    she's negative enough
and she's rough, Lord the language
    and the volume.
she tells me can't
    but she can
She tells me won't
    but she will
her actions often betray her
an ordinary person
    faced with extraordinary
        circumstances
        her failed marriage of 37 years
        her only daughter's suicide
        her eldest son's death from a boating accident
        her MI
        a stroke at the same time
not familiar or comfortable with
        words like
        grief
        depression
        cope
        mourn
        insight
a woman who always just DID
    now what? and why?
        she asks.
Frustrated and loved by her son John
    who loves and frustrates
        her.

They go round
amazingly they let me see them
    love/hate
        one another.

III

So, how about me?
    I am enriched, touched, seized with emotion
        by these experiences
        who wouldn't be?
    I feel a need in
        myself to be less
        guarded
    less in control
the rawness of my nature
        felt
        but rarely shared
what I learned from them.
I thank them all for letting me
        into their lives
they say, "really?"
        doubtful that I
        mean this
    —boy do I mean this.
And hope for us all
        reveals itself to me again
        hope that comes from the
        real lives of
        real people
letting me in
        so briefly
        and so completely
    I look the same
but walk away
        changed.

—Margaret Dodson, RN, 3 May 1990

ized or unstandardized surveys, questionnaires, or checklists (Thomas, Barnard, & Sumner, 1993). Home health nurses may focus more on client assessment than on family assessment, but both are important regardless of whether the family or the individual is the primary client.

Interviewing

Community health nurses interview both individuals and families or segments of families: most commonly, committed partners or parent and child. When individuals in families are interviewed, it is important to remember that only one point of view is being represented. Whenever possible, the nurse should make an effort to meet with all family members, either as a group or individually, in order to get an idea of the total family perspective. Although family interviews are more complex than one-on-one interaction, they do elicit data unobtainable in any other way. For instance, the reaction of one family member to another can be observed only in a group interaction.

✑❂ REFLECTIVE THINKING ❂✑

Home Visit Experience

• Have you ever had a nurse visit your home? If so, what were some of the thoughts and feelings you had about the experience? If you have not had such an encounter, how do you think you would react to such a situation?

• As you think about your own actual or imagined experience with a nurse who is making a health visit to your home, what issues can you identify that would have an impact on your own behavior as a nurse making a home visit?

Before family assessment of any kind is possible, the nurse must establish a trusting relationship with the family. Trust is a critical component of all work with the family (Zerwekh, 1992a). Initially, family members perceive the nurse as a stranger. Unless they are in extreme stress, family members are unlikely to share their most personal concerns with the nurse. The nurse can expect that initial information obtained may not reflect deeper issues. In addition, cultural factors may cause undeclared stress because family members either do not recognize that they are experiencing stress or do not consider the possibility of getting aid from outside the family to help alleviate the burdens that are causing stress (see the accompanying Research Focus) (D'Avanzo, Frye, & Froman, 1994).

As family members become more confident that the nurse is trustworthy, they will reveal more of their real concerns. In addition to their natural reticence to share personal issues and feelings with a stranger, they may have specific reasons to not trust the nurse. If they are taking drugs, are in the country illegally, or have some stigmatizing condition that causes them to fear that their secret will be revealed to a punitive authority, they cannot afford to trust without testing to see whether confidentiality will be maintained. Unless family members come to believe that they can trust the nurse not to report them, they may change residences to avoid further contact. Such an event is undesirable because it prevents them from getting the health care they need.

Observation

Assessment through observation is an ongoing process during each home visit. The nurse can easily observe the condition of the home, the interactions among family members, and the status of the neighborhood and larger community. These observations help the nurse determine the quality of life of the family, identify safety issues, and recognize problems that put the family at risk. See Figure 15-4 for a list of selected observations to make during a home visit.

Figure 15-4   List of Selected Home Visit Observations

Neighborhood

Facilities conveniently available to family (schools, stores, churches, parks, transportation, etc.)

Quality of streets (busy, quiet, well maintained)

People in neighborhood (drug dealers, prostitutes, many or few people, friendly neighbors, children, elders)

Quality of property (well maintained, clutter in yards)

Type, condition, and quantity of animals in the area

Home

Floors and walls: uneven or slippery, loose rugs, cleanliness, heavy articles on top shelves or inadequately hung on walls, unsecured tall book shelves

Walkways and stairways: uneven, broken, or loose sidewalks or paths; absence of or insecure handrails; congested or cluttered hallways or other high traffic areas; toys or other items in places where people might trip over them; adequacy of night lighting inside and outside

Furniture: hazardous placement of furniture with sharp corners, chairs or stools that are unstable or too low to get into or out of or that provide inadequate support

Bathrooms: presence or absence of grab bars around tubs and toilets, nonslip surfaces in tubs and shower stalls, adequacy of night lighting, need for raised toilet seat or bath chair in tub or shower, presence in medicine cabinet of medications no longer used or out of date

Kitchen: pilot lights in need of repair, inaccessible storage areas, hazardous furniture

Bedrooms: availability of night lights and accessibility of light switches

Electrical: unanchored and/or frayed electrical cords, overloaded outlets or outlets near water, uncovered electrical outlets in places where children can reach them

Fire protection: presence or absence of smoke detectors, fire extinguisher, and fire escape plan; improper storage of combustibles or corrosives; accessibility of emergency telephone numbers

Toxic substances: medications kept beyond date of expiration, improperly labeled cleaning solutions, cleaning materials in unlocked cabinets accessible by children

Family

Children watching TV rather than playing with one another

Parents having similar or different views of a given incident when discussing family health or interpersonal problems

Availability of family members for interviews

Quality and quantity of discipline of children

Family constellation (single parent, three generation, etc.)

Adapted from Fundamentals of Nursing: Concepts, Process, and Practice *(5th ed.) by B. Kozier, G. Erb, K. Blais, & J. M. Wilkinson, 1995, Redwood City, CA: Addison-Wesley. Copyright 1995 by Addison-Wesley. Adapted with permission.*

RESEARCH 🔍 FOCUS

Stress in Cambodian Refugee Families

STUDY PROBLEM/PURPOSE

To improve understanding both of the beliefs of Cambodian refugee women about stressors that affect their families and of the ways that these women handled the resulting stress.

Research questions were as follows:

1. What behaviors are culturally recognized as indicating a stressful state?
2. What are the perceived causes of stress?
3. What taboos are imposed by the culture when a person is in a stressful state?
4. What coping strategies for stress does the culture dictate?
5. What can a family do to help a person who is experiencing stress?
6. What is the role of women in the management and prevention of stress?

METHODS

A comparative descriptive study involving interviews of Cambodian women from one West Coast location and one East Coast location—60 from each site—was employed. A trusted female Cambodian was used to provide entry and translation. Network sampling was used. Data were collected during a two-hour structured interview; questions were asked in the Cambodian language with alternate translation and clarification. Demographic data were summarized for the whole sample and the two subgroups using descriptive statistics and tests of difference. Responses were analyzed by determining the most frequently recurring responses and the rank order of same by frequency. The two subgroups were compared for similarities of ranking of responses.

FINDINGS

The most commonly cited response to stress was headaches followed by shouting, chest pain, pressure or palpitations and shortness of breath, markedly increased sleep, and being quiet. Less frequently cited responses were sickness, loss of appetite, and neglecting religious or spiritual needs. Use of alcohol and prescription or street drugs, hitting or perpetrating violence on others, and neglecting family or friends were denied as being associated with stress.

The most commonly perceived causes of stress were thoughts about the war in Cambodia, concerns about money, and concerns about other issues including infidelity, loneliness, grief surrounding family left behind, cultural losses, and health status. Women from the East Coast were more concerned about money and language problems (having been in the United States a shorter time and being less educated); women from the West Coast experienced stress related to recalling the war, "other" individual concerns, and family conflicts. The East Coast group more frequently reported taboos against street or prescription drugs and excessive sleeping. The West Coast group reported taboos against thinking sad thoughts or being alone when under stress. Both groups opposed excessive use of alcohol in response to stress. Responses to the last three questions "indicated that while the traditional role of the Cambodian woman is to be the 'stress bearer,' she often feels unable to bear it and is resigned to a stressful state for herself and others" (p. 104).

IMPLICATIONS

Cambodians are reluctant to seek mental health services; even when they do, they often present with symptoms not recognized as stress related. Both groups believed that women and families should help stressed family members by providing company and encouragement; but women, particularly those with children, felt unable to take constructive action to reduce family stress. They felt responsible for the emotional equilibrium of their families yet ineffectual in understanding stress. "This state, accompanied by the process of acculturation, limited social supports, and low income, may produce a cycle of stress that cannot be managed without culturally sensitive health care" (p. 105). Those who had been in the United States the longest (10 years or more) were able to cite the most coping strategies.

This study emphasizes the need for nurses and other health care providers to be aware of undeclared problems.

SOURCE

From "Stress in Cambodian Refugee Families" by C. E. D'Avanzo, B. Fryer, & R. Froman, 1994, Image: Journal of Nursing Scholarship, 26, pp. 100–105. Copyright 1994 by Sigma Theta Tau International.

Other Assessment Tools

Assessment tools help in the organization of family data and provide information to remind the nurse about areas to explore with the family. Family genograms and ecograms, discussed in Chapter 18, can be used to depict the structure of the family. The Wright and Leahey (1994) family assessment model, also discussed in Chapter 18, provides direction for gathering information about the structure, function, and developmental aspects of the family. Murray and Zentner (1997) have developed a family assessment tool that assesses family lifestyle and needs. The assessment tool lists many dimensions of family life that the nurse can observe during the home visit, such as crowding, access to the phone, expression of ideas, and relationship patterns. Other aspects of the tool can be used to generate questions to ask the family. For instance, the nurse could inquire about the family's knowledge or use of food stamps or about their child-rearing practices. The nurse may use this assessment tool either in whole or in part to obtain needed information about one particular aspect of the family (see Figure 15-5).

Figure 15-5 Family Assessment Tool

MEETING OF PHYSICAL, EMOTIONAL, AND SPIRITUAL NEEDS OF MEMBERS

Ability to Provide Food and Shelter

- Space management as regards living, sleeping, recreation, privacy
- Crowding if over 1.5 persons per room
- Territoriality or control on the part of each member over lifespace
- Access to laundry, grocery, recreation facilities
- Sanitation including disposal methods, source of water supply, control of rodents and insects
- Storage and refrigeration
- Available food supply
- Food preparation, including preserving and cooking methods (stove, hotplate, oven)
- Use of food stamps and donated foods as well as eligibility for food stamps
- Education of each member as to food composition, balanced menus, special preparations or diets if required for a specific member

Access to Health Care

- Regularity of health care
- Continuity of caregivers
- Closeness of facility and means of access such as car, bus, cab
- Access to helpful neighbors
- Access to phone

Family Health

- Longevity
- Major or chronic illnesses
- Familial or hereditary illnesses such as rheumatic fever, gout, allergy, tuberculosis, renal disease, diabetes mellitus, cancer, emotional illness, epilepsy, migraine, other nervous disorders, hypertension, blood diseases, obesity, frequent accidents, drug intake, pica
- Emotional or stress-related illnesses
- Pollutants to which members are chronically exposed, such as air, water, soil, noise, or chemicals that are unsafe to health

Neighborhood Pride and Loyalty

Job Access, Energy Output, Shift Changes

Sensitivity, Warmth, Understanding Between Family Members

- Demonstration of emotion
- Enjoyment of sexual relations

    Male: Impotence, premature or retarded ejaculation, hypersexuality

    Female: Frigidity (inability to achieve orgasm); enjoyment of sexual relations; feelings of disgust, shame, self-devaluation; fear of injury; painful coitus

    Menstrual history, including onset, duration, flow, missed periods and life situation at the time, pain, euphoria, depression, other difficulties

Sharing of Religious Beliefs, Values, Doubts

- Formal membership in church and organizations
- Ethical framework and honesty
- Adaptability, response to reality
- Satisfaction with life
- Self-esteem

CHILD-REARING PRACTICES AND DISCIPLINE

Mutual Responsibility

- Joint parenting
- Mutual respect for decision making
- Means of discipline and consistency

Respect for Individuality

Fostering of Self-Discipline

Attitudes Toward Education, Reading, Scholarly Pursuit

Attitudes Toward Imaginative Play

Attitudes Toward Involvement in Sports

Promotion of Gender Stereotypes

Communication

- Expression of a wide range of emotion and feeling
- Expression of ideas, concepts, beliefs, values, interests
- Openness

Continued

Figure 15-5 Family Assessment Tool *(Continued)*

- Verbal expression and sensitive listening
- Consensual decision making

Support, Security, Encouragement

- Balance in activity
- Humor
- Dependency and dominance patterns
- Life support groups of each member
- Social relationship of couple: go out together or separately; change since marriage mutually satisfying; effect of sociability patterns on children

Growth-Producing Relationships and Experiences within and outside the Family

- Creative play activities
- Planned growth experiences
- Focus of life and activity of each member
- Friendships

Responsible Community Relationships

- Organizations, including involvement, membership, active participation
- Knowledge of and friendship with neighbors

Growing with and through Children

- Hope and plans for children
- Emulation of own parents and its influence on relationship with children
- Relationship patterns: authoritarian, patriarchal, matriarchal
- Necessity to relive (make up for) own childhood through children

Unity, Loyalty and Cooperation

- Positive interacting of members toward each other

Self-Help and Acceptance of Outside Help in Family Crisis

Adapted from Health Assessment and Promotion Strategies (6th ed.), (p. 183) by R. B. Murray & J. P. Zenter, 1997, Norwalk, CT: Appleton & Lange. Copyright 1997 by Appleton & Lange. Adapted with permission.

Many other tools are available for assessing specific aspects of the family, such as the family support scale, which assesses the family's perception of the social support they receive during parenting, the Infant Care Survey, which assesses the mother's comfort with and knowledge of caring for her infant, the Family Hardiness Inventory, which assesses the internal strengths of families in meeting challenges and stress, and the Community Life Skills Scale, which measures the mother's ability to use community and interpersonal resources (Thomas et al., 1993).

DECISION MAKING

Home Visit Assessment

You are visiting Mrs. Richards and her daughter, Alison, to assess Mrs. Richards's self-care abilities. Mrs. Richards has recently returned home following a mastectomy. She tells you that Alison, age 14, is very upset because a friend of hers has committed suicide. Alison has been unable to sleep for two days and has no appetite. She cannot study and is not sure she can go to her friend's funeral, which is tomorrow.

- Review figure 15-5. What would be come areas to explore based on this assessment tool?

- What are your priorities for this home visit? Why?

- What questions might you ask and observations might you make to gain further understanding of the family's emotional status? Physical status?

Janosik (1994) has developed a crisis assessment tool and has suggested questions to raise with family members to facilitate assessment and provide anticipatory guidance (see Figure 15-6).

Use of these tools helps the nurse provide objective, family-centered care through the assessment of family processes, parenting, family coping, health maintenance and management, and home maintenance and management.

Cultural Health Practices

An important component of family assessment is the consideration of cultural health practices. These practices influence all aspects of the nursing process, and understanding them helps the nurse to understand client behavior and to more effectively plan interventions that are consistent with client health beliefs. Selected health practices and cultural assessment tools important to the family are discussed in Chapter 6.

Nursing Diagnosis and Planning Care

On the basis of the assessment, the nurse establishes the nursing diagnoses. These diagnoses may be for the entire family or for individuals within the family. In comparison with other community health nurses, home health nurses may assign more circumscribed diagnoses that focus exclusively on the client. Long-term and short-term goals are established in conjunction with the family. Together, expected outcomes that include measurable results within

Figure 15-6 Crisis Assessment Tool

Initial Steps

1. Using various sources of information, collect data that indicate the dimensions of the problem.

2. Formulate a dynamic hypothesis concerning the problem and the coping responses of the client.

3. Assess the problem in terms of intrinsic and extrinsic factors and determine a therapeutic approach.

4. Involve the client in problem-solving activities.

5. Negotiate a contract that sets clear, reachable goals.

6. Explain that treatment will be terminated according to the terms of the contract.

General Procedures

1. Obtain demographic data.

2. Define the problem in realistic terms.

3. Assess the mental status of the client(s).

4. Assess the physical status of the client(s).

5. Assess the psychosocial status of the client(s).

6. Assess coping skills of the client(s).

Coping Skills Assessment

1. How does the client deal with anxiety, tension, or depression?

2. Has the client used customary coping methods in the current situation?

3. What were the results of using customary coping methods?

4. Have there been recent life changes that interfered with customary coping methods?

5. Are significant persons contributing to continuation of the problem?

6. Is the client considering suicide or homicide as a way of coping? If so, how? When?

7. Has the client attempted suicide or homicide in the past? Under what conditions?

8. Assess the extent of suicidal or homicidal risk presented by the client. Hospitalization may be necessary as a protective measure.

Planning and Problem Solving

1. Is the present crisis new or a reenactment of similar events that occurred in the past?

2. What alternative methods might have been used to prevent development of the present crisis?

3. What new methods might be used to resolve the present crisis?

4. What supports are available to strengthen new problem-solving methods?

Anticipatory Guidance

1. What sources of stress remain for the client?

2. Using the current repertoire of coping skills, how might the client deal with problematic issues in the future?

3. How might the current repertoire of coping skills be maintained or expanded?

4. Upon termination of the contract for crisis intervention, is further referral or follow-up care necessary?

From Crisis Counseling: A Contemporary Approach *(2nd ed.) by E. H. Janosik, 1994, Boston: Jones & Bartlett. Copyright 1994 by Jones & Bartlett. Reprinted with permission.*

---

a specific time frame are established. A useful way to confirm these decisions is through the use of a contract.

Contracts

A **contract** is a critical component of family care. It is most useful for a nurse–client relationship that lasts more than two visits (Humphrey & Milone-Nuzzo, 1991). A family contract promotes self-care and facilitates a family focus on health needs. Although this type of contract is not legally binding, a pledge of trust and commitment is implicit. The most important component to contracting is the concept of **partnership**: the shared participation and agreement between client and nurse regarding mutual identification of needs and resources, development of a plan, division of responsibilities, time limits, evaluation, and renegotiation (Sloan & Schommer, 1991).

Contracting provides the framework for the relationship. It keeps the nursing process goal directed and focused (Humphrey & Milone-Nuzzo, 1991). The nurse and family must be clear on the responsibilities of each to the relationship, the purpose of the relationship, and any special limitations. For student nurses, one limitation is the length of time that the nurse will be available to the family. Thus, the time frame, which usually ranges from 4 to 14 weeks, must be made clear, and consideration must be given to the follow-up care that will be provided. In such instances, referral to other community health nurses or to a specific community agency is not unusual. In home health care, a home health nurse is assigned responsibility for the client when the student is no longer available.

The structure of the contract facilitates the termination of the relationship and helps prevent the family from becoming dependent. Because it focuses on the client's unique needs and promotes development of problem-solving skills and autonomy, the process promotes self-esteem in the client. Clients are motivated to do that which is needed to achieve their health goals.

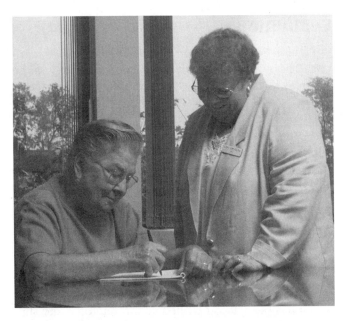

A contract developed in partnership between the client and nurse keeps the nursing process goal directed and focused.

Contracts can be as formal or informal as the partners wish. Some nurses and families develop a written document that both parties follow. More common is an oral contract that is reviewed at each visit. The main consideration is the mutuality of the complete process of client care between nurse and client (Sloan & Schommer, 1991).

Humphrey and Milone-Nuzzo (1991) have identified the following eight steps to the process of contracting in nursing:

1. Exploration of a need: Identified in collaboration with the client.

2. Establishment of goals: Should be realistic, attainable, and open to renegotiation.

3. Exploration of resources: Nurse and client work together to identify resources, such as significant others and community resources.

4. Development of a plan: Develop a prioritized list in collaboration with the client.

5. Division of responsibility: Nurse and client together decide who will be responsible for which activities.

6. Agreement on a time frame: For frequency of home visits and for the accomplishment of specific goals.

7. Evaluation: Evaluate progress to date of both the interventions and outcomes.

8. Renegotiation: On the basis of the evaluation, together determine whether the plan should be modified or terminated.

A well-developed contract that follows these steps provides distinct direction for nursing intervention. It also provides standards for evaluation because it clearly delineates the expected outcomes (Balzer-Riley, 1996).

Interventions

In conjunction with the client, nursing intervention begins on the first visit as decisions are made in the planning process about those health needs that should be addressed first and the responsibilities of both the nurse and the client. The timing of the next visit is based on the needs of the client and is mutually agreed on. In home health care, there may be assigned times for nursing visits based on the particular client health problem. A home visit should be planned to last $\frac{1}{2}$ to 1 hour. Family members can absorb only a limited amount of information before they are overloaded and unable to take in more. Similarly, the nurse takes in a great deal of information through observation and interview and can easily become overloaded. It is better to arrange a second visit to continue assessment, review that which has been taught, and evaluate progress toward goals rather than trying to accomplish too much at one visit. The home health care nurse usually must accomplish certain activities in relation to the client and may therefore be limited in the amount of time that he or she has available to work with the family. Incorporating the family members in the care of the client, however, allows many opportunities for teaching and for further assessment of family concerns and needs.

Three of the most common interventions are teaching about various health considerations (discussed in Chapter 8), helping families deal with the stress created by health problems, and making referrals for community services.

Family Stress

Some specific considerations related to developing interventions directed toward reducing family stress have to do specifically with parental and caregiver stress. Because parents are usually the family members who determine the ways that the family copes with stress, it is important to address parental anxiety. Although the tendency of the nurse may be to directly protect vulnerable family members such as children or elders, it is equally important to support and educate the caregivers so that they can provide appropriate care to other vulnerable family members. Davis and Grant (1994) found that, although caregivers of stroke survivors developed their own management skills, they were most helped by the opportunity to talk with health providers. The health provider, working in concert with the caregiver and client, can therefore facilitate the development of strategies that work for the family.

Referrals

In making referrals, the important issues to be considered are the three As: availability, acceptability, and accessibility. Perhaps the most important consideration is the acceptability of the service. If the client is not will-

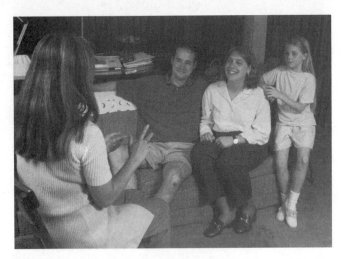

It is important not to overload a family with too much information all at one time.

ing to use the resource, its availability and accessibility are of no consequence. Similarly, no matter how acceptable the service may be to the client, it is of no use if it is inaccessible in terms of available transportation or client eligibility. In some settings, particularly in some rural areas, a service is simply not available, regardless of its acceptability to the client or the client's eligibility.

Promoting Family Strengths

Another intervention is to promote family strengths, thereby allowing family members to focus on their growth-producing dynamics rather than only on their problems. Zerwekh (1997) identifies emphasizing positives as one of the dimensions of expert connecting. While this intervention is important for all families, it is especially important for vulnerable families. In addition to emphasizing positives, the nurse can also reframe a negative behavior to highlight a positive aspect of the behavior. Alternatives that would facilitate positive behavior can then be considered. For example, if a client does not adhere to the established schedule for taking medications, the deviation can be depicted as an attempt to maintain autonomy rather than as client noncompliance. Emphasizing this positive characteristic supports the client's self-esteem, encouraging the client to reconsider the medication regime and respond in a way that is in his or her best interest.

Evaluation

Evaluation is an ongoing process that begins prior to each visit. The nurse and family must continually assess the progress of the family toward achievement of expected outcomes and must consider needed modifications to the plan. When goals are achieved, the nurse and client terminate the visits, making sure that the client and family know how to access community resources if needed.

Termination

Termination takes two forms: the ending of each home visit and the final cessation of services. The latter constitutes an important milestone that must be planned well in advance. Termination begins with the first visit. Although the structure of the contract sets the parameters of service, it is important to review with the family that which has been accomplished and to reinforce and support the family's progress. By the time of service cessation, family members will have come to value the nurse's input and will need reassurance that they themselves can make decisions that will positively affect their health care. The focus on partnership emphasizes this perspective and provides the family with the strength to make independent decisions.

Sometimes, goals are not completely met because the nurse has to terminate service before the client is ready. For instance, the nurse may have to reallocate time to families who are at higher risk, may take another job, or, in the case of a student, may have completed clinical rotation. In the case of home health, the number of visits is usually prescribed. Whenever possible in such circumstances, the nurse must ensure either a smooth transition to another community health nurse or the provision of an appropriate referral.

A successful termination is one in which both client and nurse feel satisfied that goals have been met or appropriate referrals made. To prepare family members for the last visit, the nurse should spend several weeks working with the family, reviewing client progress, and discussing any remaining issues in order to avoid leaving unfinished business. The nurse should also express and discuss her or his own feelings about ending the relationship. The association of nurse and client typically involves the expression of deep feelings. Disconnecting such a relationship takes much time and effort and should not be performed hastily. Figure 15-7 summarizes the components of the home visit as discussed here and within Byrd's (1995) framework.

Figure 15-7   Summary of Components of the Home Visit Using Byrd's (1995) Framework

Contacting Phase

Antecedent Event

Client self-refers or agency receives referral from another source.

- Clarify reason for referral.

Phone contact or unscheduled visit with family to arrange home visit.

- Clarify purpose of home visit and who referred family and why.
- Get directions to the family's residence.
- Determine whether any special equipment is needed or is available in the home.

Going-to-See Phase

Prepare for Home Visit

Collect information that will be needed about the family.

- Name, address, and phone number
- Map with directions to residence
- Telephone number of agency
- Emergency phone numbers: police, fire, ambulance (in many places, 911 covers all)

Identify any safety precautions that may be needed.

For a first visit, devise a plan for working with the family; for a subsequent visit, review prioritized plans from the previous visit.

Have a list of community resources that may be needed.

Have necessary equipment in nurse's bag and prepare any assessment or permission forms or teaching aids that may be needed.

Leave information with faculty or agency about your planned visit and expected length of stay.

Journey to the Residence

Have adequate gas in your car or adequate money for public transportation.

Observe the neighborhood where the family lives; check for safety, community facilities, people, animals, etc.

Observe the outside of the residence for environmental hazards and general quality of home environment.

Entry Phase (Seeing Phase)

Knock on the door or ring the bell. Stand where you can be seen.

Identify yourself; state your name and agency affiliation.

Ask for the person with whom you made the appointment.

Continue to be alert to your own safety.

Notice who is present and introduce yourself to them.

Allow the family to direct you where to sit. If they do not indicate a preference, ask if you may sit.

On an initial visit, explain the purpose of your agency and the reasons that you have come to their home. On a subsequent visit, review plans made during the previous visit and begin as planned unless the family indicates another priority that takes precedence.

Probable activities during the visit:

- Obtaining signatures on permission forms
- Performing health assessment of client or all family members, as indicated
- Washing hands before and after any direct physical contact
- Providing health education as indicated and written instructions as necessary
- Completing treatments as required
- Reviewing plans of care for the family, assessing for changes, and identifying and problem solving barriers to successful completion
- Identifying health needs of all household members
- Referring family members to appropriate community resources
- Identifying environmental hazards; reviewing concerns and problem solving together with family to find solutions

Conduct all visits in a caring way, providing comfort, support, information, and counseling, as indicated.

Termination Phase (Telling Phase)

Summarize accomplishments of the visit and, with the family, determine that which remains to be completed.

Discuss plans for the next home visit and the work to be completed in the interim by both family and nurse.

Ensure that the family has written documentation of your name, phone number, and agency affiliation.

Discuss referrals with the family and ensure that they have written documentation of the referral agency's name, phone number, and, if available, the name of a specific contact person.

As soon as possible after the visit, document the visit in the format used by your agency. Try to arrange time immediately after the visit to complete the written report.

COMMUNITY NURSING VIEW

Dan Jewell has been home from the diabetic teaching center for two days. He was diagnosed with adult-onset diabetes two weeks ago. Prior to that time, he had never heard of the disease. His wife, Roberta, attended some classes with him but is still confused about meeting his dietary needs. At the teaching center, Dan learned to give himself insulin injections, but he is very unsure of his technique. Given that he has a friend who has diabetes but who does not have to take insulin, Dan wonders whether he can avoid taking insulin if he is very careful about his diet. His two children, Jerry, 16, and Martha, 13, have been asking questions about diabetes. They are worried about their father's health and also are afraid that they might get the disease. They have read about diabetes and know that it can run in families.

Nursing Considerations

ASSESSMENT
• What issues do you think must be explored with this family?

• Which aspects of care lie in the realm of primary prevention? Secondary prevention?
• What assessment tools might be effective with this family.

DIAGNOSIS
• What nursing diagnoses are appropriate for this family?
• How would you set priorities with regard to the diagnoses?

OUTCOME IDENTIFICATION
• Given the diagnoses you have identified, what outcomes do you expect?

PLANNING/INTERVENTIONS
• How might you go about developing a contract with this family?
• How might you involve the family in contracting to facilitate self-care?

EVALUATION
• What might you do if an intervention were not working?
• How might you know when to terminate with this family?

Key Concepts

• The home visit is an important way of providing service to clients. While it has advantages and disadvantages, the home visit offers a dimension of health care that can be provided in no other setting.
• The nursing process is carried out in the home setting just as it is in any other setting.
• Nursing assessment of the family begins before the first home visit and includes interviewing, observation, use of a variety of assessment tools, and an awareness of cultural health practices.
• Contracting promotes self-care and facilitates a family focus on health needs.
• The major emphasis of the community health nurse is on primary prevention, including teaching, counseling, and referral to appropriate resources.
• Termination is an important part of the home visit.

Care of Infants, Children, and Adolescents

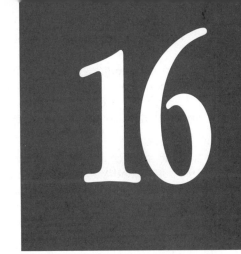

Relda Robertson-Beckley, PhD
Phyllis E. Schubert, DNSc, RN, MA

I believe that our only national treasure is our children. The one thing that we all have in common is a childhood. This period in our life comes only once, and if someone ruins that, disrupts it, or rapes it, there is no replacement for it.

—Gill, 1995, p. 31

COMPETENCIES

Upon completion of this chapter, the reader should be able to:

- Discuss maternal–child and adolescent health status in the United States.
- Recount developmental theories and conceptual frameworks applicable to infants, children, and adolescents.
- Discuss the relationship between fetal development and the need for prenatal care.
- Cite the respective indicators of infant, child, and adolescent health status.
- Detail the major health risks of infants, toddlers, and school-age populations in the United States.
- Describe the major health risks to adolescents in the United States.
- Discuss nursing's role as it applies to family-centered nursing practice and healthy development during the prenatal period, infancy, childhood, and adolescence.

Community health nurses serving families and communities are in unique positions to provide and teach caring behaviors that support healthy development. Child health care focuses on preventing acute and chronic illness while promoting normal growth and development. This chapter focuses on the care and nurturance of children from conception until passage into adulthood and on the roles of community health nurses in serving these populations.

HEALTH STATUS OF CHILDREN IN THE UNITED STATES

Although most children grow up strong and healthy, many others suffer from poverty, abuse, violence, disrespect, hunger, serious injury or chronic illness, family disintegration, inadequate parenting or child care, and limited or no medical insurance. At the Stand for Children Day held on March 12–15, 1997, Miriam Wright Edelman, president of the Children's Defense Fund (CDF) in the United States, introduced the CDF's annual report, *The State of America's Children Yearbook 1997,* by saying:

> If America's children are to grow up educated and productive, they must have a healthy start in life—with the health coverage they need to grow and thrive,

healthy communities that allow them to walk safely to school, and the opportunity to learn unimpaired by untreated vision, hearing, and health problems and violence, abuse, and neglect (Edelman, 1997, p.1).

In their study of childhood mortality trends from 1950 to 1993, Singh and Yu (1996) found an overall decline in the rate of childhood deaths, with the exception of death rates among male African American, American Indian, Hawaiian, and Puerto Rican children and children in the lower socioeconomic strata, which increased. The overall decline was related to substantial decreases in the number of deaths due to unintentional injuries, cancer, pneumonia, and congenital anomalies. Yet, this decline has almost been offset by a substantial increase since 1968 in the number of deaths due to suicide and homicide among children. This study reveals trends of increasing mortality from violence, firearm injuries, and human immunodeficiency virus (HIV)/acquired immunodeficiency syndrome (AIDS). The authors note that childhood mortality continues to be higher in the United States than in most of its international peers because of higher rates of medical problems, injury, and violence. In comparison with Japan and Sweden, for example, childhood mortality from homicide, suicide, and unintentional injuries is two to four times higher in the United States. To facilitate further decline in childhood mortality, Singh and Yu recommend improved access to health care and a reduction in socioeconomic disparity. Figures 16-1 and 16-2 illustrate the reality for today's American children.

Figure 16-2   Moments in America for Children

Every 1 second	A public school student is suspended.*
Every 9 seconds	A public school student is corporally punished.*
	A high school student drops out.*
Every 10 seconds	A child is reported abused or neglected.
Every 15 seconds	A child is arrested.
Every 25 seconds	A baby is born to an unmarried mother.
Every 36 seconds	A baby is born into poverty.
Every 47 seconds	A baby is born without health insurance.
Every 1 minute	A baby is born to a teen mother.
Every 2 minutes	A baby is born at low birth weight (less than 5 lb, 8 oz).
Every 3 minutes	A baby is born to a mother who received late or no prenatal care.
Every 5 minutes	A child is arrested for a violent crime.
Every 10 minutes	A baby is born at very low birth weight (less than 3 lb, 4 oz).
Every 18 minutes	A baby dies.
Every 2 hours	A child is killed by a firearm.
	A child is a homicide victim.
Every 4 hours	A child commits suicide.
Every 8 hours	A young person under age 25 dies from HIV infection.

Based on calculations per school day (180 days of seven hours each).

From CDF Report, Vol. 19, No. 1. by Children's Defense Fund, January 1998. All rights reserved. Used with permission of the Children's Defense Fund, Washington, DC.

Figure 16-1   Children's Defense Fund Report on the Health Status of Children

The State of America's Children Yearbook 1998 and *Poverty Matters: The Cost of Child Poverty in America,* state the following facts:

- In 1996, 11.3 million children through age 18 had no health insurance—the highest number ever recorded by the Census Bureau.

- In 1996, 3.1 million children were reported abused or neglected, and the reports were substantiated for at least 969,000.

- An average of 14 children die each day from gunfire in America—approximately one every 100 minutes.

- 14.5 million (more than one in every five) children live in poverty.

- In 1996, poor children were one-third less likely to attend a 2- or 4-year college than nonpoor children and one-half less likely to earn a bachelor's degree.

From The State of America's Children Yearbook, 1998, and Poverty Matters: The Cost of Child Poverty in America, 1998 by Children's Defense Fund, 1998, Washington, DC: Author. Used with permission of the Children's Defense Fund, Washington, DC.

In a study of adolescent morbidity and mortality trends for the years between 1979 and 1994, Sells and Blum (1996) found a 13% overall decline in mortality during the teen years. Significant reductions were noted in motor vehicle deaths; alcohol, cigarette, and illicit substance use; and gonorrhea and syphilis infection. The reduction in unintentional injuries, however, was offset by increases in teenage homicide, while worsening poverty and risk-taking behaviors negatively influenced morbidity rates among teens. Violence, suicide, and teenage pregnancy continue to be overwhelming problems for young people.

Chapter 7 illustrated that health indicators such as infant mortality, child abuse and poverty, adolescent drug use, and teenage suicides reflect deterioration of social health in the United States even as the gross domestic product (GDP), an economic indicator generally used as a significant measure of human welfare, continues to rise.

The Youth Risk Behavior Surveillance System (YRBSS) (Centers for Disease Control and Prevention [CDC], 1996b)

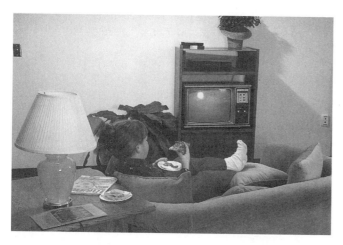

What suggestions might you offer to parents to encourage physical activity on the part of their child?

monitors six categories of priority health-risk behaviors among adolescents and young adults that contribute to morbidity and mortality among these groups: tobacco use, alcohol use, other substance use, sexual behaviors, unhealthy dietary behaviors, and physical inactivity. Seventy-two percent of all deaths in these age groups are due to motor vehicle crashes, other unintentional injuries, homicide, and suicide (CDC, 1996b).

Health Care Coverage of Children

Family income and employment status determine access to health care services and health insurance coverage. Children from low-income and poor families are the least likely to be privately insured because their parents are more likely to be unemployed or employed without health insurance benefits. Some children whose families lack health insurance are covered by Medicaid, a federal/state program for low-income and poor families.

The Wehr and Jameson (1994) study showed families with higher incomes and at least one employed parent to be twice as likely as were single-parent families to have private insurance. Approximately 35% of children lived in single-parent households headed by women, and children ages 6 to 17 were more likely to have private health insurance than were those age 5 or younger.

Immigration Status

Approximately 3 million immigrants have been given amnesty through the Immigrant Reform and Control Act of 1986. Children under 14 years of age represent an estimated 4.9% of this population; adolescents between ages 14 and 17 years represent 5.5%. These immigrant children and their families face problems with regard to health care access. In addition, health indicators reveal increased infant mortality, low birth weight, poor nutrition, congenital anomalies, and HIV/AIDS among this population (Mendoza, 1994).

THEORETICAL AND APPLIED PRINCIPLES OF CARING

Concepts related to caring, the family, and human development provide the framework for community health nursing practice in the care of individuals and families. The characteristics of an environment that supports health and healing (Chapter 7) also supports normal developmental processes of children. These characteristics—including safety, respect, nurturance, order, and beauty—reflect caring on the part of those responsible for children (Schubert & Lionberger, 1995). When children live in a caring environment, they are more apt to fulfill their potential as adults (see Chapter 7).

Family-Centered Nursing Perspectives

Family-centered nursing practice is based on the perspective that the family is the basic unit of care for its individual members and for the unit as a whole. In addition, the family is seen as the basic unit of the community and of society, representing all of human diversity—cultural, racial, ethnic, and socioeconomic. Application of family theory involves consideration of social, economic, political, and cultural factors when conducting health assess-

DECISION MAKING

Family-Centered Nursing Practice in the Community

Imagine that you are a home health nurse who has been referred to an 8-year-old boy with asthma. He is an African American child living in subsidized housing, a government-owned complex for urban poor in a large city. His mother died from asthma six months ago, and he does not want to take his medicine because of his wish to die and be with his mother. He is living with his grandmother and several other family members—adults and children. He receives medical care at a large university medical center. Consider the following questions and determine whether you would interview the child, family members, or health workers in the community.

• Who would you interview to gather data and identify problems?

• Who would you interview to assess the child's problem?

• With whom would you talk in formulating a plan for intervention?

• With whom would you communicate in evaluating the intervention outcomes?

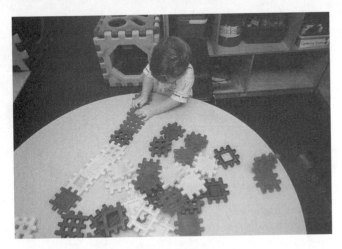

It is imperative that the nurse have a strong background in human development in order to recognize developmental delays and to teach developmentally appropriate care.

Developmental Processes

The study of **human development** involves the search for principles that address patterned, orderly changes in structure, thought, and behavior over the life span. These changes evolve via an integration of physiological characteristics; environmental forces; psychological mechanisms such as perception of self, others, and the environment; and acquired coping behaviors (Duvall & Miller, 1984). Developmental processes are influenced by **growth** (increase in body size or changes in body structure and function) and **maturation** (the emergence of genetic potential for changes in physical and mental patterns) (Dacey & Travers, 1996).

Community health nurses need strong foundational knowledge in human development in order to guide and teach parents and family members to give children developmentally appropriate care. A brief overview of the principles related to developmental theory is presented in Figure 16-3.

The major theories related to childhood and adolescent development are summarized in Table 16-1 (Wong, 1997). The theorists identified in this table cite psychosexual, psychosocial, cognitive, and moral judgment as the areas of concern during the stages of child development. Developmental theories provide tools for understanding child behavior patterns.

ments and planning, implementing, and evaluating care of children and families. Although family developmental theory and family functioning are not explored in detail until Chapters 18 and 19, this chapter assumes that the family provides the context for the care of infants, children, and adolescents. Family-centered nursing practice also acknowledges the role of the community, including community agencies and institutions that support and nurture children and their families (Gilliss, 1993).

Figure 16-3 Basic Assumptions of Developmental Theory

- Childhood is the foundational period of life; the first five years determine, to a large extent, attitudes, habits, patterns of behavior and thinking, personality traits, and health status.

- Development follows a definable, predictable, and sequential pattern and occurs continually through adulthood, but with individual differences related to the integration of many maturational factors.

- Growth and development are continuous, although a person may appear to stay in one place or regress developmentally.

- Growth is usually accompanied by behavior change, although certain traits may remain with certain adaptations related to maturation..

- Behavior has purpose and is goal directed.

- When one need or goal is met, a person has energy to pursue another need, interest, or goal.

- Critical periods in human development occur as specific organs and other aspects of a person's physical and psychosocial growth are undergoing rapid changes and the capacity for adaptation to stress is weak.

- Mastering developmental tasks of one period is the basis for mastering those of the next developmental period, both physically and emotionally.

- Progressive differentiation of the self from the environment results from increasing self-knowledge and autonomy.

- The developing person simultaneously acquires competencies in four major areas: physical, cognitive, emotional, and social.

- Readiness and motivation are essential to learning. Hunger, fatigue, illness, pain, and lack of emotional feedback or opportunity to explore inhibit readiness and reduce motivation.

- Many factors contribute to the formation of permanent characteristics and traits—genetic inheritance, undetermined prenatal environmental factors, family and society during infancy and childhood, nutrition, physical and emotional environments, and degree of intellectual stimulation in the environment.

- The young child achieves increasing ability to regulate behavior, to think and act in an individual and unique way, and to become more autonomous.

Adapted from Health Assessment and Promotion Strategies through the Life Span *(pp. 261–263) by R. Murray & J. Zenter, 1997, Stamford, CT: Appleton & Lange. Adapted with permission of Appleton & Lange.*

The early life of the person is usually divided into periods according to chronological age: the prenatal period (from the moment of conception to birth), infancy (birth–1 year), toddlerhood (1–3 years), preschool (3–6 years), school age (6–12 years), and adolescence (13 to 20 years).

Although somewhat arbitrary, these divisions serve as aids to understanding patterns that apply to most people most of the time (Murray & Zentner, 1997), and thus to understanding normal development.

FETAL DEVELOPMENT AND PRENATAL CARE PRIORITY

Certain events prior to and during the prenatal period are critical to the life of the child. These prenatal influences on development may be identified as normal inherited traits, parental age, prenatal endocrine and metabolic functions, maternal nutrition, **teratogenic effects** (environmental hazards to the fetus), maternal and fetal infections, immunologic factors, maternal emotions, and birth defects transmitted by the parents (Murray & Zentner, 1997). The community health nurse may be involved in prevention related to all of these potential or real hazards by assessing, planning, intervening via counseling and/or teaching, and monitoring results. Certain of the prenatal influences determine risk and priority status for prenatal care.

Prenatal care helps to prevent problems related to childbirth, such as prematurity and **low birth weight (LBW)** (birth weight below 2,500 grams). These events affect infant development in vital ways and account for the high cost of infant care to society. One analysis of the

REFLECTIVE THINKING

The High Cost of Prenatal Care

Imagine that you are a community health nurse in a health center funded by state and federal monies. The budget for public health services is being reviewed, and preventive services are being threatened. You are asked to testify at a hearing and justify prenatal care expenditures in your area. Present your position and your arguments for continuing to provide prenatal services to those who do not have health care insurance and cannot afford private payment.

cost related to LBW stated that "LBW accounts for 10% of all health care costs for children, and the incremental direct costs of LBW are of similar magnitude to those of unintentional injuries among children and in 1988 were substantially greater than the direct costs of AIDS among Americans of all ages" (Lewit, Baker, Corman, & Shiono, 1995, p. 1).

Given this information, it is easy to see that women who receive prenatal care beginning in the first trimester have more positive **pregnancy outcomes** (health status of mother and infant at birth) than do women who have

Table 16-1 Summary of Personality, Cognitive, and Moral Development Theories

STAGE/AGE	PSYCHOSEXUAL STAGES (FREUD)	PSYCHOSOCIAL STAGES (ERIKSON)	COGNITIVE STAGES (PIAGET)	MORAL JUDGMENT STAGES (KOHLBERG)
Infancy (birth–1 year)	Oral–sensory	Trust vs. mistrust	Sensorimotor (birth–2 years)	
Toddlerhood (1–3 years)	Anal–urethral	Autonomy vs. shame/doubt	Preoperational thought, preconceptual phase (transductive reasoning, e.g., specific to specific; 2–4 years)	Preconventional (premoral) level; punishment and obedience orientation
Early childhood (3–6 years)	Phallic–locomotion	Initiative vs. guilt	Preoperational thought, intuitive phase (transductive reasoning; 4–7 years)	Preconventional (premoral); level naive instrumental orientation
Middle childhood (6–12 years)	Latency	Industry vs. inferiority	Concrete operations (inductive reasoning and beginning logic; 7–11 years)	Conventional level; good-boy/nice-girl orientation; law and order orientation
Adolescence (12–18 years)	Genitality	Identity and repudiation vs. identity confusion	Formal operations (deductive and abstract reasoning; 11–15 years)	Postconventional or principled level; social-contract orientation; universal ethical principle orientation (no longer included in revised theory)

From Essentials of Pediatric Nursing *5th ed. (p. 91) by D. Wong, 1997, St. Louis, MO: Mosby-Yearbook. Printed with permission of Mosby-Yearbook.*

late or no prenatal care. Lack of prenatal care exacts a high price, both economically and in human terms.

Prenatal care comprises three basic components: early and continued risk assessment, health promotion, and medical and psychosocial evaluation, care, and follow-up. The **prenatal risk assessment** includes a complete history, a physical examination, laboratory tests, and fetal assessment to determine whether any factors place the pregnancy in jeopardy. **Health promotion** consists of counseling to promote and support healthful behaviors and of prenatal and parenting education. Interventions might address behavior modification related to nutrition (see Chapter 26); substances to avoid, such as alcohol and other drugs, tobacco, and pesticides; treatment for any existing illness such as diabetes; and referral to community services and resources, both social and financial.

Medically Related Risk Factors

Most women experience pregnancy with few complications to themselves or their infants. For some women, however, pregnancy holds serious risks. These risks may be related to maternal age (adolescents and women over age 35), preexisting medical conditions, socioeconomic status that contributes to poor general health and lack of access to care, or the pregnancy itself. These women are at greatest need of early intervention and continued assessment during pregnancy.

Diabetes Mellitus

During normal pregnancy, endocrine and metabolic adjustments, especially those related to the pituitary, adrenal cortex, and thyroid, occur and affect the developing fetus (Wong, 1997). Related conditions such as diabetes mellitus may exist prior to pregnancy or may develop during pregnancy (gestational diabetes). Either form of diabetes can jeopardize the health of mother and baby if proper diet, exercise, and insulin levels are not maintained. Infants of diabetic mothers (IDM) tend to be large (9 lb or more), and deliveries are often complicated by hypoglycemia, hyperbilirubinemia, and respiratory distress. The community health nurse can help clients avoid these problems by providing continued screening, education, and counseling during pregnancy.

Reproductive History

A woman's reproductive history often helps identify potential risks of pregnancy. A prior history of preterm delivery is the single best prediction of preterm birth (Joffe, Symmas, Alverson, & Chilton, 1995). Pregnancy before age 15 and after the age of 40 may carry increased biological risks and the potential for psychosocial consequences such as increased stressors related to early parenting and to educational and employment responsibilities. Short intervals between pregnancies may not allow for replacement of maternal nutrients, thereby compromising health during pregnancy (Joffe et al., 1995).

Maternal Infections

Infections during pregnancy can have a major impact on maternal and infant health. Cytomegalovirus (CMV), HIV, syphilis, chlamydia trachomatis, gonorrhea, herpes simplex, rubella, rubeola, mumps, smallpox, viral hepatitis, and toxoplasmosis are among those infections that can have detrimental effects on pregnancy outcomes. The community health nurse has a key role in the screening, counseling, immunization, and/or treatment related to these infections and, thus, in reducing the associated risks to both mother and fetus (Murray & Zentner, 1997).

Pregnancy-Induced Hypertension

Formerly called toxemia, pregnancy-induced hypertension can lead to organ damage in and even death of the mother and impaired development of the fetus. **Pregnancy-induced hypertension (PIH)** is a multisystem disorder characterized by hypertension, proteinuria, and edema. Unless treated, PIH can lead to pre-eclampsia in the third trimester. Pregnancy-induced hypertension most often occurs in first pregnancies and is most common among adolescents, women over age 35, African American women, and poor women (Cunningham, MacDonald, Gant, Leveno, Gilstrap, Hankins & Clark, 1997). Women with pre-eclampsia require weekly monitoring and may need to be hospitalized for closer observation.

Fetal and Maternal Abnormalities

Poor pregnancy outcomes can also be caused by malposition, early separation of the placenta, or other placental abnormalities. The position and size of the fetus and the condition of the cervix are variables to consider when assessing for possible complications in delivery.

Psychosocial Factors and Health Behavior

Psychosocial risk factors include socioeconomic status, psychological factors, and unhealthy lifestyle. Low socioeconomic status is linked directly with poor health, including increased maternal and infant morbidity and mortality. Crowded, often unsafe and unsanitary living conditions, inadequate nutrition, and limited access to health care all have negative effects on the expectant family. Psychological factors that may affect both the mother's understanding of and attitude about her pregnancy and the mother's health-seeking and parenting behaviors include high stress levels, low self-esteem, emotional instability, and domestic violence.

Maternal Stress

Current research indicates that the fetus is affected by maternal stress, although the effects of maternal elation, fear, and anxiety on the behavior and other developmental aspects of the baby are poorly understood (Murray & Zentner, 1997). Folklore has long indicated a link between maternal stress and infant health, but research in this area is quite recent.

Maternal Nutrition

Maternal nutrition is an extremely important variable in fetal health and prevention of complications. Approximately 60 nutrients are known to influence fetal health, and a lack of these nutrients may depress appetite, encourage disease, and retard growth and development, including causing mental retardation (Murray & Zentner, 1997) (see Chapter 22).

Cigarette Smoking

Nicotine is an environmental hazard for the developing fetus and has been associated with premature birth, low birth weight, delayed mental and physical development, and spontaneous abortion (Murray & Zentner, 1997). The more the woman smokes, the greater the risk of harm to the fetus. Thus, smoking-cessation programs take on new importance during pregnancy. Because **secondhand smoke** (passive smoking) is also known to be harmful to the developing fetus, the pregnant women should also avoid situations where others are smoking (CDC, 1996a).

Substance Abuse

Pregnant women should avoid alcohol during pregnancy in order to prevent fetal alcohol syndrome, a cluster of permanent birth defects that include mental retardation, delayed motor function, low birth weight, and craniofacial abnormalities. Use of opiates and other psychoactive drugs during pregnancy can lead to addiction in the infant and poor parenting behaviors in the mother (Wheeler, 1993). Many drugs used by prescription for medicinal purposes also create environmental hazards for the fetus and should be evaluated carefully for their potential for causing developmental problems (Murray & Zentner, 1997).

Environmental Hazards

Environmental hazards including radiation, chemical waste, contaminated water, heavy metals such as lead and mercury, some food additives, and various pollutants have teratogenic effects, adversely affecting the genetic structure of the fetus and causing developmental abnormalities (Murray & Zentner, 1997). (See Chapter 7 for a discussion of the role of the community health nurse in relation to environmental health issues.)

INDICATORS OF INFANT AND CHILD HEALTH STATUS

Community health nurses play an important role in the prevention of infant mortality and morbidity. By assessing and counseling pregnant women and referring them to perinatal resources for care and education, community health nurses help ensure positive pregnancy outcomes. By monitoring and referring infants to pediatric care, these nurses help improve the health of children. Because they serve as assessment tools for program planning of primary, secondary, and tertiary prevention services, various statistical indicators of child health in the community aggregate of concern are watched carefully. These indicators include the infant mortality rate of the aggregate and both individual and aggregate assessment related to the incidence of low birth weight infants, nutritional health status, and immunization status.

Infant Mortality Rate

The **infant mortality rate** is the number of infant deaths during the first year of life per 1,000 live births. This rate is used as a measure of community and national health status. Compared with other developed countries, the United States ranked eighteenth in the world in terms of infant mortality (Children's Defense Fund, 1996). In 1995, the

DECISION MAKING

Prenatal Nutritional Care

You have been referred to the home of a 20-year-old Caucasian woman who is three months pregnant by her boyfriend. The boyfriend comes around from time to time, but the woman does not know where he goes or what he does at other times. She has a sister living in a neighboring town, but they do not see each other because neither of them has transportation. She works part time at a fast-food restaurant down the street. She receives slightly above minimum wage and is barely able to pay her rent. She gets some food at the restaurant, and her boyfriend buys a few groceries when he is around. She says she is okay because she really does not feel like eating that much. You must make a care plan and decide the immediate focus of attention. Should you:

- Provide nutritional counseling and teaching?
- Refer her to available resources in the community for food stamps and services?
- Ask to include the father of the baby in the planning?
- Give her materials and teach her about prenatal growth and development?

Prioritize your selections and provide a rationale.

infant mortality rate in the United States reached a record low of 7.5 per 1,000 live births (U.S. Department of Health and Human Services [USDHHS], 1996c). This rate is higher among communities of color and among the poor, however. For example, the infant mortality rate of African American infants is 2.4 times that of Caucasian infants, and the infant mortality rate among Puerto Ricans has been rising. These striking differences are believed to be related more to socioeconomic status than to ethnicity. The goal of Healthy People 2000 is to reduce the infant mortality rate to no more than 7 per 1,000 live births (USDHHS, 1996d).

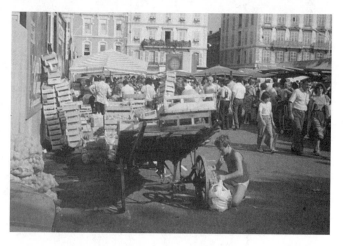

Cultural influences often affect food purchases. Reflect on your own food-buying habits. How does your cultural background affect your purchases?

Low Birth Weight and Child Health

Because they are more likely to die during the first year of life, premature infants and those having low birth weights contribute significantly to infant mortality and morbidity. They are also at risk for long-term health problems such as cerebral palsy, mental retardation, developmental delays, learning disabilities, attention deficit disorder, and/or sensory deficits (McCormick & Richardson, 1995).

Low birth weight and **very low birth weight** (less than 1,500 grams) survival rates have increased recently as a result of medical and technologic advances in respiratory medicine. In 1992, approximately 7.1% of all babies in the United States had low birth weight, and 1.3% had very low birth weight. The incidence of low birth weight is nearly twice as high among African Americans: Approximately 13% of African American infants had low birth weight, and 3% had very low birth weight (USDHHS, 1996d). The Healthy People 2000 goal is to reduce the incidence of low birth weight by 28%, to no more than 5 per 1,000 (USDHHS, 1996d).

Nutritional Needs and Child Health

Nutritional status is a very important aspect of nursing assessment in the care of infants, children, and adolescents. Needs change as the child grows, but the need for good nutrition remains constant. Nutrition is the key to maximizing child health and development. Beginning with the preconceptional period, sound dietary habits are important in establishing lifelong health patterns (Worthington-Roberts & Williams, 1996). Nutrition is influenced by socioeconomic, cultural, racial, and ethnic factors, as well as by individual and family food preferences. All of these factors must be considered when assessing child and family nutritional status.

Assessing a child's nutritional status involves obtaining a 24-hour dietary recall, taking comprehensive histories, and measuring height and weight. In adolescents, it is important to evaluate lifestyle and food preferences. The community health nurse may refer the client and family for nutritional and medical follow-up; counsel and educate about nutritional requirements related to specific stages of child development; and screen for nutritional

disorders such as failure to thrive, lactose intolerance, obesity, anorexia, bulimia, hypertension, and cardiovascular disease. Table 16-2 summarizes physical signs of health and malnutrition.

Infant Nutrition

The first year of life is characterized by rapid growth and development, with the birth weight typically doubling in the first 6 months and tripling by the end of the first year (Lankford, 1994). Such rapid growth requires increased protein and calories. Breast milk serves as the ideal source of nutrients and energy for the first 4 to 6 months. When the mother chooses not to breastfeed, commercial formulas constitute a reasonable alternative. Breast milk also contains important antibodies against infections that enter through the gastrointestinal tract. Breastfed infants have fewer infections and allergic reactions than do formula-fed infants. Breastfeeding offers many other advantages including promotion of maternal–infant attachment, more rapid involution of the uterus and return to pre-pregnancy weight, and lower cost. If the mother's own nutritional status is compromised, however, her ability to produce milk with the appropriate nutritional content may be impaired. Women who consume alcohol, caffeine, nicotine, or psychotherapeutic drugs must be informed that those substances are transmitted in breast milk.

The addition of semisolid foods to the infant's diet at 4 to 6 months of age and of finger foods in the latter part of the first year provides the nutrients essential to growth and oral and fine motor development (Table 16-3). Healthy full-term infants who are fed on demand tend to regulate their intake appropriately for growth and development and establish their own feeding schedules (Worthington-Roberts & Williams, 1996).

Although total energy requirements (kcal per day) increase during the first year, energy requirements per unit of body weight decline in response to changes in growth

Table 16-2 Physical Signs of Health and Malnutrition

	HEALTHY	MALNOURISHED
Hair	Shiny; firm in the scalp	Dull, brittle, dry, loose; falls out
Eyes	Bright, clear-pink membranes; adjust easily to darkness	Pale membranes; spots; redness; adjust slowly to darkness
Teeth/gums	No pain or cavities; gums firm; teeth bright	Missing, discolored, decayed teeth; gums bleed easily and are swollen and spongy
Face	Good complexion	Off-color, scaly, flaky, cracked skin
Glands	No lumps	Swollen at front of neck and cheeks
Tongue	Red, bumpy, rough	Sore, smooth, purplish, swollen
Skin	Smooth, firm, good color	Dry, rough, spotty; "sandpaper" feel or sores; lack of fat under skin
Nails	Firm, pink	Spoon shaped; brittle; ridged
Behavior	Alert, attentive, cheerful	Irritable, apathetic, inattentive, hyperactive
Internal systems	Heart rate, heart rhythm, and blood pressure normal; normal digestive function; reflex and psychological development normal	Heart rate, heart rhythm, or blood pressure abnormal; liver and spleen enlarged; abnormal digestion; mental irritability, confusion; burning tingling of hands and feet; loss of balance and coordination
Muscles/bones	Good muscle tone and posture; straight long bones	"Wasted" appearance of muscles; swollen bumps on skull or ends of bones; small bumps on ribs; bowed legs or knock-knees

Note: The physical signs noted here are consistent with but not diagnostic of malnutrition.

From Understanding Nutrition *(7th ed.) by E. N. Whitney & S. R. Rolfes, 1996, St. Paul, MN: West. Printed with permission of Wadsworth Publishing Co.*

rate. The recommended energy intake drops from 108 kcal/kg in the first 6 months to 98 kcal/kg in the second 6 months of life (Worthington-Roberts & Williams, 1996).

Toddler and Preschooler Nutrition

From infancy to toddlerhood, the appetite decreases. The toddler requires small portions of food, particularly nutri-

tious finger foods. Table 16-4 summarizes a recommended food pattern for adequate toddler nutrition.

The preschooler continues to require small portions of food; however, a greater variety of food sources may be

Table 16-3 Suggested Schedule for Introduction of Solid Foods

MONTH	FOOD
4	Cereal
5 to 6	Strained vegetables
6 to 7	Strained fruits
6 to 8	Finger foods (crackers, bananas, etc.)
7 to 8	Strained meat
10	Strained or mashed egg yolk
10	Bite-sized cooked foods

From Foundations of Normal and Therapeutic Nutrition *(2nd ed., p. 262) by T. Lankford, 1994, Albany, NY: Delmar.*

Table 16-4 Recommended Food Pattern for Toddlers

FOOD GROUP	NUMBER OF SERVINGS	PORTION SIZE
Milk	3	Cup
Meat/meat substitutes	2	1 to 2 oz
Fruits/vegetables	4	½ c. for vegetables ½ c. for fruits
Bread/cereal	4	½ to 1 slice bread ½ c. ready-to-eat cereal ¼ to ½ c. pasta
Fat	3	Pats of soft margarine
Nutrient-dense snacks		As desired for necessary kilocalories

From Foundations of Normal and Therapeutic Nutrition *(2nd ed., p. 265) by T. Lankford, 1994, Albany, NY: Delmar.*

required. It is essential that parents offer a wide variety of food sources, to promote adequate development throughout this phase. Parents also must set a good example by eating an appropriate diet themselves.

Nutrition of School-Age Children

School-age children grow more slowly than do infants and toddlers, and they eat less in proportion to their size. By the time children reach school age, their eating patterns are generally established. Because snacking is common, especially after school, nutritious snacks are important. To meet the needs of children from low-income families, many school lunch programs have been expanded to include breakfast.

Food choices of school-age children are heavily influenced by their peers. Although school-age children gradually increase the amount of food they eat, the range of foods they accept may be small. Sugar contributes approximately one-fourth of the calories in the average school-age child's diet. Milk, sweetened soft drinks, fruits, fruit juice, and desserts also contribute a great many calories.

Adolescent Nutrition

As children approach puberty, differences in the amounts of food consumed by boys and girls become increasingly apparent. During adolescence, the difference is striking, with boys consuming much greater quantities of food than do girls (Worthington-Roberts & Williams, 1996).

Adolescence is characterized by rapid growth and development. Because peers and the social environment have a powerful impact on adolescent eating patterns, nutrition education is important during this period. Foods that provide adequate carbohydrates, vitamins, proteins, and minerals should be emphasized. Iron, calcium, and zinc are necessary for growth of the skeletal system, sexual maturation, and overall body growth.

Eating disorders are common among adolescents, particularly females who have too often heard that thin is beautiful and fat is ugly. It is estimated that 30% of adolescents are obese and that at least 10% experience anorexia or bulimia. See Chapter 26 for more information on these disorders.

Immunization Status

Immunization provides immunity, the ability to destroy a pathogen either actively or passively. Active immunity is produced as a result of the invasion of a pathogen: for example, the varicella zoster virus that causes chicken pox. The virus may invade through accidental transmission from one child to another or may be injected as a vaccine. Either way, active antibodies are developed and may last throughout the person's life span. Passive immunity, which occurs as a result of maternal transmission of antibodies across the placenta to the fetus, is temporary, lasting only several months.

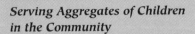

DECISION MAKING

Serving Aggregates of Children in the Community

In your capacity as the community health nurse at a local clinic, you discover that only 10% of the infants enrolled in the clinic have been immunized.

• What key decisions must be made by clinic administration and staff in order to address the problem?

• What steps should be taken to address this problem?

• What other aspects of the data must be considered before any action can be taken?

• What clinic and community strategies might be needed?

• What role might community health nurses play in addressing the problem?

Lack of knowledge and lack of access to care have resulted in increasing numbers of children not being vaccinated. The community health nurse has a major role in screening for infectious diseases, determining immunization status, and educating parents and caregivers about the need for routine immunizations, specific vaccines, and the side effects of same. The immunization schedule developed by the Centers for Disease Control and Prevention (CDC, 1998) is summarized in Figure 16-4.

Family Cultural Health Practices

Community health nurses working with immigrant populations must provide care within the cultural context of ethnic customs and belief systems related to health, nutri-

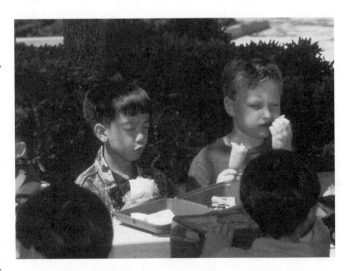

Children base their food preferences on what tastes good rather than on nutritional value. Many of children's favorite foods contain too much salt.

Figure 16-4 Recommended Childhood Immunization Schedule—U. S., January–December 1998

Vaccines[1] are listed under the routinely recommended ages. ⟦Bars⟧ indicate range of acceptable ages for immunization. Catch-up immunization should be done during any visit when feasible. Shaded ⟨ovals⟩ indicate vaccines to be assessed and given if necessary during the early adolescent visit.

Approved by the Advisory Committee on Immunization Practices (ACIP), the American Academy of Pediatrics (AAP), and the American Academy of Family Physicians (AAFP).

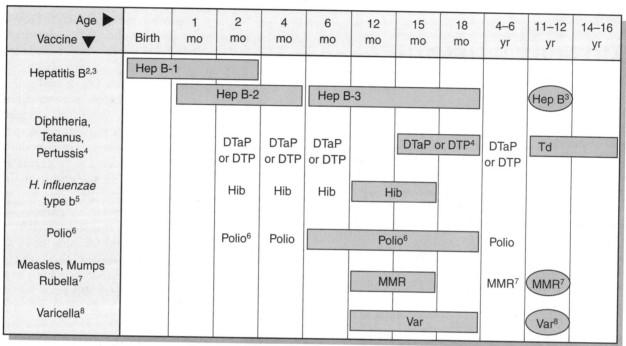

Age ▶ Vaccine ▼	Birth	1 mo	2 mo	4 mo	6 mo	12 mo	15 mo	18 mo	4–6 yr	11–12 yr	14–16 yr
Hepatitis B[2,3]	Hep B-1										
		Hep B-2			Hep B-3					Hep B[3]	
Diphtheria, Tetanus, Pertussis[4]		DTaP or DTP	DTaP or DTP	DTaP or DTP		DTaP or DTP[4]		DTaP or DTP	Td		
H. influenzae type b[5]		Hib	Hib	Hib		Hib					
Polio[6]		Polio[6]	Polio		Polio[6]				Polio		
Measles, Mumps Rubella[7]						MMR			MMR[7]	MMR[7]	
Varicella[8]						Var				Var[8]	

[1]This schedule indicates the recommended age for routine administration of currently licensed childhood vaccines. Some combination vaccines are available and may be used whenever administration of all components of the vaccine is indicated. Providers should consult the manufacturers' package inserts for detailed recommendations.

[2]*Infants born to HBs Ag-negative mothers* should receive 2.5 µg of Merck vaccine (Recombivax HB®) or 10 µg of SmithKline Beecham (SB) vaccine (Engerix-B®). The 2nd dose should be administered at least 1 mo after the 1st dose. The 3rd dose should be given at least 2 mos after the second, but not before 6 mos of age.

Infants born to HBs Ag-positive mothers should receive 0.5 mL hepatitis B immune globulin (HBIG) within 12 hrs of birth, and either 5 µg of Merck vaccine (Recombivax HB®) or 10 µg of SB vaccine (Engerix-B®) at a separate site. The 2nd dose is recommended at 1-2 mos of age and the 3rd dose at 6 mos of age.

Infants born to mothers whose HBs Ag status is unknown should receive either 5 µg of Merck vaccine (Recombivax HB®) or 10 µg of SB vaccine (Engerix-B®) within 12 hrs of birth. The 2nd dose of vaccine is recommended at 1 mo of age and the 3rd dose at 6 mos of age. Blood should be drawn at the time of delivery to determine the mother's HBsAg status; If it is positive, the infant should receive HBIG as soon as possible (no later than 1 wk of age). The dosage and timing of subsequent vaccine doses should be based upon the mother's HBsAg status.

[3]Children and adolescents who have not been vaccinated against hepatitis B in infancy may begin the series during any visit. Those who have not previously received 3 doses of hepatitis B vaccine should initiate or complete the series during the 11-12 year-old visit, and unvaccinated older adolescents should be vaccinated whenever possible. The 2nd dose should be administered at least 1 mo after the 1st dose, and the 3rd dose should be administered at least 4 mos after the 1st dose and at least 2 mos after the 2nd dose.

[4]DTaP (diphtheria and tetanus toxoids and acellular pertussis vaccine) is the preferred vaccine for all doses in the vaccination series, including completion of the series in children who have received 1 or more doses of whole-cell DTP vaccine. Whole-cell DTP is an acceptable alternative to DTaP. The 4th dose (DTP or DTaP) may be administered as early as 12 mos of age, provided 6 mos have elapsed since the 3rd dose and if the child is unlikely to return at age 15-18 mos. Td (tetanus and diphtheria toxoids) is recommended at 11-12 years of age if at least 5 years have elapsed since the last dose of DTP, DTaP or DT. Subsequent routine Td boosters are recommended every 10 years.

[5]Three *H. influenzae* type b (Hib) conjugate vaccines are licensed for infant use. If PRP-OMP (PedvaxHIB® [Merck]) is administered at 2 and 4 mos of age, a dose at 6 mos is not required.

[6]Two poliovirus vaccines are currently licensed in the US: inactivated poliovirus vaccine (IPV) and oral poliovirus vaccine (OPV). The following schedules are all acceptable to the ACIP, the AAP, and the AAFP. Parents and providers may choose among these options.
 1) 2 doses of IPV followed by 2 doses of OPV; 2) 4 doses of IPV; 3) 4 doses of OPV.
The ACIP recommends 2 doses of IPV at 2 and 4 mos of age followed by 2 doses of OPV at 12-18 mos and 4-6 years of age. IPV is the only polio virus vaccine recommended for immunocompromised persons and their household contacts.

[7]The 2nd dose of MMR is recommended routinely at 4-6 yrs of age but may be administered during any visit, provided at least 1 mo has elapsed since receipt of the 1st dose and that both doses are administered beginning at or after 12 mos of age. Those who have not previously received the second dose should complete the schedule no later than the 11-12 year visit.

[8]Susceptible children may receive Varicella vaccine (Var) at any visit after the first birthday, and those who lack a reliable history of chickenpox should be immunized during the 11-12 year-old visit. Susceptible children 13 years of age or older should receive 2 doses, at least 1 month apart.

From Centers for Disease Control and Prevention, January 1998.

tion, and parenting. Language difficulties and socioeconomic barriers may create additional stresses on the family system, particularly on the children. Because it may determine health care resources available, immigration status is an important aspect of child and family assessment. See Chapters 6 and 19 for discussions of transcultural family-centered nursing.

MAJOR CHILD HEALTH PROBLEMS

The health of today's infants and children is threatened by many factors that did not exist 50 years ago: HIV/AIDS, gun violence, drug trafficking in schools and neighborhoods, and increasing levels of environmental contamination. Other major health problems are related to parental behaviors, such as smoking, abuse of alcohol or other drugs (see Chapter 25), and family violence (see Chapter 24). Socioeconomic conditions such as poverty and homelessness (see Chapter 27) further jeopardize children's physical and emotional health.

Some of the major problems for which infants and children are at risk are discussed in this section. Children of all ages are at risk for most of these problems; however, developmental stage determines to a large extent both the response of the child and clues to appropriate intervention. The nurse most often works with the parent(s) to solve child health problems.

Failure to Thrive

When an infant falls below the 3rd percentile for both weight and height on standard growth charts, the condition is termed **failure to thrive** (FTT) (Wong, 1997). There are three general categories of failure to thrive based on causation: organic, non-organic, and idiopathic. **Organic failure to thrive (OFTT)** is caused by physical health problems such as cardiac defects or infections. **Non-organic failure to thrive (NFTT)** is usually due to psychosocial factors such as inadequate parenting skills or lack of emotional attachment to the child (Wong, 1997). **Idiopathic failure to thrive (IFTT)** is unexplained by the usual organic and non-organic causes and may also be classified as NFTT.

Failure to thrive and children at risk for this condition must be identified early to prevent serious long-term problems. If the infant is temperamental, irritable, or at high risk for medical problems at birth, the parent(s) may physically or emotionally detach from the infant, leading to psychological abuse and neglect.

Growth and development tools help the nurse assess the physical status of the child, and observation of the parent–child relationship provides clues to emotional health. By providing emotional support to the parent(s) and by teaching about child development, parenting, and

child care, the nurse can prevent parental detachment from the child and help provide a healthy environment for normal infant growth and development.

Cigarette Smoking

Many studies have shown that direct and indirect exposure to tobacco smoke has deleterious effects on health, particularly during pregnancy and childhood. Environmental exposure to tobacco smoke (ETS) is associated with increased rates of respiratory disease, reduced lung growth in children, increased rates of lung cancer, and exacerbation of asthma in children (CDC, 1996a).

The screening of children whose parents smoke should focus special attention on respiratory complications. Health education of parents must emphasize the direct and indirect effects of smoking, especially during pregnancy. Referral to smoking-cessation programs and other resources helps protect the health of both children and parents.

Educational and support programs for parents who want to stop smoking are an important aspect of child and family health care. See Chapter 8 for teaching and learning theories, teaching strategies, and health counseling that can help people change behaviors destructive to the health status of themselves and their children.

Unintentional Injuries and Child Health

Unintentional injuries, or accidents, are the leading causes of morbidity and mortality in children ages 14 and under. Children are primarily at risk of death from unintentional injury related to: motor vehicle and bicycle-related accidents (as occupants and pedestrians), drowning, fire and burns, suffocation, poisoning, choking, falls, and unintentional shootings. Injury rates vary with a child's age, gender, race, and socioeconomic status. Younger children, males, minorities, and poor children suffer disproportionately. Causes and consequences of injuries vary with age and developmental level, reflecting differences in children's cognitive, perceptual, and motor and language abilities as well as in their environments and exposures to hazards (National SAFE KIDS Campaign, 1996). The National SAFE KIDS Campaign was launched in 1988. Since that time, unintentional injury–related childhood mortality has decreased in several areas (see Figure 16-5). The National Center for Injury Prevention and Control (1997) has identified a particular demographic pattern for childhood injuries to aid providers in assessing for risk factors.

Community health nurses play an important role in injury prevention by providing both educational programs for families and communities and screening programs to assess environmental and related medical risk factors. Children at different phases of development are at risk for different injuries, but a child who is developmentally

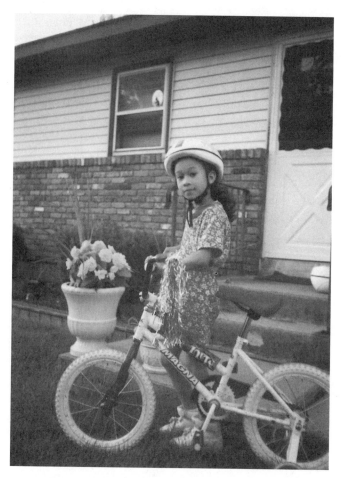

The use of equipment such as safety helmets helps to protect children from injury. What other measures can nurses implement and promote to help children protect themselves from harm?

delayed may be at greater risk for accidental injury than another child of the same age (see Chapter 22).

Lead Poisoning

One of the most common pediatric health problems in the United States, lead poisoning, or **plumbism**, was addressed briefly in Chapter 7 as a major environmental issue affecting children. Plumbism occurs in both urban and rural areas and is found most often among toddlers and preschool children. Lead poisoning is likely most prevalent among young children because they engage in the most hand-to-mouth activity; live closer to the floor, where the air holds more lead-containing dust and dirt particles; and have the most rapidly developing nervous systems, which in itself makes them more vulnerable to the effects of lead (CDC, 1994b).

The most common sources of lead ingested by children are dust and soil contaminated with lead from paint that flaked or chalked with age or that was disturbed during home maintenance and renovation. Other sources are "take home" exposures related to parental occupations and hobbies, water, and food (CDC, 1994b). Older buildings still contain lead-based paint, which has not been used in residential structures since the 1950s. Lead poisoning can also occur as a result of environmental contamination by gasoline or industrial waste.

Elevated lead levels interfere with the ability of red blood cells to metabolize iron, resulting in anemia and possible damage to the brain, liver, and other organs. Even low levels of lead exposure, determined by blood levels, can result in mental retardation and behavioral problems (Institute of Medicine, 1995). Symptom severity ranges from no symptoms to a decrease in play activity, lethargy, anorexia, sporadic vomiting, intermittent abdominal pain, and constipation, to loss of acquired skills, hyperactivity, bizarre behavior, seizures, and coma. Lead encephalopathy is almost always associated with a blood lead level exceeding 100 µg/dL but occasionally has been found in conjunction with a level as low as 70 µg/dL.

The CDC (1994b) estimates that most children in the United States have lead poisoning to some extent and advises that all children under 6 years of age receive capillary screening. Figure 16-6 lists groups at highest priority for screening. Screening and assessment generally focus on children less than 72 months of age and especially on those younger than 36 months of age. In general, children who have blood lead levels greater than or equal to 10 µg/dL receive a repeat test; those with levels above 15 µg/dL are scheduled for follow-up; and those with levels greater than 70 µg/dL and with symptoms receive immediate treatment in a medical center.

A critical aspect of treatment for lead poisoning of any degree is to drastically reduce the child's exposure to lead. Interventions may include removing the child from the environment, removing the lead source, and using chelating therapy in cases of lead levels greater than 30 µg/100 mL.

Figure 16-6   Priority Groups for Lead Screening

- Children ages 6 to 72 months who live in or are frequent visitors to deteriorated housing built before 1960.

- Children ages 6 to 72 months who are siblings, housemates, or playmates of children with known lead poisoning.

- Children ages 6 to 72 months whose parents or other household members participate in lead-related occupations or hobbies.

- Children ages 6 to 72 months who live near active lead smelters, battery recycling plants, or other industries likely to result in atmospheric lead release.

From Summary of 1991 Report: Preventing Lead Poisoning in Young Children *(p. 7) by Centers for Disease Control and Prevention, 1994, Washington, DC: Author.*

Other important nursing interventions include ongoing advocacy for any needed environmental modifications, follow-up for children with lead levels greater than 10 µg/dL, and education focusing on the risk of lead poisoning in the home.

According to the CDC (1994b), primary prevention has always been the goal of childhood lead poisoning–prevention programs, yet most programs focus exclusively on secondary prevention: that is, dealing with children who have already been poisoned. Programs must shift their emphasis to primary prevention and efforts directed toward identification and remediation of environmental sources of lead. "The purpose of community-level intervention is to identify and respond to sources, not cases, of lead poisoning" (p. 20).

Poverty and Homelessness

Poverty is increasing in the United States, and the gap between rich and poor continues to widen. In 1994, the top 20% of households in the United States received 46.9% of the nation's income, up from 40.5% in 1968 (U.S. Census Bureau, 1996). Nearly one-fourth of the nation's children, approximately 16 million, live in poverty (Center on Budget and Policy Priorities, 1994). Poor children are at greatest risk for the physical, social, and emotional effects of living in poverty (Sidel, 1996). Some of the effects of living in poverty are listed in Figure 16-7. Children in communities of color are disproportionately poor. More than 46% of all African American children and 41% of all Hispanic children lived in poverty in 1993, compared with 14% of all non-Hispanic white children. More than 50% of children living in families headed by a woman live in poverty, compared with only 12% of children who live in married, two-parent families (U.S. Census Bureau, 1996).

As poverty increases, so does homelessness. **Homelessness** can be defined as residing with relatives, living on

the streets, or living in shelters during hard times (see Chapter 27). Since the 1970s, homelessness has increased faster among families with children than among any other group (Jahiel, 1992). It is estimated that 1 million people are homeless in the United States and that nearly 40% of them are children under 18 years of age and 40% are persons in families with children (U.S. Conference of Mayors, 1997).

The statistics on poverty and homelessness do not adequately communicate the toll that poverty takes on children. Poor children often face hunger or poor nutrition; limited access to quality health care; and inferior, often unsafe, schools, all of which ultimately affect health. In the words of one author:

> Poverty wears down . . . [children's] resilience and emotional reserves; saps their spirits and sense of self; crushes their hopes; devalues their potential and aspirations; and subjects them over time to physical, mental, and emotional assault, injury and indignity (Sherman, 1994).

Poor children are also two or more times as likely as other children to experience problems such as physical and mental disabilities, severe asthma, iron deficiency, and fatal accidental injuries (Sherman, 1994). Awareness of the major threats to the health of children from low-income families helps the community health nurse focus assessment and interventions.

Child Abuse

Child abuse, the willful infliction of physical injury or mental anguish on a child (see Chapter 24), is a major child health problem in the United States. Child abuse may be categorized as physical, emotional, sexual, or a combination of the three. Abuse of as many as 23 out of 1,000 children is reported annually, and 2,000 children die from child abuse each year (U.S. Advisory Board on Child

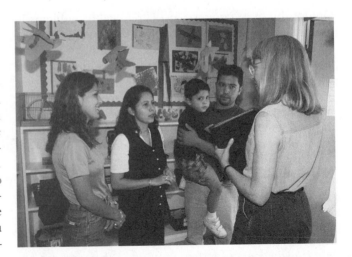

Cultural sensitivity and good communication skills will assist community health nurses in working with children and their families to help prevent child abuse and to protect the children in their care.

Figure 16-7 Children in Poverty

Low-income children are:

- Two times more likely than other children to die from accidents.
- Three times more likely to die from all causes combined.
- Four times more likely to die in fires.
- Five times more likely to die from infectious diseases and parasites.
- Six times more likely to die from other diseases.

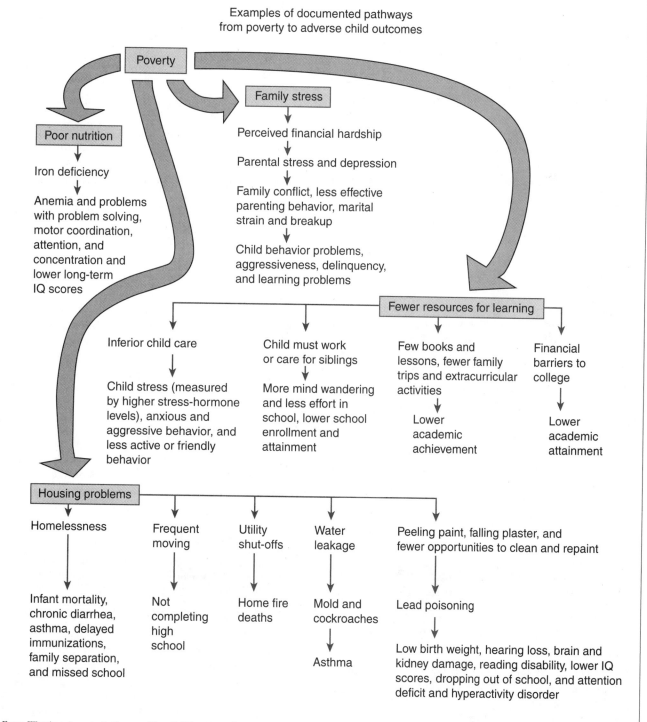

From Wasting America's Future: The Children's Defense Fund Report on the Costs of Child Poverty *by A. Sherman, 1994, Boston: Beacon. Used with permission of the Children's Defense Fund, Washington, DC.*

RESEARCH FOCUS

Managing Health Problems among Homeless Women with Children in a Transitional Shelter

METHODS

"To describe health problems among homeless women with children living in a transitional shelter, analyze how they managed various ailments, and when and how they sought care" (Hatton, 1997, p. 33) The number of families headed by single women with pre-school children is increasing and this population is expected to become the most of the homeless in the U.S. in the future. Transitional shelter is offered in most communities and single women with pre-schoolers are known to make the most frequent requests for shelter. There is little known about how single mothers in the U.S. manage health problems in these transitional shelters.

Thirty homeless women (28 with children and 2 who were pregnant) living in a shelter were given a semi-structured half-hour to two-hour interview, depending on the time the participant wished to talk to the interviewer. The shelter was considered *transitional* in nature, in that the women were involved in activities that would help them return to more conventional living situations. In the shelter, the women prepared food and cared for themselves and their children and attended school and/or rehabilitation programs during the day. In the beginning, the researchers audiotaped the interviews, but this practice was stopped after the participants reported that they did not want to be audiotaped because they were ashamed of those things they were sharing and were afraid to be audiotaped. After this point, note taking took the place of audiotaping. Grounded Theory analysis was applied; transcriptions and field notes were coded line by line and analyzed according to this method (Strauss & Corbin, 1994). As repeated areas of concern emerged during the course of the interviews, the questions were changed so that these specific areas of concern could be explored in depth.

FINDINGS

Major areas of concern that kept emerging were mental health problem management, sexually trans-

mitted diseases, and substance use. These mothers reported alcohol and other drug use, bipolar disorders, depression, suicidal behaviors, self-mutilation, and anxiety related to repeated physical and emotional abuse from male partners. The physical health of themselves and their children seemed to be of less concern and was essentially ignored.

Four conditions contributed to the reluctance of these women to seek help for health problems: shame, fear, lack of information, and lack of eligibility. The women reported a sense of shame linked to the presence of drug and alcohol abuse, sexually transmitted disease (STD), and psychiatric problems. They reported fear that they would be unable to retain custody of their children and that they would be locked up in a psychiatric facility and their children left with no one to care for them. They lacked information about basic preventive care such as the need for Pap tests for themselves and/or immunization for their children. Because they had not had prenatal care in their countries of origin, pregnant immigrant women did not consider prenatal care a priority. The aforementioned conditions plus a sense of futility created a situation in which these women felt that they had to overcome their health problems alone. The sense of futility stemmed from their past unsuccessful attempts to get help within the fragmented health care system. They did not seek preventive care and sought help only when they encountered emergencies.

IMPLICATIONS

Clinical nursing interventions for homeless mothers and children that take shame, fear, lack of information, and lack of eligibility for services into account could improve health outcomes among women and children living in transitional shelters.

SOURCE

From "Managing Health Problems among Homeless Women with Children in a Transitional Shelter" by D. C. Hatton, 1997, Image: Journal of Nursing Scholarship, 29(1), pp. 33–37.

Abuse and Neglect, 1995). Child abuse is increasing at all levels of U.S. society. Because they often see clients in the home, community health nurses are in an ideal position to detect abuse and neglect and to counsel and educate parents who are at risk for these behaviors.

Nurses and other health professionals are legally required to report suspected child abuse, both physical and sexual. Those who fail to do so are subject to possi-

ble fine or licensure loss. Many health care institutions and community-based agencies have specific procedures and guidelines for identifying and reporting child abuse. Community health nurses must be aware of such protocols. Abused children may suffer disproportionately from anger, noncompliance, low self-esteem, depression, and guilt. In addition, as adults they may abuse their own children or may have poor parenting skills.

Parenting Education

Parenting in and of itself is difficult enough; but coupled with multiple health problems, financial difficulties, and lack of education, parenting becomes an extraordinary challenge. Parenting education and skill building can have long-lasting positive effects on child and family health. Basic parenting education covers parenting roles, child develop-ment (infancy through adulthood), health promotion, nutri-tion, behavior modification, and stress management.

Through careful screening and assessment, the com-munity health nurse identifies parents or caregivers in need of improved parenting skills and helps them gain access to parenting-education resources. The nurse also works to reinforce positive parenting behaviors and mon-itors the development of parenting skills.

Figure 16-8 Positive Discipline Guidelines

- Misbehaving children are "discouraged children" who have mistaken ideas about ways to achieve their primary goal—to belong. Their mistaken ideas lead them to misbehavior. We cannot be effective unless we address the mistaken beliefs rather than just the misbehavior.

- Use encouragement to help children feel that they "belong" so that the motivation for misbehaving is eliminated. Celebrate each step in the direction of improvement rather than focusing on mistakes.

- A great way to help encourage children is to spend special time "being with them." Many teachers have noticed a dramatic change in "problem" children after spending five minutes simply sharing those things that they both like to do for fun.

- When tucking children into bed, ask them to share with you their "saddest time" and their "happiest time" of the day. Then share yours with them. You will be surprised what you learn.

- Have family meetings or class meetings to solve problems via cooperation and mutual respect. This is the key to creating a loving, respectful atmosphere while helping children develop self-discipline, responsibility, cooperation, and problem-solving skills.

- Give children meaningful jobs. In the name of expediency, many parents and teachers do things that children could do for themselves and for one another. Children feel that they belong when they know they can make a real contribution.

- Decide together those jobs that must be done. Put them all in a jar and let each child draw out a few each week; that way, no one is stuck with the same jobs all the time. Teachers can invite children to help them make class rules and list these rules on a chart titled "We decided." Children feel ownership, motivation, and enthusiasm when they are included in decisions.

- Take time for training. Make sure children understand what "clean the kitchen" means to you; to them, it may mean simply putting the dishes in the sink. Parents and teachers may ask, "What is your understanding of what is expected?"

- Punishment may "work" if all you are interested in is stopping misbehavior for the moment. Sometimes, we must beware of what works in the present when the long-range results are negative resentment, rebellion, revenge, or retreat.

- Teach and model mutual respect. One way is to be kind and firm at the same time: kind to show respect for the child, and firm to show respect for yourself and "the needs of the situation." This is difficult during conflict, so use the next guideline whenever you can.

- Proper timing will improve your effectiveness tenfold. It does not "work" to deal with a problem at the time of conflict: Emotions get in the way. Teach children about cooling-off periods. You (or the child) can go to a separate room and do something to make yourself feel better and then work on the problem via mutual respect.

- Abandon the crazy idea that in order to make children do better, you must first make them feel worse. Do you feel like doing better when you feel humiliated? This suggests a whole new approach to "time out." Tell children in advance that we all need time out sometimes when we are misbehaving, so when they are asked to go to their room or to a time-out area they can do something to make themselves feel better. "When you are ready, come back and we will work together on solutions."

- Use logical consequences when appropriate. Follow the Three Rs of Logical Consequences: ensure that consequences are (1) *r*elated, (2) *r*espectful, and (3) *r*easonable.

- During family or class meetings, allow children to help decide on logical consequences for not keeping their agreements. (Remember not to use the word *punishment*, which does not foster long-range "good" results.)

- Teach children that mistakes are wonderful opportunities to learn. A great way to do so is to model this yourself by using the Three Rs of Recovery after you have made a mistake: (1) *R*ecognize your mistake with good feelings, (2) *r*econcile by being willing to say "I'm sorry, I didn't like the way I handled that," and (3) *r*esolve by focusing on solutions rather than blame.

- Ensure that the message of love and respect gets through. Start with "I care about you. I am concerned about this situation. Will you work with me on a solution?"

- Have fun! Bring joy into homes and classrooms.

Parents often abuse their children in attempts to teach and discipline simply because they know no other way of approaching these tasks. Figure 16-8 offers some suggestions for positive approaches to the disciplining of children.

MAJOR ADOLESCENT HEALTH PROBLEMS

Beginning with the junior high school years, the adolescent period is characterized by dramatic physiological and psychosocial changes. Rapid body growth, changes in body appearance, and surging hormones create an often unpredictable mixture, difficult for parents and children alike. Adolescents make a shift from family orientation to peer-group orientation, seeking both independence from parents and opportunities to broaden their social horizons. This period is marked by an increasing sense of personal identity and progress in defining social roles, value systems, and life goals. Because adolescents tend to live in the present and with little thought of future consequences, risk-taking behaviors also increase during adolescence, particularly among males. Driving fast and/or under the influence of alcohol, experimenting with controlled substances, and engaging in unprotected sex are examples of potentially fatal risks that adolescents take.

Adolescence in late 20th-century America has become a minefield of problems waiting to explode. Today's adolescent is confronted by an epidemic of sexually transmitted diseases, the most deadly of which is HIV/AIDS, and a world grown increasingly more violent. Family violence, homicide, and suicide rates have skyrocketed in the past 20 years. Teenage pregnancy rates continue to climb as do the rates of teen suicide. The community health nurse who works with adolescent clients faces a difficult challenge in promoting health and preventing disease and injury in this troubled and troubling population.

The Youth Risk Behavior Surveillance System (YRBSS) monitors priority health-risk behaviors among youth and young adults: behaviors that contribute to unintentional and intentional injuries, tobacco use, alcohol and other drug use, sexual behaviors, unhealthy dietary behaviors, and physical inactivity. The YRBSS (CDC, 1996b) reports that 72% of all deaths among school-age youth and young adults result from four causes: motor vehicle crashes, other unintentional injuries, homicide, and suicide. A summary report of several national, state, and local surveys cited the following statistics related to health-risk behaviors known to increase the likelihood of death: 21.7% of adolescents had rarely or never used a safety belt; 38.8% had ridden with a driver who had consumed alcohol during the 30 days preceding the survey; 51.6% had consumed alcohol during the 30 days preceding the survey; 25.3% had used marijuana during the 30 days preceding the survey; and 8.7% had attempted suicide during the 12 months preceding the survey.

Substance Abuse: Tobacco, Alcohol, and Illicit Drugs

Data from several sources including federal agencies, private organizations, and published literature were reviewed, analyzed, and cross-validated by Sells and Blum (1996). These data addressed health behavior trends related to the use of tobacco, alcohol, and illicit drugs among high-school seniors from 1979 through 1994. Findings are summarized in the following paragraphs.

First-time tobacco use usually occurs prior to high-school graduation. Teens at highest risk are those who have low school achievement, friends who smoke, and low self-esteem. Although smoking in adults has decreased in recent years, adolescent use of tobacco has been increasing since 1992. The sale of tobacco to minors is prohibited in 48 states and the District of Columbia, yet most teen smokers reported buying their own cigarettes (Sells & Blum, 1996). Cigarette advertising aimed at adolescents and children has recently been banned.

Nearly all high-school seniors reported experience with alcohol. Daily consumption and intoxication was reported more often among males than females. African American seniors reported the lowest rates, and the consumption rate of all teens varied with region (Sells & Blum, 1996).

A survey conducted by the Institute for Social Research indicated that illicit drug use declined from 54% in 1979 to 27% in 1992 but then increased to 42% by 1997. The findings that illicit drug use started to rise (1997) is particularly discouraging in light of announcements made to the public beginning in 1992 of study results revealing the destructive effects of illicit drugs. Figure 16-9 illustrates the survey results (Institute of Social Research, 1997). On the whole, decreases in mortality and morbidity seemed consistent with attempts by society to encourage behavioral changes via educational efforts. Chapter 25 addresses substance abuse in greater detail.

Teen Pregnancy

Approximately 1.1 million girls between the ages of 15 and 19 become pregnant each year in the United States. Nearly half carry their pregnancies to term, resulting in more than one-half million live births each year. Another 57,000 pregnancies occur in girls under 15 years of age. Approximately one-fifth of the births in the United States are to adolescent mothers (U.S. Department of Commerce, 1993). One in 15 teenage males fathers a child (Hatcher, 1994). These alarming statistics represent children having children—teenagers becoming parents when they are physically, socially, emotionally, and financially unprepared.

Pregnant adolescents are at high risk for pregnancy-induced hypertension, iron deficiency anemia, preterm and low birth weight newborns, cephalopelvic disproportion, STD, and stillbirth. They also face the difficult developmental tasks of adolescence and pregnancy at the same time. The pregnant adolescent often lacks access to

Figure 16-9 Long-Term Trends in Annual Prevalence of Use of Various Drugs for Twelfth Graders (Based on Last 12 Months)

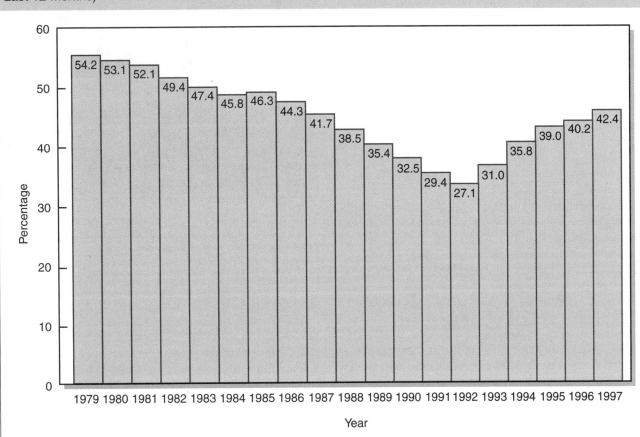

SOURCE: *The Monitoring the Future Project, at the Institute for Social Research, the University of Michigan, under Research Grant No. 3 RO1DA01411 from the National Institute on Drug Abuse. National Institute on Drug Abuse. Printed 1997.*

prenatal care and the support of family or the baby's father, increasing risks to her own physical and emotional health as well as to the health of the infant.

Adolescent mothers are at risk for many problems having long-term consequences. Although 70% do complete high school, teenage mothers are much less likely to attend college than are women who wait to become mothers in their twenties. Teenage mothers also have lower future incomes than do women who give birth in their twenties. In 1993, of the 3.8 million mothers who were welfare recipients, 55% had become mothers when they were teenagers (The Alan Guttmacher Institute, 1994).

Community health nurses play a crucial role in the prevention of teenage pregnancy via their work in school- and/or community-based pregnancy-prevention programs. Among those interventions that have proven effective in reducing pregnancy rates in such programs are counseling to delay sexual intercourse for sexually inactive teens and education and assistance to obtain contraceptive methods for those teens who are sexually active. Screening for teen pregnancy, counseling related to prenatal care, and referral to available resources are also part of the community health nurse's role. After the child is born, continued follow-up for health promotion, family

DECISION MAKING

Adolescent Developmental Needs and Pregnancy

You are a community health nurse working at a school-based community clinic serving families of children and adolescents. A 15-year-old Mexican American girl named Maria has been referred for follow-up after treatment for herpes. The referral indicates that she is sexually active and refuses contraception. Upon interview, Maria states that she wants a baby to love and to love her. Although she has a family, Maria states that she feels alone and is therefore trying to get pregnant. One of her former classmates brought her 6-month-old baby to a football game, prompting Maria to decide that she wanted a baby.

• What developmental needs are involved in this situation?

• How might you proceed with a plan of care for Maria and her family?

planning, and well-child care, including immunization, take on primary importance. Adolescent parents need the support of health professionals and access to social, educational, and vocational resources.

Sexually Transmitted Diseases

During adolescence, teens begin to explore sexual identity and gender roles and to experiment with sexual activity. Sexual identity encompasses identification with a specific gender orientation (male, female) and sexual orientation (i.e., heterosexual, homosexual, or bisexual). Gender role identity involves the identification of roles attributed to men and women. For instance, traditional roles for men are sports oriented and men are expected to be the family breadwinners, whereas women are expected to express feelings, to cry freely, and to nurture children. Gender role identification may be influenced by personal choice, society's definitions, and/or moral standards.

The proportion of young women who have sexual intercourse prior to age 18 has steadily risen from 35% in the 1970s to 56% in the late 1990s; the statistics for males are 55% in the 1970s and 73% in the late 1990s (Child Welfare League of America, 1997). The proportion of teens who are sexually active is 9% among 12-year-olds, 23% among 14-year-olds, 42% among 16-year-olds, and 71% among 18-year-olds (Child Welfare League of America, 1997).

Increased sexual activity among adolescents has led to dramatically increased rates of STD. Each year, between 2.5 and 3 million young people become infected with STD such as gonorrhea, syphilis, herpes, and chlamydia (CDC, 1990). Community health nurses play a critical role in providing screening, preventive education, counseling, and referral for STD. Sex education must be age appropriate and build on the premise that adolescents need to understand their own physiological and psychological development and the risks of unprotected sex. For example, teens need to understand that genital herpes infection is incurable and may affect a woman's ability to have a healthy baby. They also need to know that genital warts caused by the human papillomavirus (HPV) have been associated with cancers of the cervix, vagina, vulva, penis, and anus.

Human Immunodeficiency Virus and Acquired Immunodeficiency Syndrome

Infection with the human immunodeficiency virus, the virus associated with AIDS, is increasing among adolescents. Almost one-half of the 14 million people infected with HIV/AIDS worldwide acquired the infection between the ages of 15 and 24 years of age. The three largest studies of youth in the military, college health services, and the Job Corps report overall HIV infection rates of 1/1,000, 2/1,000, and 3/1,000, respectively (Weiss, 1993). In the mid-Atlantic region of the United States, HIV rates are highest among adolescents (Weiss, 1993). As in adults, the primary means of transmission are sexual activity and

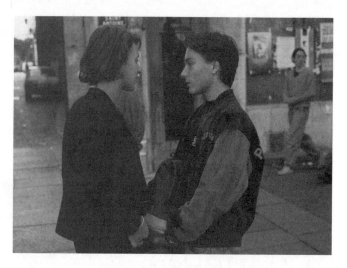

Educating adolescents about sexually transmitted diseases is critical. How might you handle this sensitive issue? Photo courtesy of Owen Franken/Corbis.

intravenous drug use. Many infected adolescents acquire HIV through heterosexual transmission. Among 13 to 19-year-old males, hemophilia/coagulation disorders and homosexual transmission represent the largest category of risk. Heterosexual transmission is the largest category of risk among adolescent girls who are 13 to 19 years of age (CDC, 1993). Because of the 7- to 9-year latency period between infection and the onset of AIDS-defining illnesses, many teenagers remain asymptomatic until they reach adulthood (Weiss, 1993). A higher percentage of infected teens are of African American, Latino, Asian, or Native American descent.

Adolescents need to understand the social, medical, psychological, and legal consequences of learning whether they are HIV negative or positive. Community health nurses who offer pretest counseling for adolescents must assess the client's developmental stage and individualize the counseling to the client's developmental needs. For example, the adolescent may be in denial, using magical thinking, or feeling invulnerable. Figure 16-10 lists some suggested elements of pretest HIV counseling for adolescents. Because some states require specialized training for HIV pretest counseling, it is important to contact the local or state health department about protocols and policies (Moon, 1995).

Teenagers who are HIV positive provide many legal and ethical challenges. Consent for HIV testing and treatment, limited access to clinical trials, and disclosure of HIV status are all legal issues that confront infected teens, their parents, and health care providers. Laws vary from state to state. Laws related to confidentiality of medical information may not extend to minors, depending on whether the condition presents imminent danger to the young person or others. Treatment may or may not require parental involvement.

Care of the HIV-positive teen involves comprehensive social and medical histories, physical examination, and laboratory tests. The nurse also must follow up with the adolescent who is HIV positive concerning signs and

Figure 16-10 Elements of Pretest HIV Counseling for Adolescents

- Establish rapport.
- Ensure confidentiality.
- Assess developmental stage.
- Conduct risk assessment.
- Discuss the meaning and implications of the HIV test.
- Conduct a risk/benefit analysis.
- Investigate the adolescent's coping history and develop future strategies.
- Forecast and role-play possible reactions to a positive test result.
- Forecast and role-play possible reactions to a negative test result.
- Discuss the waiting period.
- Investigate and help develop the adolescent's support systems.
- Discuss notifying partners.
- Discuss confidentiality and determine the adolescent's capacity to consent.
- Assist in reading and signing the consent form.

From HIV/AIDS: A Guide to Nursing Care (3rd ed., p. 233) by J. Flaskerud & P. J. Ungvarski, 1995, Philadelphia: W. B. Saunders. Used with permission of W. B. Saunders.

symptoms of HIV-related diseases, types of immunizations given, laboratory values, contraceptive practices, liver function, anemia, and medication regimens (Futterman & Hein, 1992). The nurse also must be aware of community resources and agency policies targeting this population.

To help control the spread of HIV/AIDS, community health nurses must understand adolescent development and potential barriers to care. Nurses can participate in community health fairs and school health programs offering HIV/AIDS education that targets teens. Lewis, Battisich, and Schaps (1990) suggest that an effective school-based prevention program should be:

- Clearly derived from theories that recognize the multidimensionality of risk behaviors
- Directed at influencing the general social milieu of the school, not as a separate entity but as an integral part of school life
- Focused on promoting positive influences on social development rather than counteracting negative social norms
- Comprehensive and long lasting, because socialization is a continuous process
- Incorporated into the overall mission of the school to produce a widespread and enduring effect
- Implemented early enough to precede the emergence of problem behavior, because it is harder to change established attitudes and behaviors than to prevent their initial formation

- Monitored and evaluated carefully to ensure that implementation reflects planning

Teens themselves are asking for better AIDS education—straight answers about AIDS and ways to protect themselves. The National Youth Summit on HIV Prevention held in 1995 brought teens together with federal health officials and politicians to discuss preventive measures. Politicians admitted that adults find it difficult to talk about intercourse, much less AIDS.

Non-AIDS Sexually Transmitted Diseases

Department of Health and Human Services (USDHHS, 1997) reports address concern that the intense and important national and international attention focused on HIV/AIDS during the 1980s diminished the emphasis on non-AIDS STD. Partially as a result of this decreased emphasis, rates of non-AIDS STD have soared. Adolescents (10 to 19 years of age) and young adults (20 to 24 years of age) are at a higher risk for acquiring STD for a number of reasons: They may be more likely to have multiple (sequential or concurrent) sexual partners rather than a single, long-term relationship; they may be more likely to engage in unprotected intercourse; and they may select partners who themselves are at higher risk. In addition, for some STDs such as *Chlamydia trachomatis*, adolescent women may have a physiologically increased susceptibility to infection. Age of initiation of sexual activity has steadily decreased, and age at first marriage has increased, resulting in increases in premarital sexual experience among adolescent women and in an enlarging pool of young women at risk. In addition, the higher prevalence of STDs among adolescents reflects multiple barriers to quality STD prevention services: for example, lack of insurance or other ability to pay, lack of transportation, discomfort with facilities and services designed for adults, and concerns about confidentiality.

Studies of various clinic populations have shown that sexually active adolescents have high rates of chlamydial infection and gonorrhea, with female adolescents generally having the highest rates of chlamydia. The rate of gonorrhea in males, however, decreased 36% during 1993–1996.

Although caused by a variety of organisms, STDs have at least four characteristics in common (Lemone & Burke, 1996):

- Most can be prevented via use of latex condoms.
- Transmission can occur during heterosexual and homosexual activities.
- Effective treatment requires treatment of sexual partners as well as of the infected person.
- Two or more often coexist in the same person.

Community health nurses play a key role in the prevention of STD by educating adolescents about these diseases, including prevention, treatment, and potential lifelong or life-threatening complications.

Violence

Adolescents in the United States are coming of age in an increasingly violent society. Homicide, suicide, rape, assault, and domestic and international terrorism are standard fare on the evening news, in movies, and on television programs. Far too many adolescents have grown up in violent family environments. In such environments, adolescents learn that violence is a way to resolve conflict. As they seek independence from parents and search for their own identities, adolescents imitate that which they have learned: in this case, that violence is a way to get what you want when you want it. Easy access to guns has made violence increasingly deadly.

Violent crime among adolescents is increasing in the United States. According to the Criminal Justice Institute, of the 100,000 juveniles who were incarcerated as of January 1, 1994, approximately one-fourth had committed crimes against other persons. Violence among adolescents is also increasingly related to gang involvement. Although around from the beginning of society, gangs have recently received widespread attention because of the violent behavior often associated with gang involvement. Gangs, whether they be violent or nonviolent, satisfy a number of normal needs for adolescents. One such need is that for peer approval and acceptance. Gangs also provide adolescents with an emotional base, rituals and rewards, and, in some cases, a replacement for family. Violent acts committed by gangs and individual gang members may reflect enactment of gang rituals, retaliation for violent acts performed by other gangs or community members, and the need for acceptance by members of the gang to which the adolescent belongs (Earls, 1994).

The community health nurse must be aware of the many risk factors associated with youth violence, including neighborhood environment, school-related problems, peer network, family, and individual and familial psychological and physical problems. In addition, knowledge of available resources and ways to help deal with the problems of violence are critical in adolescent health care.

Teen Homicide

The drop in the accidental teen death rate has been offset by an increase in death by homicide among this group (National Center for Health Statistics, 1994). In 1995, 21% of all deaths among youth and young adults (ages 5 to 24) were due to homicide (CDC, 1996b). Between 1985 and 1994, the greatest increase was among African American teen males (ages 15 to 19): The homicide rate among this group jumped from 46.4 deaths per 100,000 teens in 1985 to 128.5 deaths per 100,000 teens in 1992 (USDHHS, 1996b).

The increase in death by homicide among teens seems to be linked to the increased use of firearms and the increased reliance on weapons by teens. In 1995, as part of the YRBSS, the CDC conducted a national school-based Youth Risk Behavior Survey among a representative sample of 10,904 high-school students in grades 9–12. The data from that survey indicated that 20.0% of those interviewed had carried a weapon such as a gun, knife, or club during the 30 days preceding the survey. On average 7.6% reported carrying guns, but African American (10.6%) and Hispanic (10.5%) students were significantly more likely than Caucasian students (6.2%) to have carried a gun. Male students (12.3%) were more likely to have carried guns than were females (2.5%), and students in grades 9 (22.6%) and 10 (21.1%) were more apt to have carried weapons than were students in grade 12 (16.1%) (CDC, 1996c).

The 1995 survey also indicated that 51.6% of teens had used alcohol and 25.3% had used marijuana during the 30 days preceding the survey (CDC, 1996c). Having guns or weapons available while under the influence of alcohol and/or drugs presents a grave danger to adolescents and those around them. In the United States, a powerful lobby against gun control exists, and gun control is seen by some as an infringement on individual rights protected by the Constitution. Efforts to protect citizens from guns via legislation and gun control measures have been met with resistance and opposition. In 1997, legislation supported by the National Rifle Association and enacted by Congress barred the CDC from using funds to advocate or promote gun control. The CDC's stated position, however, is that the collection of data on firearms injuries neither advocates nor promotes gun control, and the agency intends to continue to conduct and publicize research on firearms (Children's Defense Fund, 1996b).

Teen Suicide

The suicide rate among adolescents exceeds the rate of homicide among this group. Each year, more than 6,000 adolescents take their own lives. Suicide rates among children and adolescents tripled between 1960 and 1990 (Koop, 1992). Rates are highest among 15- to 19-year-old males, although females in this age group attempt suicide more often. Primary risk factors include low self-esteem, chronic depression, incest, and extrafamilial sexual and physical abuse (Eggert, 1994). Other risk factors may include isolation, family crises, poor school performance or other behavioral problems, and obsession with death and dying.

The community health nurse must be able to recognize the potentially suicidal adolescent, provide emergency counseling, and make referrals to appropriate resources. Peer counseling, often as part of a school suicide-prevention program, may be helpful for some adolescents. Many programs include a peer-counseling hot line. Figure 16-11 summarizes clinical manifestations of suicidal youth. Additional information is available from the American Association of Suicidology, 2459 Ash, Denver, CO 80222, (303) 692-0985. See Chapter 23 for more information on suicide and suicide prevention and Chapter 24 for further discussion of family and community violence.

Figure 16-11 Clinical Manifestations of Suicidal Youth

Mood/Affect

Marked, persistent depression

Feelings of hopelessness, helplessness, isolation

Deteriorating schoolwork

Consistently distant, sad, remote demeanor

Flat affect ("frozen" facial expression)

Persistently sad and unhappy tone of voice

Description of self as worthless

Feelings of self-hatred or excessive guilt

Feelings of humiliation, often brought on by inadequate performance at school

Sudden cheerfulness following deep depression*

Wish to be punished

Behavior

Changes in physical appearance (e.g., a previously neat and well-groomed child stops bathing and begins to look slovenly)

Loss of function due to illness or trauma

Loss of energy (loss of interest, listlessness, exhaustion without obvious cause)

Sleep disturbances (difficulty going to sleep, excessive sleep, voluntary napping during afternoon or evening)

Increased irritability, argumentativeness, or stubbornness

Physical complaints (recurrent stomachaches, headaches)

Repeated visits to doctor's office or emergency room for treatment of injuries

Antisocial behavior (drinking, drug use, fighting, vandalism, running away from home, sexual promiscuity)

Preoccupation with death (a focus on morbid thoughts; repeated mention of people getting killed*)

Possible references to own death

School and Interpersonal Relationships

Resistance or refusal to go to school

Truancy, class cutting; failure to complete assignments

Social withdrawal from friends, activities, interests that were previously enjoyed

Desire to give away cherished possessions*

Lack of an effective social support system

Coping Skills

Loss of reality boundaries

Withdrawal and isolation of self

No use of support system

View of self as totally helpless, a victim of fate

*Absolute "red flag," or danger signal

From Essentials of Pediatric Nursing 5th ed. by D. Wong, 1997, St. Louis, MO: Mosby-Yearbook. Used with permission from Mosby-Yearbook Inc.

Parent–Adolescent Relationships

Because the child is moving toward adulthood, making more decisions, depending more on peers for support, and seeking to find an individual identity separate from parents and family, adolescent years are often difficult for both teens and parents. The parent–teen bond continues to be critical during these years, however, and is much less difficult for both teens and parents when communication is maintained. Listening is a skill that has major importance for parents during this period. Figure 16-12 provides some tips that may be useful for parenting education during these years.

IMPLICATIONS FOR COMMUNITY HEALTH NURSING PRACTICE

It is imperative that nurses work in partnership with all segments of society to deal with the problems of aggregates as well as of individuals. Aggregate nursing requires community assessment, planning, and intervention as well

as activism and leadership in social and political arenas. Yet, among their variety of roles (see Chapter 14), community health nurses are the major primary health care providers for maternal–child and adolescent care. Careful monitoring and support during these periods of rapid growth and development are essential. During these most vulnerable periods of life, nurses have great opportunities to improve lifelong health. The accompanying perspectives box, written by a public health nurse serving children and families, demonstrates the need for advocacy.

Assessment and Diagnosis

Knowledge of normal growth and development from conception to adulthood is the basis for nursing assessment. Physical examinations, weights and measures, and thorough health histories serve as indicators of health status and give clues to areas of concern. The health history and the child's responses during the examination provide more clues. Close attention is paid to psychosocial factors such as parental expectations of the child, impaired attachment, previous history of abuse or neglect, family violence, and homelessness.

Figure 16-12   Fourteen Tips for Parents of Teens

1. **Let teens know you are willing to just plain listen** to their ideas without making judgments. Talking is a way they think things out.

2. **Be accessible.** Teens often blurt things out or want to talk at strange or inconvenient times. Be ready to listen anytime, anywhere.

3. **Use questions sparingly.** Resist the urge to know *everything* your teen is thinking or planning. Show some trust; you would expect the same.

4. **Try not to be defensive.** When they make generalizations or critical remarks, do not take them personally but as opportunities for discussion.

5. **Give straightforward advice or feedback on important issues** such as sex, drinking, and drugs, but do not keep repeating it. They need to hear you, and they do hear you, even if they pretend indifference.

6. **Talk about yourself sometimes instead of the teen.** They hate to be the only topic under discussion. Tell them about your own teen memories and mistakes.

7. **Set up and use family meetings to full advantage.** Get input from each person on rules, curfews, and the like, as well as on the consequences of breaking rules. Sign agreements, try them out, and modify them as needed.

8. **Show intimacy.** Teens are still kids inside; they need the warm feelings of belonging that come from good touches and hugs.

9. **Give lots of praise and positive feedback.** Teens need to hear the "good stuff," just like the rest of us. They need to know you love them for who they are inside, as well as what they can do.

10. **Give them responsibilities with every privilege:** that is real life.

11. **Teach them to make decisions,** and make them accept the consequences of each choice they make.

12. **Teach them to deal with information.** Teach them to think critically about those things they see or hear, as well as ways to sort out and prioritize information.

13. **Take time to relax and have fun.** Teens need to learn positive ways to manage stress; enjoying each other will build lifetime relationships.

14. **Make them earn what they want,** and teach them the difference between wants and needs. Instant gratification does not teach life skills.

From Evelyn Petersen, 1995. Reprinted with permission from The National Parenting Center—www.tnpa.com. Evelyn Petersen's nationally syndicated parenting column is carried in over 200 newspapers twice each week. As a family/parenting consultant, early childhood educator, Head Start consultant, and host of a series of parent training audio and video tapes, Ms. Petersen employs an approach of providing hands-on, nuts and bolts advice to parents across the country. You can read more from Evelyn at her web site: http://www.askevelyn.com

Developmental assessment tools are useful in screening for developmental delays and helping to assess progress. The most common tool used by community health nurses is the Denver II, which screens for delayed gross and fine motor skills, adaptive language, and personal/social skills in children from birth to 6 years of age. Developmental assessment tools also serve as useful guides for teaching parents those things that a child may be ready to learn but is not yet able to do. A variety of developmental assessment tools are available for infants and preschoolers.

Assessment of family developmental processes and the interrelationship of the child/adolescent and the family is also necessary. Family developmental processes are addressed in Chapters 18 and 19 and provide the context for individual development of the child. A family torn by abusive behavior, alcoholism, drug addiction, or poverty cannot provide an environment where children can reach their developmental potential.

School performance is a crucial aspect of school-age child health and is part of the assessment. If the child is performing poorly academically, further assessment is needed to determine the problem. Testing for vision, hearing, cognitive functioning, and learning disabilities; follow-up medical examinations; and psychological and psychiatric evaluation and testing may be indicated. Poor nutrition and lack of sleep may be overlooked in the search for a cause of poor school performance. Sometimes, children are unable to perform academically and suffer because they are overwhelmed by something that is easily solved.

Assessment of the family–community relationship is also essential because this aspect is critical to the child's growth and development. Family–community relationship determines many factors such as whether the child has health care insurance, transportation services, encouragement and positive support at school, access to churches and other community groups, access to recreational facilities, and the like.

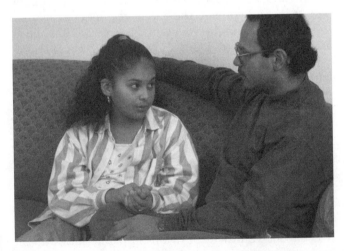

Effective communication between parents and their children is key—and often difficult to achieve. Photo courtesy of Laura Dwight/Corbis.

Perspectives...

Insights of a Public Health Nurse

I work as a public health nurse for a large county health department serving poor children and their families. One of the most important things I do is serve as an advocate. Advocacy has become even more important recently because families do not know how or are not able to navigate the health care system and need someone who can help with the managed care process. Because there are so many problems in the changing system, families often need an advocate to help them get needed services. Agents of vendoring services often do not tell clients about available services, and the nurse has to seek out the information for families.

Being an advocate for my clients is so very important. A non-English-speaking family was referred to me because the physician wanted to remove an 8-year-old daughter from the family home. The girl had cystic fibrosis, and failure to thrive had been an issue. The physician was accusing the parents of not giving the child her nighttime feedings containing medication and nutrition. The social worker from Child Protective Services and I made a home visit and found everything in place for the feedings. The mother showed me her equipment and supplies, demonstrated how she gave the feedings, and showed me the records. There was no problem, and the child seemed to be doing very well.

I made an appointment with the mother and child and went with them to see the physician. Everything checked out fine, and the child had gained weight. A resident physician who spoke Spanish saw the child and was very kind to the mother. But the primary physician came into the room after the resident physician had left and continued to insist that the child was not being fed and must be removed from the home. The mother cried all the way home, and I could not comfort her very well because I do not speak Spanish.

I checked out the medical records and talked with people to put the story together. A note posted to the medical record by a physician indicated that the child needed night feeds but that the physician assumed the vendoring agency would not approve because of the cost. As a result, the night feeds had not even been requested! The child had eventually been hospitalized due to weight loss but gained back the weight while in the hospital. Because the child had gained weight during the hospital stay, the physician assumed the child was not getting the night feeds because of negligence on the part of the mother. After the confusion had been cleared up, the physician decided against removing the child from her home, and she is doing well. I am really glad we were there for her and for her family. The language barrier makes things even harder.

I see a lot of children in foster homes who are really suffering. These children *really* need advocates. Because the licensing agencies are not allowed to make unannounced visits to these homes, I have to be their ears and eyes when I make home visits. Probably about half of the foster parents care about the children and are doing a good job. But the other half do not care at all and are just doing foster care for the money: The kids are a commodity. They were probably better off with their biological parents. We need an organization of health care workers just to be advocates for the foster kids in this county.

—Paula, RN, PHN

Nursing diagnoses related to child health problems are based on careful, thorough nursing assessment and focus on physical and/or psychosocial factors. Examples of NANDA nursing diagnoses include: *Altered nutrition: less (or more)* *than body requirements due to disorganized infant behavior*, and *Risk for altered parent/family/child attachment*.

Planning and Intervention

Planning is done with the child and/or the family. In a situation where a child needs help in learning to use his combination lock, for example, planning and intervention could be done with the child alone. More complex matters, however, require total family involvement. There

COMMUNITY NURSING VIEW

A referral is sent to the public health clinic requesting a public health nursing follow-up visit for a 17-year-old Korean parent of a 2-month-old infant. The teen mother is monolingual and resides with distant relatives.

The community health nurse brings a translator on the home visit. A family assessment is conducted and yields the following information:

- Family strengths are that the mother has support from distant relatives; the mother and infant are bonding well; and the mother is highly motivated to learn how to care for the infant.
- Areas of concern are that the infant has not gained weight since birth; the infant is breastfeeding only three times per day; the mother has only a sixth-grade education; and the father of the baby is not in the household.

Nursing Considerations

ASSESSMENT
- How would you obtain the information needed for a family assessment in this situation?

DIAGNOSIS
- What nursing diagnoses would be made for the infant? For the mother?

OUTCOME IDENTIFICATION
- What outcomes would be evidenced for the infant? For the mother?

PLANNING/INTERVENTIONS
- What nursing interventions would be appropriate? Who would you involve in the interventions? What referrals would you make?

EVALUATION
- How would you monitor and evaluate the results of your interventions?

may be a need for teaching or counseling, and the planning for these interventions should be done with the family. There may be a need for referral to community resources or for advocacy on the part of the nurse. In such cases, the family and the nurse together plan that which is to be done and by whom. It is critical that family members be involved in assessment, planning, intervention, and evaluation processes. Other community work may need to be done through social or political action to provide a healthy environment for families and children.

The nursing process is applied in the care of children at all levels of society. First, the nurse can help children within their individual developmental abilities—no more and no less. Second, the nurse can work with the family of the child within the family's developmental ability—by teaching, supporting, or serving as advocate. Third, the nurse can apply the same principles and work with the community to serve the aggregate of children represented by a particular child that happens to be in the caseload.

Evaluation

Evaluation of outcomes for child and adolescent clients must be a part of the planning and the ongoing reassessment. Evaluation of growth is done by weighing and measuring and by keeping track on growth charts. Evaluation of developmental progress is done via use of tools such as the Denver II or other tools considered

appropriate for the situation during the first 6 years of life. School progress is an important evaluative measure during the school-age and adolescent years. Behavior is a strong indicator of the child's well-being and self-esteem.

Key Concepts

- While improving in certain areas because of medical advances, child health in the United States is deteriorating in other areas because of social and environmental health problems such as poverty and violence.
- Knowledge of those developmental processes associated with the early years of life provides the foundation for identification of health risk factors and health assessment.
- Prenatal care involves careful teaching, guidance, and support of the mother as the fetus experiences this critical period of life.
- The aggregate health status of infants and children is determined statistically by keeping records of infant mortality rate, low birth weight, and immunization. Growth and development measurements serve as indicators of nutritional need and environmental health needs.
- Major health needs of children today are related to family and community environment, challenging

community health nurses to address environmental issues in the home and community.

- Major health needs of adolescents in the United States are associated with health risk behavior in the areas of sex, violence, and substance abuse.

- Community health nurses apply the nursing process using developmental theory as the basis for understanding, as principles are applied to work with individual children, families, communities, and governments.

Care of Young, Middle, and Older Adults

Judy J. Miller, BSN, MSN

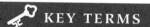 **KEY TERMS**

ageism
crystallized intelligence
ego integrity versus
    despair
empty nest syndrome
era
fluid intelligence
generation gap
generativity versus
    stagnation
homogenize
inner aspect of aging
intimacy versus isolation
male climacteric
maturity
menopause
midlife crisis
outer (or social) aspect
    of aging
presbycusis
presbyopia
sandwich generation
structure building
transition

"Life's Rainbow"
Beginnings are lacquer red
    fired hard in the kiln
    of hot hope;
Middles, copper yellow
    in sunshine,
    Sometimes oxidize green
    with tears; but
Endings are always indigo
    before we step
    on the other shore.

—Banani, 1987, p. 181

COMPETENCIES

Upon completion of this chapter, the reader should be able to:

- Discuss growth and development theories for the adult years.
- Describe the stages of adult life and tasks to be accomplished in young, middle, and older adulthood.
- Identify the risk factors and conditions most prevalent in each adult stage of life, in terms of emotional, mental, physical, spiritual, and social impact.
- Detail the relationships necessary for healthy existence in each stage of adulthood.
- Describe the nursing process as it applies to each stage of development in adult life.

The adult years have long been viewed as a stable, nonchanging period of life. Today, however, growth and development are recognized as lifelong processes. The adult years can be as exciting and full of change as are the years from birth through adolescence.

Nurses have always been aware of the developmental stages of the clients to whom they provide care. At all levels of nursing education, a common objective on evaluation forms is related to whether nursing care was appropriate to the developmental stage of the client. The nurse must understand common theories of growth and development in order to determine whether the client is exhibiting behavioral patterns appropriate for the client's given stage of life.

This chapter discusses growth and development of the adult as the basis for assessment, planning, intervention, and evaluation with regard to clients. Just as nursing itself is based on a strong commitment to caring, the nursing process is based on caring (Anglin, 1994). This chapter begins with a review of some of the growth and develop-

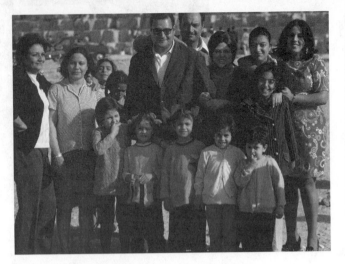

The community health nurse must remember to deliver nursing care appropriate to the developmental stage of the client. Photo courtesy of Nik Wheeler/Corbis.

ment theories for young, middle, and older adults. It examines some of the risk factors and conditions prevalent at each stage of adulthood. The discussion includes consideration of healthy environments as well as healthy relationships with self, partner, family, friends, and neighbors.

THEORIES OF GROWTH AND DEVELOPMENT

Theories about growth and development have been around for many years. Most of them concentrate on those years between infancy and adolescence. One theorist, Daniel Levinson, claims that the study of adult development is just beginning. He has concentrated on the adult years and determined a series of **eras** (periods or stages of development) and **transitions** (periods of approximately five years during which the adult is moving to the next era) through which the adult progresses (Levinson, 1978).

Erik Erikson's theory of development as a series of potential crises also covers the adult years. His stages of life are related to resolution of crises related in some way to the environment (Erikson, 1963). Tables 17-1 and 17-2 outline developmental stages as envisioned by Levinson and Erikson, respectively.

Because Erikson and Levinson devoted more time to adult development than did other theorists, their theories are more applicable to this chapter. The stages of adult life discussed in this chapter are young adult, ages 20 to 40 years; middle adult, ages 40 to 65 years; and older adult, age 65 years to death. Because human development is not always a linear process, such arbitrary divisions based on chronological age are not always the best way to view adult development. It must also be kept in mind that with the increasing numbers of older adults, especially adults over 80 years of age, an additional developmental stage of old-old adulthood may be necessary. There have already been further definitions of old age as young-old (ages 60 to 74 years), middle-old (ages 75 to 84 years), and old-old (ages 85 years and older) (Smith & Smith, 1990, p. 465).

DEVELOPMENTAL STAGES AND TASKS OF ADULTHOOD

Like the years of childhood and adolescence, the adult years have definite developmental stages. In recent years,

Table 17-1 Levinson's Developmental Stages of Adulthood

AGE	SEASON (PHASE)	CHARACTERISTICS
18–20 years	Early adult transition	Seeks independence by separating from family
21–27 years	Entrance into the adult world	Experiments with different careers and lifestyles
28–32 years	Transition	Makes lifestyle adjustments
33–39 years	Settling down	Experiences greater stability
45–65 years	Pay-off years	Is self-directed and engages in self-evaluation

From The Seasons of a Man's Life *by D. Levinson, 1978, New York: Knopf. Used with permission.*

REFLECTIVE THINKING

Gender and Adult Developmental Processes

Many developmental theorists have completed their research using only male subjects.

- How do you think growth and development are different for men and women?

- What changes might occur in adult development of women as society moves toward a position of gender equality?

more emphasis has been placed on lowering the death rate among young and middle adults and lowering the number of days of restricted activity among older adults (U.S. Department of Health and Human Services [USDHHS], 1990). These objectives are part of the goals of the

Office of Disease Prevention and Health Promotion. Policymakers and citizens are looking at each developmental stage and setting priorities for achieving optimal functioning at each level. The nurse, as a member of the health care team, must be familiar with each stage of adult development to promote appropriate healthful behaviors.

Young Adult

The young-adult stage may be the most dramatic of the adult years. These are the years of growing independence and freedom from parental guidance. Most formal education is finished. Some tasks of this life stage include establishing a career, entering into a close relationship and forming a family unit, making friends and taking part in a social group, beginning to take on social responsibilities, perhaps becoming a parent, and, finally, arriving at some philosophical view of life (Sims, D'Amico, Stiesmeyer, &

Table 17-2 Erikson's Stages of Psychosocial Development

STAGE	AGE	TASK TO BE ACHIEVED	IMPLICATIONS
Trust vs. mistrust	Birth–18 months	To develop a sense of trust in others	Consistent, affectionate care promotes successful mastery.
Autonomy vs. shame and doubt	18 months–3 years	To learn self-control	The child needs support, praise, and encouragement to use newly acquired skills of independence. Shaming or insulting the child will lead to unnecessary dependence.
Initiative vs. guilt	3–6 years	To initiate spontaneous activities	Give clear explanations for events and encourage creative activities. Threatening punishment or labeling behavior as "bad" leads to development of guilt and fears of doing wrong.
Industry vs. inferiority	6–12 years	To develop necessary social skills	To build confidence, recognize the child's accomplishments. Unrealistic expectation or excessively harsh criticism leads to a sense of inadequacy.
Identity vs. role diffusion	12–20 years	To integrate childhood experiences into a personal identity	Help the adolescent make decisions. Encourage active participation in home events. Assist with planning for the future.
Intimacy vs. isolation	18–25 years	To develop commitments to others and to a life work (career)	Teach the young adult to establish realistic goals. Avoid ridiculing romances or job choices.
Generativity vs. stagnation	21–45 years	To establish a family and become productive	Provide emotional support. Recognize individual accomplishments and provide appropriate praise.
Integrity vs. despair	45+ years	To view one's life as meaningful and fulfilling	Explore positive aspects of one's life. Review contributions made by the individual.

From Childhood and Society *by E. Erickson, 1968, New York: Norton; and* Psychiatric and Mental Health Nursing Certification *by N. Randolph, 1993, Springfield, PA: Springfield. Used with permission.*

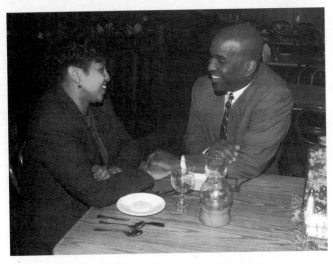

Some of the tasks of the young adulthood stage include establishing a career, beginning to take on social responsibilities, and entering a close relationship. Photo courtesy of Tom Stock.

Webster, 1995). Figure 17-1 lists developmental tasks of young adulthood.

Physical Development

Physically, the young adult is at the peak of efficiency in terms of muscle tone and coordination and has a high energy level. Growth is finished at this stage, and attention

---

Figure 17-1 Developmental Tasks of Young Adulthood

Self

- Stabilize self-concept
- Accept body image
- Formulate philosophy of life
- Establish own residence
- Achieve economic independence

Vocation/Profession

- Attain personal satisfaction
- Achieve economic stability
- Manage time schedule and job stress

Relationships

- Learn to love responsibly
- Establish intimate bonding
- Form congenial social groups
- Become involved with community

Adapted from Health Assessment in Nursing *by L. K. Sims, D. D'Amico, J. K. Steismeyer, & J. A. Webster, 1995, Redwood City, CA: Addison-Wesley.*

---

must be paid to nutritional needs. If a sedentary lifestyle is adopted, some caloric adjustment is necessary to avoid weight gain. All systems have matured, including the neurological system, which matures at around 30 years of age (Murray & Zentner, 1997). Although visual and auditory sensory perceptions are at a peak, the lens of the eye is already losing its elasticity, and close vision is becoming more difficult. Sexual maturity has been achieved, sex drive remains high, and females are well equipped for childbearing, having fully mature female organs.

Cognitive Development

Cognitive functioning of the young adult is more advanced than during adolescence. The young adult uses systematic and sophisticated problem-solving techniques and achieves new levels of creative thought with less egocentrism than is seen in younger individuals. Thinking is more reality based, and mental activities are proficient (Lefrancois, 1996). Although most formal education is complete at this time, job training, military education, or continuing education are often a part of life. Education is usually directed toward employment, an important part of the young adult's identity. Performing meaningful, rewarding work produces feelings of worth and accomplishment in the young adult.

Psychosocial Development

Psychosocially, young adulthood is a time of maturing. Erikson (1963) details the crisis as **intimacy versus isolation**. Identity was established in adolescence, and the urge now is to seek love and commitment in a close relationship. To cope with the demands of adult relationships, the individual needs a considerable degree of **maturity**. Developmentally, maturity is a relative state—a state of complete growth or development. Levinson (1986) calls this period **structure building**, when a lifestyle is fashioned. The transition period is one during which the lifestyle is evaluated and modified. This first lifestyle links the individual to adult society, and conflicts may develop when the individual later balances the exploration of new possibilities and options with the need for stability. In the later years of young adulthood, settling down becomes the main issue. Often, the decision to have children is made during this stage, necessitating another adjustment period as new parenting roles are learned and internalized.

Young-Adult Risk Factors

While living in general holds many risks to human life and health, there are risk factors more or less specific to each life stage. These risks can be emotional, mental, physical, spiritual, or social in nature.

A major consideration in looking at risk factors is cultural background. The ways that an individual reacts to the changes associated with each life stage are direct

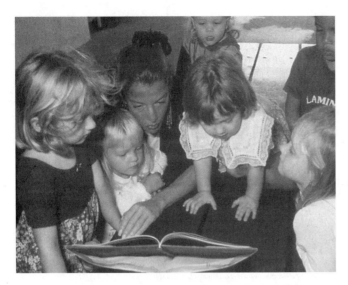

This young adult is beginning her career as a teacher. Establishing a career is an important part of young adulthood.

results of cultural variations in upbringing. For example, self-sufficiency is a highly valued trait among the Japanese—a trait that results in the absence of emotional display. Nonverbal communication and facial expression in a Japanese person may not convey serious concerns about life issues (Ebersole & Hess, 1994). A common problem when dealing with ethnic minorities is lumping them into general groups. For example, although Asians as a group may share some characteristics, there are widely diverse Asian subgroups that have very little in common and, in fact, may conflict with each other because of historical events (Ebersole & Hess, 1994).

Substance Abuse

Young adulthood is a time of major life decisions and life planning. The rigors of career choice, educational opportunities, choice of a mate for life, and decisions about childbearing and child-rearing exert considerable stress during this life stage. Rapid, continual advancements in technology and science also contribute to feelings of pressure and inadequacy. A common reaction to the stress of daily life is the use and possibly the eventual abuse of drugs or alcohol. Many young adults have learned to use alcohol to cope with problems or frustration (Milgram, 1993). Cocaine and methamphetamines have become drugs of choice for young adults and are often considered by this population to be harmless recreational drugs. Alcohol is seen as a means of relaxation, and addiction to this common substance is often not recognized until well advanced. Binge drinking, having five or more drinks on one occasion in one month, is reported in 15% of young adults over the age of 18 (DeBuono, 1996).

The use of tobacco, an addictive drug, causes disease and death. The prevalence of cigarette smoking among adults in New York State was 21% in 1994, a rate that has not changed during the 1990s (DeBuono, 1996).

The pressures of the young adult years can also result in problems with self-esteem and self-image. Low regard for self often results in eating disorders. The nurse can identify these inappropriate reactions to stress by conducting a nutritional assessment, a thorough physical examination, and a health history that includes questions about drug, alcohol, and tobacco use.

Suicide

Another reaction to life stress is depression and thoughts of suicide. Suicide is the fourth overall cause of death in young adults in the United States (USDHHS, 1990). The nurse's role in dealing with the risk of suicide in young adults includes both educating the public to the needs of young adults and identifying those at risk. The nurse can also encourage participation in groups as well as express caring concern for the client.

Sexuality

Young adulthood is the time when sexuality reaches its peak. Varieties of sexual patterns are prevalent among young adults, ranging from heterosexuality to bisexuality to homosexuality to masturbation to abstinence (Murray & Zentner, 1997). The individual's reaction to earlier sex education and sexual experience can dictate whether a rewarding sexual relationship is achieved or discomfort and frustration in the sexual role result. Researchers have found that the community can influence how early a person begins having sexual intercourse and whether contraceptive devices are used when sexual activity has begun. If the community offers a variety of opportunities for advancement in education and employment and has formal prohibitions against early sexual behavior and unwed parenthood, a person is less likely to engage in the latter activities. Young women in poor neighborhoods are less motivated to avoid or delay sexual activity than are those in neighborhoods of higher socioeconomic status. Brewster, Billy, and Grady (1993) found that the availability of family planning services failed to influence contraceptive use, and community religiosity did not have a significant effect on either intercourse or contraceptive behavior.

Incest or sexual abuse as a child may result in less than optimal adjustment as an adult. Research shows that the most common coping mechanisms of abused children, namely denial and suppression, are associated with poor long-term adjustment (Leitenberg, Greenwald, & Cado, 1992). Incest experiences in childhood or adolescence interfere with self-esteem and social development throughout adulthood, affecting the scope and quality of social relationships (Cole & Putnam, 1992). When these developmental transitions are adversely affected by incest, there are risks of serious psychopathology.

Acquired immune deficiency syndrome (AIDS) is a growing health concern because of its prevalence among young adults, especially women, who constitute the fastest growing population with AIDS in the United States (U.S. Centers for Disease Control [CDC], 1992). More recently, the CDC (1998) reports that between 1995 and 1996, there was a 3% increase in initial HIV diagnoses among women, while HIV diagnoses declined 3% among men during the same period. Needed are improved care, education, and outreach targeting these young adults at high risk. Both unprotected sexual intercourse and drug use—two factors most closely associated with the increase in AIDS cases—are prevalent among this age group (Wendell, Onorato, McCray, Allen, & Sweeney, 1992). Although research is ongoing to slow the progress of the disease and develop a vaccine to protect against it, AIDS is at this time a fatal disease. (See Chapter 20 on communicable diseases.) The nurse can evaluate the sexual health of the young adult via a careful, discreet sexual history. The community health nurse is in a unique position to uncover sexual problems through caring interactions and to help the young adult find the necessary therapy.

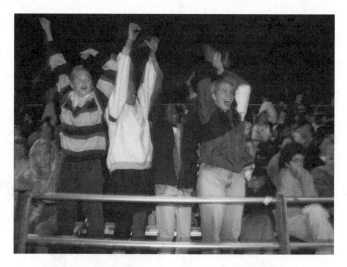

Experiences of childhood, adolescence, and the teen years affect self-esteem and social development throughout adulthood. Photo courtesy of Paul A. Souders/Corbis.

Reproductive Health Problems

Unwanted pregnancies and sexually transmitted diseases are two major health risks among young adults. The nurse should be involved in providing education about sex and family planning options. Educating clients about primary prevention of pregnancy and making referrals to agencies that are appropriate to the client's beliefs and values are two ways the nurse can help the client. A nonjudgmental attitude is vital for community health nurses dealing with sexually active adults. The nurse must be able to disperse factual information about sexually transmitted diseases.

Infertility is a growing concern of young adult couples. As many as 15% of young couples fail to conceive after a year of unprotected intercourse (Dawson & Whitfield, 1996). Investigation into both partners is important to determine the source of the problem.

Violence

Violence is a major physical risk factor in the young adult stage of life, especially violence of African American against African American. Violence can be self-directed, as discussed earlier, or directed toward others. Nurses can directly address the issue of violence by helping young adults develop healthy parenting techniques and helping young children develop nonviolent conflict-resolution skills. See Chapter 24 for further discussion of family violence.

Accidents

Accidents are a leading cause of death in both male and female young adults. Most common are motor vehicle accidents, but other unintentional injuries such as falls, poisoning by solids and liquids, fires and burns, and drownings constituted the sixth highest cause of death in the United States in 1995 (Rosenberg, Ventura, Maurer, et al., 1996).

Community health nurses work to prevent injuries in their communities, in homes, schools, workplaces, and wherever there are people. Injury prevention requires acute observation skills in noticing potential safety hazards and colloborative skills in working with others to rectify unsafe conditions. Safety education is also provided in community settings to promote personal safety.

Cancer

Cancer deaths among 25- to-44-year-old adults constituted 26.4% of total deaths in 1995 (Rosenberg, Ventura, Maurer, et al., 1996). Cancer of the testes and cancer of female reproductive organs occur in young adults. Testicular cancer has shown an alarming increase in recent years, and the risk of breast cancer in females increases steadily after age 30 (Edelman & Mandle, 1994). The nurse can teach breast and testicular self-examination and make recommendations for pelvic examination and Pap smears. It is important at this time to educate young adults about early signs of cancer. Even with education, young adults are often oblivious to danger signs and need to be reminded often. Table 17-3 lists risk factors and symptoms of common cancers.

Teaching about life habits that contribute to cancer is part of the nurse's role. Cessation of cigarette smoking for the individual and reduction of parental smoking for children's health are important, as are dietary considerations.

Employment and Housing

Social risk factors are related to the community where the individual lives, which is determined by several factors. Insufficient education or employment opportunities limit choices. The individual remains in an environment that is stifling and without the conditions necessary for successful functioning. In cases in which the individual does not leave the parental home, co-residence restricts social development. Research on co-residence has raised more questions than it has answered about outcomes and direct

Table 17-3   Risk Factors and Symptoms of Common Cancers

SITE	RISK FACTORS	SYMPTOMS
Lung	Cigarette smoking Exposure to substances causing chronic tissue irritation and inflammation Exposure to passive or sidestream smoke Occupational exposure to industrial pollution and other carcinogens	Persistent cough Hoarseness Rust-colored sputum or frank hemoptysis Recurrent lung infections
Colon	Family or personal history of colon cancer Inflammatory bowel disease Polyps Diet that contains carcinogens and foods that decrease bowel transit time	Bleeding from rectum Blood in stool Change in bowel habits Anemia
Breast	Being female and older than age 50 Early menarche, late menopause, or both Family history	Breast changes: lump, thickening, swelling, dimpling, nipple retraction or discharge Pain or tenderness

Skin	Excessive sun exposure
	Fair complexion
	Repeated irritation or injury
	Genetic predisposition
	Exposure to carcinogens
	    Coal tar
	    Arsenic
		Change in size or color of mole.
		Darkly pigmented or ulcerated lesions
		Lesion that bleeds easily

Cervix	Early sexual activity Multiple sexual partners Viral infections of cervix Intrauterine exposure to diethylstilbestrol (DES) Low socioeconomic status	Painless vaginal bleeding following intercourse or douching Spotting between menstrual periods
Prostate	Being male and older than age 50	Hard, nodular, fixed prostate Difficulty initiating urination Weak stream with dribbling Urinary frequency and urgency Nocturia Urinary retention Recurrent bladder infections

Adapted from Nursing Care of Adults *by F. D. Monahan, T. Drake, & M. Neighbors, 1994, Philadelphia: W. B. Saunders; and* Medical-Surgical Nursing *by D. D. Ignatavicius, M. L. Workman, & M. A. Mishler, 1995, Philadelphia: W. B. Saunders.*

consequences for well-being of both parents and adult children (Ward & Spitze, 1992).

The community health nurse is involved in the well-being of the young adult and is concerned about public policy involving much more than just physical health. The allocation of funds, the amount spent on prevention, and those person who make decisions regarding allocation of tax dollars are only a few of the many social issues that are of importance to nurses.

Middle Adult

Middle adulthood approximately covers the ages of 40 to 65. This period was once considered old age; but as life expectancy has lengthened, middle age has replaced and pushed old age up into the seventies and eighties. These middle years are the years of stability and structure. Some of the tasks during these years are: adapting to the phys-

ical changes of aging; reviewing and perhaps redirecting career goals and performance; accepting responsibilities associated with being a member of the **sandwich generation** (i.e., having responsibility for both increasingly

⚙ REFLECTIVE THINKING ⚙

Your Own Young Adulthood

Reflect on your own period of young adulthood, keeping in mind the risk factors of substance abuse, suicide, sexuality, violence, and accidents.

- Of these factors, which ones affected you?
- How did these factors shape your life as it is now?
- How will they affect your life in the future?

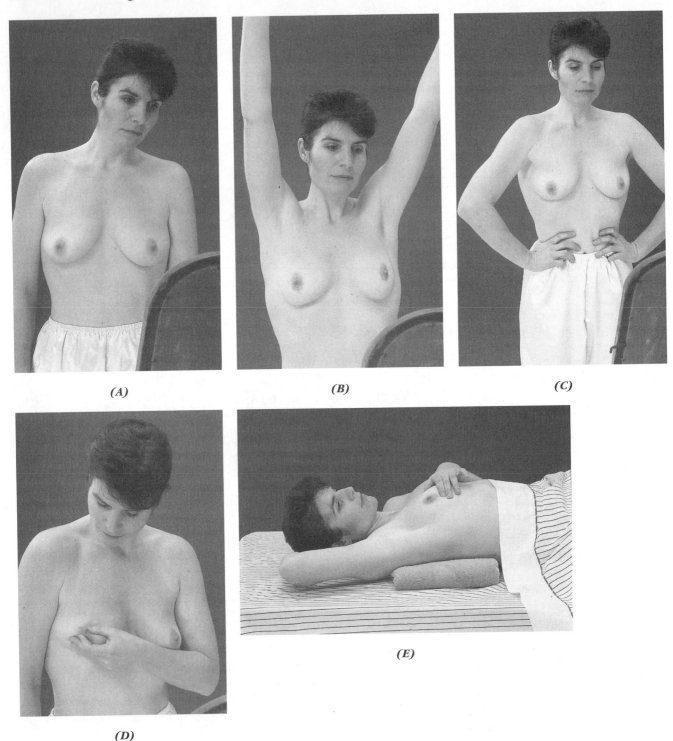

(A)   *(B)*   *(C)*

(D)

(E)

Breast self-examination: (A) before mirror, arms at side; (B) before mirror, arms over head; (C) before mirror, hands pressed into hip; (D) before mirror, compressing nipple; (E) lying down, palpating breast.

dependent parents and still-dependent children); and developing leisure-time activities of interest (Edelman & Mandle, 1994). Figure 17-2 lists developmental tasks of middle adulthood. Middle-aged adults are the stable, mature slice of society responsible for the day-to-day functioning of the world. This is a time of relatively good health, personal freedom, excellent command of self, and some influence over the social environment (Lefrancois, 1996). Most of the power in our society—in politics, busi-

ness, education, and religion—rests with middle-aged individuals.

Physical Development

Physically, middle age reflects the progression of the aging process. The skin loses its tautness, and wrinkles along with pouches and sagging begin to show on the face and neck. Hair becomes thinner or loses color. Mus-

Figure 17-2 Developmental Tasks of Middle Adulthood

Self

- Establish healthful lifestyle
- Accept physical changes of aging
- Use leisure time wisely and with satisfaction
- Continue developing philosophy of life
- Develop new hobbies and interests

Family

- Encourage increasing intimacy and support with mate
- Provide support and love to offspring
- Provide care and attention to aging parents
- Create and maintain a pleasant, comfortable home

Society

- Enjoy work, provide leadership, and prepare for retirement
- Be aware of civic responsibility
- Maintain membership in organizations
- Treasure old friends and make new ones

Adapted from The Lifespan *(5th ed.) by G. R. Lefrancois, 1996, Belmont, CA: Wadsworth Publishing.*

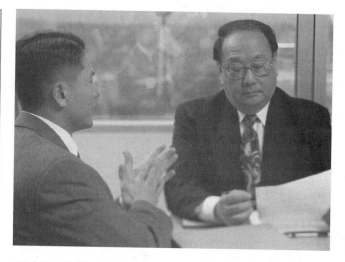

Middle adulthood developmental tasks include acting as a leader and mentor for less experienced people, whether in the workplace or in the community. Photo courtesy of PhotoDisc.

Changes in body shape in middle adulthood are often compounded by obesity. The prevalence of sedentary lifestyles and unaltered dietary patterns result in overweight adults. Most people no longer participate in the regular programs of physical exercise more common in the younger years, while attending elementary and secondary school. At this stage of life it is necessary to reduce caloric intake and adjust the amounts of fat, fiber, protein, and carbohydrates. Also extremely important for cardiovascular health as well as weight maintenance is a program of regular exercise.

Cognitive Development

Cognitive development in the middle adult is fairly constant. As at any age, intelligence is difficult to define and even more difficult to measure. Intelligence quotient (IQ) tests are designed to predict academic achievement and are not good measures of adult intelligence. **Fluid intelligence**, mental functioning based on organizing information to be used to solve problems, is different from **crystallized intelligence**, or drawing on life experiences and learned abilities. Crystallized intelligence generally increases with age as fluid intelligence decreases (Dacey & Travers, 1996). There are many variables to consider in measuring intelligence in middle adults, such as motivation, deliberation, caution, and anxiety. Such variables often result in slowed reaction times, but not in decreased intelligence levels. Middle age is considered by some to be the height of intellectual endowment, as memory and problem solving are maintained and learning continues (Sims et al., 1995). A stimulating environment plays a large part in maintaining intellectual functioning.

Memory changes are another area of concern for middle-aged adults, but recent findings show that individual cognitive development must be considered and that memory loss is highly individualized. Some middle-aged persons will experience memory loss, but many will not.

cle tone diminishes, and additional adipose deposits result in a thickened midsection and thinner extremities. Decreased bone density and decalcification of bones lead to a change of posture and the beginning of loss of height, especially in the female (Jarvis, 1992). Gradual losses in nerve conduction and muscle function slow movement and impair sensations. Blood vessels are less elastic and lead to cardiovascular disorders and hypertension. **Presbyopia**, or decreased accommodation due to lessened elasticity of the lens of the eye, leads to the necessity for reading or bifocal lenses for close visual acuity. **Presbycusis**, or diminished hearing, begins in middle age, with acuity for high-frequency sounds being first to be lost (Dacey & Travers, 1996).

✺✺ REFLECTIVE THINKING ✺✺

Physical Signs of Aging

- Which, if any, of the physical signs of middle age do you have?

- What symptoms of aging can you recognize in your parents? In your acquaintances?

- What differences can you identify in the ways that men and women cope with signs of aging?

Psychosocial Development

The middle-adult years are a good example of the blending of developmental factors. During these years, physical changes affect psychosocial and, sometimes, cognitive abilities. The ways that a person reacts to these changes affects the personality and personal development (Jarvis, 1992). Psychosocial development during these years is typified by self-assessment and introspection. Erikson (1963) defines the developmental task of this life stage as a resolution of the crisis of **generativity versus stagnation**. Individuals have the urge to contribute in some way to the next generation, by either producing that generation or producing something to pass on to that generation. If that goal is not achieved, stagnation or self-absorption results, with a reversion to adolescent self-centered behavior or psychological invalidism. Levinson (1978) defines this life stage as beginning with a transition period of reassessment by the middle adult. Various degrees of searching and self-assessment go on before the individual proceeds to making choices and building new structures. This midlife transition is handled differently by males and females. Men are more involved in reassessing life in the work or career world, whereas women concentrate more on family issues. This distinction may blur as women become more involved in career and work outside the home and men become more involved in child-rearing and family issues.

One final phenomenon in this stage of life is the **empty nest syndrome**, launched by the last child's leaving home. This period requires adjustment as the couple learns to live alone as a couple again. Some couples react negatively, discovering that, with the children gone, they have nothing in common. Such couples no longer "know" each other after years of involvement with their children's activities, or their relationships have no meaning without the children. For other couples, this is a positive time, and their relationships deepen and become stronger.

Middle-Adult Risk Factors

The middle adult faces many of the same risks as does the young adult. Life stresses continue and, in fact, may actually escalate. The risk of turning to alcohol or drugs to relieve and cope with those stressors remains present.

Midlife Crisis

Unique to this stage of life are several age-related factors. The first of these is the **midlife crisis**, a transition first identified by Carl Jung (1933). At approximately 40 or 50 years of age, the individual begins to lose the sense of purpose and responsibility that has been a part of life. A sense of uselessness and incompletion takes over, resulting in a feeling that some crucial element is missing. Some individuals endure these years of struggle and emerge as stronger, more mature people. Others resist the honest appraisal and examination of life necessary to survive and make drastic career and marital changes in an attempt to

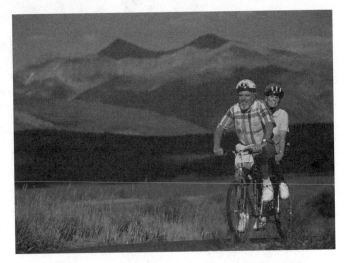

After children have left home, a couple must adjust to being "just a couple" again. Photo courtesy of Bob Winsett/Corbis.

bring meaning back into their lives (Murray & Zentner, 1997). The nurse can be instrumental in assisting the client through this phase of development by using good communication techniques and crisis-intervention tactics. Referrals can be made to counseling centers and support groups. The nurse recognizes that this crisis or transition is a part of the development of the middle adult years and can be used for positive growth and change.

Generation Gap

Another risk factor of the midadult years is the conflict between parents and adolescents. Called the **generation gap**, this conflict results from the need for young adults to move out and away from the world their parents have created. This move toward independence involves experimentation and, often, revolt against the parents' world. The parents respond with resentment and insistence on conformity, and the battle lines are drawn. Again, the community health nurse is in a unique position to assist the client in resolving these difficulties. Recognition of the developmental stage and acceptance of the necessity for tolerance are two strategies that can be used. Humor can also be used to lighten the discussion and to make a point without offending either parent or teenager (Schulman & Sperry, 1992).

Along with the responsibility for the adolescent, many middle adults face special problems associated with their aging parents. As parents age and experience losses, the middle adult often moves into a caretaking role. Depending on the relationship between parent and adult child, this new role can be rewarding or a burden (Schulman & Sperry, 1992). The nurse can assist the adult child to accept the fact that the parents' dependence may be appropriate for their point of life. The nurse can assist the client in recognizing those things that must be done and finding the necessary resources. This sandwich generation, responsible for both children and parents, faces increasing stress as their aged parents decline in ability. The stress on all can be reduced if caregiving situations are regarded as a function of families, not just of individuals (Mellins, Blum, Boyd-Davis, & Gatz, 1993). The eventual death of parents can be a relief or another source of stress, depending on how well the middle adult has resolved the child–parent relationship. Again, as in the young adult years, depression can be a reaction to the accumulated stresses of middle adult years. The nurse must be aware of the symptoms of clinical depression, such as changes in appetite and sleep patterns, loss of interest in all activities, fatigue, indecisiveness, or recurrent thoughts of death (Johnson, 1993). Suicide is a concern at any age, and care must be taken to recognize the symptoms and help the individual.

Accidents

Physically, the middle adult is at risk for accidents connected to occupation or lifestyle. Fractures and dislocations are the most common injuries at this age. These injuries may require not only medical care but also extensive recuperation and disability (USDHHS, 1990).

Health Problems

No single disease or illness is unique to these years, but health problems do occur. Cardiovascular disease, cancer, pulmonary disease, diabetes, obesity, alcoholism, and glaucoma are major problems of middle adulthood. Cancer ranks as the number one cause of death among people 45 to 64 years of age. Heart disease is the second leading cause, and chronic pulmonary disease the third (U.S. Bureau of the Census, 1995). Better maintenance of health is required at this age, and careful assessment must be performed by the nurse to identify potential health problems. Different ethnic backgrounds determine different health problems. The nurse must be aware of health risks particular to certain cultural groups. The African American client, for example, is at higher risk for hypertension than is the Caucasian client. Among those over 18 years of age and both sexes, 21.3% of African Americans are hypertensive compared with 15.9% of Caucasians (Dorgan, 1995). In the Native American population, Type II diabetes is four times more common than in the general population (Andrews & Boyle, 1995).

The female climacteric, better known as **menopause**, occurs during the middle adult years. The associated decline in hormone production produces a wide variety of physical and psychological effects, many of which are undergoing scientific study. Although many women experience no ill effects, menopause is often viewed as a disease treated by estrogen-replacement therapy, other hormones, and various medications (Wasaha & Angelopoulos, 1996). The usual symptoms of menopause include hot flushes, vaginal and libido changes, increased risk of osteoporosis and cardiovascular disease, skin changes, and mood alterations. For women who are unwilling to take replacement estrogen and other medications, alternative therapies include exercise, dietary changes, and herbal preparations (Wasaha & Angelopoulos, 1996).

The **male climacteric** usually occurs in the late fifties or early sixties. Less noticeable than menopause, this period may entail some episodes of dizziness, hot flashes, sweating, or headaches. Although males do not lose their reproductive power, sexual hormone production does diminish, and sexual response changes. Some hypertrophy of the prostate gland can begin in these years, resulting in urinary frequency and nocturia (Sheehy, 1995).

Sexuality

Sexual behavior in the middle adult varies between males and females. Males peak in desire in the late teenage years and early twenties, whereas females peak in the late thirties or early forties (Dacey & Travers, 1996). A close, loving relationship, however, is vital in promoting and sustaining a satisfying sexual relationship.

Financial Concerns and Relationship Problems

Major social risk factors of this age include financial concerns, meaningful employment, and relationship problems. Financial concerns often result from rising inflation and cost of living. A job where output is valued over the employee as a person can lead to dissatisfaction and despair. At this time of life, attention becomes focused on the remaining productive work years and whether retirement funds are going to be sufficient to allow a satisfactory lifestyle in the later years.

At this middle stage of life, divorce and all its resultant problems constitute an increasingly common occurrence. Whether the divorce is amicable or acrimonious, major life changes of this type result in stress. If young children are involved, custody questions arise; with older children, problems of behavior and supervision. New living arrangements are a source of stress as attempts are made to recreate a stable home and community. Another increasingly common occurrence is the return of adult children. When adult children move back into family homes with their aging parents, there are questions of who benefits most (Speare & Avery, 1993). Research is focusing on whether the adult child always benefits or whether the aging parent also is positively affected by the arrangement. Family or cultural beliefs about family structure often dictate the success of alternative living arrangements. The community health nurse can be helpful to all parties in resolving conflicts and helping the individuals work through problems. Communication skills and a sense of humor, again, are valuable tools in helping adults through the risks of middle-adult life.

Older Adult

Late adulthood, from age 65 to death, is more prone to negative stereotyping than is any other life stage. The

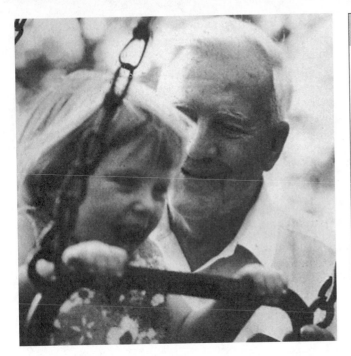

An elderly grandparent can have a very positive effect on grandchildren. In your own life, did you have a grandparent who had a positive effect on you?

Figure 17-3 Developmental Tasks of the Older Adult

Self

- Recognize and accept changes and limitations of aging
- Plan living arrangements for remaining years
- Practice healthy lifestyle including diet and exercise appropriate to status
- Pursue activities that give a feeling of satisfaction and a sense of being needed
- Face the inevitability of one's own death as well as the deaths of loved ones

Family

- Continue warm relationships with spouse and family
- Maintain connection with children and grandchildren

Society

- Establish affiliation with same age group
- Maintain close friendships and social connections
- Incorporate civic activities to maintain social responsibilities

Adapted from Health Assessment in Nursing *by L. K. Sims, D. D'Amico, J. K. Stiesmeyer, & J. A. Webster, 1995, Redwood City, CA: Addison-Wesley.*

stereotypes surrounding aging are partly a result of our cultural emphasis on youth and beauty and partly a reflection of our own anxieties about aging and death. The older adult faces the last years of life with few role models, fewer societal definitions, and even fewer directions for dealing with death, the final stage of life. This portion of our population is the most rapidly growing segment, and older adults are beginning to be seen as a diverse group with widely differing opinions and needs. The developmental tasks of the older adult include adjusting to physical and health changes; forming new family roles as in-law and grandparent; facing retirement with reduced income; associating with own age group; and developing enjoyable and meaningful postretirement activities. Figure 17-3 lists the developmental tasks of the older adult.

⊛⊛ REFLECTIVE THINKING ⊛⊛

Aging and Perception of Aging

- At what age do you think a person is old?
- Can you identify behaviors in a person over 70 years of age that would make him seem much younger than his age?
- Imagine yourself in your eighties and enjoying a relationship with someone of the opposite sex. How would that relationship be different from a relationship at a younger age?

Physical Development

Aging does not occur at the same rate for all people. In fact, aging manifests in widely divergent ways in different individuals. The external, or visible, signs of physical aging are most obvious in posture, skin, hair, and teeth (Lefrancois, 1996). The vertebral changes of age result in loss of stature and bowing of the spine. These changes give the elderly person a stooped look that can be overemphasized in women with osteoporosis. Elderly skin loses elasticity, subcutaneous fat layers diminish, and the skin becomes wrinkled. These changes lead to a decrease in the body's ability to regulate temperature. Hair becomes thinner and loses color and luster. Men grow coarser eyebrows and nose and ear hair. Women have greater problems with facial hair, especially on the upper lip and chin. Teeth problems are often a result of poor dental hygiene, but certain changes are age related. Reduced saliva results in decay and periodontal or gum disease leading to tooth loss. Years of brushing can result in enamel loss, and years of chewing and grinding can leave the older person with worn, flattened teeth (Edelman & Mandle, 1994).

Systemic Changes

Internally, or systemically, the signs of aging are many and involve all body parts. Cardiovascular and respiratory systems are less efficient because of a reduction in strength and adaptability of related organs. Blood vessels

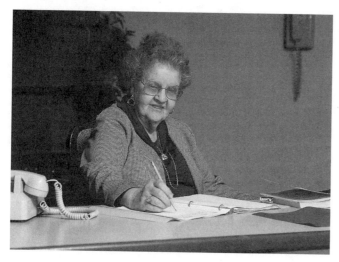

This older adult is able to maintain her independence and self-esteem through volunteer work. Describe the importance of incorporating information such as the ability and desire to make a contribution to society to an older adult's nursing care.

harden and react more slowly, causing the heart to work harder and less effectively. The gastrointestinal and urinary systems may also decrease in efficiency, with associated decreased peristalsis and less effective excretion of toxins and wastes from the body. Constipation, a common problem of the older adult, and urinary frequency reflect these systemic changes of aging (Jarvis, 1992).

Reduced blood flow to the brain as well as reduced oxygen and glucose use begin at approximately 60 years of age. However, age-related brain atrophy varies widely and is not uniform in all older adults (Roussel, 1995). Muscle mass and muscle strength diminish in older people, but some of this loss can be counteracted by regular exercise. Bone density is reduced in elderly persons, and bones become more brittle. Synovial fluid is less abundant, possibly resulting in increased arthritic pain and stiffness (Pattillo, 1995). Last, the immune response in the older adult is faulty and responds less efficiently to eliminate foreign material from the body (Wiersema, 1995). As the immune system fails, it tends to turn against the body in an autoimmune response. This results in an increase in autoimmune diseases among elders, such as rheumatoid arthritis and allergies to foods and environmental factors (Stanley & Beare, 1995).

Sexuality

Sexuality in the older adult shifts in emphasis from procreation to companionship, intimate communication, and a pleasurable physical relationship (Ebersole & Hess, 1994). Physical changes that influence coitus include decreased vaginal lubrication in the female and a less intense and slower erection in the male. As with most aging changes, there are wide variations, even at a biological level, and many older adults lead full, rich sexual lives. A common problem in Western society is the in-

creasingly large number of older females in proportion to fewer older men. The nurse can address sexuality when doing an assessment and give the older adult the support and advice necessary in this sensitive area.

Sensory Changes

Sensory capacities change in the elderly person. Visual acuity declines due to age-related changes in the eye. The lens continues to lose elasticity, becomes cloudy, and admits less light. The pupils become smaller, and the eyelids sag and interfere with vision. Hearing loss continues, with further reduction in hearing of higher frequencies and eventual trouble discerning consonant sounds (Gallman, 1995). Taste and smell sensitivity decline with age, resulting in lessened appetite and enjoyment of food. The skin is less sensitive to touch, and the older adult is less aware of changes in pain and temperature sensation.

Because these systemic and sensory changes are considered inevitable, some people regard aging and the older adult years as an overwhelming, rapid decline into sickness, incapacity, and death. The older adult takes longer to recover from illness, suffers from a greater number of chronic diseases, and has less resistance to disease. However, the older adult is capable of enduring the changes of aging and functioning very ably. Age-related changes differ greatly in time of onset, and the individual's attitude toward aging often influences the extent to which these changes affect function. Most older adults continue their activities and lifestyles with minimum adjustment to the changes of aging.

Research by Burlew, Jones, and Emerson (1991) examined the effects of an exercise program on elderly persons and whether a group approach enhances participation and compliance in exercise programs. The study showed that the combination of an exercise program and group counseling can address the problem of physical aging along with the psychological well-being issues of elderly clients.

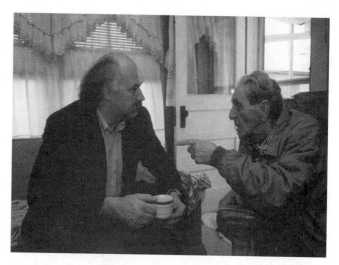

The community health nurse must exercise sensitivity when discussing sexuality with the older adult. Photo courtesy of Philip Gould/Corbis.

Many health problems of older adults are improved by exercise. Regular exercise reduces weight and stress, lessens the risks of hypertension and atherosclerosis, and improves glucose metabolism among older adults. Improved physical mobility and balance lead to fewer accidental falls. Last, elderly individuals who exercise are more inclined to change other lifestyle factors related to heart disease, such as high-fat diet and smoking.

Cognitive Development

The cognitive development of the older adult shows a reduction in reaction time, but, as with the middle adult, no decline in intellectual function. Again, certain variables affect the measurement of the older person's intellectual functioning: decreased visual and auditory acuity, slowed responses to stimuli, loss of recent memory, and altered motivation, among others (Staab & Hodges, 1996). Cultural differences can also influence measurement of intelligence. For example, because Hispanics are very concerned about hurting someone's feelings, they might respond politely even when they do not understand. Reaction times will often be slower under stress, and many older adults have endured social and environmental losses that cause stress. Other factors that can influence the measurement of cognitive ability in older adults are isolation, level of education and length of time since school attendance, interest, and the conservation of

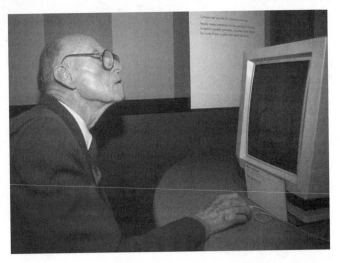

An older adult may minimize memory loss by remaining mentally active. Photo courtesy of Joseph Sohm. ChromoSohm Inc./Corbis.

time and energy for other more meaningful tasks (Wold, 1993). One important factor to consider when making any judgment about cognitive development in the older adult is the fact that the process of aging is unique to the person. Aging does not occur in the same way in all individuals. This is especially true with regard to mental abilities.

RESEARCH FOCUS

The Impact of Continuing Education on the Health of Older Adults

STUDY PROBLEM/PURPOSE

The purpose of this study was to determine whether participation in continuing education positively affects the health of older adults. In order to meet this objective, a more specific question was asked: Does participation in four different non–health-related continuing education activities positively affect the health of older adults in terms of variables such as depression, self-esteem, social satisfaction, personal control, and symptoms of aging?

METHODS

A quasi-experimental design was used with 114 subjects in four groups of participants ranging in age from 60 to 69 at a community college. The independent variable was continuing education, and the dependent variable was health.

FINDINGS

At the end of the instruction period, the three health factors of depression, social satisfaction, and symptoms of aging showed significant changes from baseline measures. Some changes represented improvement and others decline in health. Changes found at the end of instruction, however, did not persist six weeks after the programs had ended.

IMPLICATIONS

Although it could be anticipated that the benefits would be diverse, some common themes emerged. An exploration of the dynamics of active participation in continuing education by older adults can lead to a better understanding of the effects of continuing education on their health. The most obvious implication is that stimulation needs to be ongoing.

SOURCE

From "The Impact of Continuing Education on the Health of Older Adults" by K. G. Panayotoff, 1993, Educational Gerontology, 19(1), pp. 9–20.

Memory and Memory Loss

One major area of concern in the mental health of the older adult is memory and memory loss (Wold, 1993). The older person who is mentally active and well educated will not show the same problems with memory as will those adults without similar opportunities to use their minds. Research is showing that active participation in education may benefit older people's health (Panayotoff, 1993). Long-term memory seems to remain intact longer than does short-term memory, possibly because of the frequency of recall of these memories. It is difficult to measure memory in this population because there are so many variables that can affect the measurement. Memory changes or alterations in mental functioning usually result from physical or mental disorders often found among elderly people and are generally not a normal part of the aging process.

Psychosocial Development

The psychosocial development of the older adult is an interesting phenomenon. This is a time for assessment of self and life, a time to look back over that which has been achieved and to prepare for the end of life. Erikson describes the task of this stage as **ego integrity versus despair** (Erikson, 1963). Ego integrity means the coming together of all aspects of the past and an acceptance that this life was the only life to be lived. Without this sense of ego integrity, the individual suffers despair, a sense of futility, and the feeling that life was too short and that nothing was accomplished. With despair comes a fear of death, anger at the whole aging process, resentment of younger people, and feelings of inadequacy and worthlessness (Erikson, 1963).

Levinson's (1986) theory of development proposes a transitional period at this stage of life wherein fundamental changes in body and personality lead to fear that the individual has lost all identity and must find a new inner energy with which to survive these last years. The individual in this period has suffered losses, either death of peers, serious illness, or other catastrophes, and is forced to look for new inner strength. In the late years of adulthood, the individual becomes more turned inward, less involved in family and society, and more concerned with inner resources. The last tasks are concerned with the meaning of life, making peace with self, and dealing with the prospect of dying (Jarvis, 1992).

Death is considered the final developmental stage and, as such, requires careful preparation. Attitudes toward death have changed over time. In earlier days, dying was an event that took place at home in the company of friends and family. Today, over 70% of deaths in American cities occur in institutions (Angelucci & Lawrence, 1995). This tendency has made death remote and, in some cases, a fearful experience. The hospice movement has begun to affect this picture by providing support for the client and family to face death in the home. The community health nurse is often the person who assists the family and the client to come to terms with the approaching death. It is vital that the nurse, as the principal caregiver, provide support and leadership during this process (Angelucci & Lawrence, 1995).

Retirement and Life Review

Two important events in this stage of life are retirement and performing a life review. The way an individual responds to retirement depends largely on the relationship with the job or career. If the work was meaningless, repetitive, and boring, retirement may be a relief and a pleasure. However, many occupations are satisfying and fulfilling and carry high status and power. In such an instance, retirement may be devastating. Care should be taken to preplan leisure activities or new careers to perpetuate feelings of self-worth and usefulness. Adjustments in relationships are also necessary, as job-related social opportunities often are no longer available. Marital relationships need time to adjust to this new way of life as previous roles are eliminated and new roles become more clearly defined. Financial conditions must also be considered, especially if retirement brings a reduction in income. Figure 17-4 lists anticipatory actions for the retiring person.

There is no mandatory retirement age in the United States, and most older adults are still highly qualified to perform their jobs. Some people choose to retire in their fifties or sixties. Others choose to retire from one position or career and take on another career at age 60 or 70. Older people often express a need for achievement and challenge. Nonmonetary rewards are more significant to older persons than to those who are younger: 69% as compared with 48% (Ebersole & Hess, 1994).

DECISION MAKING

The Age to Retire

Imagine you are a community health nurse working with the family of a frail 85-year-old woman. She lives with her daughter and her husband. The son-in-law is 68 years old, has a chronic heart problem, and receives a disability stipend. The daughter is 62 years old and has been employed as a bookkeeper at a fruit cannery for many years. She states she has not been feeling well and is finding it difficult to work all day and come home to care for her mother, who is needing more and more help. She says she would like to retire so she could stay at home with her mother but is afraid there will not be enough income to keep their home and maintain their lifestyle.

- What factors must be considered in her decision?

- How can you assist her in making this decision?

Figure 17-4   Preparing for Retirement

- Make financial arrangements early to ensure adequate income.
- Anticipate the effect that role loss will have on self-esteem and one's close relationships.
- Form friendships outside the workplace.
- Perform assessments of living arrangements and, if relocation is planned, form new social networks in the new location.
- Form support and social groups other than family and spouse.
- In the last work years, decrease time at work by increasing vacations, working shorter days or weeks, and working part-time.
- Prepare self for initial exhilaration followed by ambivalence before the setting in of satisfaction with life.
- Plan age-appropriate exercise programs including walking, swimming, or biking.
- Plan routines to replace the work-day structure.
- Be realistic in planning retirement activities in terms of energy and money.

Adapted from Family Dynamics by B. K. Haight & K. Leech, 1995. In M. Stanley & P. B. Beare (Eds.), Gerontological Nursing *(p. 365), Philadelphia: F. A. Davis.*

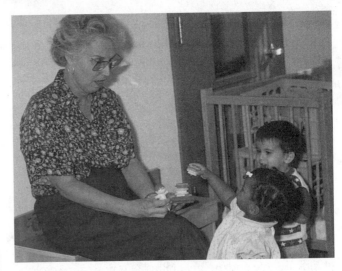

Volunteering to work with young children offers rewards to both this older adult and the children. What other types of volunteering might you suggest to an older adult who is not necessarily looking for monetary rewards?

All of these life changes remind individuals that time is limited and they are approaching the end of their lives. Thus, one last task necessary at this stage of life is life review. Most of one's life's work is accomplished. Contri-butions to society and family are complete. Now is the time to look back over the achievements and failures, to catalogue life events and gain some sense of perspective regarding life. The individual needs to acknowledge and accept that not all goals were accomplished, not all wrongs were set right, and it is too late to go back and do it over (Levinson, 1986). Acceptance of these facts and the final making of peace with the self are important to the individual in accepting the inevitability of the approaching death.

Perspectives...

Insights of a Nursing Student

"Oh my, this man is 98 years old!" I thought to myself when my first client was assigned to me during my community health rotation. My interest is in maternal/child nursing, my experience is in labor and delivery as a doula. I had limited experience with older clients and now I was assigned one to visit at his home. My concern was not so much in providing care. I knew I was capable of performing physical, functional, and environmental assessments. I knew how to look for potential risk factors in each of these areas and was confident I could perform at an appropriate level. No, this was not my concern. I was concerned that I would be unable to facilitate therapeutic communication with a 98-year-old man. Both of my grandfathers died when I was very young, and I had never had the opportunity to get to know any other elderly gentleman. I was not quite sure if I would be able to be relaxed and supportive with Raymond G., a 98-year-old widowed and retired college professor, as I was capable of being with new mothers and their infant children.

Continued

Continued

The first lesson I learned about communicating with an older person is to talk slowly. This I discovered during my first phone call to Raymond to set up our first appointment. "I'm sorry, could you repeat what you just said?" was his response to most of my statements during that first phone call. It was a course in patience and enunciation. By the end of the conversation I managed to keep my remarks brief, slow, and loud. As a result we were able to schedule a visit for the following Tuesday in the early afternoon. I spent the next week rereading chapters on working with the elderly in my community health nursing text and outlining my plan for our initial visit.

The days flew by and Tuesday morning arrived. After preconference, I reviewed my initial plan then called Raymond to confirm our appointment. At the agreed-upon time I walked up the path to his front door. I was able to look through the screen as I walked up the steps, and I saw an elderly gentleman, dressed in khaki pants and a cardigan sweater, sitting in a chair right inside the door. He looked up and smiled, then invited me in. Our visit was short, about 30 minutes, and we spent the time sitting across from each other in chairs he had carefully placed in the living room. I enjoyed hearing about his life, his deceased wife, his grown children, and his fondness for gardening. He explained that he was "eight plus ninety, that's 98" and that he didn't expect to live to see 100, nor did he want to. He introduced me to his companion, Tiffany. "She's a good cat," he said, "she loves to sit with me and never talks back." He and Tiffany had been together for eight years, and Raymond made it clear that she was quite special to him. Although I didn't want to seem too familiar, I did want to begin a general assessment of the surroundings. I asked Raymond if I could take a look around before I left. He told me to feel free to do so, and I was able to make a first assessment of the home environment before leaving.

I sat in my car for a few minutes reflecting on our visit and was surprised to discover I had really enjoyed visiting with Raymond in his home. Raymond was very easy to talk with, very appreciative of the visit, and had many interesting things to say. I looked forward to getting to know him over the course of the semester. Unfortunately, I was able to

visit with Raymond only three times before he suffered a massive MI, which resulted in his death one week later. I had been in touch with Raymond's son, John, and his wife, Sheila, regularly during the course of our relationship, and in the two weeks following Raymond's death we continued to keep in contact. I was able to assist them in finalizing the relationship they had with our student community health group (Raymond had been our client for many years) and even found a new home for Tiffany. This was a great relief for the family, because they were unable to keep her but were devastated at the idea of putting her down.

As I said earlier, my emphasis is in maternal/child health. I have worked with many women and infants during the first few weeks of life, a position I have found to be both invigorating and rewarding. I didn't expect to gain, so soon, the experience of assisting someone through the last days of life, but I know my life was enriched because of it. I know I made Raymond's last week a little more pleasant for him. Both he and his son, John, told me how much my visits meant, and I know Raymond would be pleased that Tiffany has a nice new home. I gave Raymond the gift of caring, but he gave much to me as well.

My life has been enhanced as a result of my short, but meaningful, relationship with Raymond. I have gained valuable insight into the practice of community nursing and into the final stages of life. For Raymond, life had become mundane. He was homebound and had few visitors. Yet he had a mind filled with rich memories and wondrous experiences that he was willing to share with me during our visits. He enjoyed talking about his life and told me more than once that, although it had been a good life, he was ready to "go see my wife." Raymond taught me that the final stage of life is not to be feared, but embraced. He taught me that it's ok to look back at life and rejoice while preparing for death, that just having someone there to listen who cared about what he had to say was one of life's pleasures. I will always remember fondly my relationship with Raymond, and I promise to be a good companion to Tiffany, who, by the way, is adjusting nicely to life in my home.

—*Pamela Rasada*
Student Nurse

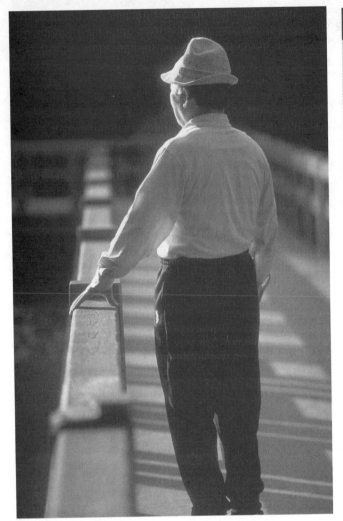

Reviewing one's past successes and failures and accepting those things that cannot be changed is a necessary part of preparing oneself for the inevitability of death. Photo courtesy of Kevin R. Morris/Corbis.

losses. These can be loss of loved ones, loss of job status and prestige, loss of income, and loss of an energetic and resilient body (Staab & Hodges, 1996).

Depression

Depression is the most common psychiatric disorder among older adults and is often a reaction to the losses experienced during these years (Johnson, 1993). The disease is characterized by intense sadness, hopelessness, pessimism, and low self-regard. Somatic complaints are more common than mood disturbance in elderly persons. Depression may lead to suicide, and the older adult communicates his intentions less frequently and is usually more successful at committing suicide than the younger adult (Johnson, 1993). Suicide is the ninth highest cause of death among the elderly, ranking higher than among any other group (CDC, 1997). The nurse needs to follow up on symptoms of depression to determine whether suicidal intentions are present.

Isolation and Loss

Isolation can result from physical barriers such as curbs, steps, and the weather or emotional barriers such as fear of crime. In either case, the older adult is often unable to access appropriate services, act as his own advocate, or coordinate the care he needs (Haight & Leech, 1995). Although community health nurses can neither reverse the process of aging nor make the associated losses less painful to the older adult, they can listen to the client's complaints, act as a liaison between client and other professionals, and support the client and family in many ways. Because the older adult often relies heavily on family members for assistance, it is important for nurses to work with families as well as individuals. Intergenerational bonds seem to constitute an important factor in the older adult's capacity to survive. Although there are still questions about whether affectionate relationships with adult children extend life, the research suggests that close relationships between child and parent help the older adult cope with the death of the spouse and promote the well-being of the parent (Silverstein & Bengston, 1991). The nurse, again, is invaluable, not only in identifying

Facing Death

Dying and death are unavoidable parts of living. Dying can be a positive experience and an opportunity for self-actualization (Angelucci & Lawrence, 1995). The community health nurse can assist the client in a growth-producing experience until death actually occurs. The client must be assessed for level of knowledge and acceptance and then supported in the process of accepting death. An atmosphere of open honesty and trust is vital during this last stage of life (Angelucci & Lawrence, 1995).

Older-Adult Risk Factors

The risk factors faced by older individuals are many, but most older adults live healthy, productive lives. These individuals, well elders, will grow in number and provide our society with a rich source of experience and wisdom (Lefrancois, 1996).

Some of the mental and emotional risk factors at this age are depression, isolation, dementia, and dealing with those individuals who are at risk for isolation but also in serving as an advocate to obtain necessary services.

Dementia

Although the majority of older adults experience little or no cognitive impairment, the fear of losing mental capacity is often expressed. Dementia, especially dementia of the Alzheimer's type, is feared most of all. Because this disease often covers a 6- to 20-year course, it has an especially devastating impact on older adults. The community health nurse is often the individual who serves as support and liaison for the family of the Alzheimer's victim. The nurse can act as a resource to the family in locating respite services, home care assistance, and, eventually, long-term care placement options (Johnson & Johnson, 1995). See Chapter 21 for more detailed information about chronic conditions.

Sensory Impairment

Sensory impairment is a factor affecting all elderly persons. Visual and auditory problems accompany progressive aging. Blindness and deafness are real risks and require special care to ensure that communication is maintained. Older adults who are hearing impaired have been shown to adapt to the stresses of late life more poorly than those who are not impaired (Stein & Bienenfeld, 1992). Figure 17-5 lists guidelines for helping persons who are blind. Figure 17-6 lists guidelines for communicating with individuals who are hearing impaired.

Reduced pain and temperature sensations can cause safety problems. Older adults need to have more covering on their beds, keep their thermostats higher in the winter, and be aware of ways to prevent hypothermia. Reaction to pain is a warning system, and care must be taken when pain sensation is reduced. Burns or frostbite can occur without warning. Foot care must be meticulous, as there is reduced sensation in the lower extremities.

Older adults are much more likely to suffer from chronic disease than are younger individuals. These chronic conditions can affect any body system and are rarely cured, only symptomatically controlled. Some of the more common chronic diseases of elderly persons are Parkinson's disease, dementias, congestive heart failure, chronic obstructive pulmonary disease, arthritis, and diabetes mellitus. See Chapter 21.

Cancer

Cancer in older adults accounts for over 85% of all cancer diagnosed in the United States (Sarna, 1995). These cancers have a variety of causes, signs, symptoms, treatments, and prognoses. The most common types of cancer in the older adult are colorectal, breast, lung, prostate, ovarian, pancreas, and stomach (Sarna, 1995). Reasons for the increased risk of cancer in elders are currently being researched. One possible reason is the accumulated exposure to carcinogens over time. Another might

Figure 17-5 Guidelines for Helping Persons Who Are Blind

- Talk to the person in a normal tone of voice. The fact that sight is impaired is no indication that hearing is also impaired.

- When offering assistance, do so directly.

- In guiding the person, permit the person to take your arm. Never grab the person's arm.

- In walking with the person, proceed at a normal pace. Hesitate slightly before stepping up and down.

- Be explicit in giving directions to the person.

- There is no need to avoid use of the word *see* when talking with a person who is blind.

- When assisting the person to a chair, place his or her hand on the back or arm of the chair.

- When leaving the person after conversing together, advise that you are leaving so that the person does not continue the conversation when no one is listening.

- Never leave a person who is blind in an open area. Lead him or her to the side of a room, to a chair, or to some landmark from which he or she can obtain direction.

- A half-open door is one of the most dangerous obstacles that people who are blind encounter.

- When serving food to the person, identify each item as you place it on the table. Call attention to food placement by using the numbers of an imaginary clock. For example, "The green beans are at two o'clock."

- Be sure to make the person aware of other guests.

Adapted from Nursing Assessment and Promotion Strategies through the Lifespan *(6th ed.) by R. B. Murray & J. P. Zentner, 1997, Norwalk, CT: Appleton & Lange.*

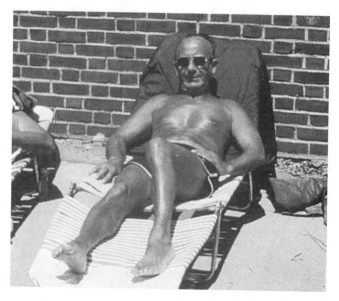

Cancer caused by sun exposure may take years to appear. *Courtesy of the Phoenix Society for Burn Survivors, Inc.*

Figure 17-6 Guidelines for Communicating with Persons Who Are Hearing Impaired

- When you meet a person who seems inattentive or slow to understand you, consider the possibility that hearing, rather than manners or intellect, may be at fault.

- Remember that persons who are hearing impaired may depend on reading your lips. You can help by always trying to speak in a good light and by facing the person and the light as you speak.

- When in a group that includes a person who is hearing impaired, try to carry on your conversation with others in such a way that your lips can be seen.

- Speak distinctly but naturally. Try not to speak too rapidly.

- Do not start to speak to the person abruptly. Attract the person's attention first by facing the person and looking straight into his or her eyes. If necessary, lightly touch one of the person's hands or shoulders.

- If the person to whom you are speaking has one "good" ear, always stand on that side when you speak. Do not be afraid to ask a person who has an obvious hearing loss whether his or her hearing is better in one ear than in the other.

- Facial expressions are important clues to meaning.

- In conversation with a person who is very deaf, jot down key words on paper.

- Many people who are hearing impaired are sensitive about their disability and will pretend to understand you even when they do not. Repeat your meaning in different words until it gets across.

- Teach family members that they do not have to exclude the persons who are hearing impaired from all forms of entertainment involving speech or music. Even persons who are profoundly deaf can feel rhythm, and many are good and eager dancers.

- Use common sense and tact in determining which of these suggestions apply to particular persons.

Adapted from Nursing Assessment and Promotion Strategies through the Lifespan *(6th ed), by R. B. Murray & J. P. Zentner, 1997, Norwalk, CT: Appleton & Lange.*

be the long latent period some cancers require before appearing; for example, skin cancer due to sun exposure may appear 40 years after exposure (Sarna, 1995). Yet another theory regarding increased cancer rates in elders is that aging changes the immune system, resulting in a decreased ability of the elderly body to detect and eliminate cancer cells.

The community health nurse's role remains as advocate, educator, support, and resource person. The nurse holds a unique place in this relationship with the client, family, and those resources needed to maintain optimal health in the client.

Ageism

Ageism is a major social risk for the older adult. This term refers to discrimination based on age. Older adults are characterized as senile, useless, dependent, and sick (Jarvis, 1992). Although publicly denounced by gerontologists, ageism continues to affect society. There have been some advances in improving the image of older adults, but there is still a tendency, even among those who work with elders, to **homogenize** this population (Ferraro, 1992). This notion that all older individuals are essentially the same is a form of ageism and is more difficult to correct than blatant prejudice. Older people themselves are often as guilty of ageist attitudes as are younger adults (Tyler & Schuller, 1991). The medical profession is also guilty of ageist assumptions when making decisions about treatable conditions. Too often incontinence, memory changes, sexual dysfunction, or preoccupation with death are considered a normal result of aging and are either not treated or are not treated vigorously (Jecker, 1995).

Closely connected with ageism is the issue of independence. Although only 5% of older people are in institutions and only 10% show even mild to moderate memory loss, the misconception continues that old people are incompetent, sick, senile, and dependent on others to function successfully (Murray & Zentner, 1997). Because of the societal orientation to youth and the fast pace of today's world, older adults often feel they are not respected or valued. Without clear guidelines regarding their role in society, many older adults opt out and become dependent, relying on others to make decisions for them. One of the nurse's roles in caring for the older adult is to promote the client's abilities and potential and to assist in promoting optimal functioning.

When an elderly person becomes unable to remain at home because of the need for extensive nursing care, however, the community health nurse can be of great assistance in helping the family or individual choose a nursing home or convalescent care center. This is one of the most dreaded decisions a family makes regarding an elderly family member. Often, the family has maintained the client for years in an informal caretaking situation with some assistance from friends, home health agencies, and other organizations. Research shows that the caregiver burden contributes to an increased risk of institutionalization in the United States (McFall & Miller, 1992). When the decision is made, the caregivers need as much support and guidance during the transition as does the client.

Loss and Bereavement

The last social risk factor for the older adult is the risk of the death of a spouse or partner. This can occur in other life stages but is more common in older adulthood. Usually, bereavement does not permanently affect the health of an older adult, but it can produce physiological symptoms (Alford, 1995). Although suddenly single status disrupts established couple-based relationships, the changes can sometimes produce positive results. Relatives and friends may become closer and more supportive; a move to a smaller residence may involve the individual in more neighborhood socializing; and being alone may stimulate the client into making new contacts and broadening life interests.

Spirituality

The nurse is in a unique position to address spirituality with the older adult. Older adults often express a desire to discuss spiritual matters. More than religious affiliation or rituals, spirituality reaches the deeper aspects of an individual's capacity for love, hope, and meaning (Ebersole & Hess, 1994). A large number of elderly individuals see religion as a means of coping with life's difficulties and turn to their clergy and church community in times of need. Recognition of this aspect of a person's life is important.

Aging Successfully

Aging successfully is difficult to define. There is the **inner aspect of aging**, one's relationship and contentment with self, and the **outer** (or **social**) **aspect of aging**, one's relationship with society as one ages. Successful aging means to age in relative contentment and happiness (Lefrancois, 1996). No one theory of aging explains the process completely. Common theories are considered to represent only some of many possible patterns of aging. Some researchers prefer to look at successful aging with regard to the individual's personality makeup. Although there have been several definitions of personalities and how successfully or unsuccessfully they age, the emerging truism for personality and aging seems to be that older people become more of who they were (Sims et al., 1995). Persons continue to develop and grow, but personality characteristics are only emphasized, and drastic changes in basic personality are not made. The talkative, flexible, social personality will become more so in older age as appropriate to physical status and life situation. If the older adult is rigid, conservative, and opinionated, it is probable that those same traits were present in younger life, but to a lesser degree. Perhaps the younger individual sublimated these traits to make them more acceptable or less obvious than they are in old age.

This final stage of life, then, is the end of the life cycle when "one must come finally to terms with the self— knowing it and loving it reasonably well, and being ready to give it up" (Jarvis, 1992, p. 42).

HEALTHY RELATIONSHIPS

Each stage of growth and development has specific environmental needs above and beyond the common needs of all ages. Chapter 7 explores environment in more detail. The relationships in each developmental stage constitute important aspects of environment. These relation-

ships may be necessary to lesser degrees at some life stages and assume greater importance at other stages of life. These relationships are explored next.

The young adult begins to establish a social support group separate from family. The needs are for friends, potential mates, and coworkers in whose presence the individual can grow and mature. Beyond this circle of support is the older, mentoring individual who can assist in the growth process. The social community offers opportunities for education and expansion of interests. Worship is another area of support often first explored as a young adult.

Middle adults are the stable support of today's society. Their needs differ from those of younger adults, centering more on the greater society. Their circle of support, besides families of several generations, include friends with similar interests, professional contacts and coworkers, as well as acquaintances in the greater society of the state, nation, or world. They are likely to be mentors to younger adults and serve as support to a variety of worthy causes. Participation in worship is a common activity at this stage of life.

Because older adulthood is the time when major losses occur, it is vital that older adults have good social support in their personal environments. Family members who love and respect the older individual are important, especially when death and disease have decimated the circle of friends and perhaps taken one's spouse. A better quality of intergenerational interactions usually results in more satisfied elders (Harvey, Bond, & Greenwood, 1991). Often, grandchildren form special relationships with the elderly person and share activities that are very satisfying to both parties (Kennedy, 1992). Sibling relationships among older adults have not received enough attention, although for many older people, siblings are the only surviving support system (Moyer, 1992). Because the older-adult stage of life spans such diverse conditions and abilities, care must be taken to include an array of support

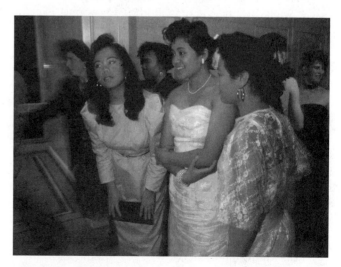

This group of young adult friends offer support to each other. Who are the nonfamily support individuals in your life? Besides your clients, to whom do you offer support? Photo courtesy of Kevin Fleming/Corbis.

systems for all older adults, from the young-old to the old-old.

Community health nurses operate within the environment of the client and must be aware of the importance of the relationships within that environment. They must be aware of all the issues that affect the well-being of clients and must take an interest in social issues, community concerns, and civic matters in addition to health-related issues.

THE NURSING PROCESS AND THE ADULT YEARS

The community health nurse provides care to adult clients in all three developmental stages. It is helpful to use the nursing process in addressing health and well-

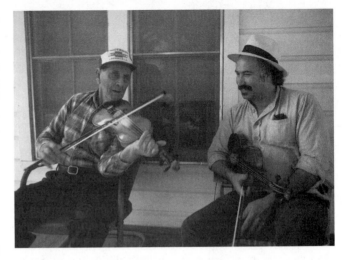

An older adult can serve as a mentor to younger adults.
Photo courtesy of Philip Gould/Corbis.

COMMUNITY NURSING VIEW

Pilar, a 55-year-old woman, comes to a blood pressure clinic operated by a community health nurse. She complains of vague headaches, feeling tired all the time, and having no energy. She has not had a menstrual period for two years and has occasional hot flashes and sweating. She recently began wearing bifocals and has had some trouble adjusting to them. She states she feels "blue" and uninterested in her usual activities, including sexual activity with her husband.

Pilar works for an insurance company in a sedentary job that is not particularly challenging. She does not exercise regularly: "Walks around the neighborhood now and then." She states that she loves to cook and misses having her two children home to cook for. The children are attending college some distance away. Because he is unable to safely live alone, her 87-year-old father recently moved in with her and her husband. Her father is on a restricted diet and cannot eat the type of food Pilar enjoys preparing, such as casseroles and meats and poultry with heavy sauces.

Nursing Considerations

ASSESSMENT
• In assessing this client, what data can be drawn from the interview to assist the nurse in the care plan?

• What additional questions might the nurse ask in order to formulate the nursing care plan?
• In what developmental stage is this client? Can you identify the developmental tasks she is trying to accomplish?
• In the review of the client's problems, which of her statements requires top priority? Why?

DIAGNOSIS
• Do any of this client's problems cluster around and pertain to a single nursing diagnosis?
• Can you identify four nursing diagnoses from the information presented in the case study?

OUTCOME IDENTIFICATION
• What outcomes can the nurse expect if the plan is successful?

PLANNING/INTERVENTIONS
• What should be the nurse's first step in forming a plan to assist this client?
• Identify interventions for each of the nursing diagnoses you have listed.

EVALUATION
• Identify evaluation methods that would enable the nurse to determine whether Pilar is succeeding or failing with regard to the nursing plan.

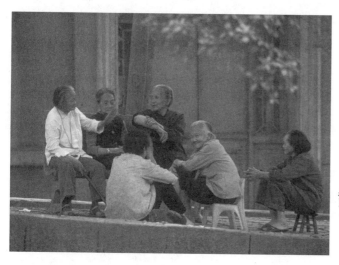

The support of friends and family is very important to the older adult, as often the spouse and many friends have died. Photo courtesy of Kevin R. Morris/Corbis

being and determining those nursing functions that are most common to each of the developmental stages of adulthood.

The nursing process contributes to the prevention of illness as well as the restoration and maintenance of health (Doenges, Moorhouse, & Burley, 1995). It is a scientific approach and requires the skills of assessment, problem identification or nursing diagnosis, planning, implementation, and evaluation. Although these terms are used separately, this process actually is a "continuous circle of thought and action" (Doenges et al., 1995, p. 3) that is an effective method of providing nursing care.

The nursing process provides the community health nurse with a scientific method for effectively planning and providing care for clients. When seen in the context of family and community, the client, by growing and developing through the adult years, offers a challenge to the nurse.

Key Concepts

- Several theories of growth and development must be considered because no one theory adequately explains the adult years.

- Adults in each stage of development—young, middle, and older—proceed through tasks and accomplish age-related skills before progressing to the next stage of adulthood.

- Particular risk factors and conditions apply to each life stage, including emotional, mental, physical, spiritual, and social risks. Some risk factors are present through all stages of adulthood.

- Healthy relationships in the adult years are a vital part of successful aging.

- The stages of adult development give nurses valuable information for applying the nursing process to young, middle, and older adults.

Frameworks for Assessing Families

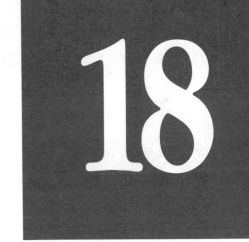

Janice E. Hitchcock, RN, DNSc

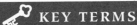
It is within the emotional connections family members have with each other that commitment to others, the capacity for shared intimacy, and personal well-being are nurtured.

—*Hanson & Boyd, 1996, p. vii*

COMPETENCIES

Upon completion of this chapter, the reader should be able to:

- Identify the difference between family as context and family as client.
- Recount definitions of family including a definition that encompasses the changing family structure.
- List a variety of family forms.
- Detail nursing theories that provide guidance for understanding families, including those of Neuman, King, Roy, and Rogers.
- Discuss social science theories that help to explain family dynamics, processes, and tasks, including developmental theory, systems theory, structural–functional framework, and interactional theory.
- Explain the contribution of family system theories to the understanding of the family.
- Describe theories that focus on the interaction between family and community.
- Discuss the difference between the nurse as caregiver and the family as caregiver to family members.
- Detail cultural aspects of the family and their impact on family life.
- Explain the importance of working in partnership with families.
- Delineate the dimensions of the nursing process—assessment, diagnosis, planning, intervention, and evaluation—as they apply to family nursing.

Families are society's most basic small group. Each person's perception of life and the world is the product of both interactions within the cultural milieu of family and the individual's innate patterns and characteristics. Until recently, most nurses had worked primarily in inpatient settings and with individuals rather than with the total family constellation. Much of the emphasis in nursing education has been on the individual rather than on the family or community. With the changes anticipated in health care, nursing will direct more of its energies toward work with families in home or community settings.

Gilliss (1993) describes two ways that nurses identify families. The first is family as context; the second is family as client. When families are treated as the context within which individuals are assessed, the emphasis is primarily on the individual, keeping in mind that he or she is a part of a larger system, the family **(family as context).** Conversely, when the nurse treats the family as a set of interacting parts and emphasizes assessment of the dynamics among these parts rather than the individual parts them-

KEY TERMS (Continued)

focal system	morphostasis	social environment
general systems theory	negentropy	structural–functional framework
genogram	network therapy	subsystems
hierarchy of systems	nuclear family	suprasystem
input	openness/closeness	surrogate mother
integrated bicultural family style	output	system
internal family structure	patterns	traditional family
macrosystem	physical environment	traditional-oriented nonresistive
marginalized family style	psychological environment	style
mesosystem	residual stimuli	transactional field theory
microsystem	rules	wider family
morphogenesis	separatist family style	

selves (family members), the family as a whole, rather than the individual members, becomes the client **(family as client).** The nurse must grasp the interacting aspects of the family, whether to understand the context within which the individual lives and to which he or she reacts or to work with the family as client.

The purpose of this chapter is to give the nurse direction, via the understanding of family theories, for family assessment, planning, intervention, and evaluation. Caring, both for families and in families, is explored as are **patterns** (family behaviors, beliefs, and values that together make up the uniqueness that is the family) and structure of the family in U.S. society; family system concepts; life cycle development; and variations on family forms and developmental patterns. The impact of culture on the family is also addressed. The reader also can expect to receive new insights into his or her own family system. Although much of this chapter is theoretical, it is important that nurses use theory in conjunction with an understanding of the subjective perspectives of families. The lived experience of the family must be the basis of care.

✺ REFLECTIVE THINKING ✺

Family Patterns

Perhaps the first time you became aware of your family's patterns occurred when, as a child, you visited a friend or relative and noticed the patterns and characteristics of this other family. Remember such an occasion now.

• Did the family eat foods that were different from those to which you were accustomed?

• How did parents and children interact?

• What were forbidden and permitted topics of conversation?

• What else about the family seemed different from life in your family?

DEFINITION OF THE FAMILY

Families are defined in many ways. Definitions of **traditional families** usually cite the presence of children, legal marriage, blood kinship bonds that include inheritance transfers ensuring intergenerational continuity, and a lifestyle that has its genesis in the family (Marciano & Sussman, 1991). The U.S. Bureau of the Census (1995) reflects this tradition, defining the **family** as "a group of two or more persons related by birth, marriage, or adoption and residing together in a household" (p. 6). However, this narrow definition does not address the many variations of family structures present in today's society. To address these changing family forms, Marciano (1991) has introduced the concept of **wider family**, a family that "emerges from lifestyle, is voluntary, and independent of necessary biological or kin connections" (p. 160). Wider families do not always share a common dwelling, although some do. Kin (those related by blood) families and wider families can coexist together. A wider family may be time limited and exist only to meet a particular need: for instance, a foster mother who cares for a child with AIDS. This concept of family accommodates such configurations as two divorced mothers and their children living together, gay or lesbian couples with or without children, group homes that may or may not provide individual living areas, some Big Sister/Big Brother relationships, and many self-help groups. In summary, a wider family is voluntary, unstructured, and family oriented; is not rule bound; and may be time limited. Craft and Willadsen (1992) offer a definition of family that encompasses this perspective:

> The family is a social context of two or more people characterized by mutual attachment, caring, long-term commitment, responsibility to provide individual growth, supportive relationships, health of members and of the unit, and maintenance of the organizational and system during constant individual, family, and societal change (p. 519).

This definition reflects the perspective of family to be presented in this text: It does not insist on or exclude blood kinship ties or the presence of children, and it acknowledges the subjective nature of family for many groups. Some other terms associated with definitions of the family and to which the literature frequently refers are as follows:

Nuclear family. Composed of husband, wife, and their immediate children (natural, adopted, or both).

Family of origin (or **orientation**). The family unit into which a person is born.

Family of procreation. The family created for the purpose of raising children.

Extended family. Traditionally, those members of the nuclear family and other blood-related persons, usually from family of origin (grandparents, aunts, uncles, cousins), called "kin." More recently, people who identify themselves as "family" but are not necessarily related by blood or through adoption. An example might be a group of lesbians and perhaps some male friends who have agreed to share in the responsibility of raising the child of one of their members.

Blended (or **binuclear**) **family.** The combination of two divorced families through remarriage.

Varieties of Family Forms

Until recently, the nuclear (traditional) family was considered the most common. Macklin (1987) defines the traditional family as a "legal, lifelong, sexually exclusive marriage between one man and one woman, with children, where the male is primary provider and ultimate authority" (p. 905). Terminology commonly used in conjunction with divorce and remarriage has negative connotations (e.g., stepchild, broken home, failed marriage, stepparent, exspouse), and members of families that have been generated through remarriage, called blended families, are not routinely accorded the courtesies afforded to members of the original nuclear family (e.g., invitations to open school night, weddings, and other family and community events).

Households with more than two adults living in intimate relationships or with homosexual couples are often denied legal rights that most citizens take for granted (e.g., insurance coverage, recognition as next of kin in health care situations). The historical bias toward viewing the nuclear family as the only legitimate form of family has led many health care workers and researchers to form negative stereotypes of other family forms and to treat individuals in other kinds of families in both subtly and overtly demeaning ways. Instead of working with the needs and perceptions of the family, they consider their task one of facilitating family adjustment to the system. Although social systems are slowly catching up with family changes, the daily experience of millions of children and adults often continues to be one of alienation.

Harway and Wexler (1996) encourage health professionals to look for the strengths and resources of nontraditional families rather than for their pathology. They propose a taxonomy of normative families that is not dependent on a traditional family perspective. The dimensions of their taxonomy are: biological relationship (both, one, or neither parent related), marital status (single, married, or cohabiting parents), sexual orientation (heterosexual, gay, or lesbian), and gender roles/employment status (traditional or nontraditional). When this perspective is used, all family forms become normative.

Studies point to the probability that families will continue to vary from the nuclear configuration. Aerts (1993) notes that, in addition to common differences such as single-parent and blended families, at the levels of social and legal considerations, at the very least, recent advances in reproductive technologies have created an artificial distinction between a **surrogate mother** (a woman who, for someone other than herself, carries a child conceived from an egg not always her own) and **biological mother** (a woman who gives birth to and raises her own children). The option to have a pregnancy via a surrogate mother leads to additional forms of family variation. A same- or opposite-sex couple may have a child that is

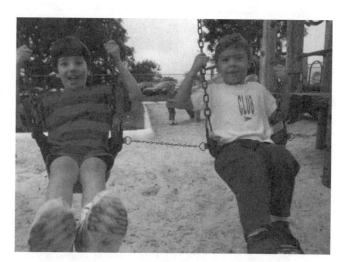

Through remarriage, these boys became members of a blended family.

conceived from their own or another person's or people's sperm and egg and nurtured in someone else's uterus. Such possibilities give rise to new considerations. For instance, problems can arise when the surrogate mother refuses to give up the child or when the growing child wants to know about his or her biological parents. In today's world, almost any imaginable combination of family form is possible and is practiced somewhere. Figure 18-1 lists some of the more common configurations.

Figure 18-1   Varieties of Family Forms

Legally married
Traditional nuclear
Binuclear or blended
- Co-parenting
- Joint custody
- One member of the original family remarried
- Both members of the original family remarried

Dual-career
Both in same household
Commuter

Adoptive

Foster

Voluntary childlessness

Unmarried
Never married
- Voluntary singlehood, with or without children
- Involuntary singlehood, with or without children
Cohabitation, with or without children
Same-sex relationship

Formally married
Widowed
Divorced
- Custodial parent
- Joint custody of children
- Noncustodial parent

Multi-adult household
Communes and intentional communities
Multilateral marriage, in which three or more people consider themselves to have a primary relationship with at least two other individuals in the group (Macklin, 1987)

Extramarital sex
- Swinging
- Sexually open marriage
- Coprimary relationships, in which one or both members maintain a primary relationship with at least two partners who may or may not know about the other (Macklin, 1987)
Home-sharing individuals, with or without children

Extended family (e.g., grandparents, parents, and children; adult children moving home; siblings living together, with or without partners or children)

Staples (1989) summarizes the expected trends for families for the next 25 years as follows:

Sexual relations will precede marriage: people will have a trial period of cohabitation before entering into marriage, and they will increasingly delay marriage until their late twenties or early thirties; the divorce rate will continue to increase, and remarriage will occur more slowly; couples will limit their families to one or two children; and the dual wage earner family will be the norm for almost all households (p. 167).

Her predictions are proving to be accurate. Thus, while many family options will be available, most individuals will continue to marry and bear children. Lesbians, more often than gay men, come to their relationships with children or give birth to children in the context of the homosexual relationship. Hare and Richards (1993) found that when one or both partners bring children into a lesbian relationship, lesbian families resemble heterosexual step-families. They also noted that children born in the context of a lesbian relationship resembled those born in the context of a nuclear family. If such a marriage/partnership dissolves, the children of the lesbian partners may go on to spend most of their lives in single-parent or blended families.

Such family changes create many issues. For instance, divorce has several stages. Before the actual divorce is the decision to divorce. Then the breakup of the system begins, first with discussion and planning of the divorce and then with the separation. The final stage is the actual divorce and all the related legal considerations (Danielson, Hamel-Bissell, & Winstead-Fry, 1993). Figure 18-2 identifies some of the issues that must be addressed in blended families.

DECISION MAKING

Domestic Partnerships

Some counties in the United States have domestic partnership registration bills that allow any couple living together in a committed relationship, including same-sex couples, to register as domestic partners. These partners have three specific rights: (1) the right to visit each other in the hospital, (2) the right to will property to one another, and (3) the right to conservatorship if one partner becomes incapacitated (Associated Press, 1994). Without these assurances, unmarried people, particularly gay men and lesbians, who cannot legally marry, may face difficulties related to their partners' not being considered next of kin. For instance, a gay man may lose all access to his partner during severe illness and may be ineligible to inherit when his partner dies.

- Should unmarried people in a committed relationship be allowed to legally register their partnership?

Figure 18-2   Major Issues in Remarriage

1. Initial Family Issues

- Name for the new parent
- Affection for the new parent and the absent parent (conflict between biological parent and stepparent)
- Loss of the natural parent (grief for the previous family structure)
- Unrealistic belief in instant love of new family members
- Fantasy about the old family structure (reconciliation fantasy)

2. Developing Family Issues

- Discipline by the stepparent
- Confusion over family roles
- Sibling conflict
- Competition for time
- Extended kinship network
- Sexual conflicts as result of more sexually charged atmosphere of the new family
- Changes over time (at least two years needed for basic remarriage reorganization)
- Exit and entry of children (visits to noncustodial parents [exit] and returns to custodial home [entry])

3. Feelings about Self and Others

- Society's concept of the remarriage family
- Familial self-concept
- Individual self-concept (whether person feels an accepted part of the family)

4. Adult Issues

- Effects of parenting on the new marital relationship
- Financial concerns
- Continuing adult conflict
- Competition of the noncustodial parent

From "Twenty Major Issues in Remarriage Families" by W. M. Walsh, 1992, Journal of Counseling and Development, 70, *pp. 709–715. Copyright 1992 by American Counseling Association. Used with permission.*

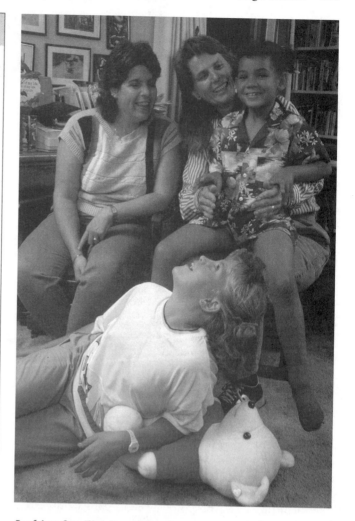

Lesbian families have been found to resemble heterosexual stepfamilies. Photo courtesy of Shelley Gazin/Corbis.

family processes. There are also several theories that provide insight into the interrelationship between the family and the larger community. These theories are important to understand because they give direction to the nursing care of families. Although no one theory completely addresses all dimensions of the family or fully explains family dynamics and behaviors, knowing the basic precepts of these theories helps the nurse to effectively assess families.

THEORETICAL FOUNDATIONS IN FAMILY NURSING

All families share certain characteristics. Every family can be characterized as a social system with certain structures and functions that move through recognizable stages. A number of theories in nursing, social sciences, and family systems theory give insight into these family dynamics and

Nursing Theories

Some nursing theories and conceptual models address the family either directly or indirectly. Although most nursing theories began with a focus on the individual, with the family being viewed as only a part of the client's context, some have enlarged their conceptual bases to include the family as client.

Neuman's System Model

Neuman's system model "is philosophically consistent with the perspectives of a family systems approach and

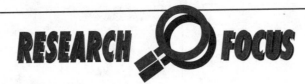

Children Raised by Lesbian Couples

STUDY PROBLEM/PURPOSE

The qualitative purpose of this study was to examine father and lesbian involvement with children in terms of the contexts of the children's birth/adoption" (p. 250), the hypothesis being that paternal involvement and parental involvement of the lesbian partner would differ depending on the context of the child's birth/adoption.

Qualitative questions posed were: Does the mother's perception of the father's involvement or of the partner's feelings for the child vary with the context of the child's birth/adoption and Does the mother's perception of the father's involvement or of the partner's feelings for the child vary with the child's gender?

METHODS

Generated were qualitative data from open-ended questions developed by the researchers and asking the subjects to discuss the involvement of the partner and father (or surrogate father) in the life of each child. Partner involvement was also explored. A second interview, conducted by telephone, asked for in-depth information regarding the father's and the lesbian partner's responsibilities and participation in the lives of the children.

FINDINGS

The family context into which a child is born or adopted is an important variable. Lesbian families resemble heterosexual stepfamilies, although the lesbian partner is in a different position from a heterosexual partner because of both lack of social recognition and homophobia. Children born in the context of a lesbian relationship resembled those born in nuclear families. When compared with heterosexual single mothers, lesbian mothers have more congenial relations with ex-spouses and more regularly include men in their children's lives. Fathers were perceived by mothers as being more involved with sons than with daughters. Partners felt significantly closer to boys than to girls. There was difficulty in finding the appropriate words to describe the partner's relationship with the child.

IMPLICATIONS

Practitioners should be sensitive both to the history of each woman in the relationship, particularly as the history relates to parenthood, and to assigning language to label relationships between child and partner. Practitioners should demonstrate understanding by inviting both women to conferences, learning about the benefits and drawbacks of known and unknown donors, and finding out about lesbian family support groups.

SOURCE

From "Children Raised by Lesbian Couples: Does Context of Birth Affect Father and Partner Involvement?" by J. Hare and L. Richards, 1993, Family Relations, 42, *pp. 249–255. Copyright 1993 by National Council on Family Relations.*

can be expanded to include the family as a client" (Tomlinson & Anderson, 1995, p. 133). The ways that each family member expresses his- or herself influence the whole and create the basic structure of the family. All transactions take place vis-à-vis this structure and are directed toward keeping the structure stable as it moves between stability (wellness) and instability (illness). The major goal of the nurse, therefore, is to help stabilize the family system within its environment (Neuman, 1983). Tomlinson and Anderson, who have developed a family health systems model that operationalizes Neuman's model, note that in the future, a family system focus will become necessary as nursing interventions are increasingly directed toward families rather than individuals.

King's Open Systems Model

As do most nursing theorists, King views the family as context (environment) but also recognizes it as client. She believes that nurses are partners with families (King,

1981). Her theory of goal attainment is useful for nurses in helping families set goals and solve problems (Ackermann, Brink, Clanton, Jones, et al., 1994). Mutual goal setting requires decision making, which King (1994) sees as a collaborative process "between nurse and nurse, nurse and physician, nurse and family, and allied health workers" (King, 1994, p. 31).

REFLECTIVE THINKING

Family and Nursing Theory

• Choose a nursing theory. How would you explain your family in terms of that theory?

• Do some theories or models fit your family life better than others, or do they all seem to have relevance to your life experiences?

Perspectives...

Insights of a Nursing Faculty Member

The community health nursing (CHN) practicum is a challenging course to teach and, from a student perspective, a difficult course to take because of the generalist nature of this practice setting. Students often comment on the difficult nature of the course and the amorphous feeling of being held accountable for diverse content areas. I also remembered this feeling as a nursing student and as a practitioner in CHN. Therefore, as a clinical professor in CHN, I decided to examine this problem and try a new way to facilitate student learning.

I believed the CHN practicum would be enhanced by using a nursing theory, as it would provide more structure and parameters to the course. As an educator, I had participated in incorporating nursing theory into classes and curriculum design. However, I had never employed a non-eclectic approach of using one nursing theorist in a course or curriculum. I wanted to use just one theorist because I believed using an eclectic approach or expecting students to use a theorist of their choice would increase the difficulty of this course.

Five years ago I began using the theory of Imogene King in teaching the CHN practicum. My rationale for using King's theory of goal attainment was three-fold: (1) Goal attainment and quality outcomes have become almost synonymous in the health care field; (2) King's theory provides a framework for looking at both the dynamics of interacting systems and mutual interactions or transactions between client, client's family, and the health care system; and (3) King assumes that the client has the right to self-determination. All of the above are consistent with principles and concepts in CHN practice, and all three provide parameters for the practitioner. By using Kings's theory, the student is provided with a perspective from which to practice. The theoretical base for nursing process demonstrates a way for students to interact purposefully with clients. The student learns that the theory involves a process focused on the goal or outcome that is an effective way of measuring nursing care.

The metaparadigm of Person has special significance for students in the CHN practicum. Fre-

quently, values of client and student conflict, and priorities for prevention and promotion activities differ. For example, the student, wanting to educate about healthful living and to see change occur, may not understand why a mother will not keep medical appointments for her children, whereas the mother is more concerned about how she is going to feed and clothe her children. Inherent in King's theory is a basic respect for the capacity of human beings to think, acquire and use knowledge, make choices, and select courses of action (King, 1986). By using King's model, the student incorporates these beliefs about the rights of clients. Students become partners in health care with their clients and respect clients' decisions.

Feedback from the students has been very positive. They find that they can more easily organize their thinking about client assessment, planning, and interventions. They also use King's framework to evaluate their work and as a reminder to focus on client needs and the implications of client interactions and transactions. As one student said, the theory acknowledges "clients as able to set goals and make decisions about their care, which are right for them, without creating value judgments over what is 'right or wrong'" (Baker, 1996, p. 20).

—*Laurel Freed, RN, CPHN, MSN*

Insights of a Nursing Student

I was introduced to King's theory of nursing as a senior student in the RN–BSN program at Sonoma State University and began to use the theory in my nursing practice during my community health nursing practicum. Applying this theory to my practice helped in organizing my care and clinical decision making. It also freed me to provide the education, instructional support, resourcing, and referrals that were truly going to make a difference in my clients' lives. It was not just a "Band-Aid" approach, but one wherein clients participated and were empowered to make decisions regarding their lives and health and the lives and health of their families.

Continued

Continued

As nurses, we must remember that our clients are biopsychosocial, spiritual individuals, rather than a series of tasks that must be completed in a given period of time. They are sentient beings, bringing with them pasts full of experiences and views of the future that are uniquely their own. These experiences and views will color the present choices they make. An experience I had illustrates this concept and how the application of King's theory of nursing helped in the establishment of a therapeutic relationship with a young developing family.

The referral came from an OB/GYN physician at the county hospital. He was concerned that Susan was not keeping her routine OB appointments. She had been drinking prior to her last appointment, and the physician had arranged for her to be driven home. She was at approximately 32 weeks' gestation with twins. She was 24 years old, para III, gravida I, unmarried, but living with her boyfriend. Her young son was almost 2 years old.

Upon attempting a home visit at the address noted on the referral, I found that the family had recently moved, leaving a large pile of debris behind. The next week another referral came from the county hospital as a result of the premature birth of female twins at 35 weeks' gestation. I was able to locate the mother at the new address noted on the hospital referral. They had no telephone. The first visit was extremely strained. Susan came to the door of the large house in front of the studio apartment where she, her boyfriend, and young son lived. She did not invite me in or volunteer any personal information, although she did briefly respond to questions. I introduced myself and offered community health assistance in preparing for bringing her twins home from the hospital. I told her I would visit with her again the next week and asked her to be thinking of questions she might have or areas where she would like my help. She immediately responded that she needed assistance with obtaining car seats in which to bring home the girls. I was elated! This was a good start. We had developed mutual goal number one!

As the weeks went on and the infants came home, she showed no evidence of drinking, and we continued to explore the problems of parenthood, birth control, cramped living space, lack of transportation, and available educational opportunities. We set several mutual goals. She liked the infants to be weighed and measured. It was encouraging to see their weekly growth. She needed respite care for her toddler son. We set goals around finding him a Head Start program and arranging transportation for him to get there and back home. Toward the end of my semester with her, we even began exploring ways for her to obtain her high-school graduate equivalency diploma.

During our visits, it was important for me to take cues from Susan and to be sure that I was not imposing my agenda on her. The goals we set had to be ones that she valued and that would empower her to take charge of her own decision making, for both herself and her children. As a nurse, I could guide her with information, but, ultimately, the choices she made were her own. Without this approach, I believe I would not have gotten a foot in the door, much less made any permanent difference in this young family's life.

This example illustrates on multiple levels the natural fit of King's theory of nursing in a community health setting. It shows use of her concepts of interaction, transaction, and mutual goal setting and demonstrates the interrelatedness of personal, interpersonal, and social systems. The use of King's theory in community health nursing helps to organize and guide nursing decisions along the continuum of care and facilitates recognition of the client's right and responsibility to actively participate in the decision-making process.

—*Deborah Baker, RN, BSN*

Roy's Adaptation Model

Roy (1983) believes that the family can be the unit of analysis and the adaptive system that is assessed. Studies have supported this assertion (Blue, Brubaker, Fine, Kirsch, et al., 1994). Enhancement or modification of the **focal stimuli** (factors that precipitate an adaptive response), **contextual stimuli** (all other factors that contribute to the behavior), and **residual stimuli** (factors that may affect behavior but for which effects are not

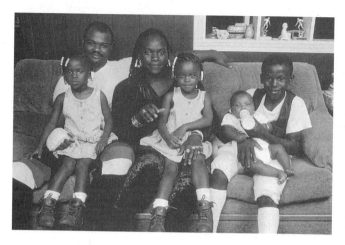

(A)

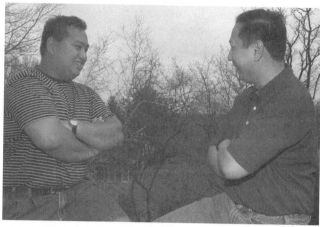

(B) *Courtesy of Laura Dwight/Corbis.*

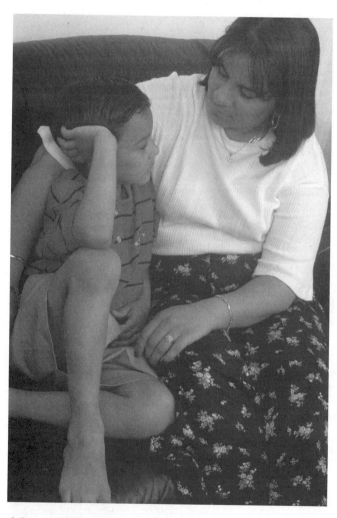

(C)

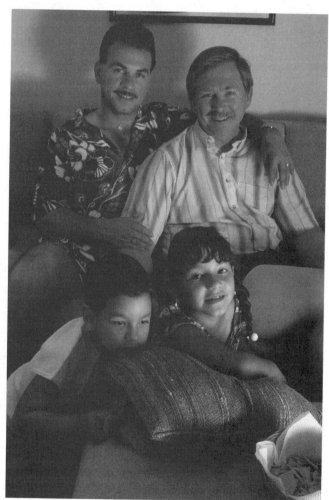

(D) *Courtesy of Shelly Gazin/Corbis.*

Different family configurations.

validated) promotes adaptation of the family system. For example, the nurse's assessment of a family's coping skills and the environmental context within which the family faces the death of a member provides the data needed to facilitate a positive adaptation to the changes engendered by the crisis.

Rogers' Life Process Model

Rogers' (1992) concepts of integrality (the continuous, mutual human field and environmental field process), resonancy (continuous change from lower- to higher-frequency wave patterns in human and environmental fields), and helicy (the continuous, innovative, unpredictable, increasing diversity of human and environmental field patterns) can be used to describe the family as well as the individual. She describes the family as an "irreducible, pandimensional, negentropic [see Figure 18-5] family energy field" (Falco & Lobo, 1995, p. 240). Thus, the energy generated by family dynamics influences all family members. Family members learn from one another in ways that are unique to that family.

Social Science Theories

A number of theories that come out of social science research help explain families. For purposes of this text, four will be examined: developmental, general systems, structural–functional, and interactional. When using these theories as frameworks for nursing care, the nurse must take into account cultural and ethnic differences that may be present. For instance, the developmental tasks identified by the theorists do not take into account the impact on 4- to 8-year-old girls (including the lifelong effects on their familial relationships) of the ritual of female genital mutilation. This rite, practiced primarily in Africa, is practiced by some immigrants from African countries who live in the United States (Allgeier & Allgeier, 1995).

Developmental Theory

Developmental theory, also known as the life cycle approach, purports that families evolve through typical developmental stages and experience growth and development much in the same way as do individuals: Each stage is characterized by specific issues and tasks. The ways that tasks at each stage are resolved help determine the family's capability for handling the challenges of the next stage.

The life cycle approach is useful because it assists the nurse in planning client care that is family oriented and appropriate to the family's stage of development. Perhaps the best-known formulation of the developmental stages comes from Duvall (1977; Duvall & Miller, 1985). Each stage has certain requisite tasks that must be completed before movement to the next stage is possible. Her model has limited value, however, because it presupposes a two-parent nuclear family and begins with marriage. Her perspective maintains that the nuclear family is the norm

and that most young adults marry in their early twenties before or instead of developing a career of their own. Life cycle changes are linked primarily to child-rearing activities. Today, the majority of family forms do not fit this configuration.

In the past, women moved from their families of origin directly to marriage. If there was a break between the two, women worked only while waiting to marry. Now, women often begin their careers before marriage and continue them after the birth of children (Rubin & Riney, 1994). Child-rearing today occupies less than half of the adult life span prior to old age (Carter & McGoldrick, 1989) such that child-rearing is no longer the central focus of the life cycle. Today's women must think about career goals in ways that past generations of women never even considered. This change in life situation has prompted women to insist on a new phase in the life cycle, that "phase in which the young adult leaves the parent's home, establishes personal goals, and starts a career" (p. 11). Carter and McGoldrick describe six stages of the family life cycle that take into account the reality of today's young adult. Table 18-1 compares Duvall and Miller's (1985) and Carter and McGoldrick's (1989) stages of family development and lists the accompanying tasks of each stage.

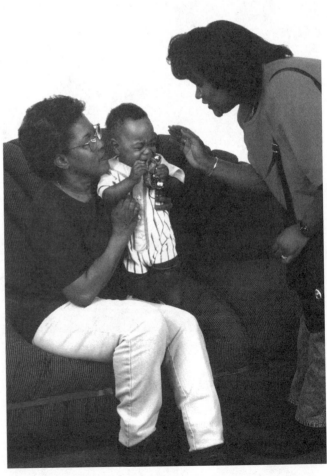

As this woman comforts her son, she must balance the tug of war between home life, career, and finding time for herself. Photo courtesy of Laura Dwight/Corbis.

Table 18-1 Comparison of Duvall and Miller, Carter and McGoldrick Family Life Cycle Stages and Tasks

STAGES		TASKS
DUVALL AND MILLER (1985)	**CARTER AND McGOLDRICK (1989)**	
No stage identified, although Duvall considers this the time of "being launched."	1. The unattached young adult	Successful separation of parent and young adult from one another
1. The beginning family or the stage of marriage	2. The newly married couple	Committing to a new family system
2. Childbearing families	3. Families with young children	Accepting new members into the system
3. Families with preschool children		
4. Families with school-age children		
5. Families with teenagers	4. Families with adolescents	Allowing the children independence through boundary modification
6. Families launching young adults	5. Launching children	Accepting many exits or entrances into the family
7. Middle-age parents (empty nest up to retirement)		
8. Retirement to death of both spouses	6. Families in later life	Accepting shifting generational roles and death

Adapted from Family Nursing: Theory and Practice *(4th ed., pp. 83) by M. M. Friedman, 1998, Stamford: CT: Appleton & Lange;* Families in Health and Illness: Perspectives on Coping and Intervention *by C. B. Danielson, B. Hamel-Bissell, & P. Winstead-Fry, 1993, St. Louis, MO: Mosby-Yearbook;* Marriage and Family Development *(6th ed.) by E. M. Duvall & B. C. Miller. Copyright © 1985 by Harper & Row. Reprinted by permission of Addison-Wesley Educational Publishers, Inc.; and* Overview: The Changing Family Life Cycle, *by B. Carter & M. McGoldrick. © 1989 by Allyn & Bacon. Adapted by permission.*

Wallerstein (1995, 1996) and Wallerstein and Blakeslee (1995), from Wallerstein's research designed to "illuminate the interior domains of happy marriages" (Wallerstein, 1995, p. 640), suggest psychological tasks that couples must address early in marriage and again during developmental milestones of their lives together. These tasks are stated here in the form of questions that the nurse can use when assessing the psychological health of the family. Each one is then briefly discussed.

1. Has the couple separated psychologically from their families of origin and begun to "create a new and dif-

ferent kind of connectedness that will maintain the generational ties" (Wallerstein, 1995, p. 642)? Women tend to have a more difficult time separating from their families of origin. Particularly if the woman is a child of divorce, there is often overdependence of the mother on the daughter and resulting guilt, compassion, and love that cements the two together. Dysfunctional family dynamics also generate guilt about separation. While a connectedness should remain between parents and adult children, it must be redefined together by the couple. These issues reemerge with pregnancy and the arrival of children and at the time of the death of a parent.

2. Is the couple able to build a marital identity? The task is to develop a sense of "we-ness." The partners identify not only with each other but also with the marriage. They create an empathy with one another whereby they listen to and are concerned about each other's needs. At the same time, the partners must maintain autonomy and set boundaries to allow themselves private and protected space. We-ness, then, does not mean merging with one another. There is a continued tension between togetherness and autonomy, and differentness is acknowledged and welcomed.

೧೦ REFLECTIVE THINKING ೧೦

Family Development

• Did you have an opportunity to live and learn as a single young adult, or did you move directly into a committed relationship? How have life choices in this regard affected your life?

• How well do you think you and your family have completed your family tasks of development?

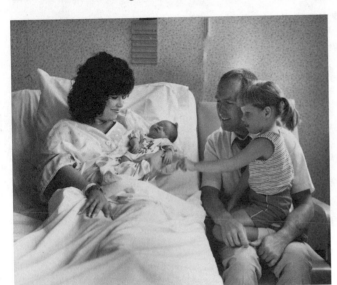

Often, a baby brings the family together. Photo courtesy of Ed Eckstein/Corbis.

3. Have the partners established a sexual life as a couple? Partners need to develop their own patterns that gratify both people, restore the core relationship, renew love, and counter the stresses and disappointments of life. The couple's sex life is the most vulnerable part of the relationship because it is "uniquely sensitive to events and mood changes that originate in all the other domains of individual and family life" (Wallerstein & Blakeslee, 1995, p. 223), such as work, childbirth, responsibilities to children, illness, and fatigue.

4. Is the marriage a zone of safety and nurturance, where the partners can express all the dimensions of feelings and experience aging and being human? Development of this safe place involves working out that which is unsafe as well as coming to understand and accept one another: "Learning to disagree and to stand one's ground without fear of dire consequences" (Wallerstein, 1996, p. 224) is important. Trusting one another is crucial.

5. Can the couple expand to psychologically accommodate children and at the same time safeguard their own private sphere? The couple must work to keep their own relationship alive. The parents' inner psychological and emotional lives are forever changed when the dyad becomes a triad with the birth of a baby. The couple must face their internal conflicts and make room for the child yet not allow the child to take over the marriage (Wallerstein & Blakeslee, 1995).

6. Has the couple built a relationship that is fun and interesting for them? Boredom can debilitate a relationship, as can constant serenity. A certain tension is necessary to prevent tedium, but not to the degree of generating anxiety.

7. Is the couple able to confront and master life crises and maintain the strength of the marital bond during adversity? There are several dimensions of coping with crisis. First, the partners must realistically acknowledge and think about the consequences to self and other family members in order to make rational plans. They must also protect one another from blame and self-blame. Another important dimension is keeping perspective by letting in some pleasure and humor so that the crisis does not totally dominate. Equally important is making a strong effort to keep destructive impulses from getting out of control. It is important to recognize that the impulses are responses to the crisis. Finally, it is important that the partners intervene at an early stage, when the potential for a crisis is first seen (Wallerstein & Blakeslee, 1995).

8. Is the couple able to nurture and comfort each other? Partners need to be able to accurately assess the cause of each other's suffering and make genuine efforts to relieve or head off that suffering. It is important to provide for a partner's dependency needs and help bolster battered self-esteem (Wallerstein & Blakeslee, 1995).

9. Is the couple able to maintain a "vision of the other that combines early idealizations with a firm grasp of the present reality" (Wallerstein, 1995, p. 649)? An important way to mute the disappointments and rage inherent in all close relationships is to maintain the ability to associate the past with the present. This ability increases in importance over time.

Although there seems to be a beginning and an end to the family life cycle (i.e., beginning with leaving home and ending with death), it is important to remember the continuity that characterizes families. Among some families, behavior is influenced by belief in life after death. Others believe that people live on through the acts they commit in life. Young adults are part of a family with a long ancestral history; the couple's children constitute the couple's link with the future. The interaction and complementarity that exist between the different generations constitute another set of factors that contribute to the patterns, behaviors, and relationships in the contemporary family.

The complementary nature of the **developmental tasks** (the work that must be completed at each stage of development before movement to the next stage is possible) of the different generations makes it useful to conceptualize family as a three-generation system moving through time. Combrinck-Graham (1985) describes a family life spiral whereby the life cycle is not seen as linear (see Figure 18-3). She defines death as a life change event rather than a life cycle event, acknowledging that death can happen at any time during the life cycle. She notes that life cycle events in different generations frequently happen concurrently. For example, the middle years of childhood occur at the same time that parents are settling down in marriage and that grandparents are planning for retirement. Marriage courtship generally occurs during the middle adulthood of parents and late

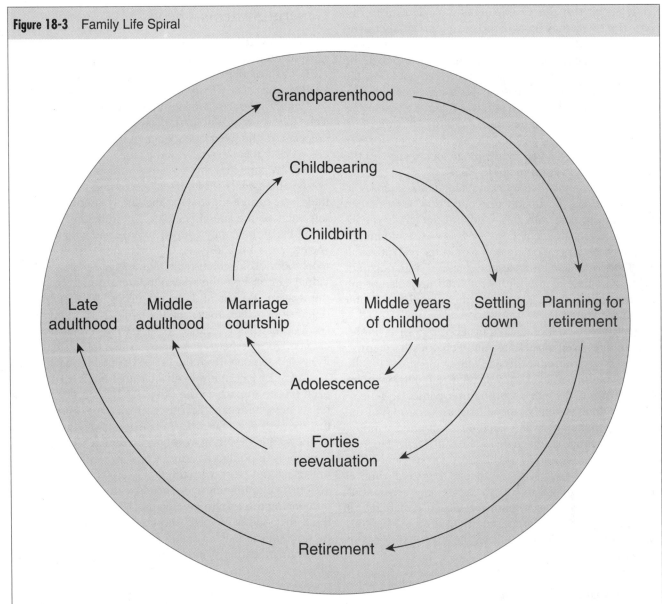

Figure 18-3 Family Life Spiral

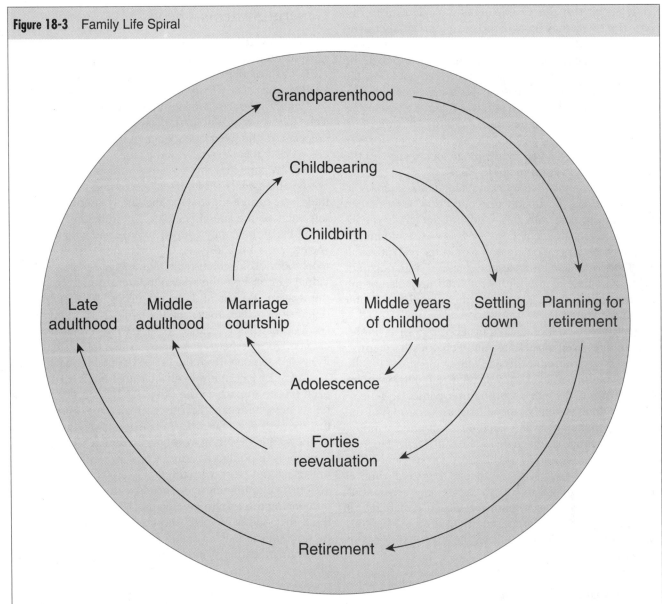

Grandparenthood

Childbearing

Childbirth

Late adulthood | Middle adulthood | Marriage courtship | Middle years of childhood | Settling down | Planning for retirement

Adolescence

Forties reevaluation

Retirement

From "A Developmental Model for Family Systems," by L. Combrinck-Graham, 1985, Family Process, 24, *pp. 139–150. Copyright 1985 by Family Process. Reprinted by permission of Family Process, Inc.*

adulthood of grandparents. When a child begins life, the roles of parent and grandparent emerge. The first two phases tend to distance the generations because each member is working on his or her own changes. The third phase, which involves childbirth, tends to bring families closer together, however.

Resolution of Developmental Tasks

The degree to which developmental tasks are successfully resolved by the family in different generations affects the functional and dysfunctional aspects of family life. Anxiety is generated when developmental tasks are resolved poorly; this anxiety is cumulative over generations in a family and, like heavy baggage, is carried from one generation to the next. Anxiety within the family is a continuous drain on the energy available for meeting the

challenges of family life. Dysfunctional perceptions and behavior perpetuate. For example, a family for which pregnancy and birth have been problematic may discover during the process of examining its history that there is a

🌀 REFLECTIVE THINKING 🌀

Life Cycle Events

• What has been your experience with life cycle events? Did they bring your family closer together or move it more apart?

• Did the birth of a child bring your family closer together?

family secret that the grandparents are reluctant to discuss. The secret may involve the great grandmother, who had a child before she was married and who was ostracized by her family and the community. Even though the family members of ensuing generations did not know the details of the traumatic incident, the anxiety generated by the event was passed down and was felt in different ways by the women during pregnancy and birth. Difficult labor, excessive bleeding, or sickness during pregnancy or crises in the family when a member is pregnant are some of the ways this phenomenon might manifest.

When a family is experiencing simultaneous crises in two generations, the anxiety generated may be more than the family can deal with at one time. If the family is conceptualized as a large emotional web, it is easier to understand how reverberations in one part of the web affect all the other parts. For instance, the death of a grandparent at the same time as the birth of a child may disrupt the closeness of the three generations and manifest at a later time in the life cycle.

Predictable developmental transitions as well as unpredictable life events such as untimely death, divorce, severe illness, war, and the like, all create stress for the family. The stress level in a particular family involves stressful events that are occurring in a particular generation over time as well as those that are occurring in the different generations at the same time. An understanding of the interactions between these stressful events can help explain why a seemingly small stress in one generation (e.g., a child's starting school) can lead to great disruption in the system if there is intense stress between generations (e.g., serious illness in a grandparent and remarriage of and relocation to a different state by a divorced parent). Stress and dysfunction in family life are considered in greater detail in Chapter 19.

Developmental Theory and Adoption

Adoption is another aspect of family development having certain phases, tasks, and emotional issues that must be addressed (Rosenberg, 1992). Birth parents, adoptive parents, and adoptees each have their own developmental tasks. Birth parents must make a decision to give up the child, prepare for the adoption, and relinquish the child for adoption. Next, they must resume their lives and mourn the loss of the child. Later, they may decide to search for the child, allow themselves to be found by the child, or finally accept their loss with tranquillity. Adoptive parents must first make the decision to adopt and go through the adoption process. Once they receive the child, they must accept the new member into the family. They then deal with adoptive issues throughout the life of the child, from acknowledging the adoption to considering finding the biological parents. Adoptees must separate from their biological parents and bond with their adoptive parents. They, too, deal with adoptive issues throughout life and must come to terms with whether to seek out their biological parents. With their own family of procreation, they must also decide whether to disclose their adoptive status.

General Systems Theory

General systems theory, also called cybernetics, was introduced nearly 50 years ago by Ludwig vonBertalanffy (1950) to describe the way units interact with larger and smaller units. The theory is used here to explain the way the family interacts with its members and with society. This theory is useful in family assessment because it emphasizes the interdependence of the family's parts and asserts both that the whole of the family is greater than the sum of its parts and that whatever affects the family as a whole affects each of its parts. According to this theory, then, one cannot understand the family simply by knowing each of the members. The interrelationship of the members of the family with each other and with the larger society must be addressed. As originally conceived, systems theory is mechanistic in that it suggests that an individual can observe the system in interaction from outside the system. Becvar and Becvar (1996) present another dimension, which they call "cybernetics of cybernetics" (p. 75), that has relevance for nurses in interaction with clients. This perspective emphasizes that the system (family) is not separate from the observer (nurse), who is also a system. In fact, there is no objective observer because each has an impact on the other. There is a mutual connectedness between the observer and the observed so that the system is really the "interaction of the two systems as they both exist within a larger context" (p. 75). This concept is important because it highlights the notion that nurses cannot work with the family system (or any other system) without being influenced by the system and also influencing the system (see Figure 18-4). It is a fallacy to think that one is "seeing" the family objectively. Nurses must recognize that "meaning is derived from the relation between individuals and elements as each defines the other. . . . Responsibility or power exists only as a bilateral process, with each individual and element participating in the creation of a particular behavioral reality" (p. 64). This

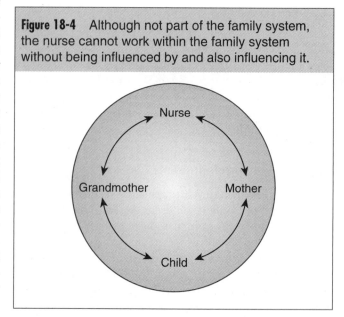

Figure 18-4 Although not part of the family system, the nurse cannot work within the family system without being influenced by and also influencing it.

perspective is consistent with Martha Rogers' (1990) theory, which characterizes human–environment transactions as a continuous repatterning of both humans and environment. Figure 18-5 lists definitions of the major components of systems theory as applied to families.

Structural–Functional Conceptual Framework

Families can also be understood in terms of their patterns of interaction, which suggest their basic structure and organization, as in the **structural–functional framework. Family structure** refers to family organization, arrangements of family units and the relationship of family units to one another. Wright and Leahey (1994) identify three dimensions of family structure: **internal family structure** (family composition, gender, rank order, subsystems, and boundaries), **external family structure** (extended family and larger systems), and **contextual family structure** (ethnicity, race, social class, religion, and environment). **Family functions** are interdependent with structure. They have to do with the ways individuals behave in relation to one another. Family functions are discussed in Chapter 19. Although the structural–functional approach does not address the importance of growth and change within a family over time, it more fully explains the relationship between family and environment than does developmental theory.

Family Interactional Theories

Family interactional theories focus primarily on the way that family members relate to the family and on internal family dynamics. These dynamics, which are further discussed in Chapter 19, consist of role-playing, status relations, communication patterns, decision making, coping patterns, and socialization. This approach, while useful in assessing and explaining these dimensions, is limited because it does not take into account the way the family interfaces with society.

Family Systems Theories

Family systems theories, which arise from sociology and psychology, are related to general systems theory, the structural–functional framework, and developmental theory. But family systems theories tend to focus on ways to change "dysfunctional" families (Whall, 1991). Whall identifies three therapeutic approaches. In the first, Haley proposes approaching the family as a unit. He emphasizes "the need for discovering the social situation which makes the problem possible" (p. 323). He considers the "family a living and somewhat open system that must accommodate growth needs" (p. 323).

Minuchin's approach is directed more toward open systems (Whall, 1991) and family structural concerns. He believes that the individual is influenced by and influences constantly recurring sequences of interaction; the

individual is reflective of the family system of which he or she is a part; stress in one part of the system affects other parts of the system (see Figure 18-6); and changes in family structure contribute to changes in the behavior of individuals within a given system.

Finally, Framo, as discussed in Whall (1991), is interested in the way the past affects the present. His is a closed-system perspective, the focus being on the way that family history affects the family in all of its facets. Family environment is not extensively addressed.

Much research is still needed to identify ways that family systems theories can be utilized in nursing practice. At present, the theories that originated in the social sciences (developmental, systems, structural–functional, and interactional) continue to offer the best guidance for the community health nurse in the provision of health care.

Interaction between the Family and the Social System outside the Family

Three approaches provide focus primarily on interactions between the family and the larger community. They are the ecological approach, network therapy, and the transactional field approach (Spiegel, 1982).

Ecological Approach

The **ecological approach** incorporates developmental, systems, and situational perspectives. This theoretical perspective emphasizes the interrelationship of these dimensions. Bronfenbrenner (1977) has delineated the ecology of human behavior. The **ecosystem** is composed of four systems. The first is the **microsystem**, which is the immediate setting within which the person fulfills his or her roles (family, school, business, and the like). The next system is the **mesosystem**, which is the interrelationships of the major settings of the person's life. The

REFLECTIVE THINKING

Status of Women and Work

Feminist thought has encouraged women's equity and has led to efforts to create new arrangements for managing family tasks such as child care, household work, and economic support.

- Will improvement in the status of women improve the quality of family life or create system conflict within the family?

- What issues emerge for women? For men?

- Why is it that, although many women work outside the home, most still carry the primary responsibility for household tasks including child-rearing?

Figure 18-5 Definitions of the Major Components of Systems Theory As Applied to Families

Boundaries. Each system has an imaginary demarcation line that is made up of rules and separates the focal system from its environment. This boundary may be more or less open. Families with open boundaries can utilize information and energy from their environment to maintain greater equilibrium or to grow. If the boundary is too porous, however, there can be so much input that the family may lose its identity (e.g., be so involved with community agencies that they depend on the agency to direct their lives). If the family boundary is too closed, the family is isolated from their environment and cannot use the services of the community to support them in times of need.

Differentiation. Refers to a living system's capability to "advance to a higher order of complexity and organization" (Friedman, 1998, p. 159). A normal social system has a natural tendency to grow (called morphogenesis), but a balance between stability (morphostasis) and morphogenesis is needed for the system to differentiate.

Energy. Energy is needed to meet the demands for system integrity. The more open the system, the more input needed from the environment to maintain high energy levels.

Entropy. Tending toward maximum disorder and disintegration. Occurs when the system is either too open or too closed, causing family dysfunction.

Equifinality. The quality of there being a characteristic final state regardless of initial state. For instance, people tend to develop habitual ways of behaving and communicating so that whatever the topic, their way of dealing with it will be the same.

Equilibrium. Self-regulation, or adaptation that results from a dynamic balance or steady state. Because the balance is dynamic, it is always reestablishing itself.

Equipotentiality. The quality of different end states being possible from the same initial conditions.

Feedback. The process of providing a circular loop so that the system can receive and respond to its own output. A self-corrective process whereby the system adjusts both internally and externally: internally by making changes in the subsystems as necessary and externally by modifying boundaries.

Feedback can be negative or positive. Positive feedback refers to input that is returned to the system as information that moves the system toward change. Negative feedback promotes equilibrium and stability, not change. An analogy would be a laboratory test labeled "negative" that indicates no body changes or "positive" that indicates a change from the normal.

Flow and transformation. The process whereby input flows through the system either in its original state or, in some cases, transformed so that the system can use it.

Hierarchy of systems. The level of influence of one system with respect to another. The closer the supra- or subsystem to the focal system, the greater the influence. With the family as a focal system, each of the suprasystems and subsystems must be considered. For example, the individual member's system would be a close subsystem of the family, and the community would be a closer suprasystem than the system of the universe.

Input. Energy, matter, and information that the system must receive and process in order to survive.

Morphogenesis. Process of growth, creativity, innovation, and change. In a well-functioning system, cannot be separated from morphostasis.

Morphostasis. A system's tendency toward stability, a state of dynamic equilibrium. In a well-functioning system, cannot be separated from morphogenesis.

Negentropy. Tending toward maximum order; appropriate balance between openness and closedness is maintained.

Openness/closedness. Extent to which a system permits or screens out input, or new information, into the system.

Output. The result of the system's processing of input. It is released into the environment as matter, energy, or information.

Rules. Characteristic relationship patterns by which a system operates. They both express the values of the system and the roles appropriate to behavior within the system and distinguish the system from other systems and, therefore, form the system boundaries.

Subsystems. The smaller units or systems of which a system (the family) consists (i.e., individual members, sibling, spouse, parent–child, extended family relationships).

Suprasystem. The larger system, such as the community (churches, schools, hospitals, businesses, clubs) of which smaller systems (the family) are a part.

System. "A goal-directed unit made up of interdependent, interacting parts that endures over a period of time" (Friedman, 1998, p. 156). Systems are made up of a hierarchy of systems that consist of suprasystems and subsystems. The particular system under study at a specific time is called the **focal system**. In this chapter, the focal system is the family.

Adapted from Family Therapy: A Systematic Integration *(3rd ed., pp. 64–69) by D. S. Becvar & R. Becvar, 1996, Needham Heights, MA: Allyn & Bacon; and* Family Nursing: Theory and Practice *(4th ed., pp. 156–159) by M. M. Friedman, 1998, Stamford, CT: Appleton & Lange. Becvar and Becvar copyright 1996 by Allyn & Bacon; and Friedman copyright 1998 by Appleton & Lange.*

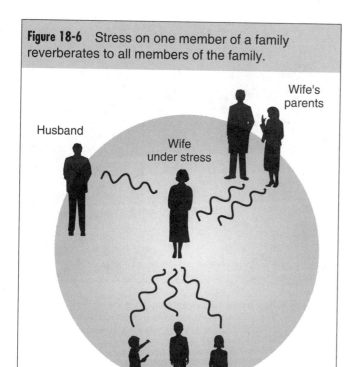

Figure 18-6   Stress on one member of a family reverberates to all members of the family.

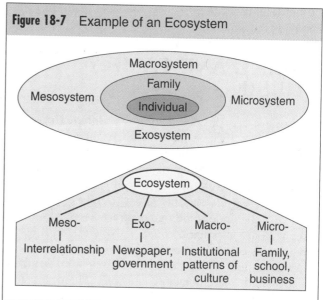

Figure 18-7   Example of an Ecosystem

third system is the **exosystem**, which includes the major institutions of the society (neighborhoods, mass media, and all levels of government). The final system is the **macrosystem**, which "encompasses the overarching institutional patterns of the culture" (p. 24). The family is viewed as nesting within the larger systems and actively influencing and being influenced by them (see Figure 18-7). Szapoeznik and Kurtines (1993) have taken the concept one step further. They use the term **contextualism** to explain the idea of understanding the individual in the context of the family and the family in the context of the culture. This concept reflects a true ecological perspective. It is a particularly useful concept for community health nurses to keep in mind.

꩜ REFLECTIVE THINKING ꩜

Work/Family Issues

Whereas many businesses continue to ignore work/ family issues, the Los Angeles Department of Water and Power has developed a number of services including a father support group, lactation programs for new mothers, and child care services. The services were developed after the department realized it was losing approximately $1 million per year because of child care problems (Solomon, 1992).

- Should businesses provide such services as child care and support groups for their employees? Why or why not?

Network Therapy

Network therapy, or social networking, focuses on the natural relationship systems of individuals and families. The family network is a relatively invisible but real structure within which the family is embedded. Networks can be either functional or dysfunctional. "A well-functioning network mediates stress, facilitates communication, and interprets the environment in an effective manner. Dysfunctional networks tend to be rigid and constraining and are characterized by depersonalization and alienation" (Becvar & Becvar, 1996, p. 304). Family networks can be mapped. Members include people within the household, emotionally significant people outside the household, casual relationships, and distant relationships. A distinction is drawn between family and nonfamily members and those people whom one dislikes or with whom one feels uncomfortable and those about whom one feels more positive. In a therapeutic setting, the goals are to resolve the family crisis through resolution of problems with the network and to ensure that the network is a positive resource for the family.

Transactional Field Approach

Transaction "denotes system in process with system, where no entity can be located as first or final cause" (Spiegel, 1982, p. 35). In the **transactional field theory** the individual is viewed in the context of his transactional field (made up of all aspects of the person's life, including physical, psychological, social, and cultural) and the family group in interaction with other social groups and in interaction with the universe. Spiegel believes that institutions are culturally anchored. In terms of his theory, he defines culture as a "set of beliefs and values about the nature of the world and human existence" (p. 36). An awareness of the system's culture, particularly the values of the dominant culture versus the value patterns of the family, is thus important.

CARING AND FAMILY NURSING

Caring must be considered from two different points of view when the focus is the family: the nurse as caregiver and the family as caregiver to family members. Pepin (1992) points out that nursing, in its quest for recognition in the scientific world, has distanced itself from nonprofessional caregivers such as family members. She notes that, while the understanding and practice of professional caregiving are important, collaborative work with family caregivers is equally important.

As described in Chapter 1, caring encompasses both affective and instrumental dimensions. There is a tendency in the caring literature to focus on the affective dimension when the subject is the caring nurse and on the instrumental (work) dimension when the subject is the family caregiver (Pepin, 1992). Davis (1996) discovered that family caregivers need affective support as well as family behavioral-management skill training to become actively involved in the management of cognitively impaired family members.

Watson believes that the caring nurse relates to individuals within the context of the family (Talento, 1995). Therefore, the nurse when caring for a family will exhibit the same behaviors as when caring for an individual. Given the complexity of the family context, the implementation of these behaviors is crucial to accurate and adequate assessment of the family and to implementation of appropriate interventions. Many times, it is the caregiver and other family members, rather than the client, on whom nursing care will be focused.

Family caregiving usually involves a primary **caregiver**, often a woman, who cares for the chronically ill spouse, child, or parent. Care may be intermittent, such as shopping or financial management, or may include in-home assistance requiring a regular time commitment. Often, intimate personal and health care are necessary activities. The more time consuming the care, the less likely it is that the affective aspects of daily living will be addressed (Pepin, 1992).

Lindgren (1993) has defined a caregiving career that gives a perspective for the lived experience of a family caring for a member with dementia. She describes three stages: encounter, enduring, and exit. These stages provide important information for nursing assessment and the development of appropriate interventions for the caregiver. The first stage, the encounter stage, is characterized by "the need for rapid adjustment to major changes and losses in the life, for information about pathologies and illness characteristics, and instruction on providing quality care" (p. 219). The second stage, the enduring stage, is the "long-term, heavy-duty caregiving phase where coping with everyday stress is the norm, and supportive interventions are more likely

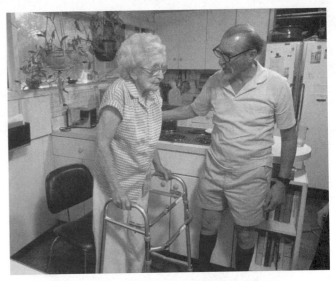

Offering supportive interventions to a caregiver in order to prevent the caregiver's physical exhaustion is imperative. Photo courtesy of David H. Wells/Corbis.

needed to prevent the caregivers' physical exhaustion" (p. 219). The exit stage, often not thought about by caregivers, has to do with "assisting caregivers in ending or reducing their career demands by either institutionalization or increased help in the home" (p. 219). Lindgren's stages can also be applied to other health-related concerns besides dementia. An excellent illustration of this process in action is provided by Givens and Fortier (1992). In their journals, they describe the process of caring as they move from Givens's diagnosis of cervical cancer to her death.

In such situations, all of a family's patterns and routines are disrupted, not just those of the caregiver and the person who receives the care. The nurse must work to develop an informed understanding of the family situation and the meaning of that situation to all the members of the family. In addition, the nurse must evaluate the impact of the situation on the family dynamics. Magilvy, Congdon, and Martinez (1994) describe a particular form of support, termed the "Circle of Care," for rural older adults not needing around-the-clock care. Nurses who were friends, neighbors, or family watched out for the elderly persons and their families and provided support, interventions, or referral to community resources as needed to facilitate "their independence and engagement in rural life" (p. 30). While caring is applicable to all of the nursing process, two specific aspects that are expressions of caring are attending to family cultural perspectives and working in partnership with the family to provide family care.

CULTURAL CONSIDERATIONS

The cultural milieu within the family develops from the blending of patterns of the two families of origin in the context of the larger society. Although it is helpful to understand the beliefs and values of the traditional culture of the families of origin and those of the dominant society, caring nurses recognize the importance of allowing the uniqueness of the family to become evident and of presenting oneself as a learner in the process of understanding the family as a cultural system. Cuellar and Glazer (1996) have hypothesized five types of **family acculturative styles**. They are as follows:

Traditional-oriented nonresistive style. First-generation parents and children "who are traditionally oriented with regard to that culture and have minimal exposure to the majority culture" (p. 20). They are open to acculturation but have had little association with the host country.

Integrated bicultural family style. Fairly equal integration of elements of both cultures resulting in a balanced orientation and acceptance of two or more cultures.

Assimilated family style. Full assimilation within the host culture with little residual traditional orientation or character.

Separatist family style. Discomfort with assimilation and active resistance and opposition to acculturation forces and pressures.

Marginalized family style. "Some or all of the family members seem to have lost their identity with both the traditional and the majority culture" (p. 21).

Most traditional cultures see health as "a state of balance with the family, community, and the forces of the natural world" and see illness as a state of imbalance (Specter, 1996). Ways of maintaining or restoring this balance vary from culture to culture. Within families where different cultures are represented, many variations on health beliefs and practices may exist. Spector notes that "ethnic beliefs and practices related to health and illness of the family are more in tune with the mother's family than with the father's" (p. 47), because the nurturer of the family tends to be the mother. Knowledge of factors such as family health practices (discussed in Chapter 19), socioeconomic status, political and historical background, and migration patterns can assist the nurse in balancing his or her general understanding of the family's culture with the unique patterns and experiences of the actual human network.

People who are secure and comfortable in their own cultural identities are more likely to be flexible and open to people of different cultural backgrounds. Respectful and sensitive behavior by the nurse can help shape the family's self-perceptions and minimize the possibility that the family will themselves participate in discriminatory behavior in the future. A basic requirement for the caring nurse is to develop the sensitivity and respect necessary for successful relationships with clients of different ethnic and socioeconomic backgrounds.

Nurses should be wary of believing they have expertise simply because they have cognitive understanding of a particular culture's traditional values. A certain amount of knowledge can be helpful, but without the openness to learn about the uniqueness of a particular family from the family itself, cognitive knowledge can become a barrier and a deterrent. The possibility of overidentification with the client family on the part of the provider must also be kept in mind, especially if family and provider are from similar ethnic or socioeconomic backgrounds.

Families are not immune to stereotyping the behavior of the human service provider. Families may also present caricatures and exaggerations of their ethnicity in their interactions with providers, a phenomenon that can be viewed as another manifestation of the family's themes and patterns.

Knowledge of socioeconomic factors is also helpful in understanding people of different cultures. For example, families from rural areas will be different from urban families within the same culture. And some families have more in common with families from other cultures than they do with families of their own culture.

The family's migration experience is another important dimension to be considered. Millions of individuals in

✺✺ REFLECTIVE THINKING ✺✺

Family Differentness

Some families move from one country to another or from one section of the country to another for employment or because they are in the military.

• Whom do you know who has moved here from another country?

• What were their reasons for moving?

• How have they adapted to their new environment?

• Do you see differences between those who chose to come here versus those who were forced to do so for political or economic reasons?

• How does cultural, ethnic, or religious background facilitate or impede a family's adjustment and adaptation to a new living situation?

• In what ways is their way of life similar or different from yours?

• How comfortable are they about their move?

• Are they different from you in ways they express themselves?

• What is your reaction to these similarities or differences?

• How do their health beliefs and practices differ from your own?

• From where did your health beliefs and practices come?

• Do your health beliefs and practices have a scientific basis?

different parts of the world migrate each year. For some, the move is the result of a lengthy planning process; for others, it represents a rapid uprooting necessitated by turmoil and crisis in their native land. Migrants differ in other ways as well. Some may come from cultures in which mobility is common and may move within the boundaries of the same culture; others may leave a society that has been highly sedentary for generations. These factors and others affect the process and problems the family experiences in the new environment. There are often generational differences regarding the place of cultural beliefs in family life. Children and grandchildren of immigrants tend to take on many of the values and attitudes of the dominant culture, values that may conflict with the cultural beliefs of the parents. For instance, there may be a great deal of conflict if a child plans to marry an individual who is from another cultural or ethnic background.

Many immigrants have had little or no experience with Western medicine. They enter our health care system with their own health beliefs and customs for preventing and dealing with illness. In order to effectively treat and educate these clients, the nurse must understand their points of view. The ability to integrate Western interventions with traditional cultural therapies is an important skill for nurses to have.

PARTNERSHIPS IN FAMILY NURSING

Family-centered care is defined by Thomas, Bernard, and Sumner (1993) as "helping the family achieve their best possible condition for promoting growth and development of individual members of the family" (p. 127). The emphasis is on the central role of the family rather than on any individual within the family. It is not enough to identify the family member who plays a central role; one must also identify the interaction among the members in relation to one another. To provide effective and acceptable care, the nurse must work in partnership with the family in an atmosphere of mutual respect and cooperation. He or she must recognize the "family's rights and responsibilities and their central role in guiding the person's selection and use of health care services" (p. 127).

FAMILY ASSESSMENT

Family assessment includes assessment of internal family functioning and of the relationship of the family to community resources and activities (Reutter, 1991). It also includes assessment of the impact of the community on the family and of the family on the community. The nurse enters the family system with the intent of assisting the family in its quest to promote health and alleviate illness. Problem solving is accomplished through application of the nursing process, with the family, rather than the individual, being the unit of focus.

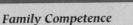

DECISION MAKING

Family Competence

Consider each of the 10 ways that nurses assist the family toward competent behavior (as noted in Figure 18-9).

• What questions could you ask of family members to elicit related information?

Wright and Leahey (1994) have developed a family assessment guide for use by nurses. As illustrated in Figure 18-8, the model consists of three major categories: structural, developmental, and functional. These categories reflect major components of family theories previously described. Each category is made up of several dimensions (external, internal, etc.), each of which has several subcategories. Although assessment of every element is not always necessary, following this guide ensures that data about the family are not presented as isolated facts. The nurse is able to develop an integrated picture of the many dimensions of the family.

Petze (1991) notes that most nursing care deals with family transitions, such as losses, occupational changes, parenthood, adulthood, retirement, or illness. Nursing care acts as a bridge to facilitate family reflection, problem solving, planning, and evaluation of outcomes, enabling the family members to regain their sense of competency and control of the situation or events for both the present and the future. Figure 18-9 lists ways that nurses assist the family toward competent behavior.

Family Environment

Major components of family assessment are the physical, psychological, and social dimensions of the environment within which the family lives. The community health nurse has a responsibility to assess each of these aspects because each has an impact on the family. A more extensive discussion of community assessment is presented in Chapter 12.

Physical Environment

The **physical environment** includes the dwelling and the conditions both inside and outside. Size, number of rooms, orderliness, cleanliness, condition of the yard, furnishings, plumbing, heat, health and safety hazards, and presence or absence of smoke detectors and fire extinguishers all provide important information regarding the status of the family. Some families may have spacious homes but be unable to buy food or to pay for telephone service or basic utilities such as heat and lights. Other families may have homes that are small and crowded but

Figure 18-8 Family Assessment Guide

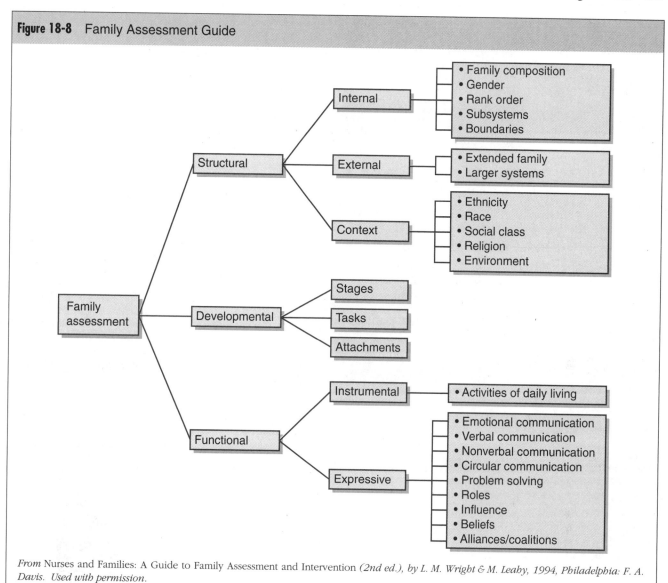

From Nurses and Families: A Guide to Family Assessment and Intervention *(2nd ed.), by L. M. Wright & M. Leahy, 1994, Philadelphia: F. A. Davis. Used with permission.*

Figure 18-9 Ways that Nurses Assist the Family toward Competent Behavior

1. Help members to clarify goals and needs.

2. Introduce or reinforce effective communication patterns, coping skills, and behaviors.

3. Encourage a safe and nurturing environment for communication activities.

4. Guide toward congruence between individual and family goals, needs, and activities.

5. Discuss and enumerate the behaviors, statements, and actions that are evidence of both functional and dysfunctional coping.

6. Provide direct physical and emotional care when needed.

7. Foster educational and informational exchange.

8. Identify additional appropriate resources.

9. Offer compassionate but honest support.

10. Help family members identify contributions they are able to make to the family process and the ill family member and contributions they expect to receive from others.

From Health Promotion for the Family *by C. F. Petze, 1991. In B. W. Spradley (Ed.),* Readings in Community Health Nursing *(4th ed., pp. 355–364), New York: J. B. Lippincott. Copyright 1991 by Lippincott. Used with permission.*

꩜ REFLECTIVE THINKING ꩜

Your Family's Competence

Think of your own family.

• How does your family deal with stress?

• How do your family activities influence your nutritional status?

• Who works in the family? How much?

• How do family work patterns affect the family's level of functioning?

• What is the use of alcohol, tobacco, caffeine, or other legal or illegal drugs in your family?

• Are rest and sleep patterns consistent and adequate, or are there frequent interruptions or barriers to adequate rest?

• Does your family exercise adequately and make appropriate use of leisure activities?

• How well do they follow appropriate safety practices?

where everyone feels secure and comfortable. An important component to assess is the presence of safety hazards and family plan for emergencies such as fire or earthquake. Figures 18-10 and 18-11 identify some of the more common hazards for which the nurse can look when assessing the family's home.

Other physical aspects of the environment to be assessed are the neighborhood and air and water quality. Information about the neighborhood can be obtained via observation when driving in the area and by asking questions of family members.

Are schools, churches, hospitals, stores, and the like easily accessible?

Is public transportation available?

What types of homes occupy the area?

How well do family members know their neighbors?

What is the crime rate in the neighborhood?

Air and water quality also can be assessed by asking questions.

What are the air, water, and noise pollution levels?

What is the quality of sanitation?

Figure 18-10 Some Common Indoor Hazards for Children

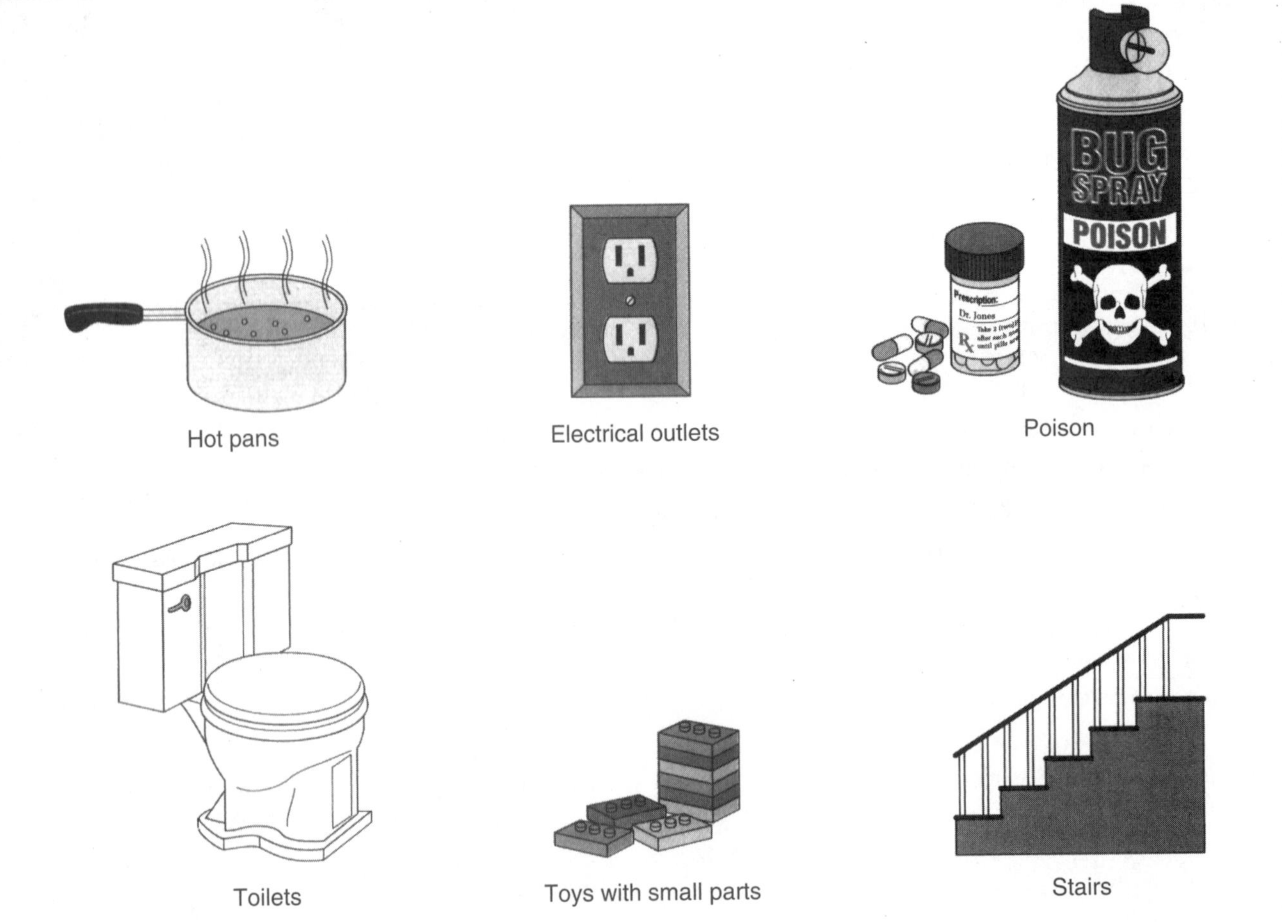

Hot pans

Electrical outlets

Poison

Toilets

Toys with small parts

Stairs

Figure 18-11 Potential Physical Environmental Hazards for Families

- Lack of barriers to stairs or upper story porches when children are in the environment
- Swimming pools without barriers to prevent children or animals from falling in
- Presence of lead-based paint (usually in older homes)
- Loose throw rugs
- Broken furniture, stairs, stair railings, or floorboards
- Hazardous materials, such as cleaning materials or medications, within children's reach
- Plumbing that does not allow for sanitary disposal of human wastes
- Toys in walkways
- Overcrowding
- Absence of fire alarms in the home, lack of a fire plan
- Lack of a disaster plan for earthquake, tornado, hurricane, or other disaster
- Lack of a poison control plan (posted telephone numbers)
- Numerous house pets such as cats, chickens, or dogs
- Lack of fenced-in yard for small children
- Lack of childproof electrical outlets
- Proximity to a heavily traveled highway

Each of these areas should be addressed according to the needs of the family. In addition, family members should be asked about their perceptions and knowledge of these issues. It is the family's perspective about the environment that will most influence both the way the family functions within that environment and the degree to which family members will respond to nursing interventions.

Psychological Environment

Significant aspects of the **psychological environment** include developmental stages, family dynamics, and emotional strengths, already discussed in this chapter. Communication patterns, including verbal and nonverbal communication, both within and outside the family, family roles, and coping strategies also provide important clues to the health of the family. These factors are discussed in Chapter 19.

Social Environment

Social environment includes religion, race, culture, social class, economic status, and external resources such as school, church, and health resources. It is important to learn about the family's perception of these areas.

- What is the kind and level of religious involvement of the family?
- How do the family's cultural values affect family members?
- What is the pattern of the family's social relations?
- What is the family's financial status?
- How involved is the family in organizations and institutions outside of the family?
- How does the family manage health and illness experiences?

Such questions help clarify the context of the family and provide information regarding family strengths and resources and well as family deficits.

Family Strengths

Often, the health provider—as well as the family itself—tends to look only at the problems and conflicts within a family. To know the full extent of the way a family functions, however the nurse must also assess **family strengths.** Otto (1963) identified family strengths as follows:

- The ability to provide for the physical, emotional, and spiritual needs of a family
- Sensitivity to the needs of family members
- The ability to communicate effectively
- The ability to provide support, security, and encouragement
- The ability to initiate and maintain growth-producing relationships and experiences within and outside of the family
- The capacity to create and maintain constructive and responsible community relationships in the neighborhood, the school, and town, local, and state governments
- The ability to grow with and through children
- The ability for self-help and the ability to accept help when appropriate
- The ability to perform family roles flexibly
- Respect for the individuality of each family member
- The ability to use a crisis or seemingly injurious experience as a means of growth
- A concern for family unity, loyalty, and interfamily cooperation

Although all these strengths are important to healthy family functioning, it is unlikely that any given family will have all of them. The degree to which they do manifest these behaviors, however, gives the nurse clues as to how well the family is managing its life. Some families may be dealing with many serious problems, but if they exhibit a number of the aforementioned strengths, they can cope with little or no outside intervention. Other families may need extensive help, even in the face of fewer or less serious problems, because they have fewer strengths.

REFLECTIVE THINKING

Assessing the Home Environment

Look at your own home environment.

• How would you assess its physical components? Psychological components? Social components?

Figure 18-12 Commonly Used Symbols for Genograms and Family Health Trees

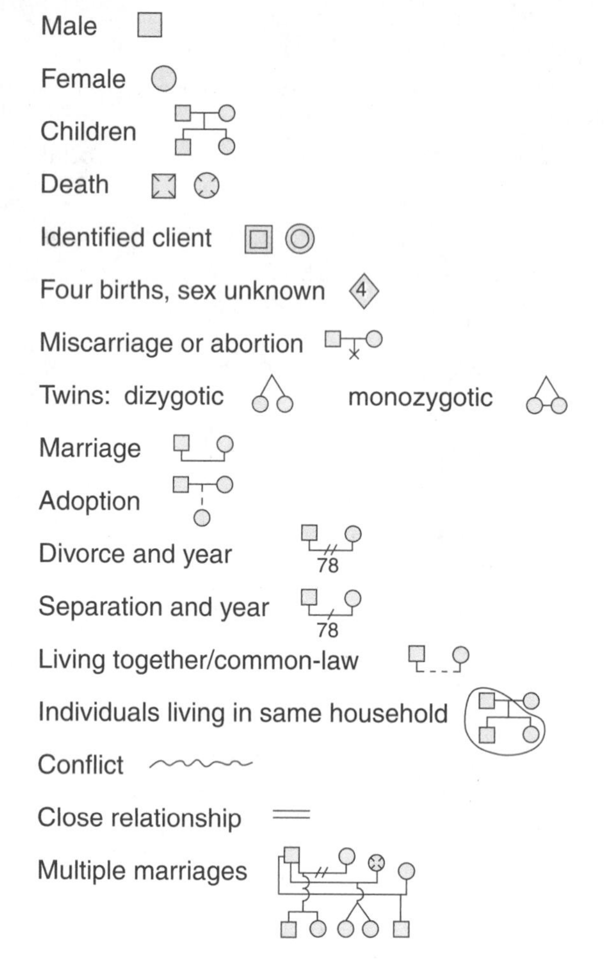

Male
Female
Children
Death
Identified client
Four births, sex unknown
Miscarriage or abortion
Twins: dizygotic   monozygotic
Marriage
Adoption
Divorce and year
Separation and year
Living together/common-law
Individuals living in same household
Conflict
Close relationship
Multiple marriages

Assessment Tools

Two of the most useful and most commonly used family assessment tools are the genogram and the ecomap. A **genogram** is a graphic picture outlining a family's history over a period of time, usually three generations (Richards, Burgess, Petersen, & McCarthy, 1993). It is a way to map the structure of the family, to record family information (e.g., significant life events, cultural and religious identification, occupations, place of residence), and to delineate relationships. By adding major dimensions of the family's health history, the genogram becomes a **family health tree** from which knowledge can be gained about genetic and familial diseases. Environmental and occupational diseases; psychosocial problems such as obesity, anorexia nervosa, and mental illness; and infectious diseases also can be noted. Family risk factors and strengths can be added to the genogram by soliciting information from the family regarding things such as the way the family manages stress and leisure and the frequency of physical exams, testicular exams, Pap smears, and exercise among family members. Resulting information can help the nurse identify areas of risk and ability, facilitate the family's awareness of the situation, and work with the family to plan appropriate interventions (Friedman, 1998; Richards et al., 1993). Figure 18-12 identifies the common genogram symbols. Figure 18-13 is an example of a genogram/family health tree.

The **ecomap** is a visual depiction of the organizational patterns and relationships of the complex family system in which the balance between the demands and resources of the family system can be identified (Holman, 1983). After the nurse develops an ecomap with the family, she or he can use the information to identify interactive family strengths, conflicts in need of mediation, connections to be made, and resources to be sought and mobilized. Figure 18-14 shows symbols and forms used in a ecomap. A completed ecomap, based on the Community Nursing View, can be found in Figure 18-18.

Both the genogram and ecomap are useful tools during an early interview with a family. The whole family can become engaged in completing each tool so that family members' involvement in their own health care is facilitated from the beginning of the relationship. Wright and Leahey (1994) note that the visual gestalt conveyed through the use of these tools provides information more simply and usefully than can words.

Other tools that are vitally important to nursing assessment are observation of the family and their environment and the family interview. The previous discussion of family environment addressed the many aspects of the family that can be assessed through observation. The family interview within the context of the home visit is explored in Chapter 15. Analysis of the information gained from all the tools together provides the basis for the identification of nursing diagnoses.

FAMILY DIAGNOSIS

There are two major systems of nursing diagnosis. The North American Nursing Diagnosis Association (NANDA) has been developing nursing diagnostic labels and defining characteristics since the 1970s. The Omaha system, which also began development in the 1970s, focuses more directly on the needs of community health nurses.

The NANDA System

Family nursing diagnoses are not yet well developed. At present, they can be best used to identify problems of the

Figure 18-13   Genogram and Family Health Tree

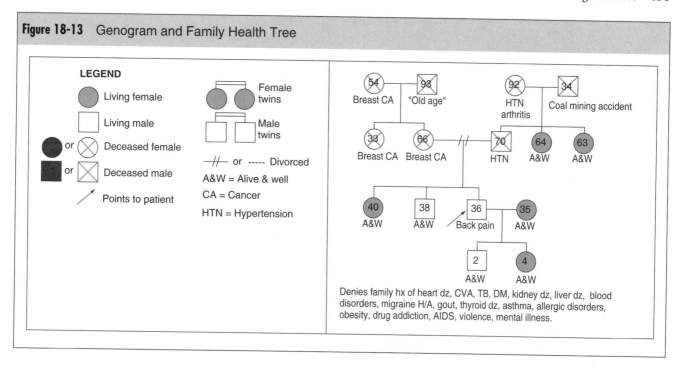

Denies family hx of heart dz, CVA, TB, DM, kidney dz, liver dz, blood disorders, migraine H/A, gout, thyroid dz, asthma, allergic disorders, obesity, drug addiction, AIDS, violence, mental illness.

individual within the family. Nurses should be prepared to devise their own diagnoses when the focus is on the family as client. Donnelly (1993) notes that few of the NANDA-approved diagnostic categories address family

Figure 18-14   Symbols and Forms Used in a Family Ecomap

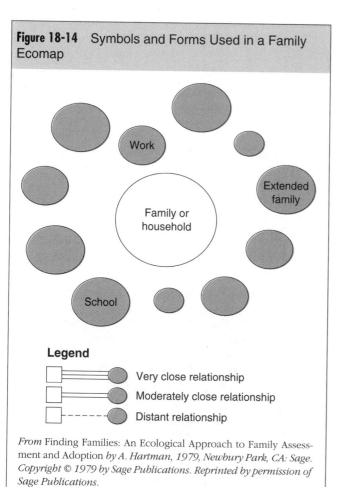

Legend

Very close relationship
Moderately close relationship
Distant relationship

From Finding Families: An Ecological Approach to Family Assessment and Adoption *by A. Hartman, 1979, Newbury Park, CA: Sage. Copyright © 1979 by Sage Publications. Reprinted by permission of Sage Publications.*

concerns, although some can be adapted to address family issues. Only one, *Family coping: potential for growth,* implies health-promoting concepts. Further, Geissler (1991) and Andrews (1995) note that the diagnostic categories do not facilitate culturally sensitive nursing care. For example, *Impaired communication related to foreign language barrier* assumes that the recipient of health care is at fault; there is no acknowledgment that the nurse is equally unable to communicate with the client. Andrews suggests that it might be more appropriate to discuss the nurse's "knowledge deficits" of the client's culture. Figure 18-15 lists selected NANDA nursing diagnoses related to the family.

The Omaha System

The Omaha system is particularly appropriate for use in community health nursing. The system was developed by community health nurses to specifically meet their needs for accurately diagnosing problems and strengths and for consistently documenting findings. The Omaha system consists of three parts: the problem classification scheme, the intervention scheme, and the problem rating scale for outcomes (Martin & Scheet, 1992). The problem classification scheme is divided into four levels. The first level is called the *domain* and includes the four general areas of community health practice: environmental, psychosocial, physiological, and health-related behaviors. The second level, called the *problem,* consists of 40 nursing diagnoses that nurses are licensed to assign and treat and that are amenable to nursing intervention. They are stated from the client's perspective and are accompanied by one modifier from each of two sets. The third level identifies *modifiers,* or terms used in conjunction with the problems. The first set describes the degree of severity of such aspects as risk factors and

Figure 18-15 NANDA Family Diagnostic Categories

- *Altered family processes*
- *Altered parenting*
- *Anticipatory grieving*
- *Compromised family coping*
- *Decisional conflict*
- *Dysfunctional grieving*
- *Family coping: potential for growth*
- *Health-seeking behaviors*
- *Impaired home maintenance management*
- *Impaired social interaction*
- *Impaired verbal communication*
- *Ineffective family coping: disabling*
- *Knowledge deficit*
- *Parental role conflict*
- *Sexual dysfunction*

From NANDA Nursing Diagnoses: Definitions and Classification 1999–2000 by North American Nursing Diagnosis Association, 1999, Philadelphia, PA: Author. Copyright 1999 by NANDA. Reprinted with permission.

DECISION MAKING

Developing a Diagnosis

You are visiting the Klee family for the first time. You know from the referral that they have no health insurance and that Ida Klee is a single parent with a 6-year-old daughter, Patty, who has asthma. Ida is two months pregnant and is undecided about whether to terminate her pregnancy. She says she is always tired and that her daughter gets on her nerves. She has slapped her daughter a few times. Patty is in the first grade and is having trouble reading and concentrating. Ida has little time to help her and spends a lot of time in bed when she is not working as a waitress.

- Using the NANDA nursing diagnosis system, identify one or two applicable nursing diagnoses.
- Using the Omaha nursing diagnosis system:

  Which domains would you address?

  What problems can you identify?

  Which modifiers would you use?

  If you have identified active problems, what are the signs and symptoms?

- With which of the two systems did it seem easier to work?

signs and symptoms (i.e., Health Promotion, Potential Deficit/Impairment, and Deficit/Impairment/Actual). The second set identifies ownership of the problem: that is, whether it is an individual or a family problem. *Signs and symptoms* are the fourth level. They are used only with actual deficits. Signs are the objective evidence of a client's problem, and symptoms are the subjective evidence of a client's problem reported by the client or another significant person. Each domain includes a number of problems and each includes one problem identified as "other" in order to accommodate a problem not in the classification. Figure 18-16 lists some of the 40 problems along with the modifiers and some problem-specific signs and symptoms.

The intervention scheme arranges nursing actions or activities in a systematic way at three different levels. All interventions include a "category," a "target," and, usually, "client-specific information." The categories are the first level and are divided into "four broad areas that provide a structure for describing community health nursing actions or activities (i.e., Health Teaching, Guidance, and Counseling; Treatments and Procedures; Case Management; and Surveillance)" (Martin & Scheet, 1992, p. 84). The targets are "the 62 objects of nursing actions or activities that serve to further describe interventions" (p. 84). These include such things as coping skills, family planning, and ostomy care. The third level, client-specific information, is generated by the community health nurse or other health care practitioner and is the detailed portion of the care plan. For more detailed information, see Martin and Scheet (1992).

The problem rating scale for outcomes "provides a framework for evaluating the client's problem-specific knowledge, behavior, and status at regular or predictable time intervals" (Martin & Scheet, 1992, p. 93). These components can be assessed on a continuum that provides five degrees of response, from the most negative to the most positive state of a problem.

PLANNING AND INTERVENTION

Perhaps the most important aspect of the planning and intervention part of the nursing process is planning in partnership with the family. As previously stated, it is critical that the nurse work with the family members to identify their concerns and to plan intervention strategies. It has long been noted, and is important to recognize, that for the health provider, "empowerment of clients and changing their victim status means giving up our position as benefactors" (Pinderhughes, 1983, p. 337). It is not always easy to let go of the wish to rescue the family, but it is in the family's best interest to do so. Lapp, Diemert, and Enestvedt (1993) agree that life and health choices ultimately reside with the client family. They see the main responsibility of the professional as "ensuring that those

Figure 18-16 Examples of Omaha System

Environmental Domain

Problem 04

Neighborhood/workplace safety. Freedom from injury or loss as it relates to the community/place of employment

Modifier

Health Promotion   Family

Potential Deficit   Individual

Deficit

Signs/Symptoms

01. high crime rate

02. high pollution level

03. uncontrolled animals

04. physical hazards

05. unsafe play areas

06. other

Psychosocial Domain

Problem 11

Grief. Keen mental suffering or distress over affliction or loss

Modifier

Health Promotion   Family

Potential Impairment   Individual

Impairment

Signs/Symptoms

01. fails to recognize normal grief responses

02. difficulty coping with grief responses

03. difficulty expressing grief responses

04. conflicting stages of grief process among family/individual

05. other

Physiological Domain

Problem 28

Respiration. The exchange of oxygen and carbon dioxide in the body

Modifier

Health Promotion   Family

Potential Impairment   Individual

Impairment

Signs/Symptoms

01. abnormal breath patterns

02. unable to breathe independently

03. cough

04. unable to cough/expectorate independently

05. cyanosis

06. abnormal sputum

07. noisy respirations

08. rhinorrhea

09. abnormal breath sounds

10. other

Health-Related Behaviors Domain

Problem 38

Personal hygiene. Individual practice conducive to health and cleanliness

Modifier

Health Promotion   Family

Potential Impairment   Individual

Impairment

Signs/Symptoms

01. inadequate laundering of clothing

02. inadequate bathing

03. body odor

04. inadequate shampooing/combing of hair

05. inadequate brushing/flossing/mouth care

06. other

From The Omaha System *by K.S. Martin & N. J. Scheet, 1992, Philadelphia: W. B. Saunders. Used with permission.*

choices were made on the basis of the most complete information possible while facilitating self-discovery of strengths and resources already existing for a family" (p. 282). From this perspective, partnership with the family is necessary at every step, and assessment and intervention occur simultaneously in a dynamic process. Further, interventions are planned taking into account family priorities and filling information gaps in the family's knowledge base so that intervention decisions are made from a position of knowledge. Interventions address primary, secondary, or tertiary levels of prevention.

Primary Prevention

Primary prevention encompasses health promotion and disease prevention. It identifies actions taken to prevent the occurrence of health problems in families. One of the major nursing activities in this realm is that of anticipatory guidance. Activities might include, for example, providing information about normative changes that can be expected in a child's growth so that parents are prepared for the changes and are ready to deal with them when they occur. Another activity might be helping a family

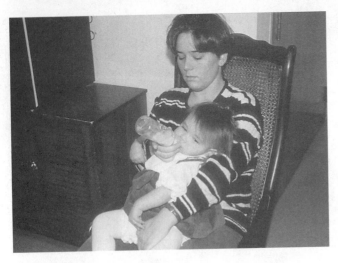

Teaching this young mother how to care for her infant child is an important part of primary prevention.

Figure 18-17   Perez Family Genogram and Family Health Tree

prepare for the changes that will occur when a member returns home after a period of time spent in a mental institution or prison. Healthy People 2000 (U.S. Department of Health and Human Services, Public Health Service, [USDHHS-PHS] 1995) addresses primary prevention for families in most of its objectives. While the emphasis of the plan is more on individuals, the impact for families is great. For instance, the implementation of programs to reduce teenage and unintended pregnancies or alcohol-related motor-vehicle–accident deaths have important implications for family life.

Secondary Prevention

Secondary prevention has to do with the early recognition and treatment of existing health problems. A family per-

spective requires examining the interactive problems that suggest family dysfunction as well as the concerns of individuals within the family. Healthy People 2000 (USDHHS-PHS, 1995) emphasizes screening exams that can detect problems early and prevent long-term and costly care that drains families resources. Such screening exams include mammography, Pap smears, and fecal occult blood testing.

Tertiary Prevention

Tertiary prevention has to do with the rehabilitative level of health care. In families, the focus is on preventing the return of the problem. An example might be helping a homeless family, through facilitating the family's connection to appropriate community services, find permanent housing as well as employment that will enable the family to maintain housing.

EVALUATION

Evaluation begins with an examination of the outcomes of the objectives of care defined in the planning and intervention phase and identification of additional data needed for further assessment. If measurable objectives have been developed, they provide the criteria for measuring the effectiveness of the outcome of the intervention. This process is ongoing in that every new piece of data adds a dimension to that which is already known and forces a new evaluation of the status of needed family care.

DECISION MAKING

Sibling Rivalry

When assessing a family composed of a single parent with two girls, ages 1 and 5 years, you recognize that the mother is devoting all her time to the 1-year-old, who has spina bifida. The mother states that the 5-year-old is driving her crazy with constant "unnecessary" demands for attention. You identify that the mother needs help in recognizing the impact of her younger child's illness on her older daughter.

• In discussion with the mother, what strategies would you propose that would enable her to attend to both children in a more equitable way so that more extensive acting out by the older child is averted?

• What level of prevention does this example illustrate?

COMMUNITY NURSING VIEW

Maria Perez is a 22-year-old mother of three children: Manuel, age 5 years, Mae, age 3½ years, and Rosarie, a 1-week-old newborn who is still in the hospital because of a chronic lung problem. When she goes home in a few days, Rosarie will need oxygen PRN. Maria has expressed concern that she will not be able to manage the oxygen equipment and will not know when Rosarie needs oxygen. Maria and her 25-year-old husband, Jamie, live in a three-room house. Maria and Jamie sleep in one bedroom, where Rosarie will also stay when she comes home. The other children, along with their grandmother, Maria's mother, sleep on a daybed in the living room. Alice, the grandmother, is 47 years old and has lived with the family since her husband's death three years ago from complications of diabetes. He was 51 years old. Maria's husband has been unable to work for the past month because of a back injury incurred in his work as a farm laborer. They do not know when he will recover enough to return to work. He is very depressed and worried about his condition and, although he does not hit Maria or the children, he frequently lashes out verbally in anger when the children become noisy or Maria reaches out to him with affection. His parents live a few blocks away and visit frequently. Maria wishes they would come less often. They spoil the children and often disapprove of the way Maria cares for the household. Manuel and Mae have a yard in which to play, but it is mostly dirt, and an old refrigerator is lying on the ground. The yard is not fenced in, and the family lives on a rather busy street. The children are friendly and playful. Manuel, who is in kindergarten, is very serious and watchful of his sister. Maria says he has become more protective since her husband became disabled. Maria has two sisters and three brothers. Jamie has one brother and three sisters. They live too far away to visit often, but both Maria and Jamie are close to all their siblings. Figures 18-17 and 18-18 illustrate a genogram and an ecomap, respectively, for the Perez family.

Nursing Considerations

ASSESSMENT
- What is the Perez family form?

- According to Duvall and Miller (1985) and Carter and McGoldrick (1989), in which stage is the Perez family? What are their developmental tasks?
- Where would you place the Perez family in terms of Combrinck-Graham's (1985) family life cycle?
- Describe the family in terms of systems definitions.
- How well do you think the Perez family is carrying out their family functions?
- What environmental hazards can you identify in the Perez family?
- What family strengths can you identify?
- What cultural considerations must you address in order to work effectively with the Perez family?
- Using Wright and Leahey's (1994) family assessment guide, identify the structural, functional, and developmental dimensions that are important to the understanding of the Perez family.

DIAGNOSIS
- What family nursing diagnoses would you assign to this family? Provide your rationale.

OUTCOME IDENTIFICATION
- Given the diagnoses you have identified, what outcomes do you expect?

PLANNING/INTERVENTIONS
- How would you begin to develop a partnership with the Perez family in order to identify the family's health goals?
- What aspects of their situation might put you at risk for wanting to "rescue" the Perez family?
- Identify primary, secondary, and tertiary interventions for the Perez family.

EVALUATION
- Given the interventions identified previously, what might you look for that would enable you to assess the effectiveness of your interventions?
- In order to answer all the preceding questions more fully, what additional information do you need?

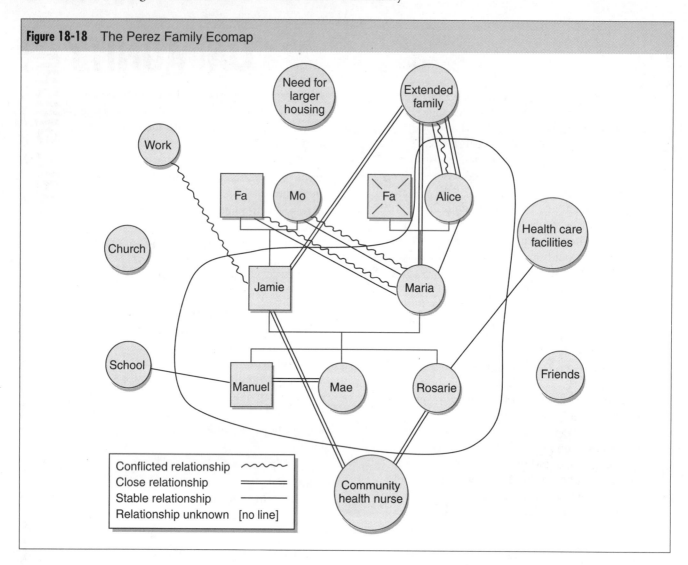

Figure 18-18 The Perez Family Ecomap

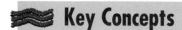

Key Concepts

- Families can be identified in two ways: family as context and family as client.

- The wider family concept addresses changing family forms and takes into account lifestyles that are independent of biological or kin connections.

- It is important to understand a variety of family theories because they give direction to nursing care of families, and no one theory addresses all dimensions of the family or fully explains family dynamics and behavior.

- Some nursing theories have enlarged their conceptual base to include the family as client.

- Four theories from the social sciences have major relevance to nursing. They are developmental, general systems, structural–functional, and interactional theories.

- The stages of family development and the accompanying tasks of each stage guide the nurse in assessing the family.

- Rather than a linear event, the family life cycle can be conceptualized as a life spiral wherein family members move closer together or farther apart depending on the life events that are occurring.

- Ecological approaches to the family focus on the way the family interacts with their environment.

- The cultural milieu within the family develops from the blending of patterns of the two families of origin within the context of the larger society.

- Family caregiving must be considered from the point of view of both the nurse as caregiver and the family as caregiver to family members.

- To provide effective and acceptable care, the provider must work in partnership with the family in an atmosphere of mutual respect and cooperation.

- Family assessment includes an assessment of internal family functioning and of the relationship of the family to community resources and activities.

- In order to understand the way a family works, the nurse must assess family strengths as well as problems and conflicts.

- Two of the most useful assessment tools for families are the genogram and the ecogram.
- The Omaha system of nursing diagnoses is more useful to community health nurses working with families than is the NANDA system of nursing diagnoses.
- It is critical that the nurse work with family members to identify their concerns and to plan intervention strategies, rather than focusing on concerns from the nurse's perspective.
- Evaluation is an ongoing process in that every new piece of data adds a dimension to that which is already known and forces a new evaluation of the status of needed family care.

Note: The author acknowledges Dr. Joan Heron, retired Professor of Nursing, California State University, Fresno, for her significant contributions to the development of this chapter.

Family Functions and Processes

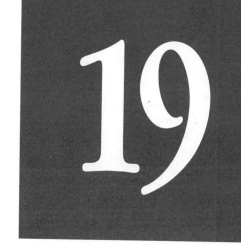

Janice E. Hitchcock, RN, DNSc

We need to move beyond the myth that one type of family is the paragon of virtue to be emulated by all families and that all others are inherently deficient. . . . It is . . . family processes—the quality of family relationships—that make the difference.

—Walsh, 1993, p. 19

COMPETENCIES

Upon completion of this chapter, the reader should be able to:

- Identify the characteristics of a healthy family.
- Discuss five functions of the family.
- Identify components of family process, including roles, values, communication, and power.
- Understand the Resiliency Model of Family Stress, Adjustment, and Adaptation.
- Identify three types of family crisis.
- Explain the dynamics of vulnerable families.
- Define four specific behaviors that occur in dysfunctional families: family myths, scapegoating, triangling, and pseudomutuality.
- Understand the Circumplex Model of Marital and Family Systems.
- Understand the McMasters Model of Family Functioning.

In Chapter 18 family structure (composition, type, size, marital status, and social network) was discussed. This chapter considers the functions and processes of the family. Family roles, communication patterns, power structures, values, and family functions in both healthy and dysfunctional modes are considered, and family stress and crisis theory are also explored.

THE HEALTHY FAMILY

Understanding the characteristics of a healthy family is helpful in understanding the many dimensions of the family in its adaptive and maladaptive states. Pratt (1976) refers to families that exhibit healthy characteristics as the "energized family" (p. 3). Curran (1983) and, more recently, the U.S. Department of Health and Human Services (1990) and Walsh (1993) have conceptualized traits of healthy family processes that support Pratt's description. Some of the major characteristics reflecting the multidimensional nature of a healthy family are:

- Flexible and egalitarian family relationships concerning power, divisions of tasks and activities, role patterns and organization of family tasks, affirmation, support and respect for one another, and trusting relationships among members.

KEY TERMS (Continued)

role accountability	role flexibility	second-order change
role allocation	role strain	socialization
role complementarity	role stress	triangling
role conflict	rules	vulnerable families
role enactment	scapegoating	

- Sense of play and humor; joint participation in structured and unstructured events. There exists a balance of interaction among family members whereby work and other activities are not allowed to infringe routinely on family time.

- Respect for individual differences, autonomy, separate needs, and privacy. The development and well-being of members of each generation are fostered. Members' contacts are supportive and facilitative, not overwhelming and limiting.

- Connectedness and commitment of members as a caring, mutually supportive unit. Cliques within the family are discouraged. Rituals and traditions are important. There are parental leadership and authority, as well as nurturance, protection, and socialization of children and caretaking of other vulnerable family members. There are adequate resources for basic economic security.

- Communication patterns that foster conversation with family members and effective listening skills; characterized by clarity of rules and expectations, pleasurable interactions, and a range of emotional expression and empathic responsiveness.

- Family coping skills developed by the family for creative problem solving. Effective conflict-resolution processes master normative and non-normative challenges and transitions across the life cycle. The family is able to admit the need for and seek help with problems.

- Shared belief system that includes a spiritual core and an ability to teach a sense of right and wrong and that fosters mutual trust, connectedness with past and future generations, ethical values, and concern for the larger community.

- Links with the broader community, such as membership and leadership participation in groups and activities that bear on family needs. The family receives enrichment from outside sources and initiates growth-producing relationships in the neighborhood, town, and the wider society. Adequate resources for psychosocial support are available from extended kin and friendship networks and from community and larger social systems. The family values service to others (Pratt, 1976; Curran, 1983; Walsh, 1993).

Although it is important to understand these healthy characteristics, it is equally important to remember that each family is unique and addresses these components in its own way. The nurse must not be quick to assume dysfunction in a family because the family's interaction seems different from that of the nurse's family. On the other hand, nurses should not normalize behavior because it seems familiar or represents that which they believe to be "good" behavior. For example, an interpretation of conflict avoidance as family harmony prevents the nurse from exploring the family's concerns regarding conflict.

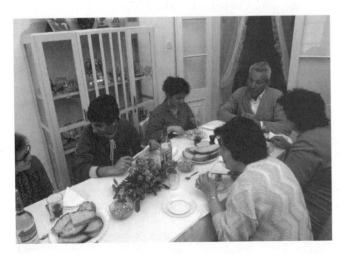

A sense of connectedness is important for a family. Photo courtesy of Bob Krist/Corbis.

FAMILY FUNCTIONS

Family functions refer to "how families go about meeting the needs of individuals and meeting the purposes of the broader society" (Hanson & Boyd, 1996, p. 152). They can be divided into two basic aspects of instrumental and expressive (Wright & Leahey, 1994). **Instrumental functions** are those that pertain to activities of daily living. **Expressive functions** have to do with the affective dimension of the family. Friedman (1998) identifies five major family functions important for nurses to understand in their work with families. These functions incorporate both instrumental and expressive components. The functions are:

- Affective
- Socialization and social placement
- Reproductive
- Economic
- Health care

Affective Function

The **affective function** has to do with affirmation, support, and respect for one another (Curran, 1983). It is one of the most vital and rewarding functions for the formation and continuation of the family unit. The family is able to express a full range of emotions (Janosik & Green, 1992). Although the affective function is important to all families, families who must focus on the more basic functions of physical maintenance may have little energy to give to it (Friedman, 1998).

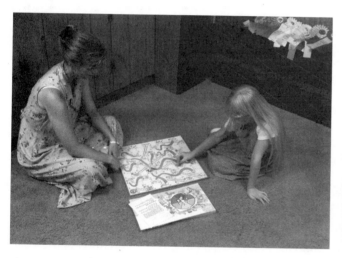

(A)

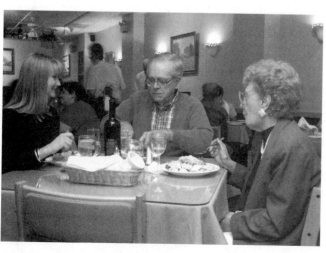

(B)

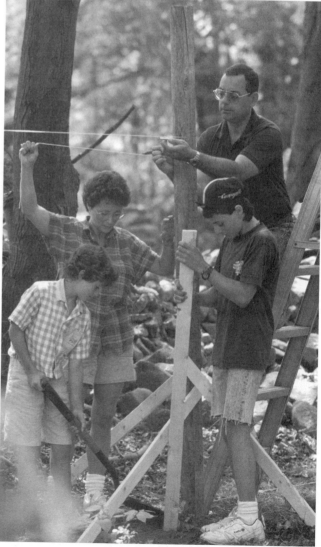

(C) Photo C courtesy of Bob Krist/Corbis.

Working and playing together are important for a healthy family.

Socialization and Social Placement

Socialization is a lifelong process of assuming the norms and values for the many family roles that are required of family members. These roles include those of child, teenager, parent, grandparent, employed person, bride or groom, and retired person. The family is the major setting and parents are the primary agents of socialization (Gelles, 1995). The family is responsible for transforming the infant into a social being who can assume adult social roles. In today's world, this function is shared with many institutions outside the family, such as school, day care centers, churches, and health and human service agencies. However, the family continues to play a crucial role in the transmission of the family cultural heritage and the indoctrination regarding controls and values related to what is right and wrong.

Studies have delineated some important implications of these socialization functions with regard to the health of families. Bisagni and Eckenrode (1995) found that a strong work identity helped divorced women adjust to their changed marital status. A study of the coping strategies of older Mexican Americans and of Anglo widows revealed that, although most tended to cope by themselves during the early days of loss rather than turning to others for help (value placed on self-sufficiency), the health of both groups benefited more from actively seeking advice for general problems during early widowhood (value placed on interdependence) (Ide, Tobias, Kay, Monk, & de Zapien, 1990).

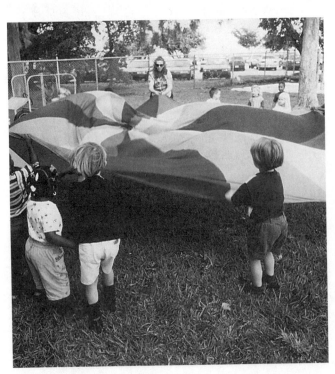

Day care often shares the responsibility with the parent of transforming a child into a social being.

Reproductive Function

The continuity of both the family and society continues to be ensured through the **reproductive function,** although this function is carried out very differently today than in previous generations. Whereas people of earlier generations considered it their responsibility to marry, have many children, and not raise children outside of marriage, today there are many single-parent families (U.S. Bureau of the Census, 1995) and couples without children. Many parents and children have come together through adoption, artificial insemination, or other technological means that may or may not include a second parent. Procreation will continue to be a family function; but it is increasingly being seen as irresponsible to bear more than two children, particularly in developing countries, and many couples are choosing to have no children.

Economic Function

Achievement of economic survival, known as the **economic function,** although important to any family, has changed in the way it is accomplished (Hanson & Boyd, 1996). At one time, the family was its own economic unit, in which all members worked together to meet their basic needs. Children were an economic resource because they could work the land and care for aging family members. In contemporary times, families, at least in developed countries, do not need each other in the same ways. There are many community resources from which they can seek help to meet their financial obligations until they are able to fulfill that responsibility themselves (e.g., Medicaid, Medicare, and Aid to Families with Dependent Children). Women no longer must depend on marriage for economic security. Children do not contribute economically as they did in the past. Two-earner families are becoming more common. In the past, such couples might have considered the possibility of both working but usually agreed that they would have children and one parent would stay home with the children. Now, such couples

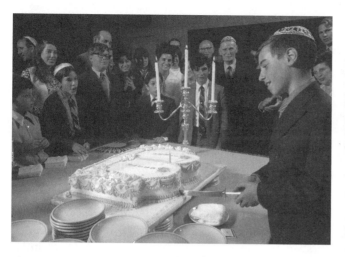

The family often is the vehicle by which cultural heritage is passed down to future generations. *Photo courtesy of Ted Spiegel/Corbis.*

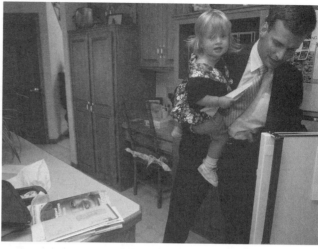

Family roles must be flexible when parents work outside the home. *Photo courtesy of Annie Griffiths Belt/Corbis.*

are more likely to question whether to have children rather than whether to work (Strober, 1988). Studies (Moorehouse, 1993) suggest that this change is a positive one when family roles become more flexible and there is cooperation among family members to complete family tasks. In many families, however, the woman who works outside the home has most of the domestic work waiting for her when she comes home (Voydanoff, 1993; Acock & Demo, 1994).

Health Care Function

The **health care function** involves both the provision of physical necessities to keep the family healthy, such as food, clothing, shelter, and protection against danger, and health care and health practices that influence the family health status. Conceptualization of health and illness varies widely among cultures, regions, and families (see Chapter 6). The more education a family has, the more health knowledge the family is likely to have (Babcock & Miller, 1994). Healthy families manage their own health care in collaboration with health professionals. "Energized" families are assertive in seeking and verifying information, making appropriate decisions, and negotiating assertively with the health care system. The nurse can assist families in this respect by reinforcing their right and responsibility to be actively involved in their own health care. Other factors important in determining the family's health are exercise; dietary, sleep, and rest practices; recreational patterns; self-care practices; and the family's health environment, which includes exposure to smoke, herbicides and pesticides, asbestos, noise pollution, and other potential hazards (Hanson & Boyd, 1996).

Healthy families participate in preventive measures to protect their health and prevent illness. They observe good dental health practices; have periodic screening proce-

dures such as mammograms, Pap smears, breast and testicular examinations, and vision and hearing examinations; and keep their immunizations up to date.

FAMILY PROCESS

Hanson and Boyd (1996) describe **family process** as "the ongoing interaction between family members through which they accomplish their instrumental and expressive tasks" (p. 67). They point out that, although families may have the same structure and may function in similar ways, they interact very differently in terms of roles, communication, power, decision making, marital satisfaction, and coping strategies. For purposes of this chapter, discussion will focus on roles, values, communication, power, and coping strategies.

REFLECTIVE THINKING

Personal Health Beliefs

Consider your own health beliefs.

• From where did they come? What influence did your family have on their development?

• With several classmates, preferably representing different cultural backgrounds, share your health beliefs and practices. How does your understanding of healthy behavior compare with theirs?

• Which of your health beliefs differ from those of a family with whom you have worked or are working? Discuss this experience with your classmates.

Family Roles

Family roles can be described as the "repetitive patterns of behavior by which family members fulfill family functions" (Walsh, 1993, p. 146). Role allocation and role accountability are two important aspects of role functioning. **Role allocation** is "concerned with the family's pattern in assigning roles" (p. 148), and **role accountability** "looks at the procedures in the family for making sure that functions are fulfilled" (p. 148). In a healthy family, allocation is reasonable, and accountability is clear. For instance, a 7-year-old son is expected to clean his room every week to earn his allowance. An inappropriate allocation would be if this child were expected to care for a 3-year-old sibling.

Other important concepts are role enactment, role stress, role strain, and role conflict. **Role enactment** concerns that which a person actually does in a particular role position. **Formal roles** consist of activities commonly assigned to a specific role (e.g., mother as nurturer). An **achieved role** includes activities not ordinarily assigned (e.g., daughter taking on the role of a deceased mother) (Janosik & Green, 1992). **Role stress** occurs when the family creates difficult, conflicting, or impossible demands for a family member. **Role strain** is generated from the stress and reflected in feelings of frustration and tension. **Role conflict** occurs when one is confronted with incompatible expectations (Friedman, 1998). As an illustration of these concepts, consider the following. Julie works full-time, has a 4-year-old child, and is taking classes to become a teacher (role enactment as mother and student). Her husband, Jim, is a fireman who is at work for several days at a time. When Jim is away, Julie has difficulty taking her daughter to preschool and getting to work on time (role stress). Because she is sometimes late to work, she is unable to leave to get to class (role conflict). She is feeling discouraged about passing her course (role strain).

In a healthy family, there must be mutual agreement about a role or modification of a role **(role complementarity).** The family must be open to shifts in role behavior to keep the family equilibrium **(role flexibility).** If one member of the family is ill or away, other members must be willing to carry out the functions usually performed by that member. For instance, when the mother is sick, the father or a friend must take the children to school, and older children must be enlisted to do some of the household chores usually carried out by the mother.

Role allocation must be clearly delineated and reasonable, with accountability clear.

Family Position

In families, individuals have a formal place (e.g., mother or father) that is associated with related roles. Examples of attached roles include, traditionally, father as breadwinner and mother as homemaker or, more currently, both parents as breadwinners and homemakers. Each family develops its own roles that meet the family's needs. Single-parent families require that the parent play the parts of both mother and father. Gay and lesbian families often work out individualistic positions within the family that do not fit traditional categories. Blended families have one blood parent and one stepparent. Some of the conflict that occurs in these families results from lack of clarity about family positions. "You're not my mother [or father]!" is a frequent comment in blended and gay and lesbian families.

Formal and Informal Roles

There are standard formal roles in every family. These are roles explicitly given to family members as needed to keep the family functioning. They include breadwinner, child-rearer, homemaker, cook, and financial manager. **Informal roles** are covert and are used to meet the emotional needs of the individual and to maintain the family equilibrium (Friedman, 1998). Informal roles can be adaptive or detrimental to the well-being of the family, depending on the unconscious purpose of their use. Examples of these roles are *harmonizer* (mediates the differences that exist between other members by jesting or smoothing over disagreements), *blocker* (tends toward the negative regarding all ideas), *dominator* (tries to assert authority or superiority by manipulating the family or certain members), *martyr* (wants nothing for self but sacrifices everything for the sake of other family members), *caretaker* (member who is called on to nurture and care for other members in need), *coordinator* (organizes and plans family activities), and *go-between* (family "switchboard" [often the mother], who transmits and monitors communication throughout the family) (Friedman, 1998).

Role expectations can be quite different depending on the culture of the family. Garbarino (1993) notes the wide variability of the role of fatherhood in different cultures. Whereas some cultures bind fathers to children, others hardly acknowledge the necessity of fathers with regard to child-rearing, leaving that role to mother.

Values

Family values are principles, standards, or qualities believed to be right, desirable, and worthy of respect (Carey, 1989; Gelles, 1995). Values, along with attitudes and beliefs, are fundamental to all that people do. Values influence family members' understanding of the world, their place in the world, and the ways to reach their goals and aspirations (Friedman, 1998). As families grow and change over time, so, too, do their values. Family values are an amalgam of society's values and the family's own subculture and are passed on by the family of origin down through the generations. Problems arise when there is a conflict between either society and subculture values or subculture values and the realities of the family's life. For instance, in a family in which the homemaker role is valued but, because of economic necessity, the wife must work outside the home, the husband may feel less of a man because he cannot, by himself, provide for the family. His wife may in turn resent the disruption to her preferred way of life.

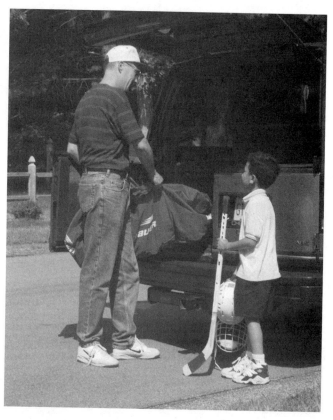

Coordination of children's extracurricular activities may be considered a formal role in some families.

Communication

Family communication "is a transactional process in which meanings are created and shared with others" (Arnold & Boggs, 1995, p. 298). Every family provides a context for learning to communicate. Our communication skills include both the general cultural language (e.g., English in the United States) and continuously created shared meanings (e.g., nicknames for family members, funny words for familiar things, particular ways to express feelings or conflict). Each family has learned these things differently. For example, whereas one family may consider it natural to hug people upon initial meeting, another may find such behavior to be personally invasive and may instead prefer to shake hands.

Communication is symbolic, and family members must have a shared understanding of which behaviors represent

---

DECISION MAKING

Family Roles

Mrs. Strong has told you that her husband is very strict with their children. He is angry that their 5-year-old son likes to play with his sister's dolls and has told him not to do so any more. She would like to discuss the situation with her husband, but because he makes all the family decisions, she does not think she should bring it up.

• How would you describe the family roles? Role flexibility? Role strain?

• How would you explore the situation with Mrs. Strong?

• Should an attempt be made to help Mrs. Strong become more assertive in her marital relationship?

✪✪ REFLECTIVE THINKING ✪✪

Family Values

• Identify some values that a family might have that would conflict with your own values about families.

• As a nurse, how would you work with a family whose members held such values?

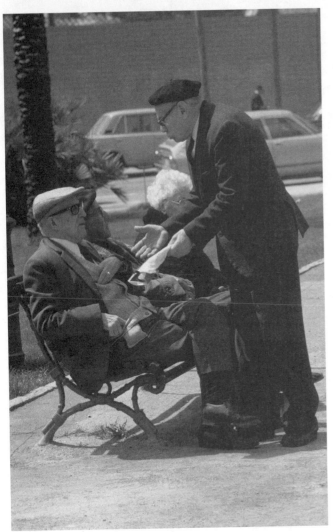

The handling of emotions differs from family to family. Is anger an acceptable emotion to be expressed in your family? Photo courtesy of Stephanie Maze/Corbis.

love, anger, fun, and the like. If meanings are not shared, disagreement and confusion will result (Galvin & Brommel, 1986; Arnold & Boggs, 1995). See Chapter 8 for more information regarding the communication process.

Family Communication Rules

All families have rules that help the family organize itself. **Rules** are the specific implicit or explicit regulations regarding what is acceptable or unacceptable and to which the family is expected to adhere. Some rules are about communication. For instance, a common rule has to do with management of anger. The rule in one family might be that anger is to be avoided at all costs and that it is considered a breach of family loyalty to express anger to a family member. In another family, anger might be an acceptable and respected emotion to be expressed as openly as possible in order to deal with the issue that precipitated the anger. These are opposing rules by which to

live, and problems could develop if members from these two families tried to resolve a conflict. In order to achieve conflict resolution in such a circumstance, the individuals must understand the rules that they have brought with them from their families of origin.

Communication rules sometimes carry anxiety and shame (Carson & Arnold, 1996). Most families have taboo topics that either cannot be discussed at all or can be discussed only under special circumstances. Sexual or financial topics often fall in one of these categories. Severely problematic behaviors such as incest or alcoholism are also frequently taboo topics. Some topics can be discussed only at certain times, in certain places, or in certain ways. "Don't bother your father while he's reading the paper" is a statement that illustrates this rule.

Sometimes, certain members of the family are not allowed to know family information. Statements illustrative of this rule include "You can talk to me about the fact that you're gay, but don't tell your father" and "We don't want Jenny to know that she's adopted until she's older."

Family Communication Networks

Family networks are the patterns of communication that families develop in order to deal with the needs of family living, particularly needs of regulating time and space, sharing resources, and organizing activities. They are a vital part of the decision-making process and are related to the power dynamics of the family (Galvin & Brommel, 1986). Networks take many configurations, but, in reality, most communication takes place in subsystems (e.g., parent, child, siblings, and spouses) (Friedman, 1998). It is therefore important to recognize family coalitions. Nurses must identify the family communication network in order to pinpoint the key communicators in the family. If these members are ignored, interventions are unlikely to be effective.

Power in Families

Family power (e.g., influence and dominance) takes two forms: the experience of closeness without coercion and the power of control over one's self and others (Walsh,

1993). **Power** is the reflection of unwritten family rules and values and is crucial in establishing and maintaining family communication channels and networks. Power structures vary greatly from family to family and may be functional or dysfunctional; however, they all involve a relationship whereby one member exerts greater control in the relationship than do other members (Friedman, 1998). In a well-functioning family, there is a clear hierarchy of power, whereby the parents take leadership in an egalitarian coalition. Children's contributions influence decisions and become more nearly equal as the children grow toward adulthood (Beavers & Hampson, 1993).

Decision making and authority are important components of power. **Decision making** is the process of "gaining the assent and commitment of family members to carry out a course of action or to maintain the status quo" (Friedman, 1992, p. 267). Authority, or **legitimate power,** refers to the shared agreement among family members to designate a person to be the leader and to make the decisions. Legitimate power is held only when other family members willingly confer authority on a member. **Nonlegitimate power** may be characterized as "domination" or exploitation, which suggests power against another's will.

Friedman (1998) identifies three areas of assessment regarding power. These are **power bases** (sources from which family members' power is derived), **power outcomes** (who makes the final decisions or ultimately possesses the control), and **power,** or decision-making, **processes** (processes used in arriving at family decisions). Figure 19-1 summarizes power bases, and Figure 19-2 summarizes decision-making processes.

Some situational changes affect the power structure of a family. For instance, chronically ill members are often left out of the decision-making process (Charmaz, 1991).

Feminist theorists look at power issues in heterosexual families in terms of male domination, seeing this behavior as a reflection of male domination in the larger society. They believe domination to be neither natural nor inevitable but recognize its prevalence in society. Male authority over women is believed by some social scientists to be one of the universal truths regarding families across cultures and over time (Gelles, 1995). The prevalence of male control over women is reinforced by Ball, Cowan and Cowan (1995), who discovered that during discussions, husbands and wives influenced different parts of the interaction. Whereas women tended to take the lead by raising issues and drawing men out, men controlled the content and the emotional depth of discussion and, usually, the outcome.

Power configurations change over time as a result of family developmental changes. As children grow, they can manage and demand more power. Adolescents, who by definition are attempting to develop individual identity, tend to challenge the family power status quo by rebelling against the family system. Such changes in children affect parents, who must adjust their patterns of power interactions with their children. Families have varying abilities to make such adjustments (McGoldrick, Heiman, & Carter, 1993). Power struggles develop when an issue becomes

---

Figure 19-1 Family Power Bases

Legitimate power or authority. Shared belief and perception of family members that one person has the right to control another member's behavior.

Helpless or powerless power. Power of the powerless; based on the generally accepted right of those in need or of the helpless to expect assistance from those in a position to render it.

Referent power. Power persons have over others because family members positively identify with them.

Resource and expert power. Power related to having the greater number of valued resources in a relationship.

Reward power. Expectation that the influencing, dominant person will do something positive in response to another person's compliance.

Coercive or dominance power. Based on belief that the person with power will punish (through threats, coercion, or violence) other individuals if they do not comply.

Informational power. An individual is convinced of the "rightness" of the sender's message because of a careful and successful explanation of the necessity for change; similar but more limited than referent power.

Affective power. Power derived through the manipulation of a family member by bestowing or withdrawing affection and warmth.

Tension management power. Control that one person achieves by managing the present tensions and conflicts in the family.

From Family Nursing *(4th ed., p. 195) by M. M. Friedman, 1998, Stamford, CT: Appleton & Lange. Copyright 1998 by Appleton & Lange. Reprinted with permission.*

Figure 19-2 Power, or Decision-Making, Processes

Decision making by consensus. Course of action mutually agreed on by all involved. Equal commitment to the decision and satisfaction among all family members.

Decision making by accommodation. One or more of the family members make concessions, either willingly or unwillingly. Some members assent in order to allow a decision to be reached.

De facto decision making. Things are allowed "to just happen" without planning.

From Family Nursing *(4th ed., pp. 197–198) by M. M. Friedman, 1998, Stamford, CT: Appleton & Lange. Copyright 1998 by Appleton & Lange. Used with permission.*

---

important to one or more family members. If exploration of alternatives does not work, various power maneuvers result, and family intimacy is affected. Variables affecting family power structures include all components of family structure, function, and process (e.g., power hierarchy, communication network, family coalitions, developmental stages, cultural and religious backgrounds).

FAMILY STRESS AND COPING

Although all families face stressful situations, families vary in how well they cope with stressors. All families "fight to remain stable and resistant to systematic changes in the family's instituted patterns of behavior" (McCubbin & McCubbin, 1989, p. 38). Family adjustment is usually minor, but some events necessitate drastic changes.

One of the most studied life events requiring substantial family change is the birth of a child. Although Tomlinson (1996) found that marital satisfaction did not significantly decrease after childbirth, Mercer and Ferketich (1990) discovered that it took at least 8 months after birth for many families to even begin to resume their normal activities. Depression was a common factor, caused by low self-esteem regarding the parenting role and a lack of a sense of mastery regarding the control of one's life.

Family Resiliency Model

McCubbin and McCubbin (1989, 1993) and McCubbin (1993) have explicated the **Resiliency Model of Family Stress, Adjustment, and Adaptation.** This model emphasizes family adaptation and enumerates family types and levels of vulnerability. The model is depicted in Figure 19-3.

In this model, there are two phases of family response to life events and changes. In the first phase, the Adjustment phase, the stressor (A) (in Figure 19-3 it is illness, but it could be any stressor) interacts with the family's vulnerability (V). The stressor can be at any level of severity, and the level of family vulnerability will depend on the pileup of family stresses and changes that are occurring at the time the new stress emerges. The family vulnerability interacts with the family's typology (T), which is manifested by the family's established patterns of functioning. These components interact, in turn, with (B) the family resistance resources: that is, their capabilities and strengths; (C), the family's appraisal of the stressor; and (PSC), the problem-solving and coping strategies used by the family. For instance, a family in which the mother becomes ill

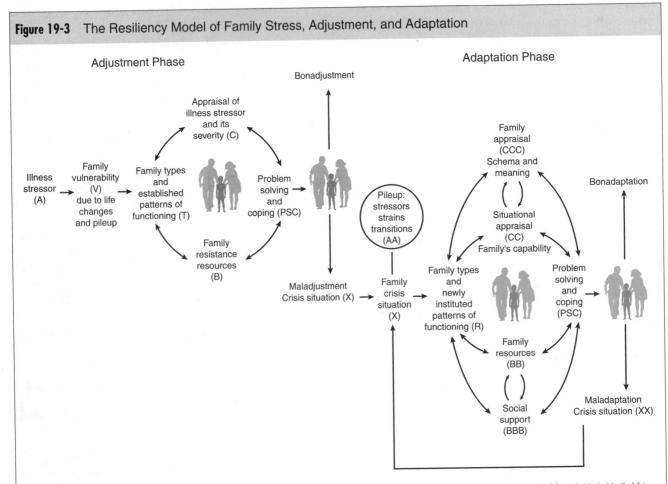

Figure 19-3   The Resiliency Model of Family Stress, Adjustment, and Adaptation

From Families Coping with Illness: The Resiliency Model of Family Stress, Adjustment, and Adaptation by M. A. McCubbin & H. I. McCubbin, 1993. In C. B. Danielson, B. Hamel-Bissell, & P. Winstead-Frye, Families, Health, and Illness *(p. 23), St. Louis, MO: Mosby-Yearbook. Reprinted with permission.*

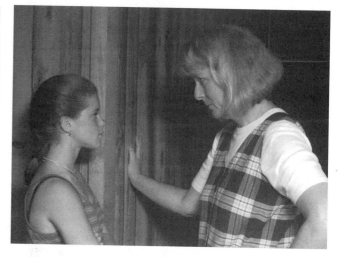

Making small adjustments in family power configurations is necessary to provide opportunities for children to develop their own identities.

and unable to work or to care for the children (stressor) will be more vulnerable (V) if she is the sole adult in the family than if there are other family members who can carry out those family functions. The family will manage better in either case if their established pattern of functioning (T) is to seek support outside the family when necessary. Their ability to communicate with one another openly about family needs (B) will affect how well they can deal with the changes in the family activities. All of the above affects their appraisal of the family stressor (C). Is it a catastrophic change with which the family can't cope, or is it a manageable situation that requires some feasible shifts in family responsibilities? If the shifts needed to accommodate the mother's illness are relatively simple, the family will adjust and move on. Most often, more-complex changes must occur. For instance, a severe or chronic illness creates a crisis or a maladjustment situation (X) that initiates the Adaptation phase (McCubbin & McCubbin, 1993).

In the Adaptation phase, the stressors (AA) from the illness and other family difficulties interact with (R), the family's level of resiliency. That is, their established patterns of functioning combined with the new patterns they may have established in response to the new stressor (the mother's illness). (R) interacts with (BB), the family resources, which are supported by the degree of support from outside the family (BBB) and the family's appraisals. A situational appraisal (CC), is determined by how the family perceives the relationship between the family's resources and the demands of the situation. For instance, if the mother's illness lasts long and she has no health or disability insurance, the family may believe that their financial resources are not adequate to support the family because they are not willing to turn to others for help, or they may see that this situation is not overwhelming because they realize that they can seek agency assistance or help from family members to get them through this difficult time. This situational appraisal (CC) interacts with the family's schema appraisal (CCC), which consists of their values, goals, priorities, and rules. These interactions create the meaning the family gives to the illness and the changes it has produced. The family problem-solving and coping repertoire (PSC) interacts with the family resource and appraisal components to facilitate family response to the crisis situation (McCubbin & McCubbin, 1993).

In health care settings, the model serves to assist health providers in assessing what "family types, capabilities, and strengths are needed, called on, or created to manage illness in the family" (McCubbin & McCubbin, 1993, p. 22) The model allows for a systematic diagnosis and evaluation of the family functioning under stress and for the development of intervention strategies. Interacting personalities, individuals, and family unit characteristics influence each other to shape the family's course of changing itself. The result may be successful adaptation **(bonadaptation),** whereby the family is able to stabilize itself in a growth-producing way, or unsuccessful adaptation **(maladaptation),** whereby the result is a more chaotic state, family growth and development are sacrificed, and the "family's overall sense of well-being, trust, and sense of order and coherence becomes very low" (McCubbin & McCubbin, 1993, p. 25).

Although the nurse's first intervention response is likely to be a focus on problem solving to deal with the immediate crisis, all the interactive factors in the family must be considered if the family is to make the needed changes in its system and if the nurse is to facilitate family adaptation to its changed circumstances. Specific ways to intervene in crisis are discussed in Chapter 23.

VULNERABLE FAMILIES

Vulnerable families are those whose physical and emotional resources are so insufficient that critical tasks and family functions are threatened. All families lose their equilibrium from time to time, often because of illness or disability. Sometimes, crisis can be overwhelming for even the healthiest family. Healthy families, however, take appropriate actions to solve their problems. Vulnerable families have few resources to help them maintain balance in the family so that even appropriate actions are usually not enough. Vulnerable families' attempts to offset their difficulties tend to be inappropriate or distorted and do not serve to solve their problems (Janosik, 1994). For instance, a healthy family having a parent diagnosed with Alzheimer's disease would reach out to community resources and friends. The family would be assertive in seeking out needed support. A marginal family would marshal all family members to take care of the diagnosed member. Although the family members do a good job of caretaking, they hesitate to use community resources or, in many cases, are unaware of those resources available to them and tend to burn out before trying other things. Disorganized families may tend to blame others for their problems, and some members may drink heavily to avoid dealing with their difficulties. These are the families in which addiction, violence, low stress tolerance, and impulsivity further strain meager resources (Janosik, 1994). As a result, they live from crisis to crisis, never really learning from their experiences. They use community services only when their crises reach such magnitude that they have to seek outside help.

Friedman (1998) has delineated adaptive strategies of dysfunctional families. She notes that such families: (1) deny problems and exploit one or more family members in physical and or nonphysical ways, using scapegoating, threats, child abuse and neglect, abuse of parents, or spousal violence; (2) deny family problems and use adaptive mechanisms such as family myths, threats, emotional distancing, triangling, and pseudomutuality that impair the family's ability to meet their adaptive function; (3) separate or lose family members (via abandonment, institutionalization, divorce, physical absence of family members, substance abuse); and (4) exhibit submission to marked domination.

Family myths are longstanding family beliefs that shape family members' interactions with one another and with the outside world (Carson & Arnold, 1996). The beliefs are unchallenged by family members, who distort their perceptions, if necessary, to keep the myth secure. Myths are established early in the life cycle to defend against the unpleasant realities of life. The more myths the family has, the less effectively family members can perform family tasks and functions because they judge family situations in terms of the myth rather than reality. Statements reflecting common myths include "We're a happy family," "We like to do things together," and "Gina needs to be protected because she is the weak child in the family." The function of family myths is to cement the cohesiveness of the family. However, myths cause the family to respond to life events in a stereotypical manner. In times of crisis, alternative approaches to problem solving are not used, and family growth is stifled.

Triangling is bringing a third person into a difficult dyadic relationship to absorb and reduce the tension (Janosik & Green, 1992). Although triangling occurs in all families to some extent, it is dysfunctional if of long duration. Conflicts are not addressed, and long-term emotional needs of family members are harmed. An example of this dynamic would be two parents' focusing on a child's misbehavior rather than addressing their own conflicts. In this situation, the effects of triangling would likely surface when the child leaves home and the parents are forced to deal with one another. Divorce may occur if the parents continue to be unable to resolve their problems with each other. Of particular concern to the community health nurse is the potential for being drawn into the family as the third member of a triangle. One member of the family may seek out the nurse to tell her or him of the problems in the family or of a particular conflict with a family member. The nurse may be asked to keep the information a secret or to be the problem solver. Although the nurse may be tempted to do as asked in order to maintain a positive relationship with the client, such an approach is not effective and undermines the family's ability to manage its own problems. The nurse must make it clear to clients that they must deal with family members directly. In some instances, it may be necessary for the nurse to act as mediator, but never as a member of the triangle (see Figure 19-4).

Scapegoating is avoiding threatening issues by blaming a family member rather than dealing with the issues (Antai-Otong, 1995). One member of the family is "chosen" to be negatively labeled and stigmatized while the rest of the family achieves unity and cohesiveness. "The identified patient" is an example of a scapegoat; all the pathology is placed on one member, and that member is identified as the cause of all the family's problems. Scapegoating hides actual family problems such as marital conflict. Children are the most common choices to be

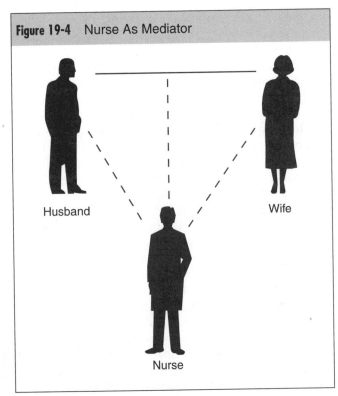

Figure 19-4 Nurse As Mediator

Husband

Wife

Nurse

scapegoats because they are less significant to family survival than are parents. The scapegoat internalizes the role and behaves as expected. As a reward, he or she gets much attention, albeit negative attention, and is exempt from all responsibility except playing the role. If the scapegoat leaves the family or refuses to play the role, the family will choose another scapegoat to maintain family balance.

Pseudomutuality is a long-term dysfunctional adaptive strategy that maintains family homeostasis at the expense of meeting the family's affective function. Families totally focus on the whole. Although the family presents a face of solidarity and cohesiveness, individual identity is viewed by the family as a threat to the family. These families lack humor and spontaneity, and their roles are rigidly assigned and maintained. Problems are denied, and the family believes in the desirability and appropriateness of this role structure (Becvar & Becvar, 1996). A member who does not wish to participate is seen as a threat to the family solidarity and is coerced into staying involved.

Heiney (1993) has outlined characteristics useful in assessing vulnerable families with regard to their functional and dysfunctional dimensions (see Table 19-1).

MODELS OF FAMILY FUNCTIONING

Through years of research, models have been developed that depict the range of family functioning. Two are discussed here because of their pertinence to community health nursing. They are the Circumplex Model of Marital and Family Systems and the McMaster Model of Family Functioning (MMFF).

Circumplex Model of Marital and Family Systems

The Circumplex Model of Marital and Family Systems identifies three critical variables that influence family adaptation (McCubbin, 1989; Olson, 1993). It is useful for the nurse to understand this model because it provides a conceptual frame of reference for assessing the family. Unfortunately, like most studies, it has focused on two-parent, middle-class, Caucasian families (Moriarty, 1990; Crosbie-Burnett & Helmbrecht, 1993). However, the dynamics presented have relevance for all family structures.

The Circumplex model (see Figure 19-5) provides a map of 16 types of marriages and family system attributes that, throughout the life cycle, characterize patterns of family life that mediate or buffer stressors and demands (McCubbin, 1989). It illustrates four types of balanced relationships and four types of unbalanced relationships.

The three critical variables that influence family adaptation are the dimensions of cohesion, flexibility, and communication. **Family cohesion** is the emotional bonding among family members (Olson, 1993). Cohesion can be measured in terms of emotional bonding, boundaries, coalitions, time, space, friends, decision making, interests, and recreation. There are four levels of cohesion, ranging from disengaged to enmeshed. Optimal family function is in the middle. Optimally functioning families are able to

Table 19-1 Assessment Summary for Functional versus Dysfunctional Family Characteristics	
FUNCTIONAL	**DYSFUNCTIONAL**
Emotional System	**Emotional System**
Independence encouraged	Dependence encouraged
Positive self-esteem prompted	One person "identified" as problem
Positive conflict resolution	Negative conflict resolution
Adapts to change	Repetitive, rigid use of ineffective coping
Differentiation	**Lack of Differentiation**
Relationships foster emotional maturity	Emotional immaturity encouraged
Thoughts separated from feelings	Thoughts and feelings enmeshed
Sense of separateness among family members	Sense of fusion
Differences of opinion allowed and encouraged	Differences of opinion unacceptable
Problem solving used to generate solutions to concerns	Family members do not think through alternatives to problems
Absence of Triangling	**Triangling**
Patterns of interaction among family members are flexible and adaptive to the situation	Patterns of interaction among family members are fixed and rigid

From Assessing and Intervening with Dysfunctional Families by S. P. Heiney, 1993. In G. D. Wagner & R. J. Alexander (Eds.), Readings in Family Nursing (p. 362), Philadelphia: J. B. Lippincott. Copyright 1993 by J. B. Lippincott. Used with permission.

Figure 19-5   Circumplex Model: Couple and Family Map

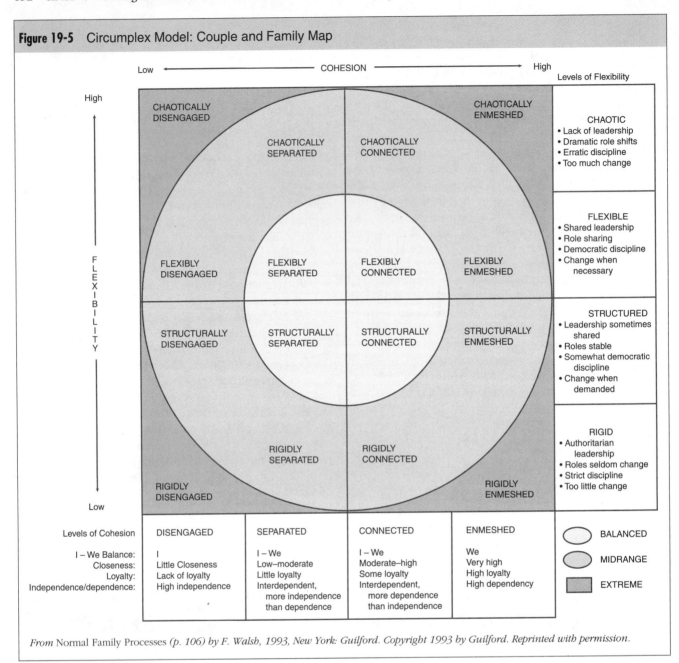

From Normal Family Processes *(p. 106) by F. Walsh, 1993, New York: Guilford. Copyright 1993 by Guilford. Reprinted with permission.*

experience and balance a degree of separateness and connectedness. That is, members need and want time apart, but times together are also important.

The second dimension of the Circumplex model, **family flexibility,** refers to the amount of change in the family's leadership, role relationships, and relationship rules (Olson, 1993). Functional families have the ability to change when necessary, whereas unbalanced (dysfunctional) families tend to be either rigid or chaotic.

Family communication is considered a facilitating dimension. As one would expect, balanced systems tend to have good communication, whereas extreme systems do not.

Olson (1993) identifies two ways that families change. **First-order change** is change in the degree of family

functioning but not in the family system. An example would be allowing an adolescent to stay out later at night and to use the family car, thus increasing his or her autonomy and independence but not significantly changing the family system.

Second-order change occurs in times of stress or crisis and is change in established family patterns. Change is greater in the balanced system, which is more flexible and able to make appropriate changes. For instance, when a breadwinner dies, another family member must take on this role. If no one is willing or able to do so, the very survival of the family is threatened.

Zacks, Green, and Marrow (1988) note that lesbian couples report higher satisfaction on the variables of cohesion, flexibility, and communication than do hetero-

RESEARCH FOCUS

The Strengths of Families Coping with Serious Mental Illness

STUDY PROBLEM/PURPOSE

To document the strengths of families with members suffering from serious and persistent mental illnesses and to identify the characteristics of these families with regard to the variables of family stressors, family coping, and family health.

METHODS

Eighty-five families of the mentally ill were compared with normative family results from previous studies on measures of family stressors, family coping, and family health. A set of questionnaires was mailed to the families. Family stressors were measured against the Family Inventory of Life Events and Changes scale (FILE) (McCubbin, Patterson, & Wilson, 1987). This measurement "is a self-administered questionnaire with nine subscales that functions as an index of family stress, seeking to evaluate the pile-up of normative and nonnormative family stressors" (Doornbos, 1996, p. 216). Family coping was operationalized by means of the Family Crisis Oriented Personal Scales (F-COPES) (McCubbin, Olson, & Larsen, 1987). This is a self-administered questionnaire of 30 items "designed to identify problem-solving and behavioral strategies used by families in difficult situations" (Doornbos, 1996, p. 216). Family health was operationalized by four instruments in terms of the subconcepts of adaptability, cohesion, satisfaction, and conflict. Adaptability measured the family's ability to adjust to stressors; the other three subconcepts measured the family's ability to function in its social roles. The first two instruments used were the cohesion and adaptability scales (measure the amount of cohesion within a family unit and the family's ability to adjust to stressors, respectively) of the Family Adaptability and Cohesion Evaluation Scales (FACES III). Each is a self-administered, 10-item questionnaire (Olson, Portner, & Lavee, 1985). The family APGAR, a self-administered five-item questionnaire (Smilkstein, Ashworth, & Montano, 1982), was used to assess members' satisfaction with family functioning. The Family Environment Scale (FES) (Moos & Moos, 1981), which is a nine-item, self-administered questionnaire, was used to measure the amount of openly expressed anger, aggression, and conflict among family members.

FINDINGS

The research question was addressed by use of descriptive statistics and *t*-tests. The families reported significantly more stressors than did the normative sample. The families relied more on the coping strategies specified in the F-COPES instrument than did the normative sample. Sample families experienced significantly less cohesion within their family units, but they had a significantly greater degree of adaptability. APGAR scores showed that the sample families scored lower than normative families, indicating a lesser level of satisfaction with the functioning of their family units. Sample families reported significantly less conflict than did the normative sample.

IMPLICATIONS

The families of the mentally ill demonstrated several areas of strength. These strengths were all in the area of functional abilities: that is, the capacity to do that which is necessary to function and to preserve integrity as a family unit. Documented strengths included the functional abilities of family coping and the family health subconcepts of adaptability and conflict management. The affective variables (members' feelings about their families) that were affected by the mental illness of a loved one were the family health subconcepts of cohesion and satisfaction. There was increased use of specific problem-solving and behavioral strategies, including reframing (changing one's viewpoint by looking at an experience in a different way, thereby changing its meaning), seeking social support, and using community resources beyond those used by normative families. It may be that the greater use of these coping strategies was related to the higher number of stressors; however, it is also true that the families responded by using a variety of positive, healthy coping mechanisms. The sample showed overall adaptability greater than that of normative families. They were "flexible and able to change in response to the various situational and developmental stressors with which they were confronted" (p. 218). These findings suggest that the "task of the professional nurse is to enhance these abilities and assist in mobilizing them in the face of the unique challenges and stressors posed by mental illness" (p. 218).

The level of conflict in the sample families was lower than that in the normative families. "These results provide validation of the strength and resiliency of these families who face the crisis of serious and persistent mental illness with highly developed skills around conflict management" (p. 219).

(Continued)

(Continued)

The results of this study suggest that mental illness in the family influences the affective rather than the functional abilities of the family unit. The sample families felt less cohesive and, thus, perceived themselves to be "less connected to one another and less bonded as a unit than normative families" (p. 219). They also felt less satisfied with the functioning of the family. The "vast stressors confronting these families may reduce the time and energy available for the

family to bond and connect" (p. 219). These findings suggest that the development of and referral to respite programs may be useful in allowing family members to spend more quality time together and, therefore, to feel more connected to and satisfied with their family.

SOURCE

From "The Strengths of Families Coping with Serious Mental Illness" by M. M. Doornbos, 1996, Archives of Psychiatric Nursing, 10, *pp. 214–219. Copyright 1996 by W. B. Saunders & Co.*

sexual couples. They suggest that this outcome may be the case because, as women, lesbians have superior relational skills and more egalitarian relationships. In addition, because there are no legal sanctions against ending dysfunctional relationships, these couples are more likely to separate and it may be more likely that it is the well-functioning relationships that endure.

Doornbos (1996), using measures developed by McCubbin, Olson, and others, identified strengths in families that had severely mentally ill relatives. Doornbos noted that these families had good flexibility and problem-solving skills but often felt affectively disconnected from one another (see the accompanying Research Focus).

Nursing interventions based on using the Circumplex model would focus on moving rigid or chaotic families closer to the center of the model. That is, in rigid families, the nurse would promote interaction flexibility through improved communication and negotiated decision making. The nurse must be careful not to push for change too fast, because doing so could increase the family's resistance to a nursing action perceived as threatening. Members of a **chaotic family** will need help in developing structure, order, and predictability in their interactions. These families tend to be crisis prone: Members rebound from one crisis to another. Emphasis would be on helping the adults to accept their leadership roles in the family and to become consistent and democratic with regard to demands and discipline.

A **disengaged family** is distanced or totally cut off from family relationships. Intervention would be directed toward the separated level of the cohesion dimension of family functioning, facilitating much separateness but some connectedness and some joint decision making among family members.

Enmeshed families sacrifice individual needs for the group. Little personal separateness or privacy is allowed. Boundaries are blurred, sometimes to the extent of fusion, so that the individual has little sense of self. Attention is focused inside the family, and there are few outside friendships or interests. Intervention would be directed toward the connected level of the cohesion dimension of family functioning, facilitating a balance between emotional closeness and respect for separateness and encouraging outside friendships. The enmeshed family may try to involve the nurse in family activities and may have difficulty understanding why the nurse cannot meet with the family as often as the family would like.

DECISION MAKING

Example of the Circumplex Model

The Martin family leads a very busy life. Both parents work, and all three children go to school and are active in a variety of school activities. On some days, the Martins see one another only in the morning, when they are preparing for the day's activities. Meals are often eaten on the run. Mrs. Martin, who is attending school part-time, tells you she is feeling overwhelmed and wishes that the family would help her more with the household tasks.

• Where would you place this family in the Circumplex model?

• How would you advise Mrs. Martin regarding her concerns about managing the household?

The McMaster Model of Family Functioning

The **McMaster Model of Family Functioning (MMFF),** named for the university where work on the model took place, is based on a systems approach. It describes a set of positive characteristics of a healthy family, focusing on "the dimensions of functioning that are seen as having the most impact on the emotional and physical health or problems of family members" (Epstein, Bishop, Ryan, Miller, & Keitner, 1993, p. 139). Each characteristic can range in quality from "most ineffective" to "most effective." The model acknowledges that judgments of health and normality are relative to the culture of the family and that family values must be taken into account in the assessment of each dimension. Focus is on the following six dimensions:

- *Problem solving:* A family's ability to resolve problems to a level that maintains effective family functioning (Epstein et al., 1993). Problems are either instrumental (mechanical in nature, such as provision of money, food, housing, and the like) or affective (emotional in nature, such as anger or depression). Families with instrumental problems rarely deal effectively with affective problems. Those with affective problems, however, may deal adequately with instrumental problems. A sequence of seven steps describes effective problem solving: (1) identifying the problem, (2) communicating with appropriate people about the problem, (3) developing a set of possible alternative solutions, (4) deciding on one of the alternatives, (5) carrying out the action required by the alternative, (6) monitoring to ensure that the action is carried out, and (7) evaluating the effectiveness of the problem-solving process (see Figure 19-6). These steps become less systematic and fewer are accomplished as functioning becomes less effective.

- *Communication:* Exchange of information within a family (Epstein et al., 1993). As does problem solving, communication has instrumental and affective areas. Two other aspects that are assessed are the clarity of communication (whether messages are clearly stated or camouflaged, muddied, or vague) and the directness or indirectness of communication (whether messages go to the appropriate targets or tend to be deflected to others).

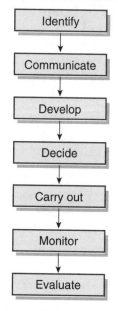

Figure 19-6 The Seven Steps of Effective Problem Solving

Adapted from The McMaster Model: View of Healthy Family Functioning by N. B. Epstein, D. Bishop, C. Ryan, I. Miller, & G. Keitner, 1993. In F. Walsh (Ed.), Normal Family Processes *(2nd ed., pp. 138–160). New York: Guilford. Copyright 1993 by Guilford.*

- *Role function:* Repetitive patterns of behavior by which family members fulfill family functions (Epstein et al., 1993). Five family functions similar to those described earlier are identified as the basis for necessary family roles: (1) provision of resources, (2) nurturance and support, (3) adult sexual gratification, (4) personal development, and (5) maintenance and management of the family system. The fifth function includes decision making, boundaries and family membership, behavioral control, household finance functions, and health-related functions. Two additional aspects of role functioning, role allocation and role accountability, were previously described.

- *Affective responsiveness:* "The ability to respond to a given stimulus with the appropriate quality and quantity of feelings" (Epstein et al., 1993, p. 149). There are two dimensions to responsiveness: responding with a full spectrum of feelings and experiencing feelings consistent with the stimulus or situational context. Also to be considered is the degree of affective response along a continuum from absence of response through reasonable or expected response to overresponse. Although overall patterns of family response are considered, this dimension focuses on the behaviors of individual members more than the other dimensions do. Two categories of affect are identified: welfare emotions (affection, warmth, tenderness, support, love, consolation, happiness, and joy) and emergency emotions (anger, fear, sadness, disappointment, and depression). A healthy family can express the full range of emotions and experiences those emotions appropriately, with responses being of reasonable intensity and duration.

- *Affective involvement:* "The extent to which the family shows interest in and values the particular activities and interests of individual family members" (Epstein et al., 1993, p. 150). The focus is on the amount of interest as well as the manner whereby interest is shown and the quality of investment in one another. Styles can range from a total lack of involvement to extreme involvement. Six types of involvement are identified, with empathic involvement being considered optimal for health. Moving away from empathic involvement in either direction results in less effective family functioning in this area. The six types of involvement are:
  1. Lack of involvement: no interest or investment in one another.
  2. Involvement devoid of feelings: some interest and/or investment in one another, although interest is primarily intellectual in nature.
  3. Narcissistic involvement: interest in others only to the degree that their behavior reflects on the self.
  4. Empathic involvement: interest and/or investment in one another for the sake of the others.
  5. Overinvolvement: excessive interest and/or investment in one another.
  6. Symbiotic involvement: extreme and pathological interest and/or investment in others; seen only in very disturbed relationships characterized by

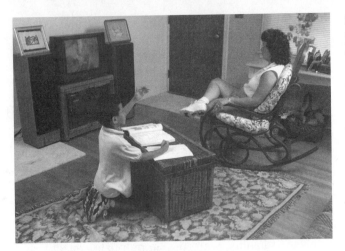

Lack of interested involvement may result in less effective family functioning.

marked difficulty in differentiating one person from another.

- *Behavior control:* "The pattern a family adopts for handling behavior in three areas: physically dangerous situations, situations that involve the meeting and expressing of psychobiological needs and drives; and situations involving interpersonal socializing behavior both between family members and with people outside the family" (Epstein et al., 1993, p. 152). The focus is on standards or rules the family sets and the freedom allowed around the standard. Four styles of behavior control are identified: (1) rigid—narrow and specific standards and minimal negotiation or variation; (2) flexible—reasonable standards with opportunity for negotiation and change (considered the most effective style); (3) laissez-faire—no standards held and total latitude allowed regardless of context; (4) chaotic—unpredictable and random shifting between other styles such that family members do not know which standards to apply or how much negotiation is possible (considered the least effective style).

Stevenson-Hinde and Akister (1996) note a seventh dimension, *general functioning,* which is an independent encapsulation of the other six dimensions. In a formalized way, these dimensions can be assessed through the use of two psychometric tools, the Family Assessment Device (FAD), which is a self-report measure that can be completed by families and scored on each of the MMFF dimensions, and the Clinical Rating Scale (CRS), which can be rated by observers during a semistructured family interview. Although these measurements are more suited for research purposes, the dimensions themselves provide useful guidelines for nurses when doing family assessments. Figure 19-7 lists suggested questions to raise with family members in order to assess the family on the basic six dimensions of family functions. These questions only propose general themes to explore. Each nurse must find wording that feels comfortable. Questions would be raised as appropriate and in no specific order. Each family is different. Specific questions will depend on the

focus and needs of the assessment. Family responses can provide data that enable the nurse to assess the family's overall general functioning.

These models provide information about important dimensions of family dynamics. The community health nurse can use this information to evaluate family needs and determine both problems and strengths in families. With the data obtained, nursing diagnoses can be made and appropriate plans and interventions developed with the family.

DECISION MAKING

Example of the McMaster Model of Family Functioning

The Ming family is an Asian American family consisting of Peter and Martha, parents of Jennifer (13 years old) and Ben (9 years old). Peter's widowed mother, Amelia, lives with the family. Peter works long hours during the week but is home on the weekends. There is some conflict between Martha and Amelia because Amelia tends to favor Ben and ignore Jennifer. Martha has discussed her concerns with Peter, and he understands but is not willing to talk with his mother about the issue. Other than that, the family identifies no ongoing family problems. The usual conflicts of daily living come and go, but the family works them out. Because Peter is essentially unavailable during the week, family members have an agreement that they will spend every Saturday together in some family activity. They realize that this pattern will change as Ben and Jennifer grow older and want to spend more time with their friends. Although family members express love for one another, their expressions tend to be reserved. There is little hugging or kissing in front of others, although Martha does express affection to her children. The children know that they are loved.

- How would you assess the problem-solving abilities of the family?

- How would you describe the level of instrumental and affective communication in the family?

- How do the Mings manage their family functions and family roles?

- How would you describe the affective responsiveness and involvement in the Ming family?

- How would you describe the standards and rules of the family?

- What is your overall assessment of the general functioning of the Ming family?

- What additional information do you need to more fully assess this family in the six dimensions of family functioning?

Figure 19-7   McMaster Model Family Assessment Questions

Problem Solving

- What do you think are your most important family problems?
- Do you discuss these problems with anyone? If you do, with whom do you discuss them?
- How do you resolve problems?
- Can you give me an example of one family problem and how you resolved it?

Communication

- How would you describe the ways you communicate with one another? Could you give me an example?

Nursing note: Observation of family interaction is important. Observe how members communicate. Do they communicate clearly or masked, directly or indirectly? Do they communicate the same way or differently with different family members?

Role Function

- How would you describe your ability to provide for your family in terms of food, clothing, money, and shelter? (Although you may observe the family situation with regard to these factors, it is important to also learn the family's perspective.)
- How do you experience and provide nurturance and support within the family?

To adults in the family:

- Do you have any sexual concerns? How satisfied are you with your sex life? What are your plans for educating your children about sexuality?
- What concerns do you have about raising your children? (Consider their responses in terms of physical, emotional, educational, and social development.)
- How are you managing regarding your job, career, recreational activities, and social activities?
- What concerns do you have regarding the discipline of your children? How do you discipline your children?
- Who makes the decisions in the family? Who takes care of the family finances? Who makes health-related decisions?
- Describe your relationships with people outside of the family. How are these relationships decided on among family members?

Nursing note: Through the answers of family members and your own observations, you can identify the family's pattern of assigning roles, their procedures for ensuring that functions are fulfilled, and whether they are in fact fulfilling the necessary family functions.

Affective Responsiveness

- How would you describe your family regarding its ability to express and receive feelings such as affection, warmth, anger, and sadness?

Nursing note: Observe the degree to which their verbal statements reflect their actual behaviors.

Affective Involvement

- How do family members show interest in and value activities and interests of other family members?

Nursing note: Observe the degree to which their verbal statements reflect their actual behaviors.

Behavior Control

- What kinds of standards and rules does your family have about socializing with others, managing potentially dangerous situations (such as children's speaking to strangers), and expressing feelings and needs.

Nursing note: Observe the degree to which their verbal statements reflect their actual behaviors.

Perspectives...

Insights of a Nursing Student

There is so much to learn and much joy to be found in sharing the knowledge acquired in nursing school. Although I recall several experiences that provided me the opportunity to share this knowledge, one in particular stands out. During my community health rotation, I was assigned to a teenager in her eighth month of pregnancy with her first child. With my heart's desire focusing on this particular population, I was delighted to take on this case. My eagerness to learn everything possible about teenage pregnancy encouraged me to search for and study all materials and information on pregnancy and adolescence that I could locate.

When it came time to make my first home visit, I felt extremely nervous because I had no idea what to expect. My mind became preoccupied with various questions such as did I know enough material about teenage pregnancy to teach about it, was I prepared to answer pertinent questions, and would my teaching style be compatible with her learning style? Despite these questions and self-doubt, my enthusiasm and determination continued. I approached this first visit with the goal of establishing a caring, trusting, and helping relationship. I realized that obtaining a complete and thorough family assessment would be essential to providing quality care and would also enable me to view the world through the eyes of my client.

As we exchanged relevant information, we identified many of her questions, concerns, and desires encompassing family and maternal health issues as well as issues surrounding the growth and development of her baby. Her primary concern focused on nutrition and the growth of her baby. I agreed that nutrition is an important aspect of prenatal education geared toward maintaining the health of the adolescent and her baby. The girl's diet must be sufficient to provide the nutritional needs of her own changing body as well as the additional nutritional needs of her growing baby. Nutrition education is a significant factor in contributing to the prevention of complications associated with teen pregnancy, such as iron deficiency anemia and low birth weight infants. Nurses working with this pop-ulation play an instrumental role in providing such prenatal education.

Another significant concern she disclosed included all of the emotions she was experiencing during her pregnancy. Although some of her feelings were normal and associated with physical and hormonal changes during pregnancy, most of them were brought on by external factors such as family difficulties. Upon listening to her express her profound emotions, the effects these feelings were having in her relationships with her mate, parents, relatives, and friends became apparent. During this visit, we discussed sources of stress, feelings associated with stress *and* with pregnancy, and several techniques she could implement to reduce stress. After our discussion, it was apparent that my client and I had developed trusting, open lines of communication, with her sharing her complicated family dynamics and fluctuating feelings toward her pregnancy. I felt honored that my client would confide in me regarding this part of her life and that I could have a positive influence on her pregnancy and the health of her baby. What a reward!

As the visit progressed, I presented her a list of topics related to health maintenance and pregnancy— topics that I had planned to cover during our home visits. However, I soon realized that not all of these topics were compatible with her unique needs. To meet these needs and motivate learning, I thus had her choose from the list those topics about which *she* desired more education. Once I gained a better understanding of her learning desires, I constructed an outline of the topics she had chosen. I prioritized the contents of this teaching plan in order of importance and to correspond with her stage of pregnancy. During our first visit, we discussed fetal development during the eighth month, feelings associated with pregnancy, stress-reduction techniques, and maternal–fetal nutrition. In the weeks that followed, I provided her an abundance of information, from exercises for childbirth preparation to ninth-month fetal development. During our last visit, which was approximately a week and a half before her due date, we discussed the labor-and-delivery process, newborn information (feed-

(Continued)

(Continued)

ing and safety issues), and normal growth and development after birth. From this experience, I quickly learned the importance of flexibility, understanding the client's needs, and client involvement in planning of care.

This first experience provided me with increased confidence in my communication skills and personal abilities. I conquered my anxieties by allowing my self-determination and devotion to this particular population to empower me. With this motivation, I was able to fulfill my goal to build a trusting relationship with my client and to provide her the best quality of care by first assessing her learning needs and then effectively meeting those needs. I believe that maintaining confidence in oneself is an essential component of goal attainment. To all students who explore community health nursing, you *do* possess the knowledge and capabilities to overcome any new and unfamiliar challenges and to attain your goals. Best of luck!

—Alisa A. Muir, Sonoma State University,
BSN Nursing Student

COMMUNITY NURSING VIEW

When making a second visit to the Perez family (Chapter 18), you notice some bruises on Manuel's (the son's) back. The mother, Maria, is not sure how the bruises got there but says that Manuel was complaining of a stomachache the night before and that Alice (the maternal grandmother) thought he might have some food stuck in his stomach. Maria further states that Alice may have pinched Manuel's back to loosen the food. Maria seems distracted and unconcerned about the bruises.

Maria's main concerns today are the family's finances and Jamie's (her husband) depression. She says that Jamie's disability payments do not provide enough money to make it through the week. Neither she nor Jamie wants to borrow money from their parents, although Alice does contribute to the household expenses. Maria realizes that she needs to return to work as soon as Rosarie, her newborn, is settled at home and Alice is comfortable caring for her. Maria looks forward to working, but the idea seems to contribute to Jamie's depression, although he will not talk about it. Maria asks you to tell Jamie that it would be a good idea for her to go back to work because they need the money.

When you talk with Jamie, he has little to say except that he wants to get back to work. He knows that Maria is thinking about going back to work, but he wants her to stay home and care for the children. He does not believe that Alice can do the job as well as Maria. He also wants to be more involved with Manuel. He believes that the boy needs more male influence, particularly living in a family that is primarily female.

Nursing Considerations

ASSESSMENT
- What elements of a healthy family can you identify?
- How well is the Perez family carrying out the five major functions of the family?
- What impact does the Perez family's level of functioning have on the family's ability to effectively manage the lives of the family's members?
- What information do you have about the internal, external, and contextual family structure of the Perez family? What additional

(Continued)

(Continued)

information do you need? How will you elicit this information from the family? Which family members do you need to talk with?

• What are some of the role issues in the Perez family? What are some power issues? How do they affect the family?

• What family values can you identify? How do they affect the family's health and health care practices?

• What are some of the communication patterns in the Perez family? Which are functional? Dysfunctional?

• What additional information do you need to evaluate the meaning of the bruises on Manuel's back?

• How would you assess the family in terms of the Family Resiliency model? The Circumplex model? The McMaster model?

• Do you think your assessment of the priorities for the Perez family are the same as those of the family? Why or why not?

DIAGNOSIS

• Identify at least three nursing diagnoses that you consider to be a priority for this family.

OUTCOME IDENTIFICATION

• What outcomes can you expect for this family?

PLANNING/INTERVENTIONS

• What might you do to resolve differences?

• Over time, what other issues would you want to work on with the Perez family?

• What aspects of family dynamics would be important to consider when implementing a plan of care so as to avoid undermining the care provided?

• What specific interventions would you want to implement for each of the nursing diagnoses?

EVALUATION

• How will you know if your interventions have been successful?

〰 Key Concepts

• The healthy family has certain identifiable characteristics that reflect its multidimensional nature. It is important to keep in mind that each family is unique and addresses these dimensions in its own way.

• Five major family functions are important in the nurse's work with families: the affective, socialization, economic, reproductive, and health care functions.

• Family process comprises several interacting dimensions that facilitate the development of family life. The major structural components are role, communication, values, power, decision making, and coping. Each of these is multifaceted.

• The Resiliency Model of Family Stress, Adjustment, and Adaptation emphasizes family adaptation and enumerates family types and levels of vulnerability. This model helps nurses deal with families in crisis.

• Vulnerable families are those who have lost their equilibrium. They are vulnerable to life stresses to a greater or lesser extent depending on whether they usually function at a healthy, marginal, or dysfunctional level.

• A typology of dysfunctional family strategies can be delineated. Four behaviors of particular interest are family myths, scapegoating, triangling, and pseudomutuality.

• The Circumplex Model of Marital and Family Systems characterizes patterns of family life that mediate or buffer stressors and demands. The three critical dimensions of this model are cohesion, flexibility, and communication.

• The McMaster Model of Family Functioning provides a view of healthy family functioning. It centers around the following six dimensions of family functioning: (1) problem solving, (2) communication, (3) roles, (4) affective responsiveness, (5) affective involvement, and (6) behavior control.

Caring for Vulnerable Populations

Unit VI provides insight into a variety of vulnerable populations with whom the community health nurse works including those populations suffering from communicable disease, chronic disease, developmental disabilities, mental illness, family violence, substance abuse.

Communicable Diseases

Rebekah Jo Damazo, RN, MSN

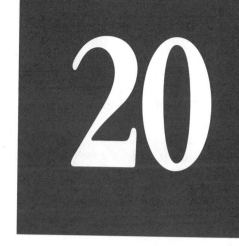

20

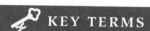
Disease can never be conquered, can never be quelled by emotion's wailful screaming or faith's symbolic prayer. It can only be conquered by the energy of humanity and the cunning in the mind of man. In the patience of a Curie, in the enlightenment of a Faraday, a Rutherford, a Pasteur, a Nightingale, and all other apostles of light and cleanliness, rather than of a woebegone godliness we shall find final deliverance from plague, pestilence, and famine.

—*O'Casey, 1949, pp. 383–384*

COMPETENCIES

Upon completion of this chapter, the reader should be able to:

- Recount the history of communicable diseases and identify efforts throughout history to control these diseases.
- Understand the reasons for the emergence of new viruses and drug-resistant bacteria that are reversing human victories over infectious disease.
- Identify modes of transmission for communicable diseases.
- Explain the difference between acquired, natural, and active immunity.
- Delineate the three levels of prevention as they pertain to sexually transmitted diseases.
- Recognize the causative agents and signs and symptoms of common sexually transmitted diseases.
- Describe appropriate nursing interventions for controlling human immunodeficiency virus (HIV) infection.
- Summarize barriers to the control of communicable diseases.
- Recognize the importance of a global perspective on communicable disease control.

The discussion of **communicable disease,** illness in a susceptible host and caused by a potentially harmful organism or its toxic products, has moved from the public health journal to the evening news and from the microscope to the big screen as new killer strains of both viruses and bacteria appear to be winning the war aimed at disease eradication. **Eradication** is the extermination of an infectious agent and, thus, the irreversible termination of that agent's ability to transmit infection (Centers for Disease Control and Prevention [CDC], 1993b). Only a few years ago, after eradicating smallpox from the planet, epidemiologists promised to move forward on eradicating other fatal communicable diseases. This battle rages on as scientists attempt to gain the high ground in the fight with microorganisms.

This chapter presents the background for nurses' involvement in the control and monitoring of communicable disease. One of the earliest functions of community health nurses was caring for individuals with communicable diseases. This focus later changed to prevention of diseases through early treatment, reporting, and immunization. This chapter also presents an overview of some of the emerging infections as well as of those infectious **agents** (organisms that transfer disease from the environment to the host) that have been known to people for centuries. Also included is a review of the natural history of communicable disease and a discussion of prevention measures effective in controlling transmission. Finally, the chapter summarizes disease transmission, immunity, disease reporting, and the characteristics of select communicable diseases. The beginning community health nurse will be able to utilize the specific principles presented as they pertain to communicable diseases in general and to those diseases reviewed in particular.

HISTORICAL PERSPECTIVES ON COMMUNICABLE DISEASE AND COMMUNITY HEALTH NURSING

Community health nursing and communicable diseases share a long history. As discussed in Chapter 2, tracking case contacts, monitoring infectious disease, and recording disease statistics have been a part of the nurse's responsibilities from the earliest years of professional nursing. Case **contacts** are persons who have been exposed to an infectious agent or environment and who thus have the potential for developing an infectious disease. For years, nurses have been dedicated to improving the health of individuals, families, and communities. The control of the spread of disease plays a large role in this task.

With the growth of urban areas in the early part of the 19th century, epidemics swept through communities. An **epidemic** exists when the number of cases of an infectious agent or disease is clearly in excess of that which is normally expected. Hospitals were unsanitary hotbeds of infection and often were considered places where people went to die. The terrible conditions in the nation's hospitals, the growing fear of epidemics, and the improved understanding of disease origins brought about health care reform efforts in the late 1800s. Just as the cities in the United States began to gain a grasp on infection, a new wave of immigrants poured into the country from Europe.

Because of the number of immigrants settling in East Coast cities, overcrowding and sanitation once again became an issue. Despite public health efforts to control the emergence of new diseases and epidemics, communicable diseases were once again on the rise. Community health nurses were fearless in their pursuit of disease. They carried the black satchel containing necessary equipment wherever there was reported illness. Responsible for keeping everything from measles to diphtheria in check, community health nurses exposed themselves to virulent infections in an effort to assist the sick and prevent further spread of disease.

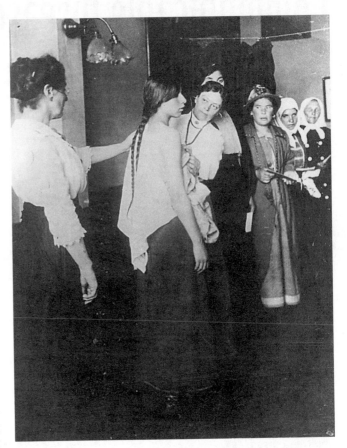

Immigrants were required to pass a physical exam while at Ellis Island to interrupt the spread of infection between countries. Photo courtesy of the Ellis Island Immigration Museum.

In 1900, epidemics of communicable disease ravaged U.S. communities and were the leading cause of death in the United States and throughout the world. Although infectious diseases have taken a backseat to heart disease, cancer, and stroke in the United States, they remain the leading cause of death worldwide. An army of new and reemerging diseases is today threatening the health of the world's citizens (WHO, 1997b).

Community health nurses are taking action to become knowledgeable about the types of diseases that threaten the health of communities in order to play a role in the diagnosis, treatment, control, and prevention of infectious disease.

CHANGING WORLD OF INFECTIOUS DISEASE

Within the past decade, human beings have been forced to focus on their vulnerability on the planet. As people, we must recognize that we are not unlike all other living things when it comes to basic survival instincts and desires, including fundamental needs such as shelter, food, and safety as well as the desire to perpetuate our species. Microorganisms that cause disease in humans neither seek special revenge against nor hold any malice toward humans; they are merely engaged in a struggle for survival and species perpetuation. Many of these organisms have simply found the human body to be a convenient halfway house well suited for their biological life cycles (Hanlon & Pickett, 1979). In the past 20 years, at least 30 new disease-causing organisms have been identified, including the human immunodeficiency (HIV), hepatitis C, and ebola viruses, and the bacterium that causes Lyme disease. Microbial predators are everywhere, and there exists a constant struggle for individual survival.

Today's hospitals are considered a breeding ground for infection. **Nosocomial infections,** infections that develop in a health care setting and that were not present in the client at the time of admission, are feared among clients and health care professionals alike. Super strains of extremely virulent bacteria and viruses make a hospital stay potentially lethal. Hospitalized individuals are more than normally susceptible to infection, are exposed to more infectious agents from both hospital staff and other clients, are given more broad-spectrum antibiotics and immunosuppressive drugs, and are subjected to more invasive procedures and surgeries that make them vulnerable to disease. Nosocomial infections cause substantial morbidity and mortality, prolong the hospital stay of affected patients, and increase direct patient-care costs

(Mandell, Bennett, & Dolin, 1995). Since 1970, the National Nosocomial Infections Surveillance System (NNIS) has collected and analyzed data on the frequency of nosocomial infections in U.S. hospitals.

Striking episodes of deadly infectious-disease emergence have become commonplace in the past two years. One need only pick up the latest news magazine or turn on the television to hear reports of "flesh-eating" bacteria, multidrug-resistant tuberculosis, hantavirus, and food or waterborne illnesses such as the infamous "fast-food bacteria," *Escherichia coli* O157:H7. These microorganisms will take every opportunity possible to develop a biological association with the human host and are spreading with astounding vigor. Communicable disease organisms require a continuous commitment to their control. It has become evident that **mutation,** organism adaptation that results in a modification in the makeup of subsequent generations of the organism, and change are "facts of nature" and that the human species will continue to be challenged by mutant microbes with unpredictable manifestations (Morse, 1993). The **Centers for Disease Control and Prevention (CDC)**—the governmental agency with the mission of promoting health and quality of life by preventing and controlling disease, injury, and disability—has stated that emerging infections lead the list of urgent threats to the world's population (CDC, 1994). Figure 20-1 shows the global microbial threats in the 1990s.

United States citizens take a measure of assurance in existing public health programs that have led to high immunization rates, early detection methods, and readily available pharmacological agents useful in the control of infectious disease. It should be recognized, however, that because of relatively inexpensive, rapid travel opportunities, disease can disseminate quickly around the globe. New patterns of human movement, growing populations and urbanization, climate changes, and changing sexual mores have set in motion a perfect situation for the development of emerging infectious disease. The Institute of Medicine has defined **emerging diseases** as: "new, re-emerging or drug-resistant infections whose incidence in humans has increased within the past two decades or whose incidence threatens to increase in the near future" (CDC, 1994). It is imperative that public health agencies maintain the infrastructure necessary for early detection and treatment of emerging infectious disease. Experts believe that the existing public health infrastructure is overtaxed and not prepared to deal with new health threats (Cassel, 1994).

HEALTHY PEOPLE 2000 OBJECTIVES FOR COMMUNICABLE DISEASE

On September 6, 1990, the U.S. Department of Health and Human Services released the Healthy People 2000 report, the national public health goals and objectives for the 1990s (CDC, 1990). This document is a comprehensive

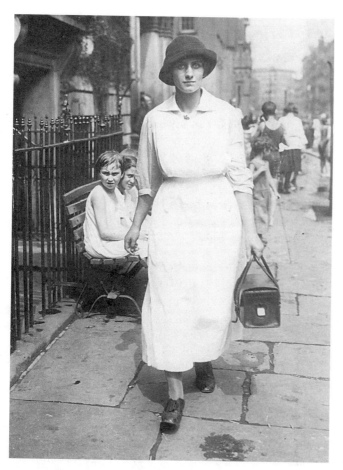

The visiting nurse service served as a first line of defense in the fight against communicable disease.
Photo courtesy of the Visiting Nurse Service of New York.

Figure 20-1 Global Microbial Threats in the 1990s

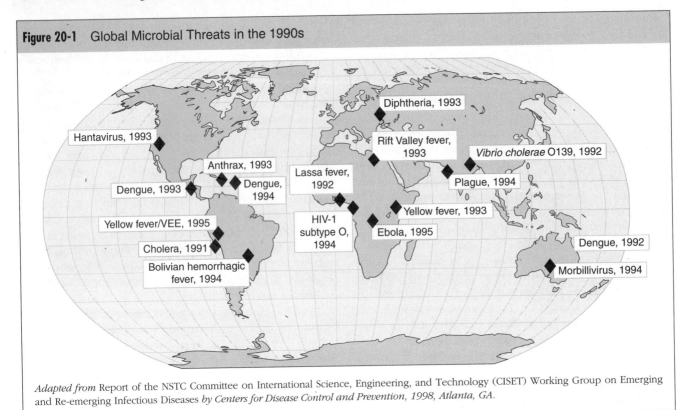

Adapted from Report of the NSTC Committee on International Science, Engineering, and Technology (CISET) Working Group on Emerging and Re-emerging Infectious Diseases *by Centers for Disease Control and Prevention, 1998, Atlanta, GA.*

agenda with 319 objectives organized into 22 priority areas. The overriding goals are to increase years of healthy life, reduce disparities in health among different population groups, and increase access to preventive health services.

More than 10,000 individuals and organizations contributed to the formation of these national goals. Five of the 22 priority categories are directly related to communicable disease: Priority Area 18—HIV Infection; Priority Area 19—Sexually Transmitted Diseases; Priority Area 20—Immunization and Infectious Diseases; Priority Area 21—Clinical Preventive Services; and Priority Area 22—Surveillance and Data Systems (CDC, 1990). Refer to Appendix A for details of Healthy People 2000.

Healthy People is the prevention agenda for the United States. It is a statement of national opportunities—a tool that identifies the most significant preventable threats to health and focuses public and private sector efforts on addressing those threats. Achievement of these objectives is dependent on the ability of health care providers and agencies at all levels to be aware of, assess, and report objective progress.

Development of national health objectives for 2010 has already begun. Through focus-group sessions, public meetings, and a Web site, people from across the country have been able to make their voices heard. To be forward-looking and positive, Healthy People 2010 will address emerging issues such as changing demographics, advances in preventive therapies, and new technologies. Healthy People 2010 will be released in January 2000 (CDC, 1998b).

MODES OF DISEASE TRANSMISSION

The **mode of transmission** of a particular disease is the mechanism by which an infectious agent is transferred from an infected host to an uninfected host. Recall the epidemiologic triangle from Chapter 11. Communicable diseases occur as a result of the interaction between an agent, the causative organism, and a **host** (a person or living species capable of being infected) in a supportive environment. **Environment** is the physical setting that provides the context for agent–host interaction. Community health nurses must be aware of different modes of transmission to be able to understand the most efficient and effective methods to interrupt disease occurrence and to prevent transmission between hosts.

Disease transmission can take place either horizontally or vertically (Gordis, 1996). In **vertical transmission,** disease is transmitted between parent and child. In some cases when a parent has an infectious disease, the disease may be spread to offspring via sperm, placenta, breast milk, or contact with the vaginal canal at birth. Examples of organisms and diseases transmitted vertically include: HIV, herpes, and syphilis. **Horizontal transmission** is the transport of infectious agents from person to person. The transport of infectious agents between hosts can be accomplished in a number of ways: direct transmission, indirect transmission, airborne transmission, and fecal/oral transmission. Figure 20-2 illustrates the concepts of vertical and horizontal transmission.

Figure 20-2 Modes of Transmission

Vertical Transmission

Infection from parent to child via sperm, placenta, breast milk, or contact in the vaginal canal at birth

Horizontal Transmission

Person-to-person spread of infection through one or more of the following routes:

- Direct
- Indirect
- Fecal/oral
- Airborne

Direct Transmission and Indirect Transmission

Direct transmission is the immediate transfer of disease from the infected host to the susceptible host. Transmission of sexually transmitted disease is a prime example of direct transmission. Direct projection of droplet infection into the conjunctiva or mucous membranes of the nose, mouth, or eye during sneezing or coughing is also considered direct transmission. Direct transmission can be implicated in the spread of numerous communicable diseases such as impetigo, scabies, and anthrax. Direct inoculation is the direct transfer of infection from a host via a vehicle that penetrates the susceptible host's natural barriers to disease, such as the skin. An example of direct inoculation would be a needle stick received by a health care worker caring for an infected person.

Indirect transmission occurs when the human host has contact with vehicles or vectors that support and transport the infectious agent. Lyme disease is a classic example of indirect transmission, where the organism is transported to the host via the deer tick. Fleas were the vectors that transmitted bubonic plague from infected rats to the human host, another example of the indirect transmission of disease.

Airborne Transmission

Airborne transmission occurs when microorganisms are suspended in the air and spread to a suitable port of entry. This type of transmission occurs primarily through droplet nuclei or aerosols. Particle size influences how long the organism can remain airborne. The longer the particle is suspended, the greater the chance it will find an available port of entry to the human host. An example of an organism that relies on airborne transmission is measles. Contaminated droplets containing the measles virus are contained in the spray from sneezing. The droplet can find a portal of entry through the mucous membranes or conjunctiva. Droplets that do not remain airborne or settle out are excluded from this category (Benenson, 1995).

Fecal/Oral Transmission

Fecal/oral transmission of an infectious agent occurs directly when the hands or other objects are contaminated with organisms from human or animal feces and then placed in the mouth. Fecal/oral transmission can also occur indirectly via the ingestion of water or food that has been contaminated with fecal particles, as when a restaurant worker fails to properly clean hands and under nails after defecation and before returning to work. Oral–genital sexual activity can also result in fecal/oral transmission of disease. Good handwashing and thorough washing and cooking of food help to decrease the potential spread of disease. Examples of diseases spread through this method of transmission are hemolytic uremic syndrome (caused by the bacterium *Escherichia coli* O157:H7) and hepatitis A.

IMMUNITY

Immunity refers to the resistance of the host to disease. One of the ways communicable diseases are controlled is through efforts directed at strengthening the host. There are three ways that the host may develop immunity, or protection from infectious diseases:

- **Acquired immunity.** The transfer of antibodies from mother to child via the placenta or breastfeeding. If a mother has developed antibodies to particular agents, she can pass on short-term immunity to the newborn child. This ability to provide immunity to neonates, who typically are vulnerable to infectious disease, is an important reason for the community health nurse to educate women about the benefits of breastfeeding.
- **Natural immunity.** The development of antibodies that protect against subsequent infections as a result of the host's having acquired an infection. Diseases such as diphtheria, measles, and pertussis are good examples of diseases that produce lifelong immunity. Not all organisms, however, produce natural immunity in the host. Most sexually transmitted diseases do not provide natural immunity. Thus, without appropriate treatment, reinfection is common.
- **Active immunity.** Vaccination of the host. Properly administered immunizations provide the host with lifelong protection from disease. United States policy requires documentation of active immunity in children prior to school entrance. Recommendations for immunization of HIV-infected children and adult immunization are listed in Tables 20-1 and 20-2, respectively. The CDC's pediatric immunization schedule can be found in Appendix J.

Table 20-1   Recommendations for Routine Immunization of HIV-Infected Children

| VACCINE | HIV INFECTION | |
	KNOWN ASYMPTOMATIC	SYMPTOMATIC
DTP	Yes	Yes
OPV	Contraindicated	Contraindicated
IPV	Yes	Yes
MMR	Yes	Yes*
Hib	Yes	Yes
Pneumococcal	Yes	Yes
Influenza	Yes	Yes
Hepatitis B	Yes	Yes

*Should be considered.

From The Manual for the Surveillance of Vaccine-Preventable Diseases, by Centers for Disease Control and Prevention, 1996, Atlanta, GA.

VACCINE-PREVENTABLE DISEASES

History is full of colorful examples of individuals who were victims of infectious diseases that were rampant around the world until the mid-1950s. Franklin D. Roosevelt was infected with paralytic polio at the height of his political career, and it is reported that Wild Bill Hickock's only son was a victim of diphtheria. Few households escaped the wrath of the "hard" measles (rubeola), German measles (rubella), and mumps. Hospitals had entire wards dedicated to the care of whooping cough (pertussis) victims. It is easy to forget the devastation these diseases caused before the widespread development of vaccines that now prevent their occurrence. National immunization programs have been so successful that parents today no longer fear these diseases.

Authorities in virtually every nation of the world recommend routine immunization of children as the best way to prevent illness and death caused by certain infections. Some individuals have not taken advantage of the availability of vaccinations at relatively low cost throughout the United States. Missed opportunities for vaccination have also impeded progress in the national campaign to have every child immunized by age 2. Missed opportunities for immunization occur when a child in need of immunization seeks health care but does not receive needed immunizations.

Contraindications to Immunization

Community health nurses must be aware of the relatively few contraindications to immunization (see Table 20-3) and must take advantage of every possible opportunity to provide immunizations to individuals seeking care. There are only two permanent contraindications to vaccination:

- Severe allergy to a vaccine component or following a prior dose of a vaccine
- Encephalopathy without a known cause and occurring within 7 days of a dose of pertussis vaccine

Four vaccine contraindications that are generally temporary:

- Pregnancy
- Immunosuppression
- Severe illness
- Recent receipt of blood products

Live vaccines should not be given until these conditions are resolved (CDC, 1996c). Mild common illnesses such as otitis media, upper respiratory infections, colds, and diarrhea are *not* contraindications to immunization. In communities with poor immunization rates, barriers to successful immunization should be assessed and, where possible, removed. Vaccination status should be assessed at all health visits in an effort to complete necessary immunizations. Health departments and clinics should be flexible in scheduling appointments and should not penalize individuals who do not have transportation or adequate financial resources. Community health nurses play a vital role in ensuring that all infants and children

Table 20-2   Vaccines and Toxoids Recommended for Adults, by Age Group, United States

| AGE | VACCINE/TOXOID | | | | | | |
	INFLUENZA	PNEUMOCOCCAL	MEASLES	MUMPS	RUBELLA	VARICELLA	Td[1]
18–24			X	X	X	X	X
25–64			X[2]	X	X[3]	X	X
65	X	X				X	X

[1]Td = Tetanus and diphtheria toxoids, absorbed (for adult use), a combined preparation containing <2 flocculation units of diphtheria toxoid.
[2]One dose for all persons born in 1957 or later; two doses for health care workers, college students, and travelers born in 1957 or later.
[3]For persons born after 1956.
Adapted from The Manual for the Surveillance of Vaccine-Preventable Diseases, by Centers for Disease Control and Prevention, 1996, Atlanta, GA.

~~REFLECTIVE THINKING~~

REFLECTIVE THINKING

Adults and Immunization

Many adults forget their vulnerability to disease and may fail to take necessary precautions to protect themselves from infection and, possibly, death and to interrupt the spread of disease.

- When was the last time you had a tetanus immunization?
- Have you been protected against hepatitis A and B?
- Should you have a flu shot?

are given the opportunity to be protected from unnecessary illness.

Development of a National Immunization Program

The first support for a national immunization program developed after the licensure of inactivated poliomyelitis vaccine (IPV) in 1955. In the two-week period following the successful field trial of this important vaccine, approx-imately 4 million doses of vaccine were administered, primarily to elementary school children. On April 25, 1955, however, an infant with paralytic poliomyelitis was admitted to a Chicago hospital. The disease case was important because it occurred exactly nine days after the child was immunized with the IPV vaccine. Five additional cases of poliomyelitis were reported the following day. All of the children received vaccine that was produced by one manufacturer. In each case, the paralysis developed first in the limb where the vaccine was administered. On April 27, 1955, the surgeon general asked the manufacturer to recall all remaining lots of vaccine (CDC, 1996c).

As a result of these vaccine-related events, state health officers were asked to designate a polio reporting officer responsible for reporting cases of poliomyelitis among vaccinated persons. Case reports were sent to the poliomyelitis surveillance unit, where the data were analyzed and disseminated via poliomyelitis surveillance reports. The first report was published only three days after surveillance activity began. Case data confirmed suspicion that the problems were confined to one vaccine manufacturer. Without the rapid instigation of a surveillance program, the manufacture of poliomyelitis vaccine might have been halted entirely. Important aspects of modern public health surveillance include data collection, data analysis, and rapid dissemination of information (CDC, 1996c).

Table 20-3 Guide to Contraindications and Precautions to Vaccinations (True and Not True Contraindications)

VACCINE	TRUE CONTRAINDICATIONS AND PRECAUTIONS	NOT TRUE (VACCINES MAY BE GIVEN)
General for all vaccines [DTP/DTaP, OPV, IPV, MMR, Hib, HBV]	Anaphylactic reaction to a vaccine contraindicates further doses of that vaccine Anaphylactic reaction to a vaccine constituent contraindicates the use of vaccines containing that substance Moderate or severe illnesses with or without a fever	Mild to moderate local reaction (soreness, redness, swelling) following a dose of an injectable antigen Mild acute illness with or without low-grade fever Current antimicrobial therapy Convalescent phase of illnesses Prematurity (same dosage and indications as for normal, full-term infants) Recent exposure to an infectious disease History of penicillin or other nonspecific allergies or fact that relatives have such allergies
DTP/DTaP	Encephalopathy within 7 days of administration of previous dose of DTP **Precautions*** Fever of ≥40.5°C (105°C) within 48 hrs after vaccination with a prior dose of DTP Collapse or shocklike state (hypotonic-hyporesponsive episode) within 48 hrs of receiving a prior dose of DTP	Temperature of <40.5°C (105°F) following a previous dose of DTP Family history of convulsions** Family history of sudden infant death syndrome

Continued

Table 20-3   Guide to Contraindications and Precautions to Vaccinations (True and Not True Contraindications) *(Continued)*

VACCINE	TRUE CONTRAINDICATIONS AND PRECAUTIONS	NOT TRUE (VACCINES MAY BE GIVEN)
	Seizures within 3 days of receiving a prior dose of DTP (see footnote** regarding management of children with a personal history of seizures at any time)	Family history of an adverse event following DTP administration
	Persistent, inconsolable crying lasting ≥3 hrs, within 48 hrs of receiving a prior dose of DTP	
OPV***	Infection with HIV or a household contact with HIV	Breastfeeding
	Known altered immunodeficiency (hematologic and solid tumors; congenital immunodeficiency; and long-term immunosuppressive therapy)	Current antimicrobial therapy
	Immunodeficient household contact	
	Precaution*	
	Pregnancy	Diarrhea
IPV	Anaphylactic reaction to neomycin or streptomycin	
	Precaution*	
	Pregnancy	
MMR***	Anaphylactic reactions to egg ingestion and to neomycin****	Tuberculosis or positive PPD
	Pregnancy	Simultaneous TB skin testing*****
	Known altered immunodeficiency (hematologic and solid tumors; congenital immunodeficiency; and long-term immunosuppressive therapy)	Breastfeeding
		Pregnancy of mother of recipient
	Precaution*	
	Recent (within 3 months) IG administration	Immunodeficient family member or household contact
		Infection with HIV
		Nonanaphylactic reactions to eggs or neomycin
Hib		
HBV		Pregnancy

*The events or conditions listed as precautions, although not contraindications, should be carefully reviewed. The benefits and risks of administering a specific vaccine to an individual under the circumstances should be considered. If the risks are believed to outweigh the benefits, the immunization should be withheld; if the benefits are believed to outweigh the risks (for example, during an outbreak or foreign travel), the immunization should be given. Whether and when to administer DTP to children with proven or suspected underlying neurologic disorders should be decided on an individual basis. It is prudent on theoretical grounds to avoid vaccinating pregnant women. However, if immediate protection against poliomyelitis is needed, OPV, not IPV, is recommended.

**Acetaminophen given prior to administering DTP and thereafter every 4 hours for 24 hours should be considered for children with a personal history of convulsions or with a family history of convulsions in siblings or parents.

***There is a theoretical risk that the administration of multiple live virus vaccines (OPV & MMR) within 30 days of one another if not given on the same day will result in a suboptimal immune response. There are no data to substantiate this.

****Persons with a history of anaphylactic reactions following egg ingestion should be vaccinated only with extreme caution. Protocols have been developed for vaccinating such persons and should be consulted (J Pediatr 1983;102:196–9, J Pediatr 1988;113:504–6).

*****Measles vaccination may temporarily suppress tuberculin reactivity. If testing can not be done the day of MMR vaccination, the test should be postponed for 4–6 weeks.

This information is based on the recommendations of the Advisory Committee on Immunization Practices (ACIP) and those of the Committee on Infectious Diseases (Red Book Committee) of the American Academy of Pediatrics (AAP). Sometimes these recommendations vary from those contained in the manufacturer's package inserts. For more detailed information, providers should consult the published recommendations of the ACIP, the AAP, the AAFP, and the manufacturer's package inserts.

From Standards for Pediatric Immunization Practices, by Centers for Disease Control and Prevention, 1997, Atlanta, GA.

The National Immunization Program (NIP) at the CDC performs national surveillance for measles, mumps, rubella, congenital rubella syndrome, diphtheria, tetanus, pertussis, poliomyelitis, and varicella. The National Center for Infectious Diseases at the CDC is responsible for surveillance of other vaccine-preventable diseases such as hepatitis A and B, *Haemophilus influenzae* type b (Hib) invasive disease, influenza, and pneumococcal disease. Cases are reported to state health departments and then to the National Notifiable Diseases Surveillance System. The collected data are analyzed and then published in the *Morbidity and Mortality Weekly Report (MMWR)*. Reported cases of selected vaccine-preventable diseases from 1990 to 1996 are shown in Table 20-4.

Development of New Vaccines

Campaigns to promote the widespread vaccination of children, as well as school entrance requirements, have resulted in tremendous decreases in the morbidity and mortality related to vaccine-preventable diseases in the United States. Diseases that in recent history were recognized as leading causes of death and disability among children, such as diphtheria and congenital rubella syndrome, are now almost nonexistent.

Until the development of the Hib vaccine in the 1980s, *Haemophilus influenzae* type b was the most frequent cause of bacterial meningitis among children and resulted in approximately 900 deaths each year (CDC, 1996c). Until 1995, most individuals expected to develop varicella (chicken pox) at some time in their life. There were an estimated 4 million cases of varicella in the United States in the early 1990s (CDC, 1996c). Although varicella has

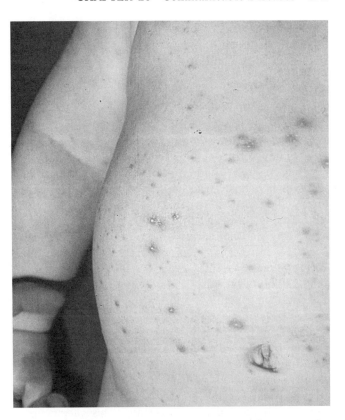

A vaccine to prevent varicella was licensed for use in the United States in 1995. Photo courtesy of Robert A. Silverman, MD, Clinical Associate Professor, Department of Pediatrics, Georgetown University.

traditionally been considered a mild illness with predictable outbreaks among school children each spring, 100 deaths with varicella as the underlying cause were reported annually. In March 1995, the live attenuated

Table 20-4 **Reported Cases of Selected Vaccine-Preventable Diseases, 1990–1996**							
DISEASE	**1990**	**1991**	**1992**	**1993**	**1994**	**1995**	**1996**
Measles	27,786	9,643	2,237	312	963	309	508
Rubella	1,125	1,401	160	192	227	128	238
Poliomyelitis, paralytic[+]	6	9	6	3	8	6	5
Diphtheria	4	5	4	—	2	—	2
Tetanus	64	57	45	48	51	41	36
Haemophilus influenzae invasive disease (aged <5 yrs)[φ]	nn	1,540	592	435	329	290	1,170
Pertussis	4,570	2,719	4,083	6,586	4,617	5,137	7,796
Mumps	5,292	4,264	2,572	1,692	1,537	906	751
Hepatitis B	21,102	18,003	16,126	13,361	12,517	10,805	10,637

Confirmed and unknown case status only.

[+]*No cases were wild virus–associated. Data from previous years subject to change due to delayed reporting.*

[φ]*Invasive disease including type b, other types, untyped, and untypable strains; only cases due to type b are preventable by vaccine. nn = not nationally notifiable*

Adapted from The Manual for the Surveillance of Vaccine-Preventable Diseases *by Centers for Disease Control and Prevention, 1996, Atlanta, GA.*

varicella vaccine was licensed for use in the United States. Immunity has been shown to persist in 20-year follow-up studies in Japan and 10-year follow-up studies in the United States. Studies have also shown fewer and milder cases of shingles, a reblossoming of infection from the dormant virus (Plotkin, 1996).

Another vaccine recently (1995) licensed for use in persons 2 years of age and older is the hepatitis A vaccine. This vaccine provides long-term protection against the hepatitis A virus. Children and adults need a two shot series of hepatitis A vaccine in a six-month interval for sustained protection. Two inactivated hepatitis A vaccines are currently commercially available: HAVRIX® (SmithKline Beecham Biologicals) and VAQTA® (Merck and Company). Surveillance will be important to monitor the impact of these vaccines.

In addition to the availability of new vaccines, recommendations for administration of standard vaccines have changed. Recommendations for the use of IPV for the first two doses of polio vaccination come as a direct result of the eradication of "wild polio" virus from the Western Hemisphere and as a result of potential vaccine complications from previous vaccines (CDC, 1996c). A new acellular pertussis vaccine is now available in combination with diphtheria and tetanus (DTaP). This vaccine produces fewer reactions (Peters, 1997a). Appendix J lists the recommended immunization schedule as of 1998.

Centers for Disease Control and Prevention Disease-Reduction Goals

The CDC's 1996 and 2000 disease-reduction goals (see Table 20-5) represent remarkable progress toward the eradication of vaccine-preventable diseases. In order to consolidate national efforts and promote further reductions in disease incidence, the Childhood Immunization Initiative (CII) established goals for the elimination of indigenous acquisition of six vaccine-preventable diseases by 1996. The goals established by the CII were interim milestones toward the Healthy People 2000 health objectives for the United States. The Healthy People 2000 objectives include disease-elimination objectives for diphtheria and tetanus (among persons 25 years of age and younger), polio, measles, rubella, and congenital rubella syndrome. Also included are disease-reduction goals for mumps, pertussis, and hepatitis B. Although no specific disease-reduction or -elimination goal for *H. influenzae* type b infection was established by the Healthy People 2000 objectives, there is a goal for the reduction of bacterial meningitis, to no more than 4.7 cases per 100,000 people, from a baseline of 6.3 per 100,000 in 1986. Refer to Appendix A for more information on Healthy People 2000.

Great challenges remain in meeting the disease-reduction and -elimination goals established by Healthy People 2000. Achievement of disease-reduction goals depends on several factors including maintenance of high vaccination coverage among children, development of improved strategies to encourage appropriate vaccination of adults, accurate and timely diagnosis and reporting of suspected cases, and thorough case investigations (CDC, 1996c). Community health nurses can take an active role in ensuring the success of immunization programs by working to eliminate barriers to immunization.

Table 20-6 summarizes the clinical descriptions, laboratory criteria for diagnosis, and case classifications of the most common vaccine-preventable diseases. Immunization is the most effective disease-control measure in

Table 20-5 Disease Reduction and Elimination Goals: 1996 and 2000			
DISEASE	**1996 GOALS**	**1996 ACTUAL**	**2000 GOALS**
Measles	0	508	0
Rubella	0	238	0
Polio*	0	5	0
Diphtheria	0	2	0[β]
Tetanus	0[ξ]	36	0[β]
Hib	0**	1,170	No goal established[ββ]
Pertussis	No goal established	7,796	1,000
Mumps	1,600	751	500
Hepatitis B		10,637	40 per 100,000 population

*Wild-type disease

[β]*Among persons ≤ 25 years of age*

[ξ]*Among persons <15 years of age*

**Among children <5 years of age*

[ββ]*Although no goal was established specifically for Hib, there is a goal for reduction in the incidence of bacterial meningitis from 6.3 per 100,000 population (1986) to no more than 4.7 per 100,000 by the year 2000.*

From "Provisional Cases of Selected Notifiable Diseases United States," MMWR, 46(51), Dec. 26, pp. 1236–1239, by Centers for Disease Control and Prevention. Atlanta, GA.

Table 20-6 Summary of Case Definitions for Selected Vaccine-Preventable Diseases

DISEASE	CLINICAL DESCRIPTION	LABORATORY CRITERIA FOR DIAGNOSIS	CASE CLASSIFICATION
Diphtheria	An upper respiratory tract illness characterized by a sore throat, a low-grade fever, and an adherent membrane of the tonsil(s), pharynx, and/or nose without other apparent cause.	Isolation of *Corynebacterium diphtheriae* from clinical specimens	*Probable:* meets the clinical case definition, is not laboratory confirmed, and is not epidemiologically linked to a laboratory confirmed case. *Confirmed:* meets the clinical case definition and is either laboratory confirmed or epidemiologically linked to a confirmed case.
Haemophilus influenzae invasive disease	Invasive disease due to *Haemophilus influenzae* may produce several syndromes including meningitis, bacteremia, epiglottitis, or pneumonia.	Isolation of *H. influenzae* from a normally sterile site.	*Probable:* a clinically compatible disease with detection of *H. influenzae* type b antigen in cerebrospinal fluid. *Confirmed:* a clinically compatible illness that is culture confirmed.
Measles	An illness characterized by the following clinical features: • A generalized rash lasting three days or longer • A temperature of at least 38.3°C (101°F) • Cough, coryza, or conjunctivitis	• Isolation of measles virus from a clinical specimen, or • Significant rise in measles antibody level as measured by any standard serological assay, or • Positive serological test for measles IgM antibody.	*Suspect:* any rash illness with fever. *Probable:* meets the clinical case definition, has no serological or virological testing, and is not epidemiologically linked to a probable or confirmed case. *Confirmed:* a case that is laboratory confirmed or that meets the clinical case definition and is epidemiologically linked to a confirmed or probable case. A laboratory-confirmed case does not have to meet the clinical case definition.
Mumps	An illness with acute onset of unilateral or bilateral tender, self-limited swelling of the parotid or other salivary gland that lasts two days or longer and has no other apparent cause.	• Isolation of mumps virus from a clinical specimen, or • Significant rise in mumps antibody level as measured by any standard serological assay, or • Positive serological test for mumps IgM antibody.	*Probable:* meets the clinical case definition, has no or noncontributory serological or virological testing, and is not epidemiologically linked to a confirmed or probable case. *Confirmed:* a case that is laboratory confirmed or that meets the clinical case definition and is epidemiologically linked to a confirmed or probable case. A laboratory-confirmed case does not have to meet the clinical case definition.
Pertussis	A cough illness that lasts at least two weeks and has one of the following: paroxysms of coughing, inspiratory "whoop," or post-tussive vomiting, all without other apparent cause.	Isolation of *Bordetella pertussis* from clinical specimen	*Probable:* meets the clinical case definition, is not laboratory confirmed, and is not epidemiologically linked to a laboratory confirmed case. *Confirmed:* a clinically compatible case that is laboratory confirmed or epidemiologically linked to a laboratory-confirmed case.*

Continued

Table 20-6 Summary of Case Definitions for Selected Vaccine-Preventable Diseases (Continued)

DISEASE	CLINICAL DESCRIPTION	LABORATORY CRITERIA FOR DIAGNOSIS	CASE CLASSIFICATION
Poliomyelitis, paralytic	Acute onset of a flaccid paralysis of one or more limbs and decreased or absent tendon reflexes in the affected limbs, all without other apparent cause and without sensory or cognitive loss (as reported by a physician)		*Probable:* a case that meets the clinical case definition. *Confirmed:* a case that meets the clinical case definition and where the patient has a neurological deficit 60 days after onset of initial symptoms, has died, or has unknown follow-up status.**
Rubella	An illness with all of the following characteristics: • Acute onset of generalized maculopapular rash • Temperature more than 37.2°C (99°F) • Arthralgia/arthritis, lymphadenopathy, or conjunctivitis	• Isolation of the rubella virus, or • Significant rise in rubella antibody level as measured by any standard serological assay, or • Positive serological test for rubella IgM antibody	*Suspect:* any generalized rash illness of acute onset. *Probable:* a case that meets the clinical case definition, has no or noncontributory serological or virological testing, and is not epidemiologically linked to a laboratory-confirmed case. *Confirmed:* a case that is laboratory confirmed or that meets the clinical case definition and is epidemiologically linked to a laboratory-confirmed case.
Tetanus	Acute onset of hypertonia and/or painful muscular contractions (usually of the muscles of the jaw and neck) and generalized muscle spasms without other apparent medical cause (as reported by a health professional)		*Confirmed:* a case that meets the clinical case definition.
Varicella	An illness with acute onset of diffuse (generalized) papulovesicular rash without other apparent cause (as reported by a health professional)	• Isolation of varicella virus from clinical specimen, or • Significant rise in varicella antibody level as measured by any standard serological assay	*Probable:* a case that meets the clinical case definition, is not laboratory confirmed, and is not epidemiologically linked to another probable or confirmed case. *Confirmed:* a case that is laboratory confirmed or that meets the clinical case definition and is epidemiologically linked to a confirmed or probable case.*

Two probable cases that are epidemiologically linked would be considered confirmed even in the absence of laboratory confirmation.
**All suspected cases of paralytic poliomyelitis are reviewed by a panel of expert consultants before final classification occurs. Only confirmed cases are included in Table 1 in the MMWR. Suspected cases are enumerated in a footnote to the MMWR table.*
Adapted from The Manual for the Surveillance of Vaccine-Preventable Diseases *by Centers for Disease Control and Prevention, 1996, Atlanta, GA.*

limiting the spread of these diseases. Educational measures are important to inform the public of the hazards of vaccine-preventable diseases and the necessity for immunization. Preventing and controlling the transmission of vaccine-preventable diseases into the next century will require the continuous efforts of public health personnel.

SEXUALLY TRANSMITTED DISEASE

Sexually transmitted diseases (STDs) are caused by more than 25 infectious organisms whose primary mode of transmission is through sexual activity, although it is believed that more than 50 diseases are capable of being transmitted sexually (CDC, 1992). The close physical contact and sharing of fluids associated with sexual activity provide perfect conditions for the direct transmission of infectious organisms. In 1996, STDs held the distinction of occupying five of the nation's 10 most frequently reported diseases (CDC, 1997i). Today's STD epidemic developed in the 1960s, when postwar baby boomers explored new-found freedoms. Birth control pills came into widespread use, and barrier contraceptives and the disease protection they offered were cast aside for the freedom and assurance that came with the oral contraceptive. Venereal disease appeared to be well controlled by the use of antibiotics. No one could have predicted the vengeance with which STDs would again explode onto the infectious-disease scene. Although AIDS would draw the attention of the nation as thousands became infected with the deadly disease, other STDs such as hepatitis B, herpes virus, and human papillomavirus spread silently until they began to be reported in epidemic proportions in the 1990s.

The spectrum of consequences related to this national epidemic range from mild symptoms to serious and long-term problems such as cervical, liver, and other cancers; reproductive health problems; and death. Societal problems, behavioral and social stereotypes, and unbalanced mass media messages present barriers to the prevention and control of STDs at all levels. These barriers contribute to the "hidden" nature of these diseases and impede important dialogue that would facilitate primary prevention efforts for risk reduction (Donovan, 1993; Eng & Butler, 1996).

The rates of curable STDs in the United States are the highest in the developed world and are higher than in some developing regions. In the United States, 12 million new STD cases are reported to the CDC annually (Donovan, 1993; Anderson, 1994). Despite these astounding figures, it is believed that STDs are underreported (CDC, 1995). Community health nurses can support STD-control programs via case contact notification and effective case management of individuals affected by disease.

Populations at Increased Risk

Adolescents, young adults, women, minorities, substance abusers, and persons of low socioeconomic status are listed among those at the greatest risk for the development of STDs and AIDS. Sexually transmitted diseases are most prevalent among teenagers and young adults under age 25. Teenage girls are particularly vulnerable to infection because of immature reproductive systems (Donovan, 1993). Women are more likely than men to acquire an STD after exposure to infection because of anatomical differences that augment transmission and support "silent" infection. In addition, women tend to suffer more devastating consequences of untreated infection, such as infertility and cervical cancer (Donovan, 1993). Intravenous drug use and heterosexual contact are responsible for the greatest proportion of AIDS among women (see Figure

20-3). Increased rates of infection among African American and Hispanic women are remarkable. Although African American and Hispanic women made up only 21% of all U.S. women, they constituted 77% of reported AIDS cases among women in 1996 (CDC, 1997f).

The use of illicit drugs and the STD epidemic have expanded together in the United States. Blood-borne diseases such as hepatitis B and AIDS can be transmitted when needles are shared. Poverty tends to create an environment that supports the spread of disease: Crowded neighborhoods with high rates of drug use, infection, and delayed health-seeking behaviors contribute to the spread of STDs in this population.

Prevention of Sexually Transmitted Disease

Sexually transmitted diseases significantly impact health care costs in the United States. In 1994, experts estimated that the health care costs associated with a select group of STD other than HIV/AIDS carried a $10 billion price tag, with HIV/AIDS adding an additional $6.7 billion (Eng & Butler, 1996). Costs could be decreased significantly via effective primary prevention, including education about ways to prevent the spread of infection and the availability of immunization for some diseases, and via secondary prevention efforts that support detection, treatment, and effective case management of STDs in their early stages. Tertiary prevention to support appropriate long-term

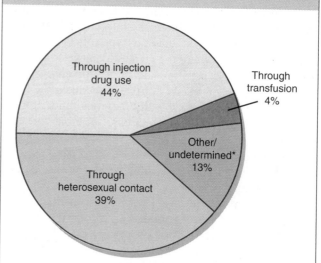

Figure 20-3 AIDS Transmission to Women—Reported Cases through June 1997

Includes clients under investigation; clients who died, were lost to follow-up, or who refused to interview; and clients whose mode of exposure to HIV remains undetermined after investigation.

Adapted from "Female/Adult/Adolescent AIDS Cases by Exposure and Ethnicity" by Centers for Disease Control and Prevention, 1997, HIV/AIDS Surveillance Report, 9(1), p. 10.

treatment and management of chronic infection will provide the most optimal health outcomes. This approach is especially important with viral STDs, which may present lifelong symptoms. Prevention of STDs will be discussed in more detail in the section "The Role of the Community Health Nurse in the Prevention of STDs."

Sexually transmitted diseases are classified into two main categories: viral and nonviral. Whereas nonviral STDs can usually be treated without long-term consequences, viral illnesses have no cure.

Viral Sexually Transmitted Diseases

When viral STDs are diagnosed, individuals face a lifetime of outbreaks and the need for both infection and symptom management. Public health efforts focus on primary prevention, with the goal of preventing disease occurrence. The emergence of AIDS in the 1980s forced a reluctant public to face the deadly consequences of viral STD infection. Research shows that STDs appear to increase in areas where AIDS is common (Henderson, 1997). Although AIDS has received the most attention in this category because of its mortality statistics, other viral infections such as hepatitis B, herpes simplex 2, and human papillomavirus are epidemic within world populations and account for larger numbers of infected individuals.

Acquired Immunodeficiency Syndrome

Human immunodeficiency virus (HIV) is responsible for the development of AIDS (acquired immunodeficiency syndrome), a devastating illness that was first recognized in 1981 (Benenson, 1995). A retrovirus, HIV infects a cell and uses an enzyme called reverse transcriptase. This enzyme then transcribes the viral genome onto the cell's DNA, resulting in viral replication by the infected cell. Although the virus is able to attack numerous types of cells, the CD4, or helper T-cell, is where the greatest damage from infection occurs. These cells are the body's defense against infection and cancer. In HIV-positive individuals, the numbers of CD4 cells decrease with time, thus rendering the infected person vulnerable to disease. Without the CD4 cells, the body becomes a host for opportunistic infections. Several opportunistic infections and cancers were considered specific indicators of AIDS and were included in the initial case definition published by the CDC in 1982. This definition was revised in 1987 and again in 1993 (CDC, 1993a) as more information about the disease became available. The disease causes a gradual destruction of the immune system and progresses at a different pace in each infected person. Opportunistic infections often occur only in the advanced stages of AIDS, causing a delay in diagnostic classification of the disease. With the revision of surveillance case definitions in 1993, a CD4 cell count of fewer than 200 cells/mm^3, regardless of an individual's clinical status, is now considered an AIDS case (CDC, 1993a; Benenson, 1995). Most individuals who die from

AIDS do so as a result of opportunistic infections or cancer rather than the virus itself. Because of their associated low resistance to disease, persons with AIDS have become "incubators" for diseases once thought to be controlled, such as tuberculosis (TB).

Human immunodeficiency virus can be subdivided into two types of infection: HIV-1 and HIV-2. Although the two types of infection have similar characteristics, the pathogenicity of HIV-2 appears to be less than that of HIV-1. **Pathogenicity** is the ability or power of an infectious agent to produce disease. Individuals infected with HIV-2 take longer to develop AIDS, and the disease progresses at a slower pace. United States blood centers have been testing for HIV-1 infection since 1985 and for HIV-2 since 1992. Those individuals listed in Figure 20-4 should request an HIV-2 enzyme immunoassay, or EIA.

Transmission

Early in the epidemic, AIDS was thought to be a disease of homosexual men. First documented with rare manifestations of *Pneumocystis carinii* pneumonia and Kaposi's sarcoma in previously healthy, young homosexual men in San Francisco and New York, AIDS is now recognized as a disease and has been recorded in almost all countries. It affects men, women, and children of all races and sexual orientation and from all social classes with equally devastating consequences (Benenson, 1995). No cure has been found, and no vaccine is available to prevent this fatal disease, which is currently the leading cause of death

Figure 20-4 Persons for Whom HIV-2 Testing Is Indicated

- Those who have sex with or share needles with West Africans
- Persons who have received blood transfusions in West Africa
- Children born to HIV-2–infected mothers
- Those with conditions suggestive of HIV infection (such as an AIDS-associated opportunistic disease) for whom HIV-1 testing is not positive
- Persons whose blood specimens are reactive on HIV-1 EIA testing and exhibit certain unusual indeterminate patterns on HIV-1 Western blot

RESEARCH FOCUS

Attitudes, Concerns, and Fear of AIDS among Registered Nurses in the United States

STUDY PROBLEM/PURPOSE

This study examined nurses' attitudes, fears, and concerns toward persons with AIDS. The study investigated nurses' willingness to interact with or provide nursing care to persons with AIDS.

METHODS

Nurses in four hospitals and two schools of nursing were recruited to participate. The sample consisted of 35 nurse assistants, 211 registered nurses, 58 nurse supervisors, and 28 faculty members employed at two schools of nursing, as well as 44 other nurses working at various institutions.

Nurses' attitudes, concerns, and fear of AIDS were measured on an 84-item AIDS questionnaire that was distributed to contact persons at each institution and collected through voluntary participation. The questionnaire was anonymous, and subjects were assured that their identity would not be revealed.

FINDINGS

Seven factors emerged as principal components in determining attitudes toward AIDS clients; the three highest-ranking scores related to fear of AIDS all involved situations that may require nurse contact with the blood of clients with AIDS. Fear-of-AIDS scores were correlated strongly with the nurses' duties and potential contact with blood or physical closeness to persons with AIDS. An additional finding, based on the nurses' choice of duties, was that clients with hepatitis were also considered undesirable clients, again probably because nurses considered blood a primary source of contracting AIDS. The study showed that nurses who were less sympathetic toward gay men had a correspondingly increased fear of contracting the disease through caring for AIDS clients.

IMPLICATIONS

Nurses who come in contact with HIV-positive persons may perceive themselves to be at great risk for contracting the disease in the routine care of AIDS clients. Some nurses believe they have the right to refuse to care for persons with AIDS. By recognizing fears, becoming educated in AIDS prevention methods, and increasing knowledge, nurses may improve negative attitudes.

SOURCE

From "Attitudes, Concerns, and Fear of Acquired Immunodeficiency Syndrome among Registered Nurses in the United States" by J. F. Wang, 1997, Holistic Nursing Practice, 11(2), pp. 36–50.

---

by any cause among adults ages 25 to 44 (Anderson, Kochanek, & Murphy, 1997).

Human immunodeficiency virus is found in the blood, semen, and vaginal secretions of an infected person and is not transmitted via casual contact such as hugging, touching, or shaking hands. Transmission from blood transfusions has been rare since HIV screening of all blood and blood products was instituted in March 1985. All blood collected in the United States is now screened for six infectious agents: HIV-1, HIV-2, HTLV-1 (human T-cell lymphotropic virus), hepatitis B virus, hepatitis C virus, and the syphilis spirochete. All potential donors are interviewed before they are tested and are informed that if they have a risk factor for HIV, they should not donate. Every unit of blood with a positive result from HIV-antibody testing is discarded, and future donations are not accepted from those persons. It is estimated that the risk of acquiring infection from a blood transfusion is now 1 in 225,000 units (CDC, 1997b).

Transmission of HIV can occur via:

- Sexual contact involving exchange of body fluids with an infected individual
- Blood transfusion prior to 1985
- Exposure to blood products or tissues of an infected person
- Perinatal transmission from an infected mother to the fetus during pregnancy, delivery, or breastfeeding
- Sharing needles or syringes with an infected person

It is important that the community health nurse be aware that the HIV virus is principally spread via unprotected sex and needle sharing with an HIV-infected person. All pregnant women should be informed about the risk of HIV transmission to their babies and of treatment options that have been shown to be effective in preventing the vertical transmission of the AIDS virus. Although blood transfusions served as a mode of transmission when the virus was first discovered, persons who received blood transfusions after 1985 have a very limited risk of acquiring the infection. It is equally important that community health nurses be able to dispel the myths surrounding this disease by informing the populations they serve that HIV is not transmitted via casual contact or insect bites or stings. Figure 20-5 shows the HIV-exposure groups that account for most cases of AIDS in the United States. Studies conducted by the CDC show no evidence of HIV transmission via insect vectors. Reasons transmission

Figure 20-5 HIV Exposure Groups

Exposure Category	No.	%
Men		
MSM[1]	111,860	48
IDU[2]	48,000	20
MSM-IDU	14,660	6
Heterosexual	12,300	5
Total	**191,040**	**81**
Women		
IDU	19,700	8
Heterosexual	22,660	10
Total	**44,440**	**19**
Total[3]	235,470	100

Note: Estimates are presented rounded to the nearest 10 because they do not represent exact counts of persons with AIDS but are estimates that are approximately ±3% of the true value.

[1]*Men who have sex with men.*

[2]*Injection drug users.*

[3]*Includes persons aged ≥13 years with hemophilia/coagulation disorders, transfusion recipients or with other or no risks reported. The sum of the estimates for men and women may not equal total annual estimates because of rounding.*

Adapted from "Update: Trends in AIDS Incidence—United States, 1996" by Centers for Disease Control and Prevention, 1997, MMWR, 46, pp. 165–173.

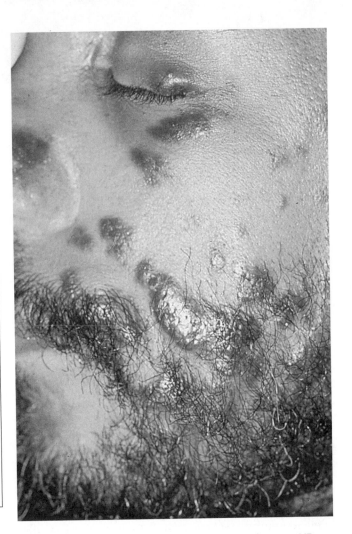

Kaposi's sarcoma. *Photo courtesy of Robert A. Silverman, MD, Clinical Associate Professor, Department of Pediatrics, Georgetown University.*

via insects is unlikely include the following: The amount of virus circulating in the blood of HIV-infected individuals is very low compared with levels observed for other viruses known to be transmitted by insects; mosquitoes do not regurgitate blood into the next victim they bite; and the saliva of mosquitoes does not contain the virus (CDC, 1997c). Furthermore, the virus cannot reproduce in insects.

Symptoms

Within the first two to four weeks, persons infected with the HIV virus experience a flulike illness. Reported symptoms include fever, sore throat, swollen lymph nodes, headache, muscle and joint pains, and nausea and vomiting. Some individuals report open ulcers in the mouth and a viral rash. As antibodies are produced to combat the initial infection, infected persons enter a symptom-free phase. The time from HIV infection to the development of AIDS varies from less than one year to more than 10 years. During the symptom-free phase, individuals often feel completely healthy. Those individuals who are carrying the virus but are not symptomatic are the most dangerous for the spread of infection. It is during this period that individuals are either unaware of their infection or are in denial (Healy, 1995). Transmission of the virus is possible even in the symptom-free period. Recognition of

early symptoms is critical to control the spread of infection. The virus lies dormant until the disease weakens and destroys the immune system and the body is unable to combat opportunistic disease.

Onset of AIDS is usually insidious, with vague symptoms such as anorexia and lymphadenopathy. Individuals typically experience one symptom and then, as the disease progresses, tend to develop clusters of symptoms that indicate the presence of AIDS. The percentage of individuals infected with the HIV virus who go on to develop AIDS is not known. Approximately 20% of infected persons have developed AIDS within 5 years of the initial infection. Seventy percent will develop AIDS by the 15th year following exposure. The long dormant phase characteristic of the infection has changed the focus from acute illness care to chronic disease management of the infection.

Diagnosis

The ELISA (enzyme-linked immunosorbent assay) and Western blot antibody tests are the most common tests used to diagnose HIV infection. Testing can be done in most doctors' offices or health clinics and should be accompanied by counseling. If they have particular concerns about confidentiality, individuals can be tested anonymously at many sites. Antibodies to HIV generally do not reach detectable levels until one to three months following infection and may take as long as six months to be generated in quantities large enough to show up in standard blood tests. Persons exposed to HIV should be tested as soon as they are likely to have developed HIV antibodies to the virus. Secondary prevention is dependent on early diagnosis and appropriate treatment in the early stages of infection. High-risk behaviors may be averted in individuals who test positive for the HIV virus.

All babies born to HIV-infected mothers carry their mothers' antibodies to HIV for several months. If these babies lack symptoms, a definitive diagnosis of HIV infection via the use of standard antibody tests cannot be made until after 15 months of age. By then, babies are unlikely to still carry their mothers' antibodies and, if they are infected, will have produced their own.

Treatment

Medical treatments for AIDS have improved dramatically since the disease was first identified. In the mid-1990s, protease inhibitors were first marketed. Researchers subsequently discovered that a combination of protease inhibitors and reverse transcriptase inhibitors could eliminate traces of the HIV virus from the blood (Leccese, 1997). This combination therapy has resulted in remarkable improvement in individuals infected with HIV. Members of the International AIDS Society published an article that described how to implement treatment with a combination of three anti-AIDS drugs (Carpenter, Fischl, Hammer, Hirsch, et al., 1997). A drawback to the combination therapy regime is cost. Combination therapy is estimated to cost approximately $15,000 per client per year (Leccese, 1997). The high cost of therapy may hinder availability of the drugs to individuals with limited financial resources. As a result of new treatment modalities, the AIDS death rate was down 19% in 1996 as compared with 1995 figures. Unfortunately, despite new treatment options for AIDS, individuals continue to become infected. As of June 1997 (CDC, 1997a) 612,078 AIDS cases had been reported to the CDC.

Because of the increase in cases of HIV/AIDS among women of childbearing age, there has also been an increase in cases among infants and children. Most of these children were infected via vertical transmission during pregnancy, delivery, or breastfeeding. In June 1994, a U.S. Public Health Service Task Force recommended AZT (zidovudine) for pregnant women infected with the AIDS virus. Research has shown that treatment with AZT can substantially reduce the risk of mother–child transmission of HIV. Treatment during pregnancy can help an HIV-infected woman protect her baby from becoming infected. Without treatment, more than one-third of all babies born to HIV-infected women will have the virus and eventually will get sick (Bloom, Curran, Elsner,

Gwinn, et al., 1995). Community health nurses must educate pregnant clients about the substantial decrease in the risk of mother–child transmission associated with AZT therapy during pregnancy. Women who fall into risk categories for HIV infection should be tested during pregnancy to decrease the possibility of vertically transmitting the disease.

For a number of years, postexposure treatment (PET) has been available to health care workers who are stuck with needles contaminated with HIV-positive blood. The results have been promising, with the CDC reporting that as many as 79% of health care workers who utilized PET did not develop HIV infection. The general populace is questioning why PET is not being made routinely available to individuals at high risk for developing HIV infection. In some areas, PET is offered to rape victims. The CDC published guidelines for the use of PET in 1998. Postexposure treatment consists of a combination of zidovudine and lamivudine for four weeks. In some cases, a protease inhibitor such as indinavir is added to the treatment regime. Controversy surrounds the potential widespread use of PET because it is feared that individuals will abandon safe-sex practices (Leccese, 1997).

Prevention

The only way to absolutely prevent HIV infection is to abstain from sexual intercourse or to maintain a mutually monogamous sexual relationship with an uninfected person (see Figure 20-6). Primary prevention measures include education about the need to use barrier methods such as condoms (male and female) to curb the potential spread of infection between sexual partners. Secondary prevention measures include increased availability of low-cost AIDS testing. Because of the high number of drug-addicted individuals at risk due to needle sharing, drug treatment facilities should be increased. Needle-exchange programs have been effective in certain areas; such programs are not widely accepted, however, despite evidence that their presence dramatically decreases the rates of HIV infection. All pregnant women should be informed about the risk of HIV transmission during the perinatal period and offered HIV testing and treatment when indicated (Bloom et al., 1995). Health care workers should protect themselves from occupationally acquired HIV infection by using Universal Precautions (see Figure 20-7). All individuals who test positive for HIV should be checked for other STDs. Researchers have demonstrated that when STDs are present, HIV transmission is two to five times greater than in populations where other STDs are not present. Further, evidence is increasing that when STDs are treated, there is a reduced risk of HIV transmission (Henderson, 1997). Tertiary prevention includes connecting clients with appropriate support agencies and informing clients of new treatments and programs that improve long-term health outcomes of infected individuals.

Surveillance and prevention measures associated with infectious diseases include partner or contact notification. Experts have opposing opinions about how HIV should be

Figure 20-6 Preventing the Spread of HIV

The following prevention measures apply to personal sex practices and intravenous drug use:

- To prevent sexual transmission of HIV, abstain from sex with an infected person.

- Ask about the sexual history of current and future sex partners.

- Reduce the number of sex partners to minimize the risk.

- Always use a condom from start to finish during any type of sex (vaginal, anal, or oral). Use latex condoms rather than natural-membrane condoms. If used properly, latex condoms offer protection against sexually transmitted disease agents including HIV.

- Use only water-based lubricants. Do not use saliva or oil-based lubricants such as petroleum jelly or vegetable shortening. If you decide to use a spermicide along with a condom, it is preferable to use spermicide in the vagina according to manufacturer's instructions.

- Avoid anal or rough vaginal intercourse. Do not do anything that could tear the skin or the moist lining of the genitals, anus, or mouth and cause bleeding.

- Condoms should be used even for oral sex.

- Avoid deep, wet, or "French" kissing with an infected person. Possible trauma to the mouth may occur, which could result in the exchange of blood. It is safe, however, to hug, cuddle, rub, or dry kiss your partner.

- Avoid alcohol and illicit drugs. Alcohol and drugs can impair your immune system and your judgment. If you use drugs, do not share "injecting drug works." Do not share needles, syringes, or cookers.

- Do not share personal items such as toothbrushes, razors, and devices used during sex, which may be contaminated with blood, semen, or vaginal fluids.

- If you are infected with HIV or have engaged in sex or needle-sharing behaviors that lead to infection with HIV, do not donate blood, plasma, sperm, body organs, or tissues.

Adapted from HIV/AIDS Prevention, Update December, 1997 *by Centers for Disease Control and Prevention, 1998, Atlanta, GA.*

Figure 20-7 Universal Blood and Body Fluid Precautions

- Special training and education programs
- Use of protective equipment such as gloves, gowns, eye protection, and face masks
- Handwashing after each patient contact
- Proper handling and disposal of sharps
- Engineering control, such as special sharps containers and safety cabinets for biologicals
- Programs of immunization, such as hepatitis B vaccine for employees
- Proper contaminated waste disposal
- Use of disinfectants
- Proper labeling and signs

Adapted from "Universal Precautions for Prevention of Transmission of HIV, Hepatitis B Virus and Other Bloodborne Pathogens in Health Care Settings" by Centers for Disease Control and Prevention, 1998, MMWR, 37, pp. 377–382.

ment, which has been proven to extend life, and may unknowingly be infecting others. Coburn and Pelosi (1997) comment that "never before in medical history have we given the responsibility of controlling an epidemic to the individuals infected with the disease" (p. 24).

Human Papillomavirus

Genital warts are caused by the human papillomavirus (HPV), the name for a group of viruses that includes more than 60 different types, approximately 20 of which infect the anal and genital areas. Experts estimate that as many as 20 million Americans are infected with HPV, and the incidence of the diseases it causes appears to be increasing (Gerchufsky, 1996).

Transmission

Genital warts are highly infectious, with two-thirds of individuals who have sexual contact with infected individuals developing the disease. As many as a million new cases are diagnosed each year (Gerchufsky, 1996).

Symptoms

Most HPV infections have no visible signs or symptoms. The fact that many people infected with HPV are asymptomatic contributes to the rampant spread of this infection, particularly among young people. Only approximately one-third of women experience symptoms with the HPV infection. Warts start to appear approximately two months after initial exposure to an infected person. The warts are typically small and may occur in clusters around the genital area and anus. In women,

managed in the United States. Some experts believe that the federal government has indirectly contributed to the growth of the AIDS epidemic by forgoing recognized public health practices, including partner notification. Instead, individuals' privacy rights have superseded accepted public health procedures. AIDS activists have asserted that AIDS testing and reporting are civil rights issues rather than a public health issue. The stigma associated with HIV and the fear of discrimination have led gay rights organizations to keep routine testing and mandated reporting politically charged issues. However, because of voluntary testing and notification, thousands of individuals who are unaware of their HIV status are being denied early treat-warts may develop in the vagina, where they are hard to detect, and they may also appear on the vaginal lips (see Figure 20-8). In men, warts typically are detected on the penis but may be found on the scrotum or around the anus. Rarely, genital warts also can develop in the mouth or throat of a person who has had oral sexual contact with an infected person. Genital warts often occur in groups and can be very tiny or can accumulate into large masses on genital tissues. Warts may spontaneously resolve, but recurrence is common. In some cases, warts may eventually develop fleshy, small, raised growths with a cauliflower-like appearance. As the warts shed their outer layer, they spread infection. People who develop genital warts have a high risk for developing certain cancers such as cancer of the cervix, anus, penis, and vulva. In both developed and developing countries, more than 90% of the new cases of cervical cancer are due to sexually transmitted human papillomavirus infection of the cervix (WHO, 1997a).

Diagnosis

Health care providers conducting routine exams of clients should check for abnormal tissue or the presence of genital warts. Clinical observation can be enhanced via the use of acetic acid stain and colposcopy or androscopy for the detection of subtle lesions. Individuals with documented HPV infection should be encouraged to have frequent screening exams so that if cancer does develop, it will be diagnosed in the early stages. The Pap smear is designed to detect precancerous changes in the cervix of women and may show changes caused by HPV infection.

Treatment

Genital warts can be removed or destroyed via chemical applications, cryotherapy, laser, or electrosurgery. Removal of genital warts does *not* constitute a cure, and new outbreaks may occur months and years after the initial treatment. Removal of warts does, however, reduce the risk of transmitting the disease to uninfected sexual partners.

Herpes Simplex Virus 2 (HSV-2)

Herpes is recognized as a chronic, lifelong infection. Genital herpes is a contagious viral infection that affects an estimated 23% of adult Americans. Genital herpes is the most common cause of genital ulcers in the United States. An estimated 40 million individuals are affected by this disease, and there are approximately 500,000 new cases of infection each year (Eng & Butler, 1996). The infection is caused by the herpes simplex virus (HSV). There are two types of HSV, and both can cause the symptoms of genital herpes. Type 1 HSV most commonly causes sores on the lips (known as fever blisters or cold sores) but can cause genital infections as well. Type 2 HSV most often causes genital sores but can also infect the mouth. Both types of HSV can produce sores in and around the vaginal area (see Figure 20-9), on the penis, around the anal opening, and on the buttocks or thighs. Occasionally, sores also appear on other parts of the body where broken skin has come into contact with HSV. The virus remains in certain nerve cells of the body for life, causing periodic symptoms in some people.

Transmission

It is possible to become infected with HSV through oral, anal, or vaginal sex. Genital herpes infection usually is acquired via sexual contact with someone who has an active outbreak of herpes lesions in the genital area. Changing sexual practices have supported the spread of HSV-1 below the waist and HSV-2 above the waist, via oral–genital sex or self-inoculation. Because HSV lesions are ulcerative, individuals with HSV are at increased risk for contracting HIV. If lesions are present, HSV may be diagnosed via clinical examination. It is important to remember that the virus may be transmitted to uninfected individuals even when no visible lesions are present (Benenson, 1995).

Newborns may be infected with HSV-2 via direct contact with lesions during the birthing process. Direct newborn contact can result in severe consequences for the neonate, including neurological damage or death. If herpes lesions are present on the mother, exposure can be eliminated by delivering the baby via cesarean section.

Symptoms

Herpes is similar to other STDs in that many people have no symptoms of infection. Furthermore, symptoms vary in those individuals who do show signs of infection. Early symptoms include a burning sensation in the genitals, low-back pain, and dysuria. Flulike symptoms may accompany the initial outbreak. Symptoms are typically reported within 2 to 20 days after having sex with an infected individual. After the initial symptoms, small, red bumps appear in the infected area and develop into painful vesicles or blisters, which then crust over, scab, and heal. After the lesions resolve, the virus remains in the body, and recurrent episodes of active disease may occur at any time.

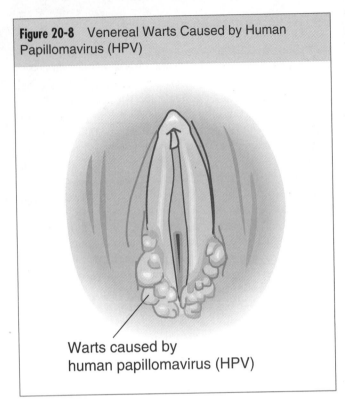

Figure 20-8   Venereal Warts Caused by Human Papillomavirus (HPV)

Warts caused by
human papillomavirus (HPV)

Figure 20-9   Genital herpes can be found in the genital area, around the anal opening, and on the buttocks and thighs.

Shallow
vesicles
on red
bases

Outbreaks are frequently associated with stress and overexertion.

Diagnosis

Confirmation of HSV infection is possible via laboratory examination of fluid from the vesicles. The most accurate method of diagnosis is viral culture. A new lesion is swabbed or scraped, and the sample is added to a laboratory culture containing healthy cells. When examined under a microscope after one or two days, the cells show changes that indicate growth of the herpes virus. Blood tests can confirm the presence of HSV antibodies but do not detect active disease.

Treatment

Herpes is a lifelong infection with no known cure. It is possible to treat the painful symptoms of herpes, however. During an outbreak, clients can speed healing by keeping the area clean and avoiding touching the lesion, remembering to wash hands after contact with lesions to prevent the spread of infection. Acyclovir (Zovirax), when taken regularly, interferes with the virus's ability to reproduce itself. It also shortens the duration of the outbreak, reduces the number of outbreaks, and reduces symptoms. Acyclovir can be taken orally or is available in a cream.

Bacterial Sexually Transmitted Diseases

Bacterial STDs, including syphilis and gonorrhea, have been documented for hundreds of years. They differ from

viral STDs in their susceptibility to treatment. Bacterial STD infections can be treated with antibiotics and, in most cases, can be cured.

Chlamydia

Genital chlamydial infection is caused by the bacterium *Chlamydia trachomatis*. More than 4 million new cases of chlamydia are reported each year. The volume of cases makes chlamydia the most frequently reported sexually transmitted disease in the United States. The annual cost of chlamydial infections and their sequelae is estimated to exceed $2 billion. The side effects of this bacterial infection can lead to pelvic inflammatory disease (PID), a leading cause of infertility (Benenson, 1995).

Transmission

Chlamydia is transmitted during vaginal or anal sexual contact with an infected partner. A pregnant woman may pass the infection to her newborn during delivery, with subsequent neonatal eye infection or pneumonia.

Symptoms

Three-quarters of the women and one-quarter of the men who have chlamydia are symptom free. If symptoms are experienced, they commonly include discharge and a burning sensation when urinating. Women with chlamydia report low-back pain and pain during intercourse. Men experience itching and burning around the penis and, on occasion, swelling of the testicles. Chlamydial infections are often acquired concurrently with *Neisseria gonorrhoeae* and may persist after the gonorrhea is treated. It is estimated that 45% of those women diagnosed with chlamydia also are infected with gonorrhea (Benenson, 1995).

Diagnosis

Chlamydia is diagnosed via cervical smear and culture.

Treatment

A single dose of azithromycin is effective treatment for chlamydia. A full 7 days of treatment with doxycycline twice a day can also kill the bacteria causing the disease. For newborns and pregnant women, erythromycin is the drug of choice. All sex partners of a person with chlamydial infection should be evaluated and treated to prevent reinfection and further spread of the disease.

Chlamydia and gonorrhea are often found together, and because their symptoms and clinical manifestation are difficult to distinguish, treatment for both conditions is recommended when one is suspected (Benenson, 1995). Because of the increasing drug resistance of many of the organisms that cause STDs, it is important that all medication be taken according to directions.

Syphilis

Syphilis is caused by a spirochete called *Treponema pallidum*. Syphilis is a serious disease that, when left untreated, can have debilitating and deadly consequences. Some historians believe that syphilis emerged as a new disease as early as the 15th century. According to one theory, early explorers like Christopher Columbus were responsible for bringing the disease from the New World and transmitting it throughout Europe. For many years, *syphilis* was a catchall term for sexually transmitted disease. Physicians assumed that gonorrhea and syphilis were the same thing until 1837, when a researcher reported differences in the two diseases. In 1906, Wasserman developed a blood test for syphilis, leading to advances in treatment including Salvarsan, an arsenic compound. With the introduction of penicillin in 1943, a once deadly infection became curable. Although syphilis appeared to be controlled for many years, there was a dramatic rise in cases of primary and secondary syphilis in the 1970s and 1980s. Like those at high risk for other STDs, people at increased risk for syphilis are those who have had multiple sex partners, have sexual relations with an infected partner, have a history of STD, and do not use condoms. Despite effective treatment, syphilis continues to be a common STD (Flores, 1995).

Transmission

The bacterium spreads from the sores of an infected person to the mucous membranes of the genital area, the mouth, or the anus of a sexual partner. It also can pass through broken skin on other parts of the body. The syphilis bacterium is very fragile, and the infection is rarely, if ever, spread by contact with objects such as toilet seats or towels. A pregnant woman with syphilis can pass the bacterium to her unborn child, who may be born with serious mental and physical problems as a result of this infection. The most common way to get syphilis is to have sex with someone who has an active infection. The rise in horizontal transmission of this disease resulted in an equally dramatic increase in the number of infants born with congenital syphilis acquired via vertical transmission. The first decline in the number of reported cases of syphilis occurred in 1994 ("AIDS Fear Brings Syphilis Decline," 1994), with a corresponding decline in the number of reported cases of congenital syphilis.

Symptoms

Syphilis is characterized by three distinct stages. The first stage, considered the primary stage, is distinguished by a painless lesion or chancre appearing at the site where the bacterium first entered the body. The sore usually appears between 10 and 90 days after contact with an infected person. The lesion may go unnoticed and is particularly difficult to discern in women because it can present inside the vagina, where it is not easily seen without a pelvic examination. The lesion can also be found on the penis or inside the mouth or anus. When syphilis goes unnoticed in the primary stage, it progresses to the second stage of infection, known as secondary syphilis (see Figure 20-10). Secondary syphilis presents as numerous, highly infectious lesions and may include flulike symptoms

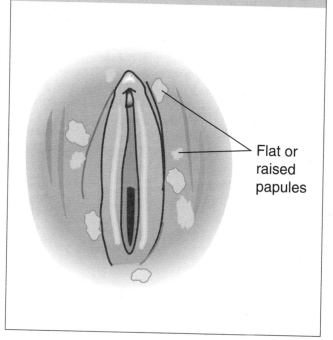

Figure 20-10 Secondary syphilis presents as numerous highly infectious lesions and may involve flulike symptoms and even hair loss.

Flat or raised papules

and even hair loss. Another recognizable feature of this stage is the characteristic rash on the palms of the hands and the soles of the feet. A generalized rash occurs in some individuals. Tertiary infection is extremely rare and appears 3 to 10 years after the initial stages of disease. Irreversible complications of this stage include mental deterioration and loss of vision, balance, and sensation.

Diagnosis

Diagnosis of syphilis can by made at any stage of the disease via the VDRL (Venereal Disease Research Laboratory) or the RPR (rapid plasma reagin) test. Both of these tests are relatively inexpensive and easy to access. Recent studies support the critical need for early diagnosis of syphilis because it seems to be a marker for the prevalence of HIV infection. Individuals who are HIV positive may present with syphilis that has already progressed to the secondary stage, with the course of the disease advancing at an accelerated pace (Hutchinson, Hook, Sheperd, Verley, & Rompalo, 1994). Because of the serious complications to the fetus of the woman with syphilis, it is recommended that all women be screened for the disease in the first trimester of pregnancy (Benenson, 1995). Annual screening is recommended for sexually active and high-risk individuals.

Treatment

Penicillin G, administered by injection, is the drug of choice in the treatment of syphilis at all stages. Other antibiotics can be used for patients allergic to penicillin. A person usually can no longer transmit syphilis 24 hours after beginning therapy. It is important to retest clients to eliminate the potential for treatment failure. Although proper treatment in all stages of syphilis will cure the disease, the damage done to organs, primarily in late syphilis, cannot be reversed.

Gonorrhea

Neisseria gonorrhoeae is a common sexually transmitted disease that affects approximately 1 million Americans each year. Because of a lack of symptoms, the disease may go unnoticed. Gonorrhea is caused by the gonococcus bacterium, which grows and multiplies quickly in moist, warm areas of the body, such as the cervix, urethra, mouth, or rectum. In women, the cervix is the most common site of infection. However, the disease can spread to the uterus and fallopian tubes, resulting in pelvic inflammatory disease (PID), which, in turn, can cause infertility and ectopic pregnancy.

Transmission

Most commonly transmitted during genital sexual activity, gonorrhea can also be passed from the genitals of one partner to the throat of the other during oral sex (pharyngeal gonorrhea). Gonorrhea of the rectum can occur in people who practice anal intercourse and may also occur in women as a result of the spread of infection from the vaginal area. Gonorrhea can be passed from an infected woman to her newborn infant during delivery. When the infection occurs in children, it is most commonly due to sexual abuse. It is important to recognize the existence of a chronic carrier state, which can develop in both men and women with gonorrhea. A **carrier** can harbor an infectious agent without showing noticeable signs of disease or infection. The carrier state can be temporary or chronic.

Symptoms

It is estimated that 25% to 80% of infected women have no symptoms of infection (Hook & Hansfield, 1990). Symptoms in women present initially as a mild cervicitis or urethritis. Men typically present with a purulent discharge or dysuria. Complications of the disease occur if the disease goes untreated. Pelvic inflammatory disease, endometriosis, and infertility are recognized complications of untreated disease. Newborns born to infected mothers and exposed to the infection in the birth canal are at high risk for the development of conjunctivitis. If not promptly treated, this infection can cause blindness in the newborn.

Diagnosis

Gonorrhea is diagnosed via a microscopic examination of exudate and via bacterial cultures. Because of the growing number of antibiotic-resistant gonorrhea strains, it is important to test organisms for sensitivity to specific antibiotics to prevent ineffective treatment and relapse of disease.

Treatment

Gonorrhea is treated with antibiotics that have been shown to be effective against the strain of gonorrhea cultured in the lab. Current antibiotics in widespread use for the treatment of gonorrhea include many of the cephalosporins and, most recently, azithromycin (Benenson, 1995). The development of antibiotic-resistant strains of *Neisseria gonorrhoeae* have complicated the treatment picture.

Trichomoniasis

Trichomonas vaginalis ("trich") causes a common STD that attacks as many as 2 to 3 million Americans each year. Trichomoniasis is found worldwide and is a frequent disease of adults. Approximately 20% of females will become infected with *T. vaginalis* during their reproductive years (Benenson, 1995).

Transmission

Transmission of the bacterium occurs via sex with an infected individual.

Symptoms

Many individuals experience no symptoms. Trichomoniasis often presents as an unusual vaginitis in women. The thin, foamy, vaginal discharge has a characteristic greenish yellow color and a very foul odor. Women with symptoms may experience vaginal or vulval redness accompanied by small petechial or punctate red spots. Other common symptoms are itching, burning, and painful urination. Men experience mild symptoms and may complain of a "tingling" inside the penis. Trichomoniasis may coexist with gonorrhea and may facilitate HIV infection. When trichomoniasis is diagnosed, a complete STD check is recommended. When symptoms occur, they usually appear within 4 to 20 days of exposure, although symptoms can appear years after infection.

Diagnosis

Either microscopic examination or a culture of the discharge can confirm the diagnosis. The infection is often diagnosed by being observed on a routine Pap smear.

Treatment

A single dose of metronidazole (Flagyl) is effective in treating most cases of trichomoniasis. Although symptoms of trichomoniasis in men may disappear within a few weeks without treatment, men can transmit the disease to their sex partners even when symptoms are not present. It is therefore preferable to treat both partners to eliminate the organism.

The Role of the Community Health Nurse in the Prevention of Sexually Transmitted Diseases

Prevention of all STDs involves educating the public about the frequency and the often deadly consequences of these diseases, both to individuals and to newborns exposed to the various infections during pregnancy or vaginal delivery. Primary-prevention efforts currently focus on educating health care providers and the public about the signs of STDs, instructing individuals on ways to avoid exposure, and emphasizing the need for regular checkups. Community health nurses can help prevent the spread of sexually transmitted infection by promoting safe-sex behavior and the need for correct and consistent condom use. Prevention efforts should also include education about immunization, when appropriate. Individuals should be educated about the potential spread of these infections via oral or anal sex and, in some cases, IV drug use or sharing of body fluids. Young people should be taught about the risks of having multiple sex partners and participating in casual sexual activity and of the health value of delaying the initiation of sexual activity. Clients should be warned about new evidence that suggests increased risk of HIV infection in individuals who have a

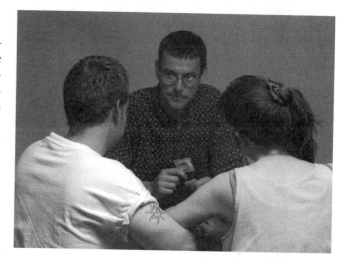

The community health nurse must take advantage of every opportunity to counsel on safe-sex practices.

history of STD. In their rush to help young clients prevent unwanted pregnancy, nurses must not forget to inform the public that oral contraceptives provide no protection against STDs and must be used with a form of barrier protection to defend against STD transmission. Secondary-prevention efforts focus on early detection and treatment of infection as well as on partner notification to prevent further spread. Encouraging pregnant women to be screened for HIV infection to prevent the vertical transmission of infection is part of secondary prevention. Tertiary-prevention efforts focus on minimizing and managing the effects of chronic STDs such as herpes, HIV infection, and untreated syphilis. Information provided to the public should take into consideration cultural differences: Educational materials and the manner whereby information is discussed should always be culturally appropriate. Table 20-7 summarizes selected sexually transmitted diseases.

EMERGING INFECTIONS

In the United States, documented emerging infections include a variety of bacterial, parasitic, and viral diseases. In addition to infections classified in these documented categories, other types of agents, such as prions detected in the investigation of "mad cow disease," provide a constant challenge to disease investigators. The recent occurrence of Ebola-Reston virus in a quarantined population of primates located in a Texas holding station indicates the importance of understanding **zoonosis,** the transmission of infection from animals to humans, and the related potential threat to human survival (Strausbaugh, 1997). Other cases support the disregard agents have exhibited for geographic boundaries and barriers. "Raccoon rabies," once thought to be confined to the eastern United States, has spread westward (Deasy, 1996), and Lyme disease, once recognized only in Connecticut, has spread via the

Table 20-7 Summary of Selected Sexually Transmitted Diseases

DISEASE (AGENT)	INCUBATION PERIOD	SYMPTOMS	DIAGNOSIS	TREATMENT	NURSING ROLE
Bacterial					
Chlamydia (*Chlamydia trachomatis*)	7 to 14 days	Women: vaginal discharge; itching; burning of the vagina; pelvic inflammatory disease (PID); often asymptomatic. Men: penile discharge; dysuria; burning or itching at the urethral opening; epididymitis; often asymptomatic	Vaginal culture; Gram stain of endocervical or urethral discharge	Tetracycline, doxycycline, or azithromycin	Partner notification; educate client regarding barrier methods to prevent reinfection, avoiding sex until therapy is complete and both partners are asymptomatic, and the importance of following medication instructions and completing therapy; recommend HIV testing
Gonorrhea (*Neisseria gonorrhoeae*)	3 to 21 days	Women: abdominal pain; dysuria; possibly asymptomatic Men: urethritis, discharge, dysuria and frequency, epididymitis	Culture	Doxycycline, spectinomycin, or ceftriaxone	Partner notification and screening; educate client regarding barrier methods to prevent reinfection, avoiding sex until therapy is complete and both partners are asymptomatic, and the importance of following medication instructions and completing therapy; recommend HIV testing; reevaluate if symptoms persist
Syphilis (primary) (*Treponema pallidum*)	10 to 90 days	Painless chancre	VDRL (reactive 14 days after appearance of chancre)	Benzathine penicillin G	Partner notification and screening; recommend HIV testing; reevaluate at 3- and 6-month intervals
Syphilis (secondary)	6 weeks to 6 months	Fever, malaise, headache, sore throat, rash	Clinical signs and symptoms	Benzathine penicillin G	Partner notification and screening; recommend HIV testing

Continued

Table 20-7 Summary of Selected Sexually Transmitted Diseases (Continued)

DISEASE (AGENT)	INCUBATION PERIOD	SYMPTOMS	DIAGNOSIS	TREATMENT	NURSING ROLE
Syphilis (tertiary)	Within 1 year of infection (early latency period)	Often asymptomatic; however, lesions may reoccur	VDRL	Benzathine penicillin G	Partner notification and screening; recommend HIV testing
	After 1 year from date of original infection (late latency period)	Asymptomatic; noninfectious except to fetus of pregnant woman	Examine cerebral spinal fluid cell count and VDRL		
	2 to 40 years after infection (late active period)	Gummas of skin, bone, mucous membranes, heart, liver; paresis; optic atrophy; aortic aneurysm; aortic valve insufficiency			
Chancroid (*Haemophilus ducreyi*)	3 to 7 days	Irregular papule progressing to deep, very painful ulcer that drains blood or pus; inguinal tenderness; dysuria	Examine lesion	Azithromycin, erythromycin, or ceftriaxone	Partner notification; educate client regarding barrier methods to prevent reinfection, avoiding sex until therapy is complete and both partners are asymptomatic, and the importance of following medication instructions and completing therapy; recommend HIV testing
Viral					
Hepatitis B (hepatitis B virus)	4 weeks	Vary from subclinical infection to cirrhosis or liver cancer	Serum IgM alpha HBc	Hepatitis B immune globulin within 14 days of last exposure, followed by immunization series	Partner notification; educate client regarding barrier methods and the importance of immunization; recommend HIV testing

Continued

487

Table 20-7 Summary of Selected Sexually Transmitted Diseases (Continued)

DISEASE (AGENT)	INCUBATION PERIOD	SYMPTOMS	DIAGNOSIS	TREATMENT	NURSING ROLE
Genital warts (human papillomavirus)	Varies from 4 weeks to 9 months	Vary from subclinical infection to cauliflower lesions in varying numbers near vaginal opening, anus, penis, vagina, or cervix. Certain types increase the risk of cervical cancer.	Pap smear; visual inspection of lesions	No cure; lesions may disappear without treatment; removal of lesions.	Partner notification; educate client regarding barrier methods to prevent reinfection and importance of annual Pap smear; recommend HIV testing
Genital herpes (herpes simplex virus)	2 to 20 days	Vesicles that progress to painful ulcerations of the vagina, labia, perineum, penis, or anus. Lesions last for weeks, and reinfection is common. Virus may be present when individual is asymptomatic.	Presence of vesicles; viral culture if lesion is present	No cure; acyclovir may minimize symptoms and duration of lesions.	Partner notification; educate client regarding barrier methods; recommend HIV testing and annual Pap smear

Table 20-8 Emerging Diseases, by Microbial Agent, Identified between 1975 and 1992

YEAR	MICROBE	DISEASE
1975	Parvovirus B19	Fifth disease; aplastic crisis in chronic hemolytic anemia
1976	*Cryptosporidium parvum*	Enterocolitis
1977	Ebola virus	Ebola hemorrhagic fever
1977	*Legionella pneumophila*	Legionnaires' disease
1977	*Campylobacter* species	Enterocolitis
1981	Toxin-producing strains of *Staphylococcus aureus*	Toxic shock syndrome
1982	*Escherichia coli* O157:H7	Hemorrhagic colitis; hemolytic uremia syndrome
1982	*Borrelia burgdorferi*	Lyme disease
1983	Human immunodeficiency virus	Acquired immunodeficiency syndrome
1983	*Helicobacter pylori*	Duodenal and gastric ulcers
1988	Human herpesvirus-6	Roseola subitum
1989	*Ehrlichia chaffeensis*	Human ehrlichosis
1989	Hepatitis C virus	Parenterally transmitted non-A, non-B hepatitis
1992	*Bartonella henselae*	Cat-scratch disease; bacillary angiomatosis

Adapted from "Emerging Infectious Diseases: A Challenge to All" by L. Strausbaugh, 1997, American Family Physician, *55(1), p. 111. Adapted with permission of* American Family Physician.

deer tick to dozens of states and countries (U.S. Department of Health and Human Services (CDC, 1998d), constituting a dramatic example of how an organism can become global within a decade. Food-borne illnesses such as hepatitis A and cyclospora infection transmitted via food processed in countries outside the United States illustrate the fact that contamination that takes place in one part of the globe can quickly be transmitted to human hosts in other parts of the world and be responsible for widespread illness (Getty, 1997). Table 20-8 lists some microbial infections that have been discovered within the past two decades and that meet the Institute of Medicine's definition of emerging infectious disease (CDC, 1994; Strausbaugh, 1997).

Known pathogens that are resurgent (emerging with increased virulence) are listed in Table 20-9 (CDC, 1994; Strausbaugh, 1997). **Virulence** is the degree of pathogenicity of the agent. Outbreaks of ebola and plague continue to surface throughout the world, and drug-resistant strains of agents have become increasingly common in the United States.

Factors Contributing to the Emergence of Infectious Disease

Human behavior plays a critical role in creating an optimal environment for the development and spread of new organisms. International travel, changing sexual mores, and high-risk behaviors create a vulnerable human host susceptible to disease organisms. Increased population and urbanization throughout the world provide for a changing ecology and an environment that supports the zoonotic transmission of disease. As humans expand their

habitats into forests, jungles, and deserts, they come into contact with disease-causing organisms and the **vectors** (agents that actively carry a pathogen to a susceptible host) that transmit them. In many areas of the world, urban development has caused overcrowding, poor sanitation, and unclean drinking water. These conditions play a direct role in the transmission of disease (Lederberg &

Table 20-9 Examples of Resurgent, Infectious Diseases in the 1990s

YEAR	PLACE	RESURGENT INFECTIOUS DISEASE
1989–1996	United States	Streptococcal toxic shock syndrome
1990	New York	Multidrug-resistant tuberculosis
1992	California	Coccidioidomycosis
1992–1996	United States	Vancomycin-resistant enterococci infections
1993	Ohio	Pertussis
1993	Wisconsin	Cryptosporidiosis
1993–1996	United States	Penicillin-resistant pneumococcal infections
1994	India	Plague
1994–1996	Oregon	Meningococcal disease
1995	Zaire	Ebola hemorrhagic fever

Adapted from "Emerging Infectious Diseases: A Challenge to All" by L. Strausbaugh, 1997, American Family Physician, *55(1), p. 111. Reprinted with permission of* American Family Physician.

Shope, 1992; CDC, 1994). The factors in disease emergence are as follows:

- Societal events: impoverishment, war or civil conflict, population growth, migration, urban decay
- Health care: new medical devices, organ or tissue transplantation, immunosuppressive drugs, widespread use of antibiotics
- Food production: globalization of food supplies, changes in food processing and packing methods
- Human behavior: sexual behavior, drug use, travel, diet, outdoor recreation, use of child care facilities
- Environmental changes: deforestation/reforestation, changes in water ecosystems, flood/drought, famine, global warming
- Public health infrastructure: curtailment or reduction in prevention programs, inadequate communicable disease surveillance, lack of trained personnel
- Microbial adaptation and change: changes in virulence and toxin production, development of drug resistance, microbes as cofactors in chronic diseases

The CDC has developed a plan designed to prepare the United States for potential epidemics resulting from emerging infectious diseases: *Addressing Emerging Infectious Disease Threats: A Prevention Strategy for the United States.* Four goals are outlined in this plan in an attempt to revitalize our nation's ability to identify and contain infectious agents that pose a potential threat to our populace. The goals are related to surveillance and response, applied research, prevention and control, and infrastructure. Each of these areas holds equal importance in the challenging fight against emerging infections (CDC, 1994).

Emerging infections were brought into the spotlight within the medical community after the 1992 Institute of Medicine (IOM) report entitled *Emerging Infections: Microbial Threats to Health in the United States* (Lederberg & Shope, 1992). Along with the ability to recognize emerging infections, community health nurses have the additional obligation of participating in effective surveillance, treatment, and case management of these diseases.

Examples of Emerging Infections
Ebola

Ebola burst on the communicable disease frontier in April 1995, with remarkable outbreaks of severe hemorrhagic fever in Kikwit, Zaire (Rodier, 1997). The disease has a rapid incubation period, and, in Zaire, the virus had a case fatality of more than 90%. Much of what is known about the Ebola virus was developed by the CDC Infectious Disease Surveillance Team that rushed to Kikwit in an effort to track the evolution of this fatal disease.

Transmission

The virus is spread from person to person by direct contact with infected blood, secretions, organs, or semen. Epidemics have resulted from person-to-person transmis-

sion, nosocomial transmission, and laboratory infections. After infection, the virus spreads through the blood and is replicated in many organs (Benenson, 1995).

Symptoms

Infected individuals manifest bleeding in the mucosa, abdomen, pericardium, and vagina. Bleeding, shock, and acute respiratory disorder are the causes of fatality among those infected with the Ebola virus. When the illness is severe, infected persons sustain high fevers and become delirious and difficult to control (Benenson, 1995).

Diagnosis

Ebola is diagnosed via the ELISA test for the specific IgG antibody.

Treatment

There is no known cure for Ebola.

Prevention

The basic method of prevention and control is the interruption of person-to-person spread of the virus.

Multidrug-Resistant Tuberculosis

"In hospitals alone, an estimated one million bacterial infections are occurring worldwide every day, and most of these are drug resistant" (WHO, 1997b). The incidence of tuberculosis (TB) in the United States increased 20% between 1985 and 1992 (CDC, 1994) but declined from 1992 to 1997 (CDC, 1998c). The increase can be attributed to a number of factors including the HIV epidemic, the deterioration in local public health infrastructure, immigration from countries where TB is **endemic** (i.e., prevalent), and increasing poverty and homelessness. The later decline was a result of prompt identification and reporting of cases and close follow-up to ensure completion of treatment. The alarming rise in new cases of TB was particularly troubling because a growing percentage of cases are resistant to traditional drug therapy (Boutotte, 1993). When an individual has TB and does not complete the recommended course of medication therapy (6 months), resistant strains of the organisms develop. Tubercle bacillus mutations are responsible for reported drug resistance in TB. Using only one drug to treat TB disease can create a population of tubercle bacilli that are resistant to that particular drug.

Symptoms

Common symptoms of TB include fever, cough, hemoptysis, fatigue, weight loss, and chest pain.

Diagnosis

Drug resistance is confirmed by laboratory culture and sensitivity.

Treatment

Currently, a four-drug regime (isoniazid, rifampin, pyrazinamide, and ethambutol or streptomycin) is considered essential in preventing multidrug-resistant cases (NJMC National Tuberculosis Center, 1997). Direct observed therapy (DOT) has shown promising results in ensuring that individuals comply with the full course of drug therapy and, thus, in decreasing the threat of resistant organisms.

Prevention

Primary prevention measures involve educating the public about the necessity to complete drug therapy. Secondary prevention includes minimizing the disease's ability to spread within the community. The nosocomial spread of drug-resistant organisms has created the need for special isolation protocols including negative pressure rooms with sophisticated air-exchange systems that prevent the nosocomial spread of disease within the hospital population. In addition, DOT has proved useful in preventing treatment failures in individuals with poor compliance records.

Hantavirus Pulmonary Syndrome

In 1993 a cluster of deaths in New Mexico set in motion a local, state, and federal investigation that lead to the identification of the lethal hantavirus. Hantavirus pulmonary syndrome (HPS) is a serious, potentially lethal respiratory disease. The number of cases and the geographic locations where the disease is found have increased dramatically since hantavirus was first identified in 1993. A total of 350 to 400 cases of HPS has been confirmed (WHO, 1997b). Of these cases, approximately 45% were fatal. The high mortality associated with this syndrome is generally thought to be due to the sudden onset of respiratory distress and pulmonary edema in previously healthy young people. The average age of victims of this disease is 37 years.

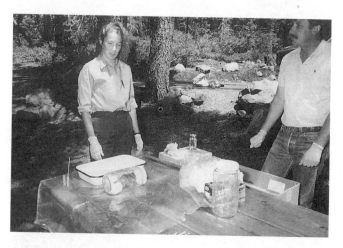

A community health field investigator before hantavirus was identified. Photo courtesy of Carl Pearson—Butte County Mosquito and Vector Control District, Oroville, CA. Used with permission.

Transmission

The disease is caused by a hantavirus that is carried by rodents, primarily the deer mouse, and subsequently passed on to humans through infected rodent feces, urine, and saliva. Breathing the virus is the most common way that the virus is spread from rodents to people. The virus enters the air in an aerosol often caused by sweeping the rodent's fecal droppings or urine in an attempt to clean an outdoor area. Transmission is believed to be primarily from rodent to person. After the investigation of outbreaks in Argentina and Chile in 1995, however, strong evidence now suggests the possibility of person-to-person transmission (CDC, 1997g). Transmission is also possible through direct contact with contaminated materials or a rodent's bite (Benenson, 1995).

Symptoms

Hantavirus infection is characterized by a febrile illness (temperature greater than 101.0°F) and bilateral diffuse interstitial edema accompanied by shortness of breath that requires supplemental oxygen within 72 hours of hospitalization, all occurring in a previously healthy person. Respiratory symptoms are often accompanied by headache; abdominal, joint, and low-back pain; and, occasionally, nausea and vomiting.

Diagnosis

ELISA and/or Western blot can establish the diagnosis of hantavirus infection by demonstrating specific IgM antibodies.

Treatment

Treatment for hantavirus infection is currently limited to supportive care. This includes controlling for fever, providing respiratory support, observing and treating for hypertension and hemorrhage, and administering medication to control pulmonary edema and other complications. Critical care unit services are essential for acutely ill clients.

Prevention

Strict barrier nursing techniques are now recommended for management of confirmed or suspected cases of hantavirus infection. Control measures focus on educating the public about the importance of rodent control in endemic areas. It is important to reduce those areas in and around buildings that may prove an attractive habitat for rodents. It is recommended that disinfectants such as chlorine bleach solution be used to decontaminate areas with potentially infectious droppings *prior* to cleaning. Surgical masks or other protective clothing may also be appropriate for cleaning high-risk areas. Figure 20-11 lists recommendations to minimize the risk of hantavirus infection. Public health workers investigating outbreaks must use caution to protect themselves during disease investigation.

Figure 20-11 Recommendations to Minimize Risks of Hantavirus Infection

- Air out abandoned or unused cabins before occupying. Inspect premises for rodents and do not occupy if there is evidence of rodent infestation.
- If sleeping outdoors, check potential campsites for rodent droppings or habitat.
- Avoid sleeping near woodpiles, garbage sites, or other areas that may be attractive to rodents.
- Avoid sleeping on the bare ground. If possible, sleep on elevated cots or mats.
- Store food in rodent-proof containers and dispose of garbage promptly.
- Do not seek out or disturb rodents, burrows, or dens.

Adapted from "Hantavirus Pulmonary Syndrome-Chile, 1997" Centers for Disease Control and Prevention, 1997b, MMWR, 46, p. 949.

The accompanying photographs show public health investigators in field dress prior to the identification of hantavirus and in field attire after hantavirus was identified.

E. coli:0157:H7

Escherichi coli is an emerging cause of foodborne illness. In early 1993, hamburgers contaminated with this bacterial strain caused a multistate outbreak of severe bloody diarrhea and serious kidney disease. More than 700 children and adults were affected, and four children died during this outbreak. After this episode, which was linked to undercooked hamburgers served at a fast-food chain in Seattle, Washington, the syndrome began to be referred to as "fast-food syndrome." *Escherichia coli* O157:H7 is one of hundreds of strains of *E. coli* bacteria. Most of the strains are harmless, but this strain is especially virulent and produces a toxin that can lead to severe illness and death.

Transmission

Transmission occurs via ingestion of contaminated foods.

Symptoms

Though sometimes asymptomatic, infection with the *E. coli* O157:H7 virus often causes bloody diarrhea and

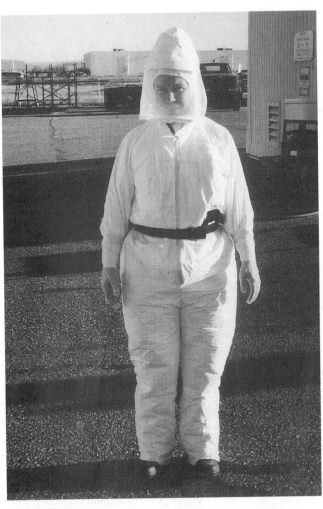

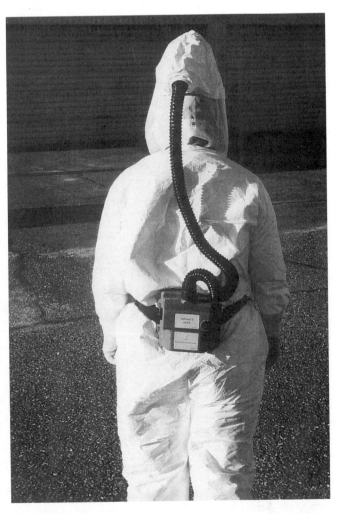

A community health field investigator after hantavirus was identified. Photos courtesy of Carl Pearson—Butte County Mosquito and Vector Control District, Oroville, CA. Used with permission.

abdominal cramps. In 2% to 7% of cases, particularly in children under 5 years of age, the infection can lead to hemolytic uremic syndrome, which can cause kidney failure. The illness resolves in 5 to 10 days. The increasing numbers of commonly consumed food items contaminated with infectious agents place large numbers of persons at risk (CDC, 1996d).

Diagnosis

Stool cultures are helpful to confirm the presence of the virus. The clinical picture assists in diagnosis.

Treatment

Treatment varies depending on the severity of the illness. Fluid and electrolyte replacement is indicated when watery diarrhea is present or if there are signs of dehydration.

Prevention

Radiation of beef has been suggested as a public health prevention measure to kill the bacteria in the nation's food supply. Adequate handwashing and proper cooking prevent the disease. Figure 20-12 lists the steps that individuals can take to prevent *E. coli* infection.

Lyme Disease

Lyme disease was first recognized in 1975 after a puzzling outbreak of arthritis in children near Lyme, Connecticut. By 1993, Lyme disease had been reported in 44 states and has become the most commonly reported vector-borne infectious disease in the United States (CDC, 1997e).

Transmission

The disease agent is carried by ticks and is transmitted when an individual is bitten by the deer tick.

Figure 20-12 Ways to Prevent *E. coli* O157:H7 Infection

- Cook ground beef or hamburger until the meat is gray or brown and the juices run clear. The inside of the meat should be hot.

- Send undercooked hamburger received in a restaurant back for further cooking.

- Consume only pasteurized milk and milk products. Avoid raw milk.

- Infected persons should wash hands carefully to prevent spread of infection.

- Drink municipal water that has been treated with adequate levels of chlorine.

Symptoms

Lyme disease is a multisystem disorder caused by *Borrelia burgdorferi,* a spirochete. This spirochete is transmitted from mammal to mammal by a small, hard tick. Erythema migrans, or the "bull's-eye" rash that has become a characteristic finding in the disease, appears at the site of the tick bite after approximately one week in some infected individuals (Walker, Barbour, Oliver, Lane, et al., 1996). This infection presents as flulike symptoms indistinguishable from those of many other illnesses. Recurrent arthritis, neurological symptoms, heart problems, and severe fatigue are commonly reported by infected individuals.

Diagnosis

Lyme disease is difficult to diagnose because many of the symptoms mimic those of other diseases. The only distinctive hallmark that seems to be unique to Lyme disease is the erythema migrans rash. However, the rash is absent in at least 25% of cases. Isolation of the agent from a skin biopsy or blood or serological evidence from serum samples confirms the diagnosis. In cases in which the diagnosis of late Lyme disease is considered, isolation of the organism from the client is rare, and laboratory support for the diagnosis depends on serological assay. The ELISA test followed by Western blot for positive or borderline reactions is the recommended diagnostic procedure (Walker et al., 1996).

Treatment

Effective treatment is essential in preventing long-term consequences of the infection. Antibiotics such as doxycyline or amoxicillin taken over a two-week period usually prevent the development of arthritis or other serious health problems. Early diagnosis is critical because the sooner the antibiotic therapy is started, the more complete the recovery. In many cases, Lyme disease is only considered after every other option has been explored, causing a delay in effective treatment.

Prevention

Prevention efforts focus on avoiding tick-endemic areas, wearing long sleeves and long pants in endemic areas, inspecting for the tiny (pinhead-sized) deer tick, and applying tick repellent when going outside. Infection usually takes place in the summer, when people venture into forested areas for recreation. People should be educated about the possibility of Lyme disease and the need to check for ticks after outdoor activity in a wooded area. Researchers believe that a tick must be attached for many hours to be able to transmit Lyme disease and that prompt tick removal can thus prevent infection (CDC, 1998a). Ticks should be removed with tweezers using steady gentle pulling. Because the infection can be transmitted from the tick's body fluids, the tick's body should not be squeezed during the removal process (Mandell, Bennett, & Dolin, 1995).

Rapid progress is being made in developing and testing vaccines that would enhance prevention efforts. In 1997, SmithKline Beecham Biologicals completed a Phase 3 trial of a vaccine developed to protect against Lyme disease. The trial enrolled 11,000 persons residing in the New England, mid-Atlantic, and Midwest regions of the United States. Data from the research trial have been reviewed by an independent Data and Safety Monitoring Board (DSMB) and suggest that the vaccine is effective in preventing Lyme's disease. After the review, the DSMB recommended that individuals who had received a placebo in the course of the trial also be vaccinated (SmithKline Beecham, 1997)

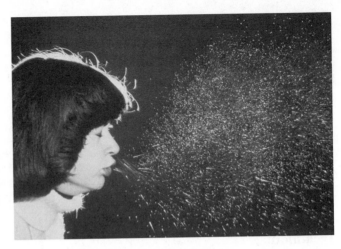

This photo illustrates how wide an area droplet nuclei from a sneeze can encompass. Photo courtesy of Lester V. Bergman/Corbis.

OTHER COMMUNICABLE DISEASES

Tuberculosis

Evidence suggests that *Mycobacterium tuberculosis* (TB) has been around for centuries. Traces of lesions from tuberculosis have been isolated from the lungs of Egyptian mummies. With the flurry of research and funding for the AIDS epidemic, tuberculosis has been called the "forgotten plague."

The incidence of TB has increased at an alarming rate in the past decade: From 1985 to 1993, the number of TB cases increased by 20% among the general population and by 36% among children. The number of infected individuals worldwide is approaching 2 billion, and an estimated 3 million people die from TB every year (NJMC National Tuberculosis Center, 1997). The prevalence of TB among persons infected with HIV has been particularly notable. Approximately 10% of HIV-positive individuals are also infected with TB.

Transmission

When an infected individual coughs or sneezes, droplet nuclei containing tubercle bacilli may be expelled in the air. For the TB organism to be transmitted, another person must inhale the droplet nuclei.

Symptoms

Symptoms of TB include fatigue, weight loss, night sweats and chills, and persistent coughing accompanied by blood-streaked sputum. Most people who become infected with the TB organism do not progress to the active-disease stage. They remain asymptomatic and noninfectious. These individuals, who have positive skin tests but negative chest x-rays, retain a lifelong risk of developing TB. Preventive therapy is recommended to minimize the risk of developing active TB. Without treatment, active TB is usually fatal. It should be remembered that TB is not exclusively a pulmonary disease; it is a systemic disease that can affect any body organ or system. Extrapulmonary

TB is most often seen in persons with HIV infection. Clients with extrapulmonary TB should be tested for the HIV virus if HIV status is unknown (Boutotte, 1993).

Diagnosis

According to the National Tuberculosis Center, there are four steps in diagnosing TB disease: medical history, tuberculin skin test, chest x-ray, and bacteriologic examination. Persons who report exposure to a TB-infected person or symptoms of TB or who have risk factors for developing TB should be given a tuberculin skin test. The Mantoux skin test is the preferred type of screening test because it is more accurate than other available skin tests. If a person tests positive on the skin test, a chest x-ray is used to evaluate whether the person has pulmonary TB disease. The bacteriologic exam of sputum is necessary to confirm active TB disease. Persons with positive smears are considered infectious. The specimen should be sent for culture and sensitivity analysis to determine whether it contains *M. tuberculosis* and, if it does, drug resistance (NJMC National Tuberculosis Center, 1997). High-risk groups that should be screened for tuberculosis are listed in Figure 20-13.

Treatment

Treatment for TB is lengthy when compared with that for other infectious diseases. Preventive therapy can be effective in preventing active disease. Skin testing can identify appropriate candidates for prevention therapy. To prevent the development of TB disease, the typical regime requires six months of chemotherapy treatment, usually with isoniazid, in persons with documented TB infection. Children should receive nine months of preventive therapy, and individuals with HIV should receive 12 months of preventive therapy.

If infection progresses to active TB disease, health care providers must prescribe an adequate treatment regime. If treatment is not continued long enough, some of the TB organisms will survive, and the potential for relapse increases (Boutotte, 1993). In most areas of the country, TB disease treatment should include four drugs: isoniazid, rifampin, pyrazinamide, and either ethambutol or streptomycin for a minimum of six months. This regime may be changed on the basis of reliable culture and sensitivity results. Clients who do not take the treatment as prescribed may relapse and develop drug resistance. Direct observed therapy (DOT) is one way to ensure that clients adhere to drug treatment requirements and has proved to be cost effective in the treatment of TB disease (NJMC National Tuberculosis Center, 1997).

Prevention

Primary prevention efforts include health promotion and education. Immunization is not widely used in the United States except in well-defined circumstances, because the incidence of TB is relatively low. Skin testing is commonly used as a control measure aimed at early detection. Chemoprophylaxis is widely used for prevention of active TB. Isoniazid (INH), an anti-tuberculin drug, is the most common form of prophylaxis. Adequate chemotherapy and instructing the person who has symptoms suggestive of TB to cover the nose and mouth when coughing, laughing, or sneezing can reduce transmission of TB. Ultraviolet light and sunlight, as well as adequate ventilation, can further reduce transmission. Secondary-prevention efforts focus on screening members of high-risk populations (see Figure 20-13) and on early diagnosis and treatment (CDC, 1988b). Tertiary prevention involves monitoring long-term health status and direct observed therapy.

The Role of the Health Department in the Prevention of Tuberculosis

Early reporting of suspected or confirmed TB cases is important for the control of TB. The public health department provides clients and clinicians with access to resources for assistance in case management and contact identification. The health department conducts contact investigations to determine who has been exposed to TB so that tuberculin skin testing can be performed and, when indicated, preventive therapy can be initiated. Figure 20-14 describes the role of the health department in TB prevention and treatment.

The Role of the Community Health Nurse in the Prevention of Tuberculosis

Community health nurses are often the individuals responsible for skin testing, reading, and referral. The nurse should be aware of persons who are at risk for infection and instigate screening clinics to facilitate early diagnosis in high-risk populations. Community health nurses have maintained growing case loads of persons with TB disease in varying stages. The nurse must understand the distinction between TB infection and disease as well as mode of

---

Figure 20-13   High-Risk Groups to Screen for Tuberculosis

- People with HIV infection
- Close contacts of infectious tuberculosis cases
- People with medical conditions that increase the risk of tuberculosis
- Immigrants from countries where TB is endemic
- Low-income populations
- Alcoholics and IV-drug users
- Residents of long-term care facilities
- Individuals living in congregate settings (e.g., shelters, prisons, and hospitals)
- Health care workers and others who provide service to high-risk groups

---

TB transmission. Identification of contacts of individuals with TB disease enables the nurse to recommend preventive therapy and interrupt the spread of infection.

The community health nurse is frequently the health professional responsible for DOT in noncompliant individuals. The importance of ensuring that the community is safe by documenting that infected individuals have completed adequate treatment cannot be overstated. Community health nurses are also responsible for educating clients regarding medications, including appropriate dosages and potential side effects. A symptoms checklist, administered periodically by community health nurses, is an effective way of documenting effectiveness of treatment and adverse side effects of medication. Community health nurses should participate with other health care workers in having annual purified protein derivative (PPD) skin tests. A checklist for tuberculin skin testing is provided in Figure 20-15.

Use of Bacillus Calmette-Guerin Vaccine

In many parts of the world, Bacillus Calmette-Guerin (BCG) vaccine is routinely used to prevent serious complications of tuberculosis. Immigrants should be asked

---

Figure 20-14   The Role of the Health Department in the Prevention of Tuberculosis

- Identify and treat all persons with TB disease and ensure that clients complete appropriate therapy.
- Identify and evaluate contacts of persons with infectious TB and offer therapy as appropriate.
- Screen high-risk groups for TB infection and offer therapy as appropriate.

Adapted from TB Reference Guide *by Georgia Division of Public Health, 1996. Adapted with permission.*

Figure 20-15 Tuberculin Skin-Testing Recommendations

Mantoux tuberculin testing is the standard used to identify persons infected with TB.

1. Inject 0.1 ml of purified protein derivative (PPD) containing 5 tuberculin units (TU) intradermally into the forearm.

2. Document the site location in the client's record.

3. Read the test 48 to 72 hours later.

4. Measure and record the induration (not the erythema) in millimeters:

   - Reactions of ≥5 mm are classified as positive in the following groups:

     Persons who are close contacts of a person with infectious TB

     Persons with known or suspected HIV

     Persons with chest x-rays suggestive of previous TB

     Intravenous drug users

   - A reaction of ≥10 mm is positive for all other persons who do not meet previous criteria but have other risk factors for TB.

   - A reaction of ≥15 mm is positive for all persons who are not in a high-risk category.

   - Persons with positive PPD skin tests should undergo a chest x-ray to rule out the possibility of active TB.

whether they have received BCG vaccine before thay are given a Mantoux skin test. The BCG vaccine is not recommended as a preventive strategy in the control of TB in the United States because of its interference with tuberculin skin testing. Although evidence is conflicting, research indicates that neither TB infection nor pulmonary TB is completely prevented by the BCG vaccine. Some studies suggest that BCG vaccination does lessen the likelihood of disseminated TB and TB meningitis in infants. Therefore, BCG may be indicated for infants and children living in households where they have close contact with an individual who has persistently untreated or ineffectively treated, sputum-positive tuberculosis, especially multidrug-resistant TB infection (CDC, 1988b).

Hepatitis

Hepatitis, an inflammatory condition of the liver, can be caused by several bacterial or viral infections, fungal or parasitic infection, alcohol, drugs, or chemical toxins. The inflammation destroys patches of liver tissue and can ultimately cause death. Despite the many origins of this disease condition, the symptoms, diagnosis, and treatment methods are similar and are discussed here in general terms.

Symptoms

Symptoms associated with hepatitis depend on the type and severity of infection. The infection may be mild and, in some cases, can go undetected, or it may be severe and life threatening. Hepatitis symptoms include jaundice, hepatomegaly, anorexia, muscle aches, nausea, vomiting, changes in taste and smell, clay-colored stools, and tea-colored urine. Physical exam may be perfectly normal, although enlarged lymph nodes, liver, and spleen are common findings.

Diagnosis

Laboratory studies reveal high liver function tests. Symptoms, physical exam, and laboratory findings cannot distinguish between the different types of viral hepatitis. Hepatitis serology lab tests are needed to make the specific diagnosis (Sjogren, 1994).

Treatment

Because hepatitis is a viral illness, there is no treatment. In mild cases, the liver is usually able to regenerate its tissue; but severe cases can lead to cirrhosis and chronic liver disease. Vaccines are now available for hepatitis A and B.

Most hepatitis infections are caused by viruses, which researchers named alphabetically as they were identified. The first hepatitis virus described was, of course, hepatitis A; hepatitis B was the next discovered. The identification of another hepatitis virus that tested negative for hepatitis type A and B was subsequently called hepatitis non-A, non-B. As researchers studied these viruses, hepatitis C was isolated and replaced the non-A, non-B classification. In recent years, hepatitis viruses D through G have been described, and the list continues to grow. Although the viruses have similar clinical presentations, each differs in etiology, prevention, and control (Benenson, 1995). Hepatitis viruses A through E are discussed next.

Hepatitis A

Transmission

Hepatitis A is caused by oral ingestion of the hepatitis A virus (HAV), which is found in the stool of persons with hepatitis A. It is usually spread from person to person by putting something in the mouth that has been contaminated with the stool of a person with hepatitis A. Because the virus is transmitted via the fecal/oral route, it is easily spread in areas where there are poor sanitary conditions or where good personal hygiene is not observed. Persons with HAV can spread the virus to others who live in the same household or with whom they have sexual contact. Casual contact, as in the office, factory, or school setting, does not spread the virus. Individuals working in day care centers or children attending day care centers, however, are at high risk for developing of the disease.

Perspectives...

Insights of a Student Nurse

Anna said she was 65, but she looked much older. Her wrinkled face, stooped posture, and tired eyes told of a hard life. Her eyes refused to brighten, even with the good news.

"Anna, I've got great news! The sputum cultures were all negative. Your tuberculosis is no longer infectious. Aren't you excited?" As I explained the results of the lab report, Anna seemed annoyed, restless. She lit a cigarette.

"I saw Hitler, heard him speak. You ever meet anyone before who actually heard Hitler speak? He was a crazy man. Even though I was only thirteen, I could tell he was crazy . . . and all those blonde German goons goose steppin' around like they were better than the rest of us! It was somethin' to see, I'll give him that." Anna's voice trailed off.

"Anna, have you been taking your medicine?" I was now becoming upset. "There are too many pills in your bottles. You should only have six left and I count at least 10. How're we gonna get rid of the TB if you don't take your meds?"

"Whatever you say," Anna replied, puffing on her cigarette. "It's a cockroach, this disease. Keeps people nosing around into a person's business, sticking their heads into my things. It's a roach I tell you!"

"Anna," I questioned as I caught a whiff of her breath, "have you been drinking?"

"Just a little brandy . . . to help the pills go down," she chuckled.

"Hey, I'm a nurse too. Fancy that . . . I was a darn good nurse, too. Worked nights for 20 years, when my Jack was small. A nurse and a mother! Now you've got somethin' to tell your friends about old Anna!"

"Anna, time to take your pills, and now I have to come back tomorrow," I scolded. "It's because you've been drinking and not taking the pills. Anna you've got to take the pills so we can keep the negative cultures. You've got to help me or we'll never get 'the cockroach' off your back! I only have two weeks of clinical left, and I'd like to end on a happy note."

"A happy note," she repeated. "Okay, I'll take my pills . . . sing a few bars too," Anna laughed. "I'll sing for the roach and you!"

It was two days before graduation when the public health nurse called. "I thought you might want to know," she said slowly. "Anna died this morning. She liked you. Well, I just thought you might want to know."

I wish I'd asked her where . . . where she'd heard Hitler speak.

—*Anonymous*

The source of infection is either contact with an infected person or direct contact with infected fecal material that has entered food or water supplies. Outbreaks have been related to sewage-contaminated water, infected food handlers (who do not wash their hands after using the bathroom), and shellfish caught in waters contaminated by sewage (Benenson, 1995). Hepatitis A is easily spread between family members if good handwashing is not a common practice before handling food and after using the bathroom.

Prevention

Hepatitis A infection typically resolves and does not result in chronic hepatitis. Deaths from HAV can occur, but they are rare. Individuals at high risk for acquiring the infection should take advantage of the hepatitis A vaccine. If persons are aware of exposure to hepatitis, immune globulin (IG) can be administered to prevent the disease or to minimize symptoms. The benefit of IG administration is protection against HAV for three to five months, depending on the dosage. It can be given before exposure to HAV or within two weeks after exposure. Travelers to areas with high rates of HAV should receive IG if they did not receive the hepatitis A vaccine. Of the more than 10 million estimated people worldwide who acquire HAV each year, most recover within three to six months (DeVincent-Hayes, 1995). Groups at high risk for contracting HAV are listed in Figure 20-16.

Figure 20-16 Groups at High Risk for Contracting Hepatitis A

- Day care workers
- Persons who work with HAV-infected animals or with HAV in a research setting. (Hepatitis A vaccine is not generally recommended for health care workers.)
- Persons with clotting factor disorders such as hemophilia
- Persons traveling or working in countries with high rates of HAV, such as Central or South America, the Caribbean, Mexico, Asia (except Japan), Africa, and southern or eastern Europe. (The first dose should be given at least four weeks before travel.)
- Persons who live in communities with high rates of HAV
- Men who have sex with men
- Persons who use illicit drugs
- Persons with chronic liver disease

High-risk individuals over 2 years of age should get hepatitis A vaccine.

Hepatitis B

Transmission

Hepatitis B is sometimes referred to as "serum hepatitis" because it is spread via direct contact with infected blood. Blood transfusions, once a common source of hepatitis B infection, are now considered safe owing to current screening tests. Hepatitis B virus (HBV) is carried in the blood and body fluids of an infected person. Considered the most prevalent of the hepatitis viruses, HBV is transmitted sexually, through shared needles, and from mother to child. The virus can pass between people through breaks in the skin, mouth, vagina, or penis. Hepatitis B is unlike hepatitis A in that a person can harbor HBV without being actively infected and can spread it to others (LaPook, 1995).

Hepatitis B is considered extremely contagious and is very hardy. Dried blood outside the body and containing HBV has been shown to be infectious up to a week or longer. Although most individuals infected with HBV recover fully, 6% to 10% of infected individuals do not completely recover and become carriers (Stein, 1993). Carriers can transmit the infection to others throughout their lifetimes. This fact is important to remember because vertical transmission remains a primary cause of new infections. Hepatitis B is potentially lethal, and it is estimated that each year in the United States approximately 150,000 persons are infected, 11,000 persons are hospitalized, and 300 to 400 persons die from acute fulminant hepatitis.

A variable portion of persons with acute HBV infection develop chronic infection. Chronic HBV infection is defined as the presence of HBsAg in serum for at least six months. The risk of developing chronic infection is age dependent and greatest for infants, who have a 90% chance of developing chronic infection if infected at birth. Overall, 30% to 50% of children and 5% to 10% of adults with acute infection will develop chronic infection (Edmunds, Medley, Nokes, Hall, et al., 1993). Persons with chronic HBV infection are at increased risk of developing chronic liver disease or primary hepatocellular carcinoma. Approximately 1 to 1.25 million people in the United States have chronic HBV infection, and 5,000 to 6,000 people die each year from HBV-induced chronic liver disease.

Chronic HBV infections are often detected via screening programs such as blood bank serological testing and refugee health screening. Cases of chronic HBV infection are not reportable to the National Notifiable Disease Surveillance System (NNDSS) (CDC, 1997j). Individuals with chronic disease are at increased risk of developing cirrhosis and liver cancer.

Persons with chronic HBV infection are a primary reservoir for transmission of HBV infections. A **reservoir** is any host or environment in which an infectious agent normally lives and multiplies. Any person testing positive for HBsAg is potentially infectious to both household and sexual contacts. These contacts should receive appropriate prophylaxis. Although chronic HBV infections are not reportable to NNDSS, all states are encouraged to make HBsAg positivity among pregnant women reportable. Pregnant women who are HBsAg positive may pass on the infection to their newborn infants, and prevention of perinatal HBV transmission requires intensive case management.

Prevention

Over the past 10 years, the most frequently reported risk factor for acute HBV was heterosexual activity (41%), followed by intravenous drug use (15%), homosexual activity (9%), household contact with a person with HBV (2%), and health care employment (1%). Many persons with

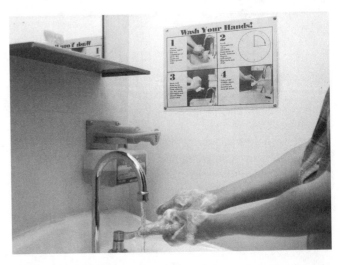

It is very important to stress handwashing to control the spread of communicable disease.

HBV do not identify risk factors (31%), and their sources of infection may be other infected persons who are asymptomatic (CDC, 1997j). Efforts at disease control focus on prevention. Primary prevention is central to the prevention of this disease. A vaccine against HBV has been available since 1982. This vaccine requires three injections at specified intervals and is now part of routine immunization schedules for children. Immunization is encouraged in adolescents prior to the onset of sexual activity. Health care workers should also take advantage of immunization to prevent HBV. Screening of high-risk populations can assist in the early detection of disease and is an important component of secondary prevention. Tertiary prevention involves minimizing the effects of the disease, primarily liver damage caused by the infection.

Hepatitis C

Transmission

Hepatitis C virus (HCV) was not identified until 1988, when researchers realized it was responsible for most of what had been known as non-A, non-B hepatitis. Specifically, HCV was responsible for most cases of post-transfusion hepatitis. The identification of the virus led to the development of a blood test in 1990, which has been useful in reducing, though not eliminating, the number of HCV infections among transfusion recipients (Stein, 1993). Currently in the United States, HCV is responsible for approximately 20% of acute viral hepatitis cases, of which fewer than 5% can be related to blood transfusions. Prevalence of HCV disease is highest among intravenous drug users and hemophiliacs (Benenson, 1995). As with other forms of hepatitis, the disease may be spread through sexual contact. It is important to note that individuals with HCV have high rates of chronic disease in more than 60% of cases (Benenson, 1995). Individuals who develop chronic disease are at increased risk for cirrhosis and liver cancer.

Prevention

Education and screening are important to prevent new cases and to minimize the effects of disease via early detection. Tertiary prevention is necessary to assist clients with chronic disease to be aware of risks, resources, and support systems. Many new support groups have formed to assist clients in living with HCV.

Hepatitis D

Transmission

Hepatitis D virus (HDV), or delta hepatitis, occurs only in clients with HBV and can cause a more serious form of hepatitis than is found with HBV alone (LaPook, 1995). Hepatitis D magnifies HBV's severity and can "co-infect" during the initial HBV episode or "superinfect" by infecting individuals with chronic HBV. Hepatitis D is considered the most severe form of hepatitis, killing 20% to 25% of those it infects (Stein, 1993).

Prevention

Prevention of HBV via vaccination will also prevent co-infection with HDV. However, neither the HBV vaccination nor hepatitis B immunoglobulin (HBIG) will protect the HBV carrier from super infection with HDV (Benenson, 1995).

Hepatitis E

Transmission

The clinical course of hepatitis E virus (HEV) is similar to that of hepatitis A. Outbreaks of disease occur most frequently in developing countries with inadequate sanitation. The disease is transmitted primarily through the fecal contamination of food or water. Hepatitis E is an acute infection that does not progress to the carrier state but can be fatal in up to 20% of pregnant women (Benenson, 1995).

Prevention

Should focus on improving sanitation and providing education about the importance of clean water supplies and proper food handling and storage. Table 20-10 compares the different types of hepatitis.

Food- and Waterborne Infections

The reporting of foodborne and waterborne diseases in the United States began more than 50 years ago when state and territorial health officers, concerned about the high morbidity and mortality associated with typhoid fever and infantile diarrhea, recommended that cases of "enteric fever" be investigated and reported. The purpose of investigating and reporting these cases was to obtain information regarding the role of food, milk, and water in outbreaks of intestinal illness as the basis for public health action. Beginning in 1923, the Public Health Service published summaries of outbreaks of gastrointestinal illness attributed to milk. In 1938, it added summaries of outbreaks caused by all foods. These early surveillance efforts led to the enactment of important public health measures (e.g., the Model Milk Ordinance) that had a profound influence in decreasing the incidence of enteric diseases, particularly those transmitted by milk and water (CDC, 1996c).

Transmission

Waterborne pathogens typically enter water supplies via human or animal fecal contamination. Americans are so accustomed to safe, clean, and plentiful water supplies that the possibility of contamination is not considered

Table 20-10 Hepatitis Facts*

TYPE OF HEPATITIS	INCUBATION PERIOD	MODES OF TRANSMISSION	PREVENTION	POSSIBLE COMPLICATIONS
A	15 to 50 days	• Fecal/oral through contaminated food or water • Poor hygiene	• Immunization • Education on proper food handling	
B	45 to 180 days	• Unsafe sex • Poor hygiene • Body secretions • Blood transfusions • Contaminated needles	• Immunization • Education to prevent exposures to blood and body fluids • Needle exchange programs • Identification of carriers	• Potential chronicity • Cirrhosis • Liver cancer
C	2 weeks to 6 months	• IV drug use • Blood transfusions	• Education to prevent exposures to blood and body fluids • Needle exchange programs • Identification of carriers	• Potential chronicity • Cirrhosis • Liver cancer
D	2 to 8 weeks	• Blood • Contaminated needles • Limited to those who have had HBV	• Immunization against HBV • Education to prevent exposures to blood and body fluids • Needle exchange programs • Identification of HBV carriers	• Potential chronicity • Cirrhosis
E	15 to 64 days	• Fecal/oral through contaminated water	• Vaccine under development • Practice of proper sanitation • Alerting travelers to the risk of infection	• Potentially fatal in pregnant women

*Hepatitis symptoms: Some individuals are asymptomatic; however, most viral hepatitis infections present as fever, chills, nausea, vomiting, diarrhea, and fatigue. Individuals also report dark urine, jaundice, abdominal pain, anorexia, muscle aches, and light (clay-colored) stool.

until a problem arises. However, a clear appearance to water does not always indicate safety as drinking water, and outbreaks of gastrointestinal illness due to contaminated municipal water still occur in the United States.

Many of these outbreaks are associated with viral and parasitic infectious agents, such as cryptosporidium (CDC, 1996b). The largest recorded waterborne disease outbreak in U.S. history occurred in Milwaukee, Wisconsin, in April 1993. The disease was cryptosporidiosis, a parasitic infection of the small intestine that can produce severe watery diarrhea. This outbreak of cryptosporidiosis affected over 400,000 people, and more than 4,400 people were hospitalized.

Symptoms

Each year in the United States, water- and foodborne infections cause mild to severe illness in millions of people and are responsible for thousands of deaths. Symptoms range from mild to violent and severe gastrointestinal symptoms.

Diagnosis

Many food- and waterborne illnesses go undiagnosed and are in many cases unreported. Diagnosis can be confirmed via laboratory culture of suspected sources of infection.

Treatment

Treatment for food and waterborne infections varies depending on the organism and the severity of illness. Fluid and electrolyte replacement is indicated in cases of severe diarrhea or vomiting.

Prevention

Preventing foodborne illness is a complex process. Despite public health efforts to maintain healthy food and water sources, many old disease scenarios have resurfaced as new challenges to health officials. Consumers obtain food after it has passed through a long chain of industrial production, with each link in the chain providing the opportunity for contamination. Investigation of disease outbreaks should focus not only on identifying the infectious organism and likely food source but also on examining the industrial process that allowed the organism to survive the food production process and, ultimately, infect the human host (Tauxe, 1997).

Although substantial progress has been made in preventing food- and waterborne illnesses in the United States, new infections are emerging that threaten the health of consumers. Approximately 400 to 500 foodborne disease outbreaks are reported each year (CDC, 1996c). *Escherichia coli* O157:H7, discussed earlier in this chapter, is one of the new foodborne pathogens that have emerged. The 1997 recall of 1.2 million pounds of hamburger that was distributed by a single processing plant in Nebraska and linked to an outbreak of *E. coli* O157:H7 infection emphasizes the potential health and economic impact of food-processing and distribution practices (Satchell & Hedges, 1997). Cyclospora was responsible for a 1996 outbreak of illness, the food source of which was traced to imported Guatemalan raspberries (Ackers & Herwaldt, 1997). Hepatitis A was transmitted to more than 150 Michigan school children and teachers after they

---

Figure 20-17   Ten Golden Rules of Safe Food Preparation

1. Choose food processed for safety.
2. Cook food thoroughly.
3. Eat cooked foods immediately.
4. Store cooked foods carefully.
5. Reheat cooked foods thoroughly.
6. Avoid contact between raw food and cooked food.
7. Wash hands repeatedly.
8. Keep all kitchen surfaces meticulously clean.
9. Protect food from insects, rodents, and other animals.
10. Use safe water.

From Control of Communicable Diseases in Man *(16th ed, p. 184) by A. S. Benenson (Ed.), 1995, Washington, DC: American Public Health Association. Used with permission.*

---

ingested frozen strawberries imported from Mexico (CDC, 1997h).

Consumer education is key in food safety and the prevention of foodborne illnesses. Foods contaminated with emerging pathogens usually look, smell, and taste normal, and the pathogen often survives traditional preparation techniques. Thorough cooking will kill almost all foodborne bacteria, viruses, and parasites and is an important step in the prevention of disease. Figure 20-17 lists 10 "golden rules" of safe food preparation.

There are several reasons for the emerging risks of food- and waterborne diseases. First, the food supply in the United States is changing. The way animals are raised has changed the picture of foodborne illness. Healthy animals have now been implicated in the spread of disease (CDC, 1996d). Second, citizens' expectation of having fresh produce all seasons of the year has led to the import of more than 30 billion tons of food each year, including fruits, vegetables, seafood, and canned goods. These food items are often raised in developing countries where sanitation is inadequate. Some of this imported food is irrigated or rinsed with contaminated water or shipped in ice made from contaminated water that has been implicated in the spread of disease (Tauxe, 1997). Third, consumers eat out more frequently and consume processed foods in higher quantities. Finally, new pathogens that can cause disease have been identified (CDC, 1996c). Policies regarding the safe handling of food should include evaluation of food production and shipping in all countries that serve as suppliers to the U.S. food stock.

Pediculosis

Few contagious situations evoke the kind of response that comes with a diagnosis of pediculosis. Simply the idea of having bugs crawling on the skin or in one's hair brings about the sensation of itching. Public health nurses and

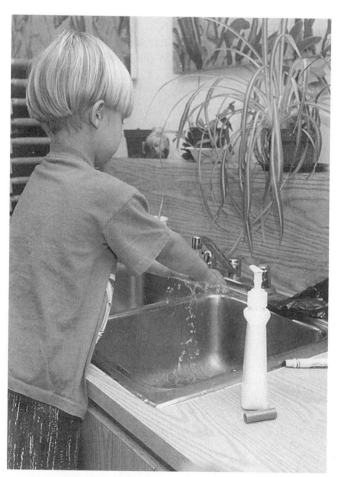

Americans are so accustomed to safe water that they do not think about the possibility of disease transmission until a problem arises.

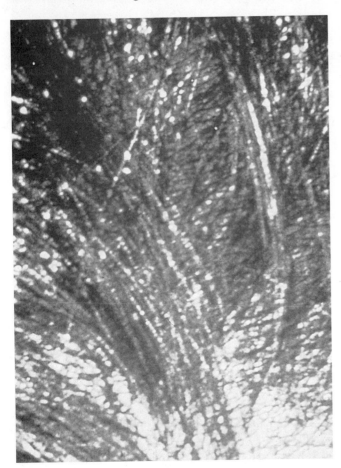

The community health nurse should counsel clients on prevention methods and the need for treatment to control the spread of head lice. Photo courtesy of Reed and Carnrick Pharmaceuticals.

school nurses are particularly familiar with the contagious nature of pediculosis and the ability of these parasites to spread rapidly.

Pediculosis refers to an infestation of lice, which are easily spread via person-to-person contact. There are three types of lice: Head lice (*Pediculus humanus capitus*) are primarily found in children who share combs or hats; pubic lice (*Phthirus pubis*), also known as pubic crabs, are frequently found in adults and are transmitted primarily by sexual contact with an infected person (Benenson, 1995); and body lice (*Pediculus humanus corposis*) are transmitted through infected clothing and linen. Poor hygiene is implicated only in the spread of body lice and is most frequently found in individuals who do not wash their clothes regularly.

Transmission

Although pediculosis infestations are considered very contagious, it is important to remember that lice do not typically jump from person to person. All three parasites are transmitted via close body contact with an infested person. They may also be transmitted by contact with shared items such as bed sheets, clothing, combs, or brushes. Younger children, who play and work closely

together and are likely to share clothing and combs, are more susceptible to disease than older children or adolescents, so outbreaks tend to be rare after grade six. Pubic crabs are found in adult populations and are transmitted by sexual contact.

Symptoms

Symptoms of infection are an itching or prickling sensation. In *Pediculus humanus corposis* infestation, the nits are laid in the seams of clothing and cause itching when in contact with the skin. *Phthirus pubis* infestation causes anogenital itching.

Diagnosis

Pediculus humanus capitis is accompanied by the appearance of nits, or white spheres, on the hair at the back of the head and neck and behind the ears.

Treatment

Pesticidal shampoos are recommended in the treatment of head lice. Products vary slightly and should be used as directed. Treatment must be accompanied by removal of the nits (egg cases) that attach to the hair shaft. Clients should be instructed in the proper treatment of this condition:

- Prior to the use of pesticidal shampoos, notify health provider if the affected individual has asthma, allergies, or neurological conditions.
- Read and follow the manufacturer's label before applying the product.
- Nit removal can be accomplished by methodical "picking" of the eggs from the hair shaft. Eggs that are not removed are likely to hatch and cause reinfestation.
- Clothing, linens, and toys should be washed in hot water and dried at a high heat; if washing is not practical, these items should be vacuumed. Upholstery (both home and car) should also be vacuumed and the vacuum bag discarded. Brushes and combs should be washed in very hot water.

Prevention

Lice can infect people of all socioeconomic groups and can infect people who take particular care to practice good hygiene as well as those who do not. In fact, some clinicians report that lice prefer clean hair. Children should be taught to keep combs, brushes, and caps to themselves. Screening of children with symptoms and isolating those infected from school populations until successful treatment is possible are recommended.

Scabies

Scabies is a parasitic disease in which tiny mites burrow under the skin. Although scabies mites are difficult to

DECISION MAKING

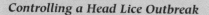

Controlling a Head Lice Outbreak

You are the school nurse at Hometown Elementary. Mrs. Jones, a third grade teacher, reports that white spots are visible in the hair of four of her students, one of whom complains of severe itching of the scalp. After examining the heads of the four children, you confirm that all four of the children have head lice. You contact the children's parents, and all four children are sent home with treatment recommendations and instructions. Each child in Mrs. Jones's class is then checked for head lice. After screening the entire class, you find three more children with visible nits in their hair. These children are also sent home with treatment recommendations and instructions.

• What primary prevention measures might have prevented this outbreak? What secondary and tertiary interventions are indicated?

• What actions will you take to protect the school community?

• What agent, host, and environmental factors may contribute to the transmission of disease in this setting?

• What social and cultural considerations may influence the effectiveness of treatment?

• Does the school nurse's responsibility stop after excluding the affected children from school?

spot, infestation can be recognized by the characteristic burrows that contain the mites and their eggs. These burrows look like tracks, or small lines that resemble scratches, across the surface of the skin. Lesions are typically visible in the webs of the fingers, on the anterior surface of the wrists, on the buttocks, on the axillae, and along the beltline.

Transmission

Scabies mites can live for only a brief time away from the host, and the infection is transmitted between persons only via close skin-to-skin contact (Benenson, 1995).

Symptoms

Scabies is characterized by intense itching, especially at night.

Diagnosis

Scabies should be suspected when clients complain of intense itching. The rash is typically found between fingers and toes and on wrists, armpits, genitals, and the lower buttocks. Dark ink applied to skin areas of sus-

pected infestation help locate the burrow sites of scabies mites. The presence of scabies is confirmed by applying a drop of sterile mineral oil to the affected area. A scraping from this area is then examined under a microscope. Scabies is often accompanied by bacterial infections and is easily confused with other skin diseases.

Treatment

Treatment is indicated for all persons who may have come into close contact with an infested individual. Over-the-counter insecticide lotion treatments are available for killing the mites. Treatment of infants, young children, nursing mothers, pregnant women, elderly individuals, and people with skin diseases requires the consultation of a physician before starting treatment. The rash may take two to six weeks to develop (Benenson, 1995). Treatment should include a thorough housecleaning, including washing all bed linens, bath towels, and clothing in hot water. Vacuuming of furniture and mattresses and immediately discarding the vacuum bag can prevent the spread of scabies from furniture and other items.

Prevention

If an infested person is in a school or institutional setting, the individual should be excluded until 24 hours after treatment has been completed. Persons who have had direct contact with the infected person should be notified and may need treatment.

Influenza

Influenza, or "the flu," is an acute viral illness, prevalent during the winter and early spring. Because of the short incubation period (one to three days), epidemics can develop rapidly, and severe complications and death have been known to accompany infection. Severe illness and death occur primarily in elderly persons and are due to viral or bacterial respiratory complications. Each flu season is unique and brings a new strain of illness (Peters, 1997b).

Three types of influenza virus are recognized: A, B, and C. Of the three types, A is the most common and is the type usually associated with epidemics, complications, and death (Hemming, Palmer, Sinnot, & Glaser, 1997).

Transmission

Influenza is commonly spread through airborne droplets, nasopharyngeal secretions, and contact with contaminated materials. Transmission is facilitated by closed spaces such as those found in schools, school buses, hospitals, and nursing homes (Benenson, 1995).

Symptoms

Influenza is an acute viral illness characterized by muscle aches, fever, fatigue, headache, sore throat, and cough. Symptoms usually last from two to four days but may linger for up to two weeks. Influenza pneumonia may develop when the influenza virus attacks the lower airways and lungs (Hemming et al., 1997).

Diagnosis

The diagnosis of influenza is clinical, based on client history and symptoms.

Treatment

Treatment of influenza is symptomatic unless complications develop. Persons at high risk for complications should seek treatment early. See Figure 20-18.

Prevention

Anyone over age 6 months who is at increased risk of developing the complications of influenza (see Figure 20-18) should have a flu shot. Changes in antigenic properties that occur from year to year, called antigenic drift, require the preparation of a new vaccine each year. Vaccines typically contain two type A and one type B virus strains. Because of antigenic changes in the virus, antibodies produced as a result of influenza infection or vaccination containing earlier strains may not protect against viruses circulating in subsequent years. Thus vaccination each year is necessary to prevent infection. When the match between the vaccine strain and circulating viruses is good, influenza vaccine is approximately 70% effective in preventing illness (Peters, 1997b). Secondary prevention involves early diagnosis and treatment of symptoms to prevent complications of the disease.

Figure 20-18   Persons Who Should Get the Influenza Vaccine

- Persons 65 years of age and older
- Residents of nursing homes and other chronic care facilities that house persons of any age with chronic medical conditions
- Adults and children with chronic pulmonary or cardiovascular disorders, including children with asthma
- Adults and children who required regular medical follow-up or hospitalization during the preceding year because of chronic metabolic diseases (including diabetes mellitus), renal dysfunction, hemoglobinopathies, or immunosuppression (including immunosuppression caused by medications)
- Children and adolescents (6 months to 18 years of age) who are receiving long-term aspirin therapy and might therefore be at risk for developing Reye syndrome after influenza
- Women who will be in the second or third trimester of pregnancy during the influenza season

---

Rabies

Over the past 30 years, reported cases of animal rabies in the United States have increased from fewer than 5,000 per year in the early 1960s to almost 10,000 per year in the mid-1990s, with 1994 recording the highest annual mortality since 1979. Most of the increase is attributable to the spread of raccoon rabies from Florida to the northeastern states (Rupprect & Smith, 1994) and the growing incidence of coyote rabies in southern Texas (Deasy, 1996). Human rabies is a preventable disease when it is recognized and appropriate therapy is initiated. If symptoms develop, rabies will invariably result in death.

Rabies is primarily an animal disease that may be transmitted to humans. Although rabies is often thought of as a disease passed from domesticated animals to humans, there has been a shift in disease prevalence to wildlife. In the United States, the most frequently reported rabid wild animals are raccoons, skunks, foxes, and bats. Because of increased urban expansion into the habitats of wild animals, humans are at increased risk of coming in contact with rabid animals. In New York and Massachusetts, where raccoon rabies is prevalent, oral immunization of these animal vectors is being tested. Areas that have instigated oral immunization programs have had decreased episodes of rabies (Uhaa, Dato, Sorhage, Beckly, et al., 1992). Bats have been implicated in several recent rabies deaths, and the CDC recommends that when a bat is physically present and the possibility of a bite exists, postexposure prophylaxis should be given (CDC, 1996a). In North America, the spread of infection follows a cycle in which the infection is passed from animal to animal via bites or scratches. In the United States, cats pose a greater risk for rabies than do dogs. In many developing countries, however, the dog is still the main vector in the spread of disease (Deasy, 1996).

Transmission

Rabies is transmitted to humans via an animal scratch or bite. A bite by a rabid animal carries a much greater risk of infection than does a scratch. The rabies virus enters the body where there is direct saliva contact with broken skin or mucous membranes.

Diagnosis

Diagnosis is based on history of exposure to infection, the occurrence of characteristic signs and symptoms, and laboratory tests.

Symptoms

The incubation period in humans ranges from five days to more than one year, with two months being the average. Initially, clients report vague symptoms that last from two to 10 days. The client may complain of fever, headache, malaise, and decreased appetite, and pain, itching, or numbness is often present at the site of the wound. As the disease progresses, clients develop difficulty swallowing and are unable to swallow their saliva. A characteristic of the infection is that the sight of water terrifies the individual. Paralysis, agitation, and disorientation are followed by coma and death from complications.

Treatment

There is no known, effective treatment for rabies once the symptoms of the illness have developed. Because of the frightening mortality associated with this disease—essentially 100%—all individuals who have come in contact with an infected animal or person should receive postexposure prophylaxis. The decision on whether to initiate postexposure prophylaxis treatment should be based on the guidelines of the Advisory Committee on Immunization Practices of the Public Health Service and should be coordinated with local health officials and animal control authorities (CDC, 1991). Management of animal bites is important and is outlined in Figure 20-19.

Prevention

Nurses can educate clients about the need to vaccinate pets to ensure a healthy neighborhood. Prevention of human rabies requires both animal control and public awareness. Consumers should be educated about the importance of rabies prevention. The public should avoid unnecessary contact with wild animals (particularly bats, raccoons, coyotes, and skunks) and should be aware of the signs displayed by rabid animals, such as daytime appearance by normally nocturnal animals. Domestic animals should be routinely vaccinated to prevent rabies.

Preexposure vaccination should be considered for individuals whose occupations, avocations, or activities place them at frequent risk of exposure to rabies virus or to potentially rabid animals. Occupations considered at risk are hunters, forest rangers, taxidermists, laboratory workers, stock breeders, slaughterhouse workers, and veterinarians.

Figure 20-19 Checklist for the Treatment of Animal Bites

- Immediately clean and flush the wound (first aid).
- Under medical supervision, thoroughly clean the wound.
- Administer rabies immune globulin and/or vaccine as indicated.
- Administer tetanus prophylaxis and antibacterial treatment when required.
- Unless unavoidable, do not suture or close the wound.

From Control of Communicable Diseases in Man *(16th ed., p. 388) by A. S. Benenson (Ed.), 1995, Washington, DC: American Public Health Association. Used with permission.*

GLOBAL PERSPECTIVES FOR COMMUNICABLE DISEASE CONTROL

Communicable diseases are a growing threat to communities worldwide. Microbes do not stop at border crossings or immigration checkpoints. Old infections such as TB, diphtheria, and cholera have resurfaced with increased virulence and drug resistance. Deadly new infections such as AIDS and hantavirus have emerged as frightening counterparts to more primitive infections. In some cases, diseases such as AIDS and TB coexist in the human host, increasing the severity and complications of infection. Because of today's mobile society, communicable diseases cannot be sealed within one country, city, or state. International travel of businesspersons, immigrants, refugees, and vacationers has assisted in the transport of deadly diseases throughout the world. Community health nurses must take a world view as they study the implications of communicable diseases in local communities. Infectious diseases should be addressed as a global issue with shared responsibility for surveillance and control.

Communicable Disease Surveillance and Reporting Guidelines

Disease reporting and surveillance have been core public health functions practiced by community health nurses (Kuss, Proulx-Girouard, Lovitt, Katz, et al., 1997). **Surveillance** is the systematic collection and evaluation of all aspects of disease occurrence and spread, resulting in information that may be useful in the control of disease. Community health nurses are among the frontline workers in the battle to detect, diagnose, and, ultimately, eliminate the communicable diseases that plague neighborhoods and communities. Community health nurses play an important role in disease surveillance by investigating sources of disease outbreaks, collecting data, reporting cases, and providing information to the public about disease morbidity and mortality within the local community.

In 1878, Congress authorized the U.S. Marine Service (forerunner of the Public Health Service) to collect morbidity reports regarding cholera, smallpox, plague, and yellow fever from U.S. consuls overseas. This information was to be used to institute quarantine measures developed to prevent the spread of disease from other countries to the United States. The law was later expanded to prevent the spread of disease among the states. Thus began the evolution of communicable disease reporting in the United States. Requirements for disease reporting in the United States are mandated by state laws and regulations. State health departments report nationally notifiable diseases to the CDC in Atlanta, Georgia. As of January 1, 1996, 52 infectious diseases were designated as notifiable

Table 20-11   List of Nationally Reportable Diseases—1997

Acquired immunodeficiency syndrome (AIDS)	Malaria
Anthrax	Measles
Botulism	Meningococcal disease
Brucellosis	Mumps
Chancroid	Pertussis
Chlamydia trachomatis, genital infections	Plague
Cholera	Poliomyelitis, paralytic
Coccidioidomycosis	Psittacosis
Cryptosporidiosis	Rabies, animal
Diphtheria	Rabies, human
Encephalitis, California serogroup	Rocky Mountain spotted fever
Encephalitis, eastern equine	Rubella
Encephalitis, St. Louis	Rubella, congenital syndrome
Encephalitis, western equine	Salmonellosis
Escherichia coli O157:H7	Shigellosis
Gonorrhea	Streptococcal disease, invasive, Group A
Haemophilus influenzae, invasive disease	*Streptococcus pneumoniae,* drug-resistant invasive disease
Hansen disease (leprosy)	Streptococcal toxic shock syndrome
Hantavirus pulmonary syndrome	Syphilis
Hemolytic uremic syndrome, postdiarrheal	Syphilis, congenital
Hepatitis A	Tetanus
Hepatitis B	Toxic shock syndrome
Hepatitis, C/non-A, non-B	Trichinosis
HIV infection, pediatric	Tuberculosis
Legionellosis	Typhoid fever
Lyme disease	Yellow fever

About this document:

In the United States, requirements for reporting diseases are mandated by state laws or regulations, and the list of reportable diseases in each state differs. In October 1990, in collaboration with the Council of State and Territorial Epidemiologists, CDC published Case Definitions for Public Health Surveillance (MMWR 1990;39(No. RR-13)[No. RR-13]), which, for the first time, provided uniform criteria for reporting cases.

This report was recently revised and provides updated uniform criteria for state health department personnel to use when reporting to CDC notifiable infectious diseases (Case Definitions for Infectious Conditions Under Public Health Surveillance (MMWR 1997;46[No. RR-10]). A revision date is listed for each case definition that has been revised. Newly generated case definitions that have not been published previously are designated as "adopted" on the specified date.

For the most current information on procedures for reporting the occurrence of communicable diseases nationally, please see the Manual of Procedures for Reporting Nationally Notifiable Diseases to CDC *(U.S. Department of Health and Human Services, Public Health Service, CDC, 1995). Note that the list of notifiable diseases varies by state, as reporting is mandated only at the state level.*

From "Case Definitions for Infectious Conditions under Public Health Surveillance" by Centers for Disease Control and Prevention, 1997d, MMWR, *46(RR-10), 19.*

at the national level (CDC, 1997d) (see Table 20-11). Community health nurses are involved in the surveillance system at many different levels including disease outbreak investigation and reporting, immunization, contact tracing, and collection of vital statistics.

COMMUNITY HEALTH NURSE RESPONSIBILITIES AND OPPORTUNITIES RELEVANT TO COMMUNICABLE DISEASE

Community health nurses must arm themselves with information about new and emerging infectious diseases. It is often the nurse who has the initial contact with clients, and an informed nurse can be instrumental in preventing the unnecessary spread of disease throughout a community. Practicing community health nurses may encounter new disease entities that have not yet been identified or adequately described. Recognizing infectious disease conditions is a challenge and responsibility of nurses working to protect the health of communities.

Community health nurses should be aware of epidemiologic principles so that they can use this knowledge to interrupt the chain of infection relative to communicable disease. Strengthening the host through immunization and education, controlling the environment through protection of food and water supplies, and controlling transmission of agents between infected hosts by promoting both barrier methods to prevent STDs and needle-exchange programs to protect intravenous drug users are part of the nurse's responsibility in the control of communicable disease.

COMMUNITY NURSING VIEW

A public health nurse is working at a local health department's sexually transmitted disease clinic. A 14-year-old girl, Amy, arrives early for her appointment at the clinic. She seems nervous and upset. While taking a health history, the nurse learns that this young woman has been sexually active for approximately 6 months. Amy reports only one sexual partner, her 21-year-old boyfriend, Jimmy. She has been using oral contraceptives to prevent pregnancy and reports reliable compliance. Two weeks ago, however, she noticed a lesion on her "privates." She says the lesion is extremely painful and causes irritation and burning when she urinates. She has also developed a "smelly" vaginal discharge, which Jimmy does not like. He says she stinks, which is what brought her to the clinic today. When questioned about the number of sexual partners Jimmy has had, she replies, blushing, "I'm his first."

On physical exam, the nurse finds the following:
- A small, ulcerated lesion, now crusted over on the labia minora
- A red and inflamed perineal region
- A greenish, foamy, vaginal discharge accompanied by a fishy odor

Cultures and a Pap test were obtained, and all other physical findings were normal.

Nursing Considerations

ASSESSMENT
- What is your initial assessment of Amy's situation?
- What additional assessment data would be useful to complete the clinical picture?

DIAGNOSIS
- What is the likely diagnosis?
- What levels of prevention are appropriate to prevent the spread of infection?

OUTCOME IDENTIFICATION
- What might be your short- and long-term goals in this situation?

PLANNING/INTERVENTIONS
- How might you involve the client in decision making?
- What are the treatment options? What nursing actions will ensure treatment compliance?
- What responsibilities do you have in this situation with regard to reporting, contact notification, and client education?

EVALUATION
- How might you evaluate your success in this situation?
- What follow-up care and referrals are indicated?

Awareness of core public health functions such as disease surveillance and reporting is key in the control of communicable diseases. Core public health functions include the surveillance of disease. In order to interrupt the spread of infection, community health nurses must rely on their knowledge of the nursing process to assess agent, host, and environmental factors that may be contributing to the development of specific disease conditions. At the same time, the nurse plans and implements control procedures that serve to protect the health of the community. Evaluation of the effectiveness of disease surveillance and control is often apparent when local, state, and national morbidity and mortality statistics are reviewed.

Educating consumers about basic sanitation principles related to food preparation as well as the importance of handwashing will help reduce the spread of infection. Information regarding Universal Precautions (see Figure 20-7) should be available to health care worker and consumer alike to assist in the fight against AIDS and other blood-borne infections. Whereas nurses in acute care settings often rely on medications and treatments to fight disease,

nurses working in the community are aware of the need to return to basic principles to keep the public healthy. Water supplies protected from contamination, appropriate waste control, knowledgeable food growers and handlers, and a public informed of barriers that can interrupt the spread of infection, such as safe-sex practices and proper handwashing and food storage and handling in the home, can go a long way toward curbing communicable disease.

Immunizations are by far the most cost effective way to prevent the occurrence of infectious diseases. Strengthening the host to resist infection interrupts the spread of infections and supports primary-prevention efforts. Community health nurses must be creative and innovative in their efforts to make immunizations available to all populations and to break down the barriers to timely immunizations.

Disease treatment, or secondary prevention, should focus on minimizing the effects of agents on both host and environment. Particularly in the age of emerging infections, nurses should be leaders in the early recognition and treatment of infection to minimize the potential long-term effects of these diseases. The recent inroads made in the treatment of AIDS illustrate how early intervention and treatment can change the natural history of disease and increase individual health potential.

Nurses can be instrumental in the development of public health policy at every level, from local to international. Awareness of community needs and issues ensures accurate information for policy development that will help maintain the public health infrastructure. Nurses can also be involved in the research and investigation of disease, leading to increased understanding and information to support disease treatment and control. Finally, it is imperative that nurses document the cost effectiveness of routine case management efforts made on behalf of the community to ensure adequate financial resources and personnel in the future.

Key Concepts

- Emerging infections pose a threat to populations throughout the world. A global perspective is necessary in addressing infectious disease concerns. Global transmission of communicable disease is a reality and must be recognized.

- Immunization is the most effective prevention against communicable disease.

- Educating clients and health care providers about the use and misuse of antibiotics in the treatment of disease is necessary to control the emergence of drug-resistant microbes.

- Sexually transmitted diseases constitute one of the most serious communicable disease problems in the United States. Community health nurses can have a direct role in stopping the spread of infection by educating clients about STD prevention.

- Early detection and case management of HIV-infected persons can help prolong the symptom-free period in AIDS. Pregnant women should be told about the possibility of AIDS transmission to the fetus during pregnancy, delivery, and breastfeeding. Testing for AIDS should be available to all pregnant women, who should also be educated about treatment to stop the transmission of infection.

- Direct observed therapy has been effective in slowing the spread of multidrug-resistant TB.

- Nurses must remain alert to new clusters of symptoms and must practice appropriate Universal Precautions.

- Nurses should be involved in policy setting related to surveillance, disease reporting, and treatment options because they are the frontline workers in disease investigation and case management.

Note: The authors would like to thank Victoria Anderson, RN, BSN for her contributions to this chapter.

Chronic Illness

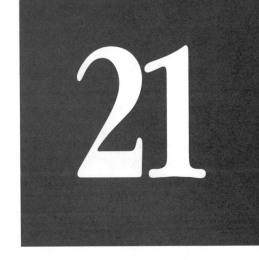

Doris Callaghan RN, MSc

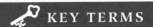

KEY TERMS

approach strategy
biographical disruption
biographical work
chronic disease
chronic illness
circular questioning
coping
insider's perspective
normalizing
power resources
powerlessness
uncertainty

Having a serious chronic illness often crystallizes vital lessons about living that otherwise may remain opaque.

—Charmaz, 1991, p. vii

COMPETENCIES

Upon completion of this chapter, the reader should be able to:

- Define chronic illness.
- Discuss the epidemiology of chronic illness.
- Identify the most common conditions that result in chronic illness.
- Discuss the concept of empowerment in the context of chronic illness.
- Understand the implications of chronic illness for ill individuals and their families.
- Describe the strategies employed by clients and families in living with a chronic illness.
- Understand the value of the perspective of the person with a chronic illness on the experience.
- Understand the health promotive role of community health nurses in relation to chronic illness.
- Identify primary, secondary, and tertiary preventive approaches for chronic illness.
- Describe the National Health Objectives for the Year 2000 that are related to chronic illness.

Chronic illness, a social phenomenon that accompanies a disease that cannot be cured and extends over a period of time, has challenged the lives of people for centuries. Major advances in health care technology and in the acute care of clients have occurred in the past few decades. During this proliferation of cure interventions, the care of people with chronic illnesses has received little attention from health care professionals and researchers. More recently, many Western nations have recognized chronic illness as an important issue in the health of their people (U.S. Department of Health and Human Services [USDHHS], 1992; Epp, 1986). This increasing interest in chronic illness can be attributed to several factors, including the increased occurrence of chronic illnesses, soaring costs of health care, and the World Health Organization's promotion of health for all.

Chronic illnesses do not respond well to prevalent curative medical interventions. Chronic illness care requires a rethinking of the traditional acute health care approaches with which health care providers are most familiar. The purpose of this chapter is to provide the nurse with an opportunity to explore the challenges faced by people who experience a chronic physical illness. The associated role of community health nurses will be discussed, as will the epidemiology of **chronic disease,** a long-term physiological disorder.

DEFINITION OF CHRONIC ILLNESS

Conrad (1987) distinguishes between a disease and an illness: A disease is "an undesirable physiological process"; an illness is "profoundly social, more to do with perception, behavior and experience than with physiological process" (p. 2). An illness may become chronic when it cannot be cured and continues over an extended period. Miller (1992c) defines **chronic illness** as "an altered health state that will not be cured by a simple surgical procedure or short course of medical therapy" (p. 4). Chronic illness represents long-term or permanent disability that hinders people's physical, psychological, or social functioning (Hymovich & Hagopian, 1992).

These academic definitions attempt to clarify the concept of chronic illness, but it is the individual experiencing the illness who can best define the meaning. Conrad (1987, 1990) labels this view as the **"insider's perspective,"** which he defines as focusing on people's lived experiences in relation to the illness. Conrad (1987) writes:

> An insider's perspective focuses directly and explicitly on the subjective experience of living with and in spite of illness. It focuses specifically on the perspectives of people with illness and attempts to examine the illness experience in a more inductive manner (p. 2).

It is important to acknowledge that many people who have a chronic illness see themselves as healthy. Being diagnosed with a chronic illness does not exclude the experience of feeling well (Charmaz, 1991; Lindsey, 1996). The highly individual nature of responses to chronic illness emphasizes the need for nurses to assess and understand the subjective experience of the client.

EPIDEMIOLOGY

The *Healthy People 2000* document classifies the specific disease processes of heart disease, cancer, stroke, lung, and liver disease and also chronic and disabling conditions such as diabetes mellitus, arthritis, deformities or orthopedic impairments, hearing and speech impair-

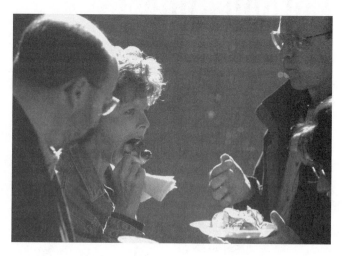

Eating high-cholesterol foods is considered a modifiable risk factor. Photo courtesy of Philip Gould/Corbis.

ments, and mental retardation as chronic illnesses (USDHHS, 1992, p. 73). As is evident in this classification, the concept of chronic illness encompasses many different disease processes. Each has its own natural history. Pathogenic processes of diseases such as coronary heart disease and some cancers begin early in life and have progressed extensively prior to clinical manifestations. Causality of chronic diseases is associated with several factors rather than a single causative agent. Causality is frequently related to factors in lifestyle, genetics, or environment and is completely unknown in some conditions. This variability of causality makes the epidemiologic study of chronic illness complex and specific to the disease being considered. The incidence and prevalence of chronic illnesses are difficult to estimate, because these conditions are not reported to official agencies as part of a disease surveillance program.

A vital part of epidemiology is risk factor identification, which can lead to risk reduction through specific interventions. Such interventions aim to reduce morbidity and mortality related to chronic illness. Risk factors can be classified as modifiable or nonmodifiable. For example,

---

꩜ REFLECTIVE THINKING ꩜

Chronically Ill Friends and Family

Think about friends or family members whom you would consider to be chronically ill.

• How do you think the chronic illness affects their lives?

• How does the chronic illness affect your perception of them?

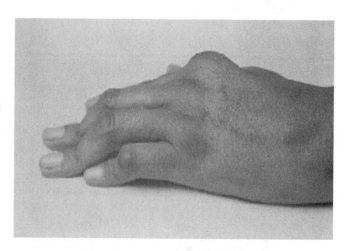

Arthritis is considered a chronic health problem. Courtesy of Arthritis Foundation.

modifiable risk factors for stroke include high cholesterol, hypertension, cigarette smoking, and obesity. The non-modifiable risks factors are heredity, race, age, and gender (Mumma, 1992). Although each chronic disease must be considered individually, the risk factors of dietary practices and smoking are significant in several common chronic diseases including heart disease and stroke, cancer, lung disease, and diabetes mellitus.

Morbidity

"Chronic illnesses are currently the prevalent form of illness in developed countries" (Harkness, 1995, p. 141). Table 21-1 identifies the 10 major causes of chronic health conditions in the United States from 1990 to 1992. The three leading causes of chronic health problems are deformities and orthopedic impairments, chronic sinusitis, and arthritis. Although many of the 10 leading causes of chronic health problems are not life threatening, they have a significant impact on people's lives and on health care costs. Life-threatening chronic conditions are also prevalent in the United States, with about 20 million people affected by heart disease. Approximately 7 million people have diabetes mellitus (Collins, 1997). Over the past two decades, the incidence of cancer has increased, with approximately 10 million new cancer cases diagnosed since 1990 (American Cancer Society, 1997). A similar picture exists in Canada, where a 1991 general survey revealed that 63% of adults, or 13.2 million people, have at least one chronic health condition (Statistics Canada, 1994). In developing countries, the incidence of chronic

illness is lower, and infectious diseases remain the major health challenge (Conrad & Gallagher, 1993).

The incidence of chronic health problems is related to gender. In the United States, the three most prevalent chronic health conditions have a higher incidence in females than in males (see Figure 21-1). The higher rate of arthritis in females is related to the higher incidence of arthritis in the population of people over 65 years of age. This reflects the longer life expectancy of females as compared with males. "In 1992 life expectancy for females was 79.1 compared with 72.3 years for males" (Centers for Disease Control and Prevention [CDC], 1995, p. 3). This same gender relationship is evident in other countries. For example, in Canada chronic health problems are overall more prevalent in females (66%) than in males (59%), for the most commonly identified chronic conditions (Statistics Canada, 1994).

The significance of chronic illness is reflected in the effect it has on the person's ability to carry out daily functions of life. Limitation of activity accompanies many chronic illnesses and presents another perspective on the prevalence of chronic illness. Table 21-2 illustrates limitation of activity according to gender and age and race and age. Although the total numbers of females and males with limitation of activity are similar, the trend is higher for females over the age of 75 years. Limitations of activity are higher for African Americans of all ages than for Caucasians (National Center for Health Statistics, 1994). Figure 21-2 shows the 10 chronic conditions with the

Table 21-1 Chronic Conditions with the Highest Prevalence Rates, in Rank Order: United States, Total Population, 1990–1992

RANK ORDER AND CONDITION	NUMBER OF CASES PER 1,000 PERSONS
1 Deformities or orthopedic impairments	140.6
2 Chronic sinusitis	135.6
3 Arthritis	135.6
4 Hypertensive disease	111.0
5 Hay fever or allergic rhinitis without asthma	96.7
6 Deafness and other hearing impairments	93.5
7 Heart disease	82.4
8 Chronic bronchitis	51.8
9 Asthma	46.2
10 Headache (excluding tension headache)	41.3

Adapted from "Prevalence of Selected Chronic Conditions: United States, 1990–92" by J. G. Collins, 1997, National Center for Health Statistics, Vital Health Statistics, 10 (1994), p. 13.

Table 21-2 Limitation of Activity Caused by Chronic Conditions, by Selected Characteristics, 1992

CHARACTERISTICS	% OF POPULATION WITH SOME LIMITATION OF ACTIVITY	
Sex and Age	**Male**	**Female**
Total	14.3	14.0
under 15 years	6.8	4.7
15–44 years	10.2	9.6
45–64 years	21.7	23.9
65–74 years	36.1	33.1
75 years and over	42.5	46.9
Race and Age	**White**	**Black**
Total	13.9	17.2
under 15 years	5.6	7.3
15–44 years	9.8	11.1
45–64 years	22.1	29.9
65–74 years	34.0	41.4
75 years and over	44.6	53.6

Age-adjusted to the 1970 civilian noninstitutionalized population.

Adapted from Health, United States, 1993 (p. 153) by National Center for Health Statistics, 1994, Hyattsville, MD: Public Health Service.

Figure 21-1 Percentage Distribution of Chronic Conditions with Highest Prevalence, by Gender and Age: United States, 1990–1992

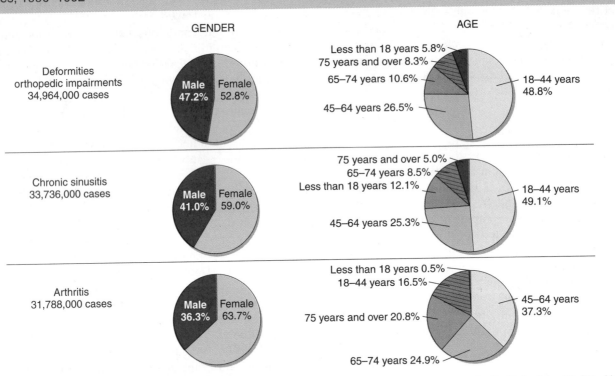

From "Prevalence of Selected Chronic Conditions: United States, 1990–92" by J. G. Collins, 1997, National Center for Health Statistics, Vital Health Statistics, 10 *(1994), p. 11.*

Figure 21-2 Percentage of the 10 Major Chronic Conditions, in Rank Order of Prevalence, that Cause Limitation in Major or Outside Activity: United States 1990–1992

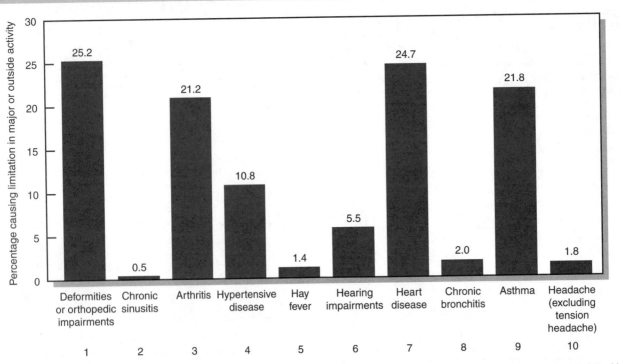

From "Prevalence of Selected Chronic Conditions: United States, 1990–92" by J. G. Collins, 1997, National Center for Health Statistics, Vital Health Statistics, 10 *(1994), p. 12.*

highest prevalence rates, in rank order, by the percentage causing limitation in major or outside activity. Chronic sinusitis causes limitations in a small number of people. Deformities or orthopedic impairments and heart disease result in the two highest rates of limitation.

Chronic health conditions are most prevalent in people with the lowest income (USDHHS, 1991, 1992; Statistics Canada, 1994). The U.S. Department of Health and Human Services (1992) states that "for virtually all of the chronic diseases that lead the Nation's list of killers, low income is a special risk factor" (p. 29). For example, heart disease and cancer have a higher-than-average incidence among people with low incomes. The relationship between chronic illness and poverty is not completely understood. Low income may contribute to the occurrence of chronic illness, or it may be the product of poor health (USDHHS, 1992, p. 31). Whatever the relationship, poverty is an important factor for the community health nurse to consider.

Although chronic illness occurs among people of all ages, the incidence increases with age (Wallace & Rohrer, 1990). In the United States in 1990–1992, arthritis, high blood pressure, hearing impairments and heart disease were the four most prevalent conditions in the population over 65 years of age (see Table 21-3). The 1991 Canadian Health Survey revealed that arthritis and rheumatism, heart trouble, hypertension, diabetes mellitus, emphysema, and emotional problems were all most prevalent in the population over 65 years of age (Statistics Canada, 1994). This relationship is especially significant in light of the "graying" of the population in the industrialized world. The U.S. population is experiencing an aging

Table 21-3   The 10 Major Chronic Conditions, in Rank Order of Prevalence, by Age Group: United States, 1990–1992

| | | | AGE | | | |
CHRONIC CONDITION	ALL PERSONS	UNDER 18 YEARS	18–44 YEARS	45–64 YEARS	65–74 YEARS	75 YEARS AND OVER
				Rank		
Deformities or orthopedic impairments	1	6	1	3	5	5
Chronic sinusitis	2	2	2	4	6	7
Arthritis	3		8	1	1	1
High blood pressure	4		6	2	2	3
Hay fever or allergic rhinitis without asthma	5	1	3	7	10	
Deafness and other hearing impairments	6	10	7	5	3	2
Heart disease	7	9		6	4	4
Chronic bronchitis	8	4	9	9		
Asthma	9	3	10			
Headache (excluding tension headache)	10		4			
Blindness and other visual impairments						8
Migraine headache				5		
Dermatitis		5				
Acne		7				
Chronic disease of tonsils and adenoids		8				
Speech impairments		10				
Hemorrhoids				8		
Diabetes				10	8	9
Cataracts					7	6
Tinnitus					9	10

Adapted from "Prevalence of Selected Chronic Conditions: United States, 1990–1992" by J. G. Collins, 1997, National Center for Health Statistics, Vital Health Statistics, 10 *(1994), p. 9.*

Note: *Shows rank by condition prevalence, not person prevalence. A person may have more than one condition in some groupings, such as deformities, orthopedic impairments, or heart conditions.*

trend. Predictions indicate that the number of Americans over 65 years of age will increase from 39 million in 2010 to 69 million in 2030. About 20% of the total U.S. population will be over 65 years of age in 2030, in contrast to 13% in 1995. The population of people over 85 years of age is growing rapidly, and predictions indicate that it will double in size by 2025 and will increase fivefold by 2050 from the 1995 rate of 3.6 million (Day, 1996). Similar demographic patterns exist in other Western nations including Britain and Canada (Central Statistical Office, 1990; McKie, 1993). Such demographic changes are likely to be accompanied by an increased incidence of chronic illnesses. There will be a corresponding increased need for nurses to work in health promotion, prevention, and acute care with people who are chronically ill, and a need for health care dollars to be allocated to chronic illness.

Mortality

Many conditions listed among the leading causes of death in both the United States and Canada are chronic diseases (USDHHS, 1992; Statistics Canada, 1994). Diseases of the heart, malignant neoplasms, cerebrovascular diseases, chronic obstructive pulmonary diseases, diabetes mellitus, chronic liver disease and cirrhosis, nephritis, nephrotic syndrome and nephrosis, and atherosclerosis are chronic conditions that were listed among the top 15 leading causes of death in the United States in 1992 (CDC, 1995). See Table 21-4. In 1992, mortality rates for each of the leading causes of death for the total population were higher for males than for females. Mortality was higher for the African American population than for the Caucasian population for most of the leading causes of death for the total population. Chronic pulmonary disease and suicide were exceptions (CDC, 1995). The leading cause of cancer deaths in 1993 for both males and females was lung cancer (American Cancer Society, 1997). See Figures 21-3 and 21-4.

Years of potential life lost (YPLL) is a measure of premature mortality that is calculated over the age range from birth to 65 years of age. Because YPLL reflects the effect of chronic conditions on the population below the age of 65, it is an important aspect of mortality rates. Table 21-5 illustrates the YPLL for deaths resulting from selected

	Table 21-4 Death Rates and Percent of Total Deaths for the 15 Leading Causes of Death for the Total Population: United States, 1992		
RANK ORDER*	CAUSE OF DEATH (NINTH REVISION, INTERNATIONAL CLASSIFICATION OF DISEASES, 1975)	RATE	PERCENT OF TOTAL DEATHS
1	Diseases of heart	281.4	33.0
2	Malignant neoplasms, including neoplasms of lymphatic and hematopoietic tissues	204.1	23.9
3	Cerebrovascular diseases	56.4	6.6
4	Chronic obstructive pulmonary diseases and allied conditions	36.0	4.2
5	Accidents and adverse effects	34.0	4.0
	Motor vehicle accidents	16.1	1.9
	All other accidents and adverse effects	18.0	2.1
6	Pneumonia and influenza	29.7	3.5
7	Diabetes mellitus	19.6	2.3
8	Human immunodeficiency virus infection	13.2	1.5
9	Suicide	12.0	1.4
10	Homicide and legal intervention	10.0	1.2
11	Chronic liver disease and cirrhosis	9.9	1.2
12	Nephritis, nephrotic syndrome, and nephrosis	8.7	1.0
13	Septicemia	7.7	0.9
14	Atherosclerosis	6.6	0.8
15	Certain conditions originating in the perinatal period	6.2	0.7
	All other causes	117.6	13.8

*Rank based on number of deaths.

Reprinted from "Advance Report of Final Mortality Statistics, 1992" by Centers for Disease Control and Prevention, 1995, Monthly Vital Statistics Report, 43(6), p. 5.

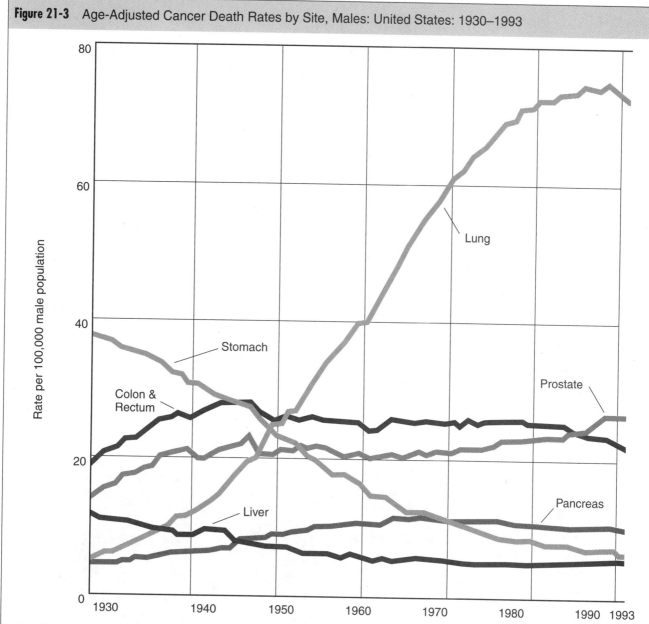

Figure 21-3   Age-Adjusted Cancer Death Rates by Site, Males: United States: 1930–1993

From Cancer Facts & Figures—1997 *by American Cancer Society, 1997, Atlanta: Author. Reprinted by permission of the American Cancer Society, Inc.*

illnesses in the United States in 1991. Malignant neoplasms and diseases of the heart were the chronic conditions that accounted for the greatest number of years of potential life lost as a result of premature death. However, chronic liver disease and cirrhosis, cerebrovascular diseases, diabetes mellitus, and chronic pulmonary disease also had a significant impact (National Center for Health Statistics, 1994).

Mortality figures are changing, and between 1991 and 1992 the mortality rate in 11 of the leading causes of death in the United States declined. Death rates for all of the chronic conditions declined during this time except for diabetes mellitus, which increased by 0.8%, and nephritis, nephrotic syndrome, and nephrosis, which remained unchanged (see Table 21-6). The downward trend in mor-

tality rates for diseases of the heart, cerebrovascular disease, and atherosclerosis has been observed consistently since 1950. This trend has largely been attributed to public education regarding disease risk factors, lifestyle changes, and medical advances in treatment. Although progress has been made in decreasing the death rate from these diseases, heart disease and cerebrovascular disease remain among the top three killers of Americans.

Chronic illness is a significant factor in mortality rates in many nations. A comparison of the leading causes of death in the United States with data from 36 countries for the years 1985 through 1989 revealed that chronic illness was prominent among the mortality rates of the countries considered. Although the ranking of the causes of mortality varied among nations, chronic illnesses including

Figure 21-4   Age-Adjusted Cancer Death Rates by Site, Females: United States, 1930–1993

From Cancer Facts & Figures—1997 *by American Cancer Society, 1997, Atlanta: Author. Reprinted by permission of the American Cancer Society, Inc.*

heart diseases, malignant neoplasms (all sites), and chronic obstructive pulmonary diseases and allied conditions contributed significantly to the mortality rate of all nations. This was the trend despite gender, although female mortality is generally lower than male mortality (Zarate, 1994). Heart disease and cancer were also found to be significant in the mortality rates in developing nations of the world. The World Development Report (World Bank, 1993) points out that "tobacco-related deaths from heart disease and cancers alone are likely to double in the first decade of the next century, to 2 million a year, and if present patterns continue, they will grow to more than 12 million a year in developing countries in the second quarter of the next century" (p. 3).

A CARING, EMPOWERING PERSPECTIVE

Chronic illness increases the vulnerability of individuals and groups (Charmaz, 1991; Hymovich & Hagopian, 1992). Situations such as poverty, lack of available resources, and inadequate health care coverage add to this vulnerability. The World Health Organization (1974) identified the care of vulnerable groups as fundamental to community health nursing.

The need for community health nurses is increasing as health care reform shifts the care of people with chronic illness from institutions to their own homes. Provision of

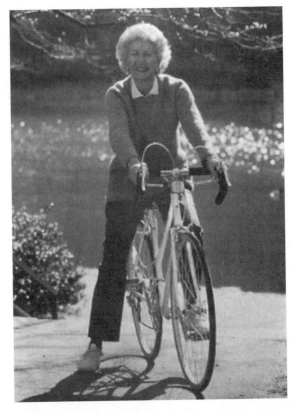

The older adult population is growing in number, and the incidence of chronic health problems is likely to increase. The community health nurse should offer primary prevention techniques, including keeping active.

Table 21-5 Years of Potential Life Lost before Age 65 for Selected Causes of Death: United States, 1991

CONDITION	YEARS LOST PER 100,000 POPULATION UNDER 65 YEARS OF AGE (ALL RACES)
Unintentional injuries	934.9
Malignant neoplasms	843.1
Diseases of heart	628.4
Homicide	394.9
Human immunodeficiency virus	347.3
Suicide	307.2
Cerebrovascular diseases	108.6
Chronic liver disease and cirrhosis	99.8
Pneumonia and influenza	80.6
Diabetes mellitus	68.2
Chronic obstructive pulmonary diseases	63.1

Adapted from Health, United States, 1993 *(p. 95) by National Center for Health Statistics, 1994, Hyattsville, MD: Public Health Services.*

Table 21-6 Age-Adjusted Death Rates for 1992 and Percent Change for the 15 Leading Causes of Death for the Total Population from 1991 to 1992 and from 1979 to 1992: United States

RANK ORDER[1]	CAUSE OF DEATH (NINTH REVISION, INTERNATIONAL CLASSIFICATION OF DISEASES, 1975)	AGE-ADJUSTED DEATH RATE FOR 1992	PERCENT CHANGE FROM— 1991 TO 1992	PERCENT CHANGE FROM— 1979 TO 1992
1	Diseases of heart	144.3	−2.6	−27.7
2	Malignant neoplasms, including neoplasms of lymphatic and hematopoietic tissues	133.1	−1.0	1.8
3	Cerebrovascular diseases	26.2	−2.2	−37.0
4	Chronic obstructive pulmonary diseases and allied conditions	19.9	−1.0	36.3
5	Accidents and adverse effects	29.4	−5.2	−31.5
	Motor vehicle accidents	15.8	−7.1	−31.9
	All other accidents and adverse effects	13.7	−1.4	−30.1
6	Pneumonia and influenza	12.7	−5.2	13.4
7	Diabetes mellitus	11.9	0.8	21.4
8	Human immunodeficiency virus infection	12.6	11.5	
9	Suicide	11.1	−2.6	−5.1
10	Homicide and legal intervention	10.5	−3.7	2.9
11	Chronic liver disease and cirrhosis	8.0	−3.6	−33.3
12	Nephritis, nephrotic syndrome, and nephrosis	4.3	0	0
13	Septicemia	4.0	−2.4	73.9
14	Atherosclerosis	2.4	−7.7	−57.9
15	Certain conditions originating in the perinatal period[2]		−5.2	−42.6

[1]*Rank based on number of deaths.*

[2]*Inasmuch as deaths from this cause occur mainly among infants, percent changes are based on infant mortality rates instead of age-adjusted rates.*

Reprinted from "Advance Report of Final Mortality Statistics, 1992" by Centers for Disease Control and Prevention, 1995, Monthly Vital Statistics Report, *43(6), p. 7.*

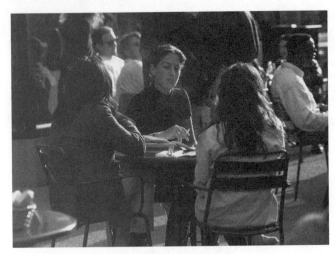

Tobacco-related deaths from heart disease and cancer are likely to increase unless preventive measures are effective in decreasing the incidence of tobacco use.
Photo courtesy of Kevin Fleming/Corbis.

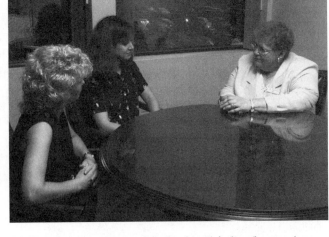

Demonstrating respect for the family's lived experience is an important role for the community health nurse.

nursing services in the community includes health education, screening, referrals, direct home care, discharge planning, and case management. To provide appropriate care, the nurse should be knowledgeable about the possible impact of chronic illness on the individual, the family, and the community. The nurse must consider the insider's perspective regarding chronic illness, whether this is the perspective of the individual, the family, an aggregate, or the community.

Important concepts underlying effective assessment, planning, and intervention by community health nurses include caring and empowerment. Valuing the client's lived experience is fundamental to caring and empowerment and moves nursing care away from a focus on technology and cure (Watson, 1988; Benner & Wrubel, 1989; Baker, 1996). Technology and cure interventions simply do not serve many people with chronic illness well. The incurability of chronic illnesses shifts the focus to the caring aspect of health care, and nurses are key providers of this care. Chapter 1 explores the foundations of a caring nursing practice.

The concept of empowerment is central to humanizing nursing care. Assumptions of empowerment that are fundamental to working with individuals and their families include the assumptions that

- People themselves are the most capable of identifying both their own problems and their own solutions to those problems.
- There are multiple ways of viewing reality, and people know their own realities best (Labonte, 1990; Fahlberg, Poulin, Girdano, & Dusek, 1991).

Developing a personal philosophy based on the assumptions of empowerment requires restructuring the traditional hierarchical structure of the nurse–client relationship to one of partnership between the individual, the family, and the nurse. In a partnership, the nurse shares power with the individual and the family.

As individuals with chronic illness, and their families, experience an extended period of time living with an illness, they become experts in their own care. They want their knowledge and ability acknowledged and respected by health care professionals (Callaghan, 1992; Corbin & Strauss, 1988; Thorne, 1993). Shifting focus to the lived experience of individuals and their families enables a nurse to recognize their expertise and their ability to make the choices that best meet their needs. This approach requires the nurse to trust that people themselves are experts about their health needs. Partnership allows individuals and their families to:

- Develop confidence in their abilities related to their own health.
- Be involved in setting their health goals thus increasing the probability that they will attend to the goals.
- Identify the best approach for attending to their health (Lindsey, 1993; Thorne, 1993).

Nurses who base their practice on the concepts of caring and empowerment support the healing of clients and their families (see Figure 21-5). These concepts are congruent with the following principles of holistic healing:

- Individuals have within themselves vast untapped resources.
- Fostering self-awareness and self-understanding can contribute to the healing process.

Figure 21-5   Tips for Nurses Working in Partnership with Their Clients

- Listen to what clients have to say.
- Respect and value what they say.
- Support them in making choices based on their own experience and their own expertise.

- Individual beliefs and values affect the healing process (Lamb, 1988, p. 12).

Participants in Lindsey's (1995, p. 303) study offer these suggestions for promoting healing in people with chronic illnesses:

"Ask me what I need, give me a sense of partnership. Don't be afraid to lose control. I would like to tell them [health professionals] to have the courage to be real with us. I wish they wouldn't hide their feelings of powerless [sic] behind their arrogance."

"The most important thing they [health professionals] can do for me is just listen, listen and try to get some sense of my story."

"The most help he [the physician] ever gave me was one day when he said 'Look, I know you will be the one to know what is right for you.' That level of respect."

"Being able to pose questions rather than give answers, to promote self-exploration and self-examination. I am talking about challenging questions that can only be done in an atmosphere of trust and respect which has to be built up over time."

"Be willing [health professionals] to take risks with people, to move into the unknown, and to be trusting."

Despite major technological advances in medical interventions during the last few decades, the incidence of chronic illness continues to have a major impact on the lives of people. When working with clients who are living with a chronic illness, nurses need to understand and acknowledge the impact the illness has on all dimensions of the lives of the individual and the family.

IMPACT OF CHRONIC ILLNESS

The experience of chronic illness permeates all aspects of a person's life, including physical, psychosocial, spiritual, and economic. King (cited in Michael, 1996), the editor in chief of the *Diabetes Interview*, tells his story of having diabetes:

Many people think diabetes is just a disease, but it's not. It is much more than that. A disease is something that happens to your body. Diabetes affects every aspect of your whole life. It's more than a medical problem, it takes over your mind too. It's more than a simple adjustment of medicine and nutrition; it requires a complete retraining of your lifestyle. Nothing is spared; no part of your life is left unscathed (p. 2).

Quality of life is a concept that appears frequently in health-related literature. Many research studies have attempted to quantify and measure quality of life. Meeberg (1993) suggests that there are as many definitions of quality of life as there are people who use the term. She

cautions that quality of life assessments are vulnerable to the individual researcher's beliefs and biases. In considering the quality of a client's life, the community health nurse must be aware of its subjective and individual nature. This concept becomes congruent with client-centered nursing if considered within a definition offered by Meeberg. She defines quality of life as "a feeling of overall life satisfaction, as determined by the mentally alert individual whose life is being evaluated. Other people, preferably those from outside that person's living situation, must also agree that the individual's living conditions are non-life-threatening and are adequate in meeting that individual's basic needs" (p. 37).

Perhaps the most important understanding of the impact that chronic illness has on people comes from accounts of people's experiences (Callaghan & Williams, 1994). The person's view of the effect illness has on his or her life may be very different from the view of health professionals, friends, and family. People living with chronic illness develop a personal knowledge of their illness. Michael (1996) found the people in her study "knew their illness better than the health care professionals did. This presented a problem, because many health care professionals were unwilling to acknowledge participants' insights and disregarded what they said" (p. 262). People's perspective on their illness will also determine how they live with it. Charmaz (1991) suggests that "how people think about and categorize their illness reflects how they treat it" (p. 67). In considering the lived experience of chronic illness, the nurse needs to recognize that each individual has a unique story of the effect of illness on his or her life.

Physical Aspects

The variety of diseases that can result in chronic illness is reflected in the complexity of physical challenges that can accompany chronic illness. Most often the onset of physi-

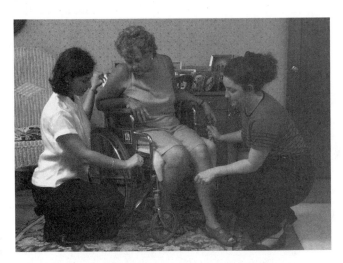

The community health nurse can help caregivers learn to care for a family member who has just returned home from a rehabilitation center.

cal symptoms is the first sign that something is wrong. The characteristics of the physical symptoms depend on the specific disease process, and, even within a specific illness, the symptoms may range from a sudden onset with accelerated progression to an insidious onset with slow progression. Corbin and Strauss (1988) suggest that chronic illness has six phases: *acute, comeback, stable, unstable, deteriorating,* and *dying.* The specific physical challenges experienced during any of these phases can be diverse, including physical immobility, pain, fatigue, disfigurement, and deformities. The physical aspects of chronic illness can limit the client's independence, and this limitation can affect self-esteem and overall life satisfaction. In addition, physical challenges may affect sexuality and may limit the individual's ability to participate in a sexual relationship.

Historically, nurses have been educated about the care of people with the physical challenges related to diseases. Besides assisting clients in living with their physical challenges, the nurse must recognize the interrelationship between physical and psychosocial aspects of an illness. One difficult facet of chronic illness is its ongoing nature. Chronic illnesses cannot be cured and do not always respond to therapeutic interventions. Physical deterioration can occur despite efforts to treat the illness. This deterioration can be challenging and discouraging for the person with the illness, the family, and the nurse.

Psychosocial Aspects

The psychosocial challenges of chronic illness have been the focus of many studies. Several concepts related to the psychosocial aspects of chronic illness have been identified. Three frequently addressed concepts include uncertainty, powerlessness, and biographical disruption (Strauss, 1975; Charmaz, 1983, 1991; Conrad, 1987; Corbin & Strauss, 1987, 1988; Thorne, 1993).

Uncertainty

"**Uncertainty** is the inability to determine the meaning of events. . . . The decision maker is unable to accurately predict events" (Mishel & Braden, 1988, p.98). Uncertainty

accompanying chronic illness can arise from the experience of diagnosis, lack of a cure, an unpredictable course, and the need for complex treatment regimes.

Diagnosis is a critical occurrence in the lives of people with chronic illness and has a major impact on them. Conrad (1987) proposed that there is prediagnosis uncertainty, when the person does not know what is wrong; medical uncertainty, when physicians try to diagnose the problem; and uncertainty that accompanies the diagnosis itself. Diagnosis is often a time when the client and family must adjust to the treatment regime and begin to integrate illness into their lives.

Commonalities in the diagnosis experience exist despite the many different diagnoses classified as chronic illness. Although for some diseases, such as diabetes mellitus or stroke, the diagnosis is usually early in the illness, others such as multiple sclerosis result in delays and prolonged prediagnosis testing procedures and even incorrect diagnoses. Thorne (1993), in her study of participants with a variety of chronic illnesses, found that often "the diagnostic testing process was an intensely difficult and confusing time, characterized by serious doubts about the benevolence or competence of health professionals as well as questions about their own [the clients'] sanity" (p. 21). Thorne suggests that the diagnostic event can mean an end to a long and frustrating diagnosis process, and many clients and families consider this a critical turning point in their lives. She writes:

Although the diagnosis represented the possibility of finally taking some action from the patient and family point of view, many found that the health care professional lost interest in their case once the diagnosis deemed the condition to be chronic (pp. 27–28).

As a way of dealing with uncertainty at the time of diagnosis, people may rely primarily on knowledge provided by professionals. However, as they live with the illness they learn about it. In her study, Michael (1996) found that for the participants' "going to the doctor, attending support group meetings and reading about the illness [were] helpful, but much of what they learned came from trial and error" (p. 262). Nurses must support clients and their families through their diagnosis experience and explore the impact it has on their lives. Listening to the client and family can help them make meaning of the experience.

Day-to-day living with a chronic illness can bring new uncertainties. The continuous ups and downs of the illness present a sense of uncertainty, which can cause people to isolate themselves (Miller, 1992a). Charmaz (1983) concluded that since many chronic illnesses have an unpredictable course, the accompanying uncertainty and fear cause some people to restrict their lives more than they need. Restrictions in the lives of people with a chronic illness are sometimes set in motion by professionals when clients are not given sufficient information and treatment.

Nyhlin (1990), in her study of people with diabetes mellitus, found that they had to come to terms with uncertainty caused by the illness and by the inadequacy of the health care system. The health care system was perceived as inadequate and causing uncertainty when it did not provide the support, advice, and information that the person was seeking. This uncertainty resulted in feelings of anger, frustration, and fear.

An understanding of uncertainty as it relates to chronic illness will help the nurse to view the client's care from a holistic perspective. Nurses need to assess the client's and the family's experience and help them in developing strategies for living with the uncertainty. Client strategies may include becoming more informed about the illness, searching for additional treatments, undertaking stress-reduction techniques, and seeking support from others including family, friends, people with the same illness, and health care professionals.

Powerlessness

The unpredictable challenges that accompany chronic illness can promote a sense of powerlessness. Miller (1992c) describes **powerlessness** as "the perception that one lacks the capacity or authority to act to affect an outcome" and suggests that in chronic illness it can be related to "remissions and exacerbations or, in some instances, to progressive physical deterioration" (p. 4). Hymovich and Hagopian

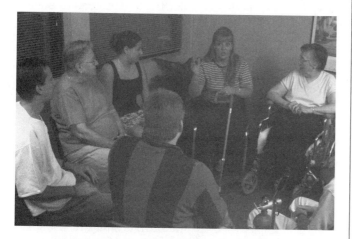

This support group of people with chronic illnesses is listening to a speaker discuss ways to relax.

DECISION MAKING

Persons with Disabilities and Society

The United States and Canada have attempted to remove barriers in the environment for individuals with disabilities (e.g., by installing ramps to buildings, leveling curbs, establishing designated parking spaces).

• What measures can society take to address the issue of psychosocial suffering of people with chronic illness?

(1992) suggest that powerlessness encompasses helplessness, hopelessness, and loss of control and can manifest as passivity, nonparticipation in care and decision making, dependence on others, and verbal expression of loss of control (p. 158). See Figure 21-6 for suggested nursing strategies aimed at decreasing feelings of powerlessness.

Biographical Disruption

Biographical disruption is a concept that has emerged from the foundational research on chronic illness (Charmaz, 1983, 1991; Corbin & Strauss, 1988). Corbin and Strauss (1988) call biography a life course: "life stretching over a number of years and life evolving around a continual stream of experiences that result in a unique identity" (p. 50). They suggest that chronic illness is often accompanied by changes or disruption in biography (biographical disruption). The changes may include alterations in clients' perception of themselves as a person; in the concept of their body, which may not function as it once did; and in their sense of biographical time. Time takes on new meaning for people, as their past abilities and performances may be very different from those of the present. Lengthy treatment regimes such as kidney dialy-

---

Figure 21-6 Nursing Strategies Aimed at Decreasing Powerlessness

- Modify the environment on the basis of ideas from the client about what can be done to increase client control.

- Increase the client's knowledge about his illness and its management.

- Facilitate the setting of realistic goals by the client.

- Increase the sensitivity of health professionals and significant others to the feelings of powerlessness that the client may be experiencing.

- Help the client verbalize feelings.

Adapted from "Decreasing Powerlessness in the Chronically Ill: A Prototypical Plan" by S. Stapleton, 1992. In J. Miller (Ed.), Coping with Chronic Illness (2nd ed.), Philadelphia: F. A. Davis, pp. 305–322.

sis impinge on a person's life routine and can disrupt biographical time (pp. 52–65). Corbin and Strauss allege that health care professionals fall short of being aware of the biographical disruptions being experienced by people with chronic illness because of the focus on the medical model and acute care. Taking a holistic approach to the care of people requires that the nurse have an awareness of the client's biographical processes.

In her study, Charmaz (1983) found that, as the participants became more dependent and immobilized as a result of chronic illness, they suffered from a loss of self in which they lost not only self-esteem but also self-identity. Their diminished sense of self resulted in the participants' leading restricted lives, experiencing social isolation, being discredited, and burdening others. These experiences occurred even when the impairments were not visible. Loss of self-esteem related to the chronic illness experience crosses ethnocultural boundaries (Anderson, 1991).

Spiritual Aspects

"Spirituality is a belief in or relationship with some higher power, creative force, divine being, or infinite source of energy" (Kozier, Erb, Blais, & Wilkinson, 1995, p. 312). Spiritual belief can influence individuals' feelings about illness and help cope with the challenges of chronic illness. It can provide a purpose for life. Spiritual resources influence the healing process, give meaning to life, and provide a sense of hope (Lamb, 1988).

Miller (1992c) describes the client's belief system that includes spirituality as a resource. She writes:

> The chronically ill person needs relief from the isolation of suffering, and having a relationship with God may alleviate this aloneness. Some individuals may find meaning in the misfortune of chronic illness through religion and faith (p. 14).

In turn, the invasiveness of chronic illness in the lives of people impinges on their spirituality. There can be a strengthening of spirituality or a turning away. Hymovich

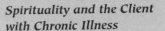
DECISION MAKING

Spirituality and the Client with Chronic Illness

Mary is a 35-year-old woman with two children: a 3-year-old and a newborn. During her recent pregnancy, she was diagnosed with breast cancer. When you make a postnatal visit to her home, you find that she is very upset. Mary tells you that she has always been a devout Christian and has in the past been able to draw strength from prayer. Now, with what has happened to her, she doubts if God exists.

- What would you do in this situation?
- What words of comfort could you offer Mary?

and Hagopian (1992) suggest that people who are chronically ill can experience spiritual distress,

> which can be characterized in ways such as questioning the meaning of suffering, the meaning of one's existence, or the moral and ethical implications of the therapeutic regimen. . . . Spiritual distress can cause nightmares and sleep disturbances or alterations in behavior and mood as evidenced by crying, anger, withdrawal, anxiety, hostility, or apathy (p. 127).

Spirituality is a concept that nurses do not always feel comfortable discussing with clients. However, it is a significant factor in how people come to live with their chronic illness. An awareness of the client's spirituality provides a basis for holistic nursing care. Walton (1996) suggests that nurses who practice holistically "can connect intimately with patients and facilitate their spiritual relationships with self, higher power, and others" (p. 247). Lindsey (1996), in her study of the experience of health within chronic illness, found that participants "attributed their experiences of feeling healthy to an awareness of their spirituality, with a sense of connectedness, wholeness, harmony and peacefulness." Nurses need to understand what experiences give meaning to life for clients and their families and promote such experiences (Miller, 1992b). In studying the meaning of spirituality to the elderly, Bauer and Barron (1995) found that participants in their study saw caring and communication skills as important aspects of spiritual care nursing interventions. The participants wanted nurses to be "attentive, respectful, caring and hopeful" (p. 277).

Economic Aspects

Chronic illness has economic implications for individuals, their families, and society. Although health care insurance covers costs such as hospitalization, doctors' visits, and home nursing care, there are many costs that the ill per-

ᐤᐤ REFLECTIVE THINKING ᐤᐤ

Sense of Self

Anderson (1991) poses two thought-provoking questions for consideration by all health care professionals. Think about these two questions:

- Why do health care providers, whose mandate it is to care for patients, interact with them in ways that sometimes reinforce the devalued sense of self?
- Why are health care services not structured to enable people to manage their chronic illness in ways that foster their feelings of self-worth? (p. 715)

son must assume. Hymovich and Hagopian (1992) refer to such costs as indirect costs, which include special diets, special equipment, vocational rehabilitation, time lost from work, travel expenses, telephone calls, and insurance.

The total amount of uninsured costs is difficult to measure, although the National Center for Health Statistics (1994) found that in 1991, 22% of all personal health expenditures were paid "out of pocket" (p. 6). The challenges faced by individuals and their families are compounded by uninsured expenses.

Chronic illness can have a direct effect on the occupation and employment of the ill individual. Equal opportunity in employment is required by law in some developed nations (Canadian Charter of Rights and Freedom, 1982; Americans with Disabilities Act, 1990). Although such laws exist to protect the individual from discrimination on the basis of disability, they do not preclude all challenges in the work environment. Symptoms associated with the illness can affect the individual's job performance and influence the attitude of coworkers. Complex treatment regimes do not always fit into work routines and may require a change of occupation. A progression of the illness can lead to unemployment. Charmaz (1991) suggests that financial pressures of the illness often force ill people to struggle to work and remain independent as long as possible, sometimes to the detriment of their health.

Chronic illness is costly to society as a whole. The increased incidence of chronic illness has contributed to the burgeoning cost of health care. In 1991, U.S. national health care expenditures, including those directed toward chronic illness, totaled $752 billion, an average of $2,868 per person. Health insurance paid for 32% of personal health care expenditures, and the federal government paid 31% (National Center for Health Statistics, 1994). Chronic illness and disability continue to be an important factor in the nation's economy. The estimated annual costs of selected conditions in the United States include: cardiovascular disease, $117 billion; cancer, $104 billion; diabetes mellitus, $91 billion (CDC, 1993).

DECISION MAKING

Employment and the Person with Chronic Illness

You have worked with Sam, a 28-year-old single man, for several years. Sam has developed rheumatoid arthritis and will require more frequent rest periods while at work. In addition, he will need to stay home and rest when the disease flares up.

• What special considerations (such as work schedules and working conditions) do you think could be made for Sam?

• Would you be prepared to make changes in your own work situation to accommodate his needs?

Governments in the United States and other developed nations are trying to contain and reduce health care costs through health care reform. One strategy is to keep people who are chronically ill at home rather than in institutions. Although such initiatives are less costly to the government, and may be more desirable to the client, there is a risk of shifting the burden of care to family caregivers.

LIVING WITH A CHRONIC ILLNESS

Chronic illness is a significant event that can affect all aspects of life, including physical, psychological, spiritual, social, and occupational (Strauss, 1975; Gerhardt, 1990). In his classic work, Strauss (1975) proposes seven key challenges faced by people who are chronically ill:

• Prevention and management of medical crises
• Control of symptoms
• Carrying out and managing prescribed regimens
• Preventing or living with social isolation
• Shaping the course of the illness
• **Normalizing** style of life and interactions with others (a coping strategy used by people to control the impact of chronic illness on their lives)
• Ensuring adequate funding

In response to these challenges, people with chronic illnesses, their families, and friends must develop basic strategies for day-to-day living. They may require the assistance of others, including health care professionals.

Corbin and Strauss (1988) have made a substantial contribution to the understanding of chronic illness. They introduced the concept of "work" to portray what it is that the client and family do in attending the challenges of chronic illness. They describe this chronic illness work as maintenance of both physical health status and emotional stability. The intensity of this work varies with the course of the illness and with the impact it has on personal relationships and personal identities. Life with a chronic illness can be complex, and clients and their families must be considered on an individual basis. The nurse must be aware of the specific **biographical work** being done by people and must support them and assist them in finding other resources to help meet the psychological challenges of their illness.

Consideration of the insider's view of illness supports beliefs related to the client's culture. Citing the work of Grace and Zola, Lubkin (1995) identifies three cross-cultural issues that may affect the way a person views his or her illness:

• Culturally perceived causes of disability. Some cultures may view the chronic illness as a form of punishment for wrongdoing. Others consider it an honor, as may be the case with Mexican Americans who have children with a chronic illness.

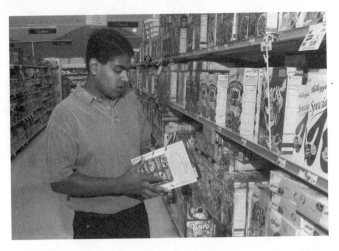

Reading labels to check for added sugars is part of this man's biographical work as he manages his diabetes.

- Expectation for survival. Cultures with limited resources may redirect resources from the person with an illness to stronger members.
- Appropriate social roles. In some cultures, family resources are not allocated to the education or achievement of girls or women. Chronic illness may reinforce this belief (pp. 36–37).

Cultural aspects of health remain important in developing countries despite an emergence of Western curative health approaches (Airhihenbuwa & Harrison, 1993; Conrad & Gallagher, 1993). A system has developed in which Western medicine is incorporated alongside the traditional approach to medicine that is rooted in the country's culture. For example, Subedi and Subedi (1993) found that the people of Nepal use Western and traditional medicine at different points of their illness. Early in an illness, the Nepalese use traditional cultural approaches. Modern health care services are, for the most part, sought only as a last resort. Nursing care that is based on the assumptions of empowerment respects the beliefs of others regardless of whether these beliefs are related to culture or religion (see Chapter 6).

Coping

Coping is a term commonly used to describe a strategy for living with a chronic illness (Nyhlin, 1990; Hymovich & Hagopian, 1992; Miller, 1992a; Lubkin, 1995). Miller (1992a) defines coping as "dealing with situations that present a threat to the individual so as to resolve uncomfortable feelings such as anxiety, fear, grief, and guilt" (p. 20). Miller suggests that coping strategies used by people who are chronically ill are more likely to be effective when they are **approach strategies**. Approach strategies signify an effort to confront the challenges of the illness and include:

- Seeking information and help
- Gaining strength from spirituality

- Using methods of diversion
- Expressing feelings, emotions, and concerns
- Using relaxation and positive-thinking techniques
- Maintaining realistic independence but being positive about depending on others if necessary
- Maintaining social activities
- Setting goals and problem solving
- Using humor
- Conserving energy
- Finding solace in the realization that other people have the same illness (pp. 36–37)

Lazarus and Folkman (1984) criticize the traditional view of coping because it focuses on successful adaptation to a stressor such as illness. Moving away from the view of coping as either an effective or an ineffective outcome, they present coping as a process. Lazarus and Folkman define coping as "constantly changing cognitive and behavioral efforts to manage specific external and/or internal demands that are appraised as taxing or exceeding the resources of the person" (p. 141). This view of coping considers what "the person actually thinks or does in a specific context" and allows for "change in coping thoughts and acts as a stressful encounter unfolds" (p. 142). The way a person copes may vary from situation to situation. They suggest that the way a person copes is determined in part by:

- Personal resources such as health, energy, existential beliefs
- Personal commitments
- Problem-solving skills
- Social skills
- Social support
- Material resources

Supporting clients and families in their efforts to cope with a chronic illness is important. The nurse must explore with them the need for referral to specific services such as counseling and stress management.

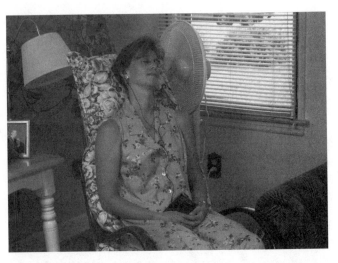

Listening to relaxation tapes is a way of coping with chronic illness.

Normalizing

"The chief business of a chronically ill person is not just to stay alive or keep symptoms under control, but to live as normally as possible despite his symptoms and disease" (Strauss, 1975, p. 58). This process of normalizing is an effort to minimize the social effects of the illness (Thorne, 1993). People with chronic illness use various strategies to normalize their lives, including:

- Making efforts to keep symptoms invisible
- Engaging in their pre-illness activities
- Maintaining social relationships (Strauss, 1975; Charmaz, 1991; Hymovich & Hagopian, 1992).

The effects of a chronic illness can be visible, such as disfigurement, changes in physical characteristics, and limitation in body functions, or invisible, such as pain or fatigue. Although having a visible illness makes it more difficult for the person to pass as being well, it does justify the need for assistance and may elicit sympathetic responses. Being visibly ill, however, can result in penalties, including stigmatization and discrimination, being labeled as disabled, and being considered less competent. Having an invisible illness may allow a person to be accepted in society. However, stigma accompanies certain chronic illnesses, such as epilepsy or acquired immunodeficiency syndrome (AIDS). In addition, the invisible nature of an illness means the person may have difficulty legitimizing the illness. Others may not take the effects of the illness seriously (Strauss, 1975; Thorne, 1993). Thorne (1993) suggests that health care professionals exhibit these same prejudices toward the chronically ill. Nurses must consider if these prejudices exist in their own practice.

Managing the Treatment

Treatment regimens can be complex and can require significant amounts of time, energy, and money. Examples include home blood glucose monitoring for diabetes and hemodialysis for renal failure. Maintaining client compliance with or adherence to treatment recommendations has long been a goal of health care professionals (Hymovich & Hagopian, 1992; Lubkin, 1995). Individuals who do not adhere to their treatment regimen risk increasing the negative effects of their illness. Nevertheless, the incidence of failure to adhere to the treatment regimen is high (Hymovich & Hagopian, 1992; Lubkin, 1995).

The client's decision to alter the treatment regimen takes on a different meaning when considered from his or her perspective (Roberson, 1992; Thorne, 1993; Lubkin, 1995). In her study, Callaghan (1992) found that participants wanted their expertise to be an integral part of their treatment plan. When health care professionals disregarded their ideas, participants who felt capable of making decisions about their care customized their treatment regimen to suit their needs, without the professionals'

consent. If a client does not adhere to treatment regimens, the client may have different expectations than health care professionals and may be making an effort to exert some control over the impact of the illness on his or her life (Roberson, 1992; Lubkin, 1995).

Wuest (1993) expresses concern about the use of the term *noncompliance* to label clients who do not follow their prescribed treatment regimen. She states that this term comes from the medical model and is grounded in a patriarchal world view. Feminist thought may offer an alternative perspective on ways to work in partnership with the client regarding the issues that arise from prescribed treatment. Wuest writes:

> This [feminist thought] requires an entrance into a dialogue with those for whom we care, a dialogue that ultimately leads to understanding personal, social, and political factors that determine what this person [the client] views as possible and desirable at this point in time (p. 23).

Considering clients' perspectives on their ability to live with their treatment regime is a vital aspect of nursing care that seeks to involve clients in the decision making. Coates and Boore (1995) advise nurses to support the efforts of people in their self-management of chronic illness. They write:

> If patients are to be given the opportunity to be active participants in care, they must also be given the right to decline to follow therapy or to modify it without recrimination. If patients and health professionals are to be partners in care, both partners must have equal power. This necessitates a change in attitude of nurses and other health care professionals which is reflected in interaction between the partners in care (p. 636).

Role of the Family

The role of the family changes and takes on new significance in the face of chronic illness. Strauss (1975) proposes that other people associated with the ill person, including the family, act as various agents:

> People act as rescuing agents (saving a diabetic individual from dying when he is in a coma), or as protective agents (accompanying an epileptic person so that if he begins to fall he can be eased to the ground), or as assisting agents (helping with a regimen), or as control agents (making the person stay with his regimen), and so on (p. 8).

Strauss submits that health professionals play a secondary role in the day-to-day lives of people with chronic illness. He advises professionals to "see with some directness and clarity the social and psychological problems faced by the chronically ill and their immediate families in their daily lives" (p. 7).

Families can enable the individual with a chronic illness to relinquish obligations such as maintaining a job,

RESEARCH ⌕ FOCUS

The Meaning of Compliance: Patient Perspectives

STUDY PROBLEM/PURPOSE

To explore the context of compliance with therapeutic regimen for 23 adult African Americans living with a chronic physical illness. Its focus was on the meaning of compliance from the informants' perspective (p. 13).

METHODS

This was a qualitative study using unstructured interviews to generate data. The researcher conducted approximately 80 hours of formal interviews with the informants in their home settings.

FINDINGS

- Informants and health professionals had different treatment goals.
- Informants and health professionals defined compliance differently.
- Informants defined compliance in terms of the successful results of their self-management practices as shown by feeling in good health and by receiving positive comments about their illness management from their physicians.
- Informants sought treatment approaches that, from their view, were manageable, liveable, and effective.

- Informants developed self-management practices that suited their lifestyles, belief patterns, and personal priorities.
- Health professionals viewed many informants as noncompliant; the informants, however, saw themselves as managing their illness and treatments effectively.

IMPLICATIONS

Clients' choices about compliance are theirs to make. Health professionals need to put less emphasis on the identification of noncompliance rates and ways to alter them and focus more on enhancing people's efforts to live well with chronic illness and its treatment.

Health professionals should consider clients' perspectives on their illness and treatment and respond to these perspectives appropriately. For example, if the treatment regime is too restrictive, consideration should be given to changes that the client believes will make treatment more acceptable.

SOURCE

From "The Meaning of Compliance: Patient Perspectives" by M. H. B. Roberson, 1992, Qualitative Health Research, *2(1), pp. 7–26.*

---

getting an education, and providing child care. (Charmaz, 1991). Charmaz states that the family can provide a major buffer against social isolation from friends, associates, and neighbors. Families can help fill the time and break the routine of the day to day challenges of the illness.

Family Caregivers

Family members often become caregivers for the ill person. Caring for a loved one can be a rewarding experience. Enjoyment can result from keeping the care receiver at home and from fulfilling a sense of duty and love (Cohen, Pushkar Gold, Shulman, & Zucchero, 1994). Home can be perceived as a place of healing. A challenging aspect of family caregiving, however, is the demanding nature of the commitment. Spousal relationships are tested, as an intrusive illness often affects the ability of the ill person to share in the partnership of the marital relationship. Mobilizing, bathing, dressing, and feeding the ill person can be physically demanding. The caregiver role is sometimes carried out in addition to employment, child rearing, and other household tasks. *Caregiver burden* is a term

commonly used to describe the challenges that accompany the caregiving. In their study, Boland and Sims (1996) found that the 24-hour commitment of the caregiver experience strained the physical and mental health of the participants. Caregivers become vulnerable to injuries, exhaustion, social isolation, and despair (Lubkin, 1995). Financial hardship is another risk as the family caregivers spend their time in this unpaid labor. This aspect of caregiving receives little political attention, because the family caregiver role is predominantly a female one and society may view this as a natural role for women.

Rutman's (1995) study of women caregivers revealed that they experienced powerlessness when:

- Their competence and expertise as a caregiver were not recognized or respected
- There was a lack of control (either over the care receiver's disease process or over the care choices) or a need to relinquish control
- They were unable to prevent harm from befalling the care receiver

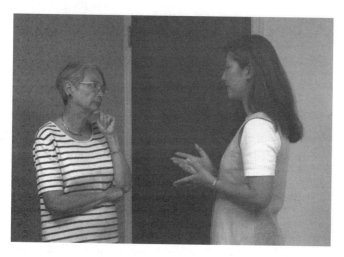

Offering support to the caregiver of a chronically ill client is important.

> **REFLECTIVE THINKING**
>
> ***The Caregiver of a Chronically Ill Client***
>
> • Think of someone you know who is caring for a chronically ill family member. How do you think the experience has influenced his or her life?
>
> • Imagine that a member of your family has become ill and you are required to provide the care. How would this situation affect your life?

• The system was bureaucratic and lacked resources; the needs of caregiver and care receiver apparently did not come first (p. 22)

The caregivers in Rutman's (1995) study provided the following suggestions for improving the caregiving experience:

• Enhanced resources to ensure quality care facilities and environments
• Enhanced public recognition for caregiving work
• Respect for caregivers
• Access to education and information
• Enhanced communication and working in partnership—families, parents, and professionals
• Support for caregivers—developing and strengthening peer support and networking within communities

Understanding the family's perspective is fundamental to an effective partnership between health care professionals and family caregivers. Some families rise to meet the challenge that illness presents. The stresses and difficulties overwhelm others and consequently can lead to neglect, abuse, or disintegration of the family unit. With an increasing number of caregivers in the community, nurses must recognize their needs in addition to those of the recipient of care. The principles of empowerment discussed earlier in this chapter are a sound basis for working in partnership with the caregiver, the care receiver, and other family members. The knowledge and expertise of caregivers in caring for their family member must be acknowledged and valued. Community resources such as support groups and respite care can help the caregiver with the challenges of the role.

HEALTH PROMOTION AND DISEASE PREVENTION

Community health nursing can be guided by the global commitment to achieve health for all by the year 2000

(World Health Organization [WHO], 1978). The United States and Canada have been among the leaders in this movement, as evidenced by the *Healthy People 2000* document (USDHHS, 1992), the Epp Report (Epp, 1986), and the Ottawa Charter (WHO, 1986). The Ottawa Charter identifies the prerequisites to achieving health for all as peace, shelter, education, food, income, a stable ecosystem, sustainable resources, social justice, and equity (WHO, 1986).

The 1993 World Development Report highlights the importance of the "good" health of citizens for the economic well-being of a country. Although many of the world's developing countries have made a commitment to health for all, the challenges are enormous. The report states:

> Rapid progress in reducing child mortality and fertility rates will create new demands on health care systems as the aging of populations brings forth costly noncommunicable diseases of adults and the elderly (World Bank, 1993, p. 3).

However, in developing nations the toll from childhood and infectious diseases remains high and adds to the health care demands that accompany a significant increase in life expectancy. The problems of controlling health care costs and ensuring the accessibility of health care to the overall population are common to both developing and developed nations.

In the United States, the Department of Health and Human Services, with extensive input from the American people, determined national health-promotion and disease-prevention objectives for the 1990s. These objectives were first reported in the document *Healthy People 2000* (USDHHS, 1992) and were updated in the *Healthy People 2000 Midcourse Review and 1995 Revisions* (USDHHS, 1996). The focus of these objectives is health promotion and disease prevention through lifestyle and environmental changes and changes in health care services. Although these objectives were written with the American public in mind, they can guide the work of community health nurses internationally.

The *Healthy People 2000* report recommends health promotion and preventive services at primary, secondary, and tertiary levels of prevention (USDHHS, 1992). The recommended services include education, counseling, screening, immunization, and chemoprophylactic inter-

Perspectives...

Insights of a Caregiver

My wife, [Louise], has Huntington's disease. It is an inherited disorder affecting the nervous system. It causes progressive deterioration of physical and mental capabilities, leading ultimately to severe incapacitation and eventual death, usually 15 to 20 years after the onset. Louise also has irritable bowel syndrome. This means most of her day at home is spent in the bathroom, a behavior she has great difficulty controlling on her own. Louise is 60 years old.

Onset for my wife occurred about 10 years ago. She can no longer perform the role of homemaker. Maintaining our home requires a reasonably reliable income. I am self-employed and work as a home-based businessman. It is essential I continue to be the breadwinner. This is becoming most challenging and stressful. Having my work in the same place as where I carry out most of my caregiving definitely has its shortcomings. Work often takes a back seat.

Without full daytime care for my wife, I am unable to generate full-time earnings. I am working to about 50% capacity. Every hour not worked is an hour of lost income plus the deterioration of my reputation of getting the job done on time.

I cannot complain about the caliber of home care and assistance we are presently receiving. But what is not available is full-time care to enable me to work away from home and to expand my business. Admission to a care facility is at least a year away. As my wife's disease progresses, my opportunity for full employment decreases. She cannot be left alone without an element of risk. If she were to require more assistance because of an accident, I would definitely be unable to care for her. To hire full-time help would cost me most of any additional income from full-time work. Unemployment is not a choice. Caregiving and working are full-time jobs. There is only one of me.

Abandonment is a choice. Then I know she will be looked after. But the outcomes, for me, are not what I want. The percentage of male caregivers of those with Huntington's disease who make this choice is very high. I don't want to be part of that statistic. In all honesty though, the thought has occurred to me.

Huntington's disease has affected our whole family. It has put a great emotional and physical strain on my wife and me. Our children are at risk as well. One has been tested positive as carrying the Huntington's gene, one tested negative, and two are undecided about being tested. We have 10 grandchildren. Seven are at risk. Is caregiving ever going to be over for me? I do know I have to continue earning a living for a long while yet.

—*Henry Ficke (1995)*

ventions. Priority care should focus on the most prevalent chronic conditions: heart disease and stroke, cancer, diabetes, and chronic disabling conditions. Specific objectives are presented in Appendix A. Community health nurses must work toward the implementation of measures to attain these objectives. The *Healthy People 2000 Midcourse Review* for 1995 shows progress toward meeting the 1995 objectives for heart disease, stroke, cancer, and unintentional injuries, with more than 65% of the objectives in those areas showing improvement. The objectives covering diabetes and other chronic conditions are among those showing the least progress (National Center for Health Statistics, 1996).

Health promotion is central to the work of community health nurses in caring for people with chronic illness (American Public Health Association [APHA], 1981; American Nurses Association, 1986; Canadian Public Health Association, 1990). The American Public Health Association (APHA) suggests that health promotion can be accomplished by nurses who work with individuals, families, aggregates, and multidisciplinary teams. The APHA includes identifying groups at risk for illness, disability, and premature death as a key element of the nurse's role. The nurse is responsible for directing resources toward these groups (APHA, 1981, p. 4). The Canadian Public Health Association (1990) considers the nurses' health-promotive roles from a health determinant basis. They see the nurse's role as:

1. Assisting communities, families, and individuals in taking responsibility for maintaining and improving their knowledge of, their control over, and their influence on health determinants.

2. Facilitating and mediating to enhance community, group, or individual strategies that help society anticipate, cope with, and manage maturational changes and the environment.

3. Encouraging communities', families', and individuals' ability to balance choices with social responsibility to create a healthier future.

4. Initiating and participating in health-promotion activities in partnership with others, including the community, colleagues, and other sectors (p. 7).

Community health nurses act as resource managers, planners, and coordinators as they help individuals and their families explore health-promotive and disease-preventive community resources. Resources vary from community to community; however, there are national resources related to the most prevalent chronic illnesses. In the United States, these include, for example, the American Diabetes Association, the American Heart Association, the American Cancer Society, the Multiple Sclerosis Society, the Kidney Foundation, and the Cystic Fibrosis Foundation. Equivalent resources exist internationally in Canada, Britain, and other developed nations. Many of these national organizations have local chapters in communities, making their services more accessible. These organizations address a variety of goals such as health promotion, public education at all levels of prevention, fund raising, support of research, and some direct client and family services.

Within the context of health care reform, community health nurses have a role in policy development and planning and in the delivery of preventive programs and services. In addition, they have a role in research that considers the effectiveness of health promotion and prevention and facilitation of the transfer of research into practice. Chronic illness issues are complex and varied: for example, accessibility of community resources, economic challenges for individuals and families, and availability of long-term care support services. Funding for research, screening, public education, and societal concerns such as poverty are examples of other issues that require community health nurse involvement. The Washington State Core Government Public Health Functions Task Force states "efforts to promote personal health, protect community health, and prevent disease are known to be effective. Yet, only 3% of current health system care dollars are spent on these services" (Washington Department of Health, 1993, p. 5). Nurses working in the community must raise the awareness of key policymakers in all levels of government of the need for a more equitable distribution of resources between the acute care and health promotive and preventive aspects of chronic illness.

The key to successful health promotion and disease prevention is partnership between community health nurses and members of the community. The nurse should encourage people to actively participate in identifying and taking ownership of community health issues. Issues related to chronic illness prevention may include the lack of parks and playgrounds, availability of cigarettes to underage smokers, tobacco advertising, high cost of fruits and vegetables, and need for access to land for gardens. The nurse serves as a resource by educating community members about the political process as it relates to health issues, about successful communication with the health care and political systems, and about strategies for participating in decisions concerning health issues (Canadian Public Health Association, 1990, p. 9).

Primary Prevention

Primary prevention focuses on taking measures to alter risk factors before the disease has begun. The increasing incidence of chronic illness, the lack of curative interventions, and the requirement for long-term care have resulted in great expense to the health care systems of many nations. Consequently, primary prevention is a vital approach to chronic illness.

Primary prevention strategies focus on environmental or behavioral risk factors that are modifiable. These measures need to be implemented before the disease has developed. For example, preventive measures for heart disease and stroke should be aimed at children and adolescents because physiological changes related to these conditions may begin in these age groups. Community health nurses have long been involved in a variety of strategies aimed at disease prevention. These include immunization, health education, and counseling. Immunization against infectious disease such as polio or measles prevents the associated sequelae that can lead to chronic disability. Community health nurses educate and counsel

DECISION MAKING

The Community Health Nurse and Political Involvement

Nurses are increasingly becoming involved in political action related to health care. Your city needs more green space to provide an area where people can be physically active.

• As a community health nurse what could you do to influence the local city government in addressing this issue?

• How might you gather support from other nurses in your community?

clients and their families about the reduction of modifiable risk factors related to chronic illness and disability. The nurse encourages changes in lifestyle activities not conducive to good health and supports those that are (Canadian Public Health Association, 1990). The need for adequate nutrition, exercise, sleep, stress reduction, and self-care are important aspects of this education and counseling.

It is important to apply the principles of empowerment to health education. Traditional models of teaching and learning have had limited success with the need for lifestyle and behavioral changes often associated with chronic illness prevention and with living with an illness (Fahlerg et al., 1991; Funnel, Anderson, Arnold, Barr, 1991). Education at the level of primary prevention addresses the general lifestyle issues that are considered risk factors for chronic illness. Preventive measures are very specific to the chronic illness being considered. However, dietary practices and smoking are risk factors for several chronic illnesses, including heart disease and stroke, cancer, and lung disease. Education related to the risks associated with smoking, obesity, and dietary fat intake are all important in the prevention of chronic illness.

Secondary Prevention

Secondary prevention focuses on early disease detection through screening programs as well as early treatment of the disease. For example, screening for high cholesterol and high blood pressure, in addition to implementing primary prevention strategies, has resulted in a steady decline in the number of deaths from heart disease and stroke over the past two decades (USDHHS, 1992). Education about the importance of taking advantage of available screening techniques such as mammograms, Pap smears, examinations for prostatic cancer, and regular physical examinations is an approach aimed at secondary prevention. Through early diagnosis, treatment can be implemented to slow the progression of an existing disease and to minimize damage caused by the disease. Early diagnosis is especially significant for chronic illnesses that may have an insidious onset, with a significant progression of the disease prior to the appearance of clinical signs and symptoms. Risk factor modification strategies aimed at asymptomatic adults become secondary prevention for chronic illnesses in which physiological changes leading to the disease begin in early childhood or adolescence, for example heart disease, stroke, and some cancers.

Tertiary Prevention

Tertiary prevention focuses on rehabilitation and restoration after an illness has occurred, to minimize morbidity and benefit the client's life. Rehabilitation following a heart attack or stroke, prevention of complications related to immobility in individuals with disabilities, and regular eye examinations for people with diabetes mellitus are

examples. Important aspects of tertiary prevention address the physical and psychosocial challenges associated with chronic illness. Self-help or support groups can offer clients and their families considerable psychosocial support. Such groups are an important resource, and they exist in many communities. Some examples are the Stroke Club, the Hospice Association, and the Arthritis Society.

The community health nurse assists individuals and their families in determining what resources may be of value to them and how they can use these services. Nurses become involved in the referral process, if necessary. Dialogue with clients and their families focuses on the exploration of their expectations related to these resources. Involvement with these resources takes time, energy, and sometimes money, a fact that clients and their families must consider.

Tertiary prevention requires community health nurses to work directly with people with chronic illnesses. This work involves assessment, planning, and intervention

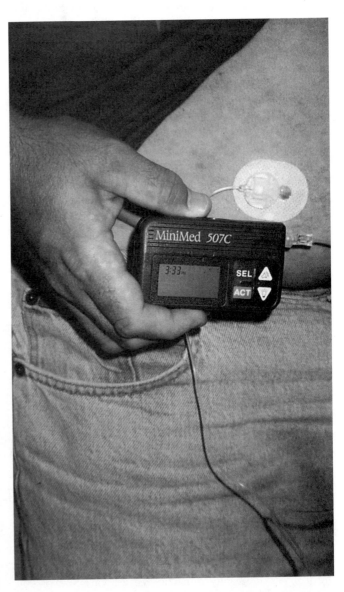

This person manages his diabetes using an insulin pump.

with individuals and their families. In all aspects of nursing care, the lived experience of individuals and their families must guide nurses as they work in partnership. In this way, the beliefs and assumptions that underlie caring and empowerment are applied.

Assessment and interventions can be focused on the individual with the chronic illness. However, this approach must be considered in the context of the family. Although individuals themselves can best elucidate the challenges they experience and the effect of the chronic illness on all aspects of their lives, it is important for the nurse to be aware of certain assessment factors that pertain to people with chronic illness. Chapters 15, 18, and 19 offer assessment tools for use with individuals and families. Assessment should reflect the whole client and seek to understand the totality of his or her illness experience, including the physical, psychological, social, spiritual, and environmental dimensions. An assessment should reveal the client's challenges as well as personal resources.

Miller (1992c) refers to personal resources as **power resources.** She advocates that nurses assess the person's power resources, which can be compromised by illness. Power resources include physical strength, psychological stamina, social support, positive self-concept, energy, knowledge and insight, motivation, and a belief system. People who are chronically ill have a vast capacity for coping, but Miller advises that nurses who do not recognize helpful coping behaviors may not adequately help clients face the challenges that accompany illness. She believes that people look to nurses to help them face the challenges of long-term health problems (pp. 9–15).

Nursing interventions need to be considered from a holistic perspective in partnership with the client. Many people with a chronic illness use healing modalities not prescribed by their physicians to assist them with the physical and psychological challenges of their illness (Lindsey, 1993; Thorne, 1993). A variety of healing modalities are used such as special diets, chiropractic care, naturopathy, stress management, biofeedback, Therapeutic Touch, and visualization. Healing modalities that are of ethnic origin are intrinsic to many cultures (see Chapter 6); for example, acupuncture is part of Asian cultures, and healing circles are part of some Native American cultures. Although research evidence is only now being accumulated on the effectiveness of these various healing modalities, people are turning to them with increasing frequency. Lubkin (1995) suggests that these therapies attract people with chronic illness for several reasons, including cultural or ethnic beliefs, frustration with the health care they are receiving, or the ineffectiveness of medically ordered treatment.

Thorne (1993) found that most of the participants in her study had pursued a course of therapy not prescribed by their physician. These therapies were often successful in helping them with symptom relief. When participants encountered negative attitudes to this therapy from health care professionals, the participants questioned the assumed superiority of traditional health care. Similarly, Lindsey (1993) found that, as participants in her study explored nonprescribed healing modalities, their relationships with health care professionals often became unsatisfactory. She suggests that these different healing modalities provide people an opportunity to "look far beyond their physical limitations, and to begin to acknowledge and embrace other important aspects of their lives" (p. 113). The community nurse needs to be aware of the wide range of healing modalities and take care not to judge or ridicule the client's use of them. Nurses must acknowledge the cultural aspects of healing that clients bring to their experience and use this knowledge in the care provided.

The fact that clients and their families seek the assistance of other therapists in no way devalues the nurse's role. The move to other therapies may signify that individuals are taking responsibility and control for their own healing (Lindsey, 1993). In this light, the nurse can be helpful in exploring other methods of healing with clients and their families when they express an interest. The nurse has a responsibility to advocate for clients and families with regard to all therapies. Lubkin (1995) recommends that nurses assist clients and their families in "identifying goals, alternatives and methods of evaluating the results of the treatment" (p. 343). This strategy should

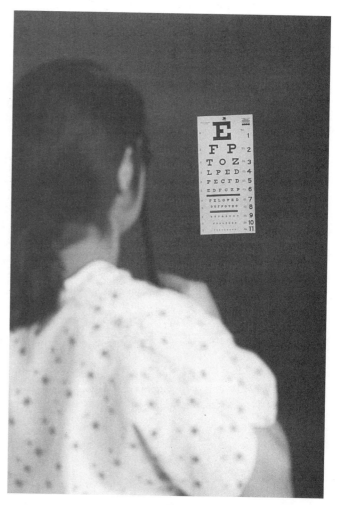

Eye exams should be encouraged for a person with diabetes as a tertiary prevention step.

apply to both prescribed medical therapies and other healing modalities.

People with chronic illnesses most often continue to live in their homes with their families and are sometimes cared for by family members. Even when the family does not become involved with the direct treatment regime or care of the ill person, each family member and the family as a unit experience the illness. A framework offered by Hartrick, Lindsey, and Hills (1994) focuses on the family's health and illness experiences and attends to the interdependent nature of assessment and intervention. Such a framework, based on health promotion and partnership, is useful for community health nurses working with families challenged by a chronic illness. Central to this framework is **circular questioning.** Wright and Leahey (1994) note that the effect of circular questions is to introduce new cognitive connections that pave the way for new or different family behaviors. Tomm (1988) describes circular questions as questions that are neutral, accepting, and exploratory. Such questions are based on the assumption that "everything is connected to everything else" and reveal patterns that connect "persons, objects, actions, perceptions, ideas, feelings, events, beliefs, context, and so on, in recurrent circuits" (p. 7). Examples of circular questions include: Who in the family is most fearful about the stroke? Who is best at helping other family members deal with the fear? How does he or she do this? What do you do when you are afraid?

The Hartrick, Lindsey, and Hills (1994) framework consists of four interdependent components, all occurring together throughout both the assessment and the intervention process (see Table 21-7). The four components are:

1. Listening to the family. The nurse listens to the family's story to gain an understanding of the family's experience with the chronic illness. Listening enables family members, including the ill individual, to become aware of important aspects of the illness. By focusing on both the individual and the family experiences, the nurse offers an opportunity for people to be experts in their own health. As the nurse and family listen to the family members' stories about their perceptions, needs, and healing experiences, they all gain a better understanding of the family's experience.

2. Participatory dialogue. Hartrick, Lindsey, and Hills (1994) advocate the use of circular questions to elicit the family's beliefs, values, and experiences of illness. Circular questions serve both as assessment questions and interventions. The questions assess each member's perceptions of relationships, experience, or beliefs. This dialogue enables the family to gain insight into how their patterns and interactions are affecting their experience with chronic illness. This awareness enables the family to "maintain or change existing family patterns and behaviors" (p. 15).

Table 21-7 Health-Promoting Family Nursing Assessment: The Framework		
COMPONENT	**STRATEGIC ELEMENTS**	**HEALTH-PROMOTION PRINCIPLES**
Listening to the family	• Eliciting different family member perceptions • Gaining an understanding of the family story • The family as experts in their own health experience	• People without power have as much capacity as the powerful to assess their own health needs. • Every person and family lives within a social historical context that helps shape their identity and social relationships. • Diversity is positively valued.
Participatory dialogue	• Posing circular questions to elucidate the taken-for-granted family patterns and interactions • Family members critically reflecting on the circular questions and posing questions of their own	• Relationships between people and groups need to be arranged to provide an equal balance of power. • Empowerment describes our intentional efforts to create more-equitable relationships with greater equity in resources, status, and authority.
Pattern recognition	• In collaboration, identifying the family's behaviors • In collaboration, recognizing the family's patterns and themes based on their beliefs and values • Co-creating the family's story	• The power of defining health problems belongs to those experiencing the problem. • Professional expertise and skills are used in new ways.
Envisioning action and positive change	• Making informed choices • Taking action • Reflecting on the action • Taking renewed action	• All people have strengths and are capable of determining their own needs, finding their own answers, and solving their own problems. • The people involved are the chief actors.

From "Family Nursing Assessment: Meeting the Challenge of Health Promotion" by G. Hartrick, A. E. Lindsey, & M. Hills, 1994, Journal of Advanced Nursing, 20, *pp. 85–91. Reprinted with permission: Blackwell Science Limited.*

COMMUNITY NURSING VIEW

Onya is a 34-year-old married mother of three children aged 10, 6, and 1. Although she has had symptoms for several years, she has been diagnosed with multiple sclerosis only recently. She is currently in remission but has some residual effects including fatigue, altered gait, and diplopia. Onya stays at home to care for the children and manage the home. The two older children attend school. Until the birth of her last child, Onya had taken responsibility for transporting the children to school and to their extracurricular activities. She finds that she can no longer drive because of her diplopia. Charles, her husband, expresses concern about Onya's condition and displays caring behaviors toward her. Charles is a company executive, and his job frequently requires out-of-town meetings. He expresses how much he values Onya's ability to manage the household when he is not at home.

Nursing Considerations

ASSESSMENT
• What psychosocial challenges do you think Onya may be facing?

• What challenges could be present for this family?
• Using the Hartrick, Lindsey, and Hills (1994) assessment framework (Table 21-7), what information do you need to gather?
• What other information would you want to assess about this family?

DIAGNOSIS
• What NANDA and Omaha nursing diagnoses can you identify?

OUTCOME IDENTIFICATION
• Given the diagnoses you have identified, what outcomes do you expect?

PLANNING/INTERVENTIONS
• Using the Hartrick, Lindsey, and Hills (1994) assessment framework (Table 21-7), how might you work with this family?
• What preventive measures would be appropriate for Onya and her family? What would be the level of prevention?

EVALUATION
• What outcome measures will tell you if you have achieved your goals?

---

3. Pattern recognition. The nurse and the family explore, examine, and create the picture of the family's experience. "Through critical reflection, the nurse assists family members to express, elaborate, and externalize their feeling and understandings about the family and about their health situation" (p. 16). In this way, the nurse can assist the family in understanding their own health story.

4. Envisioning action and positive change. With the understanding gained about their experience with chronic illness, the family is able to make more-informed health choices and to make the changes they want in their situation.

Health Education

Chronic illness often requires ongoing community health nurse involvement as clients learn to live with the illness and to manage challenging symptoms and complex treatment regimes. Funnel and her associates (1991) offer an empowering, person-centered educational model (see Figure 21-7) and a client empowerment education program (see Figure 21-8). Although these authors apply the concepts of empowerment to diabetes education, the nurse can use these models in the education of people with any chronic illness.

Figure 21-7 Empowering Person-Centered Model (Applied to Diabetes)

• Diabetes is viewed as a biopsychosocial illness.
• Relationship of provider and the person with diabetes is democratic and based on shared expertise.
• Problems and learning needs are usually identified by the person with diabetes.
• The person with diabetes is viewed as problem solver and caregiver.
• Professionals act as resources and share responsibility for treatment and outcomes.
• Goal is to enable the person with diabetes to make informed choices.
• Behavioral strategies are used to help the person with diabetes to change behaviors of his or her choosing.
• A lack of goal achievement is viewed as feedback and used to modify goals and strategies.
• Behavior changes are internally motivated.
• The person with diabetes and the professional are both powerful.

Adapted from "Empowerment: An Idea Whose Time Has Come in Diabetes Education" by M. Funnel, M. R. Anderson, M. A. Arnold, P. A. Barr, M. Donnelly, P. D. Johnson, D. Taylor-Moon, & N. H. White, 1991, Diabetes Education, 17(1), pp. 39.

Figure 21-8 Outline of Client Empowerment Education Program

1. Educator assesses current status (physical, emotional, cognitive, etc.)
   - Reviews client's actual self-care practices
   - Reviews recommended self-care practices
2. Educator provides relevant information about the chronic illness.
   - Describes various treatment options
   - Views cost and benefits for each option
3. Educator acknowledges client's responsibility for self-care.
   - Helps client clarify personal values specific to the illness
   - Helps client assess level of personal responsibility for illness care
4. Client identifies barriers and strengths related to achieving self-care.
   - Assesses chronic illness barriers and sources of support
   - Assesses life and social barriers and sources of support
5. Client assumes problem-solving responsibility.
   - Develops skills to optimize support (e.g., develops communication and assertiveness skills to enhance support from family and friends, increases support networks)
   - Identifies potential barriers
   - Learns strategies and skills to overcome barriers (e.g., negotiation, self-care agreements and plans, conflict resolution)
6. Client establishes plan with assistance from educator.
7. Client carries out plan.
8. Client and educator evaluate and review plan using problem-solving model.

Adapted from "Empowerment: An Idea Whose Time Has Come in Diabetes Education" by M. Funnel, M. R. Anderson, M. A. Arnold, P. A. Barr, M. Donnelly, P. D. Johnson, D. Taylor-Moon, & N. H. White, 1991, Diabetes Education, 17(1), p. 40.

≋ Key Concepts

- A chronic illness can affect all aspects of a person's life.

- The chronic illnesses of heart disease and stroke, cancer, and diabetes are among the leading causes of death in North America.
- The incurability of chronic illness minimizes the importance of curative approaches. The focus shifts to the caring aspect of nursing.
- Empowerment of clients and families is central to effective nursing approaches.
- The most important aspect of understanding the impact of chronic illness on people is that of the person's lived experience.
- Diagnosis is a critical time in the lives of people with chronic illness.
- Psychosocial aspects of chronic illness include uncertainty, powerlessness, and biographical work.
- Spirituality can be a resource for people with chronic illness.
- Chronic illness challenges the economic status of people through the added expense of uninsured expenditures and the effects on employment.
- Chronic illness is costly to society as a whole.
- Chronic illness has an impact on relationships and roles within the family.
- Normalization is a strategy used by individuals and families to live with the challenges presented by the chronic illness.
- Nonadherence to prescribed treatment may reflect a person's efforts to control the illness and to adjust treatment regimens to suit personal needs.
- The role of the community health nurse in relation to chronic illness includes health promotion and prevention.
- The primary, secondary, and tertiary prevention of chronic illness is a significant aspect of the community health nurse's role.
- The incurability and increasing incidence of chronic illness and the high cost of related care reinforce the need for primary prevention.
- The *Healthy People 2000* reports (USDHHS, 1992, 1995) provide guidelines for the implementation of health-promotion and preventive strategies for the most prevalent chronic conditions: heart disease and stroke, cancer, and diabetes and other disabling diseases.

Developmental Disabilities

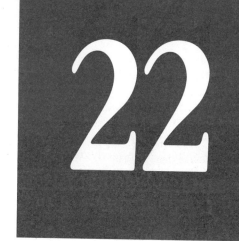

Nancy Gilien, MPH, RN

Nancy Gilien, MPH, RN

KEY TERMS

activity center
adaptive skills
attention
    deficit/hyperactivity
    disorder
autism
behavior modification
case management
cerebral palsy
continuum of care
deinstitutionalization
developmental approach
    to care
developmental
    assessment
developmental disability
developmental model of
    service
Down syndrome
dyscalculia
dyslexia
early intervention
epilepsy
fragile X syndrome
inclusion
interdisciplinary services
intermediate care facility
learning disability
mainstreaming
medical assistive device
mental retardation
newborn screening
normalization
pervasive developmental
    disorder
prenatal diagnosis
prevention
self-care
sheltered employment
small-group residence
supported employment
technology-assisted

It was as if a curtain had lifted before her eyes.
The life she had thought forever closed to her
daughter spread out its great pastoral vista.
After all, she thought, why not?

—Spencer, 1960

COMPETENCIES

Upon completion of this chapter, the reader should be able to:

- Define the term *developmental disabilities* as a legal term.
- Compare the two definitions and classifications of mental retardation. Consider the influence on the practitioner of the choice of definition and classification.
- Compare the major conditions subsumed under developmental disability and define the commonalities of care or service needs.
- Identify the attitudinal, social, and legal changes leading to improved conditions for persons with mental retardation and other developmental disabilities.
- Delineate the influence of the normalization principle on the systems of services for people with developmental disabilities.
- Explain the rationale for the developmental approach to nursing care of the developmentally disabled child, particularly the child with mental retardation. Consider the need for nursing assessment of adaptive skills through the life cycle of the person with a developmental disability.
- Describe the prevention programs and note the nursing role in primary, secondary, and tertiary prevention activities.
- Delineate the impact of developmental disability on the family. Consider the role of the community heath nurse in assisting the family.
- Describe nursing goals for family care specific to the presence of a member with a developmental disability.
- Cite the preparation needed by the person with a disability to maintain health and safety in community living.
- Cite the special supports that may be needed by parents with mental retardation.
- Outline some of the weaknesses of community health and service systems for people with developmental disabilities who are lower functioning, mentally ill, or elderly.
- Discuss the future for people with developmental disabilities and the importance of nurse advocacy to maintain their participation in the community.

People with developmental disabilities have benefited from changing social attitudes over the past 40 years of advocacy and reform. New federal and state laws were passed and funding was allocated to provide increased diagnostic services, research, health and habilitation programs, education, community residential services, and work training programs. The civil rights of all persons with disability were guaranteed. Children with significant problems entered public schools. Children and adults with disabilities left institutions for community residence. People with developmental disabilities gained opportunities formerly denied them for personal relationships, marriage, and family life. See Table 22-1 for the history of care of people with developmental disability.

Community health nurses offer support and acceptance as people with disabilities enter schools and workplaces and take up residence in the community. Nurses develop interventions with clients and their families to help maintain or improve health and functioning through the life cycle. Nurse advocacy for clients and families is important, as proposed changes in health care and reduced funding may not support the important gains made in the past four decades. This chapter offers community health nurses information, principles, and perspectives for working with people with developmental disabilities.

DEVELOPMENTAL DISABILITIES

The term **developmental disability** means any disability that is attributable to mental and/or physical impairment, manifested before age 22, that results in substantial functional limitations in three or more areas such as self-care, language, or capacity for independent living, and requires special interdisciplinary care of long duration. When the term is applied to children ranging in age from birth to 5 years, it refers to a substantial developmental delay or to a condition resulting in disability if services are not provided (Developmental Disabilities Assistance and Bill of Rights Act, 1990).

Developmental disability is a legal definition first introduced in 1970 for the purpose of identifying groups of people requiring similar services. When determining eligibility for services, states or other jurisdictions may include different combinations of conditions in their definition of developmental disability.

The most common conditions included in the legal definition of developmental disability are mental retardation, epilepsy, cerebral palsy, and pervasive developmental disorders, including autism. The legal definition of developmental disability may also include other neurological conditions of sufficient severity to require services similar to those required by persons with mental retardation. Some of these can be learning disability, attention deficit/hyperactivity disorder, and deaf-blindness. Infants and children with conditions placing them at risk for developmental disability may be included.

In 1991–1992, an estimated 48.9 million persons (19.4% of the total U.S. population) had a disability. Of these, 3.8 million (7.9%) were age 17 or younger. For the children, the leading type of disability was learning disability (29.5%). Following were speech problems (13.1%), men-

tal retardation (6.8%), asthma (6.4%), mental or emotional problem or disorder (6.3%), blindness or other visual problem (3.0%), cerebral palsy (2.7%), epilepsy (2.6%), orthopedic impairment (2.5%), and deafness (2.4%). Autism was estimated at 1.0% (Morbidity, Mortality Weekly Report, 1995).

The World Health Organization reported a worldwide estimate of the prevalence of disability as 15% to 20% of children, using differing definitions and methods of identification (Lipkin, 1996).

In one study of the causes of death for U.S. children age 1 to 19 for 1980 and for 1983 to 1989, it was found that developmental disability was the fifth leading cause of nontraumatic death for children 1 to 14 and the third leading cause of nontraumatic death for children 15 to 19. When developmental disability was listed as a related or contributing factor, the number of deaths was significantly higher (Boyle, Decoufle, & Holmgreen, 1994).

The term *developmental disability* has acquired a clinical meaning. In developmental pediatrics the term refers to a disability or disorder arising from central neurological damage, pathology, or defect that is permanent and chronic. "Developmental disorders represent lifelong differences, although not necessarily lifelong disabilities" (Capute & Accardo, 1996b, p. 21). Discussion of all developmental disabilities and their multiple causes is beyond the scope of one chapter. Four are selected for brief review to illustrate the spectrum of developmental disabilities. Two others, pervasive developmental disorder and autism, are not discussed in detail. **Pervasive developmental disorder** refers to a group of conditions characterized by qualitative impairment in the development of reciprocal social interaction, verbal and nonverbal communication skills, and imaginative activity. **Autism,** considered a severe form of pervasive developmental disability with onset before age 3, is a behaviorally defined syndrome of neurological impairment with features of impaired social interaction and communication and with restricted interests and activities. Children with autism frequently have associated problems such as seizures or mental retardation.

Mental Retardation

The person with **mental retardation** has significantly subaverage intellectual functioning manifest before age 18 with limited **adaptive skills** for his or her age in at least two or more areas of functioning, including cognition, communication, self-care, health and safety, social skills, academics, self-direction, or community use.

Community health nurses need to be familiar with two important systems of definition and classification of mental retardation offered by the American Psychiatric Association (APA) and the American Association on Mental Retardation (AAMR). Both systems employ standard IQ tests to define the intellectual level. The APA system uses an IQ of 70 or below to define mental retardation. The AAMR system defines mental retardation by an IQ of 70 to 75 or below.

There are significant differences in emphasis in the subclassifications of the two systems. The APA system classifies persons with mental retardation by the degree of intellectual impairment. Degrees of impairment are mild (IQ 50–55 to 70), moderate (IQ 35–40 to 50–55), severe (IQ 20–25 to 35–40), and profound (IQ below 20–25) (American Psychiatric Association, 1994).

The AAMR system emphasizes mental retardation as an expression of interaction between the individual and his or her environment at one point in time. Classification is by

Table 22-1 Brief History of Care of Persons with Mental Retardation and Other Developmental Disabilities in the United States	
1620–1770s	Family and community care for "feebleminded." Some stigma attached to the condition. First hospital for "idiot and lunatics" established in the Virginia Colony.
Early 1800s	Other conditions such as epilepsy confounded with mental retardation. Most care is given in the home. Children in almshouses or in a poor environment seen as needing protection. Nurse-reformer Dorothea Dix challenges states to provide care. Institutions founded and expanded.
Late 1800s	Sequin in France and later in the United States develops methods of educating children with mental retardation. Persons with mental retardation increasingly regarded as burdensome. Immigrants and the poor are held responsible for producing a disproportionate share of children with mental retardation. Directors of institutions form an organization that later becomes the American Association on Mental Retardation. Nurses join and organize a section on nursing.
Early 1900s	Mental retardation is better defined, and multiple causes are recognized. New findings on heredity and ideas on eugenics lead to view of persons with mental retardation as "menaces to society." The eugenics movement (1908–1920) leads to involuntary sterilization of persons with mental retardation and restrictions on their right to marry. Ungraded classrooms are opened in some public schools, but most families choosing not to institutionalize have few options for care and education. An organization to serve children with physical handicaps is formed and later becomes the Easter Seal Society.
1930–1950s	The Depression leads to more reliance on the institutions. Crises and scandals in the institutions lead to call for higher standards of care. The Council for Exceptional Children organizes to promote education in the community for children with disabilities. Parents begin publicly to share their experiences and concerns. Attitudes toward persons with disabilities begin to shift from regarding them as "sick," "innocent," or as the "eternal child" to viewing them as persons with special needs. Parents form the National Association for Retarded Children, now the ARC, to advocate for their children.
1961–present	President John F. Kennedy appoints the President's Panel on Mental Retardation. The findings and recommendations of the panel open a period of important legislation, funding, and social change that benefits persons with mental retardation and other disabilities. Persons with cerebral palsy, autism, and epilepsy are subsequently included by specific legislation. In 1970, the legal definition of developmental disabilities is established to include persons with needs similar to those of persons with mental retardation. Later legislation includes infants and children to age 5 who are at risk of disability. Major care changes are based on the principle of normalization and the developmental model of services. Some of the most significant services are: • Head Start, the War on Poverty, and increased preventive services in maternal and child health. Increased funding of research leads to identification of more etiologies, methods of prevention, early intervention, and treatment. New federally funded University Affiliated Programs (UAPs) are charged to develop interdisciplinary training and to provide exemplary services. Nurses are active in all of these programs and are on the faculty of many of the UAPs. • Persons with disabilities are moved from the institutions into smaller community residential facilities (deinstitutionalization). Changes in Medicaid and SSI legislation lead to establishment of smaller **intermediate care facilities** (ICF/MR or DD) in the community. Nurses serve on staff or as consultants. Nurses also serve on oversight agencies. • Free public education for all children with handicaps is mandated. School nurses begin to oversee the care of children with significant health problems. • The Americans with Disabilities Act of 1990 establishes the legal rights of all persons, prohibits discrimination based on disability, and mandates public accommodation. • Nurses work through their professional organizations to develop standards of nursing practice in different areas of service to persons with developmental disability.

From "The Nurse Whose Specialty Is Developmental Disabilities" by W.M. Nehring, 1994, Pediatric Nursing, 20, pp. 78–81; A Proposed Program for National Action to Combat Mental Retardation by the President's Panel on Mental Retardation, 1962, Washington, DC: U.S. Government Printing Office; A History of Mental Retardation: A Quarter Century of Progress by R.C. Scheerenberger, 1987, Baltimore: Paul H. Brookes Publishing; and Inventing the Feeble Mind: A History of Mental Retardation in the United States by J.W. Trent Jr., 1994, Berkeley: University of California Press.

description of present level of functioning in 10 areas, with indication of the level of support needed to maintain the person's highest level of functioning. Levels of support are denoted as intermittent support for a nearly independent person, limited support, extensive support, and pervasive support for the most impaired person. The level of support is not equivalent to the level of mental retardation: A person with mild retardation may need extensive or pervasive support depending on associated problems. The system promotes the view of the individual as capable of changing and improving. This model emphasizes the use of culturally appropriate assessments and the consideration of personal strengths, and it stresses expectation of improvement in function with sustained supports (American Association on Mental Retardation, 1992).

The APA system becomes important when correlation is sought among etiology, clinical findings, and level of functioning, and objective measures are needed. The community health nurse recognizes the value of this system for medical diagnosis, clinical and epidemiologic research, and medical reevaluation. The AAMR system, with its emphasis on defining adaptive skills and identifying needed support, is valued as it provides a knowledge base for culturally appropriate nursing interventions with client and family.

The use of one system rather than the other can influence the perception of clients and approaches to care. On the one hand, a focus on the diagnosis and IQ level with failure to identify and provide the supports needed to improve skills may impede the individual's progress. On the other hand, underlying all developmental disabilities are organic conditions, some of which are expressed sequentially and a few of which are degenerative. Medical evaluation or re-evaluation rather than a change of supports may be indicated. Community health nurses weigh the influence of the two systems when providing nursing assessments.

Role of IQ Tests

Most systems of definition and classification of mental retardation rely on standard IQ tests, which do not directly measure intelligence but measure skills considered related to intelligence by a particular culture. The tester must account adequately for gender, culture, age, or race variation. The relevant characteristics of the individual being assessed should be represented in the population on which the tests are based to avoid bias. The examiner should be from the same cultural group as the person examined or at least should be familiar with that cultural group.

Controversy still exists over the use of standard IQ tests. Some researchers contend that such tests best predict achievement in Caucasian children. Other researchers assert that some tests are equally good predictors for African American, Caucasian, or Mexican American children (Kramer, Allen, & Gergen, 1995). Nurses administering standard tests or assessing adaptive skills consider cultural factors as part of the assessment process.

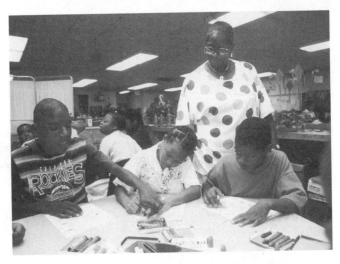

Do you know anyone who has a developmental disability? What has been done to help that person?

Characteristics

Children or adults with mental retardation learn slowly. The individual rate of learning depends on the degree of impairment. They require more repetition and instruction to learn. People with mental retardation do not generalize well and may need to learn what to do in each new situation. They do not recall information easily and have difficulty thinking abstractly or critically.

People with mental retardation are slow to develop speech and language, depending on the degree of impairment. Physical problems may inhibit clear enunciation. Motor development is also slow, and the child is late in sitting, walking, running, and acquiring self-help skills. Movements may be uncoordinated. Depending on the underlying cause of the retardation, there are often associated disorders. These can be dysmorphic features, metabolic problems, motor problems, epilepsy, speech and language disorders, vision and hearing disorders, and behavior disorders (Capute & Accardo, 1996b).

The degree of mental disability determines the level of adult functioning. In most cases, people with mild mental retardation, who constitute 85% of the total population of the mentally retarded, merge into the general population once they are out of school, and they may no longer be perceived as significantly disabled. Persons with moderate mental retardation, about 10% of the total, can learn self-care and vocational skills. Many will live independently or semi-independently with intermittent or limited support. Persons with severe retardation, about 3% to 4% of the total, may learn some self-care skills but will require close supervision and extensive support. Those with profound retardation, about 1% of this population, will continue to require pervasive support: that is, total care and supervision (American Psychiatric Association, 1994).

Both children and adults are frequently aware of their difficulties and of the stigma that society sometimes attaches to their condition. They may struggle with painful feelings of rejection or low self-esteem. With support,

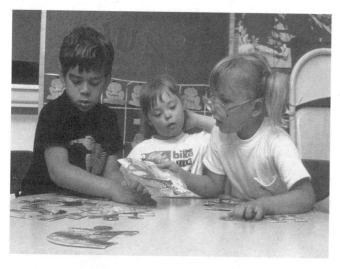

Children and adults with developmental disabilities should be encouraged to take pride in their accomplishments to promote a positive self-image.

Table 22-2 Categories of Disorders, with Examples, in Which Mental Retardation May Occur

I. Prenatal Conditions

  A. Chromosomal disorders: Trisomy 21 (Down syndrome), fragile X syndrome

  B. Syndrome disorders: Neurofibromatosis, Prader-Willi syndrome, Leeber amaurosis syndrome

  C. Inborn errors of metabolism: phenylketonuria, galactosemia, homocystinuria

  D. Developmental disorders of brain formation: anencephaly, porencephaly

  E. Environmental influences: maternal malnutrition, maternal ingestion of alcohol (fetal alcohol syndrome)

II. Perinatal Conditions

  A. Intrauterine disorders: toxemia/eclampsia, premature labor and delivery, umbilical cord prolapse

  B. Neonatal disorders: hypoxic-ischemic encephalopathy, intracranial hemorrhage, hyperbilirubinemia

III. Postnatal Conditions

  A. Head injuries: cerebral concussion, intracranial hemorrhage

  B. Infections: herpes encephalitis, HIV infection, measles encephalitis

  C. Demyelinating disorders: postinfectious acute hemorrhagic encephalomyelitis

  D. Degenerative disorders: Rett syndrome, Pelizaeus-Merzbacher syndrome

  E. Seizure disorders: infantile spasms, Lennox-Gastaut syndrome, status epilepticus

  F. Toxic metabolic disorders: Reye syndrome, lead intoxication, dehydration

  G. Malnutrition: kwashiorkor, chronic protein-calorie deprivation

  H. Environmental deprivation: psychosocial disadvantage, child abuse and neglect, social or sensory deprivation

  I. Hypoconnection syndrome

From Mental Retardation: Definition, Classification, and Systems of Support (9th ed., pp. 81–91) by American Association on Mental Retardation, 1992, Washington, DC: Author. Excerpted by permission.

however, they develop pride in their accomplishments and a positive self-image. Nigel Hunt, a man with moderate mental retardation due to Down syndrome, was taught by his mother to read and write when the schools refused to accept him. He typed his autobiography, a charming account of his positive experiences in community, travel, and family life (Hunt, 1967). His book was an important contribution, demonstrating that persons with significant cognitive impairment are capable of learning and of literary expression.

Many adults with cognitive abilities, similar to those of persons of 6, 10, or 12 years, have well-developed adaptive and social skills. They function well in familiar settings. Yet, all too often, members of their families and communities have the attitude that less than average adult intellectual functioning is unacceptable.

Prevalence

It is generally agreed that 1% of the U.S. population, or more than 2.5 million people, is mentally retarded. Prevalence is about 3% in the school-age population. Some counts are lower than 1% when people with mild retardation who no longer require special services are lost to identification (American Psychiatric Association, 1994).

Etiology

There are many causes of mental retardation, ranging from genetic disorders to infections and trauma. Any event leading to maldevelopment, injury, or infection of the central nervous system can result in mental retardation. Categories of etiologies are listed in Table 22-2.

In the majority of instances, the etiology of mental retardation is not known. In mild retardation, there are frequently few associated physical findings, although research is beginning to demonstrate subtle differences in some individuals (Capute & Accardo, 1996b).

Prevention

Many conditions leading to mental retardation are preventable. Examples are measles encephalitis prevented by immunization, fetal alcohol syndrome prevented by abstention from alcohol during pregnancy, head injury prevented by many child safety measures including abuse prevention, lead poisoning prevented by environmental sanitation measures, and genetic disorders prevented by preconception genetic counseling. Community health nurses provide services in many programs of primary prevention that reduce the incidence of conditions leading to mental retardation. See Chapter 16.

Treatment and Management

Because of the many associated problems, an interdisciplinary approach to care is considered best practice. Some conditions associated with mental retardation are treatable, such as phenylketonuria and galactosemia, in which mental retardation can be prevented by dietary treatment, or some forms of hydrocephalus, in which shunting can prevent mental retardation. If no treatable etiology is identified, management is directed to maintaining health, correcting any treatable associated conditions, and providing programs of early developmental stimulation and special education. Community health nurses working with children and adults with mental retardation, in addition to providing health care, define the adaptive skill level, help the family and client obtain services and support to enhance and advance skills, and provide health teaching adapted to the client's level of understanding.

Epilepsy

Epilepsy is a condition characterized by recurrent abnormal electrical discharges from neurons in the cortex of the brain that cause seizures. The International League Against Epilepsy classifies epilepsy as one of two major types: generalized seizures that involve the whole cortex or partial seizures that are limited to one hemisphere. The generalized seizures involve loss of consciousness. The partial seizures often do not but can proceed to impaired consciousness or generalized seizures. Within these classifications, seizures are categorized by clinical type (Batshaw & Perret, 1992).

Characteristics

People with epilepsy manifest the condition in different ways. Some may have a warning aura, lose consciousness, have clonic movement, and suffer loss of bladder control (a generalized tonic-clonic seizure). These events are often distressing to those experiencing seizures and frightening to witnesses. Others have a simple partial seizure manifested by jerking of the mouth or face, accompanied by odd movements that are involuntary but may not be understood as such by observers. Seizures in some people are only brief lapses of consciousness (absence seizure), which may be perceived as inattentiveness or rudeness. Some have sudden loss of muscle tone (atonic seizure), resulting in falls and repeated injuries. Some people may have more than one type of seizure. People with epilepsy have been misunderstood and their behavior ascribed, sometimes even today, to possession, witchcraft, divine punishment, the sins of others, mental illness, or behavior problems.

For many people with epilepsy, even those with significant developmental disability, their major problems may be more social than medical or developmental. Chil-

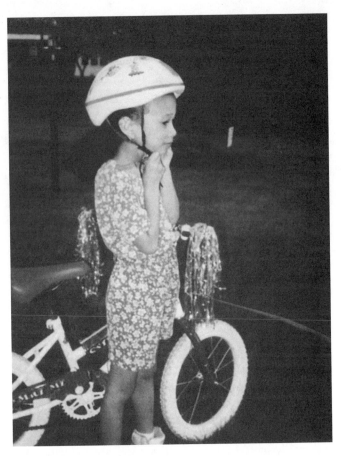

Encouraging parents to ensure their child wears a safety helmet while bike riding is a primary prevention technique that may reduce the risk for severe head injury and developmental disability.

dren with epilepsy become aware of their problem, its impact on the family and society, and the stigma that sometimes is attached to their condition. They may be denied appropriate independence and social experiences because of family fears of accidents or seizures. As adults, they may face unnecessary restriction on mobility, job opportunities, and social relationships.

Prevalence

It is impossible to estimate accurately the prevalence of epilepsy because of differences in definition, varying ages of onset, and individual manifestations of the disorder. The National Information Center for Children and Youth with Disabilities reported that 2 million Americans have epilepsy. Of the 125,000 cases that develop each year, up to 50% are children and adolescents (National Information Center for Children and Youth with Disabilities [NICHCY], 1993).

Etiology

The causes of epilepsy are legion and range from congenital malformation, hypoxia, intracranial hemorrhage, malnutrition, heredity, and infection to trauma. Many pathologies of the central nervous system may result in

REFLECTIVE THINKING

Perception of Mental Retardation

The parents and siblings of a child being provided dietary treatment for a metabolic disorder underwent psychological testing as part of the evaluation of treatment outcomes. The mother's IQ scores placed her in the moderate to mild range of mental retardation.

The young woman was beautiful, wore stylish and expensive clothes, and was well groomed. Her manner was sweetly dignified. She asked questions that encouraged the other person to talk at length while she listened attentively.

Her husband, a prominent professional man, explained that his wife's family had accepted her condition and had provided every advantage. She went to private school with no suggestion of "special" classes. She took art classes at the local community college so she could be perceived as having gone to college. Her family carefully trained her in social skills and household care.

She was unable to plan and shop for an elaborate meal or manage her child's special diet, but she had a housekeeper to assist her. She could not chair a committee meeting, but she presided well at their dinner parties.

Her husband esteemed her for what she was: a loving wife, mother, and graceful companion. Their common interests were their children, extended families, social life, and travel. Her husband helped her to avoid situations she could not handle.

• Should this woman be considered mentally retarded? Consider her ability to meet social and cultural expectations. Consider her support system.

• How might your perception of her be influenced by applying to her the system of definition and classification of the American Psychiatric Association? Of the American Association on Mental Retardation?

epilepsy. Many of the conditions listed in Table 22-2 have associated seizures. Epilepsy is associated with mental retardation in 16% of cases, with cerebral palsy in 25% of cases, and with autism in 25% of cases. In more than half the cases, the cause is not known (Batshaw & Perret, 1992).

A number of causes of epilepsy are preventable. Prevention of head trauma and brain infections would significantly reduce the incidence of epilepsy. All the nursing activities that reduce causes of mental retardation would also reduce the incidence of epilepsy.

Treatment

Treatment of epilepsy is primarily through use of antiepileptic drugs. The majority of children will have their seizures controlled by a single drug. Dietary treatment with a ketogenic diet may be offered in some cases. Surgical treatment for some partial seizures may be effective (Batshaw & Perrett, 1992). Many persons with epilepsy will have remissions of their disorder.

Nurses work with the physician and family to control the seizures of persons with epilepsy. They help the family recognize and record seizures, administer and monitor the effects of medication, and work to improve or ameliorate any associated problems. They teach the client about the disease and self-care. They encourage culturally appropriate activities and lifestyle and discourage unnecessary restrictions (Frank, 1994).

Cerebral Palsy

Cerebral palsy is a term for a group of brain damage syndromes characterized by abnormal control of movement and posture. The disorders differ with regard to the parts of the body involved and the associated difficulties experienced. The three major types are as follows:

1. Pyramidal cerebral palsy, with spasticity predominant and with hemiplegia, diplegia, and quadriplegia as subtypes

2. Extrapyramidal cerebral palsy, which includes disorders of posture and involuntary movement

3. Mixed types, which combine disorders of the two major types (Capute & Accardo, 1996a)

Associated problems can be impaired intellect (50% to 75% of cases), seizures (35% to 50% of cases), visual problems (50% of cases), hearing problems (10% of cases), speech defects, and dental defects (Dzienkowski, Smith, Dillow, & Yucha, 1996).

Characteristics

Children with cerebral palsy exhibit delays in motor development, increased or decreased muscle tone, spasticity, involuntary movement, weakness, incoordination, or paralysis. Depending on the type of cerebral palsy, a unique pattern of motor limitation emerges, as may associated problems. By school age, the child with cerebral palsy and the family usually recognize that the condition is permanent. The adolescent with moderate or severe cerebral palsy faces a challenge to achieve self-sufficiency and independence. She or he may require extensive, permanent support to live and work in the community. The older person with cerebral palsy may develop increased motor difficulties.

DeRogatis (1993), a nurse with cerebral palsy, reports that persons with cerebral palsy are rarely asked how they experience their bodies. Cerebral palsy is often experienced as a physical variation not as a deficit. It is the negative attitudes of others that make the person with cerebral palsy feel inadequate.

Prevalence

A review of studies of cerebral palsy in industrialized countries indicates a prevalence of 1.7 to 2.5 per 1,000 children of early school age. In the United States there are 100,000 persons under 18 and about 400,000 adults with cerebral palsy (Murphy, Molnar & Lankasky, 1995). Several population studies indicate an increase in the rate of cerebral palsy, particularly among infants with birth weights under 1,500 grams. The prevalence of cerebral palsy may be increased about 20% (Nelson, 1996).

Etiology

Approximately 70% to 75% of the cases of cerebral palsy are of prenatal and perinatal origin. Low birth weight, particularly below 2,500 grams, premature birth, and asphyxia are major risk factors. Some conditions that contribute to low birth weight or poor intrauterine growth are viral infections, malformations, chromosomal abnormalities, and some maternal illnesses. Inflammation of the placenta, multiple births, maternal mental retardation, and maternal hemorrhage are also risk factors. Cerebral palsy acquired after the first month of life is associated with

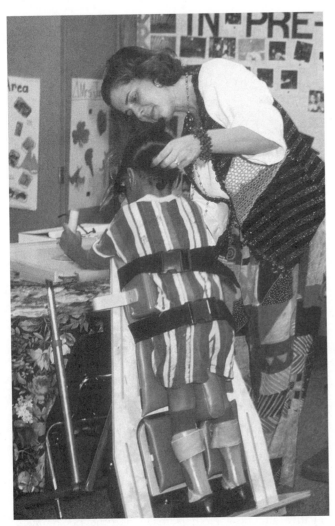

The nurse is often a member of the treatment team.

trauma, infection, seizures, and toxins (Dzienkowski et al. 1996; Nelson, 1996).

Treatment

Cerebral palsy is treated with physical therapy to maintain range of motion and to prevent contractures, inhibition and activation of postural reflexes to promote more normal movement, motor training in functional activities, and surgery to prevent or to release contractures. Drugs may be used to reduce spasticity. Associated problems are addressed as indicated. Assistive devices such as braces, crutches, wheelchairs, communication devices, computers, and special utensils are provided at the appropriate developmental level. An interdisciplinary approach to care is the best practice for persons with cerebral palsy and associated problems (Capute & Accardo, 1996a).

Community health nurses have a role in prevention, early recognition, intervention, and long-term follow-up. Depending on the level and site of practice, the community health nurse may intervene to prevent cerebral palsy by providing prenatal follow-up, teaching child care and safety, or providing immunizations. The nurse may identify the child through nursing assessment, be a member of the treatment team, act as case manager, help structure his or her environment and curriculum as school nurse, or be a nurse consultant to an adult program. With the family and members of other disciplines, the nurse works to maintain health and improve motor function to help the client compensate for limitations and maintain the maximum level of independence (Dzienkowski et al. 1996).

Attention Deficit/Hyperactivity Disorder

Attention deficit/hyperactivity disorder (AD/HD) is a behaviorally defined neurological disorder whose main features are inattentiveness, impulsivity, and hyperactivity. It is a form of **learning disability** in which the child's academic achievement is different in some areas as compared with his or her overall intelligence.

Behaviors now regarded as AD/HD have been recognized for many years. Recent research has discriminated AD/HD from other minimal brain damage conditions that can also have hyperactivity or impulsiveness as features (Blondis, 1996). Attention Deficit/Hyperactivity Disorder is also discriminated from other learning disabilities as **dyscalculia**, poor ability to learn or use mathematics, or **dyslexia**, poor ability to learn or work with visual symbols.

Characteristics

The child with attention deficit/hyperactivity disorder is unable to maintain attention. Attention mechanisms of focusing, selecting what to attend to, sustaining attention, resisting distractions, and shifting attention can break down at any point. The child may not seem to hear, may not follow through on tasks, may forget, or may be unable to organize tasks. She or he acts before thinking, interrupts, or intrudes. The young child is always on the go. In school, the child typically talks excessively, jumps about in class, and has difficulty working quietly. Associated problems can be other specific learning disabilities, such as dyslexia. Other problems can be low frustration tolerance and temper outbursts. The child's difficulties can lead to poor academic performance, peer rejection, poor self-esteem, or antisocial behavior.

There can be improvement with age. Adults who had the diagnosis as children were studied. One half of the group seemed to have resolved their difficulties; the other half continued to have problems. Problems self-reported were distractibility, forgetfulness, inability to organize, and inattention to relationships (Blondis, 1996). Many adults learn to manage their behavior and become productive and creative (Whiteman & Novotni, 1995).

Prevalence

The true prevalence is unknown. It is estimated that 3% to 5% of school children in the United States have AD/HD. Boys diagnosed with AD/HD outnumber girls by approximately 3 to 1 (Blondis, 1996).

Etiology

Genetic transmission is considered the leading cause of AD/HD. A number of conditions can be associated with AD/HD, including head trauma, extremely low birth weight, or birth hypoxia (Blondis, 1996). Parents of children with attention deficit/hyperactivity disorder who were evaluated in multiple disability clinics were studied. The parents had a high incidence of disorders including AD/HD, other learning disabilities, alcoholism, and depression (Roizen, Blondis, Irwin, Rubinoff, Kieffer, & Stein, 1996).

Treatment

With no cure, management is directed to reducing the excessive behaviors, facilitating attention and learning,

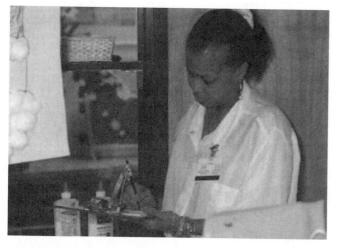

By observing and recording the behavior and actions of children, the school nurse and teacher are in a prime position to identify developmental problems.

♋♋ REFLECTIVE THINKING ♋♋

Managing Attention Deficit/Hyperactivity Disorder

The school nurse organized a meeting with Mike's teacher and mother and arranged for Mike's doctor to participate over a speaker telephone. Mike's distractibility had recently increased. He was not doing his work, and he was joining other boys in rowdy behavior at the end of the school day. Mike's mother was surprised. She thought he was improving, as his hyperactivity had decreased since he turned 12. At Mike's request his dosage of stimulant medication was being slowly decreased.

The nurse acknowledged the reduction of hyperactivity but clarified that Mike still needed help to attend and focus adequately. The nurse and his teacher knew that Mike was embarrassed about his school work and thought that he might be clowning to cover his feelings.

Mike's doctor was reluctant to increase his medication and was of the opinion that Mike was capable of better regulation of his attention and behavior. Mike's teacher and mother agreed. Mike's mother indicated that she would initiate interventions needed to get Mike back on track. She proposed to increase his time in productive activity and to decrease his time in unsupervised activity.

His mother obtained a paper route for Mike, and he began to deliver papers as he walked home from school. She took two afternoons off from work to accompany him as he learned his route. As a reinforcement, she paid a college student to meet Mike at home afterward to coach him and his friends in soccer or baseball. She sat with him for half an hour after supper to help him organize his homework and stay on task.

Mike began to complete his work. His disruptive behavior at school diminished as he participated more in school sports. Mike was proud of his ability to handle school work and his paper route. He agreed to stay on his medication until the end of the school year.

• What is the role of the nurse in assisting the child with attention disorder? The role of the family?

• How might persons not familiar with the disorder interpret Mike's behavior?

• Consider the amount and types of environmental structuring provided to help Mike. Do you think medication alone would be effective? Why or why not?

and helping the individual learn to manage his or her particular pattern of activity. Early recognition and intervention are crucial before the child and family become locked into unsuccessful interactions. A multimodal program is considered best practice, with elements including counseling of children and their parents, classroom modification, specialized instruction, and a trial of medication, usually a stimulant such as dextroamphetamine sulfate. Cognitive-behavioral training is provided to help the child develop self-regulation mechanisms to promote attention and reduce impulsive action.

A home behavioral program managed by the parents should be coordinated with the school program (Blondis & Roizen, 1996; Levy, 1996). The program requires close cooperation and communication by child, family, teacher, nurse, and physician. The clinic nurse, public health nurse, or especially the school nurse may be the one to suspect the problem and promote and organize the multimodal services. He or she may identify resources, coordinate meetings, promote communication, establish uniform observations of the child's behavior in different settings, monitor medication, and provide information and health teaching to teachers and family (Niebuhr & Smith, 1993).

Commonalities of the Developmental Disorders

There are commonalities among developmental disorders. These commonalities are addressed in the following statements:

- A significant number of conditions leading to developmental disability are preventable.
- Developmental disabilities arise from central nervous system conditions and are permanent, with effects on the individual ranging from very mild and nondisabling to very severe and seriously disabling. Associated problems may occur with a disability, appear later, increase or decrease in severity, or resolve over the life of the individual. Many interventions can prevent or treat the associated problems (Capute & Accardo, 1996b).
- Changing nature of the developmental disabilities over time requires understanding. The developmental, health, cognitive, physical, behavioral, emotional, or social issues related to the particular disability at a particular point in the person's life must be addressed.
- Persons with developmental disabilities can lead productive lives in their communities. Interdisciplinary services and support systems may be needed to maintain them in the community.
- Persons with developmental disabilities and their families require nursing care that is holistic and family-centered, empowers the client, and promotes the highest level of health and functioning (Feeg, 1994).

PRINCIPLES AND PERSPECTIVES

Changing social attitudes after World War II led to the development and dissemination of important principles of

REFLECTIVE THINKING

Individuals with Developmental Disabilities

Think about a person you know who has a developmental disability.

- How does he or she express what it is like to have the condition?
- What is the person's adaptation in the home and community?
- What system of supports is available to the person? Can you suggest other supports that would help the person become more fully integrated into the community?

service to persons with disabilities. These principles developed from the advocacy of families, particularly those with members with mental retardation, and their supporters. Their advocacy arose from their moral conviction that persons with developmental disabilities must have the same human rights and range of services as their nonhandicapped fellow citizens (see Table 22-1).

Civil Rights

The rights of people with mental retardation and other disabilities have been acknowledged in statements issued by a number of countries. In 1971, the United Nations affirmed basic and special rights for persons with mental retardation (Scheerenberger, 1987). In the United States, the civil rights of all persons with disabilities were made explicit in the Americans with Disabilities Act of 1990, which prohibits discrimination and mandates public accommodation. The intent of the law is that all persons with developmental disabilities be as fully integrated into the community as possible (Americans with Disabilities Act, 1990). Most states now have protection and advocacy agencies responsible for pursuing legal, administrative, and other remedies to protect the rights of persons with disabilities.

The civil rights of people with developmental disabilities are often unthinkingly and casually violated by family, friends, or officials. The community health nurse must be aware and prepared to intervene in situations such as the following:

- Child protection agents remove a newborn solely because one parent is mentally retarded.
- Residential service providers enforce rules that violate adult residents' rights to associate with friends, have sexual relationships, or travel in the community.
- Health care providers refuse to accept the consent to treatment of an adult with a disability although the person has no cognitive limitations.

DECISION MAKING

Normalization

A community health nurse is asked to serve on the board of a charitable organization. The organization serves adults with significant physical limitations due to conditions such as cerebral palsy and spina bifida. The board proposes to develop a facility in a rural area where clients who require wheelchairs and some attendant care may live and work. The board has purchased a van with a wheelchair lift. The sign on the van proclaims: "Serving the Handicapped."

• Review this plan for adherence to the principle of normalization. What changes should the community health nurse propose?

Normalization

The principle of **normalization** developed in the Scandinavian countries in the 1960s and was promulgated in the United States by Wolfensberger. "Normalization is utilization of means which are as culturally normative as possible, in order to establish and/or maintain personal behavior and characteristics which are as culturally normative as possible" (Wolfensberger, 1972, p. 28) This statement has had a significant influence on attitudes toward persons with mental retardation as well as toward people with other disabilities. The statement and its corollaries underlie significant positive changes in developmental disability service systems in the United States.

Acceptance of the principle of normalization requires that people with mental retardation and any other disability be permitted and encouraged to live a life that is as similar as possible to that of people without disabilities. They must have the same standard of living, similar housing, and similar routine of daily and yearly living. Acceptance requires that they have appropriate developmental experiences with the supports necessary to make the experiences available. They must be assisted to exercise their civil rights and to become self-advocates. Every effort must be made to keep them in the mainstream of their culture and to serve them in as culturally appropriate a manner as possible. Services in an institution or other restricted environment are provided only if the individual requires a level of care that cannot be developed in the community.

The principle of normalization is congruent with the nursing ethic of caring. Community health nurses should incorporate information on normalization when teaching clients and families. Understanding the principle and its implications helps the client and family formulate long-term goals for culturally appropriate life in the community.

Developmental Perspectives

Development as used in this chapter incorporates two concepts: a **developmental model of service** used to design service systems and the **developmental approach to care** of the individual. These concepts form the basis for most programs and care for people with developmental disabilities.

The Developmental Model

The developmental model of service was formulated in reaction to the medical model of care offered in institutions. The medical model was criticized as defining the person with disability as "sick" and in need of professional care. The medical model fostered dependency and failed to offer opportunities for skill development and broader social experiences (Trent, 1994). Services based on the developmental model encourage development in all areas over the life span. The goal of health services is to support development. The developmental model is widely applied in schools, work centers, day programs, and institutions.

The Developmental Approach to Care

The developmental approach to care is based on theories of normal development. The approach emphasizes the similarities between the disabled person and the nondisabled person, particularly in the early years of life. The disabled and nondisabled progress through the same stages of development, although at different rates. The broad stages of development are similar regardless of the etiology of a person's disability.

Interventions for those with cognitive impairment are, in the early years, based on the present developmental level not on the chronological age. Goals are formulated considering the expected rate of development and any associated problems. The individual's physical and social environments are structured to support development in the most positive ways.

Interdisciplinary Services, Continuum of Care, and Case Management

The complex, varied, and changing problems of many people with developmental disabilities require the services of an array of specialists over a long period of time. **Interdisciplinary services** bring the specialists to the client at one point in time to function as a team to resolve complicated issues. Interdisciplinary teams are assembled for medical diagnosis and treatment, school placement, solutions to behavior problems, vocational planning, out-of-home placement, or assistance with other complex problems. Team composition and leadership vary according to client need.

DECISION MAKING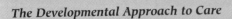

The Developmental Approach to Care

The community health nurse and family assess the skills of a 4-year-old child. John walks well and seats himself in a chair. He feeds himself with a spoon and drinks from a cup. He has just begun to use two-word sentences. He is still in diapers.

- What age child is John most like?
- What skills might he be ready to learn?

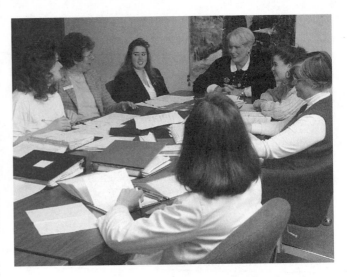

The members of the interdisciplinary team will vary depending on the needs of the client.

Continuum of care, a concern of the President's Panel on Mental Retardation, refers to the succession of services needed by the individual as he or she moves from one life stage to another. For example, many young people need to have special school services, then afterward receive vocational training, and then move into a program to learn community living skills. Implementing the continuum of care requires coordination of often fragmented services. **Case management,** whereby the individual receives personal assistance to obtain needed services, provides such coordination.

The community health nurse identifies the appropriate health and support services clients need. Also, nurses for decades have developed and implemented case management systems (Kersbergen, 1996). The nurse is in a central position to define the need for a comprehensive plan, organize an appropriate team, serve as a team member, or serve as case manager (Natvig, 1994). See Chapters 3 and 4 for further discussion of case management.

Prevention of Developmental Disabilities

The term **prevention** in discussion of developmental disabilities refers to activities to intervene in the course of a disease so that the disease does not occur (primary prevention), activities to detect and treat a disease early (secondary prevention), and activities once a disease has occurred to limit disability or associated conditions (tertiary prevention).

On the basis of the findings of the President's Panel on Mental Retardation, prevention efforts were increased in the 1960s (see Table 22-1). Today, the U.S. Centers for Disease Control and Prevention (CDC), through the Division of Birth Defects and Developmental Disability, provides prevention research and services. The CDC supports national and international public health surveillance, monitoring trends in birth defects and other disabilities and possible associated environmental factors. Personnel of the CDC perform or support epidemiologic studies to identify causes and risk factors for birth defects and developmental disabilities. They evaluate programs of treatment or support. As many states have established

developmental disability prevention plans, the CDC supports state-based prevention programs through cooperative activities or grants. A major goal is to involve local communities in prevention planning and services. Communities are assisted to replicate well-defined prevention programs, organize and plan unique programs, or address targeted needs in intensive intervention programs (Adams & Hollowell, 1992; Centers for Disease Control and Prevention [CDC], 1997).

The national health promotion and disease prevention plan, *Healthy People 2000,* has numerous objectives based on the epidemiologic work of the CDC and the states. Examples are objectives to reduce the incidence of alcohol ingestion during pregnancy, to increase immunization levels in children under age 2 to 90%, to reduce low birth weight, to prevent folic acid–preventable spina bifida and anencephaly, to increase developmental and sensory screening of young children, and to provide children at risk with early intervention and preschool programs (U.S. Department of Health and Human Services–Public Health Service [USDHHS-PHS], 1996).

Community health nurses have always been active in programs of prevention. Two examples of primary preventive services designed to prevent the occurrence of developmental disability are preconception health appraisals and prenatal care. The preconception health appraisal, often performed by the advanced practice nurse, offers an assessment of individual risks, personal and nonjudgmental education of prospective parents, and referral to specialized services such as genetic counseling (Cefalo & Moos, 1995). Early and adequate prenatal care reduces the risk of infant mortality and morbidity. Since the time of Lillian Wald, it has been demonstrated that periodic nurse contacts with pregnant women in populations of greatest risk reduce the risk of infant mortality and morbidity. Results are particularly good when contacts can be continued after the birth of the child (Deal, 1994). See Chapter 16. Secondary prevention and tertiary prevention will be discussed later in the chapter.

THE NURSING ROLE IN DEVELOPMENTAL DISABILITIES

The community health nurse provides services to the developmentally disabled client and family at any point in their lives and in many different practice settings. The goal of care is always the same: to help the client attain the highest possible level of health and social functioning (Nehring, 1994).

Prenatal Diagnosis

Prenatal diagnosis is examination of the fetus by fetoscopy, amniocentesis, maternal blood test, chorionic villus biopsy, ultrasound, or x-ray to detect abnormalities. Among the growing number of abnormalities that can be detected are inborn errors of metabolism, chromosomal abnormalities, neural tube defects, and hydrocephalus. Women are referred for prenatal diagnostic procedures because of advanced maternal age, personal or family history of a genetic disorder, or suspected problem based on history or physical findings. Evolving research in fetal surgery and gene and stem cell therapy may offer hope of future therapies to treat an affected fetus (Howell, 1994). Should a problem be diagnosed that cannot be treated, the parents are counseled about the clinical implications, prognosis, medical management, recurrence risk, and possible assistance available.

The nurse working with the family making a decision about pregnancy termination brings personal beliefs and ethics to the situation but does not impose them on the family. It is important to discuss with the family the cultural, religious, emotional, and social factors that influence their decision to continue or terminate the pregnancy and to help them explore all alternatives. In the end, the family's decision must be respected. There is no national consensus on abortion, and beliefs differ widely within cultural groups and even within families.

Early Identification of Developmental Problems

Early identification of children with variations of development or developmental delays is important in order to intervene as quickly as possible to prevent or remediate problems; a form of secondary prevention. Community health nurses, working with persons from other disciplines, provide early identification through developmental assessment, history, and examination.

Newborn Screening

All states and a number of other countries have programs that screen newborns for treatable diseases that, left untreated, lead to developmental disability. One of the

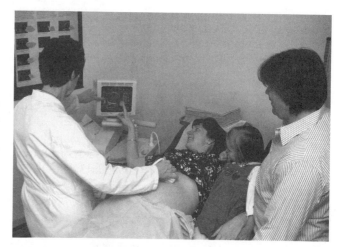

national objectives for the year 2000 is to screen at least 95% of newborns and ensure that at least 90% of the infants testing positive for disease receive appropriate treatment (USDHHS-PHS, 1996).

Newborn screening varies by state. All states in the United States screen for phenylketonuria and congenital hypothyroidism. Most also screen for galactosemia and hemoglobinopathy (e.g., sickle cell anemia and other conditions of abnormal hemoglobin). Seven additional diseases—maple syrup urine disease, homocystinuria, biotinidase deficiency, cystic fibrosis, adrenal hyperplasia, tyrosinemia, and toxoplasmosis—may be screened in some states, or on physician request, or as a pilot program (American Academy of Pediatrics, Committee on Genetics, 1996b). If screening findings are positive, the primary physician is notified and can provide further evaluation and treatment to prevent the medical and developmental problems associated with these conditions and can advise on recurrence risks. Community health nurses in public health departments, health maintenance organizations, or clinics are frequently responsible for locating and referring the family for diagnosis. Nurses follow up to assist the family with medical or dietary management. They monitor the treatment results through periodic developmental screening of the child.

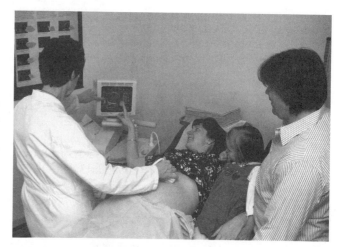

The nurse should encourage prenatal testing, as some disorders can be detected before the baby is born. Research may offer hope of future therapies to treat an affected fetus.

Nurses must be sensitive to the special issues raised for these families as well as for those families who received a prenatal diagnosis. Because most of these conditions have a genetic basis, the families may face difficult reproductive decisions relating to the risk of occurrence in subsequent children or in other relatives. For families with an affected infant, there may be no guarantee of assistance with special treatment costs. Also, although new laws may help, the diagnosis, once recorded in the health record, may expose the family to risk of loss of or increased costs of health insurance.

Developmental Surveillance

The developmental outcome for the child is a result of the interplay between the child and the physical, social, and emotional environment. A nurturing environment often leads to good outcomes. A dysfunctional environment can lead to poor outcomes, particularly if the child was initially at risk.

The child can be at risk because of biological factors, environmental factors, or both. Biological factors include conditions such as prematurity, perinatal complications, maternal drug or alcohol abuse during pregnancy, infections, chronic illness, injury, or genetic or metabolic disorders. Environmental factors can include lack of financial and social support, parental disability, temperamental differences between parent and child, abuse and neglect, or lack of parental nurturance.

Community health nurses can explore parental views and concerns about development at each contact with the family. Curry and Duby (1994) suggest that questions that elicit parental views of the child's vision and hearing, recent changes in development, temperament, activities enjoyed with the parents, favorite play activities, and recent stressful events will often elicit much information and suggest additional avenues of assessment or intervention.

Developmental Assessment

Nurses use a number of **developmental assessment** tools. The well child receives periodic screening utilizing global screening instruments such as the Denver Developmental Screening Test II, designed to identify the child needing further investigation. As long as no delays are found, the global test is an efficient means of ongoing developmental surveillance. Children with specific risk conditions, including concerns identified at the periodic screening, receive additional screening by health professionals for development, nutrition, behavior, parenting, mental health, medical status, or vision and hearing. Parent education and resource coordination are offered, often by nurses. Children who have health and development problems are monitored by some of the more comprehensive instruments suitable for children with risk conditions, such as the Bayley Scales of Infant Development II (Bennett, 1994). Table 22-3 identifies some of the instruments used by nurses.

Nurses providing developmental assessment recognize the value of parental involvement in the test situation. Parents are entitled to a careful explanation of the tests, their purpose, and how well their child performed. Parents are understandably anxious and need reassurance that they are supporting the child's development. They may need time and repeated evaluation before recognizing a delay and accepting the need for further evaluation. When the child is known to be delayed, the reassessment can be a time of disappointment and discouragement. It is important for the nurse to acknowledge parental feelings and help the parents identify all their methods that support positive development in the child.

Interdisciplinary Evaluation

Because the etiologies of developmental disabilities are multiple and diverse, there can be no standard medical evaluation. The general diagnostic elements include the medical and family history, neurodevelopmental assessment, physical examination, and appropriate laboratory tests. Additional evaluations may include psychological, genetic, speech, hearing, vision, motor status, social, or educational testing provided by relevant specialists (Farrell & Pimental, 1996). The nurse contributes health appraisal, developmental assessment, assessment of the client's special care needs and of the family's ability to provide needed care and assists the family to identify and use all available resources. The nurse also assesses cultural factors that affect care of the disabled member. The nurse has the knowledge needed to carry out the plan of care developed from all the disciplines (Nehring, 1994).

Specialized interdisciplinary diagnostic services may be identified through the local agency for the developmentally disabled, university-affiliated programs, and university medical centers.

✿✿ REFLECTIVE THINKING ✿✿

Cultural Response to Disability

A Native American couple had a baby born with congenital absence of the eyes. They refused to take the baby home from the hospital. Threats of prosecution for abandonment did not deter them, and the baby was placed in foster care. The local public health nurse told the hospital personnel that the baby's great-grandmother was responsible for the parents' decision. She had reminded all the relatives that the customary and only appropriate response to the birth of such a baby was to place it out in the desert to die, "face down in the sand." Whatever their personal feelings, the parents had accepted the decision that the baby had no place in the family or community.

• Does this family's culturally sanctioned action differ from "decision not to treat" or "do not resuscitate"?

Table 22-3   Examples of Screening and Assessment Instruments Useful to Community Health Nurses

There are many instruments now available to screen and assess children or to structure and monitor developmental programs. Listed are a few examples of instruments commonly used by community health nurses or by advanced practice nurses.

Examples of Instruments Used to Screen the Well Child

1. Denver Developmental Screening Test II (DDST). Examiner tests well child, 2 weeks to 6 years.

   Denver Pre-screen Questionnaire. Rating by parents of child, 3 months to 6 years.

   > W. K. Frankenberg, J. B. Dodds, A. Fandal, E. Kazuk, and M. Cohrs
   > ADOCA Publishing Foundation
   > 5100 Lincoln St.
   > Denver, CO 80212

2. Ages and Stages Questionnaires (ASQ). Parents respond to questionnaires (for children 4 months to 48 months).

   > D. Bricker, J. Squires, and L. Mounts
   > Paul H. Brookes Publishing Co.
   > PO Box 10624
   > Baltimore, MD 21285-0624

3. Developmental Profile II. Rating from birth to 9 years. Parents report development in physical, self-help, social, academic, and communication skills.

   > G. Alpern, T. Boll, and M. Shearer
   > Psychological Development Publications
   > PO Box 3198
   > Aspen, CO 81612

4. Home Observation for Measurement of the Environment (HOME). Birth to 3; 3 to 6 years.

   Examiner assesses home environment and parent and child interactions.

   > B. Caldwell and R. Bradley
   > University of Arkansas at Little Rock
   > 23rd and University Ave.
   > Little Rock, AR 72204

Examples of Instruments Employed with Children at Risk or with Developmental Problems

1. Bayley Scales of Infant Development II. Examiner tests child, 1 month to 42 months.

   > N. Bayley and 1993 revision team
   > The Psychological Corporation
   > 7500 Old Oak Blvd.
   > Cleveland, OH 44130

2. Mullen. An examiner offers stimulus materials to child and records child's responses.

   > E. Mullen
   > American Guidance Service
   > 4021 Woodland Rd.
   > Circle Pines, MN 55014-1796

3. Nursing Child Assessment Satellite Training (NCAST)

   Feeding scale. Examiner assesses child and parent interaction in feeding situation.

   Teaching scale. Examiner assesses child and parent interaction in teaching situation.

   > K. Barnard
   > NCAST
   > University of Washington
   > WJ-10
   > Seattle, WA 98195

4. Eyeberg Child Behavior Inventory. Parent or other adult rates child's conduct (2 to 16 years).

   > S. Eyeburg
   > Department of Medical Psychology
   > School of Medicine, The Oregon Health Sciences University
   > 3181 SW Sam Jackson Park Road
   > Portland, OR 97201

5. Achenbach Child Behavior Check List

   Rating of child's behavior (4 to 18 years).

   > T. Achenbach
   > Department of Psychiatry
   > University of Vermont
   > Burlington, VT 05401

Examples of Instruments Useful for Assessing Adaptive Skills

1. Nursing history and assessment forms.

   Numerous forms are found in nursing texts or clinical procedures manuals that guide assessment of client self-care skills, social skills, level of understanding, and mental status.

2. American Association on Mental Deficiency (AAMD) Adaptive Behavior Scales for Children and Adults. One standard scale and two school-use scales. Observation or self-report may be used. Scales designed to assess persons with mental retardation or emotional maladjustment.

   > Publishers Test Services
   > 2500 Garden Road
   > Monterey, CA 93940

3. Vineland Adaptive Behavior Scales, 1984 edition

   Observation or semi-structured interview of persons birth to 19 years. Survey form or expanded form for program planning available.

   > S. Sparrow, D. Balla, and D. Cicchetti
   > American Guidance Services Publisher's Building
   > Circle Pines, MN 55014-1796

From Forrest Bennett, M.D., Professor of Pediatrics, Clinical Training Unit, University of Washington. Used with permission.

Cultural Factors

To be effective, the nurse needs to understand the particular cultural system of the family. The family and community may not reflect Caucasian, mainstream American values, but instead may reflect the values of ethnic and minority populations. Each population has its own long-standing, distinctive cultural beliefs, practices, and support systems that determine the way members define and address the needs of persons with developmental disability. More often than not, *family* means the extended family. (See Chapter 6 for general cultural assessment.)

Groce and Zola (1993) identify three key issues that appear in almost all cross-cultural studies of chronic illness and disability. Raising these issues as questions to be explored can increase understanding and may predict how the client's care will be addressed by the family and community.

What is the culturally perceived cause of the disability? Beliefs about cause determine family and community attitudes and actions. Disability thought to be due to divine punishment for breaking of a taboo, for the sins of the parents, or for transgression in a former life may provoke shame, denial, or concealment of a problem. Families may be reluctant to seek help or to expose the disabled member. In contrast, anthropological study has identified deeply religious Mexican American communities that believe the family has been singled out by God to care for a disabled person and are esteemed by the community (Madiros, 1989).

What is the family's expectation of the individual's survival? Perception of survival will affect the care the individual receives and the effort spent on medical care, habilitation, or education. Some groups may sanction neglect or infanticide. Other groups may coddle or indulge a child or fail to provide education because the child is not expected to live long. Parents in some cultures may make more effort to help boys than girls.

What is the social role of the child or adult with a disability? Social role expectations also determine what is done for the person and the demands placed or not placed upon him or her. Mainstream U.S. culture, which values independence and self-sufficiency, may expect the adult with severe cerebral palsy to live independently and to find his or her own job and attendant care. Members of other groups would find this attitude heartless and would expect to care for the person at home. To protect the marriage prospects of siblings, a family may resist exposure of the person in school placement. Some may expect the less capable adult to live at home and work for other family members.

Respectful exploration of these questions with the family or knowledgeable members of the culture can help the nurse assess the cultural influences on individual family decisions related to care of the client. Understanding the issues enables the nurse to work more productively with the client and the family.

Planning with the Family

The goal of nursing is to help the person with a disability attain the highest possible level of health and social functioning. Nursing specific to developmental disability must: (1) help the parents to develop and follow an individual health care plan for their child, (2) help the parents teach their child self-care and appropriate social behavior, and (3) teach the adult client health self-care. Self-care is an important focus for client and family. **Self-care** is the individual's ability to engage in acts and decisions to sustain life, health, well-being, and safety.

The Nursing Health Care Plan

The child with a disability is first of all a child with the same health needs as any other. Routine health maintenance procedures can be overlooked if attention is focused on completing therapies, treating acute illnesses, or controlling seizures. The nursing plan has the goal of maintaining wellness in a person with a disability.

The nursing plan is based on assessment of the child and family and the nursing diagnoses, with measurable goals and a process for evaluation. The nursing plan may stand alone or may be part of an interdisciplinary team plan. It becomes a plan of anticipatory guidance. The basic plan can be based on published standards for well-child care. The family can be taught to develop and maintain a complete and permanent record (Steadham, 1994).

Objectives specific to the client's diagnosis should be included. For example, children and adults with **Down syndrome,** a chromosomal disorder, are at increased risk of hearing problems, cardiac problems, and obesity. Their plans should specify close surveillance for those risks (Rogers, Roizen, & Capone, 1996). **Fragile X syndrome,** an X chromosome–related disorder, can have sex differences in expression that must be taken into account in the plan. Both sexes are monitored in childhood for strabismus, flat feet, scoliosis, seizures, hyperactivity, and other conditions. Boys, in contrast to girls, may have a slowing of intellectual development in later childhood. In adolescence, anticipating such behavior changes as aggression in boys and social anxiety in girls becomes important (American Academy of Pediatrics, Committee on Genetics, 1996a).

The nursing plan should also specify removal of any barriers to the child's ability to learn. Parents may be told that glasses are not necessary for a child who cannot learn to read. This perspective is incorrect. Good vision is a developmental requirement for optimal learning, and reduced vision is a barrier. The child should have the barrier removed as soon as it is identified. Likewise, hearing aids and sign language training should be provided as early as possible to the child with hearing impairment or delayed language. Adaptive equipment should be provided to the child with motor delays so that he or she is upright and mobile at the same developmental level as other children of the same age. Resistive, hyperactive, or withdrawn behaviors that interfere with learning must be

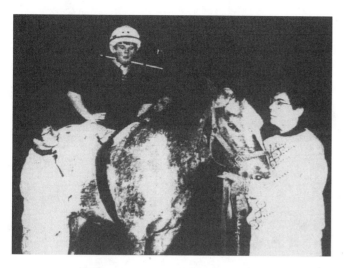

People with developmental disabilities should be encouraged to take part in new positive experiences.

addressed in the plan. Isolation from new experiences or new roles, particularly in adolescence, delays social role learning and needs to be discouraged. Nurses and families should strive to identify and include in the plan all procedures, supports, and experiences that promote health and social development.

Teaching Health Self-Care

Most parents teach their children as a matter of course, but slow development or multiple problems may disrupt the process. The nurse, by assessing the child with the assistance of the parents, can help them gain a clearer understanding of the child's current developmental level and expected rate of development and of the influence of any associated problems. Realistic parental expectations strengthen family coping and facilitate effective parental teaching. When the child is learning slowly or has behaviors that interfere with learning, the parents can be taught techniques of **behavior modification,** a system of changing behavior by reinforcing desired actions.

In working with the family, the nurse considers their attitudes, knowledge, resources, and willingness to commit to the program. The nurse can help the family define behaviors as movements that are observable, controlled by the child, and repeatable. The nurse teaches descriptions of movement and the avoidance of labels such as "hyperactive," "good," "bad," or "unmotivated" as imprecise. The nurse teaches positive reinforcement and avoidance of punishment or aversive techniques (Toleman, Brown, & Roth, 1994). Figure 22-1 presents an example of the designing of a behavioral program.

Serious and intractable behaviors require expert help and should be addressed by an interdisciplinary team that includes a physician and behavioral specialist. Some examples of serious behaviors are self-injurious behavior, rumination, extreme hyperactivity, assaultive behavior, and deeply withdrawn behavior. For example, the repetitive

and withdrawn behaviors of the child with autism usually require specialized help. All facets of the behavior can be assessed, and physical and environmental factors identified and corrected. The in-home or in-school behavior program may be conducted by a behavioral specialist who also trains the family members in the more complicated behavioral management measures (Levy, 1996).

Figure 22-1 Designing a Behavioral Program

Jean is a 4-year-old girl with mild mental retardation and a seizure disorder. Her indulgent parents report to the community health nurse that she ignores most requests and is not mastering the self-help skills that she should. They want assistance in improving her cooperation.

1. Review client and family situation.

The nurse reviewed Jean's health history and performed a developmental assessment. Jean functions near age 3 in most skills and has no physical limitations. Her seizures are controlled. She is capable of understanding and obeying simple requests. Her parents are very motivated to help her.

2. Identify target behaviors.

After much discussion, Jean's parents decide that they want Jean to comply with requests to come to them, to go to her room, and to sit at the table. They select coming when called as the first behavior to increase.

3. Obtain a baseline.

Jean's parents record the events surrounding her behavior: the parents' request to come; her response of compliance or noncompliance; and the consequences (i.e., what the parents do). They record for five days and learn that Jean complies with a request to come once in 10 times. They also learn that when she complies, they tend to take her behavior for granted. When she does not, they tend to scold or go to her.

4. Set the behavioral goal and select the reinforcement.

The parents and nurse state the goal as "Jean will come within 20 seconds of being called 95% of the time." Reinforcement for coming is a smile and a pat every time and a small food treat given intermittently. Noncompliance is ignored.

5. Schedule the plan and record results each time.

The parents specify that they will make eight trials (i.e., requests to come) per day at times when Jean is not engrossed in a favorite activity. After one week, the recording indicates that Jean is coming when called 75% of the time. The parents are pleased and are motivated to continue.

6. Review plan, evaluate, and make appropriate changes.

After two weeks, compliance is at 90%. The parents are confident that they understand how to set appropriate behavior goals and reinforce consistently. They plan to continue the program until Jean complies with their requests 95% of the time.

Family Support

Many, if not most, parents and other family members experience shock, denial, anger, helplessness, sorrow, and other strong emotions following the realization that something is wrong with their child. Depending on the circumstances, there may be feelings of guilt, shame, and isolation. The response of each family is unique and is influenced by many factors, including the child's diagnosis and gender, family belief system, attitudes of relatives and community members, and economic circumstances. The nurse offers emotional support by encouraging open discussion among family members, reflecting and helping them clarify feelings and regain a sense of control over their lives. Depending on the practice level, the nurse may offer additional counseling or refer the family to appropriate resources.

Siblings of a child with a developmental disability may need special attention. They may be confused about the cause of the disability and feel somehow to blame. They may wish to avoid any identification with their sibling or feel resentful of the time and attention the parents must devote to him or her. They will probably mirror any feeling of shame or stigma evident in the parents (NICHCY, 1994). The nurse can encourage parents to share information with the siblings and suggest ways the parents can elicit and deal with their children's anxieties or negative feelings.

The nurse helps the family identify all resources for support. Other families with a member with developmental disability can offer true understanding, emotional support, and practical advice (Smith, 1993). Organized groups of parents, such as the ARC exist in every state and most communities and can be located through the local health agency or the state developmental disability agency. Organized groups of siblings of persons with a disability can be located through the same resources. Family or individual counseling may be available through local developmental disability service programs, the family's religious affiliation, the local mental health agency, or other social service agencies.

Families need services and assistance, including financial assistance. Most states have an array of public and private resources available. Persons under 18 receive financial benefits based upon the income and resources of the family. The local health and human services agency is usually the initial source of information and service. In addition, identification of a large variety of resources useful over the life span is quickly made through the National Information Center for Children and Youth with Disabilities. The National Information Center maintains up-to-date, state-by-state information on resources for families and professional workers. See Figure 22-2 for information about this resource.

The community health nurse can anticipate points in the family life cycle when significant stressors may appear and can prepare the family to manage changes. Stress may occur when the young child receives a diagnosis, when the child enters school, when adolescent sexual interests

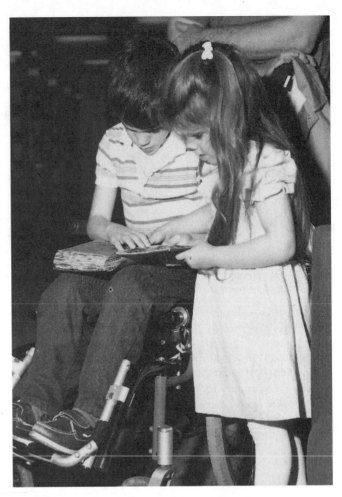

The parents of a child with a developmental disability should work to minimize the impact of the disability on their other children by sharing information about the disability and encouraging discussion of feelings.

develop, when the young adult must leave school, or when the elderly parent can no longer provide care for the adult son or daughter.

THE EARLY YEARS

The period of maximum brain growth is from birth to 3. The experiences of the child during this period influence emotional, physical, cognitive, and social development. Special supports for the child at risk or the child with a disability should be provided as soon as possible during this period.

Early Intervention

Early intervention means to provide to the infant or child and family an individual development program with associated social support services for the purpose of preventing disability, promoting more normal development, ameliorating disability, and enhancing parental skills and family adjustment. One of the objectives for the year 2000

Figure 22-2 National Information Center for Children and Youth with Disabilities

The National Information Center for Children and Youth with Disabilities (NICHCY) provides information to assist parents, educators, caregivers, advocates, and others in helping children and youth with disabilities become participating members of the school and community. Information Specialists are available to answer questions. The center provides information on specific disabilities, organizations supporting persons with disabilities, public agencies, legislation, materials for parents, resources for adults with disabilities, news digests, and other data bases. The center offers material in Spanish also. It is operated by the Academy for Educational Development through a cooperative agreement with the U.S. Department of Education.

P.O. Box 1492, Washington, DC 20013-1492
1-800-695-0285 (Toll Free, Voice/TT)
or search their web page
http://www.NICHCY.org
E-Mail: NICHCY@aed.org

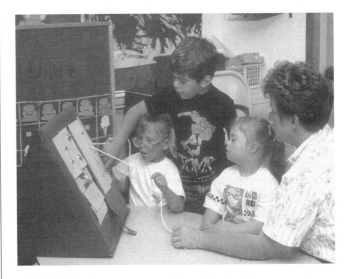

One of the objectives of Healthy People 2000 *is to provide access to preschool programs for children with developmental disabilities that will prepare them for school.*

is for all states to have service systems for children with or at risk of chronic or disabling conditions. Another is that all disadvantaged children and children with disabilities will have access to preschool programs that help prepare them for school (USDHHS-PHS, 1996).

Several federal laws and amendments mandate all state education agencies to serve children with disabilities from age 3. Part H of the Individuals with Disabilities Education Act (IDEA) permits state education agencies to provide services to children from birth to 3 who are delayed or at risk for delay if intervention is not provided. The intent of the law is to help families care for their children. Intervention services are based on an individualized family service plan (IFSP), developed by families and professionals, which states goals for the child and family and identifies child and family strengths and resources. Interagency cooperation to facilitate access for families to services and to promote comprehensive, interdisciplinary services is mandated (Individuals with Disabilities Education Act, 1990). Services may be provided by a designated agency or coalition of agencies and may take place in the home, clinic, or school. Services can include special education, family training, counseling, and appropriate related therapies such as physical therapy or language therapy. Nursing is identified as one of a number of disciplines qualified to provide early intervention service (Jenkins, Covington, & Plotnick, 1994).

Health Care

The advanced practice nurse working in these programs provides physical and developmental assessment and assessment of the family's ability to provide medical, nursing, or other health care procedures. Children who are

medically fragile or **technology-assisted** (i.e., dependent upon a device that substitutes for a body function) are also served. The home health nurse assisting the family with the fragile or technology-assisted child may also become a member of the team. With the family and program team, the nurse develops the individual family service plan, including the nursing care plan. The nurse teaches the family any needed health care procedures and may be the primary worker with the family or act as consultant to the family or primary worker. Because many early intervention procedures or therapies are provided as part of daily child care, cultural differences in practices of feeding, toilet training, discipline, sick-child care, or social training are taken into account when planning with the family.

THE SCHOOL YEARS AND TRANSITION TO ADULTHOOD

During the school years, the child with a developmental disability comes into contact with the wider community. In this setting, he or she strives to develop the skills for optimal adult adjustment.

Legal Supports

Since the passage of the Education for All Handicapped Children Act (1975), all states accepting federal funds under that act and the successor acts must provide a free and appropriate education to all children with disabilities. Related services such as transportation or physical therapy must also be provided. The school must assess the student's education needs and develop with the parents an individual education plan (IEP). The IEP must be revised at intervals and must include the transition services needed for postschool objectives such as employment, additional schooling, community participation, or independent living. See Figure 22-3.

Education must be offered in the least restrictive environment. **Mainstreaming, or inclusion,** meaning the most contact possible with children who do not have disabilities, is required. Children with physical disabilities or mild mental retardation may be served in regular classrooms with any needed physical or educational assistance. Children with significant behavior difficulties or with moderate or severe mental retardation may be served in contained classrooms with scheduled classes or activities with nonhandicapped peers. Children with the need for pervasive supports have been and may still be served in "development centers" where their special physical needs are addressed, but the trend is to place these children in classrooms attached to regular schools. Educational services may be offered until the student is age 22.

Parents have a strong position because the law outlines the rights of the child and an appeals process that must be followed if the parents are not satisfied. States and local districts vary in what is offered, so nurses should encourage the parents to examine their local programs in order to decide what is best for their child.

Figure 22-3 An Example of an Individual Education Plan

Child's Name: Tyrone S.   Age: 4 years, 2 months
Center City Public School District
September 17, 1994

Present Level of Functioning

Social development: Tyrone does not play with other children. He never approaches another child and runs away every time a child approaches him.

Annual Goals

Tyrone will learn to play cooperatively with other children.

Short-Term Objectives

Tyrone will play next to other children during highly preferred activities (for example, sandbox, sensory table, finger painting) for two 10-minute periods each day.

Special Services

School district will provide transportation to and from community preschool placement, and school district will pay Tyrone's tuition for a half-day program at the Learning Center Community Preschool.

Speech therapist will visit the preschool once a week to work with Tyrone and to meet with the teacher.

Behavior management program will be coordinated by classroom teacher and itinerant special education teacher.

Beginning and Duration of Services

Tyrone will begin attending the Learning Center on October 5. Other services will be in place by October 12. Placement and services will be reevaluated by April 5, 1995.

Evaluation

Tyrone will be reassessed on the Preschool Profile in March. A graph will be kept showing the amount of time Tyrone spent playing next to children each day.

From The Exceptional Child: Inclusion in Early Childhood Education *by K. E. Allen & I. S. Schwartz, 1996, Albany, NY: Delmar Publishers.*

Health Care

The school nurse participates in the development of the IEP and provides service in the areas of school environmental safety, health services, and health education. The school nurse works with other school staff to ensure an accessible, safe physical environment. Children with **medical assistive devices** such as gastrostomies and oxygen machines may attend school. The school nurse works with the family, physician, home health nurse, and equipment source to establish an appropriate care plan. He or she provides or arranges for the child's direct care procedures at school.

School nurses are becoming familiar with the instructive devices and computer-driven environmental controls designed to enhance the learning and function of children with physical disabilities. The school nurse works with other members of the interdisciplinary team to ensure that the adaptive technology is comfortably and safely incorporated into the school and home environment of the child (Morse & Colatarci, 1994).

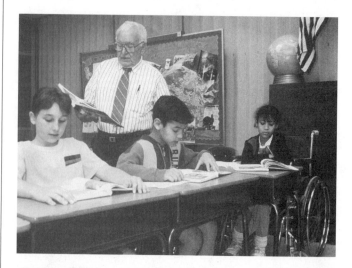

Children with developmental disabilities may be served by and encouraged to participate in traditional classrooms depending on the severity of their disability.

Self-Care Education

There are significant health education issues for children and adolescents with developmental disability. The children are learning that a condition may be permanent and that they must learn to manage it. Children with cerebral palsy or spina bifida must learn to manage orthopedic devices, skin care, or bowel and bladder routines. The child with epilepsy must learn to manage medications. A study of adults with moderate to mild mental retardation living in the community demonstrated that most could not identify their own health problems, convey their concerns to the health care provider, or follow written instructions (Edgerton, Gaston, Kelly, & Ward, 1994). The school nurse advocates for or develops general and individualized curricula that teach proper terminology, identification of common and special health problems, and appropriate health self-care. Nutrition and preventive dental care are important topics. One of the national objectives for the year 2000 targeting people with disabilities is the reduction of weight problems (USDHHS-PHS, 1996).

Sex education is often neglected because of the erroneous belief that people with disabilities are not going to be sexually active or reproduce. Early and continuing education on sexuality and family life is crucial for emotionally satisfactory adult life in the community and for prevention of unwanted pregnancies, sexually transmitted diseases, and sexual exploitation.

Many people with developmental disabilities can be vulnerable to sexual exploitation and abuse (Sobsey, 1994). See Table 22-4. Sex education content should include information on self-protection, sexually transmitted diseases including HIV infection, and safer sexual practices. Personal safety training should include training in personal rights, self-esteem, communication, social skills, and self-defense (Morse & Roth, 1994). School nurses and other community health nurses work with families to identify or develop programs of appropriate education. Curricula have been developed for children, adolescents, and adults with disabilities that can be used by parents, nurses, and teachers. Updated resources may be located through NICHCY.

Like all children and adolescents, those with developmental disabilities need education on drug, alcohol, and tobacco abuse, conflict resolution, and violence prevention. The school nurse teaches and counsels the individual student on those matters and promotes curricula for the classroom.

Table 22-4 Sexual Exploitation and Abuse of Persons with Developmental Disability

Traits of Some Persons That May Increase Vulnerability	Potential Vulnerable Situations
Normal sexual development and drives but limited social opportunities	Ability to find a suitable partner may be limited by factors beyond the individual's control such as physical attributes, societal rejection and devaluation, or restricted lifestyle. The person may tolerate someone who is exploitive or abusive in order to maintain the relationship.
Desire to be considered normal	Having a boyfriend or girlfriend or having a baby is evidence of normality. The individual may accept someone unsuitable or exploitive in order to be considered normal.
Trust and affection for the abuser	The person is easily persuaded to keep the abuse secret.
Limited ability to perceive an inappropriate social situation, limited understanding of the acts and their consequences, or socialized to be compliant and obedient	The individual is readily tricked and exploited by persons offering favors, professing affection, or exerting authority over the person.
Limited or no communication	The individual is unable to report abuse.
Physically unable to escape unwanted attention or assault	The person may have inadequate community living skills and may be unable to travel safely in the community. The living or work situation may be unsafe.
Environmental Risk Factors	
Isolated living site	Individual loses oversight protection of friends, family, or neighbors.
Multiple caregivers	Lack of attachment between individual and care providers increases risk of detachment and indifferent care and supervision.
Situation discourages independence	Individual does not learn how to resist abuse or seek help.
Individual devalued by significant people in his/her environment	Persons defined as "other," "less than," or "unworthy" are likely to become targets for abuse.

The school years can be a time when peers increasingly exclude the child with developmental disability from group activities. To compensate for this exclusion, the nurse can help the parents seek social and recreational opportunities for the client through sports such as Special Olympics, arts and crafts, parent- or church-sponsored activities, and public recreational programs. Teenagers may attend conferences sponsored by organizations for the challenged such as the Spina Bifida Association of America, Down Syndrome Congress, or United Cerebral Palsy. Many offer social and recreational opportunities for teens at the meetings as well as an opportunity to learn about their condition and its management (Johnson, 1996). Young adults may wish to join organizations, such as People First, that offer opportunities for self-advocacy. There are over 700 identified groups of people with disabilities working together to take charge of their lives and fight discrimination in the United States (Hayden, Lukin, Braddock, & Smith, 1995). Contact NICHCY for information.

Transition Services

As members of the community, persons with significant disabilities are expected to make long-term career plans, including plans for retirement (Harper, 1996; Szymanski & Maxwell, 1996). Many students will go on to college, and most, including persons with mild mental retardation, will seek competitive employment. For some, training beyond high school may be needed to prepare the young person for work and community living. Several federal laws make funds available to states for vocational training. Services are obtained through the state departments of vocational rehabilitation. An individual rehabilitation plan (IHP) that offers training and needed support services can be developed and funded. Work centers such as those supported by the Salvation Army or by parent organizations may be located through the local parent organization or state agency for persons with disability.

Graduates of special education programs are prepared for various levels of employment. Many enter competitive employment. Others obtain **supported employment** at which a job coach or other support ensures success at a competitive job. Still others train for **sheltered employment** at a work center where supports are available and individual productivity may be set at noncompetitive levels. Persons needing extensive or pervasive supports may enter an **activity center** and continue to be taught self-care, social skills, homemaking, and leisure activities skills.

One objective for the nation expressed in *Healthy People 2000* is to increase the number of worksites with a policy and program for hiring people with disabilities. Although discrimination against an employee or prospective employee solely because of disability is prohibited, the fact is that there are many young people with disabilities being prepared for work for whom there are no work programs and no jobs (Harper, 1996).

Perspectives...

Insights of a Resident in a Small Group Home

I didn't like being cooped up at the Developmental Center [large state residential facility]. I felt I was locked away in a home away from home, in a strange place. Now Pat is a nice house mother to me. I'm glad she took me in. Our house is nice and clean and I am living with my old friend Lloyd that I knew back at Bentley. He lets me help feed his dog at night. We share our dog. North Bay Regional Center helped buy our new house.

Work is wonderful. It's making me blossom into a nice woman. The workshop has plenty of windows I can see out of. I'm happy to be back in freedom-land now with no locked doors or high windows and I am surrounded by lovely dogs. I went to my first Special Olympics. I have good relaxation in my own private bedroom with my own TV and tapes. I'm glad I can go out in my electric wheelchair in my neighborhood safely.

It took me five years to get out of Sonoma. It was real hard. I won't ever have to go back again. My social worker, Blenda, helped me. Other people should get the chance to be on their own.

—*Beth Ratto*
Reprinted by permission from the North Bay Regional Center Newsletter, Napa, California, September, 1997, p. 2

ADULTHOOD

Most adults with developmental disabilities will independently and will no longer be perceived as needing services. Persons with mental retardation who are less able or persons with multiple disabilities need strong support to move from home into independent living, semi-independent living, or community residential programs. Many will continue to live with their families.

A proportion of adults with developmental disabilities who are unable to earn enough to become totally self-supporting will probably rely on some government or community benefits, in whole or in part. The standard benefits that most eligible persons may receive include Supplemental Security Income (SSI), Social Security Disability Income (SSDI), Medicare, Medicaid (in California, MediCAL), or community assistance. Obtaining and maintaining benefits can be difficult and confusing. The community nurse should help the adult identify someone to assist with application for benefits.

Residential Services

Since the 1970s programs of **deinstitutionalization** have moved persons from large institutions into smaller community settings. Many state-operated institutions have closed, and the populations in the remaining institutions continue to decrease. With deinstitutionalization there has been a growth in community residential facilities. In 1995, approximately 416,356 persons received community residential services, with over 68.2% living in settings with 16 or fewer residents (Prouty & Lakin, 1996).

Each state defines and licenses residential programs; terminology and regulations differ from state to state. Some areas have programs offering training in independent living with placement in supervised apartments or shared housing. Most areas offer licensed family care or foster care for persons of all ages. **Small-group residences,** housing with paid staff serving no more than 15 residents, are common. In some communities no more than six clients may be served in one small-group residence. Some are specialized, such as group homes for persons with autism, severe behavior problems, or special dietary needs such as diabetes. Some community facilities are licensed to give intermediate care (ICF/DD) with some Medicaid funding and usually serve multiply handicapped residents (Trent, 1994). See Table 22-5.

Health Care

Since the 1980s studies of adults with developmental disabilities living in the community and studies of people leaving the institutions indicate that many, because of associated problems, cannot be treated by the primary care physician alone. Associated problems are often hearing and vision loss and neurological, motor, cardiological, dental, behavioral, and psychiatric disorders. In addition,

it is difficult to develop adequate histories from verbally and cognitively limited clients. More time is required to work with uncomprehending and sometimes resistive persons and with changing care providers. Community health care practitioners may not be trained to serve the multiply handicapped person with developmental disability. And Medicaid, on whom most depend, often does not adequately reimburse for services. If coordinated and comprehensive health care is difficult to obtain, client health care suffers, resulting in delayed diagnoses, untreated conditions, and longer hospital stays (Minihan, Dean, & Lyon, 1993; Criscione, Walsh, & Kastner, 1995; Strauss & Kastner, 1996).

Community health nurses in most areas may find that easily accessible, comprehensive health care services for adults with complex problems associated with their diagnoses continue to be difficult to obtain. It is unclear at this writing how health care reforms may affect health care services for the more fragile clients. Under any system, the community health nurse is a key person to assess the special needs of adult clients, provide or obtain health care, and secure specialty services. The nurse may be the primary health care provider, the case manager, or the consultant to residential or work programs or to agencies serving people with disabilities. Whatever the setting, nurse advocacy for client health care may be the crucial element in obtaining comprehensive care.

Nursing Process

Although the nursing process for clients with disabilities is the same as for any client, special attention is needed for the following:

- *Communication.* Extra time may be needed to talk effectively with clients with limited understanding. Use more direct than open-ended questions. Sentences should be short and vocabulary simple. Request feedback frequently.
- *Data collection.* Make extra effort to obtain *all* prior medical records. Many clients cannot give an adequate history. Medical records are rarely transferred when clients change residence. It is not unusual to find surgical scars and never learn what procedure was done. Interview relatives, residential services providers, and friends for history and for sources of documented health history or hospital records.
- *Review latest literature on the client's particular disability.* New findings may dictate a changed approach to care.
- *Record the current level of self-care and other adaptive skills at each contact.* Physical, emotional, or degenerative conditions that the client is unable to identify may be expressed as loss of adaptive skills (see Table 22-3).
- *Nursing diagnoses.* In addition to health, diagnoses are usually needed to address self-care, motor problems, social and behavioral issues, communication, and family coping issues. Use of Orem's self-care model may be helpful. The model emphasizes developmental require-

Table 22-5 Residential Options for Persons with Developmental Disability

Residential services, terminology, and regulations differ from state to state. Services can be for-profit, nonprofit, or tax supported.

SMALL RESIDENTIAL FACILITIES: 16 OR FEWER PERSONS

Supported living	The individual lives in the same type of housing as others in the community and receives as much support as desired or needed.
Supervised living	The individual lives in regular housing, and staff from a support program monitor and continue to train the client for community living.
Child or adult foster home	The individual lives as a member of the family. Usually, the home serves no more than six residents. Some homes are licensed to care for fragile children or adults, and the service provider performs care and necessary treatments such as gastrostomy feedings. In some areas, the provider must be a licensed nurse. In others, lay providers are trained and nurses visit to consult or monitor care.
Group home	Staff provide care, supervision, and training. Some homes provide specialized care for persons with physical limitations, dietary needs, or behavior problems.
Personal care home	Staff provide personal assistance but no training.
Boarding home	Room and board are provided, but no personal care or training is offered.
Intermediate care facility (ICF/MR or DD)	Staff provide 24-hour care and training with registered nurse to supervise health care services.

LARGE RESIDENTIAL FACILITIES: 16 OR MORE PERSONS

State-supported or private developmental centers (formerly called institutions)	Staff provide 24-hour care and training with available intermediate care and often skilled nursing care.
Group homes	Offer similar services as small group homes.
Intermediate care facilities	Regular ICFs may admit a person with a developmental disability.

ments as well as health and supports normalization (Rice, 1994).

- *Nursing plans/interventions.* Confer with the client and care providers. Ensure that interventions are compatible with the normalization principle and serve also to enhance appearance, elicit age-appropriate behavior, and promote self-advocacy as well as health. Copies of the plan should go to the client and any significant person he or she indicates. Consider obtaining Medic-Alert identification.
- *Evaluation.* Update adaptive skills level as well as health status.
- *Client assistance.* Encourage the client with cognitive limitations to identify a trusted person to assist with access to health care and implementation of health care recommendations.

Behavior Disorders and Mental Illness

Clients with developmental disabilities may also exhibit behavior problems or signs of mental illness. These diffi-culties present additional challenges to the community health nurse.

Behavior Disorders

Adults with developmental disabilities who come to the attention of the community health nurse because of behavior disorders are likely to be persons with mental retardation, severe pervasive developmental disability, or multiple disabilities, or they may be persons with a behavior disorder related to the diagnosis, as in fragile X syndrome. Problem behaviors can include noncompliance, temper outbursts, regression in skills, withdrawal, aggression, repetitive behaviors, and hyperactivity.

Nurses working with clients on behavior problems need to try to communicate at length with them, interview persons who know them well in different settings, assess their environment for precipitating factors, and review the health history and adaptive behavior. Frequently, physical problems that the client cannot identify or report, such as headache, dysmenorrhea, toothache, or constipation, can be the source of the problem. Environmental changes can also evoke behavior problems. The solution could be a change of roommate or routines or a new type of recreation. A loss such as a quarrel with a friend, a change of instructor, or a death in the family can also trigger behavior problems. The person may be reacting to some form of abuse that he or she is unable to communicate. Correcting the underlying problem or instituting a short-term behavioral program with the client often can resolve the situation.

Because behavior problems can be a symptom of illness, emotional problems, or both, services of an interdisciplinary medical-behavioral team should be sought. The community health nurse can be the one to identify, obtain, and coordinate the services of the appropriate behavioral specialist and physician.

Mental Illness

Studies indicate that persons with developmental disabilities are at increased risk of psychiatric disorder. The term *psychiatric disorder* is often used for both severe behavior disorders and major mental illness. Exact figures for the prevalence of major mental illness for persons in each category of developmental disability are few. However, it is recognized that persons with mental retardation have more mental illness than persons without mental retardation. Prevalence figures range from 30% to 35% (Meyers, 1996) and from 20% to 60% (Fletcher & Poindexter, 1996). Persons with mental retardation living in the community can have all types of mental illness: psychoses, neuroses, personality disorders, or adjustment reactions. Factors influencing the risk for these disorders are associated medical, physical, sensory, and learning problems as well as family factors, restricted life experiences, and society's rejection and devaluation (Meyers, 1996).

Until recently, mental illness in persons with mental retardation was often not recognized, diagnosed, or treated but was assumed to be the expression of mental retardation. It is now understood that standardized diagnostic procedures with additional protocols to assess persons with mental retardation can provide accurate diagnoses of mental illnesses. Clients can respond to a wide range of therapies, including psychotherapy or group therapy adapted to the client's level of understanding. Drug therapy, based on the diagnosis, and behavior therapy are also effective. Ideally, acute mental health needs of persons with mental retardation and other developmental disabilities are met in the community-based psychiatric setting. Their long-term mental health care needs are met in community programs for persons with developmental disabilities with support and consultation from the mental health system (Fletcher & Poindexter, 1996; Meyers, 1996).

Nursing Care

Psychiatric nurses provide the same nursing interventions for developmentally disabled clients as those used in general mental health settings, adapted for the client's level of understanding (see Chapter 23). The nurse

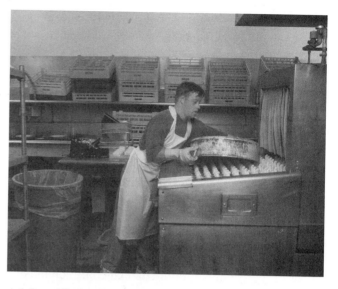

Adults with developmental disabilities work and volunteer in the community. Photo courtesy of Ed Young/Corbis.

works with family or residential staff members to provide the optimal environment for the client (Gabriel, 1994). All community health nurses promote the mental health of persons with developmental disabilities by focusing on client self-determination, establishment of a stable living arrangement satisfactory to the client, socialization opportunities, regular exercise, and recreation (O'Brien, 1994).

Family Life

Persons with developmental disabilities mature, form relationships, marry, and have children. This fact attracts little attention unless the disability is mental retardation. Public, professional, and family concerns center on parents with mental retardation. There is concern that the disability of the parent can be transmitted to the child and concern that the parents cannot care adequately for their children.

When a parent's condition is due to genetic factors, the child may be at risk, depending on the mode of transmission. When the cause of the parent's condition is not known, having one or both parents with retardation may also increase the risk for the child. The ability of the parents to care for the child is difficult to predict and depends on many factors. Community health nurses working with these families on the health care aspects of child rearing are in a key position to assess parenting skills.

Booth and Booth (1994) reviewed available literature on parents with mental retardation in the United States and England. The parents studied were not representative of all adults with mental retardation; they were identified through child protective services, residential settings, or special workshops as at risk of inadequate parenting. Nevertheless, the researchers found:

- There was no clear relationship between parental competency and intelligence; IQ does not predict parenting skills.

- Parental weaknesses included insufficient cognitive stimulation of the child, inconsistent discipline, lack of expressed warmth and affection, and inability to adjust parenting to developmental changes in the child.
- Socioeconomic effects were confounded with the effects of mental retardation. Inadequate child care was often due to poverty, unemployment, poor vocational skills, isolation, and poor health. Parents were held to an unfairly high standard of child care dictated by middle-class values rather than those of their own culture.
- Parental skills can be improved with training. The children initially assessed as normal can continue to make developmental progress. Long-term studies are needed to assess parental retention and generalization.

Community health nurses address the health care needs of these families, offer parental education in child care, and monitor the welfare and development of the children. They promote socialization by demonstrating interactions with the child, teach recognition of illness and environmental hazards, and teach preventive care and use of health care. They address the socioeconomic problems that hinder adequate child care through use of resources such as food programs. They seek social supports such as the help of a relative or friend to guide parents in the day-to-day work of child care. The children are referred to early intervention programs for at-risk children, to preschool programs, or to Head Start (Kaatz, 1992). When parental education requirements are extensive, the nurse seeks more intensive support services. Throughout the United States there are programs that offer in-home or classroom tutoring to parents with mental retardation. Help may be obtained through agencies serving persons with developmental disabilities, child protective services, or Head Start. The community health nurse can be the one to encourage work centers serving persons with developmental disability or the local adult education department to offer specialized, intensive training to parents with cognitive limitations. Young people contemplating marriage and childbirth can be

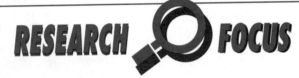

RESEARCH FOCUS

Home Environments of Mothers with Mental Retardation

STUDY PROBLEM/PURPOSE

To discriminate the risk to children's development due to maternal mental retardation from the risk to development due to poverty.

METHODS

A controlled comparison was made between two groups of mothers with children. Both groups of women were poor and on Aid to Families with Dependent Children. The Slosson Intelligence Test—Revised was administered to each woman, and results were used to create two groups. One group (N = 38) was composed of mothers with IQs of 75 or less. The other group (N = 27) was composed of mothers with IQs of 85 or greater. The two groups were matched on age, race, and parity. They were followed prospectively for two years. The Home Observation for Measurement of the Environment (HOME), an instrument designed to measure environmental supports for child development, was administered to the children at 5, 10, 18, and 24 months. The instrument has six subscales designed to measure factors of the home environment: (1) emotional and verbal responsivity of the parent to the child, (2) acceptance of the child's behavior, (3) organization of the environment, (4) provision of play material, (5) parental involve-ment with the child, and (6) opportunities for variety. There is a possible total score of 45.

FINDINGS

The mothers with intellectual limitations had lower total scores than the mothers with normal intelligence. Statistical analysis of the scores indicated the differences between the two groups to be highly significant.

Two subscales, emotional and verbal responsivity to the child and parental involvement with the child, accounted for the differences between the two groups. No significant differences between the two groups on the other subscales were found.

IMPLICATIONS

Home environments already inadequate because of poverty are made more inadequate by maternal intellectual limitations. The children from homes with lower HOME scores are at greater developmental risk owing to environmental deprivation. The results also suggest that nursing strategies promoting positive maternal–child interactions would be beneficial in assisting mothers with intellectual limitation in raising their children.

SOURCE

From "Home Environments of Mothers with Mental Retardation" by B. Keltner, 1994, Mental Retardation, 32, *pp. 123–127.*

offered family life and parent education through the same resources.

As noted in the Research Focus, Keltner (1994) conducted research to discriminate the effects of maternal mental retardation on child development from the effects of poverty. Her research also shows that nursing interventions to support mother and child interactions can be effective in helping mothers with cognitive limitations.

OLD AGE

Persons with developmental disabilities are living longer. By the year 2000 it is estimated that in the United States there will be 362,520 persons age 65 and over with a developmental disability and 672,560 such persons by the year 2040. These estimates are based on prevalence rates for cerebral palsy, epilepsy, autism, and mental retardation (Nutt & Malone, 1992) and do not take into account persons with other developmental disabilities, such as learning disabilities.

A longitudinal study of a group of institutionalized persons with mental retardation who left the institution as adults found that, as they grew older, their lives improved. Their sense of stigma lessened, and they developed confidence in their ability to manage on their own. They worked, made friends, and reported themselves satisfied with their lives. The researchers found that the greatest dangers they now faced in old age were illness and lack of adequate medical care (Edgerton 1991; Edgerton et al., 1994).

Persons with developmental disability face all the age-related health conditions of their nondisabled peers. In addition, it is known that particular developmental disorders have significant impact as the person ages. For example, older persons with cerebral palsy have greater risks of contractures, ambulation and balance decline, immobility is progressive and there may be difficulties in swallowing (Murphy et al., 1995). Persons with Down syndrome are very prone to periodontal disease and are at increased risk of dementia as they age. Elderly persons with developmental disability can become depressed. Also, what appears to be withdrawal may instead be a reaction to declining vision, hearing, or mobility. Older persons with disabilities requiring long-term medication for physical or emotional problems are at risk of overmedication and polypharmacy. In addition to specialized health care related to age and diagnoses, they need preventive care such as mammograms and prostate examinations (Edgerton et al., 1994), more and better in-home services, and family support services to prevent institutionalization (Seltzer & Luchterhand, 1994; Zigman, Seltzer, & Silverman, 1994).

Community health nurses address the health care needs of the older client through the nursing process with special attention to the diagnosis and its impact as the client ages. Particular attention is directed to assessment of adaptive skills, mental status, and the social support system available to the client. The client should be con-

DECISION MAKING

Mario

Mario, a middle-aged man with severe mental retardation and related cardiac problems, had always lived at home. The family had never sought services, and Mario was not known to any agency. After his mother died, his father assumed his care. A neighbor, aware of the father's failing health and Mario's progressively poorer care including missed medications and inappropriate diet, notified the community health nurse in the agency serving people with developmental disabilities. When the nurse called on the father to provide information about services, he became indignant. He said, "We Italians take care of our own." It was obvious, however, that extensive support was needed to maintain Mario in the family home.

- How would you proceed?
- How can the father's culture-based plan of care be acknowledged?
- Who might you enlist to talk with the father about Mario's future care?
- What resources for care can you define?

sulted about hobbies, recreation, work, and retirement plans, and the client's wishes should be respected.

At some point, both the client living at home and the client living independently may need more care and supervision. Resources for the elderly are licensed family homes, small-group residences, or the intermediate care facilities for the developmentally disabled. Those with nursing care needs may be admitted to a regular skilled nursing care facility. Not all communities have the full array of services.

The nurse provides anticipatory guidance to help the family or individual plan for the future. In addition to health care, there frequently are issues of conservatorship, inheritance, housing, financial support, or aging parents to be resolved. In addition to NICHCY, an information resource for families and professionals is the National Institute for Life Planning for Persons with Disabilities, 513 Carriage Lane, Twin Falls, ID 83301.

THE FUTURE

Persons with developmental disability, particularly persons with mental retardation, have had their civil rights acknowledged in law and have entered schools, the workplace, and the community. They have also assumed the risks of community living with perhaps less preparation than those without disabilities. Those with more serious conditions who are trying to live independently or trying to establish families will need extensive systems of support to function comfortably and safely.

COMMUNITY NURSING VIEW

Mrs. Palma has come with her daughter, Mary, to talk to the community health nurse at the local agency serving persons with developmental disability. Mrs. Palma is considering having Mary sterilized and wants the nurse to advise how to go about it. Mary, now 20, has cerebral palsy and is mildly mentally retarded. She ambulates with a cane. She has dysarthria but can be readily understood.

Mrs. Palma, 50, is a widow with two sons married and living out of the home. Her large extended family is Filipino and Catholic; they are well-educated, with ample incomes.

Mary completed high school in special classes. Her general level of understanding is similar to that of a 12-year-old. She attends a work center that offers training in workplace behavior and specific job skills. Her mother permitted her to enter the work center against family advice because Mary was lonely and bored and wanted something to do. The family objected because of unsupervised contacts with male coworkers and because they do not expect a family member with physical difficulties to work.

Mrs. Palma is very distressed because Mary has paired off with a young man at the work center. This situation is bad enough, but pregnancy would be a disgrace.

Mrs. Palma is very angry with the work center staff. They tell her that Mary is an adult and is free to choose to have a boyfriend and to be sexually active. They say it is not normalizing to expect Mary to stay home with her mother. They expect to train her in community living skills needed for apartment living and for a job. Mrs. Palma has tried to tell them this plan is inappropriate. A Filipina of good family lives at home until marriage, and, of course, Mary will never marry.

Mrs. Palma reports that Mary's judgment is poor. She has never gone out alone. She is very careless about bathing, menstrual hygiene, and dental care. She doesn't even hang up her clothes. Her mother is sure that Mary cannot manage more complicated responsibilities, and she plans to consult her attorney and obtain conservatorship. Despite her religious beliefs, she thinks sterilization is the way to protect Mary.

Mary is quietly defiant. She is proud of having a boyfriend as other girls do. She thinks she would like a big wedding like her cousins have had. She is willing to learn to improve her grooming in order to look pretty. She thinks it might be fun to have a little baby after she is married.

Nursing Considerations

Use family development theory, the principle of normalization, and the concept of self-care to develop the nursing process suitable for this case.

ASSESSMENT

- What further data from the family, Mary, and work center would be useful?
- What is the family life cycle stage?
- Has Mary's disability significantly altered the usual pattern?
- How can nursing intervention encourage the most normal pattern?
- What is normalization from the point of view of Mrs. Palma, Mary, and the work center staff?
- What is Mary capable of learning?
- What are her legal rights?

DIAGNOSIS

- What diagnoses can be formulated concerning family function?
- Does Mary have self-care deficits that can be defined and addressed by nursing interventions?
- What self-care requisites may Mary face in the future?
- What should the nursing plan include?

OUTCOME IDENTIFICATION

- What are the desired outcomes?

PLANNING/INTERVENTIONS

- What objectives can be formulated that meet the criteria for success as defined by Mary? By Mrs. Palma?
- What nursing interventions can be applied?
- How are interventions made compatible with the principle of normalization?
- What resources may be used?

EVALUATION

- How and on what time table can the plan be reviewed by the Palma family?
- Have the criteria for success been met? If they have, what new goals may be considered?

Forty years is a relatively brief time to establish the attitudes and social changes that have been so beneficial to persons with developmental disabilities. Under adverse economic and political conditions, less kindly attitudes toward persons with developmental disability may appear as they did in the past. Against that possibility, women and men with disabilities speak for themselves through organizations such as People First International or TASH: The Association for Persons with Severe Handicaps. Their families also may be active in advocacy. Community health nurses and other health professionals serve as advocates from a personal or professional platform. People thus united can retain and expand the systems of individual and family supports that maintain people with developmental disabilities in the community.

Key Concepts

- *Developmental disability* as a legal term groups people with similar service needs but with different medical diagnoses. *Developmental disability* employed as a clinical term refers to persons with permanent central nervous system conditions that vary in severity, in degree of resulting handicap, and in expression over time. The most common conditions regarded as developmental disabilities are mental retardation, epilepsy, autism, cerebral palsy, and learning disability.

- Changing social attitudes and general acceptance of the principle of normalization led to increased services, support for community living, and affirmation of the legal rights of all persons with developmental disabilities.

- A significant number of conditions leading to and problems associated with developmental disability are preventable or remediable. Community health nurses provide preventive interventions in most interactions with individuals and families.

- The goal of community health nursing is to promote the highest level of health and social functioning of persons with developmental disabilities. Nurses define and address the developmental, health, cognitive, social, behavioral, and emotional issues related to a particular disability at a particular point in the client's life. The nurse participates in or organizes the interdisciplinary services that may be needed to solve complex health problems. Individual nursing care plans are needed over the life span in response to changing health care needs.

- Early and sustained support to at-risk or delayed infants and their families promote optimal child health and development and family functioning.

- Individual education plans for school children with developmental disability must include instruction on health, self-care, family life and sex, and self-protection.

- Persons with developmental disability are at risk of behavior problems and mental illness. Nurses promote client mental health by supporting self-determination, optimal living conditions, and satisfactory social relations.

- Parents with mental retardation and other developmental disabilities can be good parents. Some may require extensive family supports to be successful. Nurses are key persons to identify the need and organize supports.

- Older persons with developmental disabilities are at risk of specific health problems related to their diagnoses as well as health problems related to aging. Specialized health and community support services will be needed in their communities.

- Current benign attitudes toward persons with mental retardation and other developmental disabilities can return to more negative ones in response to political or economic pressures. Supports may be curtailed or withdrawn. Nurses and other citizens advocate for the rights of all people with developmental disabilities.

Mental Health and Illness

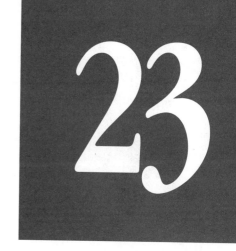

David Becker, MS, RN, CS, CNAA
Barouk Golden, MS, RN

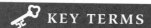

KEY TERMS

deinstitutionalization
ego
id
Mental Hygiene
  Movement
neurotransmitter
operant conditioning
psychoanaylsis
psychotherapy
stigma
superego

We cannot live for ourselves alone. Our lives are connected by a thousand invisible threads, and along these sympathetic fibers, our actions run as causes and return as results.

—*Herman Melville (1819–1891)*

COMPETENCIES

Upon completion of this chapter, the reader should be able to:

- Identify selected historical, political, and economic foundations of the concept of community mental health.
- Discuss the relationships among the various nursing, behavioral, and biological concepts and theories that guide the nurse in community mental health work.
- Identify the range of settings in which the community health nurse works with mental health clients.
- Discuss the nursing health promotion/illness prevention activities that address the continuum of mental illness in the community.
- Describe the importance of interdisciplinary teamwork in mental health nursing in the community.
- Discuss the adaptations required by clients with major mental illness in order to function in the community.

It is not supposed to work this way: The most severely ill among us not only have multiple illnesses but also are less likely to receive any treatment. The National Comorbidity Survey (Kessler, McGonagle, Zhao, Nelson, Hughes, Eshleman, Wittchen, & Kendler, 1994) discovered a much greater prevalence of mental illness in the general population than had been thought. Nearly 50% of those surveyed had or once had a diagnosable mental health disorder. Fourteen percent of the population had a history of three or more disorders over a lifetime. The majority of people with severe mental health disorders had more than one diagnosis. Most significantly, less than 40% of those who had ever had a diagnosable disorder had received any treatment. Community health nurses are uniquely positioned to reach out to those who are suffering from mental illness, uncovering and removing the barriers to mental health. Skilled and accessible, nurses are often more acceptable to clients who fear or have given up on professionals specializing in mental health.

This chapter will discuss the foundations for caring, including nursing theories, for clients who are mentally ill. The community nurse's role is disucssed, including basic screening and assessment, support interventions, and advanced psychiatric mental health nursing.

The poem in the accompanying perspectives box was written by one of the clients of a large state mental hospital as he contemplated what it might be like to enter what was to him an unfamiliar and unwelcoming place that we call "the community."

REFLECTIVE THINKING

Judging vs. Assessing

• What are my beliefs and values relating to mental health and mental illness?

• How do I know when I am being judgmental, and how do I avoid judging my clients' choices and behavior?

• How can I periodically evaluate my assumptions about a client's situation against his or her own experience of the world?

• How do I work with people who are different?

• How can I make professional assessments, as opposed to personal judgments?

Listening to our clients' voices is essential in developing, implementing, and evaluating community practice and programs. Keep listening for them, in the following pages, in other media, and in your practice.

FOUNDATIONS OF CARING

The practice of the community health nurse working with clients who are mentally ill must be guided by an understanding of history, politics, economics, and biology. Nursing theories as well as principles developed by the allied health disciplines of psychiatry, psychology, and social work also apply to mental health work.

The national health objectives for the year 2000, commonly referred to as the *Healthy People 2000* report, were developed by a consortium of over 300 national organizations, state health departments, and the Institute of Medicine of the National Academy of Sciences. They were published by the U.S. Department of Health and Human Services in 1990 and were revised in 1995, providing an agenda for the future. Community health nurses can make great contributions toward achieving the mental health objectives (see Appendix A for the details of objective 6) in a variety of ways, including, for example, reducing the incidence of depression in women (statistics show that women suffer from depression at twice the rate of men) and reducing the adolescent suicide attempt rates, which by 1995 had increased 200% from 1990 (U.S. Department of Health and Human Services [USDHHS], 1996). Nurses work in a variety of community settings, putting them in a position to identify problems and intervene, often before others in the family or the health care system are likely to recognize that there is a problem.

Historical Foundations

Attitudes toward the care and treatment of mentally ill persons have nearly always differed from those with recognized physical disease. For many people, a "sick mind" has different connotations than a sick body, and the difference has existed for centuries. Behavioral symptoms of what we now understand to be psychoneurobiological conditions were seen as evidence of demonic possession or at least grave sin. The struggles that early psychiatrists had with laypeople and the clergy for the right to treat the

Perspectives...

Insights of an Agnews State Resident

They're closing Agnews State
Where we hid empty wine bottles
In laundry baskets.
They're closing Agnews State
Where old men passed out flowers
In the canteen.
They're closing Agnews State
Where volunteers from the Red Cross
Cared enough to dance with you.

They're closing Agnews State
Where the gophers pop their heads out of lawns
And say "hi" to you.
They're closing Agnews State
Where Billy Hamilton broke a window
After every shock treatment.
They're closing Agnews State
And opening up lonely hearts' clubs.

—Yoga Bare (1974)
"Requiem for Agnews State"

mentally ill led to further isolation of both treater and the treated (Porter, 1989).

Community health nurses serving psychiatric and mental health clients are part of a historical alteration in the way humanity deals with mental health and mental illness. The current shift of mental health care to community agencies has been called the "third psychiatry revolution" (Kaplan, Sadock, & Grebb, 1998).

Moral Treatment and Psychoanalysis: The First and Second Revolutions

The first revolution occurred in the mid to late 18th century, as Western culture shifted its thinking about those who behaved in a difficult, dangerous, or worrisome way. After persecuting some and either hiding or ignoring others, society finally established asylums where rational, moral treatment was employed to restore reason. As historian Porter (1989) put it: "The madhouse should thus become a reform school." Late-19th century advances in science brought the second revolution, when the increasing power and prestige of medicine were applied to the issue. In the first half of this century, Freud and others shifted mainstream thinking about the cause of madness away from moral laxness to illnesses caused by unresolved infantile conflicts due to faulty parenting. Through all this, society tended to blame those suffering for causing the condition.

Sigmund Freud (1938) developed the concepts that explained mental illness as being caused by faulty mental mechanisms. **Psychoanalysis** offered hope in the form of a "talking cure." As a treatment technique, psychoanalysis uses free association and the interpretation of dreams to trace emotions and behaviors to repressed drives and instincts. By making the client aware of the existence, origins, and inappropriate expression of these unconscious processes, psychoanalysis helps the client eliminate or diminish undesirable affects.

By the end of World War II, the asylums begun in the 18th century had evolved to very large state hospitals. In these institutions, psychoanalysis met with limited success in the vast majority of patients with serious mental illness. Thus, the third revolution, which had begun with a pre-war **Mental Hygiene Movement,** a movement emphasizing education and public awareness techniques to promote prevention and effective treatment, gained momentum in conjunction with the great advances in the use of psychotropic drugs.

Community Mental Health Movement: The Third Revolution

This third revolution, the community mental health movement, is concerned with the prevention and treatment of mental illness and with the rehabilitation of former psychiatric clients through the use of organized community programs, including community health nursing. Some of these programs are specialized community psychiatric/mental health services, staffed by advanced practice mental health nurses. Other programs are more general, such as senior centers or home nursing agencies. The focus of this chapter is on community health nurses working with psychiatric/mental health clients in the latter type of agency. Community health nurses serve in what could be described as the area of overlap between community health nursing and community mental health. See Figure 23-1.

The historical shifts in attitudes and approaches to mental health and mental illness illustrate that physical punishment, isolation, work farms, and long-term corrective relationships with a therapist have each, in turn, been

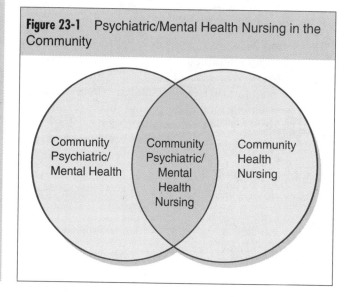

Figure 23-1 Psychiatric/Mental Health Nursing in the Community

Community Psychiatric/Mental Health

Community Psychiatric/Mental Health Nursing

Community Health Nursing

accepted as correct responses to the phenomenon of mental illness. Considering the historical perspective helps nurses understand why many clients and families of mental health clients feel shame, mistrust, or anger dealing with members of the health professions, especially those in mental health. The disgrace or reproach experienced by mentally ill persons and their families is referred to as **stigma.** Community health nurses may encounter this in the form of hostility in dealing with clients, their families, and members of the community. For this reason it is useful to emphasize the community health nurse's identification with health-promotion activities such as prenatal and well-child clinics, which are less threatening to clients and do not carry the stigma of the mental health system.

Even though science has provided a better understanding of the psychoneurobiological processes that are now thought to cause mental illness, historical attitudes based on faulty understanding continue to influence health professionals as well as the general population. The nurse, through a self-examination of prejudices and attitudes, can begin to prepare to correct the misunderstandings of clients, their families, the community, and other health care workers. From a historical perspective, a community in which families are not blamed, treatment is not feared, and clients and those who serve them are not stigmatized is long overdue.

Theories and Concepts from Allied Disciplines

Nursing practice in community mental health involves much greater interdisciplinary teamwork than in typical nursing settings. A fundamental understanding of psychiatry, psychology, social work, and rehabilitation therapies is necessary to achieve an effective interdisciplinary practice. Conversely, the nurse must be prepared to present a

theoretically based nursing view to colleagues from other disciplines. Creating or maintaining such a team is a continuing challenge in today's rapidly changing health care environment.

Psychodynamic Theories

Sigmund Freud (1938) postulated the existence of a set of mental structures: the **superego,** or conscience; the unconscious **id;** and the **ego,** which mediates between the id and the superego. Examining these can lead to uncovering unconscious conflict among them. Such conflicts, Freud claimed, are the source of mental illness. Through psychoanalysis, the client can gain insight: that is, can bring these unconscious conflicts into conscious awareness and thus be cured. Although the theories of traditional psychoanalytic treatment offer little for nurses, the vocabulary developed to explain Freud's theories is still widely used to describe clients' defense mechanisms, personality development, and relationships with others.

Social-Interpersonal Theories

Evolving from psychoanalytic theory, social-interpersonal theories emphasize the developmental influences of family and society. Mental health problems are seen to be, at their core, interpersonal problems. Improvement in interpersonal functioning is the means toward meeting psychosocial needs and decreasing mental health problems. Self-actualization is the ultimate fulfillment of a hierarchy of needs (Maslow, 1962). These ideas guide many nursing concepts and interventions. Sullivan (1953) is best known for his creative psychotherapy working with severely disturbed patients. Unlike Freud, Sullivan thought that even the most psychotic patients suffering from schizophrenia could be reached through the human relationship of **psychotherapy,** the process of addressing symptom relief, resolution of problems or personal growth through interacting in a prescribed way with a therapist. Peplau used Sullivan's concepts to develop a theory conceptualizing nursing as an interpersonal relationship (Meleis, 1997). Social theory provides nurses with a framework for personal interventions with clients and families and for community and political action.

Behavioral Theories

Many of the theories previously mentioned were of little interest to B. F. Skinner (1953) and the behaviorists who followed. In their view, observable behavior is the only certain foundation for assessing a client's state. Behavioral change is the only appropriate goal. **Operant conditioning** is the concept of seeking to discover what elicits a particular behavior in the first place and what subsequently reinforces it. These reinforcements can be manipulated to shape behavior and thereby to improve the client's functioning. Nurses use behavior theory to understand and manage behavioral symptoms and to teach appropriate life skills.

❧❧ REFLECTIVE THINKING ❧❧

A Balance of Rights and Needs

The person with a mental disorder has the same right to freedom and informed consent to treatment as any other citizen. When clients refuse treatment, their rights can conflict with our humanitarian impulse and professional obligation to relieve the suffering caused by the disorder. Their refusal can also provoke fear that untreated or unrestrained mentally ill persons in the community could behave in a disturbing, disruptive, or even violent manner.

• How do you feel about a client's refusal of treatment?

• How do you respond to some persons' fear of untreated mentally ill persons?

Neurobiological Concepts

Over time, practitioners using a medical model have used all of the foregoing theories, sometimes in combination, often with a preference for one or the other. As it is evolving, however, the medical model increasingly addresses emotional and behavioral problems as illnesses like any other. Assessment of clients is based on their symptoms. The problem addressed is an illness caused by a pathological process: lesion, toxin, or abnormality of neuroanatomy or **neurotransmitter.** The neurotransmitters are nervous system chemicals that facilitate the transmission of impulses across the synapses between neurons and are the subject of a great deal of current research. In this model, symptoms of disease are to be measured, then managed, while a cure is sought.

Nurses use these neurobiological concepts to care for clients taking powerful psychotropic drugs (and occasionally other somatic treatments) now widely used to treat mental illness. Nurses need to stay abreast of the research findings in the biological factors of mental disorders.

Nursing Theories

Nursing theories and conceptual models are often given limited attention in community mental health nursing. Nursing theorists who emphasize caring and principles of communication and relationship in their models have particular relevance to mental health nursing. These theorists (Watson, Leininger, Neuman, Peplau, Orlando, Benner) stress that care provided through the nurse–client relationship is a core component and the basis of excellence in nursing practice. Both objective and subjective (feelings and intuitions) observations by the nurse are of value (Meleis, 1997). The nurse is both an observer and a participant in the therapeutic relationship. The nurse relates to the client as a complete human being while directing nursing interventions on the symptomatic level.

DECISION MAKING

Family Disruption

You have been working with a family in which the mother has not left the house in six months and the 26-year-old single daughter is three months pregnant. The daughter wants the mother to be with her when she has her baby. The mother would like to accompany her daughter but is afraid to leave the house, let alone go to the hospital with her daughter.

• Given your knowledge of treatment of phobic disorders, what steps would you take to set mutual goals in this family?

• Do you think it is possible to meet the daughter's request? Why? Why not?

There are useful principles in most nursing theories. For the community health nurse working with mentally ill clients, the theories of Peplau and Orem may be most practical. The nurse–patient relationship is central to Peplau's (1952) nursing theory. She shifted the focus of interest from what the nurse does *for* the client to what the nurse can do *with* the client, such as mutually set goals and other interactions. She identified the stages of the nurse–client relationship as orientation, introduction, working, and termination. Orem's (1995) concepts of self-care can be easily adopted by the community health nurse, especially in addressing the needs of the chronically mentally ill.

CURRENT INFLUENCES ON COMMUNITY MENTAL HEALTH

Political, economic, and cultural events have greatly influenced the way society attempts to assist its members with mental illness. The following factors have had great impact on increasing the mental health aspects of the community health nurse's work.

Community Mental Health Reform

In response to the problems of what were seen to be expensive and dehumanizing large state mental hospitals, in 1963 Congress began to fund community mental health centers. These agencies were established to provide inpatient and outpatient services to specific geographic areas and populations of 75,000 to 200,000 as an alternative to long-term inpatient hospitalization. Twenty-four-hour emergency services and partial hospitalization options (day, evening, aftercare, halfway houses) were offered. This legislation helped to transform the way society treats mentally ill persons. Unfortunately, political and economic constraints, such as the expense of public funding for free-standing mental health centers, have always limited full realization of the intended benefits of community mental health reform.

Deinstitutionalization

In the 1960s, legal reforms making it harder to commit someone to hospitalization involuntarily, political actions limiting the budgets of the state hospitals, and the promise (which many say went unfulfilled) of the community mental health centers led to a great shift in the lives of patients with chronic, severe mental illness. The new initiative, called **deinstitutionalization,** was to discharge large numbers of patients from public mental hospitals into communities.

Deinstitutionalization requires that a range of supportive services be available and utilized. In most communities,

✿ REFLECTIVE THINKING ✿

Your Dream House

You just bought your dream house. It has all the features you want, including a quiet neighborhood, good schools, and friendly neighbors. You've settled in to raise your family and just now learn that the city is holding hearings on a plan to establish a transitional residence (halfway house) one block from your home. The facility will be in a large single-family house and will serve six psychiatric patients who need preparation for fully independent living. You understand how important and effective these programs are and that the same things that attracted you to the neighborhood make it a great choice for the program. You are concerned about its impact on your family. Your neighbors expect you to go the hearings and demonstrate against the plan.

- How do you feel about having a halfway house in the next block?

- What do you think about the idea of speaking out, pro or con, about the halfway house at a public hearing?

- What do you think about the idea of participating at a demonstration, either supporting or opposing, the halfway house?

- How does the pressure from neighbors influence your decision?

adequate services to meet the needs of the clients are not present. As a result, these former clients often regress, exhibiting increased symptoms and related problems such as homelessness and petty crime.

Economic Factors

Insurance and other third-party payors provide less coverage for treatment of mental illness and substance abuse than they do for other medical conditions. Private insurers often limit coverage to 30 to 60 inpatient days, and Medicare requires a 50% co-payment for mental health services. Recognizing that mentally ill people are stigmatized and have limited access to the services they need, the National Advisory Mental Health Council (1993), among others, has called for equitable coverage in any reform of state or federal health care finance systems.

Consumer Activism

The foremost example of effective consumer involvement in mental health is the National Alliance for the Mentally Ill (NAMI). The NAMI was formed in 1979 by people who wanted to learn how to help themselves and their mentally ill relatives. For decades, parents had been blamed for their children's mental disorders. Through the supportive networks formed by NAMI, families find the courage and hope to advocate for needed changes in public policy and attitudes. By working together, this group and those like it support one another, provide information to other consumers regarding services available, advise professionals and politicians regarding needed services, and advocate for effective humane services (National Alliance for the Mentally Ill, 1993).

Cultural Factors

Culture is an observable manifestation of inner life as displayed by manners, customs, skills, language, parent–child interactions, beliefs, and social life. Because mental health and illness are often demonstrated in terms of behavior, an understanding of cultural factors is often necessary to make sense of a client's behavior and to plan interventions that are appropriate for a particular client.

Too often, nurses with a background in the dominant culture are unaware of their own cultural heritage and especially of its unexamined customs, beliefs, manners, and so on. Keeping mindful of their own cultural heritage allows nurses to better assist clients from another culture.

Research in anthropology, ethnopsychiatry, and transcultural nursing informs nursing practice in several ways. Nurses can find data on culture-specific concepts of space, time orientation, language, and health beliefs and practices to guide their work with specific groups. (See Chapter 6).

Symptoms of the major mental disorders exist among all cultures (Kaplan et al., 1998). Although the presenting symptoms generally conform to the diagnostic categories of the *Diagnostic and Statistical Manual of Mental Disorders*, commonly called the DSM (American Psychiatric Association, 1994), clients and their families may use indigenous labels to describe their experience of a mental illness. Many of these labels have been cataloged in a Glossary of Culture-Bound Syndromes in the fourth edition of the DSM.

International Trends

Although culture, politics, economics, geography, and health systems all influence variations in the manifestation of mental illness, certain symptoms exist in all societies. These include anxiety, mania, depression, suicidal ideation, somatization, persecutory delusions, and thought disorders. Although labels and prescriptions vary, recognizing a problem and making an attempt at treatment are universal. Societies that do not stigmatize persons with mental illness have much better treatment outcomes than societies that do, because such persons are quickly reintegrated into society (Kaplan et al., 1998).

Many of the more developed nations of the world have been moving mental health activities from institution-based to community-based care for reasons similar to those of the United States. The British National Health Service has systematically employed community mental health nurses for many years. The experience of British community mental health nurses is well documented in published research about problems identified in alternatives to hospital-based mental health care (Hanily, 1995; Kwakwa, 1995), outcomes of nurses' working with families caring for a relative with schizophrenia (Brooker, Falloon, Butterworth, Goldberg, 1994; Bradshaw & Everitt, 1995), and especially in occupational stress among community mental health nurses (Brown, Leary, Carson, Bartlett, & Fagin, 1995; Carson, Leary, de Villiers, Fagin, & Radmall, 1995). Community nurses in Great Britain are expected to assume increasing responsibility for "supervision of aftercare" under provisions of the Mental Health Patients in the Community Act of 1995 (Ford & Rigby, 1996).

Some developing countries have been focusing on fostering mental health activities as an integral part of community-based care out of necessity, as well as tradition. Not only is community-based care attractive economically, but also it is more acceptable to many who have not become accustomed to the institutional approach to care more common in industrialized countries. Gournay (1995) traces the advances in the care of people with chronic mental illnesses of the recent past and how they have produced radical changes in service delivery worldwide. Frequently it has been the mental health nurse who has played a central role as community-based clinical case manager. In less developed countries, especially, it may be a generalist nurse who manages the delivery of comprehensive health care including mental health. Uys, Subedar & Lewis (1995) describe the outcomes of an innovative educational program in South Africa that prepares nurses to function in a primary health care system that fully integrates psychiatric care.

SETTINGS FOR COMMUNITY MENTAL HEALTH NURSING PRACTICE

Full participation in community mental health interdisciplinary teams can mean weaving a fabric of relationships within a nursing system, an interdisciplinary team, and, perhaps most important, a community. To that end, nurses attempt to locate themselves so as to facilitate the client's access to services and to maximize the benefit of nursing resources. Community health nurses are key because access is often enhanced when nurses operate within the client's daily social environment: home, school, or job site.

Prevention efforts located nearest to the client can best support and preserve critical family and social resource networks. Thus, nursing can be practiced in battered women's shelters, food programs for the homeless, senior centers and residences, jails, health maintenance organizations and primary care clinics, occupational health and employee assistance programs, immigrant and cultural centers, and on home visits. Some clinical nurse specialists in psychiatric or mental health nursing work in community settings. Most often, however, it is community health nurses who are found in these sites, providing comprehensive nursing care that includes elements of psychiatric and mental health nursing.

One effective model of practice has been for many nurses to work together, often with other health disciplines, at agencies organized for treatment and support of the clients. These service agencies most often work with individuals who have severe and chronic mental health disorders. Outpatient clinics in mental health centers, rehabilitation centers, and therapeutic foster care all employ nurses as part of interdisciplinary teams.

In many communities, a network of supervised living accommodations provides a range of services geared toward assisting persons in the transition from inpatient hospitalization toward full independence. Nurses play key roles in partial hospitalization programs and can be an important adjunct to such a network. Some communities provide day hospitals, sometimes called adult day treatment programs, where patients attend during business hours and return to family homes, group homes, or independent living arrangements for some meals and to sleep. Night-care serves clients who can function in supervised work settings during the day but require more structure than can be provided by other living arrangements. When psychiatric/mental health nurses are not employed within these settings, community health nurses are called on to provide care and consultation regarding clients' nursing and health care needs.

HEALTH PROMOTION/ ILLNESS PREVENTION IN COMMUNITY HEALTH NURSING PRACTICE

The goal of prevention is to decrease the onset (incidence), duration (prevalence), and residual disability of mental disorders in the community. Community health nurses can actively work toward prevention of mental disorders through primary, secondary, and tertiary prevention activities.

The range of mental health and illness phenomena of concern to nurses is illustrated in Figure 23-2. Two diagnostic classification systems, the Omaha system (Martin & Scheet, 1992) and the North American Nursing Diagnosis Association (North American Nursing Diagnosis Association, 1999) system are commonly used by community health nurses to name actual or potential client mental health problems. Advanced practice nurses certified in psychiatric nursing use the *Diagnostic and Statistical Manual of Mental Disorders-IV* (DSM-IV) (American Psychiatric Association, 1994) to diagnose mental health problems.

Figure 23-2 Mental Health and Illness: Phenomena of Concern to Nurses

Actual or potential mental health problems of clients pertaining to:

- The maintenance of optimal health and well-being and the prevention of psychobiological illness

- Self-care limitations or impaired functioning related to mental and emotional distress

- Deficits in the functioning of significant biological, emotional, and cognitive systems

- Emotional stress or crisis components of illness, pain, and disability

- Self-concept changes, developmental issues, and life process changes

- Problems related to emotions such as anxiety, anger, sadness, loneliness, and grief

- Physical symptoms that occur along with altered psychological functioning

- Alterations in thinking, perceiving, symbolizing, communicating, and decision making

- Difficulties in relating to others

- Behaviors and mental states that indicate the client is a danger to self or others or has a severe disability

- Interpersonal, systemic, sociocultural, spiritual, or environmental circumstances or events that affect the mental and emotional well-being of the individual, family, or community

- Symptom management, side effects/toxicities associated with psychopharmacologic interventions and other aspects of the treatment regimen

From Statement on the Scope and Standards of Psychiatric-Mental Health Clinical Nursing Practice *by the American Nurses Association, 1994. © 1994 American Nurses Publishing, American Nurses Foundation/American Nurses Association, 600 Maryland Avenue, SW, Suite 100W, Washington, DC 20024-2571. Reprinted with permission.*

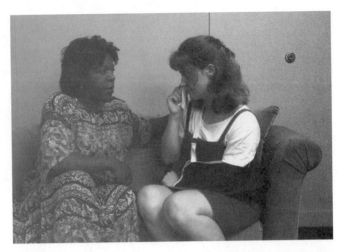

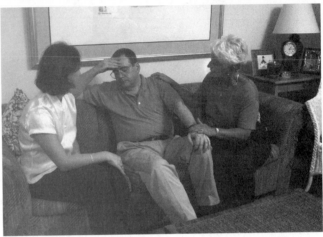

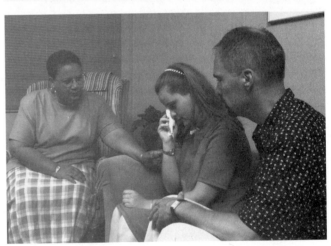

Community health nurses can be found in different settings assisting those who are in need of psychiatric help.

Primary Prevention

The goal of primary prevention is to prevent the onset of mental health disorders. Nursing primary prevention activities target groups at risk through mental health education programs. Examples include:

- Teaching parenting skills and child development to teen parents
- Teaching the psychobiological effects of alcohol and drugs to young people in schools
- Developing social support systems to reduce the effects of psychosocial stress on persons at high risk: e.g., safer sex groups for HIV-negative gay men
- Anticipatory guidance programs to assist people in preparing for expected stressful situations: e.g., training young people to run peer counseling programs at

high schools to address issues such as family abuse, street violence, date rape, peer pressure, and conflict mediation

- Crisis intervention after stressful life events, such as group disasters or the death of a child due to gang violence

Primary prevention programs also aim to eradicate stressful agents and to reduce stress. Examples of specific strategies nurses employ to help decrease the risk of mental retardation and other cognitive disorders in children include assisting families to reduce lead exposure in their housing, counseling prenatal clients to abstain from drug and alcohol use and to improve their nutrition via education.

Secondary Prevention

Secondary prevention is the early identification and prompt treatment of an illness or a disorder. The goals are to reduce the number of cases in the population at risk and to shorten the illness's duration. Secondary prevention nursing targets individuals and groups in whom a high risk for illness or illness symptoms has been assessed. Nursing activities include the provision of or referral for treatment, and other services including:

- Ongoing assessment of infants prenatally exposed to drugs and alcohol: e.g., during visits to clients' homes, residential drug treatment programs, family shelters, and foster care programs
- Provision of care to individuals through individual or group counseling, medication administration, crisis intervention: e.g., staffing suicide prevention hotlines or shelters for abused women
- Case management of emotionally ill children living with their families

Tertiary Prevention

The goal of tertiary prevention is to reduce the prevalence of residential defects and disabilities caused by severe or chronic mental illness. Nursing tertiary prevention interventions focus on client rehabilitation and the prevention of complications. Nursing activities address the medical, psychiatric, and social needs of persistently mentally ill persons. Examples include:

- Teaching clients daily living skills to support their highest level of functional capacity and independence
- Case management of the persistently mentally ill: e.g., referral to and monitoring effectiveness of various community mental health programs, making referrals to support services such as assistance with household chores and other activities of daily living, encouraging social activities

SUICIDE

Suicide, including suicide ideation or attempted suicide, is an important mental health concern, which community health nurses frequently must address.

Suicide is defined as purposely taking one's life (Frisch & Frisch, 1998). There is a high correlation between depression and suicide, which is often undetected by health professionals. While 80% of clients with depression

can be treated, less than 40% are, in fact, treated, as depression often mimics physical illness (Bonger, Berman, Maris, Silverman, Harris & Packman, 1988; USDHHS & PHS, 1996). Almost all people who commit suicide have had diagnosable mental or substance abuse disease and most have more than one of these diseases (Firestone, 1997; National Institute of Mental Health, 1998).

Rosenburg, Ventura, Maurer, et al. identified suicide as the ninth leading cause of death in the United States in 1995 and the third leading cause of death among adolescents and young adults aged 15–24 (1996). In most countries, suicide rates peak in adolescents and again in men and women over age 75. Over all, in the United States, Caucasian males account for 73% and Caucasian females for 18% of all suicides (Kachur, Potter, James, & Powell, 1995). In the United States, the highest rate of suicide is by Caucasian men over 85 years of age; the second highest rate is for Caucasian men between 20–24. The rate for African American men peaks between 20–24. Caucasian women have a higher rate than African American women but both are at least ¼ the rate of men (CDCP, 1998a, 1998b).

In 18–24 year olds, Hispanic men have the highest rate of seriously considering suicide and African American men run a close second. However, African American men have a significantly higher rate of attempted suicide than do either Hispanic or Caucasian men. Among women, Caucasian women are more likely to consider suicide but African American and Hispanic women are likely to attempt suicide (CDCP, 1997).

These figures show a growing problem among young Hispanics. This group of young people is poorly studied with regard to depression and suicide. Other high risk groups include young male Native Americans who reside on reservations, lesbian and gay teens and adults (thirty percent of teen suicides are by lesbian and gay adolescents), runaways, cult members and gang members (Center for Disease Control, 1990; Youngkin & Davis, 1998).

Death by gunshot injuries account for the majority of completed suicides while pill ingestion and lacerations constitute the majority of suicide attempts. Table 23-1 summarizes risk factors for the entire population, while Table 23-2 offers risk factors specific to adolescents and elders.

Nursing Assessment and Intervention

It is difficult to separate assessment and intervention of the suicidal client. The nurse who assesses suicidal ideation begins intervention immediately to prevent any escalation of behavior. Assessment and intervention will be considered simultaneously.

When the nurse identifies that a client is depressed and manifesting other risk factors for suicide, an evaluation of suicide potential must be completed. Warning signs which are deserving of close attention include:

- prior attempts
- escalating substance abuse

Table 23-1   Suicide Risk Factors

Gender
- Males

Race
- Caucasion—highest rate
- African American, Latino and Native American Males

Marital Status
- Widowed
- Divorced
- Separated
- Single

Age
- 80–84: highest rate in Caucasion males
- <65 in Caucasian males
- 15–19 year old

Other Risk Groups
- Gay and lesbian youth and adults
- Runaways
- Cult members
- Gang members

Method
- Firearms: 60% of suicide deaths/attempts

Family History
- Violence
- 1st or 2nd degree family member who has successfully completed suicide

Medical Diagnosis
- Cancer
- HIV/AIDS
- renal dialysis or other chronic or fatal diagnosis

- comments about suicide, such as "I am going to kill myself."
- behavior changes—particularly giving away belongings or making a will
- expressions of hopelessness or helplessness

- isolation and a preoccupation with death
- situational events, such as death of a significant other, retirement (Firestone, 1997; Frisch & Frisch, 1998; Valente, 1993)

If the client acknowledges suicidal ideation the nurse must determine if a plan exists and the degree of lethality involved. If the client has a detailed plan with no means of rescue, involving lethal methods, the means to carry it out, and a plan to do so in one to two days, she or he must be considered a high risk. Lethal methods include guns, hanging, knives, carbon monoxide poisining, drowning and jumping (Valente, 1993).

Based on the known statistics of suicide, questions to ask when assessing for lethality include the following:

- Does the client have a detailed plan?
- Does the plan include a means of preventing discovery or rescue?
- Does the method of suicide involve a gun, a knife, hanging, carbon monoxide poisoning, drowning or jumping from extreme height?
- Does the client have the means to carry out the plan (access to a gun or other weapon)?
- Does the client intend to carry out the plan within 24–48 hours?

Psychiatric referral should be sought for any high risk client and the client needs to be carefully supervised until provisions can be made for insuring safety. The nurse will save time if she is aware of the mental health laws pertaining to legal holds and hospitalization for clients who present as a danger to self.

If the client presents with low lethality the nurse may utilize a suicide contract, make referrals as indicated, develop plans for increased support, and assess the need for medications. Lethality is assessed as low when the client thinks of suicide sporadically, has a vague plan with no time frame, considers methods such as wrist cut-

Table 23-2   Risk Factors for Adolescents and Elders

ADOLESCENTS	ELDERS
• loss of family member or close friend through death, divorce or suicide	• failure to adapt to multiple stressors of aging
• lack of nurturance from parents—feeling ignored in family	• loss of partner, home or close friend
• economic insecurity in family	• severe medical illness
• low self-esteem	• chemical dependency or alcoholism
• parental alcohol	• cognitive impairment
• high parental expectations	• family history of suicide
• depression or suicide attempts in family	• major transitions (e.g., move to retirement home)
• ineffective communication in family	• phobia
• abuse—especially sexual abuse	
• suicide epidemics	
• bisexual or homosexual gender identity	

Adapted from Risk Management with Suicidal Patients *by B. Bonger, A. L. Berman, R. W. Maris, et al. (1998). New York: Guilford;* Suicide and the Inner Voice: Risk Assessment, Treatment, and Case Management *by R. W. Firestone (1997). Thousand Oaks, CA: Sage.*

ting, and has an available support system. Suicide contracts are most effective when the client has a relationship with the health care provider. A contract should be seen as an adjunct to a thorough assessment and a tool to provide an alternative to impulsive action. It is a written promise that the client will not harm himself before calling the provider. The contract should be reviewed and updated at established time intervals and at any time that the nurse observes, or the client feels, a change in emotional status or sense of safety (Firestone, 1997; Frisch & Frisch, 1998). The client may need assistance with referrals for appropriate groups or psychtherapy. Referrals are a means of expanding the client's support system and decreasing isolation. The client will benefit from examining other ways to expand his life and develop alternatives to suicide. Depression often results in tunnel vision and feelings of worthlessness. Assisting the client in identifying friends, relatives, spiritual guides or others the client has previously trusted or found to be supportive can be a first step toward the client becoming re-involved in supportive relationships. The client should also have the numbers of suicide and crisis hotlines that can be used around the clock. If the nurse assesses that there is a need for psychoactive medications, consultation with the client and a psychiatrist is indicated. Psychoactive drugs, particularly antidepressants, have varying time frames before becoming effective, they are often sedative for the first few weeks, they may have uncomfortable side effects and some have frightening adverse reactions. Thorough client education is essential to the client's sense of well-being and his willingness to remain on the medication long enough to experience its benefits. If a client is experiencing suicideal ideation and is taking antidepressants, the nurse should coordinate the dispensing of the drug with the psychiatrist to reduce the potential of a lethal overdose.

When the client returns home after a suicide attempt, the environment should be made as safe as possible. Firearms should be removed and medications assessed so that there is no possiblity of stockpiling them for a future attempt. The nurse should assess the social support system to determine how best to help reduce social isolation and to collaborate with those individuals, whether family or friends, about how they can act in the client's best interest (Frisch & Frisch, 1998).

BASIC-LEVEL PRACTICE IN COMMUNITY HEALTH NURSING

The scope of clinical practice is differentiated by the community setting and the nurse's educational preparation. Most community health nurses have a baccalaureate degree but may not have advanced or specialized training in the area of mental health. When working with clients with mental health disorders, the nurse functions at a *basic*

practice level. Nurses work in concert with psychiatric and mental health staff, some of whom are psychiatric or mental health clinical nurse specialists. The American Nurses Association (ANA) (1994) recognizes the following basic-level functions of psychiatric/mental health nurses as screening and assessment intake and evaluation.

Screening and Assessment Intake and Evaluation

Mental health evaluations are a routine component of individual and family assessment. The community health nurse may be the one to discover the compromised client and make referrals for care. Nurses practicing in the home often have access to firsthand data useful in identifying mental health disorders. Data collected by community health nurses during routine assessments of an individual's physical, functional, and nutritional status, medication and substance use, health beliefs, and domestic and family life may indicate the need to conduct more specific mental health status examinations. Although nurses at the basic level are not specifically trained to do mental status examinations, information and observations gained during client and family interactions are used to make tentative nursing diagnoses. For example, assessment of the neuromental status of all clients admitted to the nurse's caseload may identify risk factors such as long-term use of psychotropic drugs, sleep disturbance and lack of appetite in the bereaved, or symptoms of combat stress in refugees and immigrants. In these cases, follow-up using more specialized tools or referral for a more comprehensive evaluation is indicated. See Figure 23-3 for a list of general assessment areas used in a mental health evaluation. See Appendix E for an example of a mini-mental health status exam.

Many nurses use genograms or family health trees and ecomaps to assess an individual or family's general health,

DECISION MAKING

School Crisis Event

You are working in an inner city school where a third grader was shot but not killed on the playground by his stepfather in front of the other children.

• As the nurse, what can you do at a primary prevention level in response to this event? At a secondary level?

• When you learn that the child's mother has been long diagnosed as a schizophrenic and is dependent on the stepfather for her care, is there anything you can do to facilitate the situation at any level of prevention?

Figure 23-3   General Assessment Areas Used in Mental Health Evaluations

Assess the client's:

- Appearance—posture, poise, clothing, grooming
- Behavior and psychomotor activity—gestures, twitches, agitation, combativeness, gait, agility, restlessness, activity level
- Attitude toward the nurse—cooperative, hostile, guarded, evasive
- Mood—depressed, irritable, angry, sad, expansive, euphoric, frightened, anxious
- Affect—emotional responsiveness, range of facial expressions, depth of emotion, affect (for congruence with mood), dull/flat, appropriateness to the situation
- Speech—talkative, slow or rapid, monotonous, loud, whispered, mumbled, impaired
- Perceptual disturbances—visual, auditory, or sensory hallucinations
- Thought process—flight of ideas, slow or hesitant thinking, vague responses, unrelated, disconnected
- Content of thoughts—preoccupations, obsessions, compulsions, fantasies, recurrent ideas about suicide, homicide, hurting self, hypochondriacal symptoms, antisocial urges
- Alertness and level of consciousness—alert, lethargic, somnolent
- Orientation—to person, place, time
- Memory—changes in remote, recent past, and recent memories; immediate retention problems
- Environment—house cluttered, unkempt, clean

DECISION MAKING

Home Care with a Schizophrenic Client

You have made a home visit to Marie and her husband, Grant, who has recently returned home from a two-week stay in a psychiatric facility following his attempt to destroy all the electrical appliances in their home because they were "receiving messages from the government." He had stopped taking his medicine before the incident, and Marie hadn't realized how important it was for him to continue. Now that he is home, he's still not sure about the appliances and doesn't like the side effects of his medication.

- Following the suggestions for caring for the client with schizophrenia (Figure 23-7), which would be the best ways for you to work with the couple?

- How can you use the suggestions made in Figure 23-6?

functioning, and resources. Genograms help nurses identify family members with histories of mental health disorders and psychiatric-related hospitalizations and those who have been on psychotropic drugs or in psychotherapy or counseling.

The ecomap is a diagram of a family's contacts with others outside the family. It provides a visual picture of significant relationships between the person or family and others outside the immediate family and of the adequacy or lack of social support. Genograms and ecomaps are

Figure 23-4   Posttraumatic Stress Disorder Screen for Newcomer Children

Does the child/or has the child ever:

- ( ) seemed unhappy
- ( ) cried excessively (unexplained)
- ( ) tried to or actually hurt self
- ( ) had peculiar or strange behavior
- ( ) seemed excessively restless
- ( ) displayed reckless or dangerous behavior

- ( ) wet or soiled pants at night or during day
- ( ) had sleeping problem (too much or too little, frequent nightmares)
- ( ) had eating problem (too much or too little, hoarding food)

Does the child have any of these problems at home or school?

- ( ) separation problem/school phobia
- ( ) poor grades
- ( ) difficulty concentrating—gets off task easily
- ( ) has to be coaxed to play or work with peers
- ( ) difficulty making friends
- ( ) disruptive in class
- ( ) arguing or fighting with classmates, teacher, siblings
- ( ) frequent suspensions from school

- ( ) refusing to obey parents
- ( ) excessive clinging to parent or teacher, (e.g., following parent to shower, bathroom)
- ( ) lying or stealing
- ( ) running away from home
- ( ) problems with police
- ( ) engaging in inappropriate sexual behavior

Has anyone in your family ever been treated or hospitalized for emotional problems such as depression, anxiety, mood swings, suicide attempts, or alcohol or drug abuse? If YES, explain.

Figure 23-5   Caring for the Client on Antipsychotic Medication with the Abnormal Involuntary Movement Scale (AIMS)

The AIMS measures involuntary movements for clients at risk for tardive dyskinesia. The AIMS score equals the sum of the following items. Either before or after completing the procedure, observe the client unobtrusively at rest. The chair to be used in this procedure should be a hard, firm one without arms. After the client is observed, he may be rated on a scale of 0 (none), 1 (minimal), 2 (mild), 3 (moderate), and 4 (severe) according to the severity of symptoms at time of interview. Ask the client whether there is anything in his mouth (e.g., gum, candy) and if there is, ask him to remove it. Ask the client about the current condition of his teeth. Ask if he wears dentures. Do his teeth or dentures bother him now? Ask the client whether he notices any movement in mouth, face, hands, or feet. If yes, ask him to describe such movement and to what extent it currently bothers him or interferes with his activities.

0 1 2 3 4   Have the client sit in a chair with hands on knees, legs slightly apart, and feet flat on floor. Look at entire body for movements while in this position.

0 1 2 3 4   Ask the client to sit with hands hanging unsupported. If male, between legs; if female and wearing a dress, hanging over knees. (Observe hands and other body areas.)

0 1 2 3 4   Ask the client to open mouth. Observe tongue at rest within mouth. Have him do it twice.

0 1 2 3 4   Ask the client to protrude tongue. (Observe abnormalities of tongue movements.) Have him do this twice.

0 1 2 3 4   Ask the client to tap thumb with each finger as rapidly as possible for 10 to 15 seconds separately with right hand then with left hand. Observe facial and leg movements.

0 1 2 3 4   Flex and extend client's left and right arms (one at a time).

0 1 2 3 4   Ask the client to stand up. Observe in profile. Observe all body areas again, hips included.

0 1 2 3 4   *Ask the client to extend both arms outstretched in front with palms down. (Observe trunk, legs, and mouth.)

0 1 2 3 4   *Have the client walk a few paces, turn, and walk back to chair. (Observe hands and gait.) Do this twice.

*Activated movements.
From Synopsis of Psychiatry: Behavioral Sciences *by H. I. Kaplan, B. J. Sadock, & J. A. Grebb, 1998, Clinical Psychiatry 51(8), pp. 8–19. Reprinted with permission of Williams & Wilkins.*

described in more detail in Chapter 18. Other mental health screening tools and techniques are available for use by community health nurses. These tools require basic orientation, but minimal training, to use.

The Posttraumatic Stress Disorder (PTSD) Screen for Newcomer Children was developed for nurses working with immigrant and refugee children who may have developed mental health symptoms after exposure to extreme stress in their country of origin (Golden, 1994) (See Figure 23-4). Nurses may also administer standard rating scales to measure the severity of a psychiatric disorder and the effectiveness of treatment.

The Abnormal Involuntary Movement Scale (AIMS) for those at risk of tardive dyskinesia (see Figure 23-5), the Hamilton Depressive Rating Scale, and the Brief Psychiatric Rating Scale are simple, statistically reliable tools that can be used by nurses to assess clients' symptoms and to communicate findings to others.

The complex nature of a more comprehensive assessment often justifies the nurse's consultation with specialized resources. The national goals set forth in *Healthy People 2000* (USDHHS, 1991) makes it a high priority to increase the proportion of clinicians who routinely review the patient's cognitive, emotional, and behavioral functioning.

Nursing Support Interventions

Basic good listening and communication skills used to establish the therapeutic nurse–client relationship provide the foundation for counseling clients with mental illnesses. Many nurses may not recognize these support activities as significant interventions because they are so common to good nursing practice. Simple psychotherapeutic management techniques such as those outlined in Figure 23-6 do not require advanced psychotherapy training. These and other skills important to the nurse–client relationship, which are discussed in Chapter 8, can be used by nurses who are supported by ongoing clinical supervision. In the case of severe mental illness such as schizophrenia, severe depression, or bipolar disorder, such counseling is an adjunct to the primary, psychopharmacologic treatment.

Psychoanalytic concepts that the nurse may have learned should not be used to make interpretive statements about the supposed unconscious motivations of a psychotic client. Any self-disclosure and admiring or social conversation should be worded so as to avoid overtones that the client may find seductive. See Figure 23-7 for techniques on handling experiences of a client with schizophrenia.

Figure 23-6 Nursing Support Interventions

General Nursing Support Activity	Communication/Listening Intervention
Self-disclosure	Providing input regarding the nurse's personal experiences using self as a therapeutic entity. Caution! Disclosure should serve client and not the nurse's need.
Mutual sharing	Back-and-forth exchange. Focus on client. Discussion is usually on feeling level.
Active listening	Responding to content and feelings of discussion. Includes restatement, reflection, clarification of messages.
Exchanging information	Sharing information, problem solving, assisting with decision making. Often client initiated and is an active participant in exchange.
Sounding board	Using excellent listening skills, being present, taking in, but not necessarily responding.
Role modeling	By your example, demonstrating effective communication, stress management, and other healthy behaviors.
Health teaching	Teaching to provide health information. Instructions, advice, anticipatory guidance, use of teaching materials and aids.
Validation	Praise, appreciation, encouragement, positive reinforcement, feedback, or discouragement that supports healthy behaviors.
Social sharing	Interactions that give emphasis to other family members, pets, activities. Sharing tea, coffee, conversing with other family and household members.

Psychobiological Interventions

Although psychopharmacologic agents can greatly decrease or eliminate the most profound symptoms of major mental illnesses, many clients do not adhere to the optimal treatment regimen. Most often, problems with adherence can be traced to the client's experience with side effects of medication. Teaching clients about their medications and helping them to work with providers to manage the side effect symptoms is a common and very important role for the nurse.

Many home care clients referred for medical care present with mental health conditions. For example, HIV/

Figure 23-7 Caring for the Client with Schizophrenia

Patient's Experience	Nurse's Technique
Paranoia	• Maintain nonthreatening body position—side by side not face to face
	• Indirect speech content—verbal equivalent to above
	• Reciprocal emotional tone—help client to feel understood by mirroring his affect
	• Sharing mistrust—do not try to argue delusions away
	• Postpone psychoeducation until strong alliance is established
Denial of illness	• Avoid overzealous attack on denial—denial may be the best defense the client can mount
	• Provide alternative explanations—use indirect approach
Stigma	• Normalize behavior and attitudes—everyone has difficulties and struggles
	• Use your authority as a professional
	• Help client save face by tactful use of language to soften psychiatric terms
Demoralization	• Maintain a positive attitude
	• Make admiring and approving statements
	• Determine the origins of demoralization
Terror	• Reassurance
	• Companionship—offer a confident presence
	• Leave the client alone—avoid intrusive emotional reaching

Adapted from "Psychotherapeutic Management Techniques in the Treatment of Out-Patients with Schizophrenia by P. Weiden & L. Havens, 1994, Hospital and Community Psychiatry, 45(6), pp. 549–555. Adapted with permission of American Psychiatric Association.

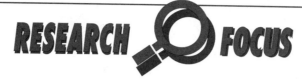

Persistent and Severely Mentally Ill Clients' Perceptions of Their Mental Illness

STUDY PROBLEM/PURPOSE

How do persistently, severely mentally ill persons perceive their illness and its effects on their lives?

METHODS

Fifteen clients in an outpatient mental health clinic at a Veteran's Administration Hospital participated in this qualitative, exploratory study. Each subject had a chronic, major mental disorder. Each subject was interviewed once according to a semi-structured format. Interviews lasted from 45 to 90 minutes.

FINDINGS

The major themes extracted from the interviews were shame and stigmatization and the resulting alienation, loss, and a pervasive feeling of distress and acceptance. Persons with mental illness perceived themselves as stigmatized, whereas persons with severe physical handicaps perceived themselves as attracting support and sympathy. The subjects perceived the loss of opportunities for relationships and jobs. The pain or "distress" persisted along with the illness. Self-acceptance and the acceptance of others led to a sense of strength and much desired normalcy.

IMPLICATIONS

The persistent pain felt by those with chronic severe mental disorders may be mitigated by addressing the stigma attached to mental illness and by supporting acceptance of the condition. Interventions include acknowledging the feelings, normalizing the client's experience, supporting self-esteem, and helping the client to "save face."

SOURCE

From "Persistent and Severely Mentally Ill Clients' Perceptions of Their Mental Illness" by B. A. Vellenga, & J. Christenson, 1994, Issues in Mental Health Nursing 15, pp. 359–371.

AIDS and elderly clients may be taking as many as 10 to 15 different medications, including a number of psychotropic drugs. A major component of home care is assessing these clients for overmedication, reviewing medications for compatibility and adverse side effects, and working with providers to address these concerns. Other psychobiological measures used by the community health nurse include relaxation techniques, diet and nutrition regulation, rest–activity cycle monitoring.

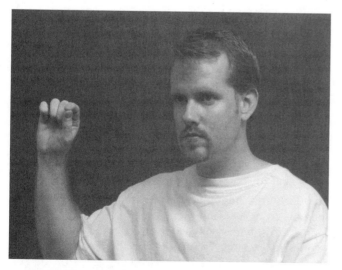

Client participating in AIMS test.

Health Teaching

Client education is recognized as an integral part of nursing practice. It is one of the most important interventions nurses use to move clients toward self-care. Unfortunately, client education is often neglected because of the pressures, time constraints, and multiple demands put on the nurse. Effective client education for the mentally ill has been lacking.

Mental illness can disrupt almost every aspect of the life of the client and the client's family. Clients and families need to be educated about mental illness. As clients are defined more as consumers of health care, the expectation is that they will have more questions and will be better informed than in the past. Providing a solid knowledge base to the client and family is essential to the client's recovery (Bisbee, 1991). Content areas should include:

- The nature of mental illness, information about different diagnoses, major symptoms experienced, variability of experiences, probable causes, treatments options, prognosis
- Medications, actions, side effects, adhering to medication regimens
- Managing stress and using coping strategies
- Communication and relationship skills
- Community resources
- Impact of illness on family members
- Support networks

Esther Stuart is a 32-year-old African American who has been living with her 19-year-old married, unemployed partner, Daryl, for the past year. She was diagnosed with insulin-dependent diabetes mellitus six months ago and is poorly controlled. Her primary care provider notes that she has a history of schizophrenia. She was referred to the public health nurse because she is considering pregnancy. Esther is preoccupied with becoming pregnant, although she is using oral contraception. Esther tells the nurse she wants a child because so many of her neighbors have young children and having a child would allow her to develop friendships in her community and feel wanted. Esther's concerns include problems sleeping at night, chronic headaches, and a recent weight gain. She is 5 feet 4 inches tall and weighs 193 pounds. Esther and Daryl live in a neat one-bedroom apartment. Her mother lives in the same building "to keep an eye on me and make sure I'm doing OK." During the visits the nurse observes that Esther is not euphoric, depressed, or sad. Her behavior appears normal, her affect is constricted, and she is anxious. She enjoys seeing the nurse and tells her openly that she is schizophrenic. When the nurse reviews Esther's medications she learns that Esther is taking Lithium 300 mg. TID, and 25 units of NPH insulin, BID; that she is followed at an outpatient mental health clinic; is not compliant taking her Lithium; and misses two out of every three scheduled appointments with her psychiatrist. Esther has been hospitalized two times within the past five months for ketoacidosis, using the emergency room for her care. When the nurse asks her about her diabetes she is very knowledgeable. She tells the nurse that she was doing home glucose monitoring until the batteries in her machine died earlier this month and that she adjusts her insulin dose depending on how she feels, "my blood sugar being too high or too low." She follows no special diet and describes poor eating habits, frequently eating frozen or fast foods. In subsequent visits the nurse learns that Esther has two school-age children living with an aunt nearby.

Nursing Considerations

ASSESSMENT
- What areas should the nurse include in the mental health assessment? Are there any specific screening tools the nurse should use? What areas of risk should the nurse focus on in the assessment?
- What medication issues need to be considered with this client?
- What individual and family strengths can be identified?
- What cultural considerations need to be addressed in order to work effectively with this client and her family?

DIAGNOSIS
- What nursing diagnoses can be assigned to this client and family?

OUTCOME IDENTIFICATION
- What measurable objectives would be used to evaluate the individual and family achievement of the best possible health outcomes?

PLANNING/INTERVENTIONS
- How will the nursing plan address mental health, as well as other health concerns?
- What community resources would be appropriate to involve with this family?
- What nursing interventions should be included in the plan to address the nursing diagnoses?

EVALUATION
- How will you know if your objectives have been met?
- In order to answer the above questions more fully, what additional information is needed?

Case Management

Case management is key to successful rehabilitation for many clients with severe and chronic mental illness. Case managers provide continuity of care by following clients through all phases of care while helping them negotiate complex and fragmented systems. Case management includes assessing each client's needs, developing an individualized service plan with objectives related to needs, identifying strategies for achieving the stated objectives, and periodically evaluating the effectiveness of the services. Availability, accessibility, cost, and quality of care

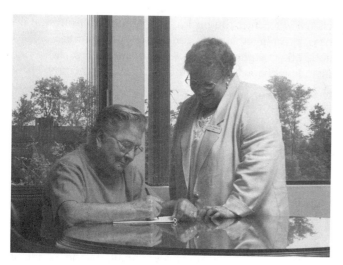

Providing encouragement to a client is an effective nursing intervention.

are central issues confronting the provision of case management services. Case managers ensure that the changing needs of their clients are addressed on an ongoing basis and appropriate choices are provided among the widest array of options for meeting those needs.

Murray and Baier (1993) describe the successful application of the concept to clients in a transitional residential program for chronically mentally ill homeless persons. Serving as coordinator, integrator, and advocate for health care needs of the chronically mentally ill is complex, given the pervasive nature of the disability. Whether serving as case manager or working with a case manager from another discipline, community health nurses employ the nursing process to periodically assess changes in clients' functional levels, medications, resources, skills and self-esteem. As these elements change, so do the interventions required to meet the goals of psychiatric rehabilitation.

Self-Care Activities

Self-care activities are often disrupted in mental illness. Alterations in thinking processes can prevent clients from learning or performing activities of daily living. Whether the client is seen in day treatment, a halfway house, an outpatient clinic, a family home, or his or her own apartment, nurses can assess and teach personal hygiene, diet, recreation, shopping, and the use of public transportation. By modeling, directing, coaching, and supporting, nurses can use the person's real-world experience to help make the transition from dependent to increasingly independent arrangements.

Home Visits

The goal of psychiatric home visiting is to assist the client to remain in the community. Hellwig's (1993) assessment of home visits as low cost and feasible is countered, however, by current reimbursement rules that are inappropriately rigid (Thobaben & Kozlak, 1990; Slay, 1993). When

typical criteria for third-party payment are used, home visits are reimbursed only for clients in "homebound status." When a client can go beyond the confines of the home, the visiting nurse's authorization for further visits is withdrawn. This constraint fosters what Slay calls a "Medicare Syndrome," referring to people whose care is not reimbursable because, although they may be best served by home care, they are not absolutely homebound. Public health nurses and others employed by governmental agencies may not be constrained in this way. Some states are nevertheless implementing programs that demonstrate the effectiveness of home visits in terms of client outcomes and cost containment (Foderaaro, 1995).

Community Action

Concern for sociocultural factors that adversely affect the mental health of population groups and taking corrective action can mean getting involved with community planning boards, advisory groups, paraprofessionals, and other key people. Because community health nurses are identified with broad health concerns, their interest in and support for mental health issues help members of the public to see these issues as worthy of support.

Disaster

Mental illness is sometimes conceived of as a severe disruption that exceeds the coping ability of an *individual*. The World Health Organization (1992) definition of disaster is "a severe disruption, ecological and psychosocial, which greatly exceeds the coping ability of the affected *community* (italics added)." When we think of disasters, we commonly think of hurricanes, floods, and the widely publicized terrorist bombing. On a slightly smaller scale, events such as the kidnapping of a child or the suicide of a popular teen can also have a serious emotional impact on a community. The disaster plan for any community should include preparing for responses to the emotional reactions to disaster. An effective response cannot only prevent many long-term effects such as posttraumatic stress disorder or major depression; it can also contribute to short-term general recovery by maintaining the abilities

REFLECTIVE THINKING

Disaster Nursing

Think about experiences you have had or have heard about in the news that describe a disaster situation.

• If you were called in as a community health nurse to participate in caring for the victims and their families, what would be your personal responses to the event?

• What concerns would you have about providing effective interventions?

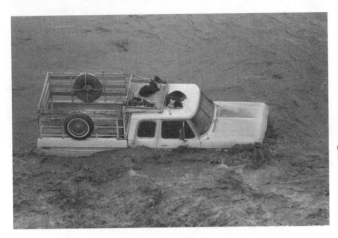

An effective response by a community health nurse can prevent long-term effects and can contribute to the relief of short-term general anxiety for the client who has experienced disaster. *Photo courtesy of UPI/Corbis.*

of a community's members to attend to themselves, their families, and their neighbors. Care for the caregivers is a priority.

A community health nurse who needs to make a referral to or consult with mental health professionals in a disaster can reach them through the Red Cross or other lead relief organization. According to the Suggested Mental Health Response Plan (American Psychiatric Association, 1993), participating mental health professionals can be expected to make themselves available to speak with groups of community workers, to visit community centers to provide direct services and backup services, and to take referrals.

ADVANCED PSYCHIATRIC/ MENTAL HEALTH NURSING

Psychiatric/mental health advanced practice nurses are prepared at the master's or higher level and are certified by a national credentialling body. They may also be referred to as clinical nurse specialists or certified specialists. Their status is designated by: RN, CS. Community health nurses will most often encounter the certified specialist as consultant-liaison. In this role, the specialist may provide direct care, from mental health promotion to illness rehabilitation, to

clients who enter the health care system with physical illness, or indirect care by consulting and educating nurses and other caregivers. Other advanced-level functions include individual, family, and group psychotherapy. Many states have granted psychiatric/mental health advanced practice nurses authority to write drug prescriptions.

Key Concepts

- Treatment of psychiatric mental health clients has gone through three historical transformations. The most recent reform is the Community Mental Health Movement.

- Historical, political, and economic factors continue to greatly influence the concept and practice of community mental health nursing.

- Various nursing, behavioral, and biological theories give direction to the nursing care of the client with mental illness, and no one theory addresses all dimensions of community mental health nursing care.

- Community health nurses practice in a broad continuum of roles in the community, from generalist to specialist.

- Basic practice level includes screening and assessment, support interventions, psychobiological interventions, case management, and teaching self-care activities.

- Nurses provide services in a variety of community settings, including the client's home, shelters, outpatient clinics, aftercare agencies, jails, and senior centers.

- Nursing health promotion/illness prevention activities target and are directed toward the highest-risk individuals and groups within the community.

- Advanced practice is differentiated by the nurse's educational preparation. The role of the clinical specialist is broad and includes consultant-liaison, direct care provider, and mental health educator.

Note: The authors would like to acknowledge Michelle Porter, RN, FNP for her contribution to the discussion of suicide in this chapter.

Family and Community Violence

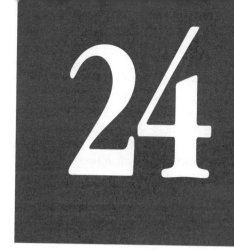

Michelle Porter, RN, MSN, FNP

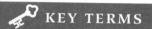 KEY TERMS

acquaintance rape
assault
battered women
batterer
child abuse
child neglect
date rape
domestic violence
elder abuse
emotional abuse
hate crimes
incest
intentional injury
intrafamilial violence
learned helplessness
partner abuse
patriarchy
rape
spousal abuse
violence against women
wife abuse

We need to all become aware of the entire continuum of family violence. We need to increase awareness, cooperativeness, and interdisciplinary networking among all researchers, clinicians, and advocates in the field.

—*Geffner, 1997*

COMPETENCIES

Upon completion of this chapter, the reader should be able to:

- Identify selected international perspectives of family violence.
- Identify four theoretical frameworks that attempt to explain violence.
- Explain the impact of community violence on children.
- Identify the various types of hate crimes.
- Identify types of violence against women and their consequences.
- Explain the impact of sexual assault on survivors, perpetrators, and partners.
- Recognize the various types of abuse under the umbrella term *domestic violence*.
- Identify the cycle of domestic violence.
- Explain the concept of learned helplessness.
- Examine common myths surrounding sexual assault.
- Explain the primary forms of child abuse.
- Identify behavioral clues of child abuse.
- Consider how social environment, poverty, family stress, and violence might be linked.
- Consider the nurse's role in working with elders and potentially abusive caregivers.
- Describe the extent of homicide in the community.
- Identify reporting laws as they pertain to violent acts against children and adults.
- Describe primary, secondary, and tertiary community nursing interventions in the treatment of family violence.
- Identify the importance of taking care of oneself when working with violent clients in order to maintain good nursing care.

The purposes of this chapter are to provide an overview of violence as it affects the individual, the family, and the community and to address the nursing process as it applies to those at risk for violence and to survivors. The chapter explores theories of violence; myths; and realities surrounding violence; patterns of physical, sexual, and emotional abuse; and risk factors associated with homicidal behavior.

"Violence is the intentional use of physical force against another person or against oneself, which either results in or has a high likelihood of resulting in injury or death" (Rosenberg, O'Carroll, & Powell, 1992, p. 3071). Former Surgeon General C. Everett

Koop (Koop & Lundberg, 1992) and Assistant Secretary for Health James Mason (1992) note that **intentional injury**, injury occurring secondary to intentional acts of violence, in the United States is on the rise. Spousal abuse, child abuse, rape, gang violence, drive-by shootings, elder abuse, hate crimes, and other forms of community and **intrafamilial violence**, violence that occurs within the family, between family members, are epidemic (Rosenberg et al., 1992).

Given that the criminal justice system generally deals with violence after the fact, it is essential that other relevant sectors of society, including nursing, develop and deliver prevention strategies. Violent and abusive behavior is one of the 22 priority areas relating to specific problems, conditions, and diseases named in the *Healthy People 2000* report (U.S. Department of Health and Human Services [USDHHS], 1990). The 1995 midcourse review shows that while suicide among adults, weapon carrying by adolescents, and rape have decreased, homicide, weapons-related violent deaths, assault injuries, and suicide attempts among adolescents have greatly increased (USDHHS, 1996).

What is the role of nursing in response to intentional violence? The definition of community health nursing given in Chapter 1 is certainly applicable to the provision of nursing care to survivors of violence as well as to interventions aimed at reducing potentially violent acts. However, Limandri and Tilden (1996) discovered that many nurses are deficient in their knowledge, particularly of older person and spousal abuse, and recommend increased education in these areas as well as providing more opportunity for nursing students to practice in real-life settings such as an abused women's shelter. In addition to providing care and prevention, there is a need for research to increase the knowledge base relevant to the community health nursing perspective in all areas of violence.

PERSPECTIVES ON VIOLENCE

Violence is making headlines across the United States. Public opinion polls evidence a growing concern regarding violence and public safety, although violence is hardly a new phenomenon. It has been and continues to be a popular theme in television, movies, music, and advertising.

Violence is embedded in our society and is not separate from us as individuals, as a community, or as a culture. Societal change begins with individual change. Community health nurses are in a position to teach nonviolent child-rearing practices, to educate families about the risk inherent in children's exposure to violent television and movie images, to counsel families at risk for violence, and to help link victims of violence to appropriate resources. Although this nursing intervention is only one aspect of addressing a complex cultural value system, it is a vital one.

REFLECTIVE THINKING

Violence

The word *violence* means different things to different people depending on their own life experiences, personal encounters, stereotypes, and conditioning. What does violence mean to you?

• When you think of violence, what images come to mind?

• Consider the following variables: sex, age, race, class, educational background, neighborhood, city, state, country, and religious group. What are your particular stereotypes with regard to violence and each variable?

• How were these stereotypes formed?

• What behaviors do you consider to be violent?

International Perspective

Internationally, research about family violence is limited. There are few estimates of the frequency of abuse worldwide. Certain cultural practices, such as female genital mutilation, dowry death, female infanticide, and forced prostitution reflect the subordination of the rights of women and children to the adult male and are accepted by many cultures as appropriate behavior. Some countries do not recognize family violence as a social problem. For instance, other countries do not regard infanticide as homicide. Only recently have Singaporean women's groups appealed to the government for support for prevention of

REFLECTIVE THINKING

Personal Experiences with Violence

• How were you disciplined as a child?

• How did your family manage anger when you were a child? Is what you do when you are angry similar to or different from what adults in your family did when they were angry?

• As a child were you taught problem-solving skills?

• How many violent images were you exposed to in the past 24 hours? Consider television, movies, newspapers, magazines, radio, advertisements, public transportation, daily life, and neighbors.

• Have you ever had a violent impulse? Did you act on it? If not, what kept you from doing so?

• Under what circumstances, if any, would you justify the use of personal violence? To what degree? What might the consequences be for you and the person upon whom you inflict violence?

spousal abuse. Some reports suggest that spouse abuse is somewhat higher in Canada than in the United States but that elder abuse is about the same in the two countries (Barnett, Miller-Perrin, & Perrin, 1997). Although there is little documented evidence outside of the United States and Canada regarding family violence, enough is known to be certain that this behavior is a worldwide phenomenon. Much remains to be done to reduce the incidence of family violence throughout the world.

THEORIES OF VIOLENCE

A variety of theories attempt to explain violence, including biological, psychoanalytic, social learning, and feminist theories. No existing nursing theory explicitly addresses violence. This area remains in need of nursing research and theory development. No one theory explains the complex reasons one person behaves violently while another person does not. It may be that a combination of theories is most helpful.

Biological Theories

The biological perspective links violence to biological dysfunction. These theories are concerned with extreme acts of violence and tend to assume that aggression is innate and lesser forms of violence are normal.

The neurophysiological effects of alcohol are frequently implicated in intentional violence such as rape, homicide, and suicide (Kelly & Cherek, 1993). In a review of 26 studies from 11 countries examining 9,304 crimes, it was found that 62% of violent offenders were drinking at the time of the crimes (Virk & Linnoila, 1993). Taylor and Chermack (1993) found that alcohol is a potent antecedent of aggressive behavior. Its effect is compounded by social pressure and the aggressive disposition of the alcohol consumer. Alcohol also plays a significant role in adolescent deaths due to homicide (Milgram, 1993). Substance use and abuse also contribute to the risk for violence.

Psychoanalytic Theories

The psychoanalytic theories of violence have been advanced by such theorists as Freud, Storr, Kaplan, and Fromme, and for the most part they explain aggression as an instinctive drive in humans. Siann (1985) and Storr (1968) expanded on Freud's theory of aggression as instinctive by theorizing that aggression exists on a continuum of behavior from a normal to a pathological response. Siann hypothesized that the aggressive response is determined by each individual's early development. Kaplan (1975) and Fromme (1977) shared the theory that aggression results from thwarting a basic human need rather than from an instinctive drive.

These theories examined mothering styles and placed less emphasis on the parenting style of fathers or the

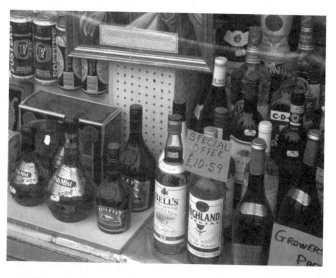

A 1993 study found that alcohol is a potent antecedent of aggressive behavior. *Photo courtesy of Michael St. Maur Sheil/ Corbis.*

effect of an absent father. Also these theories failed to explain the prevalence of violence perpetrated by men as compared with women.

Social Learning Theories

Social learning theory is a psychological theory incorporating sociological frameworks. Bandura (1973), Baron (1977), and other social scientists focus on violence as a learned response. If a child throws a tantrum whenever he wants something and the parents repeatedly give in to him, the child learns that aggressive behavior is effective. This learning can determine how the child will behave as an adult.

Modeling is another concept of socially learned behavior. When violent behavior is modeled and reinforced for children within their families, the children view it as a normal strategy to reduce stress, resolve conflicts, and get needs met. Violence can also be modeled and reinforced by aspects of the culture (school, church, neighborhood, and media). Centerwall (1992) suggests that if television technology had never been developed there would today be 10,000 fewer homicides each year in the United States, 70,000 fewer rapes, and 700,000 fewer injurious assaults.

Feminist Theory

Feminist theory views violence within the family as a gender and power issue (Bogard, 1992; Dobash & Dobash, 1992). It focuses primarily on an analysis of violence against women and identifies **patriarchy**, a male-dominated system in which males hold most of the power, as the root cause of this violence. Feminist theory rejects the notion that aspects of these roles are inherent, instead considering them socially constructed to maintain male power—not only in the family but in society at large. In this model, violence is seen as a social problem as well

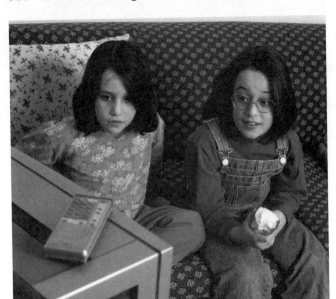

Do you think that television has contributed to a rise in violence? *Photo courtesy of Laura Dwight/Corbis.*

as a personal style of maintaining control over another person. The limitation of this model is its lack of application to other aspects of family violence such as elder abuse, sibling abuse, and child abuse.

COMMUNITY VIOLENCE

The United States is a violent country. In 1994, the murder rate was 9 for every 100,000 people, making it the highest rate in the industrialized world (Lacayo, 1996). Americans consider community violence to be the most urgent problem confronting the nation (Hart, 1994). Family and street violence are interrelated. Studies have shown that men who are violent at home are likely to be violent outside the home (Barnett et al., 1997).

Many factors have been identified that contribute to violence. These include influence of peers, unemployment, poverty, ethnic diversity, gun ownership, media violence, intrapersonal characteristics, and biological factors. However, "family influence is (arguably) the most likely determinant of an individual's level of violence" (Barnett et al., 1997, p. 4). Community violence can spill over into the workplace, including the hospital and places of worship.

Burgess, Burgess, and Douglas (1994) have defined several common types of violence that occur in the workplace. They are *nonspecific homicide,* in which there is no known reason for the behavior except to the perpetrator; *authority homicide,* which involves killing someone who has a real or symbolic authority relationship to the killer by which the killer perceives that he or she has been wronged; *revenge homicide,* in which murder is committed in retaliation for perceived wrongs; and *argument/ conflict homicide,* in which a person is killed during a dispute. *Domestic homicide* and *felony homicide* are two other types of killing. These occur when, in the former, the perpetrator kills a family member and, in the latter, when someone is killed secondary to a property crime such as robbery or murder. Unfortunately, innocent bystanders are often killed or wounded during these exchanges.

Children's Exposure to Community Violence

Many children living in urban areas are exposed to violence daily. Many have lost friends, relatives, teachers, or neighbors to homicide. Wallach (1993) cites a Chicago study of 1,000 children that found that 74% of the children had witnessed a murder, shooting, stabbing, or robbery (see Figure 24-1). Forty-six percent of the children had personally experienced at least one incident of violent crime. A six-year study of adolescents under the age of 17 living in northern Manhattan found that 79 adolescents per 1,000 per year were hospitalized or died as the result of an **assault** (Davidson, 1992). An assault is a violent attack, either physical or verbal, causing a present fear of immediate harm.

Urban children may live with the possibility of being shot in a drive-by as they walk home from school or even as they sit eating dinner in their homes. These realities rob them of any sense of safety or security. Newberger and Newberger (1992) propose that children who witness violence may develop a set of "mean-world" beliefs that places children at risk for accepting violence as normal and developing aggressive characteristics in order to survive (see Figure 24-2). Harlem junior high school students testified that their primary concerns were violence and drugs on the streets and the lack of after-school recreation programs (Davidson, 1992). The needs of urban children and the epidemic of violence affecting their lives should be a top priority for nursing education, research, and practice.

HATE CRIMES

Hate crimes are acts of violence perpetrated against people because of certain group characteristics. Common criteria for inclusion in these victimized groups include race, ethnicity, religion, sexual orientation, gender, and homelessness. Behavior may range from forms of intimidation

Figure 24-1 Children As Witnesses to Murder, Shooting, Stabbing, or Robbery

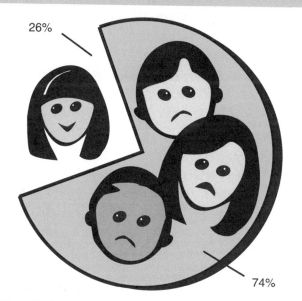

26%

74%

The Wallach Study of 1000 Children in Chicago found that 74% of the children studied had witnessed a murder, shooting, stabbing or robbery.

From "Helping Children Cope with Violence" by L. B. Wallach, 1993, National Association for the Education of Young Children, *48(4), pp. 4–11.*

such as cross burning, threats, harassment, or property damage to physically violent assaults such as rape, beatings, or murder. Martin (1995) suggests that hate crimes not only disrupt and threaten the lives of the targeted victims; they are also destructive to communities by "raising levels of fear, mistrust and hostility between groups" (p. 305). In 1996, 20 African American churches were burned to the ground in a year's time. Lesbians and gay men are also targets. It is reported that physicians some-

Figure 24-2 Mean-World Beliefs

- Relationships are defined by power: Those who have it hurt those who do not.
- If you don't have the power, those who do have it intend to hurt you in any situation that involves conflict.
- It is acceptable to use aggression to maintain power and to resolve problems.
- Aggression works to maintain power and to resolve problems.

Adapted from Treating Children Who Witness Violence by E. H. Newberger & C. M. Newberger, 1992. In D. F. Schwarz (Ed.), Children and Violence, *Report of the Twenty-Third Ross Roundtable on Critical Approaches to Common Pediatric Problems (pp. 118–125), Columbus, OH: Ross Laboratories. Copyright by Ross Laboratories.*

times fail to believe clients who say that they have been gay bashed. Physicians also tend to be especially insensitive to lesbians and gay men who have been sexually assaulted (Herek & Berrell, 1992). Martin's (1995) study of hate crimes in Baltimore County reviewed 690 reported hate crimes. Of the 346 (32%) verified crimes, 77% were found to be racial, 17% religious (primarily anti-Semitic), and less than 1% ethnic prejudice. Regardless of the basis of the hate, these violent acts threaten the well-being of the victim and are of concern to nursing.

In addition to overt acts of violence, widespread institutional prejudice also adversely affects racial, ethnic, religious, and sexual minorities. The implications for health care providers are poorly studied, and information on appropriate interventions and care is not available. This is an area in which nursing research is needed. Other issues appropriate to nursing research include motivation of perpetrators; the effect of hate on the victim's physical, mental, and spiritual health; support system needs; and prevention strategies.

VIOLENCE AGAINST WOMEN

The term **violence against women** is broad, encompassing physical violence, rape, homicide, genital mutilation, denial of rights based on gender, and female infanticide. Violence against women is often incorrectly viewed as a women's issue, but it is a community issue as well. Violence against women has emotional consequences affecting the victim and those who care about and depend on her. The financial consequence to society is high. Surgeon General Antonia C. Novello (1992) indicated that each year violence against women adds up to 100,000 days of hospitalization, 30,000 emergency room visits, and 40,000 medical office visits. She indicated that violence is the leading cause of injury to women aged 15 to 44.

Nurses are encouraged to grapple with the bigger picture as a means of unlearning biased ways of viewing female victims, to redefine the notion of prevention, to develop strategies that empower women, and to participate in solutions that will bring about long-term societal change.

SEXUAL VIOLENCE

Sexual assault exists on a continuum of violence, including behaviors ranging from staring and voyeurism to rape of children (see Table 24-1). Most women experience more than one of these behaviors over the course of their lives, and the most recent assault may trigger memories of previous unresolved or never-acknowledged events. Sexually assaultive behaviors are intrusive and nonconsensual. They disregard a person's right to freedom from harassment and are potentially intimidating. They demonstrate a profound disrespect for the victims.

Emotional response may vary widely depending on whether the assault occurs when the victim is isolated,

Table 24-1	Continuum of Sexual Assault
TYPE	**ACTIVITIES**
Nonverbal	Voyeurism; exposure; stalking; suggestive looks or facial expressions such as licking lips, thrusting tongue out, smacking lips
Verbal	Suggestive noises such as grunting, or sucking, sexist jokes; obscene phone calls
Unwanted contact	Slapping on buttocks; putting arm around a woman or a young girl and brushing her breasts in the process; touching genitals or the clothing over genitals
Harassment	Employer's negotiating job advancement on the basis of employee's willingness to cooperate in any of the activities on this continuum
Rape of adults	Sexual penetration of vagina, mouth, or rectum, without consent, using force or threat of force
Rape of children	Same as of adults, except victim is especially vulnerable because of size, age, dependency on adults, lack of power, and lack of comprehension

From Rape in America: A Report to the Nation *by D. G. Kilpatrick, C. N. Edmunds & A. Seymour, 1992, Fort Worth, TX: National Victim Center and Crime Victims Research and Treatment Center.*

whether it is ongoing or progressive, how much contact there is with the perpetrator, whether the victim has self-defense skills, and how threatening the incident seems. See Figure 24-3 for an example.

Rape

The legal definition of **rape** varies from state to state. However, it is usually defined as "sexual intercourse with a nonconsenting person by the use of force or the threat of force" (Rathus, Nevid, & Fichner-Rathus, 1997, p. 563). Figure 24-4 summarizes the findings of two nationwide studies about the ages of victims of completed forcible rapes in the United States.

Most rapes involve a man as the perpetrator and a woman as the victim. However, adult men are also raped by other men and are even more reluctant than women to report the assault. And women may be raped by

women. **Incest**, the crime of sexual relations between persons related by blood, is another underreported form of rape.

Studies indicate that only between 8% and 16% of rapes are reported to the police, making rape the most underreported violent crime in the United States. See Figure 24-5 for rape victims' common concerns (Newberger & Newberger, 1992). Some of these concerns may influence whether the rape is reported, as will the relationship of the rapist to the victim. **Acquaintance rape** or **date rape** is less likely to be reported than stranger rape (USDHHS, 1990). In acquaintance or date rape, the perpetrator is an individual known to the victim. He or she may be

Figure 24-3 Example of Sexual Assault Awareness among Female Teenagers

The author taught sexual assault awareness to senior teens. During discussions of the continuum of violence, several similar examples arose repeatedly from young women in different schools. One example was that of walking past a construction site alone and having several men yell, whistle, comment about their bodies, and shout out sexually suggestive invitations. These young women reported a variety of feelings including anger, intimidation, and fear. When asked how they handled the situation, several women mentioned that they evaluated their environment to see if other people were around, then picked up their pace and checked behind them several times to be sure they weren't being followed. Some women wanted to yell at these men but believed it was unwise because they were alone.

Figure 24-4 National Rape Statistics

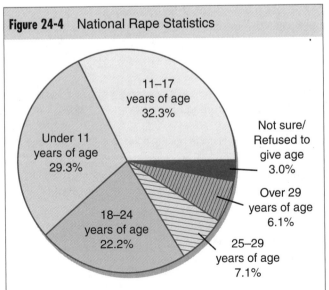

From Rape in America: A Report to the Nation *by D. G. Kilpatrick, C. N. Edmunds, & A. Seymour, 1992, Fort Worth, TX: National Victim Center and Crime Victims Research and Treatment Center. Copyright by National Victim Center and Crime Victim Research and Treatment Center.*

Sexual Assault

Popular novels, television, movies, and magazines continue to portray rape in a stereotypical manner. Answer the following questions based on stereotypes. Put aside what facts you might know. Try doing this with a partner—jot down your answers without conferring and then compare your responses.

Consider the victim.

- How old is the victim?
- Describe the victim's appearance: clothes, type and color of shoes and stockings, makeup, hairstyle and color, and race.
- What is the victim doing? Where?

Consider the rapist.

- Identify the rapist's age, race, and appearance, level of education, and employment.
- Where is the rapist? What is the rapist doing? Is there a weapon? What is it?
- Does the victim know the rapist?

Consider the circumstances.

- List the three most likely places this stereotypical rape would take place.
- What time of day is it?

Figure 24-5 Concerns Prominent among Female Rape Victims

- Her family knowing she had been sexually assaulted (71%)
- People thinking it was her fault or that she was responsible (69%)
- People outside of her family knowing she had been sexually assaulted (68%)
- Her name being made public by the media (50%)
- Becoming pregnant (34%)
- Contracting a sexually transmitted disease, not including HIV/AIDS (19%)
- Contracting HIV/AIDS (10%)

From Treating Children Who Witness Violence by E. H. Newberger & C. M. Newberger, 1992. In D. F. Schwarz (Ed.), Children and Violence, Report of the Twenty-Third Ross Roundtable on Critical Approaches to Common Pediatric Problems *(pp. 118–125), Columbus, OH: Ross Laboratories. Copyright by Ross Laboratories.*

an individual in a position of confidence (priest, therapist, etc.), an acquaintance, date, or spouse.

Attitudes toward Rape Victims

It is not uncommon for people to consider the victim as being responsible for the rapist's behavior or to claim that the allegations are untrue. This attitude continues to influence the criminal justice system, the health care system, and the culture at large. Furthermore, these attitudes affect the psychological reactions of the victim after a rape or sexually assaultive incident. When a person is raped, a self-blaming, shamed response is in part a reaction to this legacy.

Myths and Realities

The myths surrounding sexual assault serve to keep the focus and blame on the victim. Some myths also serve as defense mechanisms against the fear of sexual assault. We think that if we can identify the things the victim did wrong, we can avoid those behaviors and successfully avoid sexual assault. Although the myths listed in Table 24-2 refer to rape, they are applicable to any type of sexual assault. Figure 24-6 illustrates the psychological characteristics of rapists. As educators, nurses are in a position

to provide accurate information about these topics and to eliminate misconceptions.

Victim Response to Sexual Assault

Rape and other forms of sexual assault abruptly alter the victim's life to varying degrees depending upon the nature and extent of the actual or threatened violence. Life events involving overwhelming threats to a person's physical or psychological integrity, including sexual assault, often result in posttraumatic stress disorder (PTSD) (American Psychiatric Association, 1994). Symptoms of PTSD include hyperarousal, flashbacks of the traumatic event, and a state of surrender manifested by dissociation, detached calm, or a disconnection from the meaning of the events. In children, symptoms may include repetitive play in which themes or aspects of the trauma are expressed, frightening dreams without recognizable content, or specific reenactment of the traumatic event.

Herman (1992) sees recovery from PTSD as a three-phase process: (1) establishing safety, (2) remembrance and mourning, and (3) reconnection. Burgess and Holmstrom (1974) identified a two-stage response to rape trauma—acute and reorganization—that they labeled rape trauma syndrome; and Sutherland and Scherl (1970) identified an outward adjustment phase. Figure 24-7 delineates the stages of rape trauma syndrome.

Intervention for Survivors

Intervention during the period of crisis following the rape is vital and can help to reduce the severity of long-term consequences. The needs of the survivor are greatest during the first hours and days after the incident, but the vic-

Table 24-2   Rape Myths and Facts

MYTH	FACT
Sex is the motivation for rape.	Rape is an expression of power, anger, violence, and aggression—sex is the weapon.
Women lie about rape.	Only about 2% of all rapes and related sexual charges have been found to be false (Ehrhart & Sandler, 1985).
Rape is an isolated event, a temporary loss of control or lapse in judgment on the part of the rapist.	A rapist is likely to have raped before and to repeat the act in the future. The average number of victims per rapist is seven (Kilpatrick et al., 1992; Thobaben, 1998).
Most rapes involve men of color raping white women.	Rape is primarily an intraracial crime. The myth of black men raping white women has been perpetuated by racist and sexist sentiments. It also masks the history of white men's sexual violence against women of color.
Rapists are mentally ill or developmentally disabled and are therefore not responsible for their acts.	Rapists cover the full range of age, race, culture, class, and intelligence, and only a minority are psychotic (Quina & Carlson, 1989; Thobaben, 1998).
Women's behavior (e.g., manner of dress, makeup, use of language, walk, whereabouts, use of alcohol, etc.) evokes rape.	Persons of all ages are raped: infants, toddlers, children, adolescents, young women, middle-aged women, and elders. They are dressed in a wide variety of garb; 50% are raped in their homes; and the circumstances surrounding the rapes are as varied as the victims themselves.
The majority of rapes are committed by strangers.	The majority of rapes are committed by men known to the victim. Children are at greatest risk from sexual assaults by family members and caretakers. Adolescents and young adult women are most at risk for acquaintance and date rape. Adult women are most likely to be attacked by partners or ex-partners.

tim might return to a state of crisis months or years later. Crisis intervention focuses on the assault and gives that trauma precedence over other issues in the client's life. The goal is to help the client cope. Rape temporarily alters a victim's sense of personal power and control and inhibits decision-making skills.

As the crisis phase subsides, the nurse can discuss activities that facilitate empowerment. Many victims find it helpful to take a self-defense or martial arts class. Other helpful activities include instruction in the proper use of pepper spray or mace, assertion training classes, or even weight lifting in order to feel physically stronger.

Figure 24-6   Psychological Characteristics of Rapists

1. Power rapists—motivated by desire to control and dominate so victim cannot resist or refuse. The rapist experiences a reassuring sense of strength, mastery, security, and control. Force is used only to subdue the victim. Sexual gratification is secondary.

2. Anger rapists—motivated by need to express feelings of intense anger toward the victim and/or against the world in retaliation for perceived wrongs. Usually applies more force than needed and often coerces the victim into performing degrading and humiliating acts, fellatio, or anal intercourse. Satisfaction is derived from the discharge of anger and humiliation of the victim. Rape is perceived as revenge against the victim, not as sexual satisfaction.

3. Sadistic rapists—motivated by pleasure in ritualistic acts of violence. Attacks are often carefully planned and frequently include humiliation and mutilation. Torture and death also occur. Anger and need for control become sexualized through the pleasure obtained from the violence perpetrated on the victim.

Power rapes are most common, followed by anger rapes. Sadistic rapes account for only about 5% of rapists.

From Psychiatric-Mental Health Nursing: Adaptation and Growth *(4th ed.) by B. S. Johnson, 1997. Philadelphia: Lippincott; and* Human Sexuality in a World of Diversity *(3rd ed.) by S. A. Rathus, J. S. Nevid, & L. Fichner-Rathus, 1997, Boston: Allyn & Bacon.*

DECISION MAKING

Helping a Rape Victim

You are a nurse in a well-child clinic. A mother asks you, "What would you do if you had been raped?" She is very nervous. She has red eyes and there are tears in them.

- How would you answer her?
- What would you do?

Nurses can contact a local rape crisis center for information regarding available services. See Appendix B for a national number that connects with area rape crisis centers.

Partner Response to Rape

Rape usually has a devastating effect on the survivor's partner. While trying to deal with the survivor's emotional response, the partner must also deal with personal reactions ranging from shock to self-blame. Intimacy and sexual relations may be problematic for both partners. The survivor may have flashbacks that interfere with ability to respond to the partner or may have difficulty with sexual advances. Partners often feel that they are somehow being blamed for something they did not do, particularly if the survivor is displacing anger about the rape. The time it takes victims to recover can be surprising to partners, who want their loved ones to be able to return to their former state of being in a short time. Frequently, there is no discussion around these issues, and the two are unable to support one another. The nurse can anticipate these problems and encourage discussion between the partners. Referral to a counselor who has expertise in this area may be indicated.

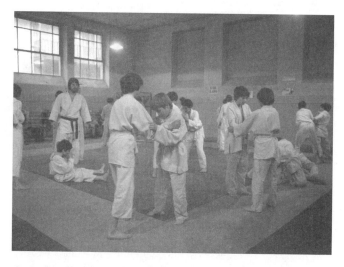

A victim of abuse may take a self-defense class to build a feeling of self-empowerment. Photo courtesy of Michael S. Yamashita/Corbis.

Figure 24-7 Rape Trauma Syndrome

Crisis Stage

Shock, helplessness, fear, anxiety

Guilt, shame

Overwrought or very controlled

Fear of making decisions

Pseudo-adjustment Stage/Outward Adjustment

Conscious forgetting

Emotional blocking

No further internal work on assault

Remains in this stage

Disturbing dreams or fantasies

Memories triggered

Reemergence Stage

No longer in denial

Experiences some crisis-stage responses

Desire to regain sense of power in life

Relives emotional experience

Desire to feel in control of sexuality

Resolution/Integration

Positively integrates assault experience

Able to cope with memories

Adapted from Trauma and Recovery *by J. L. Herman, 1992, New York: Basic Books; "Adaptive Strategies and Recovery from Rape" by A. W. Burgess & L. L. Holmstrom, 1974,* American Journal of Psychiatry, 136, *pp. 1278–1282; and "Patterns of Response among Victims of Rape" by S. Sutherland & D. J. Scherl, 1970,* American Journal of Orthopsychiatry, 40, *pp. 503–511.*

Intervention for Sex Offenders

The role of the community health nurse with regard to sex offenders includes reporting suspected child sexual abuse, working with families in which a member is an offender and has been incarcerated, having contact with offenders in institutions, or working with a family with whom an offender has been reunited. It is important to be aware of treatment options and to be familiar with the concepts of intervention.

Current research on treatment outcomes among sex offenders (particularly child molesters) indicates that, to be effective, the treatment must be cognitive-behaviorally based and must include a relapse prevention component (Marques, Nelson, West, & Day, 1994; Marshall & Pithers, 1994). Specific treatment goals are reduction of deviant sexual arousal, enhancement of nondeviant sexual interest, improvement of social skills, and modification of distorted reasoning and beliefs (Brody & Green, 1994; Marques et al., 1994).

Most often, sex offenders receive treatment through the criminal justice system during a period of incarceration or as a condition of their parole or probation (Frenken, 1994; Marques et al., 1994). Many treatment programs refuse to admit any offender who still denies having committed the offense (O'Donohue & Letourneau, 1993). Denial is a strong precursor to recidivism and as such needs to be addressed (Marshall & Pithers, 1994).

VIOLENCE IN INTIMATE RELATIONSHIPS

Violence occurring within the context of an intimate or familial relationship can be defined in many ways:

- **Domestic violence**—a broad term encompassing a spectrum of violence within a family.
- **Spousal abuse**—the physical, emotional, or sexual abuse perpetrated by either a husband or a wife against the marriage partner. This can also be referred to as marital rape.
- **Wife abuse**—the physical, emotional, or sexual abuse perpetrated by a husband against his wife.
- **Partner abuse**—the physical, emotional, or sexual abuse perpetrated by one partner in an intimate relationship against the other.
- **Battered women**—women who are in relationships in which battering is ongoing.
- **Child abuse**—physical or mental injury, sexual abuse or exploitation, negligent treatment, or maltreatment of a child by a person who is responsible for the child's health or welfare. (Child abuse will be discussed further later in the chapter.)
- **Elder abuse**—physical abuse, neglect, intimidation, cruel punishment, financial abuse, abandonment, isolation, or other treatment of an elder, resulting in physical harm or mental suffering. (Elder abuse will be discussed further later in the chapter.)

Domestic violence can take different forms but frequently involves a combination of assaultive acts, which may include sexual, physical, or emotional abuse or damage or destruction of property (see Table 24-3).

Dynamics of Partner Abuse

Partner abuse is frequently discussed in terms of males as perpetrators and females as victims, because these relationships constitute the greatest proportion of abusive relationships (Sheridan, 1993). This viewpoint does not negate or minimize violence that occurs in lesbian and gay relationships or dismiss heterosexual relationships in which men are assaulted by women (Butler, 1995). Yegidis (1992) notes that, although women commit spousal violence at about the same rate as men, the damage that men inflict is greater and "violence by wives tends to be retaliatory in nature; that is, . . . women

become abusive for reasons of self-defense" (p. 522). Figure 24-8 lists current facts concerning domestic violence against women. Table 24-4 lists numerous myths concerning partner abuse with regard to heterosexual couples in which the male is the perpetrator.

Lesbian Battering

The incidence of this violence in relationships is variously reported as from 17% to 26% (Loulan, 1987; Herek & Berrill, Lie, Schlitt, Bush, Montagne, & Reyes, 1991). There has been very little research on violence in lesbians (Crowell & Burgess, 1996). Increasing numbers of lesbians are calling battered women's shelters seeking assistance. Lesbians may be less likely to identify themselves as victims secondary to protecting the image of lesbians in the community at large. The risk of exposing oneself to a heterosexual agency may be perceived as greater than the risk of remaining silent. Battered lesbians need the same services as any other abused woman but are also dealing with the

Table 24-3 **Continuum of Violence in Intimate Relationships**	
TYPE	**ACTIVITIES**
Sexual	Any sexual act or behavior without consent, from degrading name calling with sexual implications (such as whore, tramp, or slut) to rape.
Physical	Any forceful physical behavior such as slapping; shoving; pinching; poking; punching; kicking; spitting; throwing the person bodily; wrestling; pulling hair; throwing things at the person; denying the person sleep, food or fluids, or use of bathroom or confining the person in any manner. Harming self, partner, children, pets, or property.
Emotional	Verbal or behavioral actions that diminish another's self-worth and self-esteem. Examples include belittling name calling (e.g., "You're stupid," "You're ugly") or threatening actions such as taking the children and disappearing; leaving the relationship to be with someone else; or revealing personal or intimate information to others. Other emotional violence includes forcing someone to stay awake; forcing degrading behavior such as eating out of a pet dish; constant blame or ridicule; controlling behavior such as telling a person what to or not to wear, stopping partner from seeing friends or using the phone, timing absences from home, monitoring the mileage on the car.
Property	Breaking partner's special or treasured possessions; punching holes in walls; destroying furniture, doors, windows, or partner's vehicle; throwing things.

abuse of a homophobic society and the possibility of homophobia within the agency involved. Lesbians batter for the same reasons that men batter, and threat of violence is just as traumatizing to the victims as in other situations.

Gay Male Violence

Like abuse in the lesbian community, battering between gay male partners is frequently hidden (Klinger, 1995). Abused men are often afraid or embarrassed to tell anyone about the violence in their relationship. One partner is usually more violent than the other; the fact that the victim, like any battering victim, may engage in self-defense does not mean that the partners are equally violent. The estimates of annual rates of relationship violence for gay men is from 11% to 20% (Island & Letellier, 1991; Bourg & Stock, 1994; Community United Against Violence, 1998).

Learned Helplessness

Learned helplessness, as applied to domestic violence by Walker (1979), describes the behavior resulting from learning that responses cannot control certain outcomes (Carden, 1994). Chronic feelings of powerlessness and decreasing motivation to respond ensue. These responses in turn lead to passivity, submissiveness, and helplessness.

Figure 24-8 Domestic Violence Fact Sheet

1. Domestic violence is the leading cause of injury to women.

2. Close to 4 million women are beaten by a male partner in the United States every year.

3. Women are six times more likely than men to be victims of violent crime in intimate relationships.

4. Murder of women by male partners accounts for 40% of all homicides against women.

5. Divorced and separated women constitute 7% of the population in the United States. They account for 75% of all battered women and report being battered 14 times as often as women still living with their partners.

6. Thirty-seven percent of pregnant women are abused. The escalating incidence of abuse is a leading cause of infant mortality and the escalating incidence of birth defects.

7. Battering accounts for 25% of all female suicide attempts and 50% of all suicide attempts made by African American women specifically.

8. Up to 50% of all homeless women and children in the United States are fleeing domestic violence.

From "Domestic Violence" by K. Dunn, 1995, Nursing News, 45(4), pp. 6–7; "The Pregnant Battered Woman" by P. Klaus, M. Rand, N. L. Noel & M. Yam, 1992, Nursing Clinics of North America, 27(4), pp. 871–883.

Abuse occurs randomly and is not necessarily connected to any particular action or behavior. Abuse victims learn that, regardless of how they change or try to do things differently, the abuse continues. The victim cannot predict which responses will work in a given situation and avoids any unknown situations. To a person in a state of learned helplessness, the known—even the known violence—holds less fear than the unknown. Depression is well documented as a component of learned helplessness, although abused women frequently remain functional in terms of work, caring for their children, and performing activities of daily living (ADLs). The combination of helplessness and depression places women and their children at high risk for self-harm.

Cycle of Violence

Walker (1979) proposed the cycle theory of violence. The cycle consists of three phrases: the tension-building phase, the battering incident or explosion, and the aftermath or honeymoon phase. The cycle is represented in Figure 24-9 and describes the usual process through which the individual passes.

Intervention with Domestic Violence Victims

Early identification of partner abuse is the first goal of intervention. Given the prevalence of domestic violence, routine screening of all women should be part of the health history. The nurse's approach to exploring violence among family members must be nonjudgmental and empathetic in order to facilitate trust. Sheridan (1993) documents clues and physical signs that should raise the index of suspicion for abuse. These are listed in Figure 24-10.

Once alerted to the possibility of abuse, the nurse needs to address concerns to the victim directly and in a caring manner. This discussion should take place in a safe and private setting away from the suspected assailant. Questions can be intertwined with information about abuse in order to communicate an understanding of the issue and to indicate what kinds of assistance are available in the community such as emergency shelters, counselors trained in domestic violence, male antiviolence programs, and legal services to assist with restraining orders. Urge the client to have a domestic violence plan. Preparation should consist of having the following items packed in a box or suitcase and kept in a safe and trusted place such as the home of a reliable neighbor, friend, or relative:

1. Identification: a duplicate driver's license, passport, and birth certificate

2. Cash: at least enough for a couple of nights shelter, food, perhaps a bus ticket

3. Emergency phone numbers: women's shelter, legal services

4. An extra set of car keys

5. Clothing for self and children

Table 24-4 Myths and Facts about Partner Abuse	
MYTH	**FACT**
Battering happens primarily in low-income families.	Battering and other forms of abuse occur in all income groups. Poorer people rely more often on social service agencies, police, emergency rooms, and courts for assistance, hence statistics are higher for that population. Middle-class and upper-class individuals are more able to afford attorneys, private therapists, and personal physicians, consequently avoiding reports that contribute to statistical findings.
Battered women are masochistic. Why doesn't she leave?	Such questions maintain focus on the victim's behavior and ignore the fact that the batterer has no right to abuse. Many people stay in relationships, trying one thing after another, thinking their changes will stop the abuse. Some who are economically or emotionally dependent on the batterer feel trapped.
Women of color are battered more often than white women.	This myth is often linked with the socioeconomic myth that battering occurs only in low-income families. There are few comparative research studies that specifically explore domestic violence among various ethnic or cultural groups. Lewis (1987) found that when controlling for social class, there is no difference between African American and European American couples with regard to incidence of abuse.
Men who beat women are mentally ill.	Else, Wonderlich, Beatty, Christie & Stanton (1995) report that some abusers are mentally ill, but they are of no greater proportion among batterers than in the general population.
Battering occurs because the man is drunk and out of control.	The relationship between alcohol and battering is unclear, and current research shows a widely varying range of prevalence. Many abusive men do not drink.

Intervention for Batterers

Health professionals have traditionally not specifically focused on the **batterer**, one who beats, strikes, or pounds another person, as the problem in cases of family violence (McKay, 1994). Instead the violence has been viewed as a family problem and is frequently addressed by referral for family or couple therapy. Some believe that this approach sends a message of shared responsibility, deemphasizes the batterer's behavior, and ignores the very real danger to the victim. One group that takes this perspective, Men Overcoming Violence, a San Francisco–based antiviolence program for violent men, states that they do not offer couples counseling. If the couple stays together, conjoint therapy may eventually play a role in treatment, but it is generally introduced after the batterer has addressed the violence in a treatment format (Carden, 1994).

Safety for the victims of domestic violence is the first priority in the treatment of batterers. Currently the victim and children generally leave their home and find safety in a shelter. A consideration for future treatment programs for assailants might be a shelter in which the *batterers* are confined until it is determined that they are in control of their behavior. Programs designed to treat batterers are relatively new, and research regarding effective intervention is still in its infancy. Grassroots antiviolence self-help collectives were the first wave of treatment for

batterers. These programs grew out of the feminist movement and usually combined a social analysis of domestic violence with a counseling element emphasizing nonviolent masculinity.

In the early 1990s professional organizations took their first steps toward focusing on family violence as a health issue, and opportunities for professional training have increased (Carden, 1994). Likewise, the criminal justice system has developed training programs specific to domestic violence, and some progress is being made with regard to how battering is handled by the police and the courts. One such change is the institution of mandatory arrest laws for perpetrators of spousal abuse in some areas. Programs tend to exclude batterers who are mentally ill or developmentally disabled or who cannot admit their violence. Commonalities among treatment programs are listed in Figure 24-11.

Outcome studies are lacking, and it is difficult to say which approach works in the short or long term. It is also doubtful that any one approach will work for all offenders. We need to be able to identify what constitutes progress and when programs need to be altered to meet the needs of a particular participant. Carden (1994) also notes the importance of being able to measure more subtle forms of violence that may replace physical abuse in the treated offender. Currently there are more questions than answers about what constitutes effective intervention

Figure 24-9 Cycle of Violence

Phase One: Tension Building

Batterer Behavior

Irritable.

Tense.

Minor outbursts.

Attempts to control rage or meter violence in small doses.

Victim Behavior

Avoids confrontation.

Attempts to control environment to keep batterer calm.

Makes excuses for his behavior.

May provoke explosion to get explosion over with.

Phase Two: Explosion/Battering Incident

Batterer Behavior

Rage overrides control. Battering occurs. May be progressive and last for a number of hours.

Victim Behavior

May express rage, may fight back, though usually too fearful of more serious injury. If has the opportunity to leave, may hide until she feels batterer is back in control

Phase Three: Honeymoon Phase/Hearts and Flowers Phase

Batterer Behavior

Apologetic.

Remorseful. Makes promises to get help, stop drinking, enter therapy, etc. Swears this will never happen again.

Gives gifts, helps around the house, mood lightens.

Victim Behavior

Wants to believe this is the last time.

Accepts gifts, discusses plans for getting help.

Moves into denial.

Return to Phase One—Cycles Shorten

From "Wife Abuse and the Wife Abuser—Review and Recommendations" by A. D. Carden, 1994, The Counseling Psychologist, *22(4), pp. 539–582.*

Figure 24-10 Indicators of Domestic Abuse

1. Complaints of insomnia and nightmares.
2. Passivity and lack of energy.
3. Somatic symptoms such as headaches, gastrointestinal complaints, asthma, chronic nonspecific pain.
4. Frequent emergency room visits with escalating injuries; explanations that fail to match injuries.
5. Depression, suicide attempts.
6. Substance abuse.
7. Anorexia, bulimia.
8. Sexual assault.
9. Suggestive injuries such as cigarette burns; black eyes; facial bruising or facial lacerations; injuries to the chest, back, breast, abdomen and/or genitalia; injury patterns that indicate use of belts, bites, hands, fists.
10. Anxiety, fear demonstrated when being interviewed.
11. Turning to partner before answering questions; visible fear when partner is in the room.
12. Partner consistently speaks for the person suspected of being abused.
13. The partner is overly solicitous and condescending to the partner who may be the victim of abuse.
14. One partner adheres rigidly to traditional roles and expects the other partner to meet needs and follow directions.

Adapted from "The Role of the Battered Woman Specialist" by D. J. Sheridan, 1993, Journal of Psychosocial Nursing, *31(11), pp. 31–36.*

and prevents recidivism, but the issue of domestic violence is coming more clearly into focus and is beginning to receive the attention it deserves.

Relationship Violence and Its Effects on the Family

The family is a complex system made up of individuals with multiple needs, different strengths, and varying coping mechanisms. Violence between partners was discussed earlier, but the impact on the family is deserving of further exploration.

Violence between parents or parental figures affects the children in a family. Although witnessing family violence is not always harmful, studies indicate that many children are negatively affected. Gage (1990) refers to a number of studies indicating that children who are exposed to spousal abuse have a variety of adjustment problems. Boys tend to demonstrate bullying behavior, temper tantrums, and cruel acts. Girls tend to exhibit anxiety, depression, perfectionism, and excessive neediness. When these children are adults, they will have a greater incidence of alcohol and drug dependency and will be more likely to abuse their children. Abused children are more likely than their nonabused peers to use aggression as a response to conflict or frustration, and the combination of witnessing violence and being the victim of abuse doubles the acceptability of violence as a solution to problems (Straus, 1992).

McKay (1994) cites studies showing that child abuse is 15 times more likely to occur in families where wife abuse is present. The community health nurse who identifies spousal battery must suspect abuse of children in the family. When children demonstrate behavioral problems, the nurse should obtain a careful history about family dynamics including past or present violence.

CHILD ABUSE

Child abuse includes physical and sexual abuse and child neglect. It commonly occurs within closed family systems (see Chapter 18) or is associated with substance abuse and social stressors (Blau, Whewell, Gullotta, & Bloom, 1994). Studies stress, however, that alcohol and drugs are not an excuse for violence or neglect (Yegidis, 1992). Social stressors may include poverty, unemployment, social chaos, unwanted pregnancies, and crowded living conditions (D'Antonio, Darwish, & McLean, 1993). Race and culture seem to predict violence, but research yields conflicting results. Gelles and Loseke (1993) point out that several studies found that poor children and children of color were much more likely to be both correctly and incorrectly reported for child abuse than were white and middle- to upper-income families. This discrepancy creates a risk for people of color, who may not receive needed services and referrals, and for those from middle- to upper-income families at risk of abuse, who may not be identified because of stereotypical thinking (Bourne, Chadwick, Kanda, & Ricci, 1993).

Child abuse is another area in which nurses must examine their own biases and belief systems to avoid being blinded to possibilities. Any family of any race, class, income bracket, religious background, neighborhood, or sexual orientation can be violent or neglect their children. Keep family violence or neglect as an assessment possibility regardless of the external appearance of the family and their material possessions.

Characteristics of Child Abuse

According to *Healthy People 2000* (USDHHS, 1990) the Child Abuse Prevention, Adoption and Family Services

---

Figure 24-11   Common Components of Treatment Programs for Batterers

Lethality assessment involves an assessment of the batterer's history with regard to the severity and frequency of the violence, substance abuse, psychiatric impairment, abuse toward children, current stressors, and access to victims. Higher levels of lethality may call for other forms of intervention. Lethality assessment should be ongoing throughout the course of treatment and the interventions adjusted to prevent further violence.

Group treatment is utilized because of its cost effectiveness and its potential for the batterers to gain insight into and to understand their behavior through interpersonal interaction and feedback.

Client accountability is an approach that holds the batterer accountable for past, present, and future actions. Minimization, projection of blame, and lack of motivation are addressed and challenged. If a batterer reoffends while in treatment, there must be a predictable and consistent response from the treating staff including making a report about the new offense. It is important that the legal system and the health care system coordinate their efforts.

The psychoeducational approach relies on the belief that violence is learned and can be unlearned. The goal is to teach new behaviors and attitudes that will prevent any future episodes of violence. Issues might include such things as: learning about the disinhibiting effects of drugs and alcohol; examining gender role socialization and the links to violence; defining what constitutes violence; examining the effects of violence on children; identifying how the media glamorize violence, including violence against women; learning techniques of stress management and anger management; and recognizing the covert ways in which society sanctions male violence and discourages male sensitivity.

Adapted from "Wife Abuse and the Wife Abuser—Review and Recommendations by A. D. Carden, 1994, The Counseling Psychologist, *22(4), pp. 539–582; and Perpetrators of Domestic Violence: Overview of Counseling the Court Mandated Client by A. L. Ganley, 1989. In R. A. Annernon & M. Hersen (Eds.),* Treatment of Family Violence. *New York: John Wiley & Sons.*

Act of 1988 defines child abuse as "physical or mental injury, sexual abuse or exploitation, negligent treatment, or maltreatment of a child by a person who is responsible for the child's welfare, under circumstances which indicate that the child's health or welfare is harmed or threatened." (p. 232) It is estimated that 2,000 to 5,000 children die each year as a result of assault by their caretakers. In 1986 the number of children experiencing abuse or neglect was estimated to be 1.6 million (USD-HHS, 1990). By 1992 this number had increased to 2.9 million reports of suspected physical abuse, sexual abuse, and neglect (Devlin & Reynolds, 1994). In the United States, child neglect accounts for 64% of abuse, followed by physical, sexual, and emotional abuse (Bourne et al., 1993). Table 24-5 identifies the physical and behavioral signs of abuse.

Children are frequently referred to as innocent. They are also extremely vulnerable by virtue of their size, age, basic dependency on adults, and lack of power. They are at greatest risk of being injured in their own home by a family member or other care provider. Research shows that child victims are more severely injured by male perpetrators and that perpetrators are more likely to be male (Hegar, Zuravin, & Orme, 1993). Severe child abuse resulting in permanent injury or death is most commonly perpetrated by fathers and boyfriends of children's mothers (Starling, Holden, & Jenny, 1995).

There continues to be ambivalence about what constitutes child abuse from a community perspective. Children have been viewed as the property of their parents for centuries, and the community has been reluctant to interfere in matters concerning child-rearing. Community endorsement contributes to the notion that parents have the right to use abusive forms of discipline with their own children. Buntain-Ricklefs, Kemper, Bell, and Babonis (1993) examined adult approval of varying types of punishment and found that individuals who were severely punished in their own childhood had a greater tolerance for severe punishment of children. Table 24-6 shows certain characteristics of children that increase their risk for being abused.

Nursing Assessment

The community health nurse who works with families and individuals is in a position to recognize abuse and to advocate for the child. Advocacy is difficult, however, if the nurse cannot maintain the objectivity necessary for obtaining a history. Because a thorough history taking is an important aspect of advocacy, the nurse who finds it difficult to address the issue adequately should ask for assistance and consultation from another professional. Differentiating between abuse and discipline may also pose a problem. Any suspicious finding warrants a thorough history and a complete physical assessment to provide for the ultimate safety of the child.

Although most health professionals discourage corporal punishment, the majority of American families resort to a slap or a spanking on occasion (Bourne et al., 1993).

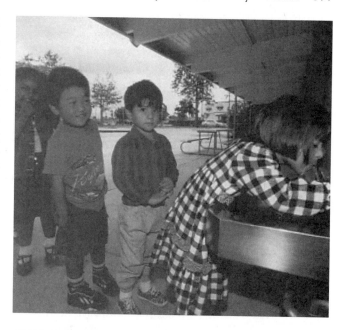

Child abuse can occur in any family regardless of race, class, income bracket, religious background, neighborhood, or sexual orientation.

Discipline may be classified as abusive when a child is struck with objects such as cords, hairbrushes, or sticks; when the adult uses a fist, knee, or foot to hit the child; or when sensitive body parts such as the head, face, or abdomen are involved. In assessing any type of child injury, the nurse must remain alert to the possibility of abuse whenever the signs and symptoms fail to match the history given by the child's caretaker or the description of the method of injury fails to match the child's developmental or motor skills.

Child Neglect

Child neglect and psychological maltreatment are diagnosed when the family fails to provide for a child's basic needs of food, clothing, shelter, supervision, education, emotional affection and stimulation, and health care. Child neglect is the most frequently reported form of child maltreatment. The majority of child neglect victims are under the age of 5 (Barnett et al., 1997).

The nursing assessment of child neglect may be problematic if the family is struggling with limited resources or physical disabilities. A careful history is important to determine if there are resources that are not being utilized to meet the child's needs. If the family does not have the resources to provide for the child's basic needs, the nurse can offer referrals to social service agencies that can assist. Depending on the particular manifestation of neglect, the nurse should assess what type of education and support the family might need to improve the care of the child. If, for instance, the neglect involves inadequate or inappropriate clothing, the nurse might explore how the parents see this problem, taking into consideration the issues raised in Figure 24-12.

Table 24-5   Indicators of Different Types of Child Abuse

TYPE	INDICATORS
Physical	History given fails to match injury Bruises on soft tissues and on multiple planes of the body: e.g., on the buttocks, lower back, cheeks, genitals Bruises in various stages of healing Finger marks on the neck indicative of choking Hand imprints on the face or body Human bites Cigarette, immersion, or scalding burns Unexplained fractures and pattern of healed fractures Bilateral black eyes Retinal detachment, dislocated lens, traumatic cataracts (shaken baby syndrome) Subdural hematoma (shaken baby syndrome) Abdominal injuries
Sexual	Child reports sexual abuse Frequent urinary tract infections Frequent yeast infections Sexually transmitted diseases Perianal bruising or tears Decreased anal tone Encopresis/enuresis at inappropriate developmental stage Genital pain or itching Genital trauma and/or bleeding Excessive masturbation Sexual acting out with younger children Age-inappropriate sexualized behavior or language Pregnancy Promiscuity, prostitution
Emotional	Failure to thrive Speech disorders Developmental delays Regression Poor social skills, antisocial behavior
Neglect	Lack of adult supervision, inappropriate supervision (e.g.; children supervising children) Poor hygiene Hunger, distended abdomen, signs of malnutrition, anemia, stealing food Teeth in poor repair Clothing inappropriate to weather conditions
All types: emotional signs	Withdrawal, depression, suicidality, anxiety, or fear Self-destructive behaviors Substance abuse Sudden changes in behavior Sudden school difficulties Dramatic mood extremes Sleep disorders Nightmares Repeated runaway Aggression

The parents' childhoods should also be explored. If they were neglected, they may be parenting in the only way they know how. These are issues that have the potential to respond to education, counseling, and support. An important nursing intervention is teaching parents specific skills for increasing positive parent–child interactions, improving problem-solving abilities, and enhancing personal hygiene and nutritional skills. Family therapy may be another helpful adjunct if the family is amenable. Cultural and religious beliefs should be assessed because some behaviors that appear neglectful may stem from a family's belief system. If those beliefs are placing the child at risk, the nurse should consult with a child abuse specialist to determine how to proceed.

Neglect can be a precursor to other types of abuse: It might exist in tandem with other abuses or as a singular

Table 24-6   Certain Characteristics in Children That Increase Risk of Abuse

CHARACTERISTIC	DESCRIPTION
Age	Young children (under the age of 3) are at greater risk for severe physical abuse and fatalities secondary to abuse (Devlin & Reynolds, 1994).
Gender	There have been inconclusive findings with regard to the relationship between the child's gender and the severity of the abuse. However, one study found that boys were more likely to be the victims of serious injuries from birth to 12 years of age, and girls were more seriously injured after the age of 13 (Hegar, et al., 1993).
Anomalies	Children who are perceived to be different, such as in the areas of developmental delays, congenital abnormalities, chronic disease, or temperamental traits, are at increased risk (Devlin & Reynolds, 1994).

From "Child Abuse: How to Recognize It, How to Intervene" by B. K. Devlin, & E. Reynolds, 1994, American Journal of Nursing, 94(3), pp. 28–32; and "Can We Predict Severe Child Abuse?" by R. L. Hegar, S. J. Zuravin & J. G. Orme, Violence Update, 4(1), pp. 2–4.

form of abuse. Though neglect is less externally dramatic than other forms of child abuse, the long-term sequelae and potential for adult dysfunction are serious (Bourne et al., 1993).

Physical Abuse

As shown in Table 24-5, certain types of injuries are characteristic of physical abuse. These include certain types

Figure 24-12   Points for the Nurse to Consider when Exploring Reasons for a Child's Inappropriate Clothing

- Is clothing too large, too small, or inappropriate for the child's developmental stage?
- Is the child dressing himself or herself without adult supervision or input?
- Is clothing being handed down and forced to fit?
- Do the parents have unrealistic expectations of the child's ability to cope with environmental realities such as cold weather?
- Is either parent abusing substances and thus depleting the family income and contributing to poor decision making?

DECISION MAKING

"Problem Child"

You are making a first home visit to a family for post-partum follow-up. Their doctor was concerned about the family situation because the mother, Mary, had expressed concern that her husband, Jim, would not like it if the new baby cried much. He was very busy at work and needed his sleep and quiet time in the evening. They returned from the hospital two days ago with a newborn boy, Robert. There is also a 3-year-old girl, Annette, in the family. Mary tells you that Robert is crying a lot and Annette is constantly bothering her and her husband for attention. She had no idea it would be so difficult. She has had little sleep since she got home. Her husband, who is Annette's stepfather, has been no help during the day. He is a stockbroker and is kept very busy. He is angry at Annette because she has been so clingy, but Mary tells you that she is relieved because Annette stayed away from him last evening. You note a large bruise on Annette's arm that looks like finger marks.

- Are there signs in this family that might suggest child abuse or potential abuse? What type of abuse?
- As the nurse, how would you proceed with the visit?
- What community resources might help?
- How would you follow up on the family after this visit?

and patterns of bruises, burns, fractures, and other injuries, as shown in Table 24-7. Bruises that are common in childhood are generally found over a bony prominence, such as an elbow, whereas bruising of soft tissue is suggestive of abuse. Scalding is the most common burn injury in children (Devlin & Reynolds, 1994). An accidental burn that occurs from a splashdown of a hot liquid generally will be more severe on the upper body than on the lower body because the liquid cools as it moves downward. Intentional burns tend to be on the feet or the hands. Devlin and Reynolds (1994) may be referred to for ways the nurse can differentiate healing cigarette burns from impetigo or other skin lesions. Some cultures use folk remedies such as hot oils, herbs, or cupping that may imitate burn marks on a child's back. It is important to explore this possibility.

Abusive head trauma in infancy is the most common type of child abuse resulting in death (Starling et al., 1995). Abusive head injury is also referred to as the shaken baby syndrome, although Starling et al. (1995) make the point that this is a misnomer because the mechanism of injury may be either shaking or impact trauma. In either event, the trauma results in central nervous system damage.

Table 24-7   Patterns of Certain Abusive Injuries to Children

TYPE	PATTERN
Bruises	On soft tissue, especially lower back and buttocks; multiple sites; or in various stages of healing. Any bruising on an infant, though bleeding disorders should be ruled out.
Burns	On the back or buttocks, cigarette burns, branding types of burns such as those from a hot iron, comb, or curling iron; or glove-stocking pattern burns from immersion of the arms or legs in hot water.
Fractures	Spiral or transverse fractures of the humerus or femur and fractures of the scapula or sternum (Bourne et al., 1993). Rib fractures in infants or children under 3 are almost always diagnostic of abuse, as are skull fractures or subdural hematomas in the first year of life, with irritability, vomiting, apnea, seizures, lethargy, poor feeding, or unexplained unconsciousness. There may be bruising on the shoulders, armpits, or abdomen where the baby was grabbed (Starling et al., 1995).
Abdominal	There may be no sign of external injury, or signs may be limited to mild bruising (Devlin & Reynolds, 1994).

From "Child Abuse: How to Recognize It, How to Intervene" by B. K. Devlin & E. Reynolds, 1994, American Journal of Nursing, 94(3), *pp. 28–32; "When You Suspect Child Abuse" by R. Bourne, D. L. Chadwick, M. B. Kanda & L. R. Ricci, 1993.* Patient Care, 27(3), *pp. 22–54; and "Abusive Head Trauma: The Relationship of Perpetrators to Their Victims" by S. P. Starling, J. R. Holden, & C. Jenny, 1995,* Pediatrics, 95(2), pp. 259–262.

Abdominal injuries are the second leading cause of death among abused children. Any abdominal injury of undetermined etiology should be assessed for abuse. These injuries may be secondary to the child's being kicked or punched in the abdomen (Devlin & Reynolds, 1994).

Sexual Abuse

Sexual abuse of children is cited by one author as "the most underdiagnosed form of child abuse and the highest unreported crime in the United States" (Van Horst, 1990, p. 44). The various terms used to discuss child sexual assault are defined in Table 24-8.

Sexual abuse of children is any sexual act with a child. It may or may not involve force or coercion. It may not be violent or involve physical contact or physical harm. Children of all ages, from infancy to adolescence, may be victims. Kilpatrick et al. (1992) note that 29% of all forcible rapes of girls occur before the age of 11. The incidence of sexual abuse of male children is difficult to ascertain because of underreporting. Various studies indicate that between 3% and 31% of male children are sexually

assaulted. Sexual abuse of both boys and girls is usually perpetrated by a male who is a family member (Black & DeBlassie, 1993). A common misconception holds that gay men have a high incidence of sexually assaulting children. In fact, child sexual abuse—including same-sex child abuse—is overwhelmingly perpetrated by heterosexual males. Only 1% of sexual abuse cases can be attributed to gay and lesbian perpetrators (Jenny, Roesler, & Poyer, 1994).

Indicators of child sexual abuse depend in part on a child's developmental stage and vary from child to child. Possible indications of sexual abuse according to the child's age (Black & DeBlassie, 1993) are listed in Table 24-9.

Table 24-8   Terms Associated with Child Sexual Abuse

TERM	MEANING
Child sexual abuse	The National Center on Child Abuse and Neglect has established the following definition of child sexual abuse: "Contact or interaction between a child and an adult, when the child is being used for the sexual stimulation of that adult or another person. Sexual abuse may also be committed by another minor, when that person is either significantly older than the victim, or when the abuser is in a position of power or control over that child" (p. 195).
Incest	Sexual behavior within the context of a preexisting family relationship. Included in this definition are family members of the same or opposite sex, stepparents and steprelatives and common-law partners of a parent.
Sexual molestation	Sexual contact that does not involve penetration. Behaviors might include exposure, masturbation, or touching (see sexual contact).
Sexual contact	The intentional touching of a child's genitalia or clothing covering the genitalia when the touching can be construed as being for the purpose of sexual arousal or gratification.
Sexual penetration	Vaginal or anal penetration, cunnilingus, or fellatio. Intrusion of any orifice of a child by any of the adult's body parts, or intrusion by objects.
Rape	Sexual penetration of a child by an adult.
Statutory rape	Sexual penetration of a child who is at least 13 but less than 18 by a person at least 4 years older.

From "Child sexual abuse" by D. Murman, 1992 Psychiatric and Adolescent Gynecology, 19, *pp. 193–207.*

Table 24-9   Sexual Abuse Indications According to Child's Age Group

AGE GROUP	INDICATIONS
Infancy	Without physical signs of abuse, it may go undetected barring diagnosed sexually transmitted disease (STD).
Preschool	May withdraw, regress, act out sexually with peers, masturbate compulsively, attempt to insert an object into the vagina or anus of self or of a pet, have nightmares, or develop recurrent urinary tract infections or STDs.
School age	May regress, withdraw, demonstrate excessive dependency, or begin to exhibit antisocial behaviors.
Adolescence	May demonstrate aggressive behavior, depression, substance abuse problems, truancy or poor school performance, running away, or eating disorders. Older children and adolescents are also at increased risk for suicide.

Adapted from "Sexual Abuse in Male Children and Adolescents: Indicators, Effects, and Treatments" by C. A. Black, & R. R. DeBlassie, 1993, Adolescence, 28(109), pp. 122–133.

Emotional Abuse

Emotional abuse is a component of all forms of abuse, in which verbal or behavioral actions diminish another's self-worth and self esteem. In itself, it is the least reported form of abuse (Barnett et al., 1997) When it exists alone it can be difficult to identify and even more difficult to validate for the purposes of reporting. Observing family dynamics, particularly how children are talked to, disciplined, and attended to, offers clues to the emotional climate. Emotional abuse includes name calling, put-downs, and isolating, stigmatizing, humiliating, or ignoring the child.

Differentiating between a child who is emotionally abused and a child who is emotionally disturbed may be challenging because presentations are so similar. To further complicate matters, characteristics such as speech disorders, learning disabilities, and failure to thrive are identified in children who *may or may not* suffer from abuse or an emotional disorder. Bourne et al. (1993) suggest that a detailed psychosocial assessment of the family may help differentiate between emotional abuse and an emotional disturbance. They generalize that parents of emotionally disturbed children tend to recognize that there is a problem and seek help, whereas parents of emotion-

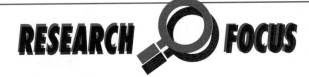

RESEARCH FOCUS

A Brief Group Treatment for the Modification of Denial in Child-Sexual Abusers: Outcome and Follow-Up

STUDY PROBLEM/PURPOSE

To determine the efficacy of group treatment to modify denial among sexual abusers of children.

METHODS

Participants in the study were 17 offenders, 15 of whom had been in complete denial for an average of two years, one who denied memory of the event but concurred it may have happened, and one who accepted responsibility but had refused individual treatment. The group met for 1.5 hours weekly for seven weeks and focused on victim empathy, irrational beliefs regarding child–adult sex, sex education, assertiveness and social skills, sex offender therapy, and the consequences of continued denial.

FINDINGS

Following treatment, eight offenders fully admitted to their crimes; five offenders maintained partial denial either by admitting to previous offenses while denying the most recent offense or by minimizing the impact of their current offense; and four offenders remained in complete denial.

IMPLICATIONS

This outcome suggests that offenders in denial may benefit from intervention focused on their denial in order to ready them for subsequent treatment. Offenders who are unable to shift from denial are a continued threat to the community and are the responsibility of the criminal justice system. Predicting the likelihood of reoffense among child molesters and rapists, treated or not, needs further research.

SOURCE

From "A Brief Group Treatment for the Modification of Denial in Child-Sexual Abusers: Outcome and Follow-Up" by W. O'Donohue, & E. Letourneau, 1993, Child Abuse and Neglect, 17, pp. 299–304.

ally abused children may deny that there is a problem and refuse help.

Parents who are emotionally abusive may benefit from nonjudgmental education and positive role modeling. They may need information about how to discourage behaviors without making the child feel like a bad person. Time-outs, loss of privileges, rewards for positive behaviors, and elimination of name calling and put-downs may be new concepts to the family. Parental education should include the impact that this type of treatment has on their child's self-esteem and emotional adjustment in later years. Parents may benefit from classes on parenting techniques in addition to family therapy.

Violence and Adolescents

Adolescents are often overlooked when family violence is assessed, yet statistics indicate that they experience disproportionately high levels of abuse (Randall, 1992). Some warning signs of possible past or present abuse include behaviors such as chronically running away, sexual promiscuity (particularly prostitution), gang involvement, truancy, substance abuse, eating disorders, and self-abusive behaviors. Adolescents demonstrating these behaviors should always be carefully and privately assessed for an abuse history.

An extreme form of violence is adolescent parricide. Parental murder often occurs in a situation in which the adolescent feels unable to escape abuse; the adolescent has often been considering the possibility of murder for years (Toch, 1995). Heide (1995) has classified adolescent parricide offenders into three typologies: the severely abused child, the severely mentally ill child, and the dangerously antisocial child. The classifications are not mutually exclusive in a particular individual. Early assessment and intervention into the family situation can do a great deal to prevent this deadly outcome.

Thirty-two percent of all forcible rapes of females occur to victims between the ages of 11 and 17. A study of 77 male victims found a median age of 8 years with a range of 1 to 15 years of age (Roane, 1992). A large number of assailants in date rape of female teens are adolescents between the ages of 12 and 20 (Kershner, 1996).

Violence is a major cause of injury and death among adolescents, with homicide ranking as the second leading cause of death for all 15- to 24-year-olds in the United States. African American adolescent males between the ages of 15 and 24 are at greatest risk for fight-related assaults and death from homicide. *Healthy People 2000* (USDHHS, 1990) notes that males between the ages of 15 and 34 are at highest risk of death from suicide and homicide, secondary to a gunshot wound. The midcourse review reported a 22% increase in the homicide rates among young men, with "young black men exceeding that of young white men in 1992 by as much as eight times" (USDHHS, 1996, pp. 61–62).

Urban youths have the highest rates of firearm-related homicides. Although nonurban areas have lower numbers of homicides, nonurban rates among teens are substantially higher in the United States than in many other industrialized nations (Fingerhut, Ingram, & Feldman, 1992). Suicide ranks as the second leading cause of death among all adolescents age 15 to 19. Cummings, Koepsell, Grossman, Savarino, and Thompson. (1997) found an association between the legal purchase of a handgun and an increased risk of violent death through both homicide and suicide.

Garrett's (1995) research review suggests that gangs give insecure adolescents a sense of security, self-worth, and respect; that the pressures of survival in poverty-stricken communities push children into gangs; and that the violence is an outgrowth of frustration stemming from the lack of opportunity for people of color. These links are presented not as an attempt to justify violence but to assist in thinking of ways to prevent the creation of another generation of frustrated, angry children with sorely inadequate coping skills.

ELDER ABUSE

The earliest research concerning elder abuse was completed in the 1970s. Current statistics suggest that between 2% and 4% of the elder population is subject to caregiver abuse (Benton & Marshall, 1991). Elders are at greatest risk of being abused by a family member who is also the caregiver and lives with the victim (Delong, 1995). Eighty percent of care in the home is provided by a woman, often a daughter. Sons are more likely to perpetrate active physical abuse; daughters are more likely to be responsible for emotional abuse or neglect. Husbands caring for their ailing wives are at high risk for caregiver overload and subsequent abuse secondary to limited nurturing experience, inadequate training, and limited support (Butler, Finkel, Lewis, Sherman, & Sutherland, 1992). In general, caregivers are at greater risk to abuse if they do not know the normal physical and cognitive changes that accompany aging. Prevention of caregiver overload is one of the primary interventions the nurse can make to avoid elder abuse.

Nursing Assessment

Caregiver stress placing the elder at risk for abuse may be generated by events that are unrelated to the role of caretaking (Benton & Marshall, 1991). Typical caregiver stressors include marriage, divorce, pregnancy, substance abuse problems, job loss, and financial problems. Role-related stressors tend to be associated with the caregiver's perceptions of the role as a burden, increased dependency of the elder on the caregiver for activities of daily living, fecal or urinary incontinence, insomnia, and intellectual impairment. Another factor is the age of abusers. Many are elderly themselves and suffer from a variety of difficulties such as mental and physical impairment, low levels of social support, and substance abuse (Barnett et al., 1997).

Table 24-10 Examples of Three Types of Elder Abuse

TYPE	EXAMPLES
Physical	Slapping, punching, hitting with belts or other objects, etc.
	Physically restraining
	Isolating
	Withholding personal care—adequate food, clothing, medical attention, hygiene needs
	Sexual assault
Psychological	Verbal assault, humiliation, name calling, belittling, intimidation, threatening harm
	Not allowing access to phone, transportation, mail, friends
	Provoking fear
Financial/material	Theft
	Manipulating finances
	Blocking access to money or property
	Extorting funds
	Failure to use elders' funds to meet their needs

From "Elder Abuse" by D. Benton & C. Marshall 1991, Clinics in Geriatric Medicine, 7(4), pp. 831–845.

Social isolation also places elders at greater risk for abuse. The socially isolated elder is not observed by others who might identify changes in behavior or appearance, and he or she has no one to talk to about possible mistreatment. The home health care or public health nurse is in a position to develop a relationship with the primary caregiver, to monitor for stressors, to assess the elder, and to promote self-care in the caretaker as well as in the elder when that is possible.

Elder abuse may be categorized as physical, financial, or psychological. Physical abuse includes physical or sexual assault, neglect, and medical mismanagement. Neglect, including self-neglect, accounts for the largest percentage of elder abuse reports, followed by physical, financial, and psychological abuse (Benton & Marshall, 1991). Table 24-10 gives examples of types of abuse in each category. Figures 24-13 and 24-14 list signs of physical mistreatment and psychological abuse in the elderly, respectively.

In cases of suspected abuse, assessment includes the elder's dependency needs, social situation, and relevant aspects of the history and physical exam. Culture, belief systems, and income must be evaluated as part of the assessment. Some folk treatments might be mistaken for abuse, and poverty may manifest in signs similar to neglect (e.g., unfilled prescriptions or inadequate diet). Certain religious beliefs involve the refusal of blood products or other medical interventions. The nurse will be challenged to respect the family's beliefs and maintain their dignity while assuring that the elder is not suffering or at risk secondary to these realities.

Assessing the potential for abuse is an important aspect of prevention. The nurse's assessment should include both the elder and the caretaker. When the caretaker is a family member, family dynamics should be explored. Benton and Marshall (1991) discuss the increase in caregiver roles by younger family members as older members live longer. This phenomenon increases

Figure 24-13 Signs of Physical Mistreatment in the Elderly

- Contusions
- Abrasions
- Sprains
- Burns
- Bruising
- Human bite marks
- Sexual molestation
- Untreated but previously treated conditions
- Misuse of medications
- Freezing
- Depression
- Erratic hair loss from hair pulling
- Lacerations
- Fractures
- Dislocations
- Oversedation
- Over- or undermedication
- Welts
- Scratches
- Decubiti
- Dehydration
- Malnutrition
- Poor hygiene
- Head and face injuries (especially orbital fracture, black eyes, broken teeth)

From Maltreatment of Older Adults by L. C. Curry & J. G. Stone, 1994. In M. O. Hogstel (Ed.), Nursing Care of the Older Adult (3rd ed., p. 492), Albany, NY: Delmar Publishers; and Older Adult by A. G. Pierce, T. T. Fulmer, & C. L. Edelman, 1994. In C. L. Edelman & C. L. Mandle (Eds.), Health Promotion throughout the Lifespan (3rd ed., p. 655), St. Louis, MO: Mosby.

Figure 24-14 Indicators of Psychological Abuse in the Elderly

- Clinging to the abuser
- Extreme guardedness in the presence of the abuser
- Wariness of strangers
- Expression of ambivalence toward family or caregivers
- Denial of abuse due to fear of retaliation
- Vague explanations for cause of injuries
- Depression
- Confusion and disorientation
- Anger, rage
- Social or physical isolation
- Conflictual interpersonal interactions
- Anxiety

From Maltreatment of Older Adults by L. C. Curry & J. G. Stone, 1994. In M. O. Hogstel (Ed.), Nursing Care of the Older Adult (3rd ed., p. 492), Albany, NY: Delmar Publishers.

the family's stress by taxing financial, emotional, and physical resources and makes the experience of caretaking a burden. This feeling of being burdened sets the stage for abusive behaviors. Families with long-term dysfunctional patterns are suspect for abuse potential as are caregivers with a history of having been abused themselves. Psychological problems and substance abuse in either the caretaker or the elder have also been found to be linked to abuse.

Evaluating the caregivers' concerns, their feelings about providing care for the family member, their ability to provide that care, and their need for support, counseling, or health care provides the nurse with the information needed to formulate prevention planning. Depending on what the family is comfortable with and is able to afford, the use of home health aides, sitters, temporary placement in an extended care facility, or intermittent respite care by alternating family members and friends might be coordinated by the nurse.

Longstanding dysfunctional family problems that create

DECISION MAKING

An Ethical Issue

If an elder is determined to remain in a situation with abusive elements rather than be removed from the home and placed in an institution, should the right to autonomy and self-determination be honored?

- What is the nurse's legal obligation?
- What is the nurse's caring obligation?
- What factors other than safety are at issue?

a potential for abuse should be identified and discussed. These may not be resolvable, but discussing them allows for supportive interventions such as counseling or shared responsibility for caregiving. The family can benefit from information about normal changes associated with aging as well as specific information about any existing illness or disability. Teaching specific skills needed to care for the elder and supervising return demonstrations can prevent passive neglect as well as reduce caregiver stress.

Nursing Intervention

Elder abuse victims are often reluctant to acknowledge the abuse. They may fear being moved to a nursing care home if authorities become involved. They may be ashamed that a child or spouse is abusing them, or they may fear retaliation from the perpetrator for reporting the violence. Abuse may also involve social isolation, and the elder may be unable to report what is happening. The fact that elders are adults with rights raises ethical issues that influence intervention strategies. The two guiding ethical principles of intervention in halting abusive acts are beneficence (to do good) and nonmaleficence (to do no harm). What the nurse determines as good (e.g., pushing for separation from the abuser or forcing institutionalization) may in fact be experienced as harmful by the elder.

Although reporting of elder abuse is mandatory in 42 states (Barnett et al., 1997), the elder may refuse to cooperate with the process. Once the nurse has met the mandated legal obligation, the range of available interventions needs to be considered, including attempting to work with the caregiver to change any abusive behaviors. It may take considerable time, consistency, empathy, and patience to establish a trusting relationship with an elder abuse victim. The nurse needs to avoid any criticism of the elder or the caretaker, even when that person is abusive. Criticism may be viewed as abusive and may reinforce the elder's distrust of others.

Once trust has been established, the elder or the caretaker or both may open up to the nurse about the difficulties experienced and be receptive to additional help. The nurse may then become the liaison between social services and the family. The long-term goals of intervention are to stop the abuse and to help the family accept help and support, thus lowering the potential for future abuse. Not all families will respond to these efforts. In some cases, the only solution may be separation of the abuser and the victim.

HOMICIDE

The homicide rate in the United States is much higher than that in any other industrialized country and doubled between 1960–1992 (Centers for Disease Control and Prevention, 1992, Flannery, 1997). Sixty-one percent of all homicides involve the use of a firearm, and firearm fatalities rank second only to motor vehicle accidents (Kellerman, 1994).

Although the United States continues to hold the lead as the most violent of industrialized countries in the world, the profile of violence has changed. Adolescents and young adults account for an increasing number of the victims and perpetrators of homicide (CDC, 1997). In fact, the United States also has the highest rate of childhood homicides among 26 industrialized countries (Fingerhut, Ingram, & Feldman, 1998). In the years spanning 1985–1994 the homicide rate for African American males aged 15–19 increased by 293%, while the homicide rates for white males in the same group rose by 214%. Homicide is now the leading cause of death among African American males aged 15–24, the second leading cause of death among white males aged 15–24, and the third leading cause of death in all children aged 5–14. Three-quarters of these homicides involve a firearm (Stanton, Baldwin, Rachuba, 1997) and according to a 1995 study, one out of twelve children now carry guns to school (Hennes, 1998).

Close to 40% of women homicide victims are murdered by an intimate—their spouse, a close acquaintance, or a family member (Kellerman & Mercy, 1992). Women make up over 50% of the U.S. population, account for 23% of all homicide victims, and commit 14.7% of all homicides. In 80% of the homicides committed by women, the victim was their spouse or an intimate acquaintance (Kellerman & Mercy, 1992). Women have a 1.3 times greater risk than men of being killed by their partner (USDHHS, 1990). Men most commonly murder a partner who is trying to leave the relationship. Women most frequently kill a partner in self-defense or in retribution for battering. Children under the age of 4 are most frequently killed by a family member or caretaker; older children are murdered primarily by acquaintances or strangers (USDHHS, 1990).

Healthy People 2000 (USDHHS, 1990) identifies socioeconomic status as a link to violence but indicates that homicide statistics have not monitored this variable. The 1995 midcourse review (USDHHS, 1996) notes a continuing serious gap in knowledge and understanding of the causes and prevention of violent behavior and recommends that individual, familial, social, and economic influences be studied to determine their impact on violent behavior. Centerwall (1995) conducted two retrospective studies examining intraracial domestic homicides among African American and Caucasian populations. When these populations were compared according to socioeconomic status, there was no significant difference with regard to risk of homicide. Several studies (Fingerhut et al., 1992; Meehan & O'Carroll, 1992; Saltzman, Mercy, O'Carroll, Rosenberg, & Rhodes, 1992) link the availability of firearms to the increase in homicide.

MANDATED REPORTING OF VIOLENCE

Currently, 45 states and the District of Columbia have laws mandating that health care professionals and others report injuries resulting from crime, intentional violence, abuse, and injuries that involve weapons. These laws vary from state to state with regard to specific provisions such as the seriousness of the crime, the type of weapon involved, and what constitutes violence. Each community health nurse should obtain a copy of local reporting statutes.

Nurses are mandated reporters of suspected child abuse in all 50 states. Reports are made to the local child protective service agency; failure to comply may result in a fine, arrest, and the possibility of civil action. Although health care professionals are protected against any liability resulting from a report made in good faith, most experience some apprehension about filing. The nurse may not be sure if a particular situation actually represents abuse or neglect. Child protective services are always willing to discuss the situation with the nurse to help determine whether it warrants reporting. It may be that not all cases reported will be investigated immediately because of the extensive number of child abuse cases handled. However, if problems continue to be reported, an investigation will become a priority. The child's safety and health are the nurse's primary concern. Reporting may be a lifesaving measure.

Bourne et al. (1993) suggest that, when possible and safe, the family be informed before a report is made and that nonaccusatory language such as "do you have any reason to suspect that anyone has abused your child" be used (p. 51). Filing procedures and time lines vary from state to state. The nurse should be aware of the local and institutional procedure. Documentation is an important aspect of reporting. Charting should be chronological and in detail. Quote any important information given by the child or the parents and note any discrepancies between the history and the injury. See Bourne et al. (1993, p. 37) for more specific details on documentation.

Most states now require health care professionals to report elder abuse. If abuse is suspected but there is not enough information to determine that it has occurred, the nurse should consult with the state agency responsible for elder abuse. The nurse will often be in the position of reporting *suspicions;* it is up to the state to investigate and determine if abuse has taken place. Elders capable of making informed decisions are free to decline any offered assistance providing they are not being coerced or threatened into refusing.

Controversy surrounding the idea of mandatory reporting of domestic violence stems from the fact that, although the goal of reporting is enhanced safety, that is not always the outcome. The risk of retaliation is high. Abusers continue to assault their partners through the period of prosecution. Even though mandatory reporting should shift the blame off of the victim, it frequently does not. Because many victims are afraid of worse treatment if the police are involved, there is the risk that if mandatory reporting becomes the norm, victims will simply stop seeking medical attention (or will be stopped by their batterers).

Will mandatory reporting result in more effective legal intervention? According to a report by Hyman, Schillinger, and Bernard (1995), the current picture is bleak. The percentage of police reports actually filed in follow-up to reports is low; if a report is made and an investigation follows, arrests occur in only 7% to 12% of cases; and women are at greater risk of reassault after criminal justice intervention. In addition, support for battered women, including community services such as shelters and low-fee legal assistance, is frequently scarce, underfunded, or unavailable. These problems are compounded for people of color, low-income women, immigrants, gays, and lesbians.

PREVENTION

This chapter has covered issues such as child abuse, child sexual assault, domestic violence, rape, and elder abuse. It is clear that the ethic of violence may need to be examined to understand the amount of violence perpetrated by people of all walks of life. Regardless of the source of violence, however, the most powerful tool we have to combat it is prevention.

Primary Prevention

Violence prevention activities by community nurses may include, but are not limited to, political activism, networking, health promotion, education, counseling, and development of agency protocols. Nursing leaders stress the need for nurses to become politically active and for nursing programs to include politics in both didactic and clinical curricula (Williams, 1993). Advocating for the community is a political act as well as a caring act. Examples of advocacy actions are listed in Figure 24-15.

Health promotion activities for female clients should include groups or classes that (1) help them identify strengths and (2) encourage personal independence and assertive behaviors. Male clients may feel threatened by the changes taking place in society. Some men express anger that women are working in fields that were traditionally male and hold women responsible for their feelings of financial insecurity. Men or adolescent boys dealing with these issues may benefit from a progressive men's support group. Advocacy for school-based programs that teach age-appropriate assault prevention techniques helps to assure that children are learning methods to reduce their vulnerability to violence.

Anticipatory guidance can begin with individual interactions such as well-child checks. There is opportunity to talk about privacy, the right of the child to be examined with a trusted parent present, and the right to say no if someone tries to touch the child's genitals or touches the child in any other way that makes him or her uncomfortable.

Children who live in communities where they are exposed to daily violence need strong family support and community involvement to assist them in coping with and processing their realities. They also need to learn that violence is not the solution to problems. Evaluate the family's method of conflict resolution. If families can learn and

---

⊘⊙ REFLECTIVE THINKING ⊙⊘

Mandatory Reporting

• Is it paternalistic to do something you consider in the client's best interest?

• If you report violence against the victim's wishes, are you putting that person in yet another situation of not being heard? Of disrespect?

• Will reporting undermine trust? Increase fear of health care providers?

• With whom can you consult about the situation before reporting?

---

model nonviolent problem-solving methods, children will carry those lessons into the world each day.

Schools also play an important role in providing a curriculum that allows children to talk about the violence they are seeing and to learn alternative solutions. If schools in the community do not offer this, nurses can work with other community groups or existing programs. Churches, police departments, boys' and girls' clubs, and other youth-oriented programs can be approached if antiviolence programs, after-school recreational activities, and child care programs do not exist. Children also benefit emotionally and physically from martial arts training.

Some communities are recognizing the need to develop an integrated program in which a city's schools,

---

Figure 24-15   Examples of Advocacy Actions

• Offering community-based classes and support groups

• Speaking about violence at schools and civic groups

• Involvement in local activities that you perceive as important to reduce violence in the community

• Networking in the community to identify resources for clients who need counseling, education, and support around aggression issues

• Participating in advisory boards for rape crisis centers, shelters, antiviolence programs, and community alternatives to gang activity

• Developing assertiveness-training groups to provide an alternative to aggression

• Screening for drug and alcohol abuse and gang activity

• Establishing mentor programs to link teens with adult role models and support people

• Developing anticipatory guidance programs regarding developmental stages, to reduce parent frustrations concerning child behavior

• Establishing parenting groups

• Modeling effective adult–child communication skills in the community churches, police, businesses, and youth organizations work closely together to develop programs for youth that emphasize prevention of crime and gang development. Boston has a model program that is being duplicated in other cities around the country in which there is zero tolerance for gangs and that contains a proactive plan. Youth service officers have been increased to teach antidrug and antigang programs in schools, take students on field trips, run sports clinics, and sponsor basketball tournaments. These activities are directed at reaching younger children before they join gangs (Freedberg, 1997).

Adolescent screening should explore family relationships, current relationships, history of violence including sexual violence, and dating violence. All teens should be asked what they know about sexual assault and relationship violence. Any misconceptions should be corrected. Explore what clients see as effective prevention and what kinds of warning signs they can identify with regard to controlling or potentially assaultive people. Teens may benefit from assertion training.

Therapy or support groups aimed at assisting students with effective anger management might be appropriate. Garrett (1995) suggests that schools screen adolescents for possible violent behaviors and set up classes and workshops to teach them how to handle conflict, frustration, and anger. He notes that assertiveness-training, whether peer or counselor facilitated, decreases anger. Nurses are in a position to screen for potential violence and to assist in establishing these types of groups. Such programs give children hope, activity, and role modeling.

Children's exposure to media violence should be explored with parents, and appropriate education provided. Discovering the family's philosophy regarding such issues as discipline, management of tantrums, and potty training is an important part of gathering a family history. Any tendency toward abusive parenting needs to be addressed and the family assisted in exploring alternative parenting techniques and nonviolent problem-solving methods. Families at risk such as teen parents; single-parent households; families with children who are physically, developmentally, or emotionally challenged; and alcohol- or drug-dependent families require frequent visits, careful evaluation, and parenting education. The nurse can assess strengths and weaknesses with the family and act as a liaison to facilitate the assistance of appropriate organizations or support people.

The community health nurse should introduce the topic of violence as part of obtaining a complete history with all adults. Clients who give you a history of sleep disturbances, eating disorders, nightmares, alcohol or drug abuse, or self-abusive behaviors should be carefully and sensitively screened for a past or current history of sexual and physical abuse. The single most important thing that health care providers can do to prevent and reduce the amount and degree of violence is to ask about it (Roberts & Quillian, 1992).

Last, established protocols for dealing with the victims and perpetrators of violence should be part of every agency setting. These protocols should include a referral list of private and public community agencies that serve victims of violence.

Secondary Prevention

Families using violence may be referred because abuse is suspected or has been confirmed or because a child is acting out violently at school. The nurse may identify symptoms of abuse when treating a family member in the clinical area. When abuse is suspected, intervention should take place as quickly as possible.

When a family member has been physically injured or a child has acted out by running away, joining a gang, or assaulting another person, or if sexual abuse has been diagnosed, an imbalance may exist between the problem and the family's available coping skills. The tension, discomfort, and anxiety resulting from the identified problem often motivate the family to seek or accept assistance and to participate in finding solutions. Crisis intervention methods are helpful at this time, as is establishment of a support network. The nurse will initially help family members identify what they individually understand about the problem and how they feel. Family members may, for instance, blame the victim for what has happened, alerting the nurse to belief systems that need to be addressed. Often in closed family systems, support networks are lacking and the nurse may need to work with the family to determine what agencies, family members, or friends would be accepted as a support system. Determining how the family has coped with past crises provides information about family strengths and helps the family identify or recall coping mechanisms that have served them before. Any healthy coping mechanisms, such as crying, expression of grief or sorrow, or comforting others in the family should be identified and supported by the nurse.

When the victim is a child, and the nurse is in the position of filing the child protective services (CPS) report, the family should be prepared for this event. Or the nurse may be working in conjunction with CPS. The crisis period is, by definition, approximately 4 to 6 weeks in length. Working with the family to establish goals and making any indicated referrals to family therapy, parenting classes, or other community support agencies should be completed as early in this cycle as possible to maximize openness in the family system.

In some cases a family member may have to be removed from the home. This person may be a sexually assaultive adult, although far too often it is the child victim who is removed to a foster home. If the nurse has the ability to maintain contact with that child it is essential to help the child understand that removal from the home is not punishment. The community health nurse may be in a position to help other children in the family understand what has happened, to monitor the progress of short-term goals, and to work toward the prevention of any further abuse. These efforts should be coordinated with other agencies such as the legal system or social services.

It was mentioned earlier that abuse victims, especially sexual assault victims, are at high risk for suicidal behavior. If the child remains in the home, the nurse should be sure to ask about weapons in the home. Suicidal risk factors need to be carefully assessed. Other family members should be educated about warning signs for suicide and given information about appropriate community resources for family support. See Chapters 16 and 17 for a discussion of suicide.

Nurses should be aware of agencies, church groups, schools, and volunteer agencies in the community that work with gangs and should encourage teens who are drawn to gang activity to utilize these services. Early identification and acknowledgment of family problems in addition to working with the family to seek solutions can avert some of the drastic outcomes. Throughout this process, the nurse should remain open, direct, caring, flexible, and nonjudgmental. To achieve this stance, the nurse needs a personal support system in addition to good consultation.

Tertiary Prevention

Tertiary prevention will involve working with families who have suffered the long-term consequences of violence. Examples include a family in which a parent or child has died as the result of violence; parents who have had children placed in foster homes; families in which a member has been incarcerated because of abuse; or a family with a child who is a runaway, a delinquent, sexually promiscuous, or substance addicted or has psychiatric problems related to abuse.

The nurse will be working with the family to maximize strengths, to heal from the trauma and loss, and to build support systems. Children and adolescents in families may need help with expressing their feelings about the violence that has altered the family, as well as their fears that the violence will be repeated. The family should be assessed for any remaining interactions that might be violent or frightening to any family member, including the use of violent language or aggressive nonverbal communication. Serious emotional effects in any family member call for appropriate referrals and follow-up.

Some male nurses have taken a proactive stance against violence and work with men who act out in violent ways. These nurses are in a position to educate men about their individual power to work against violence and the more subtle forms of approval of violence.

ISSUES AFFECTING THE NURSE

Working with clients who have been affected by violence is challenging for any helper, regardless of discipline. Nurses are well suited to address the needs of these clients by virtue of their focus on holistic care and advocacy. It is important, however, that they feel comfortable with their abilities and their support systems. Nursing education is a logical starting point for assuring that nurses are prepared to work in this arena, because contact with sexual assault survivors, abused and traumatized children, battered women, or neglected elders is inevitable.

Institutions need to provide clear protocols for dealing with community or family violence as well as clinical support and supervision for the nurses who are caring for the client or families affected by violence. Professional nursing organizations are in a position to set the tone for how nursing views violence and what the role of the professional nurse should be. Addressing these issues in publications, at conferences, and on a local level and taking a political stance are all ways of affirming nursing's central role in halting violence. This type of advocacy is also a way of supporting the individual nurse, who may at times feel isolated or afraid while dealing with some of these highly charged issues.

Dealing with violence—seeing its effects, hearing the painful stories, and caring for its victims—is emotionally challenging. King and Ryan (1989) point out that 18% of nurses they studied were themselves victims of physical and emotional abuse, and 28% reported abuse within their families. Each nurse is called upon to examine individual judgments, control issues, codependency, and sometimes past and unresolved pain. This work is not something that should be done in isolation or silence: Clinical supervision is important.

Through all this, the nurse must attend to self-care, which means different things to different nurses. Some may find that they have unresolved issues that require therapy or codependent issues that need to be addressed. Others may need to increase their exercise in order to reduce their stress level or spend more time attending to spiritual life. Replenishing their own energy and spirit is crucial to maintaining good nursing care.

Men may have a difficult time with some of the information presented. Men are often the perpetrators of violence, and it may sometimes sound as if all men are being viewed as violent. All nurses have an obligation to not laugh at sexist, racist, or homophobic jokes; to eliminate demeaning language aimed at people of other races, religions, or sexual orientation; and to verbalize disapproval of abusive actions. These are all individual actions that will help to put an end to violence.

Leaders in health care, law enforcement, government, education, and religion are acknowledging the extent of the violence problem and are willing to take part in finding solutions. Domestic violence and sexual harassment are being debated in the open, increasing consciousness about the underpinnings of violence. Efforts are increasing to divert children from joining gangs and to find real solutions to gang violence. Gun-control legislation is targeted at reducing the number of firearm-related homicides. Research efforts that address issues such as elder abuse, hate crimes, and the impact of violence on people of color may be crucial in the effort to halt violence.

Much may be learned from studying nonviolent cultures such as the Mbuti people, the Zuni Indians, and the

Perspectives...

Extinguishing the Light

Heavy laden with chains
I cannot dance.
Movement unbearable
Mired in sorrow.

Wailing from within
Yet no cry escapes

Silent tears
As silent as the voices raised
Against rape

The silence is deafening.

I am alone.

In despair
I search the depths,
There is no reservoir
I crumble, broken

My spirit once bright with brilliant hues
Like fall spattered leaves once painted
Red and orange
Withers turns black
Dies

I free fall into oblivion
The dark I welcome
It meets me where I am.

Through the silence of my broken spirit
The moaning creeps grows louder.
The wails of my sisters and brothers assail me,
Ripping shard by shard the curtain
Of despair

Wailing . . .
Hope is an illusion
Wailing . . .
Oppression is reality
Wailing

20 years
200 years

2000 years of moans
Haunting cries
Muffled wails of defiled women and men
Generation by generation
Greeted with silence
1 heart breaking
2 hearts broken
Generations of hearts heavy with the dark
memories

The heavens fill with their cries
The skies deluge with sorrowful weeping
The earth shivers with sorrow
The people turn away silently
Heavy laden with chains of impotent voice
I cannot dance

I am wounded
Struggling
I want to be deaf too
To the wailing
So like the masses.

But the moaning
The flow of tears
Unceasing
Finds me a river.
I have no strength to turn away.

Lights going out one by one
Ten by ten
Hundreds
Generation by generation
Innocence lost in bruised bodies
Broken children
Souls stolen in the night
In the daylight.

One more child moans in the darkness
One more light went out tonight.

—*Pat Stewart (1995)*
Survivor

Child Protective Services has requested a public health nurse to visit the Miceli family. They have been notified by the family's nurse practitioner that the family has repeatedly failed to bring 20-month-old Celeste in for follow-up visits. The child has had a very serious candida diaper dermatitis that failed to respond to conservative treatment. The family repeatedly has not shown up for scheduled one-week follow-up visits; instead they returned two months later when the rash was once again to the point of bleeding and secondary infection. This pattern of behavior has gone on for eight months despite prevention education from the nurse practitioner and reminder calls to the family prior to scheduled visits. There has also been a concern about spousal abuse. The father, James, a 28-year-old part-time factory worker, is very controlling. He doesn't allow his wife, Marla, to drive or to go anywhere without him or one of her parents. The nurse practitioner reported an office visit to which Marla's father brought Celeste and Marla. James called during the visit and asked what time they had arrived and what time they would be leaving. During that same visit, Marla related that James told her he would not spend money on cloth diapers, as recom-

mended, and thinks it's high time the baby started potty training.

Nursing Considerations

ASSESSMENT
• Are there risk factors for abuse? For neglect? If so, what are they?
• What information does the nurse need to complete the assessment?

DIAGNOSIS
• What nursing diagnoses would be appropriate to this family?

OUTCOME IDENTIFICATION
• Given the diagnosis you have identified, what outcomes do you expect?

PLANNING/INTERVENTIONS
• What levels of prevention need to be addressed?
• What areas of education will be needed by this family?
• What referral services might be useful for this family?

EVALUATION
• What evaluation criteria will indicate if the interventions are effective?
• What should be done if interventions are ineffective?

Utku Eskimos (Campbell & Humphreys, 1984), in whose cultures children are not physically punished and are taught that jealousy and the use of force are unacceptable. In these cultures, competition is not valued, but gentleness and cooperation are, and caution, fear, and timidity are considered healthy traits.

These values are inherent in nursing. Nursing care has the potential to teach families and individuals that we all have the right and capability to live nonviolently. "Live the change you want for the world" (Mahatma Gandhi).

Key Concepts

• Violence may affect anyone regardless of race, culture, socioeconomic status, or educational background and is not limited to any particular country.
• Violence is a community and societal issue, not merely the problem of the individual victim.

• There is no one explanation for violence in any culture.
• Knowledge of existing theories and a broad political understanding can provide direction in the care of survivors of violence and in the development of effective prevention efforts.
• It is essential that nurses address their own biases regarding violence.
• Strategies for decreasing vulnerability to rape should emphasize empowering behaviors as opposed to behaviors that restrict freedom.
• There are identifiable stages in the process of recovery from sexual assault.
• Nurses can utilize the rape trauma syndrome model to assess clients and to determine appropriate interventions.
• Physical and behavioral clues can alert the nurse to the possibility of child abuse.

- The United States has the highest rate of homicide of any industrialized country.

- Nurses are mandated reporters for all aspects of family violence.

- Theories of learned helplessness and the cycle of violence in domestic abuse provide a framework for nursing interventions.

- Preventing caregiver burnout is a crucial aspect of preventing elder abuse.

- Assessing the potential for abuse is an important aspect of prevention.

- Asking clients about violence in their lives is one of the most important things the nurse can do.

- Dealing with violence is emotionally challenging, and therefore replenishing one's own energy and spirit is crucial to maintaining good nursing care

Substance Abuse

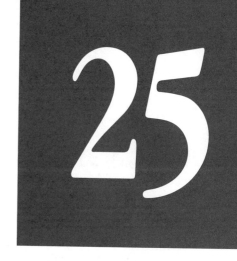

25

Linda G. Dumas, RN, PhD
Mary Beatrice Hennessey, RN, MSN

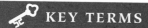 **KEY TERMS**

crack
crack babies
cutting agents
depressant
designer drugs
detoxification
fetal alcohol syndrome
freebase
inhalant substances
needle and syringe
   exchange programs
psychoactive substances
sedative

*I'd be so strung out . . . and I'd be shooting up and I'd be thinking,
My god . . . I'm frying my brains . . . I don't want to fry my brains.*
   *A formerly homeless and addicted woman talking of her
   response to a public service announcement that showed an egg
   with the message "This is your brain" and then showed an egg
   sizzling in a frying pan with the message "This is your brain
   on drugs."*

COMPETENCIES

Upon completion of this chapter, the reader should be able to:

- Identify and define six substances commonly abused in the United States.
- Identify three populations at risk for substance abuse.
- Analyze common attitudes of nurses toward people who abuse substances.
- Discuss issues related to substance abuse at the primary, secondary, and tertiary levels of prevention.
- Discuss the upstream analogy and apply it to substance abuse as a social behavioral problem in the United States.
- List settings where primary and secondary prevention can take place.
- Discuss the impact of managed care and cost cutting on tertiary-level intervention for people who abuse substances.
- Discuss differences between detoxification centers, transitional housing, and home care as referral resources for people who abuse substances.
- Be aware of the many legal issues surrounding the treatment of substance abusers and substance abuse itself.
- Discuss the concept of caring as it might apply to the care of people who abuse alcohol, tobacco, and other drugs.

The vast majority of U.S. citizens use mind-altering substances. Alcohol, caffeine, nicotine, and prescribed and illicit drugs are a part of the American culture. A love-hate relationship is often apparent. Drugs have been taxed and studied, promoted and outlawed, controlled and extolled, used and abused. Health warning labels are legally mandated on tobacco and alcohol containers, and yet debate rages regarding the marketing of these products to youth (Grube & Wallack, 1994; Mosher, 1994; Annas, 1996; Dority, 1997; Teinowitz, 1997).

The approaches of health care professionals to people who use and abuse various substances have been likewise ambivalent. Throughout history health providers have learned and relearned the same lessons. It is now clear that addictions are both preventable and treatable. Interventions, however, are often ineffective because they are based on negative and inaccurate stereotypes (Sullivan, Handley, & Connors, 1994).

This chapter is about alcohol, tobacco, and other substance abuse from a community nursing perspective. Substance abuse has been studied from a number of different perspectives, and plans for treatment often reflect the perspective studied. For example, if substance abuse is viewed as strictly a pathophysiological problem, then a medical model would seem a reasonable treatment approach; whereas if it were seen as a behavioral problem, behavioral therapy techniques would seem a better option. This chapter takes an eclectic view of substance abuse. It recognizes that there are many different pathways to the addictions and many diverse and valid treatment approaches. Individual, family, and community dimensions are identified, with special attention to certain high-risk groups. Levels of prevention are addressed, and primary, secondary, and tertiary interventions are discussed.

A BRIEF HISTORY OF SUBSTANCE ABUSE IN THE UNITED STATES

National ambivalence toward alcohol and those who consume it is evident in history. As Hewitt (1995) points out, there has been a historical inability to reach a national consensus about the role of alcohol in American society. At varying times over the past 150 years the excessive use of alcohol has been considered a sin, a crime, and a disease, and the excessive drinker a sinner, a criminal, and a victim. Alcohol was the first drug to be considered a problem in the United States, and the first attempt at controlling it took the form of an excise tax on whiskey. This law, passed in 1791, led to the so-called Whiskey Rebellion. Farmers who considered whiskey an economic necessity and a medium of exchange refused to pay the tax. President Washington called upon the militia of several states to enforce the law. This action was particularly significant as it was a test of the new federal government's ability to enforce its laws within a state (Witters & Venturelli, 1988).

Narcotic addiction first became a problem during the Civil War, when the hypodermic syringe was invented. Morphine was used widely for the treatment of pain and dysentery, and morphine addiction became known as "the Soldiers' disease" (Julien, 1985).

By the late 1800s great strides had been made related to the conceptualization of alcoholism, or the addiction to alcohol, as not only a disease but as an inherited disease with a progressive course (Palmer, 1896). The beliefs of the early founders of the Temperance Society were in harmony with those of Alcoholics Anonymous. By the turn of the century, however, the focus of the Temperance membership changed, and alcohol became a "demon." There was a campaign to rid society of alcohol, which in 1920 led to the ratification of the 18th Amendment to the U.S. Constitution, better known as prohibition. Prohibition overshadowed all the hard work that had

been done to promote the concept of alcoholism as a disease. Interestingly, the 18th Amendment is the only amendment to the U.S. Constitution that has been repealed, another incidence of national ambivalence. The repeal occurred in 1933, and the disease concept was resurrected and expanded upon. Much of the later work on alcoholism as a disease was done in the 1950s at Yale, most notably by Jellinek (Levine, 1978).

In the late 1800s and early 1900s the use of cocaine reached epidemic proportions. Cocaine could be found in patent medicines, wine, and Coca-Cola. The Pure Food and Drug Act of 1906 was actually a labeling law aimed at controlling the patent medicine industry. It required complete labeling of the contents in each container, specifically mentioning alcohol, morphine, opium, cocaine, heroin, and marijuana (Witters & Venturelli, 1988).

In the 1930s marijuana became the focus of concern. Newspaper and police reports associated crime with marijuana use, and the film *Reefer Madness* (now a cult classic) depicted high school use of marijuana as leading to murder, rape, prostitution, and madness (Ray, 1983). In 1937, concern about its effects led the federal government to classify marijuana as a schedule I substance (Gold, 1991). Under the Controlled Substances Act, the criteria by which a drug or substance is determined to be schedule I are: (1) It has a high potential for abuse; (2) it has no currently accepted medical use in treatment in the United States; and (3) there is a lack of accepted safety for its use under medical supervision (Fishbein & Pease, 1996).

In the 1960s, the Vietnam War brought new patterns of drug use (McKim, 1986). The user tended to be better educated, and the drugs of choice were those that altered mood and consciousness. "Mind-expanding drugs" such as LSD became common. There was also an increase in heroin use. In the 1970s drugs were labeled by the government as "Public Enemy No. 1" (Ray, 1983).

The 1980s brought a resurgence in the popularity of cocaine. Chemists found a way to remove the impurities and the hydrochloride from the cocaine, thereby creating a smokable and much more potent product. Initially this process required the use of highly volatile products such as ether. It was later found that a relatively pure cocaine could be prepared using baking soda. This form, known as **crack** or **freebase** cocaine, delivers a potent but short-lived high followed by a longer depression. The availability of cocaine in freebase or crack forms increased its use. Crack cocaine is widely available, cheap, and highly addictive (Flynn, 1991; Gold, 1991).

In the 1980s, some high-profile people succumbed to drugs. The death of John Belushi from a "speedball" (a mixture of heroin and freebase cocaine) brought the method of "freebasing" to public awareness. The death of Len Bias, who was celebrating his selection to the Boston Celtics with what was reportedly his first use of cocaine, compelled the attention of high school and college athletes. The death of Robert Kennedy's son David highlighted the fact that drugs can be devastating at all socioeconomic levels.

In the 1990s the use of marijuana is again making headlines (Buckley, 1996; Leo, 1996; Morganthau, 1997). More than two centuries after the Whiskey Rebellion the supremacy of federal law over states' rights is again being questioned. In late 1996 in what might someday be called "the marijuana rebellion," California and Arizona voters each approved propositions allowing prescription of marijuana for medical purposes (Buckley, 1996). This practice is in conflict with federal law. In January of 1997 federal authorities warned physicians that they might face prosecution if they prescribe marijuana (Rogers, 1997). This debate will no doubt continue into the 21st century.

Another area of debate at the approach of the 21st century is federal funding for **needle and syringe exchange programs,** in which intravenous drug users can swap used needles and syringes for new ones (Chapman, 1997; Lurie & Drucker, 1997). Such programs started in Amsterdam in 1984 (van Ameijden, van den Hoek, & Coutinho, 1995) and the concept spread throughout the United Kingdom and to other European countries without opposition (Coutinho, 1995). Several studies in the Netherlands, Sweden, Australia, the United Kingdom, and the United States have demonstrated that needle and syringe exchange programs are effective in lowering the rates of needle sharing (Watters, Estilo, Clark, & Lorvick, 1994). The sharing of contaminated injection equipment is a major route for transmitting HIV. In December of 1994, the Centers for Disease Control and Prevention reported that a little more than a third (35.3%) of reported AIDS cases were associated with intravenous drug abuse and that syringe exchange programs appear to be effective in preventing the transmission of infectious diseases (Centers for Disease Control and Prevention [CDC], 1995c).

Lurie and Drucker (1997) conclude that the absence of a needle-exchange program in the United States has contributed to between 4,000 and 10,000 cases of preventable HIV infection. Along with the costs in human suffering, they put the societal costs for treating the infections between a quarter and a half billion dollars. The idea of needle and syringe exchange programs in the United States, however, has met with considerable opposition. Despite growing evidence to the contrary, there is continued concern that needle exchange programs will increase drug abuse. Des Jarlais and colleagues (1995) express concern that, as they become more prevalent, overly restrictive government regulations will undermine the effectiveness of syringe-exchange programs.

SUBSTANCE ABUSE STATISTICS FOR THE 1990s

Since 1975 an annual survey of drug use by children and young adults has been conducted by the University of Michigan's Institute for Social Research with funding from the National Institute on Drug Abuse (NIDA). Data from this survey are used to study trends in drug use as well as attitudes toward the use of drugs (U.S. Department of Health and Human Services [USDHHS], 1994a).

The overall trend from 1980 through 1991 was a decrease in drug use by high school and college students. The annual prevalence of illicit drug use by college students dropped from 56% in 1980 to 29% in 1991. There was a similar decline in drug use by twelfth graders (USDHHS, 1994c).

There was general public concern that the decrease in illicit drug use might be accompanied by an increase in the use of alcohol. However, this was not the case. In 1981, the consumption of alcohol in the United States reached a peak of an annual average of 2.76 gallons of pure alcohol per person 14 years of age and older (USDHHS, 1990a). This was followed by a steady decline down to 2.25 gallons in 1993 (USDHHS, 1996). One goal established in the national *Healthy People 2000* report is to reduce alcohol consumption to an average of no more than two gallons of pure alcohol, per capita, per year (USDHHS, 1996). See Table 25-1.

Table 25-1   Halfway to 2000: Progress toward the Goal of Reducing the Proportion of Young People Who Have Used Alcohol, Marijuana, Cocaine, or Tobacco in a One-Month Period

SUBSTANCE	AGE	% BASELINE 1988	% 1992	% 1993	% 1994	% TARGET 2000
Alcohol	12–17	25.2	15.7	18	21.6	12.6
Alcohol	18–20	57.9	50.3	49.9	54.6	29
Marijuana	12–17	6.4	4.0	4.9	6	3.2
Marijuana	18–25	15.5	11.0	11.1	12.1	7.8
Cocaine	12–17	1.1	0.3	0.4	0.3	0.6
Cocaine	18–25	4.5	1.8	1.5	1.2	2.3
Tobacco	12–17	10.8	9.6	9.6	18.9	6

Adapted from Healthy People 2000: Midcourse Review and 1995 Revisions *by U.S. Department of Health and Human Services, 1996, Sudbury, MA: Jones & Bartlett; and* National Household Survey on Drug Abuse: Population Estimates *by U.S. Department of Health and Human Services, 1994, Washington, D.C.: Author.*

In examining the results of the 1992 Institute for Social Research survey, NIDA expressed concern in finding a decline in the perceived dangers of drug abuse as well as a decline in peer disapproval of drug use. It was feared that this softening of attitudes might presage an increase in drug abuse, and it appears that it did. The results of the 1994 survey showed a sharp increase in the use of marijuana, particularly by the younger groups interviewed. Marijuana use among eighth graders had more than doubled since 1991, with 13% saying they had used it at least once in 1994 as compared with 6.2% in 1991. Among high school seniors, 31.7% had tried marijuana at least once in 1994 as compared with 21.9% in 1991 (USDHHS, 1994b).

The 1994 survey demonstrated that attitudes about drug use have continued to soften. Students now perceive less danger in the regular use of marijuana, in smoking one or more packs of cigarettes a day, or in trying cocaine (USDHHS, 1996). They also have less-negative attitudes toward their peers who use tobacco and marijuana (USDHHS, 1994b; USDHHS, 1996).

What are the reasons for this decreased negativity? Perhaps the youth of today find it harder to identify with Belushi, Bias, and Kennedy. Perhaps they do not have concrete examples on which to base their fears. Perhaps the general public has become more complacent about drugs and has allowed the counterculture drug message to be stronger and louder than the voices against that message.

THE NATURE OF ADDICTION

Despite years of study and debate, the nature of addiction, including the disease concept, continues to be controversial (Meyer, 1996). There are a number of theories: social, biological, psychological, behavioral, and cultural explanations for addictive behavior. Many different models for understanding the addictions have been proposed, and a variety of diagnostic tools have been developed. In 1994 the American Psychiatric Association published the fourth edition of its *Diagnostic and Statistical Manual* (DSM-IV). One interesting change from its previous edition is that in discussing substance abuse it dropped the term *psychoactive*. **Psychoactive substances** are drugs or chemicals that affect the mental state. It has been demonstrated that people who abuse substances not primarily characterized as psychoactive (e.g., steroids) can also meet diagnostic criteria for dependence (Brower, Eliopulos, Blow, Catlin, & Beresford, 1990). The generic criteria for substance dependence as stated in DSM-IV are listed in Figure 25-1.

Alcoholism has been discussed as an inherited disease since the 1800s, but the first scientific evidence to support this theory did not come until the 1970s. In a classic 1973 study of twins, Goodwin and Winokur found that sons born to alcoholic fathers were three times more likely to become alcoholic than those of nonalcoholic fathers (Blum, Cull, Braverman, & Comings, 1996). Several well-designed studies carried out in the 1990s confirm the ear-

Figure 25-1 Generic Criteria for Identification of Substance Dependence

A maladaptive pattern of substance use, leading to clinically significant impairment or distress, as manifested by three (or more) of the following, occurring at any time in the same 12-month period:

(1) tolerance, as defined by either of the following:
   (a) a need for markedly increased amounts of the substance to achieve intoxication or desired effect
   (b) markedly diminished effect with continued use of the same amount of the substance

(2) withdrawal, as manifested by either of the following:
   (a) the characteristic withdrawal syndrome for the substance (refer to Criteria A and B of the criteria sets for Withdrawal from the specific substances)
   (b) the same (or a closely related) substance is taken to relieve or avoid withdrawal symptoms

(3) the substance is often taken in larger amounts or over a longer period than was intended

(4) there is a persistent desire or unsuccessful efforts to cut down or control substance use

(5) a great deal of time is spent in activities necessary to obtain the substance (e.g., visiting multiple doctors or driving long distances), use the substance (e.g., chain-smoking), or recover from its effects

(6) important social, occupational, or recreational activities are given up or reduced because of substance use

(7) the substance use is continued despite knowledge of having a persistent or recurrent physical or psychological problem that is likely to have been caused or exacerbated by the substance (e.g., current cocaine use despite recognition of cocaine-induced depression, or continued drinking despite recognition that an ulcer was made worse by alcohol consumption)

Specify if:

With Physiological Dependence: evidence of tolerance or withdrawal (i.e., either Item 1 or 2 is present)

Without Physiological Dependence: no evidence of tolerance or withdrawal (i.e., neither Item 1 nor 2 is present)

Course specifiers

Early Full Remission

Early Partial Remission

Sustained Full Remission

Sustained Partial Remission

On Agonist Therapy

In a Controlled Environment

From Diagnostic and Statistical Manual of Mental Disorders *(4th ed.) by American Psychiatric Association, 1994, Washington, DC: Author. Copyright 1994. Reprinted with permission.*

lier work, suggesting that unspecified genetic factors increase the risk of developing alcohol addiction (Meyer, 1996). Blum and colleagues (1996) propose that there is a common genetic basis involved in several disorders including alcoholism, drug addiction, attention deficit disorder, binge eating, and addictive gambling. They believe that there is an inborn chemical imbalance that alters the intercellular signaling in the brain's reward process; this alteration supplants a feeling of well-being with feelings of anxiety and anger and leads to a craving for a substance that could alleviate the negative feelings. They propose the term *reward deficiency syndrome* to describe this condition. Genetic research is ongoing and should continue to shed light on the nature of addiction.

SUBSTANCE ABUSE AND THE COMMUNITY HEALTH NURSE

Community health nurses, particularly those working in the inner city, might be surprised to hear that there was a 10-year decline in drug and alcohol use. In their daily practice they continue to witness the ravages of substance abuse on urban men, women, and children. Nurses see too many addicted babies being born; too many youngsters suffering anomalies due to **fetal alcohol syndrome,** caused by their mother's prenatal use of alcohol, struggling in school; too many young men and women showing early signs of HIV infection because they share needles; and too many stressed single mothers finding relief in drinking, smoking, snorting, and injecting drugs. Nurses also see increasing numbers of men and women in their middle years suffering the emotional and physical effects of chronic substance abuse.

The community health nurse sees firsthand that substance abuse problems are prevalent and costly. The cost is measured in dollars and, more importantly, by increases in violence, accidents, suicides, domestic abuse, physical problems, social and psychological problems, and premature death. Community health nurses are pivotal in identifying addictive behaviors and in decreasing their numerous associated problems (Talashek, Laina, Gerace, & Starr, 1994). Assessment and observation skills are employed to identify a problem, and a caring manner, good judgment, and effective communication skills influence the client's and the community's willingness to do something about it.

EFFECTS OF SUBSTANCE ABUSE ON HEALTH

Substance abuse is associated with a wide range of health problems. Types of substances that are often abused include depressants, stimulants, hallucinogens, inhalants, marijuana, steroids, and prescription drugs. A **depressant** is an agent that depresses a body function or nerve activity. Included in this grouping are alcohol, barbiturates, opioids, and opiates (heroin). Stimulants are agents that temporarily increase functional activity. These include amphetamines, cocaine, caffeine, and tobacco. Hallucinogens cause the user to have hallucinations; LSD and some designer drugs are considered hallucinogens.

The community health nurse who is aware of the associated health problems is in a better position to recognize when substance abuse might be a problem for a client. This section will review common health problems associated with the abuse of alcohol, heroin, tobacco, caffeine, marijuana, cocaine, methamphetamine, and other drugs of abuse.

Alcohol

Alcoholism has long been considered a major public health problem, resulting in increased morbidity and mortality (Miller, Gold, Cocores, & Pottash, 1988). The use of moderate amounts of alcohol has been associated with a wide range of disorders that affect all body systems (USDHHS, 1990b). Alcohol is considered a depressant **(sedative).** Alcohol is a small, water- and fat-soluble molecule that does not have to be broken down for absorption and easily reaches all areas of the body (Fishbein & Pease, 1996). Alcohol has the potential to cause great harm to all body tissues.

Alcohol exerts its effects both directly and indirectly. Harmful effects are due to the direct, irritating, and toxic effects of alcohol on the body, to the changes that take place during the metabolism of alcohol, to the aggravation of existing disease, to accidents while intoxicated, and to the irregular taking of prescribed treatments while intoxicated (Goroll, May, & Mulley, 1995; Miller et al., 1988; USDHHS, 1990a). The user feels relaxed at first and experiences a decrease in inhibitions. As drinking continues, the user develops slurred speech and lack of physical coordination. Nausea and vomiting are common responses to extensive alcohol intake. Frequently, the user becomes very sleepy and depressed (Faltz, 1998).

The signs and symptoms of alcohol intoxication vary with the blood alcohol level and individual characteristics, including tolerance to the drug. Impairment increases directly with the level of alcohol in the blood, and an overdose of alcohol can lead to respiratory depression and death (Witters & Venturelli, 1988). Withdrawal from alcohol can be dangerous. Symptoms range from mild discomfort to possibly fatal delirium tremens. High anxiety and sleep disturbances are common, and grand mal seizures frequently accompany withdrawal (Yost, 1996).

Studies indicate that between 25% and 50% of clients seen in general medical practice have significant physical and psychological problems associated with alcohol use (Goroll, May, & Mulley, 1995; Miller et al., 1988; ; Tweed, 1989). Alcohol has significant effects on the immune system secondary to liver disease, bone marrow depression, and malnutrition (Baker, Burton, & Zieve, 1998; USDHHS,

1990a; Witters & Venturelli, 1988). These effects lower resistance to pneumonia and other infectious diseases. Alcohol is known to interfere with the absorption of many nutrients including amino acids, glucose, zinc, thiamine, vitamin A, and folate, further compromising health (USD-HHS, 1990a).

Alcohol consumption is a risk factor in the development of several types of cancer, especially those of the liver, esophagus, nasopharynx, and larynx (USDHHS, 1990a). Several studies indicate a higher prevalence of breast cancer in women who drink as compared with nondrinkers (Rosenberg, Metzger, & Palmer, 1993). It is not clear as yet how alcohol consumption increases the risk for breast cancer, but there is suggestive evidence that it may be linked to increases in the estrogen levels of women who drink (Reichman, 1994). Figure 25-2 illustrates the common medical diagnoses related to alcohol intake.

Liftik (1995) states that the prevalence of alcoholism in any type of mental health setting is as high as 30% to 70%. Persistent heavy drinking is associated with anxiety, depression, psychosis, and cognitive deficits. Because treatment choices and outcomes differ, it is important to differentiate between primary psychiatric disorders and psychiatric symptoms that are secondary to alcohol intake or withdrawal. Secondary disorders will generally disappear with abstinence (Goroll, et al. 1998; Schuckit, 1983).

Depression, for example, is highly correlated with alcoholism. In 5% to 10% of alcoholics, depression may be the primary problem (Baker, et al. 1998; Schuckit & Monteiro, 1988). In the majority of cases, however, the depression is secondary to the alcoholism.

Alcohol itself is a depressant drug. Its use is associated with several types of anemia (Davenport, 1996; Wheby, 1996). There is a decreased production of red blood cells in the bone marrow accompanied by an increased loss in the gastrointestinal tract, as well as decreased storage of iron, copper, and vitamin B_{12} in the liver. Depression is a common presenting complaint with anemia. Depression is also a common symptom of withdrawal, which decreases with abstinence from the drug (Nace, 1995). The grief reaction that an alcoholic experiences as he or she faces the prospect of life without alcohol is often profound. In each of these cases it is fruitless to treat the depression without addressing the underlying alcoholism.

Figure 25-2 Common Alcohol-Related Diagnoses

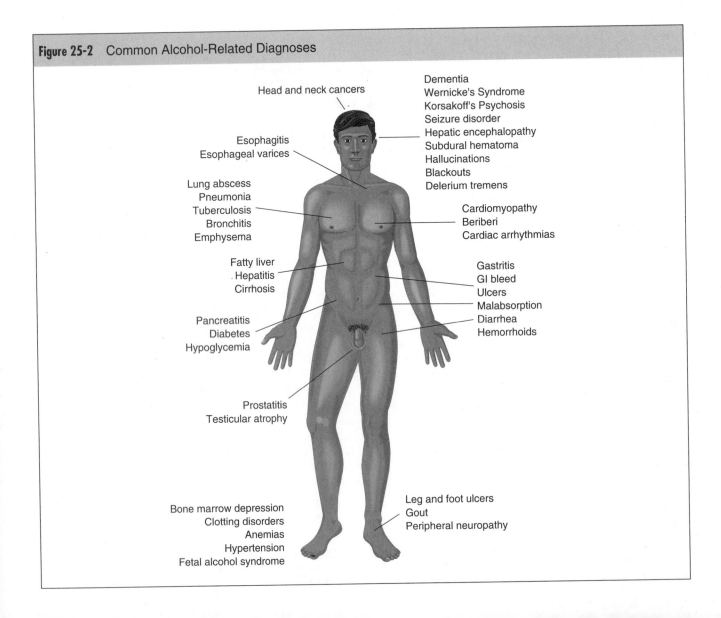

Head and neck cancers

Dementia
Wernicke's Syndrome
Korsakoff's Psychosis
Seizure disorder
Hepatic encephalopathy
Subdural hematoma
Hallucinations
Blackouts
Delerium tremens

Esophagitis
Esophageal varices

Lung abscess
Pneumonia
Tuberculosis
Bronchitis
Emphysema

Cardiomyopathy
Beriberi
Cardiac arrhythmias

Fatty liver
Hepatitis
Cirrhosis

Gastritis
GI bleed
Ulcers
Malabsorption
Diarrhea
Hemorrhoids

Pancreatitis
Diabetes
Hypoglycemia

Prostatitis
Testicular atrophy

Bone marrow depression
Clotting disorders
Anemias
Hypertension
Fetal alcohol syndrome

Leg and foot ulcers
Gout
Peripheral neuropathy

Alcohol has also been implicated in the four leading causes of accidental death in the United States—motor vehicle accidents, falls, drownings, and fires. Automobile accidents are the leading cause of death between the ages of 15 and 24 and are a significant cause of death at all ages. Studies have shown alcohol to be a factor in about 50% of all fatal automobile accidents, between 17% and 53% of falls, about 38% of drownings, and 64% of deaths by fire (USDHHS, 1992).

According to *Healthy People 2000,* the United States ranks first among industrialized nations in violent death rates. In the United States, suicide is the third leading cause of death between the ages of 15 and 24, and between 2 and 4 million people are physically battered each year by their partners. Alcohol and other substance abuse are consistently found to be associated with all forms of violence (USDHHS, 1990b).

Another major concern is the use of alcohol during pregnancy resulting in fetal alcohol syndrome. This is characterized by low birth size and weight, developmental deficiencies, facial anomalies, cardiovascular defects, cognitive problems, hyperactivity, and learning difficulties (Fishbein & Pease, 1996). Because a safe level of drinking during pregnancy has not been established, it is generally recommended that a woman abstain from alcohol during pregnancy.

Heroin

Heroin is considered an opiate, a CNS depressant. The estimated number of heroin users, which remained fixed at roughly 600,000 from the 1970s into the 1990s, almost quadrupled in the 1990s to an estimated 2 million users (Monroe, 1996). Heroin is both physically and psychologically addicting and creates a strong craving in the user. Because tolerance to the effects of the drug develops quickly, increasing amounts are needed to achieve the desired effects (Fishbein & Pease, 1996). Euphoria is the initial response to the drug but then changes to drowsiness, reduced libido, difficulties with memory and concentration, and the absence of the sense of pain (Faltz, 1998).

Because heroin is an illegal drug, there is no quality control on its manufacture or sale. The strength of the drug and what is added to it (cutting agents) are unknown to the buyer. **Cutting agents** are substances added to street drugs to increase bulk (e.g., mannitol and starch), to mimic or enhance pharmacological effects (e.g., caffeine and lidocaine), or to combat side effects (e.g., vitamin C and/or dilantin). The contamination of heroin with cutting agents, the use of unsterile equipment, and combination with other drugs can lead to serious health consequences. An unsuspectedly pure batch often results in a number of overdoses, which can precipitate respiratory depression, coma, and possibly death (Ling & Wesson, 1990).

Buyers of street drugs can never be sure of what they are buying. In 1996, the health departments and poison control centers in four eastern U.S. cities reported at least 325 cases of overdoses requiring medical intervention for people who had used heroin bought on the street that had probably contained scopolamine, an anticholinergic drug. In one hospital in Baltimore, 22 patients who had reported taking heroin were treated; testing of a specimen identified scopolamine, quinine, and dextromethorphan but no heroin (CDC, 1996b).

Historically, heroin has been mainly administered by injection leading to extremely serious health threats. Unsterile intravenous injection can cause skin abscesses, inflammation of the veins, serum hepatitis, and subacute bacterial endocarditis. All of these have serious sequelae. Sharing of needles is a leading cause of HIV infection that leads to acquired immunodeficiency syndrome (AIDS) (McCusker, Stoddard, Zapka, Morrison, et al., 1992).

The present increase in the number of heroin users is attributed to the fact that a purer and less expensive heroin is available (Monroe, 1996) particularly in the northeastern United States (L. P. Brown, 1995). This pure form allows the user to get high by smoking or snorting it, thus avoiding the dangers associated with injection.

Tobacco

Tobacco is considered a stimulant and is highly addictive. The user feels as if he or she performs better and is more alert. A decrease in appetite is experienced (Faltz, 1998). The connection between cigarette smoking and lung disease, particularly lung cancer, has been recognized since the 1950s. In 1989 the U.S. Surgeon General issued a report concluding that cigarettes and other forms of tobacco are addictive and that smoking is a major cause of stroke. Increasingly, studies are demonstrating the relationship of a wide range of illnesses to the use of tobacco in both smokable and smokeless forms, including lung cancer; cancers of the mouth, lips, esophagus, and larynx; emphysema; heart disease; stroke; and congestive heart failure. In addition, Ambrosone, Freudenheim, Graham, Marshall, and colleagues (1996) demonstrated an increase in breast cancer related to past or present smoking in postmenopausal women who genetically cannot quickly metabolize certain carcinogenic chemicals. Each year in the United States, approximately 400,000 deaths result from cigarette smoking (CDC, 1995b).

The population at highest risk for new smoking behaviors is children, in particular teenage girls (Dumas, 1992b). A lifetime of cigarette smoking will shorten a life expectancy by 10 years. Dumas (1992b) noted that 80% of lung cancers in women are caused by heavy smoking.

In March of 1997, the Liggett Group Inc., one of the country's leading cigarette makers, made national headlines by announcing at a news conference that smoking is addictive, that it causes cancer, and that tobacco marketing has been directed toward minors. The admission

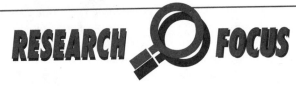

Trends in Cigarette Smoking among U.S. Physicians and Nurses

STUDY PROBLEM/PURPOSE

To determine the trends in cigarette smoking prevalence among physicians, registered nurses, and licensed practical nurses since 1974.

METHODS

Trends of smoking prevalence among physicians, registered nurses, and licensed practical nurses were tracked by analyzing data from the National Health Interview Survey from 1974 through 1991.

FINDINGS

The rate of cigarette smoking among professionals had declined since 1974, with physicians showing the greatest decline. When survey figures from 1990 and 1991 were compared with those of 1974, 1976, and 1977, the prevalence of cigarette smoking among physicians had declined from 18.8% to 3.3%, with an annual decline of 1.15%. Among registered nurses the prevalence dropped from 31.7% to 18.3%, with an average annual decline of 0.88%. Cigarette use among practical nurses dropped from 37.1% to 27.2%, with an annual average decline of 0.62%.

IMPLICATIONS

Cigarette smoking is a leading cause of death in the United States and yet its prevalence among all nurses, and particularly among licensed practical nurses, remains high. Nurses are important as educators and role models to their patients. Their practice of unhealthy behavior undermines both of these roles.

SOURCE

From "Trends in Cigarette Smoking among U.S. Physicians and Nurses" by D. E. Nelson, G. A. Giovino, S. L. Emont, R. Brackbill, L. L. Cameron, J. Peddicord, & P. D. Mowery, 1994c. JAMA, The Journal of the American Medical Association, 271(16), pp.1273–1276.

was made as part of a settlement in a law suit filed by 22 states accusing the tobacco industry of hiding knowledge of the adverse effects of tobacco use (Broder, 1997).

After an extensive review of the literature, the Agency for Health Care Policy and Research (1996) issued guidelines to assist health care workers to convince smokers to quit. In their introduction they state, "It is difficult to identify a condition in the United States that presents such a mix of lethality, prevalence, and neglect, and for which effective interventions are so readily available."

Stopping smoking is not easy. According to Beim (1995), 70% of the 46 million smokers in the United States say they want to quit, one-third actually try, and only 2.5% succeed. Daily cigarette smokers were more likely to report feeling dependent upon the substance than those who used marijuana, alcohol, or cocaine (CDC, 1995b). There is a low success rate in treatment of nicotine addiction, with 70% to 80% resuming smoking within a year after treatment (O'Brien & McLellan, 1996).

Nurses must take a proactive stance in reducing the morbidity and mortality associated with the use of tobacco products. Strategies should be implemented to further reduce the availability and social acceptability of tobacco use in order to decrease the numbers of new users, particularly adolescents. Continued and increased education at all levels is necessary along with increased access to treatment programs. Perhaps in this endeavor nurses need to begin with themselves. See the accompanying Research Focus.

Caffeine

The most ubiquitous and widely used psychoactive drug is caffeine. Caffeine, a stimulant, is found in coffee, tea, cocoa, soft drinks, and over-the-counter preparations. Over 80% of U.S. citizens consume it daily (Lamarine, 1994). The user feels stimulated with increased mental acuity and a sense that he or she can continue forever without becoming exhausted (Faltz, 1998). A 1994 study found evidence to support the existence of a caffeine dependence syndrome, which includes the development of tolerance to the effects, physical withdrawal, difficulty cutting down or controlling use, and continued use despite medical contraindications (Strain, Mumford, Silverman, & Griffiths, 1994).

Caffeine has been studied in relation to a number of health problems including hypertension (Myers, 1988), cardiac arrhythmias (Myers, 1991), increased cholesterol (Pietinen, Geboers, & Kesteloot, 1988), heart disease (Klatsky, Friedman, & Armstrong, 1990), and malignancies (Rosenberg, 1990; Rosenberg, et al., 1993). Lamarine (1994) reviewed over 100 references related to the health and behavioral effects of both acute and chronic caffeine exposure. He identified beneficial effects of improved athletic performance and increased basal metabolic rate. Regarding the health effects, he found the research results to be contradictory and concluded that the relationship between caffeine consumption and various illnesses remains equivocal. He suggested that chronically ill and pregnant women exercise restraint in their use of caffeine, although the research suggested low to nonexistent risk with moderate caffeine consumption.

Marijuana

Marijuana has been both deified and vilified, often with more emotion on both sides than hard scientific data. There is, however, increasing evidence that it is both a physically harmful and addicting drug (Goroll, et al., 1995; Miller & Gold, 1989). Use of the drug can lead to a sense of euphoria or depression and restlessness. The individual becomes relaxed and drowsy and experiences a heightened perception and awareness of color and sound. Time is distorted as are spatial perceptions. The user has poor coordination and often experiences a sense of weightlessness and tingling. Dry mouth, difficulty articulating words, and food cravings are other responses (Faltz, 1998).

Tetrahydrocannabinol (THC), the most psychologically active ingredient, is but one of more than 400 chemicals in marijuana (Fishbein & Pease, 1996). The toxicology and pharmacological action of most of these chemicals are poorly understood. Some are thought to be carcinogenic (Witters & Venturelli, 1988).

Chronic use of marijuana can lead to cardiovascular, pulmonary, reproductive, and psychological problems (Goroll, et al., 1995; Miller & Gold, 1989). Psychological effects include euphoria, distortions in space and time, paranoia, impairment in memory and concentration, and difficulties in abstraction (Goroll, et al., 1995; Miller & Gold, 1989). In view of the increased usage of marijuana in the eighth grade group (USDHHS, 1994b), cognitive effects of the drug are of particular concern. Marijuana use has long been associated with a motivation syndrome, particularly in adolescents (Gold, 1991). Its increased acceptance by youth is particularly disturbing.

Withdrawal symptoms have been identified as irritability, nausea, weight loss, insomnia, and anxiety (Witters & Venturelli, 1988). According to Gold (1991), the marijuana in use today is perhaps 30 times stronger than that cultivated in the 1960s.

Cocaine

Cocaine is a stimulant that is snorted or injected. Cocaine use can result in a number of physical problems that include inflammation of the nasal passages and damage to the nasal septum, hypertension, cardiac arrhythmias, heart attacks, seizures, strokes, and malnutrition (Taylor & Gold, 1990). In addition, the person who injects the drug is exposed to all of the problems associated with unsterile intravenous injection. Chaisson, Baccheti, Osmond, Bradie, and colleagues (1989) found that daily intravenous cocaine use significantly increased the risk of HIV infection, relative to use of heroin alone. Psychological problems include restlessness, irritability, depression, anxiety, and paranoia (Goroll, et al., 1995; Landry & Smith, 1987; Taylor & Gold, 1990).

The process of "freeing" cocaine from its hydrochloride

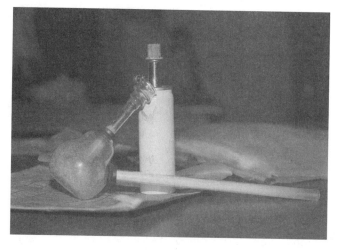

Crack, when smoked, increases the high feeling experienced by the user and increases the risk of heart attack, stroke, and respiratory problems. Photo courtesy of UPI/Corbis.

base is called freebasing. Smoking cocaine in freebase or crack form not only increases the euphoria but also increases the many associated dangers. The euphoria (or high) is rapid because the cocaine reaches the brain in seconds, but it is short-lived and lasts less than 15 minutes (Landry & Smith, 1987). Crack is a short-acting, powerfully addictive drug that is often lethal. Crack cocaine constricts blood vessels and dangerously raises the blood pressure, possibly resulting in heart attack or stroke or severe respiratory problems (Landry & Smith, 1987). The use of crack cocaine is responsible for a generation of young people who will live as cardiac cripples, with seriously damaged hearts and damaged lives.

The Drug Enforcement Administration (DEA) estimated that there were 373,000 crack babies born in 1989 (Dumas, 1992a). It should be noted that the late 1980s were a time when cocaine use had decreased. **Crack babies** have physical problems and developmental delays due to their mother's prenatal use of cocaine. Crack babies have been found to have numerous problems including abnormal electroencephalograms (EEGs), an increased incidence of sudden infant death syndrome (SIDS), visual impairments, mental retardation, delayed development, and learning problems (Gold, 1991). The children are prime subjects for abuse, because they tend to be tense infants and hyperactive children. This situation is compounded by the fact that the mother may continue her use of crack, which increases the potential for infant abuse and neglect.

As these children reach school age, they present tremendous challenges to their teachers and to school nurses. Sluder, Kinnison, and Cates (1996) have identified a complex range of cognitive, social, language, behavioral, and motor deficiencies characteristic of children who had prenatal drug exposure. School nurses need to be aware that the children might exhibit multiple disabilities and be prepared to work with the children, their teachers, and their parents. The school nurse should work with local and state agencies to develop resources to enhance the education and support of the children and their parents.

Methamphetamine

Methamphetamine is an amphetamine, a CNS stimulant manufactured chemically. Methamphetamine, variably known as "speed," "crank," and "go," has been a drug of abuse for many years. Its smokable form, usually referred to as "ice" or "crystal," has been available in the United States since the early 1980s (Beebe & Walley, 1995). In the 1990s it is replacing cocaine as a drug of choice in some areas of the country, most notably in the West, South, and Midwest (CDC, 1995a). The user experiences an initial euphoria followed by depression. The individual feels wide awake, has a decreased appetite, and experiences insomnia. With continued use, the user frequently becomes very suspicious of the actions of others, resulting in aggression (Faltz, 1998).

From 1991 to 1994, methamphetamine-related emergency department visits more than tripled, and methamphetamine-related deaths reported by medical examiners rose from 151 to 433 (CDC, 1995a). In view of the increased morbidity and mortality associated with the use of the drug, the Comprehensive Methamphetamine Control Act of 1996 was passed by Congress. This law increased the penalties for trafficking in methamphetamine and toughened the penalties for trafficking in the chemicals used to produce it.

Physical effects associated with methamphetamine abuse include weight loss, tachycardia, tachypnea, hyperthermia, insomnia, and muscle tremors (CDC, 1995a). In chronic users, the most common presentation is acute psychosis with auditory and visual hallucinations, aggressiveness, and extreme paranoia (Beebe & Walley, 1995).

The link between use of methamphetamine and violence is being increasingly documented. Its use and associated social consequences are rapidly rising in the Midwest. In North Dakota, for example, where use of methamphetamine quadrupled between 1994 and 1997, a Northeastern University research study suggested that the teen murder rate spiraled by 320 percent (Bai, 1997).

Properties of Sedatives, Narcotics, and Cocaine

Signs and symptoms of intoxication, overdose, and withdrawal from sedatives, narcotics, and cocaine can be seen in Table 25-2. The term *narcotic* has many definitions and has been commonly used to refer to a central nervous

Table 25-2   Addictive Properties of Sedatives, Narcotics, and Cocaine

DRUG	ADDICTIVE PROPERTIES	USE/ INTOXICATION	OVERDOSE	WITHDRAWAL
Sedatives (alcohol, barbiturates)	Physically and psychologically addicting; tolerance	Relaxation; decreased inhibitions, judgment, reflexes; slurred speech, clumsiness, drowsiness, psychomotor retardation, labile mood	Sleepiness, shallow respiration, apnea, difficulty in arousal, decreased or absent response to painful stimuli, loss of deep tendon reflexes, cold clammy skin, dilated pupils, hypotension, coma and death	On a continuum: slight tremors → uncontrollable shaking; insomnia → total wakefulness; mild diaphoresis → drenching sweats; frequent dreams → vivid nightmares; nausea and vomiting → dry heaves and total increased vital signs Convulsions possible
Narcotics	Physically and psychologically addicting; tolerance; craving.	Euphoria, drowsiness, respiratory depression, constricted pupils, nausea, and insomnia	Slow and shallow breathing, pinpoint pupils, clammy skin, decreased consciousness, convulsions, coma, death	Watery eyes, runny nose, yawning, decreased appetite, tremors, panic, chills, sweating, nausea, muscle cramps, insomnia, increased vital signs
Cocaine	Strong psychological addiction; strong craving	Dilated pupils, increased vital signs, anorexia, insomnia, euphoria followed by letdown, dullness, tenseness, irritability; risk of seizures, heart and respiratory failure	Hyperthermia, panic attacks, seizures, arrythmias, hypertension	Decreased energy, depression, fatigue, craving, insomnia, inability to feel pleasure

system depressant, or analgesic, or any drug that can lead to physical dependence (Lehne, 1995). Sedatives are included under the broad category of CNS depressants. Examples of narcotics are heroin, morphine, demerol, and Darvon. The mildest form of CNS depression is sedation. At low doses sedatives diminish physical and mental responses but do not affect consciousness. Benzodiazepines and anxiolytics are newer terms for sedatives. Withdrawal from narcotics, although extremely uncomfortable to the client, poses less actual threat than withdrawal from sedatives such as alcohol or barbiturates (Julien, 1985). Heroin withdrawal is often described retrospectively by the client as a very bad case of the flu.

Other Drugs Misused and Abused

Several other substances are abused and misused, most notably steroids, inhalants, designer drugs, and prescription drugs.

Steroids

Reports of steroid abuse are a relatively recent phenomenon. Steroids are used primarily by athletes in order to build muscle strength and to improve athletic prowess, but they bring with them physical and psychological risk. Associated risks include depression, aggressiveness, acne, hair loss, weakened tendons, breast development and testicular shrinkage in men, and facial hair, lowered voice, and irregular menstrual periods in women (Groark, 1992). Symptoms of dependence on steroids consistent with DSM-III-R criteria have been demonstrated (Brower et al., 1990), pointing to the need for an awareness of possible steroid dependence in clinical practice. DSM-IV includes anabolic steroids as a substance-related disorder (American Psychiatric Association, 1994).

Inhalants

The National Survey Results on Drug Use (USDHHS, 1994b) reported an increase in the use of **inhalant substances.** These volatile substances are purposely inhaled to produce intoxication. This group of drugs consists of gasoline, glues, paint thinners, cleaning fluids, aerosol propellants, lighter fluid, nitrous oxide, and ether, among others. The user experiences giddiness and euphoria. Inhalants are associated with a wide range of serious effects including organic brain syndromes; pulmonary, liver, and kidney damage; and potentially fatal cardiac arrhythmias (Witters & Venturelli, 1988).

Hallucinogens and Designer Drugs

After a 15-year gradual decline, hallucinogens appear to be making a comeback. Lysergic acid diethylamide (LSD), a drug often associated with the 1960s, is increasingly becoming a drug of the 1990s. The use of LSD by twelfth

graders increased from 4.8% in 1988 to 6.8% in 1993, and at the same time there was a significant decline in the percentage of persons seeing a risk associated with taking LSD (USDHHS, 1994b).

Designer drugs is the name given to new drugs that are created by chemically altering known drugs. Several heroin-like drugs have been created, for example, by making chemical changes in demerol and fentanyl. Serious health risks have been associated with the use of designer drugs. The risks are dependent upon what the ingredients of the drug are.

Prescription Drugs

Another problem is the misuse of drugs that have been prescribed for a legitimate purpose. This might be accomplished by seeking prescriptions from several health care providers, by taking the drug in excess of the prescribed dose, or by forging or altering prescriptions. Large quantities of prescription drugs are diverted to the illicit drug market by use of fraudulent prescriptions (Beary, Mudri, & Dorsch, 1996). An estimated 3% of the U.S. population deliberately seek psychoactive prescription drugs for the purpose of intoxication or resale (Wilford, 1990).

Although alcohol and the various other drugs are generally studied as separate entities, the common practice is to use two or more substances concomitantly (Kinney, 1991). It is difficult enough to describe the effects of any psychoactive drug, because they vary depending upon experience with the drug, increasing and decreasing blood levels, intoxication, overdose, withdrawal, and so on. When a second or third drug is added with synergistic, additive, or antagonistic properties, the results are impossible to predict.

NURSING CARE OF CLIENTS WHO ABUSE SUBSTANCES

Community health nurses are often the first to recognize the existence of a substance abuse problem. With knowledge of the addictions, nursing skills can be employed to help the client recognize and seek help for the problem.

Effect of Attitudes on the Delivery of Care

Prior experiences, personal likes and dislikes, values, beliefs, family background, peer interests, education, and knowledge all affect the choices that people make and the way that they perceive others. The dictionary defines attitude as "a manner, disposition, feeling, position, etc. with regard to a person or thing" (Flexnor & Hauck, 1993). Nurses have varied feelings or attitudes with regard to working in different specialty areas.

The same dictionary further defines attitude as "a position or posture of the body appropriate to or expressive of an action, emotion, etc." A nurse wanting to work in psychiatry but assigned to a medical unit might well express displeasure in facial expression and body posture. It is important that nurses recognize ways that attitudes manifest themselves. Attitudes or feelings about particular clients or specific diagnoses are apparent in behavior as well as in speech. In communication, nonverbal content far outweighs the power of words in communicating a message. For the most part, however, people take responsibility only for what they put into words. It is not at all uncommon for a client to receive one message verbally and quite another nonverbally.

Most nurses have had prior experiences living with, working with, or caring for people addicted to alcohol and other drugs. These experiences, together with education, will determine how they react to the next client with the same diagnosis. Attitudes affect behavior, and some may produce more therapeutic outcomes than others. That does not mean that some attitudes are "good" and others are "bad"; in fact, labeling them as such tends to be countertherapeutic. Nurses must strive to examine their own attitudes without labeling or judging. This examination may or may not result in change, but, at the very least, it should increase the nurse's awareness of nonverbal messages.

Attitudes toward people who use alcohol and other drugs tend to be inconsistent and conflicting. Although there is widespread acceptance that the addictions are treatable diseases, clients are often regarded as weakwilled, self-destructive people with little hope of change. This ingrained moralistic, pessimistic, and hopeless attitude, though often unrecognized by the nurse, affects all aspects of the nursing process. The nurse who has this attitude might be less apt to include questions regarding use and abuse in the assessment process and may miss obvious clues. If questions about substance abuse are included, they may be asked in a way that minimizes concern. This approach presents a problem, because early recognition, diagnosis, and prevention have the same value and benefits for the addictions as for other illnesses.

Some nurses view addictions as willful self-abuse or bad habits better treated by addiction specialists. These nurses might address the secondary problems created by the addiction without regard to the addiction itself. For example, a nurse who does not regard excessive drinking as a health issue might treat a client's high blood pressure, sleep disturbance, anxiety, or excessive bruising without considering the role that alcohol might be playing in causing those disorders. The planning of care becomes fragmented, and opportunities for education are lost.

The Use of Labels

A nurse may insist that a client accept a label such as "alcoholic" or "addict" when the client is neither ready nor willing to do so. Clients as well as nurses have strong ideas about what an addicted person looks and acts like. It is often easy to exclude oneself from this description. "Uncle Joe was an alcoholic. He drank straight whiskey and was often disheveled and unemployed. I've been in the same job for several years and drink only martinis and manhattans. I therefore am not an alcoholic." This client might be willing to entertain the idea that an enlarged liver is related to alcohol intake. At the same time, the label "alcoholic" might be totally unacceptable. If a nurse attempts to apply such a label, credibility in the eyes of the client may be lost. Many clients are willing to consider that some of their problems may be related to their drinking or drug-taking practices and to seek intervention without ever accepting the diagnosis (Amodeo, 1995).

When a client is unwilling to accept the diagnosis of "alcoholic" or "drug-addict," health care professionals may say that the client is "denying." Denial has long been considered a part of the addiction process. Wallace (1977) points out that diagnosing alcoholism is not easy and that professionals often have difficulty in agreeing as to how and why the diagnostic label should be applied. Wallace questions whether the clients should always be called "in denial" when they are unable to apply the label "alcoholic" to themselves.

Unrealistic Expectations

A nurse might feel that intervention that does not result in client sobriety is a failure. Evaluation of client outcome

---

৩৩ REFLECTIVE THINKING ৩৩

Client Choices

It is your first day in a new hospital, and you have your choice of client assignments. Of the following choices, which would you be most apt to choose first, second, third, fourth, fifth, and sixth?

a. An elderly man from a nursing home who has pneumonia.

b. An 8-year-old boy who has had an appendectomy.

c. A 67-year-old suicidal woman with alcoholic pancreatitis.

d. A 22-year-old postpartum Spanish-speaking woman.

e. A 26-year-old drug-addicted man with HIV infection.

f. A 35-year-old ICU patient with multiple trauma.

• What influenced your decisions?

• Were they easy or hard to make?

• If you were assigned to your sixth choice, what would your feelings be about that assignment?

• How do you think those feelings might show in your behavior?

• Do you think that other members of your class would choose the same?

should be made from a realistic appraisal of the facts. For example, clients are often labeled treatment failures when they continue to drink or to take drugs after several trips to a detoxification facility. Detoxification, however, is exactly what the name implies, a process of safely removing toxic substances from the body. If this has been done, the intervention is a success regardless of the clients' subsequent behavior. A myriad of interventions might be necessary before sobriety is achieved. If the nurse honestly and skillfully treated the clients in accordance with a sound knowledge of the disease, neither credit nor blame is associated with treatment outcome.

Identifying Populations at Risk

High-risk or target populations for substance abuse cross all race, age, socioeconomic status, culture, and gender groups (National Center for Health Statistics, 1995). It is important to note that populations at risk vary by type of addiction and sequelae. It may be easy to think of populations at risk for alcoholism and the use of street drugs but more difficult to realize that substances such as nicotine, prescription drugs, and drugs that Americans use every day present serious problems for people in terms of lost productivity and disability.

Nurses in hospital and community settings need to have a good working knowledge of diverse populations at risk. Risk means that behaviors, social roles, genetic factors, health status, family history, gender, age, race, class, and occupation may, alone or together, increase one's vulnerability to addiction. Some populations are at higher risk than others to problems of substance abuse. Poverty, race, and other barriers to care are all important variables that contribute significantly to risk. The most pervasive of all risk factors is poverty. Poverty breeds despair and hopelessness, isolation and anger. Any stressor, in particular an unremitting stressor such as poverty, can leave one at higher risk of substance abuse (Dumont, 1992; Easley-Allen, 1992).

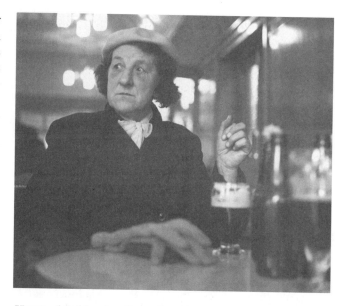

Heavy drinking has been found to be more common in white women than African American or Latino women.
Photo courtesy of Hulton-Deutsch Collection/Corbis.

Women

As many as 6 million women drink excessively in the United States, accounting for approximately a third of the problem drinkers (Oppenheimer, 1991). Much of the early work on substance abuse was conducted exclusively with male subjects, and treatment programs were designed accordingly. It has only been relatively recently that research has focused on the special needs of women. Many differences have emerged, and stereotypes have been challenged. When compared with men, women have different risk factors, different drinking and drug-taking patterns, different treatment needs, and different barriers to treatment.

Women who abuse substances are a diverse group, crossing racial, ethnic, and socioeconomic lines. Wilsnack and Wilsnack (1991) found heavy drinking among white women more common than among African American or Latino women. Despite widely held stereotypes to the contrary, national survey data indicate that white women are significantly more apt to have used any illicit drug in their lifetime than African American or Latino women (USDHHS, 1994a). Despite this fact, women of color are much more likely to be tested for drug abuse than are white women and consequently are more apt to face criminal charges and child protection interventions (Maher, 1992).

Goldberg (1995) identified major risk factors for women as childhood physical and sexual abuse, adult victimization by domestic violence, and a spouse or partner who abuses substances. Bean (1984) stresses the need for establishing an environment of safety in helping people to engage in alcoholism treatment. Women in abusive situations who feel threatened where they live will find it very difficult to engage in treatment. See also Alexander, 1995 and Hennessy, 1992.

There are important differences between the sexes in regard to alcohol. Women reach higher blood alcohol

⚭❧ REFLECTIVE THINKING ❧⚭

The Homeless Shelter

You are beginning a community clinical rotation in an urban homeless shelter. You enter the shelter for the first time and see men lying drunk on the floor of the lobby. One man vomits and passes out.

• What immediately comes to mind when you see the men?

• Do you have biases? What are they? Are you making judgments on the basis of fact or emotion?

• How do you perceive the role of your classmates in helping you and themselves become more comfortable in the shelter setting?

levels from drinking a given amount of alcohol than do men of comparable size. Women develop alcohol-related problems much earlier in their drinking careers than do men. Cirrhosis of the liver develops more quickly in an alcoholic woman, with an average of 13 years of drinking as compared with 22 years in a man (Oppenheimer, 1991).

There is an increasing body of literature concerned with the relationship between the addictions and obstetric and gynecological problems, including damage to a developing fetus. Sexual dysfunction, infertility, miscarriage, and breast cancer have all been associated with heavy drinking. Substance abuse in women of childbearing age can have tragic consequences. Fetal alcohol syndrome (FAS) refers to a pattern of anomalies occurring in infants born to mothers who abused alcohol during pregnancy. Problems in the early years of life include prematurity, developmental delays, facial dysmorphia, neurological abnormalities, and mental retardation (Abel & Sokol, 1991). Fetal alcohol syndrome is an underdiagnosed illness that has profound social and economic burdens. It is estimated that there are 1,200 infants born each year with FAS, and this may be only the tip of the iceberg. For the 1,200 cases alone, the annual cost of treating the children as they grow older is estimated at $76.6 billion. Most of this cost is associated with institutional care of mentally retarded children (Abel & Sokol, 1991). Many other drugs including cocaine, heroin, marijuana, PCP, and tobacco inflict damage to the fetus when abused during pregnancy (Calhoun, 1996).

There is widespread intellectual acceptance of the addictions as treatable diseases, yet underneath the surface deeply ingrained, stereotypical beliefs can often be found. There is stigma associated with the addictions, and this is a particularly heavy burden for women. Women may tend to be judged by harsher standards than men. Rather than recognizing the primacy of the addiction, health care providers may focus on its consequences. "How can she do that to her children?" they may ask. The same question would sound heartless, even ludicrous, if the mother were suffering from multiple sclerosis or a brain tumor. Present controversy regarding mandatory testing of pregnant women, mandatory confinement of pregnant addicts during pregnancy, and criminalization of drug use by pregnant women add to the stigma (Finkelstein, 1994).

Perhaps because of the stigma and fear that their children will be taken away, women are slower to seek treatment for alcohol and drug-related problems than are men. Often they seek help for associated depression or anxiety and are treated with psychotropic drugs that further compound their problems. Once the problem has been identified, the treatment plan often does not take into consideration the special needs of the woman.

Elders

Although problems with alcohol and other substance abuse are prevalent among the elderly, they tend to be underdiagnosed and sometimes ignored. In one study,

alcoholism was accurately diagnosed in only 37% of elderly as compared with 60% of nonelderly clients (Curtis, Geller, Stokes, Levin, & Moore, 1989). Elderly alcoholic clients can be divided into two groups: those who developed alcoholism early in life and survived to old age and those who did not manifest symptoms until in their sixties or later. The latter group are often drinking in response to situational factors such as retirement, death of a spouse, loss of friends, loss of health, or other major life changes that accompany old age. Some may have been drinking the same amount for years with no problems, but changes related to aging and or the development of chronic illnesses now make this amount troublesome. Late-onset problem drinking is more prevalent in those who are wealthier and better educated. Fewer elderly women than men drink. Problems tend to develop at a later age for women but more often include the problematic use of prescribed psychoactive substances (Gomberg, 1995)

Aging modifies the rate of absorption, distribution, and excretion of drugs including alcohol (Atkinson, Ganzini, & Bernstein, 1992). Owing to decreased fluid volume in elders, blood alcohol content may reach higher levels. Older adults have more chronic illness and might be taking any number of prescription drugs. Alcohol interferes with at least one-half of the most commonly prescribed drugs (Olsen-Noll & Bosworth, 1989; Hooyman & Kiyak, 1996).

The effects of chronic drinking in the elderly can be profound. Associated illnesses include hypertension; cancers of the mouth, larynx, and esophagus (especially when combined with smoking); cirrhosis; and malnutrition. Falls are a major concern, because they often result in hip and other fractures.

Social isolation is both cause and effect of alcoholism in elders. Treatment approaches should include both education and the development of a social support network.

Gays and Lesbians

Alcoholism is prevalent in the gay and lesbian community, with various studies reporting rates between 18% and 35% (Herbert, Hunt, & Dell, 1994). Even so, there is little literature addressing the special needs of this population. Herbert, Hunt, and Dell (1994) discuss several possible contributing factors for the high incidence. They include coping with internal homophobia, counteracting the anxiety and stress related to the "coming out" process, and the reliance of gays and lesbians on bars as places for socialization and entertainment. L. Sorenson (personal communication, June 26, 1996) points out that it is very difficult to compare alcohol use and abuse between lesbian and heterosexual women because of inconsistencies in the studies and the fact that past studies on lesbians and alcohol have sampled lesbians in bars.

Bean (1984) and Alexander (1995) stress the need to form an alliance in order to engage the client in treatment. Forming an alliance involves creating an atmosphere that allows for mutual respect and the free expression of feelings. Gay men and lesbians often face not only the negative and stereotypical attitudes associated with substance abuse but also homophobia and discrimination related to their sexual orientation. These attitudes are manifest in both subtle and overt behavior and undermine successful intervention.

Homeless and Mentally Ill Persons

The comorbidity of severe mental illness and alcohol and other drug disorders has been put as high as 50% in community mental health settings and is probably much higher among homeless people (Drake & Mueser, 1996). Often, addiction treatment facilities exclude people with mental illness, and mental health facilities ignore or discriminate against people with addictions. Thus, the dually diagnosed client is left unserved.

Particularly vulnerable and at risk are homeless men and women with both substance abuse problems and mental illness. Overall, they have more trauma, physical illness, and legal problems than do other homeless people; are more deficient in social and vocational skills; and are more apt to live on the streets than in shelters or other refuges for homeless people (Drake & Mueser, 1996).

Those exhibiting symptoms of both substance abuse and mental illness are not a homogeneous group. Some with a primary mental illness use alcohol or other drugs to combat loneliness or to alleviate psychiatric symptoms. Others have a primary substance abuse problem and exhibit psychiatric symptoms secondary to drug use or withdrawal. A third group exhibits both disorders independent of each other. In any case, research has indicated that the most positive outcomes occur when the two problems are treated in an integrated manner (Woody, 1996).

Woody (1996) expresses concern about the lag that exists between present research and health policy. Often, addiction treatment is separated from medical, psychiatric, and other interventions, undermining the development of integrated treatment approaches.

Nurses and Other Health Professionals

It is estimated by the American Nurses Association that from 6% to 8% of nurses use alcohol or other drugs to an extent sufficient to impair their professional performance (Hughes & Smith, 1994). The extent of addiction among physicians has been widely reported to be as much as 30% to 100% greater than in the general population. Kinney (1991), however, traced this figure as originating from a 1954 to 1957 study of narcotic addiction in the allied medical professions of Germany and, after reviewing the literature, concluded that addiction among physicians is on a par with the population as a whole. Alcohol and drug abuse cases account for two-thirds of complaints coming before state nursing boards (Kinney, 1991). Reasons often cited for substance abuse in the helping professions are parental alcoholism, high stress, easy access to drugs, and an underlying belief that knowledge of the drug protects the user from succumbing to addiction.

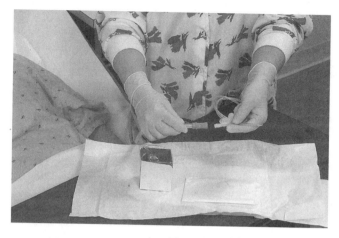

A substance-dependent health professional working with a client can be a lethal mix. If you suspect one of your colleagues to be abusing drugs or alcohol it is your responsibility to report it. It may be a matter of life or death for the client as well as your colleague.

Substance-abusing nurses and other health care professionals are often "protected" by misguided colleagues. Protecting them can be dangerous for both the impaired colleague and for clients. If impairment is suspected, colleagues need to report concerns to the supervisor, stating only the facts and not drawing conclusions. For example, "I am concerned about Miss Doe. She has missed three days of work in the past month and has returned late from lunch on four occasions in the last two weeks. She is usually well liked by the clients, but during this past week three clients complained of her being irritable and a fourth said she smelled alcohol on her breath. Yesterday, she fell asleep at the desk while writing her notes."

Some colleagues may interpret such a report as betrayal. This interpretation is rooted in the fundamental belief that substance abuse is a moral weakness or a crime, not an illness. Chemical addiction is a treatable illness and untreated can be dangerous. In one study, nearly 66% of chemically dependent nurses considered taking their lives as compared with less than 20% of nondependent nurses (Hughes & Smith, 1994). Helping a colleague to treatment for an addiction will not only protect client safety but could also save the life of the colleague.

Employee assistance programs, programs associated with professional organizations, and programs of state licensure boards can be employed to assist the impaired professional.

LEVELS OF PREVENTION

In this chapter primary, secondary, and tertiary levels of prevention provide an organizing framework for a discussion of substance abuse. It should be noted, however, that the nursing process can be just as easily categorized by using terms such as health promotion, health maintenance, and health restoration. What is important is not the terms but the need for an organizing frame of reference in both hospital and community settings.

Perspectives...

Insights of a Nurse on Alcohol Abuse

It began with binge drinking as a teenager. It progressed to more regular drinking as a young adult. Parties, liquor, music, and a general feeling of well-being came to be associated with scotch, cigarettes, and friends. It was difficult to feel good without the scotch. For years, it was "social drinking" and a lot of parties. It progressed to drinks at home, after work, alone. A drink before dinner, I would rationalize. Or two before dinner. It progressed to a pint of scotch each evening and commonly, a hangover each morning. It progressed to visiting different liquor stores each evening so that people would not know I was an alcoholic. I lived like that for 25 years. I worked, as a registered nurse; I was functional, and most people thought I just enjoyed a few drinks. I had car accidents and many "near misses." It was the '60s and '70s when cigarette smoking and heavy drinking were not only acceptable but the norm. One night, I went to dinner with friends, drank my usual, got into my car and ran into an unmarked police car. I was arrested for drunk driving with a blood alcohol level of 0.16. It was, as an officer pointed out, enough to cause a 180-pound man to pass out. I weighed 115 pounds. I went to court the next morning, was sentenced to a 60-day suspension of license and mandated to attend a three-month alcohol awareness program. I denied that I had a problem, but after three months of group work, I realized I had a big one. I was no longer drinking and driving. I was drinking and taking a cab. I realized that I was unable to stop drinking without professional help. Once I acknowledged that I had a problem, I moved slowly and sometimes painfully toward my goal—never another alcoholic drink for the rest of my life. I spent six months in an alcohol group, then two years with a support group that became my sustenance. I spent another year beginning the long road to making it on my own. It is now 10 years later and I have made it. I was one of the lucky ones. I didn't lose a job, hurt another in a motor vehicle accident, or hit the bottom. I am one of the lucky ones. I realize I can never become complacent about alcohol. I cannot stop drinking once I begin. Therefore, I will never drink again. Thank you, community support group, friends, and loved ones who helped me make it through a major life crisis. Recovery is hard work, and it never ends. Caring for others, being sober, and no longer struggling is a gift.

—*Anonymous*

Primary Prevention

The first level of prevention is health promotion and disease prevention. McKinlay's (1974) "upstream analogy" is increasingly being used in community health texts as a way to describe our health care system and how providers respond to illness. The upstream/downstream analogy has two components: the public health, or health promotion, level, where upstream endeavors take place, and the downstream dimension, where ad hoc tertiary interventions are applied. Upstream interventions prevent illness and modify behaviors before people become sick. Downstream interventions refer to short-term, crisis-focused interventions that make no difference in the long run. Downstream interventions are directed toward individuals, and upstream interventions are directed toward populations. In health promotion, where modification of un- healthy behaviors is desired, nurses need to look beyond the individual to the community and to the larger society.

Morbidity and Mortality

Morbidity and mortality patterns in the 1990s are characterized by the fact that most illnesses are social, behavioral, and environmental in origin. The addictions, AIDS, many cancers, liver disease, mental illness, cardiovascular disease, homicide, battering, motor vehicle accidents, birth defects, and work-related injuries are all examples of diseases with social or behavioral etiologies. Many of the events precipitating such problems are brought about by alcohol and drugs (Shannon, 1990; Waller, 1991; Dumas, 1992a, 1992b; Frisch and Frisch, 1998; Hennessey, 1992; McKinlay, 1993). Morbidity and mortality profiles point to the fact that substance abuse is prevalent in American society (National Center for Health Statistics, 1994). People with substance abuse and its related problems fill hospitals and home care caseloads.

Drugs and alcohol are deeply rooted in our norms, our belief systems, and our customs. Preventing addiction, preventing a child from growing to become an adult with an addiction, means uprooting the societal beliefs about alcohol, about smoking, and about prescription and street drugs that are such an integral part of American life. This is no easy task.

Currently, funding priorities, provider roles, and health education models are shifting back to the neighborhoods and communities. Nurses are reclaiming the neighborhoods to practice the primary prevention they do so well (Portnoy & Dumas, 1994). Health providers and community members should meet in the community setting to mutually identify problems and define goals. If nurses are to be effective in teaching about drug and alcohol abuse, they must first assess the community's perception of the problem. Norms and belief systems must be discussed, particularly in relation to preventive care and the potential for some widely accepted behaviors to do great harm. This approach will require compromise, negotiation, and more acceptance of cultural diversity as related to drug and alcohol use.

A community is only as healthy as the people in its neighborhoods, and, although drug and alcohol abuse occur among all classes, the poor and disenfranchised suffer disproportionately from their effects (Dumas, 1992a). In assessing the community, the nurse must ask: Who are the highest-risk community groups? What kinds of treatments and outcomes are associated with different populations at risk? What happens to the poor, the disenfranchised, and the socially vulnerable substance abuser? What are public and private distinctions between access to care, utilization, and quality of services for substance abusers in the community? The answers to these questions will provide direction toward finding solutions to an escalating substance abuse problem. Nurses have a responsibility to teach, to promote health, and to advocate for the social change that will improve the quality of life for all citizens. The community nurse role is a challenge and presents an opportunity for nurses to make a difference.

Community Settings for Primary Prevention

There are many community settings where the nurse can teach about the prevention of alcohol, tobacco, and other drug abuse. The settings are as diverse as the nursing roles within them. The common bond shared by community health providers is the philosophy of care that is based on populations rather than individuals. Community settings include the neighborhood, the home, the school, the church, the workplace, the area council on aging, the community health center, the community youth center, and the "streets" of the community. Community settings with populations at high risk for drug and alcohol problems are adult day health centers, shelters for homeless people, and the home. Table 25-3 lists community settings and typical health promotive nursing activities.

Table 25-3 Community Settings and Health-Promotion Activities

SETTING	HEALTH-PROMOTION ACTIVITIES
School	Education on common addictive substances and the relationship between alcohol and violence
	Health teaching in the classroom on smoking behaviors, street drugs, substance abuse, and AIDS
	Student health fairs; visits to school by role models such as "Girl Power" promotion by Olympic champion Dominique Dawes
	Inclusion of parents, using PTA meetings as site for education
Workplace	Seminars on alcoholism
	Woman-to-woman discussion groups about high-risk behaviors, pregnancy, smoking cessation, fetal alcoholism, HIV infection
	Education of men regarding the relationship between substance abuse and domestic violence
Clinic	
Outpatient	Health education related to primary illness and risk reduction
Community	Outreach and group work in elderly buildings, schools, and throughout neighborhoods; target groups of all ages: children, elders, teens
Shelter	Student nurse health education groups; student-run projects
Home	Health promotion education; education about over-the-counter medication, drug schedule for pain
	Identification of high-risk individuals
	Assessment of risks to women and children; assessment of safety in home
Church	Narcotics Anonymous, Alcoholic Anonymous meetings on site; outreach, teen education
	Social activities without alcohol
Neighborhood	Outreach workers, dicussion groups, family teaching
	Educating community activitists, leaders to carry on work after health providers leave
	Blood pressure screening; teaching relation of cardiovascular risk to drug abuse

Home care is an ideal place to initiate health promotion instruction relating to substance abuse of all types. The visiting nurse, who is most often referred for skilled nursing by a hospital or rehabilitation facility, can assess the client and family risk factors for substance abuse during early home visits and develop teaching plans accordingly. The public health nurse usually works out of a local health department or city hospital. Maternal–child health promotion efforts initiated by public health nurses are especially relevant to substance abuse education, because many women and their children are at high risk for problems. In visits to the home for maternal–child health promotion, the public health nurse is able to do informal teaching about abstinence or moderation with potentially addictive substances such as cigarettes, alcohol, and other drugs. Sharp assessment skills are required for all home visits, and there should be few differences between the goals of public health and visiting nurses in regard to substance abuse prevention.

As the community moves to the forefront of health delivery and as the concept of health promotion becomes more familiar to the public, broader goals emerge that address problems more difficult to solve. These are problems at the societal level, problems embedded in society and in our ways of life: for example, alcohol and smoking behaviors and the promotion of such behaviors by cigarette manufacturers and the media (McKinlay, 1974, 1993). The problem of fetal alcohol syndrome, the outcome of alcohol use in pregnancy which ruins the lives of many children, is 100% preventable (Weiner, Morse, & Garrido, 1989; Apgar, 1995).

Secondary Prevention

Secondary prevention is focused on case finding and early intervention for people with alcohol and other drug abuse problems. Early intervention can mean the difference between moving forward in good health or being threatened by chronic illness and premature death. A good assessment is the foundation of the nursing process.

Community health nurses work in a variety of settings with diverse clients. Clients with substance abuse problems are often evasive or ashamed of their problem, or they are poor historians. Using effective assessment skills, the nurse can identify individuals with substance abuse problems as well as community factors that contribute to those problems.

Assessment and Identification of Substance Abuse Problems

Assessment involves forming an alliance with the client and gathering information to determine the existence and extent of a problem. This process *precedes* diagnosis and intervention. To label a person or to offer solutions prematurely usually leads to a breakdown in communication (Hennessey, 1992).

Assessment is a mutual exploration involving the client, the nurse, and other concerned individuals. It is important

that the nurse work with the client as an ally. This approach involves treating the client with dignity, attending to the client's concerns, assessing for strengths as well as problem areas, and fostering an atmosphere that promotes mutual respect and the free expression of ideas and feelings.

Questions regarding drug and alcohol intake should be a part of every assessment interview. In order to elicit honest responses, the nurse should ask the questions in an open-ended, nonjudgmental, matter-of-fact manner (Liftik, 1995). Care should be taken not to jump to conclusions. The nurse is an explorer here, attempting to examine and understand the unknown, not a detective attempting to pin a diagnosis on a client.

Substance abuse problems are often manifested in several areas of a person's life. To get a clear and thorough picture, the nurse should not limit exploration to one area. For example, if physical findings indicate substance abuse, indicators should be sought in behavioral, occupational, legal, and social areas as well. Table 24-4 summarizes possible indicators of substance abuse.

Although there are often strong negative stereotypes about addicted people, there is no one clear picture. Addictions are prevalent in all strata of society; one addicted person can look quite different from another. There are few definitive diagnostic criteria.

Assessment should also include the client's perception of the problem and what steps, if any, have been taken to remedy the problem. Often, the client is aware that a problem exists and may have attempted to deal with it in the past, either alone or with help. What is now needed is a nonjudgmental person who is willing to listen as possible next steps are sorted out. Nurses may be surprised at how open and honest addicted people can be when the atmosphere for openness is created.

Assessment in the Workplace

The workplace is an important setting where an occupational health, public health, or visiting nurse can screen, identify, and participate in the treatment of people who abuse alcohol, tobacco, and other drugs. In a time of managed care, it is becoming a setting of choice for insurers. Early identification and treatment contain costs by preventing outcomes of chronic alcoholism or drug abuse. In the work setting, more employee assistance programs are using routine or random testing and screening for a variety of drugs. Companies in the United States and worldwide can reap the rewards of employee assistance programs. Identification of people with substance abuse problems, however, presents challenges with respect to preserving anonymity while maximizing worker safety through treatment. Drug screening and HIV testing are understandably controversial as their use in the workplace increases.

Healthy People 2000 (USDHHS, 1990b) does not directly reference substance abuse as an important occupational health focus for the year 2000. It does, however, list HIV infection and AIDS as important areas of concern.

Table 25-4 Indications of Drug- or Alcohol-Related Problems

ENVIRONMENTAL	BEHAVIORAL	PHYSICAL	EMOTIONAL
Neglected children	Secretiveness	Unsteady gait	Personality change
Inadequate living facilities	Change in friends	Slurred speech	Moodiness
Frequent moves	Missed work or school	Odor of alcohol or inhalant on breath	Irritability
Unkempt house	Poor job or school performance	Constricted or dilated pupils	Anxiety
Poor personal hygiene	Frequent job changes	Needle or track marks	Attention deficit
Presence of empty bottles or drug paraphernalia	Failing grades	Runny nose or sniffling	Restlessness
Cigarette burns on furniture or rugs	Legal difficulties	Twitchiness or tremors	Euphoria
	Increase in accidents	Seizures	Depression
		Ecchymosis	Agitation
		Excoriation from picking or scratching	Paranoia
		Weight loss	
		Red eyes	

There is a direct relationship between the use of intravenous drugs and HIV infection. The population at highest risk now and in the year 2000 will be women, particularly women of color and urban women who are poor (CDC, 1996a). As the number of women in the work force increases, emphasis on identification and case finding of intravenous drug users and partners of intravenous drug users becomes imperative. Women at risk for HIV infection because they take intravenous drugs or have sex with infected partners are only one example of a target population in the workplace.

Numbers of women in the workplace will rise significantly in the 21st century. By the year 2000, the median age of the work force will rise to 40 years, and over 80% of new entrants will be women and minorities (Population Reference Bureau, 1989b). Therefore, the workplace assumes a new significance as a site for primary and secondary prevention of diverse substance abuse problems in women.

Latinos will be the majority minority population by the new millennium, and they will be vulnerable because of poor education and low income (Apgar, 1995; Valdiviesco & Davis, 1988; Harper, 1990). Differences in values and beliefs and the cultural implications of teaching about safe sex, substance abuse, and AIDS will be a particular challenge to nurses. New program development is needed to target populations at risk, and language and cultural norms are important considerations in designing such programs. Employee assistance programs that focus on drug and alcohol abuse are best when tailored to the predominant risk group in the workplace.

The problem of fetal alcohol syndrome is also relevant at the level of secondary prevention. There is a scarcity of funded research for this preventable problem, and there are many alcoholic mothers who bear infants who qual-

ify for the FAS diagnosis. The Massachusetts Fetal Alcohol Education Program, Division of Psychiatry, Boston University School of Medicine, suggests that FAS is an underreported disorder and that its symptoms might be diagnosed as other physical or developmental problems in children (Abel & Sokol, 1991; Lewis, 1995; U.S. Bureau of the Census, 1995). Public health attention has waned over the years, but the problem has not. It is important that nurses be adept at screening, case finding, and education in both adult and pediatric settings. It is of interest to note that alcoholic pregnant women who stop drinking early in their pregnancy significantly decrease their risk of bearing an infant with FAS (Weiner, Rosett, & Mason, 1985; Weiner & Larsson, 1987; U.S. Bureau of the Census, 1995). See Figure 25-3.

Screening, casefinding, expert assessment skills, a nonjudgmental attitude, and the ability to ask the right questions at the right time are important clinical skills for nurses in community settings. The "Ten Question Drinking History" is a tool for organizing an assessment of alcohol consumption in pregnant women. The 10 questions are listed in Figure 25-4.

Assessment in the Schools

The school is a primary care setting where nurses are redefining the problems, the work, and their roles. In Boston, a model of high school adolescent clinics is being tested in the inner city, with the goals of teaching conflict resolution and reducing substance abuse. Children in middle and high schools are at risk for addiction to alcohol, tobacco, and drugs. The direct relationship between violence and substance abuse is well documented (Blumenstein, 1995; Marzuk, Tardiff, Leon, Hirsch, et al., 1995;

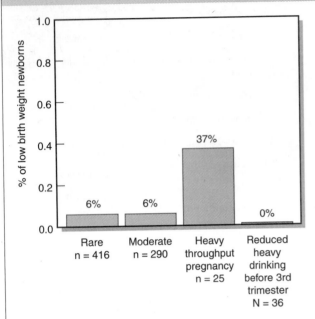

Figure 25-3   Growth Benefits Observed in Infants from Reduction of Mother Prenatal Drinking

From "Clinical Prevention of Fetal Alcohol Effects, a Reality: Evidence for the Effectiveness of Intervention" by L. Weiner & G. Larsson, 1987, Alcohol Health and Research World, *Summer, pp. 60–65.*

abuse, HIV/AIDS, and violence prevention are health-related topics that student nurses teach to inner city boys and girls. The outcomes have been positive, with students expressing more self-confidence and enthusiasm for learning. The school nurse model for baccalaureate registered nurse and non-registered nurse seniors is an exciting direction for community curricula (Igoe, 1994).

Assessment in the Home

The home is an important setting for secondary prevention such as screening and case finding. The home setting might be someone's apartment, a common living situation such as congregate housing, the community room in an elder housing complex, single-room occupancies, halfway houses, or quarterway houses.

Informal nursing clinics in community housing complexes to screen, advise, refer, and identify cases are places where nurses can educate as they screen for illness. Informal education about addictive substances, about the more common substances that can harm such as cigarettes and over-the-counter medications, and the proper use of prescription drugs can take place here. Early referral can be made that will decrease the potential of substance abuse from social isolation, depression, and the loneliness of old age.

Visiting nursing is more formal, and clients are already in the system. They are being seen for a problem for which

Rodriguez & Brindis, 1995). Studies of homicide in the United States reveal that alcohol was present in the blood of victims in about one-half of all cases. Prothrow-Stith (1990, 1996) writes that the basic scenario for a homicide begins with two people of the same race who know each other. Add alcohol, a handgun, and an argument, and a situation emerges that "tough anticrime laws" can do little about. There is a direct relationship among alcohol, drugs, and violence for all Americans, but in particular for young people. Preventing the problem of substance abuse and emphasizing substance-free conflict assumes a growing importance for nurses in school settings.

The 1993 National Household Survey on Drug Use (USDHHS, 1994b) reported that 63% of high school seniors have been drunk at least once; 62% have tried cigarettes; and for the first time in 15 years daily marijuana use had increased significantly. Decreases in cigarette use were apparent in every group except the 12- to 17-year-olds, with 19% of twelfth graders reporting daily use. In 1993 only about half of the youths aged 12 to 17 believed there was great risk in being a pack-a-day smoker, using marijuana occasionally, or trying cocaine, PCP, or heroin.

Grade schools, middle schools, and high schools are excellent settings for primary prevention, but for many students secondary prevention measures are indicated. In Boston, at the University of Massachusetts, community models are in place for senior nursing students to have a clinical experience in high schools, middle schools, and grade schools. The work is not easy, but the nurses and the students benefit from mutually rewarding relationships. Cardiopulmonary resuscitation, smoking, substance

Figure 25-4   Ten Questions to Ask in the Assessment of Drinking Behaviors

The following questions provide a systematic and objective tool to accurately report drinking behaviors. It assumes that the client consumes some alcohol and is nonjudgemental. Nurses and other professionals should adapt the tool to reflect their personal style.

Beer   How many times do you drink beer each week?

How many cans do you drink each time?

Do you ever drink more?

Wine   How many times do you drink wine each week?

How many glasses each time?

Do you ever drink more?

Liquor   How many times do you drink liquor each week?

How many drinks each time?

Do you ever drink more?

Has your drinking changed during the past year?

From "Clinical Prevention of Fetal Alcohol Effects, a Reality: Evidence for the Effectiveness of Intervention" by L. Weiner & G. Larsson, 1987, Alcohol Health and Research World, *Summer, pp. 60–65.*

DECISION MAKING

Teaching Students about the Dangers of Smoking

You are a school nurse in an inner city high school. Over 60% of the students in this school smoke cigarettes. All are under 17 years old. When you discuss smoking in your health education class, the students respond to your discussion about the dangers of smoking with laughter and disregard for potential health problems.

• How do you proceed in getting a group of uninterested students to at least discuss smoking behaviors and the dangers of the habit?

• Would you present smoking as an addiction, a substance abuse similar to cocaine, marijuana, or alcohol abuse? Or would you present it as a public health issue?

• How do you respond in what seems to be a "no win" situation in the short time you will have in the high school?

• What are the ethics that you might involve the students in discussing?

• What are the ethical issues involved with corporations that become "manufacturers of illness"?

they have been referred to the home health agency. Whatever the reason the nurse is in the home, the expert nurse will be able to make ongoing assessments of clients at high risk for substance abuse. A comprehensive assessment tool should always have questions about substance abuse potential, drinking and smoking behaviors, and over-the-counter medications. In the home, clients feel safer, more in control, and less threatened when questions are asked that are troubling or compromising to their sense of integrity.

Tertiary Prevention

Tertiary prevention is the most common mode of health delivery in the United States. It is a "downstream" mode, crisis driven and illness oriented. As health care organizations and insurers rein in costs, decreased reimbursement for interventions at the tertiary level are insufficient to meet the often complex care required by people who have social or behaviorally induced illnesses such as alcoholism or addiction. Tertiary care related to substance abuse includes treatment for liver failure from chronic alcoholism, the opportunistic infections of AIDS and intravenous drug abuse, the cardiomyopathies associated with cocaine abuse, and the emphysema and cancers due to

cigarette smoking. Tertiary care addresses the malnutrition, the neurological damage, and the cardiovascular and pulmonary disabilities that emerge after years of self-neglect while on alcohol or other drugs. Also in tertiary care are people with organic brain disorders, cerebral vascular accidents, and disabilities related to falls, accidents, and violence. Many victims of fetal alcohol syndrome also need tertiary care for profound mental retardation.

At the tertiary level, options for a person with substance abuse problems include detoxification units, transitional or halfway houses, treatment in public and private hospitals, treatment in clinics and respite units for homeless people, and home care.

Detoxification Settings

A **detoxification** unit (often referred to as "detox") is generally where a chemically dependent person is sent to safely withdraw from alcohol or other drugs. Some detoxification centers are hospital based while others are free-standing, but all must have skilled nursing care to supervise potentially life-threatening withdrawal. In a detoxification center, the client's physical status is closely monitored and medications are administered to ensure a safe withdrawal and to minimize uncomfortable symptoms. If removal of toxic substances from the body is accomplished, the intervention is a success regardless of whether the individual returns to alcohol or other drug use. Some detoxification centers are combined with longer-term treatment, usually 15 to 30 days. Facilities can be public or private, and there are significant distinctions between the two types. Private detoxification centers have quicker intake procedures, more options for longer stays, and more individualized, intensive therapy. Urban detoxification centers are usually full, and beds are frequently unavailable when the client is ready to seek treatment. Being able to pay makes a difference for people with substance abuse problems just as it does for other high-risk populations in the United States.

Transitional Housing Programs

Transitional housing programs such as halfway houses are formal programs that are between detoxification and community reintegration for the substance abuser. They are structured programs with substance abuse counseling, relapse prevention work, life skills teaching, and health education. The transitional program affords more time in a protective environment for the recovering person. Medicaid will reimburse for most of the short-term programs, as will disability insurance. Medicare does not cover transitional programs.

Ideally, pregnant women in transition are referred to programs that are focused specifically on issues of women and children. Such programs can better address their individual issues with both substance abuse and their personal relationships.

Private Hospitals and Clinics

Private hospitals and clinics abound in the United States but must be paid for by the client or a private insurer. Private insurance coverage varies, but most policies will cover the cost for a detoxification unit or a private hospital. The federal and state third-party reimbursement programs, such as Medicare and Medicaid, will not. The Betty Ford Clinic is a well-known example of an expensive private clinic for substance abusers.

Clinics and Respite Units for Homeless People

Clinics for homeless people, often nurse managed, provide care for many indigent individuals who are suffering from the long-term effects of alcohol and other drug abuse. The individual often arrives at the clinic intoxicated and seeking help for a crisis situation, such as trauma, infection, or pain. To address more than the crisis presents a challenge to the nurse and can be a slow process. Many homeless, addicted people, because of previous negative experiences, distrust the formal health care system. They are reluctant to accept referrals. Because of active substance abuse, they miss appointments and their care is often episodic. Clinic nurses work to develop caring relationships that will enable clients to return to the clinic when they are not in crisis and to engage in active treatment. When trust is present, the client is also more apt to listen to and heed teaching regarding such things as not sharing needles and cleaning drug paraphernalia with bleach.

The Barbara McInnis House is an innovative program developed by the Health Care for the Homeless Project in Boston. The program addresses the needs of the many homeless and addicted people who are too sick and too weak to manage in the shelters but are not considered sick enough to be in the hospital. Under managed care guidelines, many are discharged from the hospital to the street with complicated discharge instructions. The McInnis House gives the homeless person respite from the streets in a substance-free environment where help is available for medications, dressing changes, and other treatments.

Home Care

As clients are discharged from the hospital sooner and sicker, home care is an increasingly important community resource. Because home care is generally initiated by a referral system, it is often a setting for tertiary care.

Addicted women are a population at high risk in the home care setting. The care of addicted women and their children at home is complex and presents many challenges for the community health nurse. The nurse must balance being a support and a resource for the mother and child while, at the same time, providing structure and setting limits as needed. A woman who is actively abusing substances is generally in no condition to care for her children. Injury and neglect are common sequelae in these situations.

Dumas (1991) wrote of the tenuous relationship when caring for cocaine-addicted mothers and their children. The visiting nurse must establish a primary and trusting relationship with the client and be skilled in both the art and science of nursing. Appointments must be kept, compliance evaluated, and expectations clearly articulated by the nurse.

Effecting a balance between structure and flexibility with respect to nursing interventions is difficult at best, and the concept of "tough love" is an important one. Addicted individuals require a combination of structure, control, and compassion. Keeping these in balance is a difficult task that cannot be done alone (p. 17).

Women and their children, in particular infants, are the most common population at risk seen in the home. The women are increasingly being referred from hospitals after giving birth to premature, addicted, and overall high-risk infants. This is an excellent example of an opportunity for interdisciplinary collaboration. Nurses, social workers, physicians, therapists, maternal–child workers, home health aides, and homemakers all have an important role to play in the client's recovery.

DECISION MAKING

Chronic Alcoholism and Hypertension

You are a home care nurse who admits a client to caseload. The client is a 68-year-old woman with acute and chronic alcoholism and hypertension. She is an active alcoholic and admits to drinking a half bottle of wine daily. Her blood pressure is 172/96. She has not taken her medication in three days. She lives alone in elderly housing. Evaluate the following decisions and give a rationale for your choice.

• You tell the client she needs detoxification and that you will see about having her admitted immediately to a unit.

• You assess the client's response to her alcoholism and evaluate her receptiveness to inpatient treatment. If she is not receptive, mandate an inhospital plan of care.

• You tell her she will need outside supports to assist her in a recovery. Review what some of these supports might be. Obtain a list of informal supports (friends and neighbors).

• You give her an extra dose of medicine because her blood pressure is high.

• You telephone the nurse practitioner or physician to collaborate on a plan of care for this client. Obtain a list of her formal professional supports.

• You refer her to AA immediately.

Mutual Support Groups

Alcoholics Anonymous (AA) and Narcotics Anonymous (NA) fellowships are informal community supports for individuals in recovery. They internalize a spiritual dimension wherein the fellowship becomes an integral part of the member's life. The support extends through all aspects of daily life. The 12-step program, the foundation of AA, takes members through the most difficult days of their lives. Narcotics Anonymous (NA) uses the same 12-step program as AA. They are counterpart programs for alcoholics and addicts. These are prototypes of self-help groups. Because of the anonymity implicit in the fellowship there are few data that evaluate the effectiveness of AA and NA on recidivism rates. According to most sources, however, Alcoholics Anonymous has "the greatest rate of continuing success in helping people maintain abstinence" (S. Brown, 1995).

In summary, there are diverse treatment modalities ranging from early detoxification programs to self-help groups in the community. The treatment modalities, much like the individuals who use them, take many different forms. Methods may be modified for some addicts depending on the program. In most programs, however, strict rules and structure, a limited setting, and an authoritarian environment are norm. Families may or may not be involved in the actual programs. Much depends on the relationship between the client and the family, as well as on the rules of the program with respect to family participation.

LEGAL ISSUES

In discussions of addiction, the interface between medicine and the law is ambiguous. Drug addiction and alcoholism are highly correlated with crime and violence. The question of whether the addicted person is sick and should be treated in the health care system or is a criminal and is better dealt with by the law is a complicated debate. It covers many issues at many different levels.

Violence associated with illicit drugs is often related to the business of procuring and selling the drugs. Crime and violence are most highly correlated with the abuse of alcohol. Two million women in the United States are badly beaten every year, and alcohol is a factor in 40% of the beatings (University of California, 1994). More than half of all homicides involve alcohol (Martin, 1997). Despite laws against possession and consumption of alcohol for people under 21 years of age, one study found that 95% of violent crimes on college campuses involved alcohol or drugs or both, and about half of the assailants in courtship violence were under the influence of alcohol (Nichols, 1995). Driving under the influence is against the law, but approximately 41% of traffic fatalities in 1994 were related to alcohol, and two of every five people in the United States will be involved in an alcohol-related motor vehicle accident at some time during their lives (Liu, Siegel, Brewer, Mokdad, Sleet, & Serdula, 1997).

Other legal issues include child abuse, possession of illicit substances, underage possession of alcohol and cig-arettes, disorderly conduct, theft, the responsibility of both mother and father to an unborn child, juvenile delinquency, violation of restraining orders, and on and on. Most of these are not victimless crimes. Who should be treated? Who should be punished? What are the ramifications of these decisions? These are questions that must be considered by the community health nurse. Public health as well as individual health must be considered. Questions of policy must also be considered. Will supplying clean needles and syringes prevent the spread of AIDS, or will it encourage the continued use of drugs? Will incarcerating drug-addicted pregnant women increase the chances of a healthy child, or will it prevent addicted women from seeking prenatal care? Will denying disability benefits to individuals claiming disability due to drug or alcohol addiction provide needed incentive to sobriety, or will it condemn people on the edge to the streets or to shelters? If the addictions are diseases, should the individual be held responsible for actions while intoxicated? Should there be mandatory drug testing in the workplace?

The nurse has many roles in this emotionally laden aspect of addiction. It is important for the nurse to have access to legal assistance through different agencies. Most communities have free attorneys or legal advice for women and elders who are in the midst of domestic violence. Other legal resources for clients can be found at shelters, hospitals, and welfare agencies. Some attorneys provide free assistance for people who are unable to hire their own legal representative.

CARING AND CASE MANAGEMENT OF CLIENTS WHO ABUSE SUBSTANCES

The clinical care or case management of people who abuse substances presents difficulties under the best of circumstances. With the advent of managed care and changes in the health care system, several new problems have emerged. First, there are more cost constraints; many services relating to addiction and treatment are not covered, or are only partially covered, by third-party payors. Second, poverty, and in particular poverty among women and children, has become more of a stigma. Third, when health care is based on capitation, a predetermined cost per person, the human element is easily overlooked, as cost containment prevails. Managed care has changed the profile of health care delivery in the United States. Hospitals are downsizing; home care agencies are negotiating with insurers; and bureaucratic tasks have increased. There are escalating health care demands and fewer resources available to meet the demands. There is a lack of fit between available resources and the numbers of people who need them.

In the next decade, hospitals will be for the sickest, with increasing burdens put on home care. This trend will increase the difficulties in providing comprehensive care for addicted individuals. In the 1980s and early 1990s, the numbers of comprehensive substance abuse

DECISION MAKING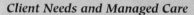

Client Needs and Managed Care

You are a nurse in a managed care organization. You have an 18-year-old client who is an amphetamine addict. You realize he will need counseling and referral for his problem; he is becoming ill because of poor nutrition and his substance abuse.

Information indicates that he will be covered for three mental health visits and that he is not covered for any long-term stay in a detoxification facility. You realize that he is not going to do well attempting recovery on his own, without supports or structure. This is a dilemma that is becoming increasingly common in nursing practice.

• How do you resolve the disparity between what he needs and what his health plan will pay for?

• What approaches would you take to advocate for this client?

• What could you do within your organization, with respect to making changes in what managed care will cover when problems are social and behavioral?

treatment centers increased with demonstrated success, but today they are reserved for the wealthy. Long-term care of the poor is for those with disease so advanced that it is unlikely that they will benefit from long-term intervention (Delbanco, 1996).

The clinical management of addicted people demands excellent medical surgical nursing skills, excellent assessment skills, a great deal of patience, a good sense of humor, and a strong sense of advocacy. It also requires a sound knowledge of community resources, admission procedures, and eligibility requirements for the different programs.

The concept of caring is an important component in working with people addicted to drugs and alcohol. Caring has traditionally been nurses' work, beginning with Nightingale and moving forward to Wald. Caring characterizes the nursing role, and it is a component that medical students are learning in their curricula from nurses who have the greatest respect for its art.

Many of the populations at high risk for substance abuse and many of the people who abuse substances have social and economic issues that are profound. It hurts to look at them, it is frustrating to try to help them, and it is easy to shame them.

The concept of "disaffiliation" that Baum and Burnes (1993) emphasize in their book about homeless people

COMMUNITY NURSING VIEW

Ayla, a 34-year-old pregnant bank vice president, had recently separated from her husband of 10 years. She was first seen by the occupational health nurse at three months into her pregnancy with complaints of fatigue and poor weight gain. She had had no prenatal care. She admitted to depression over her recent separation and unplanned pregnancy. A drinking history revealed she had three or four scotches before dinner each evening and "a brandy" at bedtime. Weekends brought more drinking, and she admitted to "occasionally" going through a fifth of scotch on Saturdays and Sundays. "My drinking is not a problem. I'm just lonely and tired." She worked a five-day week and, in view of her risk, was offered a leave for the remainder of her pregnancy. She refused the leave and did not keep appointments with the occupational health nurse. She was seen again by the occupational health nurse at six months, when she went to the bank's health clinic with fatigue and headache. Her blood pressure was 170/90, heart rate 110 regular, respiratory rate 20, unlabored and lungs clear. She had a 1+–2+ bilateral peripheral edema, and lung sounds

were diminished but clear to auscultation. She appeared bloated, her fingers were swollen, and she had some red blotches on her face. She appeared sad and nervous. She had continued to smoke 10 to 12 cigarettes daily during her pregnancy, and despite efforts to improve her nutrition, her weight gain had been poor. She was depressed and anxious and admitted to a slight hangover on this particular day. "I am drinking more, but my pregnancy is almost over." She was referred to her obstetrician for immediate attention, and the nurse asked her to return later in the week for a blood pressure check and nutritional counseling. Ayla was also advised by the nurse to stop drinking for the remainder of her pregnancy. Ayla did not return to the clinic. The nurse did not seek her out at the work setting, and her obstetrician advised her to continue with monthly appointments and to stop drinking. Ayla said to a friend, "I go to the doctor each month and I'm trying to cut down on my drinking. I don't know what more they want from me. I just want my husband home again."

Continued

COMMUNITY NURSING VIEW

Continued

Ayla delivered a premature girl at 33 weeks, and head circumference was below normal. The infant was nervous and hypertonic. The infant had some respiratory distress and was placed in the intensive care nursery. She was discharged to home after two weeks. At six months, the baby was noted to have growth retardation and facial dysmorphia. She was diagnosed at six months with fetal alcohol syndrome. At this time, Ayla was hospitalized with a major depressive episode and the baby was placed in temporary foster care. The long-range plan was for Ayla and the baby to return home together to visiting nurse services and other community supports.

Nursing Considerations

ASSESSMENT
- At which time in Ayla's pregnancy would primary prevention have been optimal?
- What would be included in the preliminary assessment of Ayla?
- What is the prevailing female alcoholic stereotype that Ayla's case refutes?
- Distinguish questions related to primary, secondary, and tertiary prevention in the data collection.

DIAGNOSIS
- List four nursing diagnoses for Ayla.

OUTCOME IDENTIFICATION
- Given the diagnosis you have identified, what outcomes do you expect?

PLANNING/INTERVENTIONS
- What kinds of health-promotion interventions would you plan for Ayla?
- What would you consider secondary prevention for Ayla?
- On what criteria will you base your nursing diagnoses?
- What kinds of skilled activities will you conduct for this dimension of care?
- How would you define tertiary prevention in this case?
- What would your nursing plan be, and how will the nursing process direct your plan?
- What would you have done differently if you had been Ayla's occupational health nurse?
- Your tertiary level of prevention will involve both Ayla and her baby. What kind of plan for restoration of the health of both mother and infant will you delineate?
- Which community facilities in your area will you use as resources when Ayla is back at home with her baby?
- What kinds of home health services will you suggest in your referral to the local visiting nurse association?

EVALUATION
- How will success or failure at primary, secondary, and tertiary levels of prevention be evaluated?
- What would be the outcome of physical therapy for the infant?

---

also holds true for those addicted to alcohol and drugs. Community health nurses must be willing to help their clients bear the burden, to provide hope, to advocate for the future, to listen, to counsel, and to assist them through the health care system with the goal of "reaffiliating" them.

Nurses have two very special gifts, a capacity to provide comfort and the knowledge to provide highly skilled clinical care. People who abuse substances have many needs, and the skilled nurse will be able to prioritize them with respect to what can and cannot be realistically accomplished.

〜 Key Concepts

- The term *substance abuse* includes alcohol, tobacco, and other drug abuse.

- Substances frequently abused include alcohol, tobacco, marijuana, cocaine, methamphetamine, opiates, and prescription drugs.

- Alcoholism and drug addiction are "equal opportunity" addictions. They occur among all class, socioeconomic, gender, race, and culture groups.

- Women, elders, gays and lesbians, and persons who are homeless and mentally ill are at higher risk than others for the development of alcohol, tobacco, and other drug addiction.

- The upstream analogy invites diverse health providers to work at individual and societal levels to promote healthy behaviors and healthy lifestyles before illness occurs.

- Nurses need to be able to analyze their own attitudes toward people who abuse substances and to identify their preexisting biases and value judgments.
- Primary, secondary, and tertiary levels of prevention are an epidemiologic method by which nurses can organize their approach to the problem of substance abuse.
- Cigarette smoking is an addictive behavior. The group at highest risk are adolescent girls.

- Poverty is a compelling risk factor for alcoholism and drug addiction.
- Education and guidance are interdisciplinary endeavors at all levels of prevention.
- Caring and clinical expertise are prerequisites for the practice of nursing with people addicted to alcohol, tobacco, and other drugs.

Nutrition

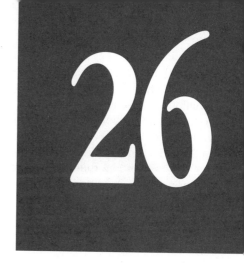

Suzanne Chubinski, RN, BSN, MA
Ruth Roth, MS, RD
Gail P. Howe, MA

Suzanne Chubinski, RN, BSN, MA
Ruth Roth, MS, RD
Gail P. Howe, MA

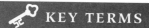

KEY TERMS

anorexia nervosa
bulimia nervosa
cachexia
foodborne illness
geophagia
obesity
pica
substance substitution

With age, your body undergoes various biochemical changes that have been mistakenly accepted as the inevitable consequences of aging when instead they are signs of deterioration and disease that can be dramatically reversed, sometimes by a modest dose of common nutrients.
—Carper, 1996, p. 4

COMPETENCIES

Upon completion of this chapter, the reader should be able to:

- Identify nutrition as a national and global concern.
- Explain the four categories of risk factors for nutritional problems.
- Explain how the risk factors affect clients in different stages of life.
- Discuss the community nutritional problems in each stage of the life span.
- Describe the types of nursing interventions for clients with specific nutritional deficits.
- Identify foodborne illnesses and practices to prevent them.
- Verbalize how a nutritional assessment can identify problems and guide the nurse in appropriate interventions.

Nutrition is an essential component to health and is necessary for growth and development. Maintaining adequate nutrition throughout the life span prevents, delays, or lessens the impact of stress and disease.

According to the World Bank (1993), poor nutrition, by itself or associated with infectious disease, accounts for a large portion of the world's disease burden. In the United States, it is estimated that 20 to 25 million people go hungry every year. That translates to one in eight American children under the age of 12 who suffer from hunger (Food Research and Action Center [FRAC], 1998).

The community health nurse is in a frontline position to identify and intervene in individual and aggregate threats to nutrition. The nurse can identify actual or potential threats to a client's nutrition with individualized levels of intervention.

This chapter discusses nutritional problems and their importance to health, explores nutritional problems across the life span, and determines risk factors that lead to nutritional problems and how these factors affect clients in each stage of life. Nursing interventions to lessen or alter these problems are examined with each problem.

A GLOBAL CONCERN

In 1977, the World Health Assembly accepted a social goal for all its member agencies of "the attainment by all citizens of the world by the year 2000 a level of health that will permit them to lead a socially and economically productive life." By 1978, the WHO, UNICEF, and 67 other organizations representing 143 countries committed themselves to this goal. Nutrition has been identified as an integral part of meeting this goal (World Health Organization, 1986).

Negative and chronic effects on health and behavior are observed when there is poor nutritional intake. Any malnourished condition among a population can increase susceptibility to illness. Infants, children, pregnant women, and elderly adults "are the most vulnerable to the adverse effects of hunger" (Davis & Sherer, 1994) Worldwide, environmental and economic conditions that are related to poverty make the largest contribution to underconsumption of nutrients, especially ones needed for building protein such as iodine, vitamin A, and iron.

RISK FACTORS FOR NUTRITIONAL PROBLEMS

The risk factors for nutritional deficits are derived from four general categories: socioeconomic, food supply, behavioral, and biological (see Figure 26-1). The presence of these risk factors increases the likelihood of developing a disease or a health problem (Green & Kreuter, 1991).

Socioeconomic Risk Factors

The socioeconomic category includes the risk factors of income, education, culture, and religious practices. These risk factors cross the life span. Income is a key factor in nutritional health for a variety of reasons. Low educational levels have been linked with increased health risks.

Culture and religious practices affect food selection from an early age. Socioeconomic factors are seen as factors that can be altered with nursing interventions.

Poverty

Income, or lack of it, is a key factor in determining nutritional health in the United States. Hughes and Simpson (1995) reported socioeconomic status as one of the most powerful factors in determining health and nutritional outcomes. The Food Research and Action Center (1998) states that poverty is the root cause of hunger. According to *Healthy People 2000* (U.S. Department of Health and Human Services [USDHHS], 1990b), one of every eight Americans lives in a family with income below the federal poverty level. In 1998, the federal poverty level for a family of 4 was $16,450 (U.S. Bureau of the Census, 1998). Table 26-1 lists federal poverty levels.

According to the U.S. Bureau of the Census, the majority of Americans living in poverty are Caucasian and live in rural or suburban communities. Forty-six percent of single female parent households are at or below the federal poverty limits. In 1997, it was estimated that 36.5 million persons with 13.7 million children (under the age of 18), or one in four children, were living at or below the federal poverty limit (U.S. Bureau of the Census, 1998). Children of poverty suffer from poor academic performance, cognitive and developmental delays, and chronically poor nutrition (Benjamin, 1996). The elderly poor are also nutritional risks. The Food Research and Action Center (1998) states that 11% of elder adults are poor, and the majority of elder poor are women (Gram, 1988).

Poor families tend to skip meals or go hungry when money runs out, eat less nutritious foods, spend 33% of their income on food (as opposed to the nonpoor, who spend 20% of their income on food), live in areas where

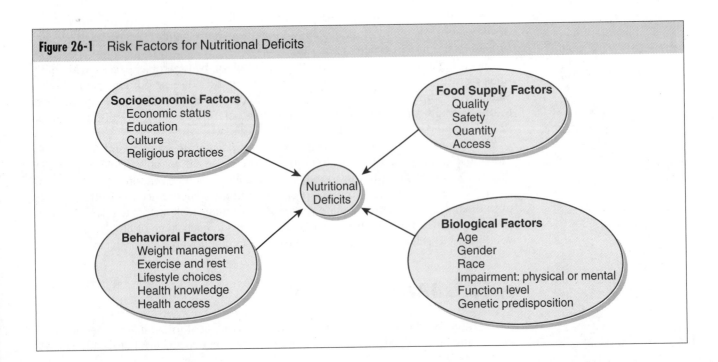

Figure 26-1 Risk Factors for Nutritional Deficits

Socioeconomic Factors
Economic status
Education
Culture
Religious practices

Food Supply Factors
Quality
Safety
Quantity
Access

Nutritional Deficits

Behavioral Factors
Weight management
Exercise and rest
Lifestyle choices
Health knowledge
Health access

Biological Factors
Age
Gender
Race
Impairment: physical or mental
Function level
Genetic predisposition

Table 26-1 1998 Poverty Guidelines for the 48 Contiguous States and the District of Columbia	
SIZE OF FAMILY UNIT	POVERTY GUIDELINE
1	$ 8,050
2	10,850
3	13,650
4	16,450
5	19,250
6	22,050
7	24,850
8	27,650

For family units with more than 8 members, add $2,800 for each additional member.

From Federal Register, *February 24, 1998, Vol. 63, No. 36.*

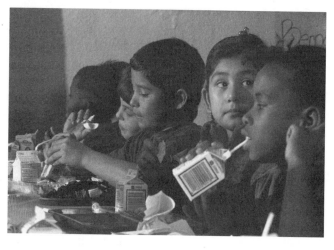

Government-sponsored school breakfast and lunch programs are designed to help poor children get proper nutrition and to combat the negative effects of hunger on learning.

food is expensive and variety is limited, and experience food storage difficulties.

Healthy People 2000: Midcourse Review and 1995 Revisions (USDHHS, 1996) reported that lower-income families continue to experience disproportionately worse health outcomes than other Americans because of their poor nutrition and increased risk for illness.

Minority Children and Elders

Poverty takes an especially heavy toll on children and elder adults. Child poverty rates remain twice as high as adult rates (FRAC, 1998). The largest numbers of children who are poor are Caucasian. One-third of all poor children are African American. The next largest percentage of poor children are Hispanic, Asian, or Native American. Children in single-parent homes are twice as likely to be poor as children in two-parent homes. In contrast to the continuing high rates for children, the rate of poverty has decreased for the elderly (U.S. Bureau of the Census, 1995). As of 1993, 3.8 million people over the age of 65 lived in poverty. But elderly African Americans are three times more likely than Caucasians to live in poverty, and elderly Hispanics are two times more likely than Caucasians to live in poverty (Wallenstein, 1992). Minority children and elders are already vulnerable to nutritional deficits because of their age and dependency on others for their food supply. Poverty raises their risk. The discussion of children and elder adults' specific risks will continue in a later section.

In 1990, when children, elders, and minorities were identified at higher risk in *Healthy People 2000,* the Office of Minority Health (OMH) was created as a part of the U.S. Department of Health and Human Services. The mission of the OMH is to develop, coordinate, and monitor a national strategy to improve minority health. One of the

major goals is to reduce the health disparity among Americans. The 1995 *Midcourse Review* indicates that in "many health measures—such as mortality, morbidity and health services utilization—differences between whites and minorities continue to be substantiated." For example, the total number of "healthy years" for blacks is 56 versus 75 for whites (USDHHS, 1996, p. 6).

Although federal and local programs exist for assistance with supplying food, Crockett, Clancy, and Bowering (1998) and *Healthy People 2000: Midcourse Review and 1995 Revisions* report that the use of food stamps falls from 4% to 17% short of the amount needed to provide adequate nutrition. The Food Research and Action Center (1998) also reports that only 63% of eligible families are using food stamps, and only 50% of women who are eligible for the WIC (Women, Infants, and Children) program are using it. Children participating in school breakfast and lunch programs are less likely to suffer the side effects of hunger that affect their ability to learn. But at the present time only 50% of schools participate in the school breakfast and lunch program (FRAC, 1998).

The Community Health Nurse's Role in Minimizing the Impact of Poverty

The community health nurse can provide intervention on a variety of levels. On the community program level, the nurse can help create and execute programs to assist the community in providing food to those who need it. The nurse who sees the problem has an opportunity to create resources to intervene in the problem such as starting a food bank where none exists, presenting data to the chamber of commerce as to the need for such a service, or persuading a local church or nursing agency to start such a service. As an advocate in the political arena at the local, state, or national levels, the nurse can provide data to lawmakers to help eliminate the root cause of hunger, poverty. The nurse has the opportunity to provide information about the human impact of poverty to legislators who can change the federal poverty income levels, alter the food stamp program, and approve funds for new programs. On the individual family level, the nurse can assess how the family is coping with the impact of poverty and can plan interventions to lessen its impact on their health.

The nurse can help clients stretch their food dollar by teaching clients how to purchase the most nutrients per dollar. See Table 26-2 for a listing of nutritional bargains. Nutrient-dense foods such as potatoes, brown rice, beans, peanut butter, liver, tofu, eggs, carrots, and powdered milk are inexpensive sources of essential nutrients. The use of meat substitutes such as beans, peanut butter, and

Table 26-2   Nutritional Bargains from the Basic Food Groups

FOOD GROUP	MORE ECONOMICAL	MORE EXPENSIVE
Milk	Fat-free and reduced-fat milk	Whole milk
	Nonfat dry milk	
	Evaporated milk	
Cheese	Cheese in bulk	Grated, sliced, or individually wrapped slices
	Cheese food	Cheese spreads
Ice cream	Ice milk or imitation ice cream	Ice cream or sherbet
Meat	Home-prepared meat	Luncheon meat, hot dogs, canned meat
	Regular hot dogs	All-beef or all-meat hot dogs
	Less tender cuts	More tender cuts
	U.S. Good and Standard grades	U.S. Prime and Choice grades
	Bulk sausage	Sausage patties or links
	Pork or beef liver	Calves liver
	Heart, kidney, tongue	
	Bologna	Specialty luncheon meats
Poultry	Large turkeys	Small turkeys
	Whole chickens	Cut-up chickens or individual parts
Eggs	Grade A eggs	Grade AA eggs
	Grade B eggs for cooking	
Fish	Fresh fish	Shellfish
	Chunk, flaked, or grated tuna	Fancy-pack or solid-pack tuna
	Coho, pink, or chum salmon (lighter in color)	Chinook, king, and sockeye salmon (deeper red in color)
Fruits and vegetables	Locally grown fruits and vegetables in season	Out-of-season fruits and vegetables or those in short supply and exotic vegetables and fruits
	Grades B or C	Grade A or Fancy
	Cut up, pieces, or sliced	Whole
	Diced or short cut	Fancy-cut
	Mixed sizes	All the same size
	Fresh or canned	Frozen
	Plain vegetables	Mixed vegetables or vegetables in sauces
Fresh fruits	Apples	Cantaloupe
	Bananas	Grapes
	Oranges	Honeydew melon
	Tangerines	Peaches
		Plums
Fresh vegetables	Cabbage	Asparagus
	Carrots	Brussels sprouts
	Celery	Cauliflower
	Collard greens	Corn on the cob

Continued

Table 26-2 Nutritional Bargains from the Basic Food Groups (Continued)

FOOD GROUP	MORE ECONOMICAL	MORE EXPENSIVE
	Kale	Mustard greens
	Lettuce	Spinach
	Onions	
	Potatoes	
	Sweet potatoes	
Canned fruits	Applesauce	Berries
	Peaches	Cherries
	Citrus juices	
	Other juices	
Canned vegetables	Beans	Asparagus
	Beets	Mushrooms
	Carrots	
	Collard greens	
	Corn	
	Kale	
	Mixed vegetables	
	Peas	
	Potatoes	
	Pumpkin	
	Sauerkraut	
	Spinach	
	Tomatoes	
	Turnip greens	
Frozen fruit	Concentrated citrus juices	Cherries
	Other juices	Citrus sections
		Strawberries
		Other berries
Frozen vegetables	Beans	Asparagus
	Carrots	Corn on the cob
	Collard greens	Vegetables, in pouch
	Corn	Vegetables, in cheese and other sauces
	Kale	
	Mixed vegetables	
	Peas	
	Peas and carrots	
	Potatoes	
	Spinach	
	Turnip greens	
Dried fruits and vegetables	Potatoes	Apricots
		Dates
		Peaches
Breads and cereals	Day-old bread	Fresh bread
	White enriched bread	Rolls, buns
	Cooked cereal	Whole grain
	Regular cooking oatmeal	Ready-to-eat cereals
		Quick-cooking or instant oatmeal
	Plain rice	Seasoned rice
	Long-cooking rice	Parboiled or instant rice
	Graham or soda crackers	Specialty crackers

From Nutrition in Contemporary Nursing Practice *by H. J. Green, 1981, Albany, NY: Delmar Publishers.*

Lack of Money

Think of a time in your life (it may be currently) that you didn't have very much money. Think about how you felt about your economic situation then.

- What emotions come to mind?

- What priorities determined how you spent your money?

- What kind of food did you buy?

- Did you ever go hungry?

cheese can stretch clients' limited dollars. Using larger quantities of grains and cereal, preparing foods from scratch, avoiding processed foods, and planning weekly menus are actions that can help stretch the food dollar.

Education

Education is linked with low income as a co-risk factor. *Healthy People 2000* (USDHHS, 1990b) states that low income, low education level, and low occupational level are linked to increased mortality, prematurity, low birth weight, and infant deaths. Education is a risk factor in two ways. First, lack of information about nutrition and managing nutrition may cause unhealthy eating habits; second, lack of formal education may make it hard for the client to secure employment.

According to *Healthy People 2000* (USDHHS, 1990b) low-education families have difficulty functioning in society. Poor families tend to live in poorer neighborhoods and attend less academically adequate schools. According to the Community Childhood Hunger Identification Pro-

DECISION MAKING

Community Resources

Find out what community resources are available for the person who is hungry and has no money to purchase food.

- What resources can you find in the phone book?

- Call two of the places you find in the phone book. What other resources do they mention?

- Go to a church and ask what resources they know about.

- Go to the downtown area of your city, and ask a stranger what resources exist in your community.

- How do you imagine someone who is hungry would find some of these resources?

ject (CCHIP), poor children are more likely to be undernourished and perform at a lower level in school (FRAC, 1998). In poor neighborhoods, the quality and level of education fall below nonpoor neighborhoods. The poor tend to be less educated and underemployed. Low income and low education levels are linked to poor health outcomes (USDHHS, 1996). The nurse has the opportunity to assist poor families in improving their housing selection, improving their employment status, and improving their nutritional intake by providing information and resources and supporting clients by linking them with those resources.

Culture

The selection of food is influenced by the cultural food patterns learned at home in the family. These patterns are established at a young age. No culture has ever been known to make food choices solely on the basis of the nutritional and health value of the food (Davis & Sherer, 1994). Culturally guided food selection may place a client at risk for a nutritional deficit. Table 26-3 lists potential nutritional problems of cultural groups in the United States.

It is essential for the nurse to be knowledgeable about the nutritional practices and health beliefs of the ethnic groups in the community. If a nutritional deficit can be traced to cultural practices, the nurse needs to recognize that changing it may be slow and difficult. The cultural practices are reinforced by behavior of the client's neighbors and family. The nurse needs to design strategies that demonstrate respect for the client yet provide remediation of the nutritional deficit. The nurse may need to work with the community, church, or community leaders to effect a change. For example, trying to persuade an older Mexican American woman to stop frying her food because of her recent diagnosis of heart disease may be more easily accomplished by having a class for at-risk women in her neighborhood sponsored by the church. Cultural competency will become even more important in the future with the trend of increasing numbers of minorities in the U.S. population. See Chapter 6 for a discussion of cultural perspectives.

Religious Practices

Religious practices are a part of an ethnic group's culture. Religious practices can affect the selection of food and eating patterns. Religion may also attach special meaning to certain foods. For example, persons from India who do not eat beef because of reverence for the cow will need to identify other sources of protein. Religious practices do not usually result in nutritional problems but may add to the effect of other cultural, social, and economic risks. The nurse needs to become familiar with religions in the area. This knowledge will enable the nurse to practice with sensitivity, caring, and respect.

Table 26-3 Potential Nutritional Problems of Cultural Groups in the United States

CULTURAL GROUP	VALUES	POTENTIAL PROBLEM	INTERVENTION
Native American Consists of 270 tribes. Each has its own language, beliefs, and customs	Value family and community; live in the present; see health as harmony with nature; use herbal medicine, some use medicine man	**Social**—poor sanitation, poverty, and crowded housing **Children**—fetal alcohol syndrome, infectious diseases, especially dysentery **Adults**—trachomatous conjunctivitis, diabetes, obesity, alcoholism, tuberculosis, and substance abuse	Address sanitation to decrease illness Identify affordable sources of food, especially vitamin A, C, and dairy Provide education for healthy eating, especially low fat, low-cholesterol diet
African American 12% of U.S. population, consists of subcultures based on geographic origin and relocation	Extended family may retain native language; may view illness as hex or punishment; may believe in laying on of hands and home remedies	**Social**—poverty and single-adult homes common, unemployment, lack of education common **Children**—twice the infant mortality as Caucasians, sickle cell anemia, malnutrition, teen pregnancy **Adults**—life expectancy of 69 years versus 76 for Caucasians, hypertension, stroke, diabetes, cirrhosis, cancer, and AIDS (50% of U.S. AIDS cases)	Education for low-sodium, low-fat, high-potassium diet Educate about solutions Encourage use of vegetables and fish Education on cooking methods
Hispanic American 9% of U.S. population, expected to reach 21% by 2050 (U.S. Bureau of the Census, 1993) includes Latinos and Chicanos	Present oriented; extended family with male patriarch; female usually self-sacrificing (Friedman, 1990); children taken everywhere with family; may retain native language; religion may be a blend of Catholic and pre-Courtesan Indian (Friedman, 1990); illness may be seen a punishment for sins; Latinos may use witchcraft and herbal healing	**Social**—violence common **Children**—malnutrition, parasites **Adults**—hypertension, diabetes, obesity, AIDS, tuberculosis, infectious diseases, and lactose intolerance	Education about diet especially use of sodium and cooking methods Education about calcium and calcium substitutes Education about parasites
Asian American Consists of people of many countries and many cultures. Chinese is the largest group, Filipino the second largest; also includes Koreans, Thais, Laotians, Vietnamese, and Cambodians	Retain native language; patriarchal family; elder adults respected; value achievement and saving face; cooperation is important; use herbal medicine. Chinese: health a balance of yin and yang resulting in qi (chee), or harmony. Filipino: health or illness an act of God.	**Social**—newest immigrants often in poorest area **Children**—parasites and malnutrition **Adults**—tuberculosis, cancers, diabetes, hypertension, lactose intolerance, suicide, and mental illness	Education about sodium and calcium, alternative cooking methods especially meats, e.g., broil rather than fry

Adapted from Fundamentals of Nursing: Concepts, Process and Practice *(4th ed.) by P. A. Potter & A. G. Perry, 1997, St. Louis: Mosby.*

Food Supply Risk Factors

The food supply risk factors include food quality, safety, quantity, and access. These risk factors affect clients at all stages of life. The safety of available food is affected by the execution of government regulations at every stage of food handling. A primary barrier to eating nutritious food is access. The quality and quantity of foods are determined by what is available to the client.

The adequacy of nutrition is, in part, a consequence of the adequacy of the food supply. A food supply is adequate if a variety of food is readily available to the client. The food needs to match the client's need in quality and quantity. The food needs to be safe, accessible, and affordable. If one of these factors or a combination of these factors are not present, the food supply may be inadequate and the client may be at risk for a nutritional problem. Food supply factors are amenable to nursing interventions.

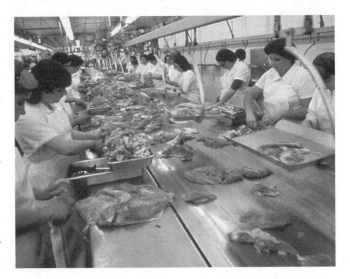

The food inspections carried out by government agencies minimize the incidence of contaminated food illnesses. It is imperative for the community health nurse to communicate safe food-handling procedures to clients.
Photo courtesy of USDA.

Food Quality

Quality refers to the freshness and nutrient value of food. For example, deep green lettuce is likely to have more nutrients than white lettuce has; large, thick, and crunchy leaves are more likely to be fresh and nutritious than are small, transparent, and soft leaves. The quality of the food supply may vary greatly within the same community depending on the source and method of handling. Smaller neighborhood stores tend to have less selection and higher prices (Davis & Sherer, 1994). It is often a challenge for a poor client to purchase a wide variety of nutritious, affordable food in a small neighborhood store (FRAC, 1998). It takes knowledge of the variety of foods needed for a balanced diet, planning, and budgeting to make food dollars stretch. The community health nurse may often find that poor clients are not familiar with the Food Guide Pyramid or how to plan nutritious meals. The client's food preferences, culture, and knowledge of the Food Guide Pyramid influence the purchase of food.

Food Safety

The nutrition of the client reflects the nutrition of the community. The nutrition of the community is influenced by the safety of food and the execution of government regulations. Safety in food refers to freedom from disease, infestation, or contamination.

Government agencies are responsible for supervising every aspect of food production. The U.S. Department of Agriculture (USDA) enforces the standards for quality and wholesomeness of grains, poultry, meat, milk, eggs, and produce produced in the United States by inspecting and grading products. This department also inspects imported foods. The Environmental Protection Agency (EPA) regulates pesticide use. This agency sets safety limits for new pesticides, and the Food and Drug Administration (FDA) enforces these limits. The FDA is responsible for ensuring the safety and wholesomeness of foods shipped from state to state (except meat and poultry, which fall under the jurisdiction of the USDA). The FDA is responsible for the inspection of seafood. Despite the presence of these agencies in the food production industry, there are periodic outbreaks of *Escherichia coli* and *Salmonella* infection.

Foodborne Illnesses

It is possible that at any stage of life a client can become ill from a **foodborne illness.** There are news reports of unsafe beef and poultry handling that threaten food safety. Keeping the food supply consistently free of contamination continues to be a government and presidential goal. With impaired or poorly developed immune systems, infants, children, and elderly adults are most vulnerable to foodborne illnesses. Food poisoning due to infectious microorganisms occurs in at least 30% of the U.S. population each year. Episodes are characterized by abdominal pain, diarrhea, vomiting, and weakness within two days of exposure to contaminated food. Often, symptoms of food poisoning are mistakenly attributed to the flu (Foulke, 1994). Older and elderly adults must be especially vigilant if they have a preexisting immune system deficit. See Table 26-4 for information about diseases that can occur as a result of unsafe food handling or contaminated foods. Safe food handling by the client can control illnesses caused by foodborne microorganisms. The community health nurse should explain safe food-handling techniques. Figure 26-2 offers recommendations for ways to prevent such illnesses.

Food Quantity

Quantity refers to the volume or amount needed to meet the client's nutritional needs. The quantity may be limited

Table 26-4   Foodborne Illnesses

BACTERIUM	TRANSMISSION	SYMPTOMS	PREVENTION
Campylobacter jejuni	Via unpasteurized milk, contaminated water, raw and undercooked meat and shellfish.	Diarrhea, fever, headache, abdominal pain and nausea	Avoid unpasteurized milk and questionable water; cook meat and fish thoroughly.
Clostridium botulinum	Home-canned foods.	Double vision, speech difficulties, inability to swallow, respiratory paralysis	Avoid bulging cans; boil home-canned green beans for 10 minutes
Clostridium perfringens	Sometimes referred to as the "cafeteria germ." Outbreaks occur when large quantities of food are served at room temperature or from a steam table. Meat, poultry, cooked dried beans, and gravies are the most common carriers.	Diarrhea and gas pains beginning between 6 and 24 hours after ingestion and lasting approximately 24 hours	Keep hot food hot (at or above 140°F) and cold food cold (at or below 40°F); leftovers should be heated to at least 165°F before serving; wash all soil from vegetables.
Cyclospora cayentanensis	Feces-contaminated food or water.	Watery diarrhea, abdominal cramps, decreased appetite, and low-grade fever; could last off and on for several weeks	Wash hands thoroughly; wash fruit before eating, use and drink only clean water.
Escherichia coli (E. coli O157:H7)	Contaminated foods such as undercooked hamburger.	Abdominal cramps, watery diarrhea, nausea and vomiting; serious complications: bloody diarrhea and severe abdominal cramps; onset within 3–9 days; duration: 2–9 days, if no complications	Cook ground meat to 160°F; eat no raw ground meat; wash all fruits and vegetables before eating.
Listeria monocytogenes	Unpasteurized milk, raw and cooked poultry, meat, seafood, and salads.	Sudden onset of fever, chills, headache, backache, and occasional abdominal pain and diarrhea	Avoid unpasteurized milk and dairy products; cook ground meats to 160°F, ground poultry to 165°F; hot foods should be kept hot and cold foods cold; wash produce thoroughly.
Salmonella	Raw or undercooked food such as eggs, poultry, unpasteurized milk or other dairy products, and meats; cross-contamination by uncooked foods.	Headache, abdominal pain, diarrhea, fever and nausea; onset: 8–48 hours; duration: 1–8 days	Avoid cross-contamination of raw and cooked foods; do not eat raw eggs; cook ground beef to 160°F; keep hot foods hot and cold foods cold; eat no unpasteurized raw or undercooked food of animal origin.
Shigella	Contamination of food by infected food handlers; primarily transmitted in cold salads such as tuna, chicken, and potato.	Severe diarrhea, nausea, headaches, chills, and dehydration	Prevented by good hygiene of food handlers and sanitary food preparation; keep hot foods hot and cold foods cold; always wash hands in hot soapy water after going to the bathroom and before preparing or eating food.
Staphylococcus aureus	Infected food handlers.	Vomiting, diarrhea, abdominal cramps; onset: 3–8 hours; duration: 1–2 days	Prevented by good hygiene of food handlers; always wash hands in hot soapy water thoroughly before preparing food; keep hot foods hot and cold foods cold.

Adapted from Safe Food Backgrounder, 1994, National Livestock and Meat Board.

by the source of food or the budget of the client. A continuous supply of food is vital. Very often, low-income clients do not have a continuous supply of income to purchase food, so they experience periods of hunger. Interruptions in food supply can put the client at nutritional risk. In the setting of low income, poor shelter, and unemployment or underemployment, obtaining affordable, nutritious food from all the food groups can be a daily challenge.

Federal programs such as food stamps and Women, Infants, and Children (WIC) were intended to close the gap between what the client can afford and what is needed to maintain health. For elders, home-based meals or congregate meals were intended to provide nutritious food. The 1995 *Midcourse Review* report (USDHHS, 1996) states that the elder programs reach only 20% of the eligible elders. In many communities, food banks, soup kitchens, and churches attempt to bridge the gap by providing food to the poor and the elderly.

Food Access

Access is the ability to easily obtain the food needed to maintain health. The ability may be impaired by physical limitations or lack of transportation or both. Access to the food supply is a common barrier for the poor, elderly, disabled, and clients with limited mobility. For the poor, if the least expensive food supply is in a large suburban supermarket and there is no public or subsidized transportation to that location, the food is not accessible to them. For the rural poor, public transportation may not exist. For the disabled or elderly with limited mobility, if the bus or special transportation does not go to the lower-priced supermarket, they do not have access either. The elderly with multiple restrictions such as low vision may not feel they can safely travel to select their own food. The community health nurse has an opportunity to assess and intervene when clients in the community, especially at-risk or more vulnerable clients, can not reach the food supply. Helping clients overcome these access barriers can facilitate nutritional health.

Fast Food

The risk of a nutritional deficit is increasing in the entire U.S. population because of the increasing consumption of fast and convenience foods. Since 1965, sales have more

Figure 26-2   Guide for Safe Food Handling

- When shopping, choose perishable foods last and store them as soon as possible. If immediate storage is not feasible, use a cooler until they can be stored.
- Note "sell by" and "use by" dates when purchasing items. Do not buy items beyond the "sell date."
- Do not buy items with holes or tears in the packaging, bulging cans or lid, or cracked jars.
- Be sure hands, equipment, and surroundings are clean.
- Use soap and hot water to wash hands before preparing food.
- Use soapy water with a disinfectant to wash cutting boards, utensils, and countertops that come into contact with uncooked meats, poultry, or fish, which can be contaminated with microorganisms. These organisms are killed only in cooking.
- Do not place cooked foods on unwashed surfaces where uncooked food has been prepared.
- Foods must be kept colder than 40° F or hotter than 140° F to avoid development of microorganisms. Potluck and picnic dishes often have temperatures in the danger zone.
- Do not cool foods to room temperature before refrigerating them. They should be refrigerated immediately after eating or cooking.
- When reheating leftovers, make sure they reach 165° F to kill any microorganisms.
- All home-canned vegetables, meats, poultry, and fish should be boiled for 10 minutes before tasting them.
- All marinades should be destroyed or boiled after marination to kill bacteria that may be present in the food being marinated.
- All meat, poultry, shellfish, and fish must be cooked to the well-done stage. Never store defrosted or partially cooked meats and poultry. Ground beef must be cooked to 160° F and ground chicken to 165° F.
- Any uncooked foods containing raw eggs, including cookie and cake batters, could contain *Salmonella*. Do not eat or taste them.
- Do not use raw eggs in any mixture to be frozen.
- Remove all stuffing from leftover foods and store separately.
- Never store cleaning supplies or pesticides in food containers or near food.

Adapted from Foundations and Clinical Applications of Nutrition: A Nursing Approach *by M. Grodner, S. L. Anderson, & S. DeYoung, 1996, St. Louis, MO: Mosby-Yearbook, and* Nutrition Handbook for Nursing Practice *(3rd ed.) by S. G. Dudek, 1997, Philadelphia: Lippincott-Raven.*

than doubled the food expense (Davis & Sherer, 1994). The cost of these foods is estimated to be from two to seven times higher than the cost of the basic ingredients. The meals are typically high in saturated fat, cholesterol, and sodium and low in vitamin A, biotin, folate, and iron.

The community health nurse has the opportunity as an educator to inform the community about the health risk of reliance on fast food. As a community program planner, the nurse can assess the community as a client and assess the risk in the community. The school nurse has many opportunities to educate about the composition of fast food and the health impact. On an individual basis, the nurse has the opportunity to educate clients, neighbors, church, and civic groups about the personal health risk associated with frequent consumption of fast foods.

The Community Health Nurse's Role

The community health nurse has the opportunity to intervene in food supply risk factors in many ways. The nurse has the opportunity to assess each client's situation and offer interventions suited to the problem. Since income and access are the most common barriers, the home health care, clinic, board of health, and school nurse frequently work on finding resources to break down those barriers. Linking the client with community food sources such as food banks and soup kitchens is one immediate action. Helping the client apply for programs such as WIC, the county Expanded Food and Nutrition Education Program (EFNEP), Aid to Dependent Children (ADC), food stamps, and local food supply programs is a longer-range solution. Government agencies that are appropriate sources of assistance include the local welfare office; city, county; or state health departments; and local social service agencies.

Once the client has been linked with food sources and income assistance, linking the client with free or low-cost transportation is the next step. If the client has Medicaid or Social Security income, the client can also get subsidized transportation. Agencies such as the local county council on aging, county trustee office, church, and social

agencies that subcontract to provide transportation to low-income clients are longer-range solutions.

One long-range intervention is teaching the client or the at-risk population about the Food Guide Pyramid, food selection, and meal planning. Taking the client to the store and showing the client how to shop and plan meals is another long-range action that the nurse or dietitian can provide. In one community in Indiana, this service is provided at no charge by nutritionists in one of the large grocery store chains and by two physician offices. In this same community, at annual community health fairs, dietitians teach nutrition information. Many local churches or schools with large low-income populations welcome such classes and will provide space and food to practice new cooking techniques. The community health nurse can work with the local neighborhood stores to encourage provision of affordable foods.

Behavioral Risk Factors

The behavioral category includes weight maintenance, exercise and rest, lifestyle choices such as use of cigarettes, alcohol, and drugs, and health knowledge and health access. These behavioral risk factors are amenable to intervention. Weight control, exercise, and rest can have an impact throughout the life span, with their greatest impact in middle adulthood. The community health nurse should explain to clients the benefits of weight control, regular exercise, and adequate rest. Counseling against the abuse of substances such as cigarettes, alcohol, and drugs is very important, as is offering support to the client to overcome the substance abuse. Weight control and substance abuse will be addressed at length later in the chapter. Late childhood is the most common period for beginning the use of substances such as alcohol, illegal drugs, and tobacco. Health knowledge is what clients understand about healthy living habits and nutrition. *Health access* is driven by income. If a client has the income, health care can be obtained to prevent and treat illness. If a client does not have the income, health care is usually not obtained until there is a severe functional or life-threatening problem. Aday, Lee, Spears, Chung, and colleagues (1993) report that low-income clients have inadequate access to health care throughout their lives and at all levels of prevention. Chronic problems are often untreated or undertreated. Goldstein (1994) reports that the poor are hospitalized three times more often than people in higher income categories. Illness puts the client at increased risk for nutritional problems.

Biological Risk Factors

The fourth category of risk factors, biological, includes age, race, gender, impairments, and genetic predispositions. Age refers to chronological years and physiological maturity. Age is a significant risk factor for the very young and the elderly. They are usually immune compromised or have immature immune systems and therefore are at greater nutritional risk. Age, race, and gender will be addressed in each subsequent stage of life discussions. Impairments refer to physical or developmental disabilities. Chubon, Schulz, Lingle, and Coster-Schulz (1994) report that physically impaired clients often experience poverty. Genetic predisposition means predisposition to illnesses such as hypertension and obesity. The factors in the biological category are considered nonmodifiable; for example, clients can not change their age or sex. Nursing interventions are designed to help the client maximize adaptation.

STAGES OF LIFE AND NUTRITIONAL PROBLEMS

At every stage of life there are nutritional problems that are common to that stage. Some nutritional problems bridge several stages of life. For purposes of the following discussion, the nutritional problems are discussed in the stage of life where they are most prevalent. The reader may refer to Chapters 16 and 17 for common nutritional needs of infants, children, and adults. At every stage of life, nutrition remains an important prerequisite to health. According to Cohn and Deckelbaum (1993), the quality of nutrition determines growth and development and the prevention of disease.

Infant Nutritional Problems

The infant may suffer nutritional deficits because of the presence of socioeconomic risk factors such as low income, low educational level of the parent, and poor food supply. Infants may also be affected by the behavioral choices of the parent, especially health knowledge and lifestyle choices. Biological risk factors such as prematurity or low birth weight put the infant, with immature immune and gastrointestinal systems, at higher risk (Davis & Sherer, 1994). When infants demonstrate a loss of weight, delay in development, signs of malnourishment, or failure to thrive (FTT), the root of the problem may be a nutritional deficit. The nutrition of an infant is essential to survival. In the home setting, the nurse, family, and neighbors have the opportunity to make observations that are critical to the survival of the infant. Identification of any of the above problems requires intervention.

The cause of a nutritional deficit may vary from a single reason such as a lack of income in the family to a cluster of causes as in the case of, for example, a low-income, first-time, teen parent who is abusing substances. The community health nurse working with infants needs to have a working knowledge of normal growth and development. Working with that framework, the nurse has the opportunity to intervene in a variety of ways. The more common nursing interventions are parent education about infant nutrition, encouragement of parent participation in parenting classes, and postnatal home visits. It is also common for low-income, high-risk or at-risk mothers to require all of the above interventions plus assistance with the food supply for mother and infant. Enrollment in programs such as WIC, food stamps, ADC, and subsidized housing may be necessary to ensure the survival of the infant.

Childhood Nutritional Problems

Children are at greatest risk for nutritional deficits because of socioeconomic risk factors, particularly poverty. According to FRAC (1998), 59% of all children under age 6 living in a single-parent female-headed household live in poverty. Poor children are typically affected by a cluster of risk factors such as limited food supply, limited food access, parental factors of limited education, unhealthy lifestyle choices, lack of health information and access, and their own poor school performance.

Poor nutritional status is more prevalent in lower socioeconomic groups because of the limited amount and variety of food available (Davis & Sherer, 1994). Children with poor nutritional status are frequently hungry. Children who are hungry suffer from unwanted weight loss, fatigue, headaches, increased school absences, poor school performance, and increased illnesses. They frequently have a low intake of iron, zinc, and protein. These children suffer from anemia, which increases their risk for infections and chronic illnesses. It is estimated that between 10% and 20% of children have iron deficiency anemia (Centers for Disease Control and Prevention [CDC], 1992). Children who are hungry suffer two to four times more health problems than children who are not hungry (FRAC, 1998, p. 4). When children are hungry, they suffer slowed growth and development, stunting of height, and decreased protein intake (World Bank, 1993).

As for infants, the definitive screening criteria for children for nutritional problems are growth and development and maintenance of weight. School-age children have the added screening criterion of school performance. Being underweight or overweight can place a child at risk for a nutritional or health problem. According to Bronner (1996), obesity can put a child at risk for atherosclerosis, non-insulin-dependent diabetes (NIDDM), hypertension (HTN), and gallbladder disease in adult years. It is estimated that 14% of children are obese. Obesity will be discussed in the section on middle adulthood.

The Community Health Nurse's Role

The community health nurse working as a school nurse has a prime opportunity to screen children and intervene. Intervention may include further assessment of child and family dietary habits and economic resources. The nurse can assist the family in applying for programs such as free or partially subsidized school breakfast and lunch. The nurse can provide nutritional education and referral to the school social worker for application for assistance such as ADC and food stamps. The child who is iron deficient can be referred to a clinic for iron and vitamin supplements. The child also needs to increase intake of vitamin C to increase the absorption of iron. Eating such foods as iron-fortified cereal, meat, beans, or rice would be helpful. The school nurse has the opportunity to continue to monitor the results of interventions.

Nutritional Problems with Substance Abuse

As discussed in Chapter 16, lifestyle choices of smoking, alcohol, and substance abuse are behaviors that threaten nutritional health. According to the National Institute on Drug Abuse, by eighth grade 67% of children have tried alcohol, 45% have smoked, 12% have tried marijuana, and 3% have tried cocaine. Alcohol threatens nutrition by its delay of gastric emptying and decreasing of food absorption. Alcohol also accelerates metabolic rate and suppresses appetite (Lieber, 1995). Malnutrition is a common result of alcohol and substance abuse. Eating is not a priority, and substance abuse increases the use of caffeine and sugar ("Dietitians Teach," 1991). Deficiencies of vitamins, iron, zinc, and protein are common (Davis & Sherer, 1994). Alcohol leads to decreased absorption of water and electrolytes, thiamin, and glucose. It contributes to anemia, clotting defects, convulsions, and small bowel dysfunction. Alcohol is the third leading cause of death in the United States after cardiovascular diseases and cancer (Johnston, O'Malley, & Bachman, 1996).

Substances such as tobacco, cocaine, and marijuana put the client at risk for nutritional deficits. Fifty million Americans smoke. Children of smokers are likely to smoke. Teens who smoke are rarely able to quit (Rasco, 1992). One of the *Healthy People 2000* goals is to decrease the number of children and teens who smoke. Unfortunately, the number of teens who smoke has increased steadily since 1980 (USDHHS, 1996). It is estimated that 6 million teens and 100,000 preteens smoke (USDHHS, 1996). In contrast, it is estimated that 20 to 30 million people use marijuana, and 60% of them are 18 to 25 years old (Doweiko, 1999). Cocaine and tobacco are appetite suppressants, and their use may lead to unplanned weight loss (Addison, 1990). According to House (1992), cocaine and tobacco users are at risk for deficiencies of vitamins, especially vitamin C and thiamin, and for gastrointestinal complaints. According to Newcomb (1992), cocaine and tobacco users are also at risk for increased consumption of alcohol, coffee, and fatty foods. In contrast, marijuana enhances appetite and may cause weight gain (Davis & Sherer, 1994). The use of substances such as alcohol, tobacco, and illegal drugs increases the nutritional risks and increases the likelihood of illness for children.

The Community Health Nurse's Role in Controlling Substance Abuse

The community health nurse has three major goals with regard to controlling the abuse of substances: assessing the impact on the client, restoring nutritious eating habits,

and referring the client to programs to eliminate the substance abuse practice. In the school setting, the school nurse has the opportunity to assess the impact on growth and development, weight management, and school performance. The nurse also has daily access to the child and can work with the parents and the school administration to restore healthy eating habits. Refer to Chapter 25 for a detailed discussion of the nurse's role in eliminating substance abuse in school-age children.

Adolescent Nutritional Problems

The community-based nutritional challenges of adolescence are insufficient nutrition, eating disorders, and nutrition in teen pregnancy. Teens who may have eaten a balanced diet as a child or may eat a balanced diet at home may not demonstrate the same behavior in the company of peers. The challenge of adults in teens' lives is to encourage and model healthy eating habits. Caucasian adolescent females are at greater risk for eating disorders and inconsistent or insufficient nutrition than their male counterparts. Female teens demonstrate more dieting behavior and verbalize more concern and dissatisfaction with their bodies and more interest in obtaining a model-like appearance (Davis & Sherer, 1994).

Eating Disorders

Eating disorders are a complex combination of physical behaviors and psychological beliefs (Davis & Sherer, 1994). Some experts believe that eating disorders occur because food is the only thing the teen can control in life (Waller, 1998). The disorders are believed to originate from a distorted self-image in which the teen sees herself as overweight, when in reality she is not (Davis & Sherer, 1994). Eating disorders have a progressive nature. Usually the changes observed by friends, family, neighbors, or teachers indicate when the disorder becomes a health threat to the teen.

A teen is at greater risk of developing eating disorders in a setting where great emphasis is placed on appearance or weight. Teens involved in certain sports such as figure skating, ballet, gymnastics, or wrestling or teens in modeling are at risk. Use of amphetamines or cocaine to lose weight may increase the risk of an eating disorder. The three most common eating disorders in teens are anorexia nervosa, bulimia, and binge eating.

Anorexia Nervosa

The term **anorexia nervosa** denotes an abnormal fear of becoming obese, a distorted self-image, a persistent aversion to food, and a loss of 25% of normal body weight in a relatively short period of time. About 5% of anorectic clients die in the first 12 years after onset. The mortality rate doubles in the following 12 years according to follow-up studies of anorectic teens. A client with anorexia is six times more likely to die than her counterparts who do not have anorexia (Hsu, 1993). The emotional, behavioral, and physical characteristics of anorexia are shown in Table 26-5.

Bulimia Nervosa

Bulimia means "ox hunger." The word *nervosa* was added to the name because, as in anorexia, the person has a nervous fear of gaining weight. **Bulimia nervosa** is also called binge-purge syndrome. It is characterized by episodes of excessive food intake followed by periods of fasting and self-induced vomiting or laxative abuse. The physical characteristics are not as obvious as those of anorexia. It is less likely to be fatal than anorexia because the person is getting some nutrition. Nine percent of chil-

dren under the age of 14, 25% of high school and college-age females, and 13% of college males report purging behavior (Wolf, 1991). The emotional, behavioral, and physical characteristics of a person with bulimia are shown in Table 26-5.

Binge Eating

Binge eating, or compulsive overeating, is habitual eating to excess due to an irresistible irrational impulse. It begins most commonly in the teen years. Overindulgence occurs at all social levels and is an increasing health risk. Binge episodes become an eating disorder when the eating is: (1) more rapid than normal, (2) done until uncomfortably full, (3) done when the person is not hungry yet eats

Table 26-5   Characteristics of Anorexia and Bulimia

TYPE	ANOREXIA NERVOSA	BULIMIA NERVOSA
Physical	• Amenorrhea • Lowered body temperature • Lowered potassium and chloride levels if vomiting • Thinning hair • Dry, flaking skin • Lowered pulse rate and blood pressure • Constipation • Insomnia • Lanugo (growth of downy body hair) • Dental caries and periodontal disease if person is vomiting • Broken, split fingernails and toenails • Significantly below ideal body weight (IBW)	• Chronic sinusitis • Swollen and infected glands in the neck and under the jaw • Chronically puffy skin under the eyes and ruptured blood vessels in the cheeks and face • Deterioration of dental enamel due to stomach acids • Gastritis, stomach ulcers, kidney damage, edema • Electrolyte imbalances • Usually at IBW
Behavioral	• Unusual eating habits: starving, bingeing, purging, food hoarding, and ritualized eating • Preoccupation with meal planning, shopping, and cooking for the entire family while not eating • Hyperactivity and excessive exercise • Chronic or excessive use of laxatives, diuretics, diet pills	• Isolation due to abnormal eating habits and affect • Excessive exercise and other ritualized behaviors • Chronic or excessive use of laxatives, diuretics, diet pills, and emetics • Extreme split between public self (competent, cohesive) and private self (chaotic, unhappy)
Emotional	• Low sense of self-worth: inferiority about IQ, personality, and appearance • Distorted thinking: "If I can't control my environment, at least I can control my body" • Low sense of self-control • High achievement from driven compulsive behaviors • Denial of hunger and delusions about food ingested • Isolation contributing to depression • Outward compliance toward others, alternating with temper tantrums	• Appears more independent and professionally successful than persons having anorexia, who act dependent and tend to be withdrawn • Extremely vulnerable to rejection, especially with men • More outgoing, socially adept, and sexually involved in relationships • Unrealistically high standards of performance and appearance and inability to relax or to savor experiences • More prone to serious personality disorders • Fear of loss of control and of getting fat • Dependence on others for self-esteem and validation

Compiled by Gail P. Howe, MA.

large amounts, (4) done alone because of the embarrassment of the volume consumed, and (5) the cause of feeling disgusted with oneself, depressed, or very guilty about eating (Edelstein, 1989). Recovery begins with meeting another recovered or recovering binge eater or with intervention by family, nurse, or physician. The nurse can play a pivotal role in facilitating this process. Figure 26-3 illustrates the spectrum of eating disorders.

The Community Health Nurse's Role in Identifying and Treating an Eating Disorder

Eating disorders can be identified by the community health nurse. The nurse, especially the school nurse, may be involved in community screening for eating disorders. The home health nurse may be involved in monitoring home nutrition of a client. An appropriate referral to a physician, treatment center, or psychiatric treatment center can be initiated by the community health nurse. The nurse can provide information to the family or client to facilitate the referral process. Eating disorders are typically treated over a long period of time by an interdisciplinary team. The treatment of eating disorders is not just a matter of education but a long process of uncovering the cause and building new coping skills for the client and family.

A good recovery program should evaluate the client's physical condition, nutritional habits, psychological problems and strengths, social situation, family relations, and school or work performance. Individual counseling provides a safe environment to express feelings that have been hidden. Group therapy helps develop new coping skills, socialization, and healthy interests. Family counseling helps educate and support the family to assist in the recovery process. Overeaters Anonymous is a resource for restoration of healthy eating habits modeled after the 12-step program of Alcoholics Anonymous.

Teen Pregnancy

Pregnant teens have special nutritional needs. Low or no income, poor nutrition, age, and lifestyle choices are some of the most common nutritional risk factors for pregnant teens. They are at risk for low birth weight babies and premature births for several reasons. Teens are often reluctant to gain weight for the safe growth and development of the infant, because of their concern about their own appearance. This behavior could be disastrous, because they must increase their calories to meet their needs as pregnant females and the infant's needs (Rees, Engelbert-Fenton, Gong, & Bach, 1992). They have not matured enough to temporarily put their own interests aside for the needs of others. Teens are usually economically dependent, disregard nutritional guidelines when with peers, act on food cravings and aversions, skip meals, and eat high-fat fast foods. They may be smoking or using drugs. The pregnancy may not have been planned, and prenatal health may not be at its best. All of these factors make pregnant teens a high nutritional risk group.

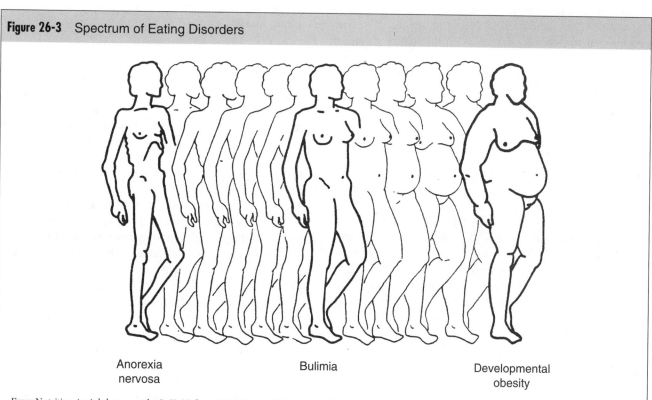

Figure 26-3 Spectrum of Eating Disorders

Anorexia nervosa   Bulimia   Developmental obesity

From Nutrition in Adolescence *by L. K. Mahan & J. M Rees, 1984. Originally published by St. Louis, MO: Mosby. Present copyright by L. K. Mahan, and J. M. Rees, Seattle, WA, 1989. Reprinted with permission of authors.*

The Community Health Nurse's Role in Guiding the Pregnant Teen

The nutritional changes that teens need to make are addressed in the pregnant adult section in the later part of this chapter. Teens can make the pregnancy a success by adhering to optimum nutritional guidelines; taking prenatal vitamins; participating in prenatal care through Planned Parenthood, a neighborhood clinic, a nurse practitioner's office, or a physician's office; having a stable support system; and maintaining optimum health. Pregnancy, especially an unplanned pregnancy, is an emotionally charged situation that can temporarily overshadow the nutritional requirements necessary for a successful pregnancy. It is essential that nutritional needs quickly take priority for a successful outcome.

The community health nurse can act as a resource person to the pregnant teen. The nurse's goal is to limit the impact of the risk factors on the teen by supporting the teen in continuing her education. As discussed earlier, low educational level is a risk factor for nutritional deficits. The teen will also need prenatal care, parenting classes, life skill classes, and counseling during the pregnancy. Postnatal needs include child care, financial support, possibly subsidized housing, and income for food and postnatal health care for mother and infant. Regular home visits support the first-time mother in her parenting efforts.

The school nurse is in a position to educate students, starting in middle school, about pregnancy prevention and delaying sexual initiation. According to the Maternal and Child Health Bureau (MCH) (1996) statistics, one in 10 teens age 15 to 19 gets pregnant. This same source reports pregnancies increasing in number since 1988 and the age of sexual initiation as young as age 12. It further reports that two-thirds of females report sexual initiation by age 18. The nurse's efforts will be directed toward one of the nation's goals in *Healthy People 2000:* that is, decreasing pregnancies under the age of 18.

Young Adult Nutritional Problems

Young adulthood, ages 20 to 40, is a relatively problem-free period of life. If young adults adopt and maintain a healthy lifestyle, they can prevent or delay the major causes of death in adults. The top five causes of death in adults are cancer, heart disease, stroke, chronic respiratory disease, and injury. This is the time to begin screening activities such as Pap smears, breast self-examinations, and testicular self-exams. The nutritional problems that young adults are at risk for are related to AIDS, hepatitis C, pregnancy, and chronic diseases such as diabetes.

Acquired Immunodeficiency Syndrome (AIDS)

Acquired immunodeficiency syndrome (AIDS) has become the leading cause of death in adults age 25 to 44 (CDC, 1996). The highest number of deaths has been among minorities (CDC, 1995b). From a nutritional standpoint, it is critical for an adult who tests positive for the human immunodeficiency virus (HIV) to prevent weight loss and avoid infections. Clients with AIDS can be nutritionally compromised with any change in their health or nutrition. Common problems are anorexia, nausea, vomiting, diarrhea, fatigue, and disorders of the mouth or esophagus that prevent eating. When the gastrointestinal system is affected, absorption may be diminished. The nurse should evaluate and monitor the client's intake to ensure that the client is getting enough nutrients to maintain the immune system at optimum level. Monitoring weight, food intake, lab values of albumin, protein, and total iron-binding capacity will ensure intervention early in any nutritional deficit. The client and at least one other adult or caregiver from the household should attend nutritional counseling with a dietitian to learn how to handle some of the acute and chronic nutritional challenges. When a fever or infection is present, dietary adjustments need to be made.

Hepatitis C

The young adult with hepatitis C, or inflammation of the liver, can have chronic nutritional problems. Hepatitis C is transmitted by blood or blood products, semen, or saliva. It can evolve into cirrhosis of the liver or liver failure. The nutritional challenge in hepatitis is to maintain carbohydrate and protein metabolism. The liver is also involved in the storage and transportation of vitamins and minerals including zinc, iron, copper, and magnesium. The community health nurse needs to educate the client about dietary challenges and monitor the client's efforts to maintain intake.

Pregnancy

The pregnant woman is at risk for nutritional deficits if she fails to meet the additional requirements of the pregnancy. Sexually active women should be taking 400 mg/day of folic acid to prevent infant neural tube defects (NTDs). If they become pregnant, the infant is also at risk, especially if the birth weight is low. The infant's mortality and developmental disabilities are linked to the infant's birth weight (National Academy of Sciences/Institute of Medicine, 1990). Two critical indicators of maternal nutrition are maternal size and weight (gained during pregnancy). Maternal size is the prepregnancy height and weight. Underweight mothers can increase their infant's survival by reaching a higher prepregnancy weight and gaining extra weight during the pregnancy (Naeye, 1990). The National Academy of Sciences (NAS) (1990) recommends a weight gain of 25 to 35 pounds for women of normal weight. The NAS also recommends routine assessment of dietary practices for all pregnant women to determine the need for improving diet and vitamin and mineral supplementation. The requirement for some nutrients more than doubles during pregnancy, whereas calorie needs increase only about 15%. The increase in calories is about 300 kcal/day. Pregnant women need more protein, usually 10 to 16 g/day, and vitamins and minerals, including vitamins A, B, C, D with calcium, phosphorus, iron (beginning in the 24th week), and zinc (Grodner, Anderson, & DeYoung, 1996). Eating appropriate foods is the best method to deliver nutrients; however, prenatal vitamin supplements of iron and folic acid are recommended for all pregnant women.

Eating small snacks throughout the day may be preferable to three meals as the woman's uterus grows. Drinking fluids between meals helps avoid a feeling of being too full. Drinking four cups of milk a day or the equivalent in dairy products is helpful to provide the additional 32 g of protein needed. The pregnant woman needs to avoid alcohol and reduce her intake of caffeine to avoid birth defects.

Pregnant women are also nutritionally challenged by some of the expected side effects of pregnancy, such as nausea and vomiting. Nausea in pregnancy is usually short lived; however, when excessive vomiting occurs, loss of protein, calories, minerals, vitamins, and electrolytes may result. Frequent small dry meals of carbohydrates are usually tolerated. Heartburn can usually be relieved by smaller, more frequent meals. The community health nurse can provide information, resources, reassurance, and meal planning at birth preparation classes during this period.

Nutritional requirements for the lactating woman are similar to those during pregnancy. Increased carbohydrate intake helps the mother maintain lactose synthesis and milk volume. Trying to lose weight on a low-fat, low-carbohydrate diet while breastfeeding can be hazardous and can increase the duration of postpartum amenorrhea (Popkin, Guilkey, Akin, Adair, et al., 1993).

Gestational diabetes, pregnancy-induced hypertension (PIH), and pica are all serious health risks with serious nutritional consequences such as malnutrition. These medical conditions require referrals to a physician and dietitian. In some cases, hospitalization is necessary.

Pica

Pica refers to the persistent ingestion of materials that have no nutritional value. Pica in pregnancy is frequently manifested in the consumption of dirt or clay, also known as **geophagia.** Other substances may include hair, matches, gravel, or ice. Pica is not limited to one geographic area or socioeconomic class. Pica is poorly understood and researched at present.

Diabetes in the Pregnant Woman

Diabetic pregnant women need to be monitored closely for adequate nutrition. Non-insulin-dependent diabetics may require insulin during the pregnancy. More frequent glucose monitoring is required. Nondiabetic pregnant women may experience gestational diabetes, which usually arises after 20 weeks. It generally requires some carbohydrate and calorie reduction and close glucose monitoring. The community health nurse can be helpful in supporting the pregnant woman in the community by teaching her how to check her glucose and educating her about diabetes and her diet.

Pregnancy-Induced Hypertension

Pregnancy-induced hypertension (PIH) is believed to be linked with low protein intake or low calcium intake or both. It is defined by a systolic pressure of 140 mmHg or a diastolic pressure greater than 90 mmHg, or both. The development of PIH is associated with poverty, poor nutrition, and lack of prenatal care (Mahan & Escott-Stump, 1996). Prevention has proven to be successful with at-risk populations, but treatment is still controversial. The nurse is in a position to prevent PIH with education and screening programs and individual client monitoring at home.

Diabetes

Insulin-dependent diabetes (IDDM) accounts for 5% to 10% of diabetes in the United States. It is usually diagnosed under the age of 30. The goal of nutrition is to maintain near-normal blood glucose of 70 to 110 mg/dl by balancing food, insulin, and exercise. The diet needs to be individualized, with adjustments for protein and fats. Increasing carbohydrates is recommended. Insulin-dependent diabetes clients need to be constantly aware of the impact of stress, exercise, and alcohol on their diabetes. A young adult with the developmental tasks of career, marriage, and family may find it difficult to manage. Non-insulin-dependent diabetes is addressed in the older adult section.

Paraplegia and Quadriplegia

The impact of physical impairment on nutrition is evident in the young adult paraplegic and quadriplegic. Paraplegic and quadriplegic adults need to constantly monitor for skin breakdown. If skin breakdown occurs, protein needs to be increased along with vitamin C and zinc for healing. As a general rule, the client's weight should be between 10 and 15 pounds below ideal body weight (Hommerson, 1992). These clients also need to monitor bowel function and to consume enough fiber and water to ensure that they do not become constipated or impacted. The nurse can be helpful with education on nutrition, bowel programs, and skin assessment.

Middle Adult Nutritional Problems

Middle adulthood, the years from 41 to 64, presents the nutritional challenge of weight control. During the middle adult years, the behavior risk factors of controlling diet, weight, exercise, and lifestyle choices can present a threat to nutrition.

Obesity

With each decade of adult life, calorie intake needs to be decreased to match decreasing metabolism in order to maintain a stable weight. Activity level and exercise become critical factors in weight management. According to Popkin and Doak (1998), obesity is the fastest-growing chronic health condition. As much as one-third of the population is overweight. The percentage is higher for women and minorities, especially African American and Mexican American women (Kuczmarski, 1994). Obesity is not just a concern for adults but also for teens—20% of teens are overweight and the trend is moving upward according to the 1995 *Midcourse Review.* Developmentally disabled teens and adults are at risk for obesity because of their limited participation in exercise regimes and limited income from Social Security for a low-fat, low-calorie diet. One of the *Healthy People 2000* goals is to decrease obesity in the population to less than 20%. Another goal is to increase to at least 30% the number of people age 6 and above who engage in regular exercise. According to the 1995 *Midcourse Review,* the number of obese persons

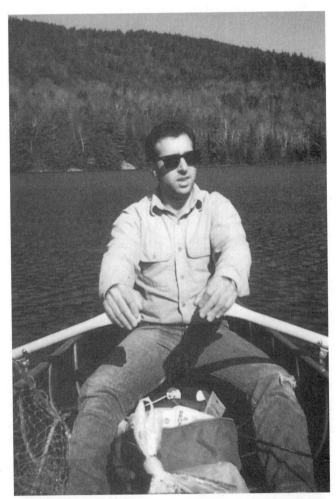

Middle adulthood is generally a healthy time, but proper exercise, nutrition, and healthy lifestyle choices must be incorporated into daily activities to ensure that good health continues into older adulthood. *Photo courtesy of Cathy Esperti.*

had increased and the number of persons eating a low fat diet had increased by only 2% (USDHHS, 1990, 1996).

Obesity is defined as the condition of being 20% above ideal body weight (according to the Metropolitan Life Insurance company tables). Severe obesity is the condition of being 40% above ideal body weight. Morbid obesity refers to being more than 100 pounds above ideal body weight (Mahan & Escott-Stump, 1996). Obesity and its health complications, such as diabetes, hypertension (HTN), gout, and hypercholesterolemia, are treatable with a medically supervised reduction of calories. Obesity also causes fatigue, shortness of breath, digestive and bowel disruptions, joint pain, and varicose veins. The treatment of obesity needs to be based on the Food Guide Pyramid for an extended period of time, such as one to three years, to achieve success. The diet should be composed of 20% protein, 25% to 30% fat, and 30% to 35% carbohydrates, with adjustments for each individual. The client should take in no less than 1,200 kcal/day, and no category of food should be totally eliminated. Once the weight loss diet plan is in place, an exercise plan shoud be started. Counseling and behavior modification are critical components of permanent weight loss. In cases in which morbid obesity is lifethreatening, there are surgical options such as gastric bypass or gastroplasty. Sugarman (1996) states that weight loss from gastroplasty has been maintained by 73% of clients for three years but only 45% for five years and 10% to 40% for 10 years. Other studies indicate that 50% to 60% of clients maintain weight loss after five years (Yale, 1989; Sugarman, Kellum, et al., 1992; Pories, Swanson, et al., 1995).

Weight Control

Persons who have been successful in weight loss share consistent methodologies. Long (1996) offers the following tips for successful weight loss:

- Believe that you can be thin for life.
- Do it for yourself.
- Set realistic goals.
- Adopt a sensible eating plan that includes your favorite foods.
- Eat high-calorie foods in small portions.
- Cut the fat.
- Get moving.
- Track your progress.
- Get organized and take the time to eat well.
- Plan for the long haul: no short-term solutions.

The community health nurse who has never had a weight problem must examine any attitudes she might have that could destroy nurse empathy and client trust in the client–nurse relationship. Nurses need to examine and possibly modify their attitudes, values, and practices to assist obese clients just as they would any other clients with a serious health problem. It is important for the nurse to take an understanding approach in encouraging the obese client's efforts to control health-related problems and to lose weight.

Chronic Illnesses

Some chronic nutritional problems for the middle-aged adult are cancer, diabetes, heart disease, hypertension, and alcoholism. The middle-aged adult who experiences these chronic illnesses is at less nutritional risk than the older adult because the middle adult has not yet experienced the compounding effect of multiple chronic illnesses, as have many older adults. The older adult, unlike the middle adult, experiences social and economic changes that increase the nutritional risk. The nutritional effect of chronic illnesses will be discussed in the next section.

Older and Elderly Adult Nutritional Problems

Older adults, ages 65 to 80, and elder adults, ages 81 and older, have multiple nutritional problems and are at greater risk of repeatedly experiencing nutritional deficits. Older adults experience multiple chronic health problems and social and economic problems that put them at risk for nutritional deficits. In this section, the common nutritional problems will be explored. Keep in mind the previous discussion of socioeconomic factors as it applies to the older and elder adult.

The average age and the proportion of older adults living in the United States are increasing. The older population itself is getting older. The Census Bureau projects that the population age 85 and older will double from 3.5 million today to 7 million by 2020, then double again by 2040. Over the next 50 years, the United States will become a mature nation in which one citizen in five will be 65 years or older (Waite, 1996; Corman, 1997).

Chronological age is not a determining factor for nutritional problems. Only persons with physiological changes caused not only by aging but also by poor nutri-

tion, disabilities, and disease states will become clients for the community health nurse. It is estimated that 85% of noninstitutionalized older persons have one or more chronic conditions that could improve with proper nutrition and that up to half have clinically identifiable problems that require nutrition intervention. The detection of nutritional risks among the elderly and referral, as needed, to appropriate nutrition services and resources are key concerns of health care professionals (Posner, Jette, Smith, & Miller, 1993).

Clinical evidence of nutritional deficiencies is more prevalent among those who are very old and frail, those who suffer from severe physical or emotional limitations, those who have multiple chronic conditions or take many medications, and those who are homebound. See Table 26-6 for clinical signs of nutritional problems. The nutrition problems that affect the elderly range from nutritional deficiencies to nutrient excesses. By far, the most prevalent nutrition-related problems of the elderly are chronic conditions that benefit from diet therapy, such as obesity, atherosclerotic cardiovascular disease, diabetes, hypertension, osteoporosis, certain cancers, and gastrointestinal disorders (American Dietetic Association, 1993).

Physiological Risk Factors

Maintenance of adequate nutritional status is an important component of preventive health care. Often in the elderly a functional change is the cause of a nutritional deficit. Some of the risk factors related to nutrition, if noted, need to be addressed by the community health nurse with appropriate referrals. They include: (1) decreased appetite and food intake, (2) poor dentition, (3) decreased sense of thirst, (4) constipation, (5) vision loss, and (6) food and drug interactions. See Figure 26-4 for a list of risk factors for nutritional deficits specific to the elderly. Some of the management or intervention strategies for these problems are listed in Table 26-7.

Table 26-6	**Clinical Signs of Nutritional Problems**	
	NORMAL APPEARANCE	**SIGNS OF NUTRITIONAL PROBLEMS**
Hair	Shiny, firm, not easily plucked	Dull and dry, thin, easily plucked
Face	Uniform color, healthy appearance, not swollen	Pale, scaling skin around nostrils, swollen
Eyes	Bright, clear, shiny, no sores, healthy pink and moist	Pale conjunctiva, dryness, dullness, white ring around eye
Lips	Smooth, not swollen	White or pink lesions at corners of mouth
Tongue	Not swollen or smooth, deep red	Purplish, smooth and atrophy or hypertrophy of the taste buds
Teeth	No cavities, no pain, no or few teeth missing	Many teeth missing or no teeth, cavities
Gums	Healthy, red, no bleeding, not swollen	Spongy, bleeding, receding

Appetite

Total food intake decreases with age, in part as a result of lower metabolic rate but primarily because of decreased physical activity. Nutrition affects aging in that lowered intake may not meet nutrient requirements and therefore can adversely influence the rate of aging. Clients with severely decreased appetites may be suffering from a recent loss of a spouse or loved one or a change in living arrangements. Clients with chronic decreased appetite and food intake may need to be referred to their physician for appetite stimulant medication. Also, nutrition education by a dietitian or a community health nurse can be a key factor in helping older and elderly adults realize the importance of not only eating, but eating a well-balanced diet. After assessing the situation, the community health nurse can recommend strategies for the client such as having neighbors come in for meals several times a week or going to a congregate meal site for lunch. The nurse can contact the client's church or local senior services agency

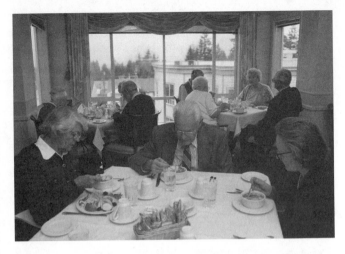

Loneliness is common in older and elderly adults as spouses and long-time friends pass away. Encouraging participation in community meals may offset the nutritional deficits sometimes found in lonely older and elderly adults. Photo courtesy of Photodisc.

or council on aging for help such as home-cooked meals, visits at meal time, and transportation. Sometimes the client's family needs to be alerted to the cause of the nutritional problem. The nurse needs to assess available options for each client and tailor the intervention accordingly.

Poor Dentition

If the client has trouble chewing because of poor dentition or no teeth, nutrition need not suffer. The client should be encouraged to eat a soft diet or ground foods until a referral can be made to a dentist. Many communities have facilities that do dental work for those who are unable to pay or are underinsured.

Thirst

Older adults and the elderly will have a diminished sense of thirst. They need to be encouraged to drink throughout the day, even if just sips, and to consciously drink a glass of water when they brush their teeth and after each meal.

Constipation

Declines in physiological function occur with aging; optimal nutrition is believed to slow these processes. Clients may suffer from chronic constipation due to lack of activity, depression, and diminished appetite, as well as physiological changes. Low income may also be a contributing factor because clients may feel that fresh fruits and vegetables are too expensive for their budget. The nurse can teach the client to watch for in-season bargain produce. To help alleviate constipation, the nurse should encourage clients to eat more foods with fiber such as fresh fruits and vegetables, oatmeal or oat bran, and prunes (no more than three times a week), and to drink more water. Products containing carbohydrates that increase bulk in the colon should not be used

---

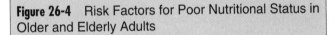

Figure 26-4 Risk Factors for Poor Nutritional Status in Older and Elderly Adults

Nutritional and Physiological Risk Factors

Diminished appetite

Chewing or swallowing problems

Recent unintentional weight loss of ≥10 lb in 1 to 2 months

Food and drug interactions

Obesity

Nausea and vomiting for ≥3 days

Poor dentition or no teeth

Psychological Risk Factors

Depression or loneliness

Mental confusion or dementia

High alcohol intake

Recent loss of spouse or loved one

Diseases and Surgeries

Diabetes

Recent surgery (any kind)

COPD (chronic obstructive pulmonary disease)

Chronic disease

Socioeconomic Risk Factors

Limited available food

Inability to cook or shop

Homebound

Eating limited to only a few foods

Low socioeconomic status

Table 26-7	Management of Nutritional Problems of Older and Elderly Adults	
CONDITION	**INFLUENCES**	**MANAGEMENT**
Poor dentition	Ability to chew food and to take in nutrients	Refer for dental work or grind meat and eat soft foods.
Reduced metabolic rate	Weight and number of calories required	Decrease caloric intake; if overweight, refer to dietitian.
Osteoporosis	Quality of life, mobility	Encourage weight-bearing exercise. Advise client to consume more calcium-rich foods and to take medication when necessary.
Decreased thirst	Hydration, electrolyte balance, orientation	Encourage drinking even when not thirsty. Advise client to eat very sweet, tart, or salty foods and to suck on hard candy.
Constipation	Transit time and development of cancer	Client should eat prunes 3 times/week, drink more water, and eat more fiber.
Vitamin D deficiency	Calcium absorption and bone density	Get ten minutes of sunlight per day or supplement during winter.
Decreased sense of taste and smell	Appetite; possible addition of too much salt	Use more herbs and spices; marinate meats.
Low intake of fruits and vegetables	Constipation; essential nutrient intake	Buy fruits and vegetables in season. Refer client to food bank if economics is the issue.
B vitamin deficiency (occurs mainly in alcoholics)	Brain function, mental ability, orientation	Use a supplement or increase intake of grains.
Anemia	Oxygen-carrying capacity of the blood	Remove cause such as medication, ulcers, or hemorrhoids. Drink orange juice with iron-fortified cereal.
Pernicious anemia	Energy level	Refer client for vitamin B_{12} injections.
Zinc deficiency	Wound healing, proper immune function, storage and release of insulin	Encourage intake of lean meat, poultry, and dairy products.

by diabetics unless the carbohydrates are counted as part of their daily diet.

Vision Changes

Clients with low vision or loss of vision are at nutritional risk because of their physical inability to get to the grocery store, to locate desired food, to read labels, and to prepare nutritious foods at home. Also, the client may be eating moldy or spoiled food because of the inability to see. Family and friends or home health aids can help with food shopping, food preparation, and discarding of spoiled food. They could also help prevent food and drug interactions by marking food that should not be taken with the client's medications.

Drug and Food Interactions

The elderly are at high risk for food and drug interactions because they are likely to take multiple prescription drugs. Common prescription and over-the-counter (OTC)

medicines alter nutritional needs in many ways, particularly in the elderly. Prescribing physicians and pharmacists have an obligation to inform clients of the dangers or imbalances likely to occur in using prescription drugs. Some common OTC medicines and their effects on nutrition are listed below:

- Diuretics and laxatives cause a loss of water, sodium, and potassium.
- Aspirin, often used to manage osteoarthritis, can produce iron deficiency.
- Mineral oil, often used as a laxative, interferes with the absorption of fat-soluble vitamins.
- Sodium bicarbonate antacids increase gastric pH, inactivating thiamin and hindering iron absorption.
- Antacids containing aluminum hydroxide cause phosphate depletion and calcium excretion thereby accelerating bone loss.

Drug-induced malnutrition can occur during long-term treatment for chronic diseases. Some drugs such as non-steroidal anti-inflammatory agents can also cause nutritional

⚙ ⚙ REFLECTIVE THINKING ⚙ ⚙

Vision Impairment

Think back to a time before you had your driver's license and you couldn't wait to drive. Now think about how driving gives you independence and control over how and when you travel. Pretend for this activity that you have suddenly lost so much of your vision that you have to wear thick glasses just to see objects within arm's length. You can no longer see well beyond the length of your arm.

• How do you feel about the situation in which you find yourself?

• How would it change your life?

• What obstacles would this condition present?

• How would you get around your community?

• Imagine if you were 80 years old, living alone, and this were your situation. How do you think you would feel?

• How do you think having a loss of vision would affect your ability to care for a client in a similar situation?

problems, including irritation of the gastrointestinal tract and bleeding and fluid retention, if not ingested with food. Clients on long-term diuretics are at risk for potassium deficiency as well as deficiencies in calcium, magnesium, and zinc. Their food intake needs to be monitored for potassium- and calcium-rich foods. See Table 26-8 for a more detailed list.

The community health nurse has a pivotal role in identifying and preventing drug and food interactions. The nurse needs to be aware of all the medications the client is taking and the possible interactions and monitor the client for potential problems. The nurse needs to educate the client about potential problems and teach the client how to avoid those problems. Periodically, the nurse needs to review these precautions with the client and family to ensure that the client is vigilant.

Homebound Meals

The Homebound Meals program was established by Congress in 1972 as the Nutrition Program for the Elderly under Title VII of the Older Americans Act. The act also addressed the problem of many elderly people who do not eat adequately for the following reasons: (1) They cannot afford to do so; (2) they lack the skills to select and prepare nourishing, well-balanced meals; (3) they have limited mobility, which may impair their capacity to shop and cook for themselves; and (4) many feel rejected and lonely, feelings that can obliterate the incentive to prepare and eat a meal alone. The nutrition program,

designed to provide nourishing meals in a social setting (congregate meal sites), was also established under Title VII of the Older American Act. Because lack of transportation tended to keep the elderly isolated, transportation services to the congregate meal sites was established in 1978.

This homebound meal will supply one-third of the recommended dietary allowance (RDA) for the client according to government regulations. The other two meals need to be supplied by the client. One problem is that many elderly persons eat only part of this meal and save the rest for their evening meal; dividing the meal gives the client fewer nutrients than needed for good nutrition, and if the food is not refrigerated and reheated properly it could cause foodborne illness.

The community health nurse, family members, case managers in hospitals, case workers, neighbors, and family doctors are often the ones who identify a need in a family for home-delivered meals. It is often necessary to explain the value of the service and to encourage the client to participate. Many people find it difficult to accept this type of service initially, believing that it is "charity." Once they are convinced that they have a right to this service and become acquainted with the person who brings the food, if homebound, or make friends at their congregate meal site, they may look forward to the personal contact as well as to a hot nutritious meal.

Food Supplementation

In the past, food consumption was virtually the only way to supply nutrients to the body. Today, however, nutrients can also be provided by food supplements such as liquid drinks, powdered drinks, vitamins, and herbs. Elders need to be wise consumers in the area of food supplements. They need to look at the utility of the supplement and the cost if they are on a limited budget. At present there is very little research for the consumer to read to evaluate whether these supplements are appropriate for their nutrition. Elders who take prescribed medications for medical problems need to consult with their physician to ensure that the supplements do not interfere with their medications. Many elders have found that herbs and supplementation assist in the control of arthritis and minor bowel and skin conditions. With the increasing interest in maintaining health by the general public, supplementation has received more attention. This attention has brought herbal, holistic, and alternative therapies into the mainstream.

The use of multiple vitamins and mineral supplements to guarantee good health is fairly common among the elderly and may indicate that the client needs guidance from the community health nurse or other qualified health professionals to make informed choices on whether to take supplements. Guidance in terms of safety and cost are also needed. The community health nurse needs to ensure that the client is making an informed choice when adding a food supplement and respect that choice if it differs from the nurse's.

Table 26-8 Drug–Nutrient Interactions

DRUG	EFFECT
Alcohol	Decreased absorption of thiamin, folic acid, and vitamin B_{12}; increased urinary excretion of magnesium and zinc
Analgesics	
Aspirin (salicylates)	Decreased serum folate level; increased excretion of vitamin C
Colchicine	Decreased absorption of vitamin B_{12}, carotene, fat, lactose, sodium, potassium, protein, and cholesterol
Amphetamines	Decreased appetite and caloric intake; possibly reduced growth
Antacids	
Aluminum hydroxide	Decreased absorption of phosphate
Other antacids	Decreased thiamin and fatty acid absorption
Anticonvulsants	
Barbiturates	Decreased vitamin B_{12} and thiamin absorption; increased excretion of vitamin C; deficiency of folate and vitamin D
Hydantoins	Decreased serum folate, vitamin B_{12}, pyridoxine, calcium, and vitamin D levels; increased excretion of vitamin C
Antidepressants	Increased appetite; weight gain
Antimetabolites	General absorptive decrease secondary to intestinal wall damage and oral mucus breakdown; specific malabsorption of B_{12}, folate, fat, and xylose
Antimicrobials	
Chloramphenicol	Increased riboflavin, pyridoxine, and B_{12} requirements
Neomycin	Decreased absorption of fat; carbohydrate; protein; vitamins A, B_{12}, D, and E; calcium; iron; sugar; potassium; sodium; and nitrogen
Penicillin	Increased potassium excretion; inhibition of glutathione
Sulfonamides	Decreased synthesis of folic acid, vitamin K, and B vitamins
Tetracyclines	Decreased absorption of calcium, iron, magnesium, and fat; increased excretion of vitamin C, riboflavin, nitrogen, folic acid, and niacin; decreased vitamin K synthesis
Cathartics	Decreased absorption of calcium, vitamin D, potassium, protein, glucose, and fat
Chelating agents	Increased excretion of zinc, copper, and pyridoxine; depression of appetite
Corticosteroids	Decreased absorption of calcium, phosphorus, and iron; increased excretion of vitamin C, calcium, potassium, zinc, and nitrogen; decreased tolerance of glucose; increased triglyceride and cholesterol absorption; increased vitamin D metabolism; increased appetite
Diuretics	
Furosemide	Increased excretion of calcium, magnesium, and potassium
Mercurials	Increased excretion of thiamin, magnesium, calcium, and potassium
Thiazides	Increased excretion of potassium, magnesium, zinc, and riboflavin
Triamterence	Decreased serum folate and vitamin B_{12} levels
Hypocholesterolemic agents	
Cholestyramine	Decreased absorption of cholesterol; potassium; vitamins A, D, K, and B_{12}; folate, fat; glucose; and iron
Clofibrate	Decreased absorption of vitamin B_{12}, iron, glucose, potassium, and sodium; decreased taste acuity; aftertaste
Hypotensive agents	Increased excretion of pyridoxine
Laxatives	
Mineral oil	Decreased absorption of vitamins A, D, E, and K; calcium; and phosphate
Phenolphthalein	Increased excretion of potassium
Levodopa	Decreased absorption of amino acids; increased use of ascorbic acid and pyridoxine; increased excretion of sodium and potassium
Potassium chloride	Decreased absorption of vitamin B_{12}
Sedatives	
Glutethimide	Increased metabolism of vitamin D
Sulfonamides	
Azulfidine	Decreased absorption of folate; decreased serum iron level
Other sulfonamides	Decreased synthesis of folate and vitamins B and K
Surfactants	Decreased absorption of fat
Tranquilizers	Increased appetite; weight gain

From Nutrition and Diet Therapy *(6th ed.) by C. Townsend, 1994, Albany, NY: Delmar Publishers.*

Chronic Illnesses

Many older and elderly people have chronic illnesses that must be medically and nutritionally managed to ensure quality of life. They can be managed through assessment, intervention, referral to a physician and a dietitian, and follow-up by the community health nurse.

Diabetes

Non-insulin-dependent diabetes mellitus (NIDDM) usually occurs after the age of 40. This type of diabetes can be controlled by diet and exercise, or by diet, exercise, and an oral glucose-lowering medication. Its onset is gradual and is exacerbated by obesity and an inactive lifestyle. Common symptoms are excess thirst, excess appetite, and excess urine output; however, a client may have none of these symptoms. Many times a diagnosis is made during a routine urine or blood test, or following a heart attack or stroke, or during hospitalization for another medical problem.

Management of diabetes is essential and can prevent hyperglycemia (elevated blood glucose), ketoacidosis (high levels of ketones in the blood), and hypoglycemia (subnormal blood glucose). For optimal control and prevention of diabetic complications, blood glucose levels need to be between 70 and 120 mg/dl. This can be accomplished by a diet specifically designed for each client. A client should be enrolled in diabetic education classes, taught by a certified diabetes educator, to obtain in-depth knowledge of the disease, its ramifications, and the best way to control blood glucose levels. The goals of medical nutrition therapy for the client with NIDDM are to: (1) maintain good control of blood glucose, (2) decrease cholesterol level (if above 200 mg/dl), (3) maintain good blood pressure, and (4) decrease weight, if necessary.

The newest method for teaching diabetics to control their blood sugar is through carbohydrate counting. Carbohydrates are starches/breads, fruits, and milk. Within one meal, clients may choose any of these food categories, as long as they stay within the number of carbohydrates they have been allowed. This method allows greater flexibility for the client. Diabetics need to utilize the "Exchange Lists for Meal Planning" published by the American Diabetes Association to accurately count carbohydrates. The biggest change in the updated version of the exchange lists is that vegetables (nonstarchy) are free up to 1½ cups cooked or 3 cups raw per meal.

Research indicates that carbohydrates from simple sugars are not digested or absorbed more rapidly than are complex carbohydrates and they do not appear to affect blood glucose control if eaten with other foods as part of a regular meal plan (Wheeler & Mazur, 1997). It is the total amount of carbohydrates eaten that affects the blood glucose levels. Being able to include foods containing sucrose increases flexibility for diabetics. Clients should be made aware that "diabetic candy" is usually manufactured with an alcohol sugar such as sorbitol, which is metabolized in the body like sucrose and must be counted as a carbohydrate.

If the client does not adhere to the diabetic diet, and blood glucose levels remain too high for optimal health, the physician may determine that the client needs an oral glucose-lowering medication. See Figure 26-5 for the most common oral diabetic agents.

If the client remains noncompliant with the diabetic diet even with the oral glucose-lowering medication and the blood glucose level runs too high, the physician will put the client on insulin injections. The community health nurse can help clients learn to give their own injections, monitor blood glucose levels, and comply with the diet, explaining the complications that can be caused by noncompliance. Excellent control of blood glucose levels can prevent the complications of diabetes such as heart disease, renal disease, retinopathy, which is the leading cause of blindness in the United States, and neuropathy, which leads to amputations of the toes, feet, and legs.

When a client is on insulin there is a possibility of hypoglycemic episodes. Some symptoms are headache, blurred vision, sweating, tremors, confusion, nausea, and unconsciousness. The community health nurse needs to make sure that the client has access to glucose tablets, orange juice, or table sugar in the event of low blood glucose levels. Because many older and elderly adults have decreased appetites, many physicians are only specifying "no concentrated sweets" for their diabetic diets such as desserts made with sugar, candy, and sugared drinks.

Osteoporosis

Osteoporosis affects both men and women. Risk factors include calcium and vitamin D deficiency, immobilization, inactivity, alcoholism, and cigarette smoking. It is most common in fair-skinned, small-boned women who are postmenopausal and not on estrogen replacement therapy (ERT).

In 1997, the Food and Nutrition Board (FNB) developed guidelines for adequate calcium intake for women

DECISION MAKING

Home Visit to a Newly Diagnosed Diabetic

This is your first visit to Mrs. S., who is an 80-year-old newly diagnosed insulin-dependent diabetic. When you arrive, she is sitting at the kitchen table with a can of Coca-Cola and half a cigarette. On the table you notice a bowl of candy, with several crumpled wrappers in the bowl. Her lunch plate is still on the table and contains chocolate frosting and cake crumbs. She proudly tells you that she ate what was on the diet plan that she got at the hospital.

- What observations are important to address?

- What does this client need to review about her diet?

- What does this client need to know about insulin?

and men 51 through 70 years old. The Dietary Reference Intake for calcium is 1,200 mg/day. This is adequate to maintain bone density at current levels. This equates to four glasses of milk per day. Other calcium-rich dairy products could also be consumed. Calcium citrate is a good calcium supplement. The calcium intake of the average American is only half of that needed to maintain healthy bones.

Postmenopausal women not on ERT should participate in weight-bearing exercises to help delay the onset of osteoporosis (Ryan, Treuth, Hunter & Elahi, 1998). Research has shown that exercise and increased calcium intake can decrease the loss of calcium from the bones (Prince et al., 1995). Even bedridden clients can do upper arm weight training, which could increase their ability to help with their activities of daily living (ADLs) (Frischnecht, 1998).

Taking 500 IU of vitamin D during the winter can reduce late-winter bone loss and increase bone density in the spine (Reid, 1996). During the summer, 10 to 15 minutes of sun, without sunscreen, is needed to stimulate production of vitamin D in the skin. A diet history, taken by a dietitian, could be used to plan a nutrient-dense, calcium-rich diet. If bone density has decreased substantially, then the physician can prescribe medication to help increase bone density. The community health nurse needs to monitor any client on this medication to determine if the medication is being taken properly.

Cardiovascular Disease

Coronary heart disease is the leading cause of death in the United States. Most deaths occur in people over the age of 65. Hypertension is also a risk factor for coronary artery disease (CAD) (Cappuccio, Cook, Atkinson, and Strazzullo, 1997). According to the American Heart Association, hypertension is highest in the following groups: (1) African Americans, Puerto Ricans, Cuban Americans, and Mexican Americans; (2) people with lower educational and income levels; (3) women over the age of 75; and (4) men younger than 55 years old.

The risk of cardiovascular disease (CVD) increases with high fat intake, increased blood cholesterol, smoking, high blood pressure, a sedentary lifestyle, and family history of CVD (Cappuccio, Cook, Atkinson, and Strazzullo, 1997). Sometimes hypertension can be managed with nutritional care if the client adheres to the nutritional recommendations, has no other major medical problems, and only slightly elevated blood pressure (Banning, 1998). The recommendations for nutritional management of hypertension by diet are found in Table 26-9.

Many clients have not only hypertension but also hyperlipidemia and must also restrict their cholesterol and fat intake. A low-cholesterol/3–4 g sodium diet is the usual recommendation. The physician may also prescribe a cholesterol-lowering medication, especially in the older or elderly adult.

Many older and elderly clients will have or will develop congestive heart failure (CHF) (Kohn, 1998). CHF can be caused by CAD, lung disease, hypothyroidism, or damage

---

Figure 26-5 Four Types of Oral Diabetes Medication

1. **Non-sulfonylureas**

   Glucophage (Metformin)

2. **Alpha-glucosidase inhibitors:**

   Precose (Acarbose)

3. **Second-generation sulfonylureas**

   Diabeta
   Micronase (Glyburide)
   Glynase Prestabs
   Glucotrol (Glipizide)
   Gluctrol XL
   Amaryl (Glimepiride)

4. **First-generation sulfonylureas**

   Diabinese (Chlorpropimide)
   Orinase (Tolbutamide)
   Tolinase (Tolazamide)
   Dymelor (Acetoheximide)

---

to the heart muscle. When the diagnosis of CHF is made, the client must be restricted to 1 to 2 g of sodium per day. Even when on the 3 to 4 g sodium diet, products labeled "low sodium" (containing no more than 140 mg of sodium per serving), such as soups, canned vegetables, and tomato products, must be used in addition to other restrictions (see Table 26-9). The community health nurse may need to recommend an appointment with a dietitian to help the client understand the restrictions and to help with meal planning. For older and elderly adults, management of the cardiac problems becomes a key issue. Good management makes the difference in quality of life.

Cancer

Cancer is the second leading cause of death in the United States. Although no specific food is known to either cause or prevent cancer, beta carotene has been associated with cancer prevention because of its antioxidant effect on the development and maintenance of cells (Weisburger, 1991). Vitamin A and beta carotene from yellow and green fruits and vegetables and cruciferous vegetables such as cauliflower, broccoli, cabbage, and Brussels sprouts are anticarcinogenic and prevent cell membrane damage. Foods rich in the antioxidants, vitamins A, C, E, beta carotene, and selenium, can help reduce the incidence of lung, breast, oral mucosa, esophageal, and bladder cancers.

Research on the intake of carotenoids (major provitamin A) and retinol (vitamin A) in relation to the risk of prostate cancer found that lycopene or other compounds in tomatoes may reduce prostate cancer risk (Giovannucci, Ascherio, Rimm, et al., 1995). One study found that vitamin and mineral supplementation was effective in lowering the incidence of esophageal and stomach cancer. The study was carried out in the Linxian province in north-central China, which reports the world's highest incidence of these cancers (Blot, Li, Taylor, Guo, et al., 1995). See the accompanying Research Focus.

Table 26-9 Nutritional Management of Hypertension

GOAL	RECOMMENDATIONS
Control weight.	Be within 15% of ideal body weight (IBW).
Maintain sodium within 3–4 g/day.	Restrict high-sodium foods: pickles, olives, bacon, ham, and other processed meats; chips; canned soups and tomato products; salted nuts; and crackers. Eat moderate portions of meat (6–8 oz/day), fish, eggs (3 per week), and dairy. Allow three months to reduce sodium intake. Do not add salt in cooking or at the table.
Maintain calcium intake at RDI for age.	Clients at risk for osteoporosis may require supplementation.
Increase potassium.	Potassium chloride may be partially substituted for sodium chloride in cooking if allowed by doctor. Eat 5 servings of fruits and vegetables. Not recommended for clients with abnormal renal function.
Restrict fat.	Use less saturated fat: animal origin, palm oil, coconut oil, cocoa butter, stick margarine, hydrogenated shortening.

Adapted from "The Treatment of Mild Hypertension Study: A Randomized, Placebo-Controlled Trial of a Nutritional Hygienic Regimen along with Various Drug Nontherapies" by Treatment of Mild Hypertension Research Group, 1991, Archives of Internal Medicine, 151(7), pp. 1413–1420.

The nutrient and caloric needs of the cancer patient are greater due to increased metabolic rate. Nutrients lost to the cancer must be replaced. Individuals with certain kinds of illnesses, particularly ones who receive chemotherapy or radiation treatment or have AIDS, can suffer **cachexia,** a severe loss of appetite that can lead to weight loss and anorexia. When cachexia leads to anorexia, feedings by intravenous or gastric tube may be necessary. Diet plans for cancer patients must be individualized. Small, frequent meals may be better tolerated and may increase intake. The community health nurse should refer to a dietitian any client who is not eating adequately to maintain weight. Care should be taken to protect compromised clients from pathogenic organisms in foods that could lead to vomiting and diarrhea, because of their already depressed immune systems (see Table 26-4).

Alcohol

Alcoholism is defined as a medical disease with congenital predisposition. Older adults are increasing their alcohol consumption and becoming vulnerable to the effects of alcoholism on the liver, heart, and pancreas. The older alcoholic experiences extreme fatigue due to insomnia. Overconsumption of alcohol leads to liver chemistry imbalance and large amounts of fat in the liver, which leads to hypoglycemia and inhibition of drug metabolism (Fink, Hays, Moore, & Beck, 1996).

The alcoholic at greatest nutritional and health risk is one who stops eating or makes non-nutritious food substitutions **(substance substitutions).** Non-nutritious substances are substances such as sugar, caffeine, and nicotine. Alcohol depresses appetite, resulting in insufficient intake. It can also cause nausea, diarrhea, ulcers, small bowel malfunction, impaired water and electrolyte absorption, anemia, clotting defects, and convulsions. Alcoholism interferes with absorption of thiamin, vitamins

B6, B12, and D, folate, magnesium, and zinc. The disease is compounded by low fiber, low protein, and high fat intake, stress, smoking, and a sedentary lifestyle.

When the client's alcoholism results in cirrhosis of the liver, the nutritional risk for the client is serious. The first goal is to ensure that the client eats if he is still drinking. A diet high in carbohydrates and protein totaling 2,000 to 3,000 kcal/day is the second goal. Restriction of sodium is necessary if the client has edema or abdominal ascites. Supplementation with vitamins and minerals is helpful (Jaffe & Skidmore-Roth, 1993).

The community health nurse can act as the client's resource and advocate by providing information about withdrawal programs such as Alcoholics Anonymous (AA) and assisting the client with the initial contact. The client's family can be provided with information about Al-Anon. In cases in which the client may be hospitalized for medical complications of alcoholism, the physician may refer the client to an inpatient detoxification program followed by participation in AA.

Depression

Depression in the aging population is often experienced as exaggerated sadness due to an event, loss of mobility, or internal conflict. It can seriously affect a person's desire to eat. Loneliness due to loss of a spouse is a leading cause of depression and anorexia. Inflation, failing health, social isolation, and medical bills on a fixed income can have a devastating effect and exacerbate depression. The food budget suffers, and most often fresh fruits and vegetables are eliminated. Many elderly may become homebound, and being homebound further increases isolation and depression.

Depression is not a natural part of aging. A person can maintain a good quality of life with optimum feelings and a healthy appetite near to death. When depression is

RESEARCH FOCUS

The Linxian Trials: Mortality Rates by Vitamin-Mineral Intervention Group

STUDY PROBLEM/PURPOSE

To assess the effects of supplementation with vitamins and minerals in nearly 30,000 participants who have a chronically low intake of several nutrients. The researchers were trying to find out if vitamin and mineral supplementation is likely to lower the relative risk (RR) and cancer mortality rate.

(1) Do 30,000 participants from the general population who daily receive four nutrient combinations: retinol and zinc; riboflavin and niacin; vitamin C and molybdenum; and beta carotene, alpha-tocopherol, and selenium, lower their RR of cancer and mortality rate? (2) Do 3,318 participants who have esophageal dysplasia, a precursor to esophageal cancer, who receive daily multiple-vitamin supplementation or a placebo, have lowered RR and cancer mortality rate?

METHODS

A factorial design was used. Qualitative data were collected to assess the effects of the four specific supplements given to the general population over a 5.25-year period. A similar design was used to collect the data for the 3,318 persons given the vitamin and mineral supplements over a 6-year period.

FINDINGS

Restoring adequate intake of certain nutrients may help to lower the risk of cancer and other diseases in this high-risk population. Small but significant reductions in total (RR = 0.91) and cancer (RR = 0.87) mortality were observed in participants receiving beta carotene, alpha-tocopherol, and selenium but not the other nutrients. The reductions were greater in women than men and in those under age 55 compared with over the age of 55; however, differences in sex or age were not significant.

In the smaller dysplasia trial, reductions in total (RR = 0.93) and cancer (RR = 0.96) mortality were not significant. The largest reductions were for cerebrovascular disease mortality: A significant reduction was observed in men (RR = 0.45) but not women (RR = 0.90).

IMPLICATIONS

The implications of this study are that vitamin and mineral supplementation may help decrease the risk of certain cancers and the mortality associated with them. A larger study may reveal how valuable vitamins and minerals are in reducing the risk and mortality of cancer.

SOURCE

From "The Linxian Trials: Mortality Rates by Vitamin-Mineral Intervention Group" by W. J. Blot, J. Y. Li, P. R. Taylor, W. Guo, S. M. Dawsey, & B. Li, 1995, American Journal of Clinical Nutrition, 62 (Supplement), pp. 1424S–1426S.

noted by the community health nurse, a referral needs to be made to the client's physician for treatment.

NUTRITIONAL ASSESSMENT

Nutritional screening is necessary to design individual interventions and programs for communities. Screening tools help the nurse identify potential or actual nutritional deficits and their severity. The nutritional database guides the nurse in the design of the appropriate intervention. Needs and nutritional risk status change as a client progresses through the life span. Prevention strategies need to be based on the stages of the life cycle and focused on the most common and avoidable nutrition problems.

Nutritional assessment can take place in a variety of settings, including the client's home, a congregate eating center, or a clinic. Health care professionals in different settings have different nutritional priorities. Some may be interested in an assessment of an aggregate group's nutri-

tional health; others may be interested in an individual client's nutritional intake.

Nutrition has not been the number one priority of community health nursing, but it needs to be brought to the forefront. Nutrition knowledge and healthy eating can help prevent acute and chronic diseases. The community health nurse must be able to assess each client's nutritional status with tools specifically designed to determine immediate needs. A useful framework for the home health care nurse in performing a nutritional assessment is the informal rule of thumb that each additional chronic or acute diagnosis raises the client's risk for a nutritional deficit. For example, an elder client who just lost his spouse and has another hospitalization for angina and a new diagnosis of congestive heart failure now has three factors that increase his risk. It is imperative that the community health nurse correctly assess the client to determine if he is at nutritional risk and to facilitate immediate intervention.

Figures 26-6 and 26-7 contain assessment tools for the community setting to assess individual clients and the

Figure 26-6 Client Assessment for Nutritional Problems

Food Access

Food availability _____

Ability to shop _____

Transportation to buy food—Any barriers? _____

Quality/quantity of food (observed in the home) _____

Financial resources—Do you feel you have enough money for food? _____

Storage and prep ability _____

Cooking ability _____

Dietary Habits

Meal frequency/pattern—How many times a day do you eat? _____

Describe what you eat at each setting. _____

Appetite _____

Ability to chew—Any barriers? _____

Likes _____ Dislikes _____

Food allergies _____ Intolerances _____

Special food issues _____

(ethnic/religious)

Health Habits

Current medical problems _____

Past medical problems _____

Recent illnesses _____

Recent hospitalizations/surgeries _____

Do you have enough money to buy your medications? _____

Recent nausea and/or vomiting _____ How long? _____

Recent diarrhea _____ How long? _____

Bowel movements—Last? _____ How often? _____

Medications _____

OTC medicines _____

Vitamin/mineral supplements _____

Dental health _____

Smoking _____

Alcohol use—How much? _____

Activity/exercise—What and how often? _____

Other health supplements/substances _____

Health Care Services

Do you feel you have adequate health care? _____

Do you feel you have enough money to pay medical bills? _____

Socioeconomic Needs

Do you have adequate shelter? _____

Do you feel you have enough money for clothing? _____

Do you feel you have enough money for personal care items? _____

Have you had a recent change in the family or your support system? _____

Are there any other factors affecting your nutrition? _____

Ht _____ Wt _____ Wt gain _____ Wt loss _____ How long _____

Figure 26-7 Nutrition Screening Initiative 10-Point Screen

The warning signs of poor nutritional health are often overlooked. Use this checklist to find out if you or someone you know is at nutritional risk. Remember that warning signs suggest risk but do not represent a diagnosis of any condition. Read the *determine* list, below, to learn more about the warning signs of poor nutritional health.

Read the statements below. Circle the number in the "yes" column for those that apply to you or someone you know. For each "yes" answer, score the number in the box. Total your nutritional score.

	YES
I have an illness or condition that made me change the kind and/or amount of food I eat.	2
I eat fewer than 2 meals per day.	3
I eat few fruits or vegetables or milk products.	2
I have 3 or more drinks of beer, liquor, or wine almost every day.	2
I have tooth or mouth problems that make it hard for me to eat.	2
I don't always have enough money to buy the food I need.	4
I eat alone most of the time.	1
I take 3 or more different prescribed or over-the-counter drugs a day.	1
Without wanting to, I have lost or gained 10 pounds in the last 6 months.	2
I am not always physically able to shop, cook, and/or feed myself.	2
TOTAL	

Total your nutritional score. If it's—

0–2   Good! Recheck your nutritional score in 6 months.

3–5   You are at moderate nutritional risk. See what can be done to improve your eating habits and lifestyle. Your office on aging, senior nutrition program, senior citizens center, or health department can help. Recheck your nutritional score in 3 months.

6 or more   You are at high nutritional risk. Bring this checklist the next time you see your doctor, dietitian, or other qualified health or social service professional. Talk with them about any problems you may have. Ask for help to improve your nutritional health.

The nutrition checklist is based on the warning signs described below. Use the word DETERMINE to remind you of the warning signs.

Disease Any disease, illness, or chronic condition that causes you to change the way you eat, or makes it hard for you to eat, puts your nutritional health at risk. Four out of five adults have chronic diseases that are affected by diet. Confusion or memory loss that keeps getting worse is estimated to affect one out of five or more of older adults. This can make it hard to remember what, when, or if you've eaten. Feeling sad or depressed, which happens to about one in eight older adults, can cause big changes in appetite, digestion, energy level, weight, and well-being.

Eating poorly Eating too little and eating too much both lead to poor health. Eating the same foods day after day or not eating fruit, vegetables, and milk products daily will also cause poor nutritional health. One in five adults skip meals daily. Only 13% of adults eat the minimum amount of fruit and vegetables needed. One in four older adults drink too much alcohol. Many health problems become worse if you drink more than one or two alcoholic beverages per day.

Tooth loss/mouth pain A healthy mouth, teeth, and gums are needed to eat. Missing, loose, or rotten teeth or dentures that don't fit well, or cause mouth sores, make it hard to eat.

Economic hardship As many as 40% of older Americans have incomes of less than $6,000 per year. Having less—or choosing to spend less—than $25–$30 per week for food makes it very hard to get the foods you need to stay healthy.

Reduced social contact One-third of all older people live alone. Being with people daily has a positive effect on morale, well-being, and eating.

Multiple medicines Many older Americans must take medicines for health problems. Almost half of older Americans take multiple medicines daily. Growing old may change the way we respond to drugs. The more medicines you take, the greater the chance for side effects such as increased or decreased appetite, change in taste, constipation, weakness, drowsiness, diarrhea, nausea, and others. Vitamins or minerals, when taken in large doses, act like drugs and can cause harm. Alert your doctor to everything you take.

Involuntary weight loss/gain Losing or gaining a lot of weight when you are not trying to do so is an important warning sign that must not be ignored. Being overweight or underweight also increases your chance of poor health.

Needs assistance in self-care Although most older people are able to eat, one of every five has trouble walking, shopping, buying and cooking food, especially as they get older.

Elder years above age 80 Most older people lead full and productive lives. But as age increases, risks of frailty and health problems increase. Checking your nutritional health regularly makes good sense.

Reprinted with permission by the Nutrition Screening Initiative, a project of the American Academy of Family Physicians, the American Dietetic Association, and the National Council on the Aging, Inc., and funded in part by a grant from Ross Products Division of Abbott Laboratories.

Perspectives...

Insights of a Home Health Care Nurse

Missy was going on vacation for a week in April, and the rest of her team had to cover her home health care patients while she was gone. I got Bessie B. and Calvin T. I had heard comments about Calvin in the office, none of them ever good. The agency had considered canceling his visits twice, something about cooperation and not being there for visits. I read Missy's file on Calvin before the first visit. An 82-year-old black male, Calvin lived alone in a rundown home in an older part of town and had multiple diagnoses. Missy was doing sterile dressing changes to stage 3 wounds on both feet. He had NIDDM, stage IV, CHF, cardiomyopathy, and nutritional deficits. She had scribbled on the side, "grumpy man."

Because Missy had been his only nurse for a while, I was prepared to win his acceptance. I brought food, homemade muffins. When I pulled up to the old house, I noticed that part of the siding was falling off, the porch was sagging, and the yard was just dirt.

As I stood at the front door for a long time, I thought about his not being home for the visit. No such luck. Calvin was yelling at me from the back of the house. I could understand the curse words and something about ringing the bell and making him come to the door. When he stood in the doorway, he blocked all the light and just looked huge to me! Then I noticed he had a shotgun in his arms; it was as long as he was tall. "Oh great," I thought, "Missy didn't say anything about any weapons." I was determined to complete all of Missy's visits that week. I waited for him to open the screen door, but he just turned and took his seat on the nearby couch. "Ok, I'll just let myself in," I thought. I introduced myself, but he just called me Missy anyway. He was still rambling on about why did I ring the bell and just get in here and he didn't have all day. So on that pleasant note, I thought I'd better be quick about the rest of the visit.

I offered him the plate of muffins. Before I could even get the words out about what kind they were, he grabbed two of them and put them on his lap and stuffed one of them into his mouth before I even set my bag down. He was grumbling something while he was eating. Then he said loudly, "Where the coffee, Missy?" He looked straight at me as if I were his hostess or his wife, so I went looking for the kitchen and the coffee. Feeling triumphant that I had made a cup of black coffee, I returned, only to be sent back for creamer. Then I was sent back for sugar. Then I was sent back for a bigger spoon. Then I was sent back for a towel. I still had not even started his dressings! The foot dressings finally got done, as did the rest of the assessment. I was finally done with Calvin and only 45 minutes behind schedule. The end of the week finally came, and I celebrated when Missy came back and I could return Calvin to her.

Two months later, our team of cardiovascular home health nurses was adjusting client assignments. I got Calvin T. again, only this time it was for the duration of his care. I was determined to make this work. It was now late June.

When I arrived at Calvin's house this time, there were green plants growing on the side of his house where there had been just dirt before. As a gardener, I couldn't help but notice how large and healthy the plants were. Those green plants were the beginnings of cabbage, zucchini, squash, tomatoes, and collard greens. One of the advantages I enjoyed about home health care was being outside. In the summer, before starting my visits, I would work in my garden. The early morning air was cool and crisp. The atmosphere was quiet and peaceful, before all the hubbub of the day started. The lighting was soft, and the dew was often still on the plants.

I didn't realize I had made it halfway down the sidewalk admiring and identifying each group of plants when I literally ran into Calvin. I screamed, and he laughed a hearty bass laugh. We talked gardening for at least 15 minutes, like two school girls sharing some new gossip. I learned he lived to tend his garden. He took great pride in his ability to provide food for himself. Gardening opened the door to getting to know Calvin and providing for his needs.

Continued

(Continued)

A routine unfolded over the rest of the summer for Calvin and me. I came to visit Calvin very early in the day so I could help him in the garden and help him get back into the house to dress his feet. I learned that Calvin could barely walk because of his neuropathy and peripheral vascular disease. He "saved his walking time for his garden." He was an early riser like me, and he had figured out that he could be in the garden longer after a night's sleep than in midday or afternoon.

He preferred to go in the garden barefoot because the soil was cool and soft and reminded him of gardening as a child. Eventually, I was able to persuade him to wear some old slip-on shoes to cover and protect the dressings while he was in the garden. The wound clinic doctor commented on how clean his feet were and how much faster the wounds were healing.

We made some progress on his nutrition. I made sure he ate breakfast. Sometimes I cooked; sometimes the aide cooked. I brought him cases of Ensure from the food bank, when they had them. He "paid for the Ensure" (he didn't take "no charity, Missy") with fresh squash, zucchini, and tomatoes, which the food bank needed. He kept a cooler near his seat on the couch where we put a couple of cans of Ensure for his lunch. I found an old ottoman for him to put his feet on through the day to decrease the edema in his legs. Within two months, he had gained 10 pounds, and he continued to gain weight slowly.

I learned that he could see only figures and had a constant buzz in his ears from some of the medications he was on. He kept the shotgun nearby because he was alone. He confessed one day that it was unlikely he could hit a target, but strangers didn't need to know that. He also kept a machete out on the kitchen table at the back of the house for the same reason. The most surprising thing I learned was what he told me on the day he got out his family album. He showed me pictures of his seven children, he ex-wife, his grandchildren, and himself. He had been a coal miner and weighed about 250 pounds in his prime! After that, if I asked, he would share little tidbits of his life and what he had learned in life.

By late that fall, his wounds were healed and it was time to discharge Calvin from home care. On my last official visit, I explained one more time that I wouldn't be coming to see him anymore. He said, "That's ok Missy, I'm gettin' along pretty good now." And I didn't mind being called Missy anymore.

—*Sue Chubinski, RN*

factors that may influence their nutritional status. Please note the inclusion of the risk factors in the nutritional assessment tool. Figure 26-6 can be used in conjunction with Table 26-6. Figure 26-7 shows the Nutrition Screening Initiative 10-point screen. It can be used for clients 60 years old and older. This ten-point screening can quickly determine nutritional risk, but it is not as comprehensive as the assessment for nutritional problems shown in Figure 26-6.

THE FUTURE FOR THE COMMUNITY HEALTH NURSE

Good nutrition management is an important part of any wellness program (Cookfair, 1996). Whether in clinics, in the home, or in community education programs, nutritional counseling is a critical component. Although problematic nutritional issues must be addressed, education about healthy nutrition throughout the life span must also occur. The 1995 mid-decade report on *Healthy People 2000* goals indicates that we still have challenges in the area of hunger, especially with children and elders. We still have disproportionate health between whites and minorities, but we are moving in the right direction on two-thirds of the nation's goals for a healthier population. These issues will continue to shape the direction of health care for the future (USDHHS, 1996).

Key Concepts

- Nutrition has been identified as an integral part of achieving health for all.

- Socioeconomics, food supply, behavior, and biology are considered factors that affect nutrition.

COMMUNITY NURSING VIEW

Evelyn is an 88-year-old widow who continued to live in her own home after her husband, Edgar, died just a year ago. Evelyn was independent and drove to the grocery store, church, and beauty shop. Evelyn and Edgar had always enjoyed the company of friends for dinner and cards. Evelyn was proud of the fact that she had stayed home to raise her children and had been a good homemaker.

For the past several months, her neighbor Hilda thought something was wrong. Evelyn forgot Hilda's birthday. Evelyn was taking her walks in baggy, rumpled old clothes. Hilda worried about what else might be going on. Hilda persuaded Evelyn to see her doctor. Hilda explained her concerns and her observations to the doctor.

After the doctor completed a physical examination and had some blood drawn, he suggested that Evelyn consider moving to a nursing home. He was very concerned about her 20-pound weight loss since her physical last year. Evelyn started to cry and stated that she wanted to stay in her own home. The doctor reluctantly agreed but only for a trial period and only with certain conditions. The doctor's conditions were that Evelyn would have a home health care nurse visit her, take daily vitamins, and work on gaining weight. He told Evelyn that Hilda would be making unannounced visits to see of she was taking better care of herself. He gave her three months to work on these conditions.

Nursing Considerations

ASSESSMENT
- What observations prompted Hilda to be concerned?
- What objective data did the doctor have?

DIAGNOSIS
- Which nursing diagnoses apply to Evelyn's problems?
- What contributed to the development of Evelyn's problems?

OUTCOME/IDENTIFICATION
- What changes do you want to see in three months for Evelyn?
- How much weight can she realistically gain in three months?

PLANNING/INTERVENTIONS
- Name at least three methods that Evelyn could use to improve her nutrition.
- How could Meals on Wheels help?
- How will the home health care visits help?
- How could friends and neighbors help?

EVALUATION
- What changes would you expect in three months with the above program?
- What would the doctor measure?
- What observations would the home health care nurse or aide make?
- What observations would Hilda make?

- Poverty has been identified as one of the most powerful factors in determining health and nutritional outcomes.
- Poverty, education, and cultural and religious practices are key socioeconomic factors that can influence nutrition.
- Food quality, safety, quantity, and access are determinants of a sufficient food supply.
- Fast food is quickly becoming a nutritional risk for many clients.
- Weight maintenance, exercise, rest, lifestyle choices, health knowledge, and health access are behavioral factors affecting nutrition.
- Nutritional risks and problems exist at all stages of life.

- To lessen infant nutritional risk, the community health nurse should educate parents about infant nutrition, encourage participation in prenatal care and parenting classes, conduct postnatal visits, and offer referral to food assistance programs as warranted.
- Childhood nutritional risk factors include poverty, limited food supply, poor education of parents, and lack of health information.
- Substances such as alcohol, tobacco, cocaine, and marijuana put a client at risk of nutritional deficits.
- Eating disorders generally start during the adolescent and teen years.
- Young adulthood tends to be a healthy time in which good nutritional habits should continue to be practiced to lessen the effects of aging.

- Obesity has been found to be a nutritional problem that spans the stages of life.
- Risk factors related to nutrition for older and elderly adults include decreased appetite and food intake, poor dentition, decreased sense of thirst, vision loss, and food and drug interaction.

- The effects of chronic illness, diabetes, cancer, osteoporosis, and cardiovascular disease can be managed with proper nutrition.
- The community health nurse should assess clients' nutritional risk and be prepared to offer assistance and referral to proper agencies and professionals.

Homelessness

Mary Beatrice Hennessey, RN, MSN

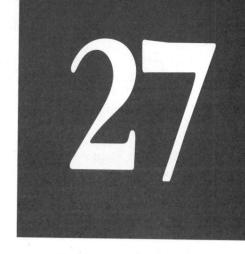

We all deserve the basics of life. Nobody should be allowed to freeze to death, to starve to death. What we need most of all is acceptance and love.

—Sullivan, 1982

COMPETENCIES

Upon completion of this chapter, the reader should be able to:

- Discuss the history and present scope of homelessness in the United States.
- Discuss at least four factors that could increase a person's risk of becoming homeless.
- Identify two ways that private groups and two ways that public agencies have attempted to deal with the problem of homelessness.
- Describe the pioneering role that nurses have played in bringing health care to the homeless.
- List and examine the features of homelessness that lead to poor health.
- Discuss five health problems that pose a particular threat to homeless people.
- Describe intervention strategies at each level of prevention.

Over the past two decades, the number of homeless men, women, and children has increased dramatically, to perhaps as many as 3 million people in the United States. Economic, political, and sociological factors have contributed to this increase. Private sector and public sector agencies have combined forces to seek innovative ways to deal with the problem. Homeless people tend to have more health problems than the general population and, once ill, to have difficulties managing their health problems.

Nurses have been at the forefront in bringing health care to homeless people. By employing strategies at the primary, secondary, and tertiary levels of prevention, the community health nurse can continue to have a powerful impact in increasing access to care and improving the general health of homeless people.

The Pine Street Inn shelter, I don't believe it! Isn't that some flophouse for drunks? Did the school run out of hospitals to send us to? I know one thing, I'm not going there. I'll quit school first.

That was the reaction of one nursing student to her community/mental health assignment in 1979. It was typical of the reactions of students assigned to a 250-bed shelter for homeless men in downtown Boston. The students were to spend a semester at a volunteer nurses' clinic established at the shelter seven years earlier. Very little had been written about homelessness. The problem had yet to attract the attention of the media or social activists.

I was so scared. I don't think it's fair to make us go out into the lobby to talk to those people. The clinic is one thing, but to just *talk* to them . . . Who knows what they're going to do? But you know, the ones I talked to were nice . . . I mean . . . . they're people!

That was the reaction of a nursing student in 1996 on the first day of her rotation at the Pine Street Inn, which now houses close to a thousand men and women. Much has been written about homelessness, and the problem has certainly received the attention of the media and social activists; yet misconceptions and stereotypes persist.

Homelessness is a complex and controversial issue. Discussions regarding definition, accurate census, causes, and solutions often lead to heated debate.

There is no general agreement on definition. Some include only the people who are living on the streets and in emergency shelters. Others include people living in abandoned buildings, in camping areas, and in single room occupancy hotels. Still others include people believed to be on the verge of homelessness because they have doubled up with families or friends in overcrowded apartments. Baum and Burnes (1993) believe that the term *homeless* is itself misleading, because it focuses on only one aspect of an individual's situation. This focus, they fear, will lead to interventions that fail to consider individual differences.

The lack of an agreed-upon definition, as well as the difficulties in counting an often transient population, has led to widely varying estimates of the numbers of homeless people. Numbers estimated by advocates are often 10 times those cited by government agencies. In the mid-1980s, for example, the U.S. Department of Housing and Urban Development (HUD) estimated the number of homeless people to be between 250,000 and 350,000, while, at the same time, the late Mitch Snyder, head of the Washington, D.C.–based Community for Creative Non-Violence, came up with an often quoted number of 3 million homeless people (Snyder & Hombs, 1986). More recently, the Federal Task Force on Homelessness and Severe Mental Illness (1992) estimated that there are 600,000 homeless people in the United States. The continuing debate was the topic of a special section of the July 1995 issue of the *American Journal of Orthopsychiatry* (Bassuk, 1995). A recent review by the Coalition of the Homeless (1997) of studies of the homeless over the years 1987–1997 found that shelter capacity had more than doubled in nine communities and three states. The number of shelter beds in demand is another measure that is used to determine need. Despite the disagreement on the actual number, however, all sources seem to agree that the number is too high and is rising.

The debate becomes even more heated when the causes of homelessness are discussed. Kozol (1988, p. 12) states emphatically that "the cause of homelessness is lack of housing." Baum and Burnes (1993) think that stance homogenizes a disparate population, confuses poverty with disabling conditions, and leads to the inaccurate conclusion that a single solution is sufficient to solve the problem.

The National Coalition for the Homeless (1998) cites the following causes of increasing homelessness: increasing poverty from eroding work opportunities and the decline in public assistance, lack of affordable housing and the inadequacy of housing and the inadequacy of housing assistance programs, lack of affordable health care, domestic violence, mental illness, and chemical dependency. These issues are addressed in other chapters throughout this book.

It is not the purpose of this chapter to resolve or even take sides in these debates. The interested student can find many compelling arguments for conflicting viewpoints in the literature. The main focus of the chapter is on the health care needs of homeless populations and the role of the community health nurse in meeting those needs. The chapter begins with a brief review of the history of homelessness, discusses its impact on individuals, families, and communities, and describes private and public responses to the problem.

HISTORICAL DEVELOPMENT OF HOMELESSNESS

In the 1950s and 1960s, the idea of large numbers of people in the United States with no permanent address, huddled in doorways, living in shantytowns or squatter settlements, begging on the streets, and searching garbage for sustenance was unthinkable. These were things that people did in developing countries, in famine- and drought-ravaged Africa, in overcrowded India, in poverty-stricken South America. Such problems, it was believed, could not exist in affluent, industrialized societies.

However, there have been homeless people in the United States throughout its history. The numbers have fluctuated in response to economic and political events. Interestingly, early efforts to deal with the problem were aimed, mainly, at providing institutional care for the mentally ill (Jones, 1983). In the first half of the 20th century, the Great Depression and the World Wars added numbers to the homeless ranks.

In 1963 the Mental Retardation and Community Mental Health Center Construction Act was passed. This led to large scale **deinstitutionalization** of patients in state mental hospitals (Bassuk & Gerson, 1978; Riesdorph-Ostrow, 1989). Supervised living arrangements and follow-up treatment were to be arranged within the community for the discharged patients released. Because community-based resources were never adequate to meet their needs, many of the deinstitutionalized people found themselves with no place to go. Concurrently, the decriminalization of alcoholism and public drunkenness left on the streets many chronic alcoholics who might have previously spent the night in jail cells.

The 1970s trend toward urban renewal led to displacement of many poor families and a sharp decline in available single room occupancy dwellings (Baum & Burnes,

1993). A dramatic rise in unemployment to 9.7% in 1982, coupled with a decrease in unemployment benefits, increased the number of families living below the poverty line (Burt, 1992). Other major factors such as condominium development, increased rents, and decreased federal funds to build or rehabilitate low-income housing further reduced the housing supply and placed decent, affordable housing out of the reach of many (Kozol, 1988).

Recent Developments and Scope of the Problem

During the 1980s, the problem of homelessness burst upon the public awareness. For example, the subject heading "Homeless Persons" is not found in the *Cumulated Index Medicus* until 1986, but in that year alone there are 39 citations under that title. As both advocates and government agencies reported an increase in numbers, the visibility of homelessness also increased.

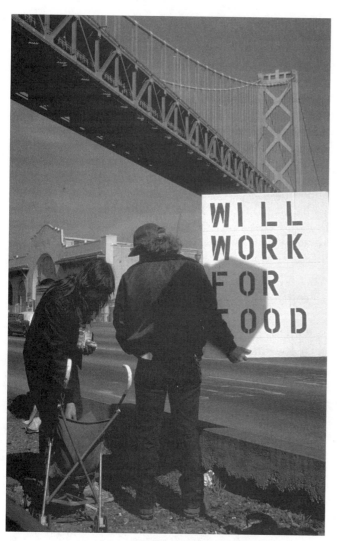

The visible homeless shape the public perception of the homeless; however, the homeless population includes diverse types of people and circumstances. Photo courtesy of Morton Beebe–S.F./Corbis.

Harrington (1962), in his classic work, *The Other America: Poverty in the United States*, spoke of "the invisible poor." He described the poor as being segregated from the rest of the populace, in both urban neighborhoods and rural settings. He warned that urban renewal would force poor people into slums and that poverty, lack of education, and lack of medical care would force people from their rural homes into the cities, where they would become misfits. He expressed concern that the poor's lack of visibility keeps them out of public awareness and therefore off the public agenda.

By contrast, some of today's homeless people make themselves quite visible in urban settings. They can be seen **panhandling**, or begging on city streets. Some wear signs saying such things as "Help the homeless" or "I am a father of two. I work for food." They might approach cars at stoplights, wipe the windshield, and ask for a handout. The visible homeless, although a small sample, often shape the public perception of the whole population.

Careful studies of the homeless population have always revealed diversity. The stereotypes, which reflect only the most visible, have never presented a true picture of the population and have often interfered with efforts to help. The generic term *homeless* implies that the individuals in this group have more in common than they actually do. This perception is especially so today, as families with young children, the majority headed by women, constitute 36.5% of the overall number (Bassuk, Weinreb, Buckner, Browner, et al., 1996).

According to Marin and Vacha (1994), poor households provide most of the housing for the homeless by allowing friends and family members to share their living space. When families who have doubled up or tripled up and families who pay more than half of their income to rent or mortgage are considered, there are an increasing number of families living on the brink of homelessness.

Although several studies have been done in an attempt to describe homeless people, care must be taken not to generalize the results, which may say more about the locus of the study than about the homeless population as a whole. Large urban shelters, for example, often serve only an adult population. A study conducted at one such shelter in Massachusetts (Bassuk, 1983) showed a median age of 34, with a four-to-one male-to-female ratio; 77% of the population was white, 22% black, and 1% Hispanic. More than two-thirds had graduated from high school. Gelberg, Gallagher, Andersen, and Korgel (1997) describe the homeless population in their study. They found that 80% were male, 63% were aged 18–41, and slightly over half were African American.

The U.S. Conference of Mayors (1995) in a 29-city survey reported that single men accounted for 46% of the homeless population; families with children, 36.5%; single women, 14%, and unaccompanied youth, 3.5%. They reported that 56% of the homeless population was black, 27% white, 13% Hispanic, 3% Native American, and 1% Asian. See Figure 27-1. Ringwalt, Green, Robertson, and McPheeters (1998) found that 5% of youth aged 12–17 were homeless for at least one night of the past year.

Delegates at the 89th National Convention of the Veterans of Foreign Wars addressed the issue of homeless veterans, describing the situation as "a grave embarrassment" and a "national disgrace." By their figures, 30% of homeless people are veterans. Of this group, 31% reported combat experience, 37.8% had served during the Vietnam era, 82% had completed high school, and 44% had a skilled or high-level occupation (Scharfman, Anderson, & Maus, 1989). In 1997, the U.S. Conference of Mayors' survey of 29 American cities found that 22% of the urban homeless population were veterans (National Coalition of the Homeless, 1998).

Etiology

The origins of the current homelessness situation are complex. Economic, social, personal, and political influences all contribute to this growing crisis.

Economic Influences

Throughout the years, persons who study homelessness and those who work with homeless people have linked the problem with the economy. Today, many U.S. citizens are unable to afford housing. Rossi (1994) states that family homelessness reflects extreme poverty precipitated by the restructuring of the American labor force. He cites widespread unemployment and underemployment, particularly among minority groups, a decline in the real value of federal Aid to Families with Dependent Children (AFDC) payments, and a reduction in the stock of inexpensive rental housing as contributing factors. As the cost of buying or renting a home increases, so does the gap between the rich and the poor. In 1993, the top 20% of U.S. households received 48.9% of the aggregate income, while the bottom 20% received only 3.6% (Bassuk et al., 1996).

Especially affected are female-headed families. Bassuk et al. (1996) report that in 1993 nearly 36% of all families headed by women were living under the federally established poverty level. This percentage was even higher for African American and Latino female-headed families, with rates of 49.9% and 52.6%, respectively.

Also affected by economic changes are many elderly men and women who, despite what had appeared to be adequate planning, find themselves on a fixed income that is insufficient to meet even their most basic needs for food and shelter. Some manage to stay in their homes, stretching their meager pension money by using soup kitchens and elderly meal sites. Others end up in shelters. These forms of support are discussed in detail later in this chapter.

Many people now in the shelter system are eligible for some sort of economic relief from sources such as Social Security, the Veterans' Administration, Workers' Compensation. Often they are unaware of their eligibility status. Even when they have the knowledge, the nature of their disability or the powerlessness inherent in being homeless, or both, may make it difficult, if not impossible, to obtain services on their own if, in fact, services are even available (NCH, 1998).

Some observers believe that the economics of homelessness has been overplayed and that a focus on economics leads to a new, but equally inaccurate, stereotype of homeless people. They express concern that this perspective will lead to the belief that housing alone is sufficient to solve the problem (Baum & Burnes, 1993).

Social Influences

The family as a social unit has undergone tremendous change and has become less stable (Bassuk, Rubin, & Lauriat, 1986). Changes date back to the Industrial Revolution, which brought a shift from rural to urban living.

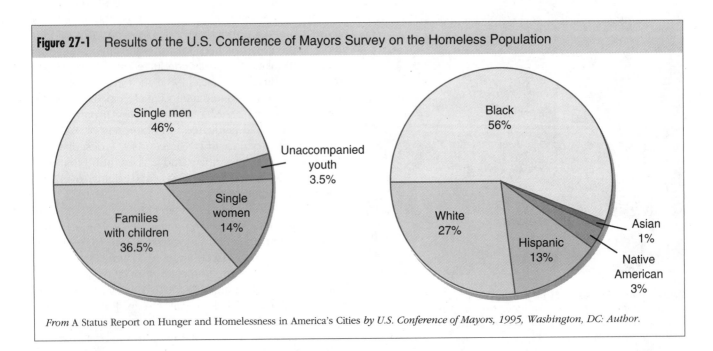

Figure 27-1   Results of the U.S. Conference of Mayors Survey on the Homeless Population

Single men 46%
Unaccompanied youth 3.5%
Single women 14%
Families with children 36.5%

Black 56%
White 27%
Hispanic 13%
Asian 1%
Native American 3%

From A Status Report on Hunger and Homelessness in America's Cities *by U.S. Conference of Mayors, 1995, Washington, DC: Author.*

Often, a nuclear family moved, leaving the extended family behind, changing roles and expectations of all family members. In the last 25 years, the role of women has changed dramatically; women are now able to make choices regarding education, employment, and childbearing. It is now quite common to have both parents working, and children are often left in the care of outside agencies.

Attitudes regarding sex and marriage have also changed, and the marriage union has become less stable. There is more sexual freedom outside of marriage for both men and women, and divorce is no longer viewed as the catastrophe it once was. For poor families, however, the disruption of family ties and the experience of divorce can be quite catastrophic. One result is an increase in single-parent homeless families. McMurray (1990) states that most studies fail to recognize the impact of family dissolution on homelessness. The loss of extended family and community support has had an especially strong impact on single mothers. Wagner and Menke (1991) found that homeless mothers experienced significantly more stressors than their domiciled counterparts. Unsafe living situations, inadequate child support and child care options, low wages, job discrimination, the stress of homelessness, and the threat of violence all add to the problems of the homeless mother (Bassuk, 1993; Shinn & Weitzman, 1996).

Personal Influences

Individual circumstances and personal characteristics place some people at a higher risk of becoming homeless. Most notable among these are the presence of physical or mental disability and addiction to drugs or alcohol (Baum & Burnes, 1993; Buckner et al., 1997). These factors will be examined more closely in the section on health issues of the homeless. Other factors include educational level, marketable skills, family violence, and availability of personal supports.

Poverty and homelessness have been tightly linked, and homeless people have been referred to as the poorest of the poor. Among the main causes of homelessness identified by the U.S. Conference of Mayors (1995) are unemployment and other employment-related problems, the lack of affordable housing, substance abuse and the lack of needed services, mental illness and the lack of needed services, domestic violence, family crises, and poverty or insufficient income. See also NCH, 1998.

Political Influences

Examples of how political policy can affect the numbers of homeless people and their access to health care can be seen at all levels of government. The allocation of funds and the rules and restrictions regarding their use determine who will be helped, and how. Thus far, much of the aid at all levels has been aimed at emergency intervention without attention to the complex and diverse needs of the population or to their need for permanent housing.

At the local level, examples can be seen in zoning legislation. These laws often prohibit transitional housing or remove the incentives for developing low-cost residential housing.

An example at the state level can be seen in the laws regarding the care of the mentally ill, which have resulted in many psychotic individuals' being left on the streets to fend for themselves. Many advocates fear that the Personal Responsibility and Work Act passed by Congress in August of 1996 will have a similar effect. This welfare reform bill replaces the federal welfare system by shifting the responsibility for administration to the states (Katz, 1996). States are awarded block grants and, with some federal guidelines, decide who receives benefits. The act limits recipients to five years of eligibility and requires that they find work within two years. At the U.S. Conference of Mayors in 1995, St. Louis Mayor Bosley expressed concern that welfare reform would lead to increased hunger and homelessness, increased stress on families and communities, fewer housing options, and less child care. Detroit officials estimated a three-fold increase in the number of families needing emergency shelter if only 1 percent of current AFDC recipients lose benefits (Worsnop, 1996).

Numerous examples of public policy that may have exacerbated homelessness have been cited at the federal level. Kozol (1988) asserts that during the early 1980s "the White House cut virtually all federal funds to build or rehabilitate low-income housing. Federal support for low-income housing dropped from $28 billion to $9 billion between 1981 and 1986" (p. 13). Redburn and Buss (1986) suggest that the reduction of federal social welfare spending, together with stricter eligibility requirements for benefits during the Reagan years, is another explanation for the rise of homelessness. Another example at the federal level can be seen in income tax laws that provide

REFLECTIVE THINKING

Homelessness

Imagine that this happened to you.

You are a new graduate nurse who, having difficulty finding a full-time job, found a part-time job on a medical-surgical unit of a local hospital. This is your first nursing job and it pays well but has no fringe benefits. A few weeks ago you moved into a very nice apartment. While moving some boxes into your new apartment, you severely injured your back. It will be well over a year before you will be able to work again. You have no health insurance.

- Will you be able to continue to afford the rather high rent on your apartment? Do you have savings or other assets to support you for a while? Do you have family or friends who will support you? For how long?

- Who is going to pay your extensive medical bills?

- What benefits might be available to you?

loopholes for the rich while putting a heavier tax burden on those with less money. There has been a decline in public assistance in recent years. The Personal Responsibility and Work Opportunity Reconciliation Act of 1996 replaced the Aid to Families with Dependent Children (AFDC) program with a block grant program called Temporary Assistance to Needy Families (TANF). TANF benefits are below the poverty level and in many states are below 75% of the poverty level (NCH, 1998).

Other industrialized countries have also reported an increase in homelessness. Within the countries of Western Europe, Great Britain has the largest and most visible population of homeless people (Toro & Rojansky, 1990; Schmidt, 1992). Cohen (1994) compared homelessness in London with that in New York City. He found numerical comparisons difficult but stated that both the government figures and those of advocates indicate that New York City has three to 30 times more street people than London. Members of minority groups tend to be overrepresented in both cities. He found remarkable parallels in government philosophy during the Reagan and Thatcher years and concluded that "although individual life experiences and personal attributes, such as mental illness, surely increase vulnerability to homelessness, this comparative analysis of New York City and London suggests that structural factors, such as government policy and socioeconomic variables, play a dominant role in the creation and mitigation of homelessness" (p. 775).

In 1986 there were virtually no people living on the streets in Japan. In 1996, according to government statistics, there were 3,300 homeless people in Tokyo. Social workers say the number is closer to 10,000. The economic recession and the decay of the family as a unit are cited as precipitants (Kakuchi, 1996).

IMPACT OF HOMELESSNESS

Homelessness has profound effects on the individual, the family, and the community. Community health nurses

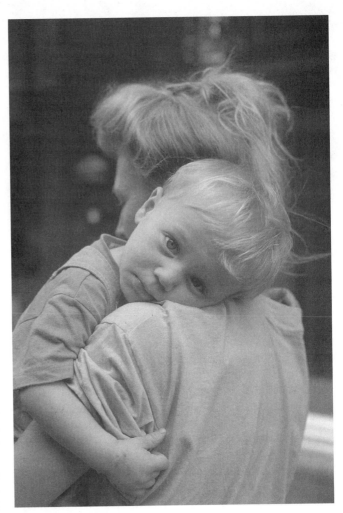

One of the faces of homelessness. *Photo courtesy of Owen Franken/Corbis.*

need to understand these effects before they can devise meaningful interventions.

Impact on the Individual

Being homeless is devastating to the individual. A sense of powerlessness and low self-esteem are reinforced time and again throughout the day. Misunderstood, feared, ridiculed, avoided, and stereotyped, the homeless suffer a continual barrage of assaults to their sense of self. The feeling of worthlessness that low self-esteem generates can block motivation to find employment, housing, and other essential needs (DiBlasio & Belcher, 1993). Sleeping in a different place every night, often with no choice as to where or with whom, leads to disorientation and dissociation. The longer the person is on the street, the more difficult it is to become domiciled again. The individual is trapped in a vicious circle. A person needs income in order to afford a place to live, but the lack of a fixed address limits employment opportunities and, in many cases, excludes the person from benefits.

In *Travels with Lisbeth*, Eighner (1993) describes three years of living on the streets, traveling between Texas and

DECISION MAKING

Factors of Homelessness

List the factors that have led to the increasing numbers of homeless people in the United States over the past 25 years.

• Take any one of the identified factors and discuss, in retrospect, how community health nurses might have intervened to lessen the impact of this particular factor.

• What actions can community health nurses take at the present time to lessen the impact of this particular factor?

California with his dog, Lisbeth. He describes his experiences of searching through dumpsters and finding places to sleep as well as his interactions with dogcatchers, police, and doctors. His firsthand stories are vivid and articulate. Despite his often humorous accounts, he describes most days on the streets as consisting of unrelenting boredom. Lack of direction and the absence of progress, he states, make time nearly meaningless.

Impact on the Family

Much has been written about the effect of homelessness on the American family. In *Rachel and Her Children*, Kozol (1988) vividly portrays the plight of the homeless family, documenting the effects of living in welfare hotels, constantly moving, losing neighborhood connections, frequently changing schools, and so on. Bassuk, Rubin, and Lauriat (1986) and Zima, Bussing, Forness, and Benjamin (1997) have shown that homeless children exhibit a wide range of psychological, social, and cognitive problems as well as lags in physical and emotional development.

An area yet to be studied is the impact on the family when one of its members becomes homeless. Parents, spouses, and children of homeless people have often tried in vain to seek help for a homeless family member. There is a stigma attached to alcoholism, addiction, and psychiatric problems. When homelessness is added to one of these conditions, it is very difficult for family members to seek and receive support.

Impact on the Community

Homelessness is a community problem. Communities suffer when so many of the members are suffering. Unfortunately many members of the community refuse to recognize and take responsibility for the problem. This disregard for the homeless and their problems can be seen in the language people use, often referring to the homeless as "those people." It can be seen in the so-called NIMBY (Not In My Back Yard) syndrome.

RESPONSES TO THE PROBLEM

Both public and private organizations and agencies are developing programs to help homeless people. The community health nurse needs to be aware of both types of programs and how they can be used individually and collectively to meet the needs of the homeless population.

Responses from the Private Sector

Until the 1960s, much of the help that homeless people received was carried out by volunteer civic and church groups who founded shelters and soup kitchens. Some

REFLECTIVE THINKING

Solutions to Homelessness: An Analogy

A woman with a severe circulatory disorder developed a blister on her left foot; without treatment, the blister became an ulcer. The ulcer frightened her so much that she ignored it, hoping it would just go away. When it didn't, she put a Band-Aid on it. Seeing no improvement, she became increasingly angry and upset. She continued to add Band-Aids until osteomyelitis developed. Her pain was so severe that by the time it became necessary, she readily agreed to amputation.

• Can you see an analogy between this story and society's manner of dealing with homelessness?

• Can you identify "Band-Aid solutions" that have been used to deal with community problems in your neighborhood?

• What strategies might be helpful to move beyond the "Band-Aid solutions?"

were small, independent efforts; others, such as the Salvation Army, had a national network (Bogue, 1963).

Shelters

Shelters vary greatly from one to another. They range from those that supply only a place to get in out of the weather to those that deliver a wide range of services, including meals, individual counseling, advocacy, health services, day programs, employment training, and rehabilitative facilities. Some shelter providers believe that the provision of a wide range of services legitimizes shelters as an acceptable alternative care system for the homeless and that this type of shelter takes the pressure off other agencies to recognize and work with homeless people. Others think that unless the shelters provide the services, homeless people will go without.

Shelters also vary in terms of who is eligible to receive their services. Some may screen by age, sex, diagnosis, or behavior. Some of this screening is clearly spelled out in written policy, and some is done by more subtle means. Shelter **guests** themselves often have a good feel for who is and who is not welcome at the various shelters. Rules and requirements also vary, making some shelters more or less acceptable to individual guests.

Some shelters are specialized, set up to deal with specific problems. One example is shelters for battered women, where women seeking refuge from an abusive situation can find protection and support for themselves and their children.

Soup Kitchens and Outreach Vans

Food services to homeless people are also provided in a variety of ways, and many are specialized to meet the needs of certain groups. **Soup kitchens** are places where food is offered either free or at a greatly reduced price. These services often provide emotional as well as physical nourishment. Soup kitchens and outreach vans try to meet the needs of homeless people where they live or where they congregate. Soup and a sandwich are generally served by a person who knows and cares about the individual being served. **Meal sites** might cater to a specific population, such as the elderly or women, by offering meals at greatly reduced prices. Being allowed to help with the preparation and serving the meals family style often help a homeless person feel that this is more than just a handout.

Day Programs

Some sites combine luncheon services with a wide range of social, recreational, and health services. Many shelters close their doors during the daytime. Day programs fill the gap and provide much needed services for many.

Responses from the Public Sector

As the homeless population increased in the 1980s, it became apparent to the private sector groups that their efforts were no longer sufficient to meet the growing demand for services. Much of the early lobbying for increased public awareness and government response was the result of the work done by grassroots organizers.

In the mid-1980s, the Robert Wood Johnson Foundation, in partnership with the Pew Charitable Trusts, provided seed money to 19 major cities to help deal with homelessness. The program was cosponsored by the U.S. Conference of Mayors. The purposes of the grants were to develop programs to meet the basic health care needs of homeless people, to improve their access to care and benefits, and to encourage citywide involvement and response. The money was earmarked to be spent in direct care to homeless people with the expectation that services would continue, supported by public funding, when private grant monies ran out. In the first four years of this program, primary care, assessment, and referral services were provided to more than 200,000 homeless persons, and all funded cities found the resources to continue after foundation funding had ended (Somers, Riml, Shmavonian, Waxman, et al., 1990).

Local Programs

Many local municipalities have now become active in providing shelter services for their homeless citizens. Both state and local funds are being used to support them. It is becoming increasingly common to have health clinics at these sites.

State Programs

Response to the crisis at the state level has varied considerably from state to state and over time. A 1984 *Newsweek*

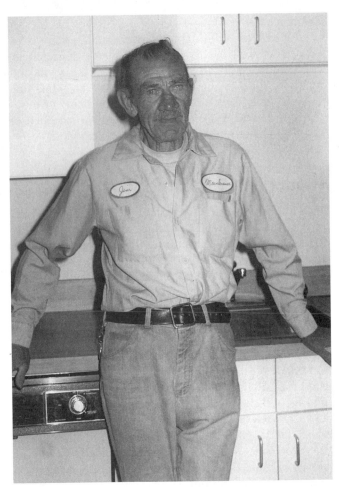

An 86-year-old man, who has lived for many years in a shelter for homeless people, proudly stands in the kitchen he keeps clean at a meal site for the elderly.
Photo courtesy of gentleman pictured.

article compared the response of Arizona with that of Massachusetts, describing them as two extremes. The article reported that Arizona simply wanted the homeless out of the state and used police to aid in this endeavor, discouraging private efforts on behalf of homeless people. An Anti-Skid Row Ordinance was adopted in Phoenix in 1981; four Arizona missions closed their doors under pressure; and a church soup kitchen was sued as a public nuisance. In Massachusetts, on the other hand, there was a commitment to provide shelter for all those needing it. Changes were made in the public welfare laws to enable those without addresses to receive benefits, and steps were taken to increase the supply of low-cost housing (Altman, Buckley, Taylor, & Doherty, 1984).

By contrast, in the results of a 27-city survey on hunger and homelessness conducted in 1990 by the U.S. Conference of Mayors, city officials from Boston expressed concern regarding state budget cuts that had severely affected all community-based programs for the homeless mentally ill and brought to a standstill services for homeless substance abusers (U.S. Conference of Mayors, 1990). In 1996, it was reported that Massachusetts Governor Weld implemented a number of rules designed to deny shelter to families that the state believed were somehow responsible for their loss of housing. These rules reduced the number of families in state-funded shelters by 43% and made it particularly difficult for families on the brink of homelessness, usually headed by single mothers (Kennedy & Reed, 1996).

Because there is such variation from state to state and over time, it is important for nurses to familiarize themselves with the laws and social policies of their particular state and how these affect both the numbers of homeless people and their access to services.

Federal Programs

The federal government has responded to the homeless crisis through a number of agencies. The U.S. Department of Housing and Urban Development (HUD) allocated funds for the expansion of shelter capacity and services. It also encouraged local housing authorities to give priority to homeless families and elderly individuals (U.S. Department of Housing and Urban Development [HUD], 1984). The Federal Emergency Management Agency provided funding for increased shelter and meals. The Department of Defense made certain military facilities available to the homeless, paid for the necessary renovation, and donated blankets and cots to shelters.

The Stewart B. McKinney Homeless Assistance Act was passed in 1987 to provide assistance to homeless people with handicaps. This law, which focuses on vulnerable populations, was designed to organize, coordinate, and enhance federal support to homeless individuals. Among other things, it has provided grant money aimed at developing and supporting a required set of mental health services for mentally ill persons who are homeless or at risk to become so (Mauch & Mulkern, 1992). Breakey (1997) points out that "the Act was intended only as a first step toward addressing the problems of homelessness in America: more far reaching responses were to follow, but have yet to occur" (p. 103). The Department of Agriculture is responsible for the Women, Infants and Children (WIC) program. This program provides shelter and nutrition assistance to families in need.

NURSING CARE OF HOMELESS PEOPLE

In *Healthy People 2000: National Health Promotion and Disease Prevention Objectives* (U.S. Department of Health and Human Services [USDHHS], 1990) a number of major health problems have been identified and objectives set which call for interventions at the primary, secondary, and tertiary levels of prevention. The focus is not only on personal health but also on targeted populations considered at risk. In this publication, it is clearly stated that attainment of the objectives "relies substantially on improved access to and increased use of clinical preventive services." It is further acknowledged that "many

Americans lack access to an ongoing source of primary care, and therefore to essential clinical preventive services as well as to episodic health care" (p. 530). These points were reaffirmed in the 1995 Midcourse Review (USDHHS, 1996).

Nurses have been at the forefront in recognizing the difficulties that homeless people experience in obtaining health care and in developing innovative ways to improve their access to care. Lenehan, McInnis, O'Donnell, and Hennessey (1985) describe the experiences of a group of nurses who, in 1972, brought nursing care to the Pine Street Inn, a large shelter for homeless men in downtown Boston. As emergency room nurses, they had treated guests from the nearby shelter. Often the men arrived intoxicated, disheveled, and unruly. They came to the emergency room for routine care. They returned a few nights later in worse shape, with dirty, unchanged bandages and unfilled prescriptions. It would have been easy to dismiss them as noncompliant and uncaring.

Instead, the nurses embarked on a 30-day experiment to meet the men on their own turf. They brought some supplies and used an office in the shelter. Timidly at first, and at times defensively, the men entered the nurses' clinic. They found that this group of health care professionals was different. They did not present themselves as all-knowing. In fact, in this setting, the nurses were more nervous and less sure of themselves than the men. They were willing to listen and learn from the men. There were communication and caring that had not been felt in the hustle-bustle of the emergency room. The men felt accepted and cared for, even when they did not keep appointments or follow advice. Clinic schedules were arranged for the convenience of the clients rather than the other way around. An attitude of acceptance and consultation helped the client to feel like a partner with the nurse rather than a passive recipient of health care and advice. The nurses' "experimental clinic" continues to this day and has become a national model for health care for the homeless. In the summer of 1995, the Pine Street Inn Clinics, which now number four, were highlighted in *Reflections*, a publication of Sigma Theta Tau, Int., the International Nursing Honor Society. Using basic nursing skills, clinic nurses handled more than 132,000 visits in 1994 (Goldsmith, 1995). They were licensed by the Massachusetts Department of Public Health as a freestanding nurses' clinic in 1996.

There are many advantages to having a nurses' clinic in a shelter for the homeless. With daily contact, the nurse becomes a trusted ally and is able to practice in a preventive role before a crisis develops. Being familiar with a client's baseline health status, the nurse recognizes health threats in the early stages and has concrete data to assist the client in understanding and accepting any need for further intervention. Being in the shelter also allows the nurse to observe trends, recognize environmental hazards, and serve as a role model to other shelter staff.

Nurses practicing in a shelter often experience first-hand the barriers that homeless people encounter in their attempts to obtain health care. They witness the labeling

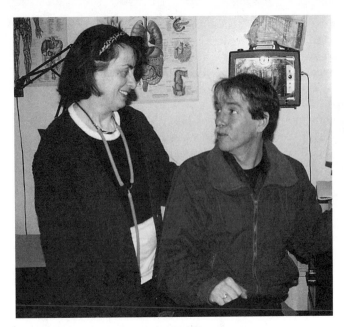

The caring relationship is apparent in this interchange between a nurse and a client in a nurses' clinic located in a shelter for homeless people. Photo courtesy of Pat O'Connor.

and demeaning attitudes a homeless client may encounter. They serve as teachers to other health care providers regarding the needs of homeless people. As advocates and teachers, they facilitate access to needed services for this often underserved population.

The Nurse's Role in Prevention

Early nursing efforts targeting homeless populations describe secondary and tertiary intervention (which was often crisis driven) delivered mainly to middle-aged, white, alcoholic men (Lenehan, et al., 1985). As the population of homeless people increased and became more diverse, the role of community health nurses expanded. They now care for homeless people across the life span and from diverse cultural, ethnic, and minority groups. Primary prevention strategies are often the focus of intervention.

Working in clinics, meal sites, outreach vans, and other places where homeless people congregate, the community health nurse often has the first and most consistent professional contact with a homeless client. Responsibilities include relationship building; triage; first-aid; ongoing treatments; monitoring of health status, medication, and therapeutic diets; health education and referral; and liaison with other health care providers. Relationship building and maintenance of self-esteem are important aspects at all levels of prevention. If a person is treated with dignity and respect, there is a much better chance that advice will be heeded, prescribed treatments followed, and return appointments kept. Efforts are made to plan care *with* rather than *for* the client, so that care plans are tailored to fit the needs and the resources of the individual.

A number of factors can lead to the breakdown of physical and mental health in homeless people. These include (but are not limited to) stress, exposure to extremes of temperature, sleep deprivation, crowded living conditions, inadequate facilities to maintain personal hygiene, poor nutrition, inadequate clothing, and ill-fitting shoes. Following are some examples of how nurses can intervene at each level of prevention in order to eliminate or minimize these risks.

Primary Prevention

In primary prevention, efforts are aimed both at preventing people from becoming homeless and at preventing morbidity in those who are. An assessment of the community will give a picture of the extent of homelessness, a determination of contributing factors, and available resources. The assessment will help the community health nurse plan where efforts will be most effective. Recognizing a client at risk and bolstering available supports might help to maintain a client in the community. Counseling and support services to homeless mothers and homeless pregnant women should help to prevent second-generation homelessness.

Valued and trusted by the community, the nurse's participation in neighborhood associations, on community boards, and in the political process can have a powerful impact on public policy. This involvement will take on particular importance as changes in the welfare regulations are enacted. There are many caring people at neighborhood, state, and federal levels who are influencing policy without understanding the full impact of the policies on human lives. Unlike the nurses, they rarely get close enough to hear the human cries of pain and suffering. Community health nurses must make those cries real to them. At the same time, community health nurses must learn to describe their observations with specific, systematic data reports, lest they be dismissed as "anecdotal."

Once a person becomes homeless, the community health nurse can be a positive influence in the promotion and maintenance of health. Examples include working to ensure safe and sanitary living quarters, the availability of a nutritionally sound diet, adequate ventilation, and the administration of vaccines against influenza and pneumonia. Educational programs can be developed regarding

ꙮꙮ REFLECTIVE THINKING ꙮꙮ

Communication with the Homeless

Accompany a homeless, poorly dressed, or intoxicated individual to a health care setting. Pay attention to both verbal and nonverbal messages that are given.

• Are the messages congruent? Discuss with classmates how verbal and nonverbal communication facilitated or interfered with the care of the client.

specific health threats. One example is programs to prevent acquired immunodeficiency syndrome (AIDS), including safer sexual practices, distribution of condoms, and cleansing of intravenous (IV) drug needles. Pamphlets and other educational materials developed must be geared to the understanding of the client with attention paid to possible language barriers, cultural practices, and illiteracy.

Secondary Prevention

Efforts at the secondary level are aimed at early detection and prevention of disability. Routine screening of shelter staff and guests for tuberculosis and administration of appropriate prophylactic medications are excellent examples of secondary prevention. Other examples include blood pressure screening; teaching breast self-examination; early detection of skin, head and neck, prostate, and other cancers; early detection and treatment of diabetes; treatment of wounds, blisters, and cuts before infection sets in; and monitoring prescribed treatments and medications.

Nurses need to be aware of shelter rules and policies that affect the health of the guests. Shelter rules should be flexible enough to allow guests with health problems, such as high blood pressure, fevers, or casts, to stay inside on days when the weather poses a threat.

Many of the conditions from which homeless people suffer are stigmatizing conditions, as is homelessness itself. The nurse's sensitivity to the client's feelings helps to facilitate trust, allowing the client to give a more complete history. Together they can then develop a care plan that is feasible. Visiting local facilities for the care of homeless people will give the community health nurse a better picture of the day-to-day situation that a homeless person faces. Networking with shelter clinics offers a better understanding of what can and what cannot be accomplished there.

Tertiary Prevention

Early case finding and treatment of chronic illness in the homeless population can minimize disability. Discharge planning that recognizes the limited resources of homeless clients can result in the development of realistic aftercare plans leading to healthier practices.

Agencies often have subtle, and some not so subtle, ways of treating a homeless person as a second-class citizen. Community resources may not be available to a person without an address. Agency expectation that the homeless client will not follow through on a treatment plan often becomes a self-fulfilling prophecy. Rehabilitation hospitals often choose who will receive their services (and who will not) on the basis of the availability of home support. Homeless people with an acute flare-up of a chronic illness should be admitted to the hospital sooner and discharged later than patients with homes. The opposite is often done. The community health nurse's involvement in discharge planning and in educating other health care providers might help to minimize the many barriers

that a homeless person faces in order to maintain an optimal level of health.

Much progress has been made in the intervention and treatment of early and middle-stage alcoholics. Nursing research is needed to find creative and innovative ways of helping the homeless alcoholic, who is often a late-stage, chronically ill individual.

Nursing Theories

Working as a nurse with homeless people is enjoyable and rewarding. It can also be challenging, frustrating, draining, difficult, and exciting. The nurses who pioneered the role at the Pine Street Inn in Boston in 1972 were visionaries. They saw themselves as primarily responsible to their clients and set up a framework based on caring and mutual respect.

They recognized the importance of relationship. They understood that success would depend not so much on what they knew as on the attitude that they conveyed. Foot soaks became a hallmark of their clinic. What better way to demonstrate caring than to soak and massage tired and aching feet? The words **compliance,** meaning a disposition or tendency to yield to others, and **noncompliance,** meaning failure to yield or obey, became taboo. The nurses realized that people might make unhealthy decisions for a variety of reasons. Sometimes there was simply no real opportunity to do otherwise. When the difficulty appeared to be a lack of knowledge, an attempt was made to create an atmosphere where clients could learn about their health condition and options for treatment (Lenehan et al., 1985).

It is easy to picture Virginia Henderson working in a clinic for the homeless. Her book *The Nature of Nursing,* (1966) could serve as a guide to nurses working with homeless people. In it she states:

> The nurse who sees herself as reinforcing the [client] when he lacks will, knowledge, or strength will make an effort to know him, understand him, "get inside his skin," . . . this process of putting oneself in another's place is always difficult and only relatively successful. It requires a listening ear and constant observation and interpretation of non-verbal behavior. It also demands of the nurse self-understanding and the recognition of emotions that block her concentration on the patient's need and helpful responses to these needs. It calls for a willingness on the nurse's part to selectively express what she is feeling and thinking so that a *mutual* understanding may develop between nurse and patient (p. 24).

Watson (1985) explores the role of human-to-human caring and its incorporation into the nursing process. She views caring as an essential part of nursing and recognizes the challenge of maintaining its importance in an increasingly technological world. Her thoughtful and scholarly work affirms and validates the work being done in shelter nursing clinics.

HEALTH PROBLEMS COMMON IN HOMELESS POPULATIONS

Homeless people are subject to the same illnesses and medical conditions found in the general population. However, as with all economically depressed groups, they tend to be sicker and to have more health management difficulties. Small problems left untreated tend to become major.

Following are examples of health problems commonly encountered in homeless populations. Prior to the discussion of each health problem, a vignette presents a real-life example. Although mainly discussed as discrete entities, several of these conditions more often occur concurrently. Where applicable, the health problems will be discussed in relation to the national health objectives identified by *Healthy People 2000* (USDHHS, 1990) and the 1995 Midcourse Review (USDHHS, 1996).

Nutritional Deficiencies

The outreach van stopped in the alleyway. It was late in the shift, and supplies had dwindled. Two men got up from where they were huddled at a heating grate; two others joined them from a nearby doorway. Together they timidly approached the van. "Whatcha got to eat?" asked one. Looking over the diminished supplies and seeing only instant soup and peanut butter and jelly sandwiches, the worker answered, "I'm afraid we're down to the daily special, soup du jour, and peanut butter sandwiches prepared with essence of grape jelly." The man grinned and replied, "Say, that special wouldn't come with coffee, would it?"

Nutritional deficiencies underlie many of the health problems found in homeless populations. In *Healthy People 2000* (USDHHS, 1990) the collection of more data on the nutritional status of homeless people is identified as a high-priority need (p. 131) although not followed up in the 1995 Midcourse Review (USDHHS, 1996). Wright (1990) reported that comparisons with national data showed that nutritional deficiencies (mainly malnutrition and vitamin deficiencies) were 20 times more prevalent in homeless populations (2% versus 0.1%). Because homeless people depend on handouts, it is extremely difficult, even for those so inclined, to obtain a well-balanced diet. Poor nutrition leads to apathy and decreased energy, further compounding the problem. Alcoholism and the use of street drugs or prescription drugs can lead to vitamin deficiencies, which in turn decrease healing ability and temperature control (Strasser, Damrosch, & Gaines, 1991).

Even when attempts are made to provide a well-balanced diet, the special needs of a significant number of homeless people are not met. The elderly, individuals with poor dentition, growing children, and those on therapeutic diets are particularly affected. Winick (1985)

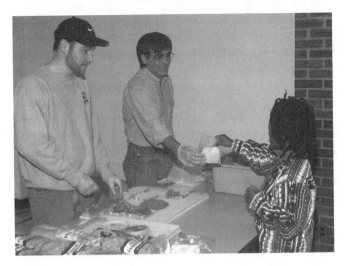

Attempts to provide a well-balanced diet do not necessarily meet the special needs of a significant number of poor homeless people.

expresses concern for the pregnant homeless woman, whose nutritional demands are often left unmet. He states that weight gain needs to be monitored; foods rich in calcium and iron should be available; and supplemental vitamin and mineral preparations should be given. He expresses particular concern regarding zinc deficiency, because zinc is essential for cell division and its deficiency in the pregnant women can lead to birth defects (p. 105).

Peripheral Vascular Disease

The clinic nurse was surprised when she saw Henry's foot. She had been treating him off and on for years, and his foot looked better than usual. The edema and hyperpigmentation were still present, but the ulcer over his ankle looked smaller with no sign of infection. He told her that he had just been discharged from a three-month stay in a veteran's hospital. Later in the day she happened to see him sitting on a park bench, shoes and socks wet and muddy, with his three heavy bags next to him.

Homeless people are frequently afflicted by foot problems, leg ulcers, cellulitis, and venous insufficiency (Goldsmith, 1995). McBride and Mulcare (1985), citing several studies, use what they call "a conservative figure of 10%," when discussing peripheral vascular disease among the homeless. The lifestyles of homeless people tend to compound the problem. They rarely have a place to sit down with their feet elevated during the day. Venous return is hampered when they spend a great deal of time on their feet or sitting on park benches with their feet down. Some homeless people sleep in an upright position. They are exposed to all extremes of weather.

Homeless people often have no change of socks and wear ill-fitting shoes, increasing the chance that their skin will break down. This situation frequently leads to infections, as their surroundings are often unsanitary and they lack the facilities to maintain hygiene. Poor nutrition hampers their healing abilities. Even feet that are not compromised by peripheral vascular disease break down and become macerated when a person wears the same damp socks for days.

Chronic Conditions

Dolores had been admitted to the hospital several times for the treatment of metastatic cancer and had received both chemotherapy and radiation. The hospital stays seemed to do her good. Upon leaving she would appear rested and better nourished, only to return two to four weeks later, cachectic, exhausted and, twice, with pneumonia. She explained that she was a single parent of four girls, ages 2 to 10. Her sister-in-law would care for the children while she was in hospital but felt that this was Dolores's responsibility once she was discharged. Concerned that Dolores did not keep an arranged appointment, the nurse decided to make a home visit. The address in the chart turned out to be that of the sister-in-law. From there the nurse was directed to an abandoned, unheated building where Dolores and her four children illegally occupied an apartment. The apartment was furnished only with mattresses on the floor. In the bathtub, there were signs of a fire, which Dolores said she lit to keep warm on really cold nights.

Dolores and her children would not be included in a census of the homeless. Indeed, she did not consider herself homeless. Her story illustrates the need to be thorough in assessment and the importance of considering homelessness in after-care planning.

In comparing data from homeless clients with national statistics, Wright (1990) concludes that "the homeless suffer from most chronic physical disorders at an elevated and often exceptionally elevated rate" (p. 27). This statement is supported by the National Coalition for the Homeless (1997) who note that the homeless have extremely high rates of both chronic and acute health problems. Chronic medical conditions commonly encountered include diabetes, heart disease, respiratory disorders, seizure disorders, hypertension, and malignancies. The control of these conditions, difficult under the best of circumstances, presents a major challenge to homeless people. Because there is no place to store medications, they are often lost or stolen. There is no safe place for diabetics to keep insulin, syringes, and needles. Concern about where to spend the night takes precedence over keeping medical appointments. The stress of having no fixed address exacerbates many chronic conditions. Living in crowded, often smoke-filled shelters, having no place to rest or to wash, and lacking a balanced diet all compound the problem. The loneliness and humiliation of being homeless, the lack of self-esteem, and the lack of a supportive person who cares often rob the homeless individual of the motivation to maintain health.

HIV/AIDS Infections

Margaret had been diagnosed with AIDS and wanted to find a place to live other than the shelter. She was asked what she found most difficult about living in the shelter with an HIV infection. She answered, "I guess I should say that I catch every little bug that comes through, or that I get real tired during the day and there's no place to lie down, or that it's real hard to stay sober here, but you know, I really think the hardest part is not having a private bathroom when I get diarrhea real bad."

Reports in the literature (Tynes, Sautter, McDermott, & Winstead, 1993; St. Lawrence & Brasfield, 1995) support the observations of shelter workers that there is a large and increasing number of homeless people with problems related to the human immunodeficiency virus (HIV). In their 1995 report, the U.S. Conference of Mayors reported that the number of homeless people suffering from AIDS or HIV-related illness had risen to 8% as compared with 5% in their 1990 report. Significant differences were found in a retrospective study in which homeless individuals with HIV were compared with housed persons (Lebow, O'Connell, Oddleifson, Gallagher, et al., 1995). The homeless group were more apt to be African American or Latino, more likely to have intravenous drug use as a risk factor, and were at greater risk of opportunistic infection.

Many persons with HIV infections find themselves with no place to go except a shelter. AIDS and AIDS-related illnesses present major management difficulties in this setting. Sharing dormitory and living space, often with hundreds of others, puts a person with a compromised immune system at high risk for tuberculosis and other communicable diseases. Spending the day with companions who are actively using alcohol and other drugs increases the likelihood that the HIV-infected person will do likewise. When intoxicated, a person is highly likely to share needles and to engage in unsafe sexual practices. In 1989, 65% to 75% of opiate abusers used contaminated drug paraphernalia. An objective of *Healthy People 2000* (USDHHS, 1990) is to decrease that to 50%, although there is no report of the decrease in the 1995 Midcourse Review (USDHHS, 1996).

Nurses working with homeless people can intervene by assisting clients to find help for their addiction problems, educating clients regarding the dangers of sharing needles and other paraphernalia (works), providing bleach and teaching how to disinfect the works, and providing information regarding needle-exchange programs.

The prevalence of HIV infection and the existence of risk factors have been examined in detail in certain subgroups. Several authors have examined runaway youth and other adolescents living on the streets (Stricoff, Kennedy, Nattell, Weisfuse, & Novick, 1991; Sugerman, Hergenroeder, Chacko, & Parcel, 1991; Bond, Mazin, & Jiminez, 1992; MacDonald, Fisher, Wells, Doherty, & Bowie, 1994; Greene, Ennett, & Ringwalt). Often, dire circumstances in the home precede life in the streets. These circumstances include extreme poverty, violence, drug and alcohol abuse, rejection, physical abuse, and sexual abuse. The stress of being on the streets, lack of self-esteem, immaturity, exploitation, and sexual abuse put the youth at high risk for HIV infection. There is a high incidence of risky behavior including intravenous drug abuse, sharing needles, prostitution, anal intercourse, unprotected sex, and sex with multiple partners. Although often knowledgeable about the risk factors, most youth see themselves at little or no risk for HIV infection (Sugerman, et al., 1991, p. 434).

Another identified group at high risk for HIV infection is homeless women. A study by Fisher, Hovell, Hofstetter, and Hough (1995) found long-term homeless women to be at particularly high risk for battery, rape, mental distress, and lack of a supportive network. Domestic violence is cited as a major cause of homelessness for women. Once a woman becomes homeless, factors associated with survival on the streets increase the risk for HIV infections. A woman might trade sex for money or team up with a male protector, often an IV drug abuser. Fear for safety, the use of drugs, and perceived dependency upon the male increase the difficulties in negotiating for safer sex.

The results of these and other studies point out the need for community health nurses to develop population-specific education and intervention strategies.

Other Infectious Diseases

Bob is a chronic alcoholic who lives on the streets. He has not been feeling very well lately. He has lost weight, and he often wakes up coughing at night. He finds it hard to get back to sleep because, for some reason, he has been perspiring a lot and his clothes have been soaking wet. He did have a Mantoux test for TB but was on a bender when he was due back to have it read. That was three weeks ago.

In 1989 the Centers for Disease Control and Prevention announced the goal of eliminating tuberculosis (TB) from the United States by the year 2010 (CDC, 1994). From 1953 through 1984 the number of reported cases of TB in the United States declined by an average of almost 5% per year (CDC, 1992). From 1985 through 1993 the number of new cases increased by 14%. The increase is attributed to at least four factors: the association of TB with the HIV epidemic; immigration from countries where TB is common; the transmission of TB in congregate settings (such as shelters for homeless people); and a deterioration of the health care infrastructure (CDC, 1994). Further complicating the problem is the recent increase in the incidence of multidrug-resistant TB, most commonly found among patients infected with HIV (CDC, 1993).

The control and management of infectious diseases among homeless people present a major challenge. Crowded living conditions, poor nutrition, substance abuse, stress, and chronic medical problems put them at high risk. Influenza and tuberculosis can spread quickly in a shelter setting. Case finding is difficult in a population that is often transient and distrustful of the health care system. Routine surveillance for tuberculosis using a Mantoux test requires that the person return to have the test read. When positive sputum is found, it might be difficult to locate a person who has no fixed address. By the time the client is located, he may have stayed at several different shelters, exposing an unknown number of people to the illness.

Case management of tuberculosis infection presents another series of challenges. It is hard to take medications for six months to a year, especially since the medications have side effects and can interfere with drinking. Cohen & Cesta (1997) stress the importance of relationship in case finding and case management. Clients are more apt to reveal contacts to a person whom they trust. They are also more apt to follow through on treatment when it is explained by a nurse who is a trusted friend, rather than by an impersonal member of the health establishment.

An objective of *Healthy People 2000* (USDHHS, 1990) is "to increase to at least 80% the proportion of people found to have tuberculosis infection who completed courses of preventive therapy." This would be an increase from 66.3% reported in 1987 (p. 525). Unfortunately, the 1995 Midcourse Review (USDHHS, 1996) notes a rise in tuberculosis rates, particularly among minorities. Taking medications might not be a high priority to homeless people, especially when they are not feeling sick. McGinnis (1995) reports that preventive therapy for TB can be successfully delivered to a mobile, homeless population using a case management model together with an incentive program. She has found the most success using cash as an incentive, paying clients for each week of directly observed therapy. When the incentive is coupled with sensitive nursing care that respects the client's right to

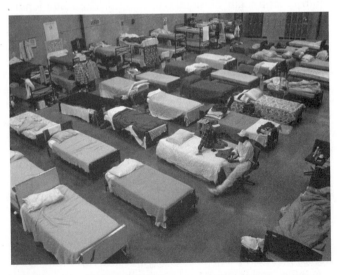

The spread of infectious disease is difficult to manage and control in the homeless population. Close quarters in shelters contributes to the spread of disease. Photo courtesy of Bob Rowan; Progressive Image/Corbis.

make decisions, the likelihood of completing the course of therapy is greatly increased.

Thermatoregulatory Disorders

Bill was telling the story from his hospital bed. "Me'n Jimmy were out, you know. We'd had a few pops and were real glad we'd managed to get ahold of a bottle of port. It was real cold I guess, but the port warmed us up good. We had one of them army blankets and we went over to the grate at the library. It didn't seem all that cold really, except for the wind. I managed to get to sleep pretty quick. Next thing I know, some security guard's waking me up and there's red flashing lights and stuff. I tried to get up but it was like my legs weren't there. I found out later that Jimmy bought it. I guess I'm lucky just to have frostbite."

Hector (1992) points out that hypothermia is not only a problem of extreme cold. It can occur in temperatures as high as 59 to 64°F, especially if the person is not sheltered or is inadequately dressed. Wind and water immersion magnify the effect (p. 785). In Moscow, 25 people died and more than 100 others were treated for frostbite in November of 1995 alone. Homeless people and heavy drinkers were identified as those most at risk (Jameson, 1995).

Homeless people have little protection from the weather and often are victims of hypothermia and frostbite. They are apt to be wet from the rain, over- or underdressed, and unprotected from the wind. Alcohol, commonly used to fend off the cold, does just the opposite. Although it gives a subjective feeling of warmth, it produces peripheral vasodilation, resulting in more rapid heat loss. Alcohol and drugs dull the perception of cold. The presence of dampness or wind hastens the development of hypothermia. Burns suffered from fires, started in an effort to keep warm, are a secondary problem related to the cold weather.

A homeless person wearing or carrying a heavy coat on a warm spring day might be viewed as "crazy" by a passerby. With no place to store the coat, the person has little choice but to carry or wear it. That same coat might be a lifesaver during the night when the wind picks up and the temperature drops into the forties.

Dangers during the warm weather are heat exhaustion, heat stroke, and dehydration.

Infestations

The student nurse was taking care of Joe, a long-term guest at the shelter. Diagnosed as a paranoid schizophrenic, Joe referred to himself as "a State Kid." This reference dated back to his early days in a state hospital for mentally ill children. Indeed, Joe had never lived independently, moving di-rectly from a state hospital into the shelter. As she took his blood pressure, the student noticed something move on his head. Looking more closely, she noticed a small grayish white bug moving through his hair. The skin around the base of his neck was reddened, and there were dandruff-like nits clinging to the shafts of his hair. Suspecting that Joe had lice, but never having seen them before, the student asked her instructor for confirmation. Hearing the question, Joe became quite upset, stating emphatically that "lice do not grow on cultured hair."

Lice and scabies have been around since biblical times and in 1983 were the two most common diagnoses in the emergency room of a large San Francisco hospital (Green, 1985). They present a major management problem in homeless populations and often go untreated and unnoticed until secondary infections are apparent.

Crowded living conditions, sleeping close together for warmth and comfort, infrequent laundering of clothing, sharing clothing and bedding, poor hygiene, embarrassment about seeking help, and difficulty locating and treating contacts all contribute to a high incidence of lice and scabies in the homeless population (Baumohl, 1996).

Alcoholism and Other Substance Abuse

The shelter nurse treated Danny's foot, noting some new signs of infection at the amputation site where he had lost three toes to frostbite. Seeing his bloated face and puffy eyes, she thought, how pathetic he looks. She had first met him 25 years earlier. He had been a handsome, young man. Drinking heavily and depressed, he had slit his wrists and was admitted to the psychiatric unit where she worked. Before discharge he was told that he was an alcoholic and that there was little that the professionals could do for him until he "reached bottom" and found some motivation. It was up to him. Looking at him now, it is hard to believe that he is only 45. He appears to be in his sixties. Clearly, he has reached bottom. Now the professionals are busy treating young men in their twenties, while they can be helped, before they lose everything.

Danny's story is typical of many of the middle-aged alcoholics dependent on the shelter system. The treatment of alcoholism has changed dramatically over the past 25 years. Previously it was thought that the individual had to lose everything in order to be engaged in treatment. Now it is believed that the sooner treatment is begun, the better the prognosis. The instillation of hope is considered the cornerstone of successful treatment of alcoholism. Danny and others like him have been given a consistent message of hopelessness.

The middle-aged and older alcoholic men have been joined by a younger group of alcoholic and polydrug abusers. Because they are homeless, alienated from their families, do not have cars, and work mainly at day labor, they are deprived of the traditional means of accessing care. Owing to their impoverished state, they are also more likely to share needles, putting them at a high risk of exposure to AIDS.

The reported extent of alcoholism and substance abuse in homeless populations varies greatly, depending on research methods and locus of study. Fischer and Breakey (1991), in a review of the literature throughout the 1980s, found the prevalence of reported alcohol-related problems ranging from 4% to 86% and for drug abuse from 1% to 70%. The higher numbers were from studies conducted in the streets or in shelters. In a comparison with a five-city household sample, the lifetime prevalence of alcohol use disorders was two to five times greater in homeless populations (p. 1118).

An objective of *Healthy People 2000* (USDHHS, 1996) is to "establish and monitor in 50 states comprehensive plans to ensure access to alcohol and drug treatment programs for traditionally underserved people" (p. 84). The financing of adequate treatment services for homeless people is identified as an intractable barrier.

Mental Illness

Rita is an intelligent, articulate woman. She functioned quite well in a responsible position until an automobile accident left her disfigured and her sister dead. Now, years after the accident, she resides at the shelter. Her disfigured appearance, her biting sarcasm, and her aloof manner present a formidable picture. She has never had a psychiatric hospitalization and refuses suggestions that she seek outpatient counseling. She was evaluated by psychiatry during an inpatient stay for kidney stones and was given the diagnosis of chronic paranoid schizophrenia.

Lately she has had problems with nocturnal incontinence. She describes this as a terrible laundry problem. "I don't know what they are doing with the laundry," she says, "but every morning when I wake up, the sheets are wet from my hips to my knees." The staff noticed that her clothes were stained during a recent bout of diarrhea. When they approached her, she looked at them sternly and stated, "I don't understand why some people find it necessary to deposit their excrement at my anus."

Perspectives...

Insights of a Homeless Person

Helen was in the shelter for eight months before finding suitable housing. She is now taking classes at a local college and plans to pursue a career in nursing. In discussing her experience, she talked about how angry labels and stereotypes make her. "Like when I was in the shelter I often wondered if I was losing my mind. I saw friends who had been pretty normal begin to act real bizarre . . . but I could understand it. It made sense. Like one woman who didn't like staying at the shelter because her old man would know where to find her. She'd stay outside. I had to stay outside a few times and it's hard to sleep. If you stay in a public place where it's safe, the police are apt to tell you to move, but you really can't sleep anyplace. Things get stolen or you could get beaten or raped so you're always sleeping with one eye open. I mean they talk about peo-

ple getting psychotic from spending time in intensive care units, but they're not labeled crazy for the rest of their lives. Even if you stay in the shelter, it's usually a different bed every night and different people (who knows what they're going to do?) next to you. And then the way you dress, like it's mainly donated clothing that might not fit or the colors don't go together and you have to carry your stuff because there's no place to store it. I can remember looking in the mirror one time and thinking, Oh my god, am I a bag lady? Am I really crazy?

It took me a while after I got my own place to get my confidence and self-esteem back. A lot of the women in the shelter aren't crazy. They're incredibly strong. I'd like to see some of the people who label them "crazy" live with the stressors that they live with."

—*Anonymous*

Studies of the extent of mental illness among homeless men and women have yielded numbers as low as 2% and as high as 90% (Fischer & Breakey, 1991). Differences are accounted for by the study methods used, specific populations studied, and location of study. For example, some studies base their results on history given by the subject, others on the judgment of the clinician, and still others by the application of strict diagnostic criteria. There appears to be a general consensus, however, that approximately one-third of the adult homeless population suffer from a major psychiatric disorder, including schizophrenia and affective disorders (Dennis, Buckner, Lipton, & Levine, 1991; Peterson, 1997). Most studies report a larger percentage of homeless women than men suffering from psychiatric illnesses.

Advocates who witnessed the increasing numbers of homeless mentally ill during the 1970s and early 1980s, and who struggle now to find adequate care for severely mentally ill clients, point to changes in the mental health system as a major cause of the problem. They believe that many of the present shelter guests would previously have occupied state psychiatric hospital beds. Now, deinstitutionalized, or never institutionalized, they are left to fend for themselves on the streets. Goodman, Saxe, and Harvey (1991) look at the homeless situation as psychological trauma and believe that many homeless people are suffering from psychological devastation brought about by the homelessness itself. The adverse effects of stress on health in general and mental health in particular are addressed in *Healthy People 2000* (USDHHS, 1990). The 1995 Midcourse Review shows a decrease in the number of people taking steps to control stress (USDHHS, 1996). The economically disadvantaged are identified as a group at higher risk for both psychosocial and psychophysiological stress reactions (p. 214).

There is increasing discussion in the literature as to whether mental illness is a cause or an effect of homelessness (Cohen, & Thompson, 1992; Buckner, Bassuk, & Zima, 1993). Client insights mirror this dichotomy. Cohen and Thompson (1992) state that mentally ill individuals are homeless for the same reasons as other homeless people: poverty, inadequate housing, and inadequate health care. They urge mental health workers to recognize the primacy of homelessness and to band together with other advocates for the homeless to deal with common issues.

Regardless of whether mental illness is cause or effect of homelessness, the mentally ill are a particularly vulnerable group. Often not street-smart, they are ridiculed and victimized by others. Many mental health professionals prefer not to work with the chronically mentally ill. Homeless chronic patients present even more challenges. They are inconsistent in keeping appointments. Many do not take prescribed medications. Some express the feeling that taking medication causes them to decrease vigilance and thus become more vulnerable. Another group of homeless mentally ill are those suffering from organic brain syndrome. Because of disorientation and memory impairment, they often have difficulty negotiating the shelter system. They are often also prey to violence.

Ferguson (1989), who has worked as a psychiatric nurse in a large urban shelter for more than 10 years, expresses frustration with the difficulties in accessing mental health services for even the neediest homeless client. She reports that the chronic, deinstitutionalized patient has been joined by a new wave of younger, chronic schizophrenic clients. This group, not affected by years of institutional living, tend to be angrier and more demanding. They are also more apt to use alcohol and other drugs and to produce children. She also stresses the importance of relationship in helping individuals to access services. See also Peterson, 1997.

Trauma

Jerry, an elderly man, limped into the shelter. He was covered with blood. He pleaded with shelter staff to go help his friend Scotty. "He's hurt awful bad," he said. "I can't wake him up." Both men were returning to the shelter and had taken a shortcut through an empty lot. They were approached by seven boys, roughly 12 to 14 years old. "Get out of here," the boys said. "We might want to play baseball here tomorrow and we don't want you messing the place up." The boys then proceeded to trip, kick, stone, and beat the men with baseball bats. Scotty had a fractured skull and a broken hip. Jerry had a fractured wrist, several broken ribs, and facial lacerations.

Trauma is a frequent occurrence on the streets. It is the presenting complaint in about one-quarter of homeless clients with acute disorders and occurs at a rate two to three times that of a domiciled control group (Scanlan & Brickner, 1990). Life on the streets is dangerous. Elderly men and women are prey to young thugs, who beat them for their possessions or because of some warped sense of entitlement. As reported in the section on HIV, domestic violence is a major cause of homelessness for women, and long-term homeless women are at particularly high risk for battery and rape (Fisher et al., 1995). Seizures, falls when intoxicated, fights, and burns account for more incidents of trauma.

Often, treatment of trauma is delayed. A homeless person who is lying on the street because of trauma is often seen as drunk and is ignored. Many street people are reluctant to go to the hospital for x-rays or stitches when they feel that they will be kept waiting for a long time. Negative experiences at the hospital in the past keep many people from seeking prompt treatment.

In 1987, only two states had emergency medical services and trauma systems linking prehospital, hospital, and rehabilitation services in order to prevent trauma deaths and long-term disability. An objective of *Healthy People 2000* (USDHHS, 1990) is to increase those services to 50 states (p. 287). By 1993, however, only seven states had increased their services (USDHHS, 1996). Reducing the delay in receiving services and coordinating the services received could go a long way toward reducing death and disability in homeless populations.

Childhood Illnesses

The 8-year-old girl was lying on a bench outside of a shelter with her head in her sister's lap. She had just vomited and complained that her stomach hurt. She wanted nothing to do with the student nurse who had come from the nurses' clinic at the mother's request. "Why won't you let the nurse see you?" the mother asked. "I don't want to," the girl answered. "I don't feel good and I want to go home." "Yes," replied the mother, "but where's that?" "I don't know," answered the girl, "all I know is that I want to go there."

The unique health care needs of homeless children deserve further attention. A New York City study (Alperstein, Rappaport, & Flanigan, 1988) showed a higher rate of immunization delay, a higher prevalence of high lead levels, and a higher hospital admission rate as compared with control groups. In a study conducted in Los Ange-

les County, California, 78% of homeless children in shelters suffered from either depression, a behavioral problem, or severe academic delay. Of these, only 15% had

DECISION MAKING

Assessment of School Children

You are a school nurse in an elementary school. A teacher tells you that she has a student who comes to school without a lunch. She is usually dirty and wears ill-fitting shoes. She seems listless and appears severely underweight. She usually has not done her homework. Her attendance is poor. The teacher wants you to talk to the child and find out what is wrong.

- From the description of this child, what signs might suggest that this child is homeless?
- What would be your first step in addressing the teacher's concerns?
- What interventions would you suggest?

RESEARCH FOCUS

Disease Patterns in Homeless Children: A Comparison with National Data

STUDY PROBLEM/PURPOSE

This study examines the differences in the patterns of illness found among homeless and uninsured children seeking help as compared with their insured counterparts. Implications for nursing care were drawn from the conclusions.

METHODS

An epidemiologic approach was used. Information from a sample of 303 uninsured children who visited a nurses' clinic at an urban shelter was compared with data from 5,403 reimbursed visits by children surveyed in the 1985 National Ambulatory Medical Care Survey (NAMCS). Diagnoses were divided into five categories: acute illness, communicable disease, chronic disease, prevention, and injury care.

FINDINGS

The homeless sample had a higher proportion of visits in the communicable disease, prevention, and injury categories and less in the acute disease category. In the communicable disease category, the large proportion of visits were for pediculosis and scabies, with fewer visits than the insured group for

pharyngitis and upper respiratory infections. The difference in the prevention category was attributed to the aggressive efforts at TB screening practiced in shelter clinics. Fewer homeless children had received immunizations. Homeless children had a significantly higher rate of injuries than the control group. Lacerations and open wounds were common. Children in the insured group were more often diagnosed with acute illnesses although serous otitis was more common in the homeless group.

IMPLICATIONS

Nurses working with homeless children need to be aware that immediate concerns for food and shelter take priority over acute problems and preventive care. In many cases, early intervention can prevent more serious consequences. The high proportion of infestations points to the need for a clean environment with facilities to maintain adequate personal hygiene. The high proportion of injuries among homeless children may reflect a greater exposure to abuse and violence as well as the need for safe play areas.

SOURCE

From "Disease Patterns in Homeless Children: A Comparison with National Data", by J. Murata, J. P. Mace, A. Streblow, & P. Shuler, 1992, Journal of Pediatric Nursing, *7(3), pp. 196–204.*

COMMUNITY NURSING VIEW

It was shortly after midnight when the outreach van stopped at the doorway of an abandoned building. A man huddled in the corner, clutching a bottle of vodka. As she approached him, the nurse noticed that his left leg was noticeably larger than the right and that the pants leg was stained with drainage.

The man gave his name as Richard Polk. In answer to the nurse's concern, he said he had been in the hospital for the leg but had signed out. He refused to allow the nurse to look at the leg or to take his temperature. When she reached to touch his forehead, he pulled back with a frightened expression and said, "You weren't in 'Nam lady. What do you think it was like watching my best friend get his head blown off? They're all around, you know. They're up in the trees now." He looked around as if expecting gunfire at any moment.

He became increasingly agitated when the nurse suggested that he be seen at the hospital. He appeared to be responding to internal stimuli and muttered about his combat experiences in Vietnam. He refused to go anywhere until he finished his bottle. The van returned at 4 A.M. The bottle was empty. The man, now quite intoxicated, refused to accept any help. There was fresh, foul-smelling drainage on the pants leg.

When they returned to the shelter, the nurse found a chart for Mr. Polk in the clinic. It had limited information. He had been seen in the clinic a week earlier for a draining infected wound on his left leg. His temperature was 99.4°F, and the area surrounding the wound was reddened and warm to the touch. There was a moderate amount of serosan-guineous drainage on the dressing. There was mention that he had signed out of the hospital three days earlier. The only personal information that he had given was his birth date (July 23, 1962) and that he was allergic to Trilafon, Artane, and Lithium.

Nursing Considerations

ASSESSMENT
- Are there any inconsistencies in the information that is presented?
- Is any information presented that would make the nurse think that Mr. Polk has a major psychiatric illness?
- What additional information is needed?
- What are Mr. Polk's strengths?

DIAGNOSIS
- What could be possible nursing diagnoses?
- Prioritize his problems.
- Would Mr. Polk be considered a danger to himself?

OUTCOME IDENTIFICATION
- Given your diagnoses, what outcomes could you expect to achieve?

PLANNING/INTERVENTIONS
- How could the nurse engage Mr. Polk in treatment?
- Are there any commitment laws in your state that could be used to bring Mr. Polk into treatment against his will?

EVALUATION
- What would determine Mr. Polk's progress in meeting his goals of treatment?

ever received mental health care or special education (Zima, Wells, & Freeman, 1994; Zima, Bussing, Forness & Benjamin, 1997).

There are inadequate resources to meet the needs of homeless children. According to *Healthy People 2000* (USDHHS, 1990), 40% of battered women and children were turned away from emergency shelter in 1987 owing to lack of space. The goal is to reduce that to less than 10% by the year 2000 (p. 569); however, according to the 1995 Midcourse Review, there has been no reported movement in this direction (USDHHS, 1996).

With the frequent moves to which homeless families are subjected and the constant stress under which the parents operate, it is not surprising that preventive health measures take a low priority and that health care is crisis oriented and episodic. A study by Murata, Mace, Strehlow, and Schuler (1992) highlights the need for community health nurses to take an active role in primary prevention and early intervention when working with homeless children (see the accompanying Research Focus).

ADDITIONAL ISSUES IN CARING FOR HOMELESS PEOPLE

Several factors to be considered by the community health nurse in assessing and planning care for homeless clients have been discussed. However, the above-mentioned health problems rarely occur in isolation. As stated earlier, several health problems may be present in the same individual, each having an effect on the course and treatment of the others.

There are several other important considerations not discussed in this chapter, or mentioned only briefly. They include cultural and religious differences, sexual orientation, legal status, criminal record, language barriers, and literacy. Each can have a powerful impact on a client's ability to accept care and follow through on a treatment plan. It is important that community health nurses be thorough in their assessments so that care plans are both acceptable and feasible.

The problem of homelessness is complex and defies simplistic solutions. Where does the nurse begin? A homeless woman answered the question this way:

> Try not to look at homelessness as a massive social, political, or public health problem. That view is discouraging. Look at it instead as a problem involving people, individual people. If each person did something to help one homeless person, the problem wouldn't be so big. When I say help, I don't mean take somebody home or buy them a meal or even give them a quarter when they're begging on the street. I mean something as simple as looking a person straight in the eye and saying, "I'm sorry, but I can't help you out today" (Anonymous, personal communication).

Key Concepts

- Homelessness is not a new phenomenon in the United States.

- Since the early 1980s, the number of homeless men, women, and children has been increasing at an alarming rate, with estimates now ranging up to 3 million people.

- Homeless individuals are a diverse group. The term *homelessness* should not imply that individuals in this group have anything more in common than the lack of a fixed address.

- Responses to the problem began with grassroots organizers and private agencies but now come from local, state, and federal government as well.

- Nurses were the first professionals to bring health care to homeless people.

- Nurses, working within the scope of basic nursing practice, can do a great deal for homeless people.

- Homeless people tend to be sicker, have more stress, and have fewer supports than domiciled individuals.

- Health problems of particular concern include nutritional disorders, peripheral vascular disease, infectious diseases including HIV infections, infestations, substance abuse, psychiatric disorders, and trauma.

- People without homes have limited access to the health care system and lack the necessary resources to follow a regimen of care.

- Intervention is most effective when nursing care plans are developed *with* rather than *for* the client and the highest priority is given to the client's concerns.

- The community health nurse is in a position to intervene at all levels of prevention.

Rural Health

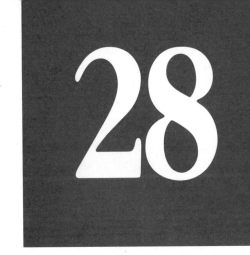

Marshelle Thobaben, RN, C, MS, APNP,
   FNP, PHN
Patricia Biteman, RN, MSN

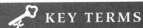
KEY TERMS

frontier area
metropolitan (metro)
   areas (MAs)
migrant farm worker
nonmetropolitan
   (nonmetro) areas
population density
rural areas
rural health clinics
rural nursing
seasonal farm worker
telemedicine
urban
urban area (UA)

A good fit of illness proves the value of health; real danger tries one's mettle; and self-sacrifice sweetens character. Let no one who sincerely desires to help the work in this way, delay going through any fear; for the worth of life lies in the experiences that fill it, and this is one which cannot be forgotten.

—*Louisa May Alcott, 1863*

COMPETENCIES

Upon completion of this chapter, the reader should be able to:

- Discuss the history of rural health.
- Compare and contrast the various definitions of *rural*.
- Identify rural and frontier values.
- Discuss the factors that influence the rural health care delivery system.
- Examine the health status of rural residents.
- Discuss key legislation and programs affecting rural health.
- Identify alternatives available to the rural community for providing rural health care.
- Discuss the various roles community health nurses play in rural communities.

Rural community health nurses are an integral part of a community's health and have potential power in influencing local health policy. They play more than one role in clients' lives. In the absence of a health center, it is the community health nurses who respond to people's concerns about cholesterol, diabetes, immunizations, and birth control, as well as medical issues. This closeness provides for increased client contact and potential for continuity of care (Ciarlo, Wachwitz, Wagenfield, & Mohatt, 1996; U.S. Department of Agriculture, Economic Research Service [USDA-ERS], 1997e). This chapter provides a historical overview of rural health and discusses definitions, legislation, health problems of rural residents, and rural community health nursing roles.

HISTORICAL OVERVIEW OF RURAL HEALTH

The 1800 census counted 5,308,000 citizens; 92.6% were rural residents and only 3.8% were living in urban areas (Grun, 1991). The care of the ill in both rural and urban areas fell to wives, mothers, and daughters. Women traded remedies handed down by their mothers and cared for the sick, with the doctor making occasional house calls with his black bag. All that was known about medicine was contained in the black bag that the doctor carried.

The first hospital in the United States was founded in Philadelphia in 1752 by Benjamin Franklin; hospitals were basically established to accommodate persons whose homes could not provide the most routine nursing care (Sharpe, 1980, p. 10). Hospitals were places of pestilence and isolation; people were admitted when there was no other alternative.

In 1841 the first wagon train left for California, opening the West to new settlers. The settlement of new territories moved nursing care farther away from hospitals and into remote outposts.

Life expectancy in the United States was 40 years in 1850. The advent of preventive medicine and pasteurization, bacteriology, and immunization did much to increase longevity over the next 100 years.

The Civil War raged from 1861 to 1865. More hospitals were built to care for wounded soldiers. Dorothea Dix supervised the training of the first 100 nurses and continued to recruit more. Louisa May Alcott was one of those temporary nurses. She was a nurse in a field hospital during the Civil War, caring for the sick and injured with scarce resources in an alternative setting. She became a nurse out of her desire to do something as the great battles were fought. Many of the first rural nurses began their practice following the same inner drive.

In the last quarter of the 19th century, the hospital became the center of medical care because of the development of new technology. Surgical, x-ray, and laboratory facilities combined with long-term nursing care made the hospital a better place to recover. The size of houses decreased, and families began living in apartments to be closer to new jobs; business and industries grew.

As the cities and hospitals grew, the distance between rural communities also grew. In the 1885 census, 64.9% of the country was rural and 35.1% was urban. Farming community residents found the transportation to large hospitals difficult. Health in the rural communities declined.

In 1908 Lillian Wald determined there was a need for organized rural nursing service. The Visiting Nurse Department was started in 1909 by the Metropolitan Life Insurance Company to furnish nursing services to Manhattan. The service expanded to other policyholders, and by 1912 there were 589 Metropolitan Life nursing centers in the Northeast. Wald continued to present the plight of isolated communities, believing that mobile nurses could reduce the rate of mortality from childbirth and infant diseases. She was instrumental in persuading the American Red Cross to establish the rural nursing service in 1912. The name was later changed to the Town and Country Nursing Service. The ranks were too small to make a big impact. The nurses reported diseases, quarantined contagious persons, cared for the acutely ill, and delivered babies. In place of adequate medical supplies, the rural nurse improvised, a characteristic that remains constant today (Bushy, 1991).

The 1920 census was the first to show growth in urban areas surpassing that of rural areas. Then 51.2% of the population was urban while only 48.8% was rural. Mary Breckinridge founded the Frontier Nursing Service in 1925 in Leslie County, Kentucky. The nurses worked primarily as midwives and reduced the rate of stillbirths by one-

third. They also offered care for infants and children. Well-child visits were augmented with lessons about diet, sanitation, and cleanliness. The rural nurses also gave inoculations against typhoid, diphtheria, and smallpox.

Two world wars increased the population in cities as the demand for industrialization grew. Women worked as nurses or teachers or in factories. The wars resulted in the growth of hospitals as technology improved. Soon, hospitals were the centers of medicine and teaching. Development continued until medical costs skyrocketed in the 1970s, resulting in federal controls in the form of Medicare and Medicaid. Reimbursement declined, and the rural hospitals were the first to close during the 1980s.

The advent of hospital reform, managed care, and reduced hospital stays has precipitated a growth in rural home health nursing care that will continue into the 21st century. Nurses working for a licensed agency make home visits to follow up on treatments started in acute care centers. Despite the passage of more than 70 years, rural nurses are still required to be experienced generalists, with a high level of resourcefulness. The future of rural nursing lies in clinics staffed by nurse practitioners and physician assistants in close contact with physicians by telecommunication (Gorman, 1997). Telecommunication will be discussed later in this chapter.

DEFINITIONS OF *RURAL*

Community health nurses need to be aware of the diverse definitions of *rural* and of the diversity of rural populations. Rural areas are often thought of as either being the Western frontier or farmlands. People imagine farms with acres of land separating farms, with rural towns located sporadically and the population as consisting of pioneers, hunters, trappers, ranchers, and Native Americans. However, rural populations include members of every cultural and ethnic group and cross all economic boundaries. There is no individual community, region, or lifestyle that can be considered representative of the entire rural population (Ciarlo et al., 1996; Mulder & Chang, 1997). Pooley (1997) states that in the 1990s 2 million more Americans will have moved to the rural areas from cities than the reverse. Rural communities now consist of retired

℘℘ REFLECTIVE THINKING ℘℘

Your Image of Rural

• When you think about clients living in rural areas, what thoughts come to mind?

• Where do they live? What does their home look like? How do they make a living?

• What are their health care problems? Where do they get their health care?

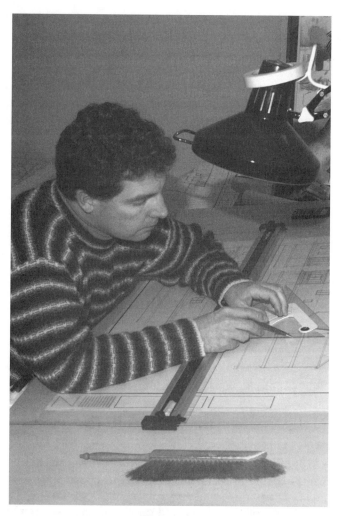

The rural population is changing with the influx of people who can use the computer to telecommute.

persons, artists, small business owners, writers, and others who can use the computer to extend their work desk.

There is no agreement among health professionals or policymakers on a single definition that best describes rural areas. The same geographic area could be considered rural by one definition and metropolitan by another. These inconsistencies affect the quality of data used to compare rural and urban areas. Whether communities are identified as rural has dramatic policy implications, including decision making about opening or closing of health care facilities, receiving federal funds, and where health personnel shortages exist (Johnson-Webb, Baer, & Gesler, 1997).

United States rural areas vary along a continuum from frontier to urbanlike. A **frontier area's** greatest defining characteristic is its isolation, having fewer than 6 or 7 persons per square mile. The frontier areas are characterized by considerable distance from central places, poor access to market areas, and people's relative isolation from each other in large geographic areas. Frontier areas contain less than 1% of the population but a prodigious 45% of the total U.S. land mass. The states with more than 15% of

their population in frontier counties or with a total frontier population of greater than 250,000 are Wyoming, Alaska, Montana, South Dakota, North Dakota, and Idaho (American Nurses Association [ANA], 1996; Ciarlo et al., 1996; Ciarlo, 1997).

Federal Agencies' Definitions

The U.S. Bureau of the Census, the U.S. Office of Management and Budget (USOMB), and the U.S. Department of Agriculture (USDA) provide the three most common federal definitions of rural. They define rural in terms of rural versus urban and metropolitan versus nonmetropolitan.

U.S. Census Bureau

The Census Bureau collects, analyzes, and disseminates statistical data on population and the economy. These data are used to determine eligibility for reimbursement of government funds, funding for research projects, and the distribution of public monies. The U.S. Census Bureau classifies urban as comprising all territory, population, and housing units in urbanized areas and in places of 2,500 or more persons outside urbanized areas (U.S. Census Bureau, 1995).

An **urban area (UA)** is defined by **population density;** that is, it includes a central city and the surrounding densely settled territory that together have a population of 50,000 or more and a population density generally exceeding 1,000 people per square mile. More precisely, **urban** consists of territory, persons, and housing units in:

1. Places of 2,500 or more persons incorporated as cities, villages, boroughs (except in Alaska and New York), and towns (except in the six New England states, New York, and Wisconsin) but excluding the rural portions of extended cities

2. Census-designated places of 2,500 or more persons

3. Other territory, incorporated or unincorporated, included in urbanized areas (U.S. Census Bureau, 1997, p. 1)

Territory, population, and housing units not designated as urban are considered rural. In other words, **rural areas** are those with fewer than 2,500 residents and open territory. In 1990, 24.8% of the U.S. population lived in rural areas (U.S. Census Bureau, 1995). See Figure 28-1 for a comparison of urban and rural populations in 1990.

U.S. Office of Management and Budget

The predominant mission of the U.S. Office of Management and Budget (USOMB) is to assist the president in overseeing the preparation of the federal budget and to supervise its administration in executive branch agencies. It classifies counties as either **metropolitan areas** (MA)

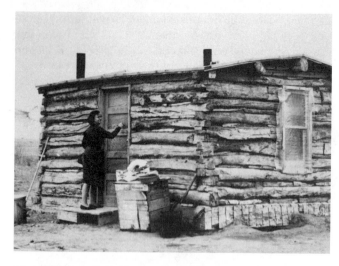

The differing definitions of rural have implications for health care funding. Photo courtesy of the National Institutes of Health/Corbis.

or **nonmetropolitan areas**. The MA classification is a statistical standard developed for use by federal agencies in the production, analysis, and publication of data. In 1999, about $86 billion in tax incentives and $141 billion in federal monies will be designated to provide direct health care services, promote disease prevention, conduct and support research, and help train the nation's health care work force. The activities of the USOMB and distribution of federal resources have allowed progress to be made in decreasing infant mortality, extending life expectancy, and reducing the fatality among persons with HIV/AIDS (U.S. Executive Office of the President [USEOP], 1998).

The MA designation includes the following considerations:

- Each MA must contain either at least one city with 50,000 or more residents or a Bureau of the Census defined urbanized area with a total MA population of at least 100,000 (75,000 in New England).

Figure 28-1 Rural and Urban U.S. Population, 1990

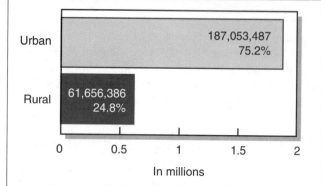

Urban	187,053,487 75.2%
Rural	61,656,386 24.8%

0   0.5   1   1.5   2

In millions

From Selected Historical Census Data: Urban and Rural Definitions and Data *by U.S. Census Bureau, September 1997, Washington, DC: U.S. Government Printing Office.*

- Each MA must include the county in which the central city is located (the central county) and additional contiguous counties (fringe counties) if they are economically and socially integrated with the central county. The county or counties that include a MA and any outlying counties that are part of the same large market area with a specific level of commuting to the central county for work and commercial activity are called metropolitan (metro). Metropolitan areas in New England are composed of cities and towns rather than whole counties.

- All counties not classified as metropolitan are by definition nonmetropolitan (nonmetro); they have boundaries outside of metro areas and have no cities with as many as 50,000 residents (USCB, 1992).

There were 61.7 million rural residents in 1990, a little more than half (52.5%) of whom lived in nonmetro counties. There were 50.9 million nonmetro county residents, 63.6% of whom lived in rural areas. Overall, 20.5% of the U.S. population lived in nonmetro counties and 24.8 percent lived in rural areas in 1990 (USDA-ERS, 1997b). Table 28-1 offers a comparison of rural-urban and metro and nonmetro residency patterns.

U.S. Department of Agriculture

The U.S. Department of Agriculture's (USDA) economic research agency, the Economic Research Service (ERS), has a classification system of nonmetro counties, known as ERS typology. This system is widely used by researchers, policy analysts, and public officials as a source of information about the economic and social diversity characterizing rural U.S. areas. The classification system is based on 2,288 U.S. counties designed as nonmetropolitan (nonmetro) in 1993. The typology consists of 11 types of nonmetro counties classified into one of six nonoverlapping economic types (farming, mining, manufacturing, government, services, and nonspecialized). It also classifies counties into five overlapping rural policy-relevant types (retirement destination, federal lands, persistent poverty, commuting, and transfer-dependent) (Cook & Mizer, 1995). Tables 28-2 and 28-3 offer examples of the ERS typology.

The ERS typology indicates the diversity and wide range of economic activities—from manufacturing to

DECISION MAKING

Defining Rurality

You are conducting a research study analyzing the rate of alcoholism among the adolescent and adult residents in a particular rural area.

- What criteria would you include in your definition of rural?

- How would you decide the criteria?

Table 28-1   Comparison of Rural-Urban and Metro and Nonmetro Residency Patterns, 1990

| County | RURAL | | URBAN | | TOTAL | |
	Population	%	Population	%	Population	%
Nonmetro	32,366,006	52.5	18,531,896	9.9	50,897,902	20.5
Metro	29,292,324	47.5	168,519,647	90.1	197,811,971	79.5
Total	61,658,330	NA	187,051,543	NA	248,709,873	NA

Share (%) of metro and nonmetro residents living in rural and urban areas

Nonmetro	63.6	NA	36.4	NA	NA	NA
Metro	14.8	NA	85.2	NA	NA	NA
Total	24.8	NA	75.2	NA	NA	NA

From What Is Rural? *by U.S. Department of Agriculture, 1997 , Washington, DC: U.S Government Printing Office.*

Table 28-2   Nonmetro Counties Based on Economy Types

TYPE	LOCATION	POPULATION SHIFT	ECONOMIC BASE
Farming-dependent (556 counties)	Concentrated in the Midwest	Declined through outmigration	Economic decline; they lost 111,000 farming jobs
Mining-dependent (146 counties)	Mostly located in South or West; distinct specialization in different types of mining activities, including coal, gas, oil, and metals	Declined through outmigration	Economic decline with a 27% loss of jobs
Manufacturing-dependent (506 counties)	Often located contiguous to a metro area; exhibit a more urban orientation; located mainly in the Southeast	More densely populated than other types	Economy grew slightly
Government-dependent (244 counties)	Scattered across the nation; specialize in federal, state, and local government activities	Grew	Economy grew with an overall gain of 433,000 new jobs
Services-dependent (323 counties)	Fairly evenly distributed across the country with a slightly higher representation in the West; service-sector jobs, which include centers for trade and services, consumer service centers for residential areas, and centers of specialized services such as recreation	Grew significantly	Economy grew with a 24% growth in earnings
Nonspecialized (484 counties)	Large majority are in the South; did not qualify for one of the activities such as construction, forestry, or fisheries	No data	Reflected both strong and weak economies; two-thirds experienced growth

From The Revised ERS County Typology: An Overview. Rural Development Research Report 89 *by P. J. Cook & K. L. Mizer, 1995, Washington, DC: Rural Research Service, Economic Research Service, U.S. Department of Agriculture.*

Table 28-3 Nonmetro Counties Based on Policy Criteria

TYPE	LOCATION	ECONOMY
Retirement-destination (190 counties)	Fifteen percent or greater increase in population aged 60 and above; over 80% are in the South or West, most prevalently in Florida and the Southwest	Served as recreational or resort sites; 60% of these counties had job growth faster than the national average
Federal lands (270 counties)	Seventy-six percent of these counties are in the western states and are federally owned; had larger land areas and are more sparsely populated than all-nonmetro counties; on average, grew faster than all-nonmetro counties	Approximately 70% of the jobs were in services or government sectors, reflecting the recreational use and land management function of the group; strong growth in service-sector jobs
Commuting (381 counties)	A majority are in the South, where counties have smaller land areas and are more apt to adjoin metro areas than all-nonmetro counties	Economies shaped by workers' commuting to jobs in other counties; the level of economic activity within the local economies was less than in all-nonmetro counties
Persistent poverty (504 counties)	Eighty-five percent of these counties are located in the South	A distinguishing feature is a disproportionate number of economically at-risk people including minorities, female-headed households, high school dropouts, and disabled persons; unemployment was considerably higher and incomes considerably lower than in all-nonmetro counties
Transfer-dependent (381 counties)	Economies were heavily based on unearned income from government transfer payments, including Social Security, unemployment insurance, Medical, Medicaid, food stamps, government pensions, and welfare benefits; the large majority are in the southern states; they are sparsely populated and usually remote from metro areas; about three-fifths of these counties were also in the persistent poverty category	They include a large number of elderly; overall economies grew more slowly with real earnings declining by 9%

From The Revised ERS County Typology: An Overview. Rural Development Research Report 89 *by P. J. Cook, & K. L. Mizer, 1995, Washington, DC: Rural Research Service, Economic Research Service, U.S. Department of Agriculture.*

recreational services—in rural (nonmetro) areas. The rural economies have shifted from being dependent on farming, forestry, and mining to experiencing a striking diversity of economic activities. Nonmetro areas vary dramatically in their health needs. Strategies to address problems in each area must fit the community. The role of the community health nurse is to match the health needs of the nonmetro community with the potential available funds for state, county, and federal programs.

RURAL AND FRONTIER VALUES

Despite the diversity of rural and frontier residents, researchers have identified that they have some common characteristics. There is a tendency for rural residents to

be independent, self-reliant, conservative, religious, work-oriented, individualist, fatalistic, and distrusting of outsiders, including new health care providers. Many residents view health as synonymous with being productive and able to work. Their attitudes, values, and health beliefs affect their utilization of the health care system and may prevent them from timely entry into the health care system if they have an illness or a condition, such as pregnancy, that they consider normal. They are more likely to obtain help through the informal system of family and neighbors than through any formal health care system (ANA, 1996).

Lee (1993) writes that health behaviors are the result of values learned during childhood. In farming and ranching environments, children grow up with values of productivity, industriousness, role performance, and independence. If they do not complete their tasks, no one is there to take the responsibility for them. In rural families, it is

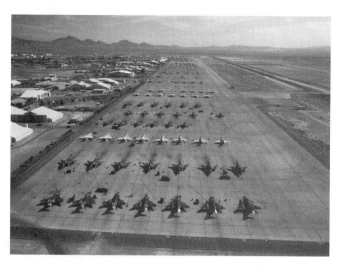

The ERS typology system is used by researchers, policy analysts, and public officials as a source of information about the economic and social diversity characterizing rural areas. The system classifies 11 types of nonmetro counties into one of six nonoverlapping economic types that include government-dependent counties. Photo courtesy of PhotoDisc.

their clients and their services will not be accepted in the community (ANA, 1996; Ciarlo et al., 1996).

The 1990s have seen a shift of urban dwellers moving to the rural open spaces. Rural America has enjoyed a net inflow of 2 million Americans this decade—that is, 2 million more people have moved from metropolitan centers to rural areas than have gone the traditional small-town-to-big-city route (Pooley, 1997). This movement is perplexing for several reasons. Racial prejudice toward urban concentrations of African Americans and Hispanics ignores rural America's large minority population. Things feared lost in urban areas—that is family, community, hard work—are in fact still there. Finally, the ills of urban society—crime, poverty, family breakdown—are also found in rural areas (Rowley, 1997).

Local residents view the newcomers with skepticism, and the urbanites must change their expectations while settling in. Without the urgent care clinics or the telenurse at the local medical center, new residents must learn to care for simple medical problems on their own and might have to commute considerable distances for complicated medical procedures.

the women's role to care for the family's health. Women take care of colds, flu symptoms, and cuts and abrasions. They determine when outside assistance will be sought. They attempt to care for the husbands' health but are often restricted by the work season (p. 25).

That rurality connotes a separate set of values and attitudes is a subject of debate. Some believe it is a myth that rural people's values are different from those of urban residents. Instead they think that systems of interstate highways and television and other mass media have largely ended the isolation of rural areas. It is conceivable that rural and urban value differences are not as great as they might have been in the past. It is more probable that the differences reflect the demographic or socioeconomic composition of the area. In either instance, community health nurses need to consider the values of rural communities and their residents when planning preventive health care and providing clients direct nursing care. Unless they do, it is likely that they will be distrusted by

FACTORS INFLUENCING THE RURAL HEALTH CARE DELIVERY SYSTEM

Factors that have affected the delivery of health care in rural areas include the reorganization of health care delivery systems; the availability, accessibility, and the acceptability of health care services; and the poverty level of some rural residents.

Availability, Accessibility, and Acceptability of Health Care

One of the great flaws of the present system of medical care is that it is not available to all segments of the population. Medical services must be available, accessible, and acceptable to clients when they decide to seek care. Availability is the existence of essential services and the necessary personnel to provide essential services. Accessibility implies that the client has access to as well as the ability to purchase needed services. Acceptability means that a service is offered in a manner that is congruent with the values of a target population (Bushy, 1993, p. viii).

Since the 1950s, the traditional method of rural health care delivery has revolved around a hospital with a laboratory for fluid and tissue examination, x-ray capabilities, surgical suites, and an emergency room. A physician needed the support of a hospital to better care for clients. The rural hospital was the center for trauma triage and acute exacerbation of asthma, diabetes, epilepsy, and other chronic conditions. The management of health care has changed in the past decade. Programs have been excised and personnel decreased in efforts to cut costs.

DECISION MAKING

Understanding Differences in Rural Communities' Values

You are organizing a preventive health care program on hypertension for the Iroquois Native Americans of the rural Northeast and the Vietnamese immigrants of rural western Kansas.

• How would your programs compare? What would be the similarities? The differences?

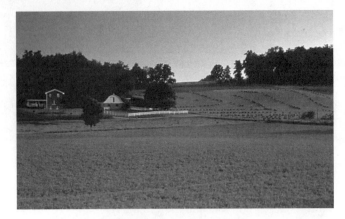

The community health nurse must always consider the values of the community when planning care. Photo *courtesy of Michael Dzaman.*

The rural hospitals that remain open have difficulty recruiting and retaining qualified staff. Sophisticated procedures learned at medical centers that require extensive technology often cannot be duplicated at small, poorly equipped hospitals.

The U.S. Department of Health and Human Services, Office of Evaluation and Inspections (1994) reported that 193 rural, general, acute care hospitals closed during the period from 1987 to 1991 in a total of 39 states. Most rural hospitals that closed were small, with an average of 39 beds. The average occupancy rate was 23% compared with an average of 37% for all rural hospitals. Hospital closures were caused by the effects of declining occupancy, poor revenues, and rising costs. The study showed that the community was not affected by the closures because alternative emergency and inpatient medical care was available within 20 miles.

The U.S. Department of Health and Human Services, Center on Budget and Policy Priorities (1991) examined the health status and availability of health care for rural residents. They concluded that rural residents are not as healthy as those of urban areas. Within the rural population, the health status of low-income residents is inferior to that of higher-income residents, and rural residents use health care services less than urban residents. The barriers to health care services for rural residents included:

- The pressure to work that prevents clients from taking the time off to seek care
- The lack of proximity to providers
- Limited resources
- Scarcities of primary care providers
- Lack of reliable transportation

The Center for Health Policy (1997b) reported that over the past 15 years, rural areas have struggled to maintain access to essential health services sites. This struggle is the result of inequitable payment rates for medical services, shortages of health care providers, and closure of hundreds of rural hospitals. Obtaining and providing any type of health and social services to rural populations can present formidable geographic, cultural, and human resource problems.

Poverty of Rural Residents

The poverty rate in the urban United States in 1994 was 14%. The rural poverty rate was 16.4%. Poverty rates differ not only between urban and rural groups but also among minorities. The poverty rate among rural African Americans was 36.4%, and among rural Hispanics 39.8%. The poverty rate for rural children was 23.0%, but for African American children the poverty rate was 48.2%. The majority of rural poor children lived in single-parent households (59.1%) (USDA-ERS, 1997b).

In 1994, unmarried mothers accounted for 31% of rural births and 33% of urban births. Those rates increased among both African Americans and caucasians, but far more among African Americans. Nationally, nearly three-fourths of African American births occurred to unmarried mothers in 1994, compared with one-fourth of caucasian births (USDA-ERS, 1997a, 1997d).

Nonmetro counties with the greatest poverty can be found in two general areas: the South and Appalachia, and in western frontier counties. These counties make up the bottom 25% of counties when ranked by per capita income. There is a strong relationship between a lower socioeconomic level, reduced access to health care, and a poorer than average health status (USDA-ERS, 1997c).

The available income for the poor must be spent on necessities such as food, heat, and clothing. Few poor families have enough money to pay cash at the doctor's office or at the prescription counter. Some physicians will not accept the indigent as clients.

HEALTH STATUS OF RURAL RESIDENTS

This section includes the types of rural health issues related to children, people who have mental health problems, farm workers, and Native Americans.

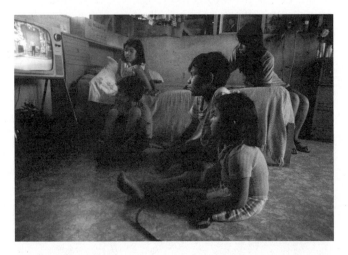

Rural children are more likely to be uninsured than urban children because their parents are self-employed and are unable to attain or afford health insurance. Photo *courtesy of Jim Sugar Photography/Corbis.*

Rural Children

Rural children are more likely than urban children to be uninsured; rural residents are likely to be self-employed and without comprehensive health care coverage because of the high cost. Rural children with treatable problems often cannot access primary care services and thus are likely to develop an acute illness. The Colorado Migrant Health Program (1998) has established a list of factors related to poverty and poor access to health care. Many of these factors could be prevented with better childhood health care. Some of these factors are dental disease, hearing impairment resulting from untreated otitis media, poor immunization status, absent prenatal care, and high-risk pregnancies.

Rural community health nurses can improve the physical well-being of rural children by developing a comprehensive preventive health care plan. It can include such activities as screening programs, mobile clinics, and health education presentations.

Nonmetro Elderly

One-quarter of the elderly population live in nonmetro areas and have characteristics and needs that differ from the metro elderly. The nonmetro elderly poor are apt to be less healthy than their wealthier counterparts because they have less access to support services, good housing, adequate nutrition, and transportation (Frenzen, 1997; USDA-ERS, 1997b). In 1996, 93% of nonmetro persons age 60 and older were caucasian, 6% were African American, and 7% were Hispanic. They were concentrated in the South and Midwest owing to out-migration of young and middle adults and in-migration of retirees. Many counties dependent on farming and mining, and with a net out-migration (Great Plains, southern Appalachian coal fields), have been aging through the loss of young adults. Some counties have in-migration of elderly residents, largely because of an influx of retirees. This changing geographic distribution of the elderly population has resulted in disparities between resources and needs, such as medical and social services, housing, and long-term care services. The lack of services causes a greater number of elderly persons in nonmetro areas to have unmet needs.

Community health nurses can reach the nonmetro elderly by documenting the need for services and establishing clinics in churches, grange halls, or mobile units that make frequent rounds of the outlying areas.

Mental Health

Few recent studies clarify the prevalence of mental illness among rural dwellers. Wagenfeld (1994) determined that rural areas in general tend to be economically unstable and that instability may have an impact on the mental health of residents because they work continuously for very little gain. Ciarlo et al. (1996) cited isolation, the economy, and poverty as the reasons why mental health problems were high in frontier areas. Isolation results in long trips for people to receive treatment for mental health problems. Transportation can be an obstacle for them to receive care, because they do not have private transportation and inexpensive public transportation is not available. Poverty is a factor in the mental health of rural residents because it is persistent and involves complex social, psychological, and cultural problems. Mental health services for inpatient mental health services, suicide prevention, crisis intervention, support groups, and individual services rely on a large volume of cases or donations from nonprofit foundations to support their existence. The volume of clients needed to support such services is often not available in rural areas. For example, fewer than one in five rural hospitals have treatment services for alcoholism and substance abuse (USDHHS-AHCPR, 1995).

Rural residents are unlikely to be offered a full array of behavioral health services. For example, whereas 95% of urban counties have psychiatric inpatient services, only 13% of rural counties have such services, and outpatient services are available in twice as many urban as rural hospitals. In addition, supportive resources such as public transportation, housing, and vocational assistance are often limited or unavailable in rural areas. Community health nurses may be the only resource available for mentally ill and substance abuse clients in rural areas. This lack of services is particularly problematic when nurses have clients who need inpatient treatment, such as a client who is suicidal. The community health nurse must work closely with other professionals and the client's informal network of family and friends to try to provide the type of care a client may need (Mohatt, 1997).

Farm Workers

The majority of the nation's most dangerous occupations are located in rural areas. Agricultural occupations including farming, ranching, and commercial fishing are among the most hazardous occupations, with a death rate approximately four times that of all other industries combined. Approximately 3.5 million full-time workers are employed in agriculture, and with the inclusion of unpaid farm workers and family members at least 15 years of age, nearly 8 million people work in agriculture. Approximately 1 million children and adolescents under 14 years of age live in farm-operator households, and another 800,000 children and adolescents live in households headed by hired farm workers (USDHHS-NIOSH, July 1996).

The agriculture work-related death rate is 24 per 100,000 workers, behind mining's 30 per 100,000, and 16 per 100,000 in construction. The agricultural rate translates into a total of 800 workers killed each year, approximately 140,000 disabling injuries, and nearly 300 deaths per year of children and adolescents caused by farm injuries. Farm vehicles account for approximately half of the fatal farm injuries, and the majority of these deaths are due to tractors. Farming injuries are underreported in standard surveillance data because published estimates for employment exclude self-employed workers. If self-employed workers were included, the actual mortality rates might be 30% to 100% greater (Klassen, 1996; USDHHS-NIOSH, July 1996; Kurtz, 1997b).

Every day, about 500 agricultural workers suffer disabling injuries, and almost half of these result in permanent impairment. They include traumatic injuries, lung diseases, noise-induced hearing loss, skin diseases, and cancers associated with chemical use and prolonged sun exposure (brain, lip, and skin cancer). Agricultural workers can experience numerous sources of stress, including financial uncertainty and losses, intense time pressure, drought and other natural disasters, intergenerational conflicts, and health and safety concerns (USDHHS-NIOSH, April 1996; Kurtz, 1997b).

Community health nurses can help reduce many of the high-risk, nonfatal agricultural injuries by the application of primary preventive nursing approaches. The preventive techniques must be understood by agricultural workers, their families, and the health personnel who treat them. They include injury prevention programs in English and Spanish on handling emergency situations, safety around animals, human factors that contribute to injury, and danger signs and symbols. They also include screenings for agricultural work-related injuries, counseling, and stress reduction techniques (Klassen, 1996; USDHHS-NIOSH, April 1996; Kurtz, 1997a).

Figure 28-2 provides a summary of the health care problems experienced with the rural population, and Table 28-4 offers a typology for health care needs of communities.

Migrant and Seasonal Farm Workers

A **migrant farm worker** is a person employed in agricultural work of a seasonal or other temporary nature

---

Figure 28-2   Brief Summary of Rural Health Care Problems

- Almost one in three rural adults are in poor to fair health and have at least one major chronic illness.

- Higher rates of occupational injuries and traumatic injuries occur in rural areas than in urban areas; clients face worse outcomes and higher risks of death than urban clients because of transportation problems and lack of advanced life support training for emergency medical personnel.

- Rural hospitals and other health care resources are unavailable, and clients lack choices; rural hospitals are shifting rapidly toward outpatient services and show a decline in admissions and lengths of stay compared with urban hospitals.

- Primary care nurses and other primary health care providers are in short supply or unavailable.

- Adequate treatment for alcoholism and drug abuse is lacking because of a scarcity of mental health professionals.

- A high proportion of rural residents have no comprehensive health insurance coverage.

Adapted from Factors Affecting Children's Health: A Rural Profile 1(2) by Center for Health Policy (CHPa), 1997.

---

who is required to be absent overnight from his or her permanent place of residence. A **seasonal farm worker** is a person employed in agricultural work of a seasonal or other temporary nature who is not required to be absent overnight from his or her permanent place of residence. The actual size of the racially and culturally diverse migrant and seasonal farm worker labor force is difficult to determine. It is estimated that a total of 3 to 5 million migrant and seasonal farm workers work in the United States (Migrant Clinicians Network [MCN], 1997).

The labor force is a diverse one, and its composition varies from region to region. It is estimated that 85% of all

Table 28-4   Typology for Health Care Needs of Communities

TYPE OF COMMUNITY	POPULATION SHIFT	NEEDED HEALTH CARE SERVICES
Aging counties	Fairly recently low fertility rates; existing population is aging	Increased demand for services for the elderly
Previous out-migration counties	Young people have migrated out in past decades leaving a smaller number of older adults needing health care. As a result of normal reproduction rates, a mostly young adult population now exists.	Increased demand for obstetric and pediatric services
Boom counties	Substantial in-migration of young adults, both single and with families	Need for obstetric, pediatric, emergency, and substance abuse services
Retirement counties	Gradual influx of elderly residents	Need for health services for the elderly and health services providers

Adapted from Rural/Frontier Nursing: The Challenge to Grow (pp. 7–8) by American Nurses Association, 1996, Washington, DC: Author.

RESEARCH FOCUS

Factors Influencing Exposure of Children to Major Hazards on Family Farms

STUDY PROBLEM/PURPOSE

The purpose of this descriptive study was to understand factors that influence parents' decisions to expose children to major hazards on family farms.

METHODS

The study involved a two-phase descriptive study that was based on planned change and using mail survey research methods. A representative sample of 1,255 Wisconsin dairy farmers was drawn from a stratified random sample of 6,000 dairy farmers. Eighty-nine percent of these farmers agreed to participate in the study. They provided data about factors that influence their decision to expose children younger than 14 years to driving a tractor with more than 20 horsepower; being a second rider on a tractor without a cab that is driven by the father; and being within 5 feet of the hind legs of a dairy cow. Fathers' behavioral intentions to expose their children to these major farm hazards and factors influencing those intentions were measured.

FINDINGS

Multivariate analyses revealed that attitudes, subjective norms, and perceived control accounted for up to three-fourths of the variance in fathers' behavioral intentions. On a seven-point scale from very likely to very unlikely, they were quite likely to allow children 10 to 14 years old to drive a tractor and less likely to allow a child to be near a dairy cow or to be an extra rider on a tractor without a cab. For all three high-risk behaviors, multivariate analyses revealed that it was the father's attitude toward the behavior that accounted for his allowing a child to engage in it. The child's grandparents and mothers exerted a little influence, and health care providers exerted only modest influences on fathers' feelings of social pressure.

IMPLICATIONS

A comprehensive approach to childhood agricultural injury prevention is needed. Strategies that may influence farmers in allowing their children to be exposed to major hazards on farms include individual counseling, educational resources, group activities, and community-based initiatives.

SOURCE

From "Factors Influencing Exposure of Children to Major Hazards on Family Farms" by B. C. Lee, L. S. Jenkins, J. D. Westaby, 1997, Journal of Rural Health, 13(3), pp. 206–215.

---

migrant workers are minorities, of whom most are Hispanic (including Mexican American, Puerto Ricans, Cubans, and workers from Mexico and Central and South America). Historically, the migrant stream has been described by three geographic locations. These are the East Coast Migrant Stream, the Midwest Migrant Stream, and the West Coast Migrant Stream. Migrant families often migrate together to maximize their income. Some families settle in a town to seek better educational or work opportunities. See Table 28-5 for a description of the three migrant stream patterns (Centers for Disease Control and Prevention [CDC], 1992).

Housing

Housing for migrant farm workers is scarce. One study indicated that about 30% of the units needed by migrant farm workers were available. Private housing is not subject to federal regulation. The housing that is available is often substandard (unsanitary, lacks safe drinking water and bathing or laundry facilities) and expensive. Workers face barriers in obtaining housing in local private housing markets because not enough rental units are available or rental units are unavailable to migrant farm workers because they cannot provide deposits or make long-term rental commitments. In the absence of affordable and available housing, migrant farm workers are forced to sleep in cars, ditches, open fields, or tents. Some states are more active in providing assistance for the development of migrant housing. Florida, for example, has a program that provides mortgages for the construction or substantial rehabilitation of rental housing that is affordable to very low income tenants (National Center for Farmworker Health [NCFH], 1997).

Health Problems

The federal migrant health care program spends $65 million a year and provides more than 100 clinics across the United States, but this is not enough to meet the needs of the migrant workers and their families. Mobile units are effective means for community health nurses to reach these isolated and transient clients, but few health centers have the resources to establish mobile programs. Most

Table 28-5   Migrant Travel Patterns

MIGRANT STREAM	CULTURAL GROUP	HOME BASE
East Coast	Hispanic, primarily Mexican Americans, Mexicans, Central American refugees, and Puerto Ricans; others include African Americans, Haitians, and Appalachian caucasians	Primary home base is southern Florida; reside in ethnically homogeneous labor camps including family unit housing or single-sex barracks; during harvest season, farm workers may change camps or move to a new location
Midwest	Mexican Americans, Southeast Asians	Primary home base is southern Texas; work crops there before moving up into the Midwestern states; may also move to East and West Coast migrant streams; family unit travels "upstream" from the home base in groups with children and other relatives; live primarily in labor camps
West Coast	Mexican Americans, African Americans, non-Hispanic caucasians, and an increasing number of Southeast Asians	Primary home base is southern California; stream runs north through Idaho, Oregon, and Washington; primary individual family, some males from Mexico; live in migrant camps when they leave their home base

From "Prevention and Control of Tuberculosis in Migrant Farm Workers: Recommendations of the Advisory Council for the Elimination of Tuberculosis" by Centers for Disease Control and Prevention, 1992, MMWR, June 6.

migrant and seasonal farm workers make annual incomes well below the federal poverty rate, and they earn below $7,500 per year. Rarely do they have access to disability benefits or occupational rehabilitation. Many who have paid into Social Security have difficulty proving their claim for benefits. Insurance coverage for seasonal workers is usually nonexistent, leaving only the choice of waiting until a condition needs to be seen in the emergency room. In addition, migrant workers often face linguistic, cultural, financial, immigration, educational, and other barriers that also make it difficult for them to obtain needed health care services (ANA, 1996; Ciarlo et al., 1996; Hornblower, 1996; Health Resources and Services Administration [HRSA], 1998; NCFH, 1997).

Migrant and seasonal farm workers are at greater risk and have more complex health problems than the general population because of poverty, malnutrition, infectious diseases, exposure to pesticides, and substandard housing. Acute and chronic respiratory distress due to conditions such as grain fever syndrome, asthma, allergic alveolitis, and chronic bronchitis from occupational exposure to grain dust have been reported. Exposure to pesticides increases the risk of cancer, dermatologic conditions, and chronic ailments. Refer to Table 28-6.

The transient nature of migrant and seasonal farm work makes it difficult for community health nurses to monitor these clients and for clients to obtain adequate treatment. This characteristic of migrant workers is particularly difficult for health care professionals working with clients who have contracted a communicable disease. For example, migrant and seasonal farm workers are approximately six times more likely to develop tuberculosis (TB) than the general population of employed adults (CDC, 1992). Rural nurses caring for clients who are suspected to have

or are diagnosed with TB face challenges in helping their clients obtain adequate care. It is the primary health care provider's responsibility to immediately notify the public health department when they know or suspect that their clients have TB. Notification permits public health officials to examine contacts and initiate other health department diagnostic, preventive, or client management services. Rural public health nurses should help ensure that the following services are available to clients and their family or other contacts:

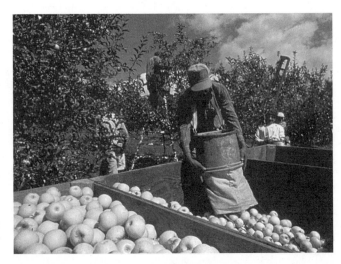

Life is difficult for many migrant workers because they work away from home, often are not supplied or cannot afford adequate housing, do not have access to health or disability insurance, are exposed to pesticides and other health risks, have difficulty obtaining needed health care services on a consistent basis, and earn below the poverty level. Photo courtesy of California Agriculture, University of California.

Table 28-6	Examples of Occupational Hazards for Migrant and Seasonal Farm Workers	
OCCUPATIONAL HAZARD	**HEALTH PROBLEMS**
Farm work	Low back pain, disc disease, arthritis, sprains, carpal tunnel syndrome, lacerations, soft tissue trauma, eye injuries
Toxic chemicals	Pesticide-related dermatitis and conjunctivitis; effects associated with chronic low-level pesticide exposure: headaches, blurred vision, malaise, anxiety, unknown risk for cancer, birth defects
Pterygium	Chronic eye exposure to wind and sun (secondary to)

From Colorado Migrant Health Program Internet Page, 1998.

- Detection, diagnosis, appropriate treatment, and monitoring for those who have TB
- Contact investigation and preventive therapy for those exposed to infectious clients, including widespread tuberculin test screening for workers and family screening (CDC, 1992)

Migrants who are placed on antituberculosis treatment or preventive therapy should be given records they can take with them when they move, to indicate their current treatment and diagnostic status. Special care should be taken to instruct them on how to take their medications and how and where to get additional medication and medical care at their new destination. Out-of-state communications regarding TB care should be routed through state health departments to ensure that the information is transmitted appropriately and that necessary follow-up is initiated (CDC, 1992).

Native Americans and Alaska Natives

The Indian Health Service is the major federal health care provider to the Native American and Alaska Native people. The original inhabitants of North America are citizens both of their tribes and of the United States. More than 350 treaties were signed between the United States and the Native American tribes between 1784 and 1800. On the basis of treaty rights, the Native American people participate in federal financial programs and other services, such as education and health care. The Indian Health Service (IHS) and the Bureau of Indian Affairs (BIA) administer services under the umbrella of the Department of Health and Human Services (DHHS).

The 1990 census identified over 2 million people of Native American heritage. Approximately 1.34 million of this group qualified for IHS and BIA services. There are 545 tribes located throughout the United States, living in villages and on reservations. The health status of Native Americans and Alaska Natives is not equal with the general U.S. population. Poor nutrition, unsafe water supplies, and inadequate waste disposal facilities have resulted in greater incidence of illness in the Native American population. Many reservations and Native American communities are located in isolated areas without accessible health care, including a lack of maternal and child health care and other types of preventive health care. The leading causes of death for the Native American population are:

- Diseases of the heart
- Accidents
- Malignant neoplasms
- Diabetes mellitus
- Chronic liver disease and cirrhosis (USDHHS-IHS, 1997)

The IHS has worked with the Public Health Service to improve the health of the Native Americans. Preventive health services are provided by clinical staff at IHS and tribal facilities and by community health personnel working directly with the Native American community. Since 1973, infant mortality has decreased by 54%, maternal mortality by 65%, tuberculosis mortality by 74%, and gastrointestinal mortality by 81%. Among the IHS programs that have been designed to reduce mortality and raise life expectancy are the Diabetes Program, the Mental Health Program, the Community Representative Program, the Dental Program, and the Accident and Injury Reduction

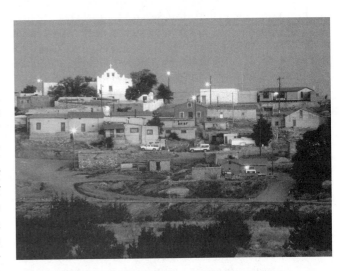

Poor nutrition, unsafe water supplies, and inadequate waste disposal facilities have resulted in greater incidence of illness in the Native American population.
Photo courtesy of PhotoDisc.

Program (USDHHS-IHS, 1997). Community health nurses who are not Native American, however, need to appreciate the difference between Western medicine and Native American healing practices. They work on reservations in the capacity of health educators, substance abuse counselors, and safety program advisors. They will need to recognize that a dual health care system exists and to learn to work cooperatively with tribal healers.

LEGISLATION AND PROGRAMS AFFECTING RURAL HEALTH

The last thirty years have been marked with an increase in legislation and public programs aimed at protecting rural health care and improving the status of farm workers.

Rural Occupational Health and Safety

The Occupational Safety and Health Act of 1970 was enacted "to assure so far as possible every working man and woman in the Nation safe and healthful working conditions and to preserve our human resources" (USDHHS-NIOSH, April 1996). It established the Occupational Safety and Health Administration (OSHA) and the National Institute for Occupational Safety and Health (NIOSH) as two distinct agencies with separate responsibilities. OSHA is in the U.S. Department of Labor and is responsible for creating and enforcing workplace safety and health regulations. NIOSH is in the U.S. Department of Health and Human Services and is a research agency. They often work together toward the common goal of protecting worker safety and health (USDHHS-NIOSH, April 1996, 1997).

NIOSH is the federal agency responsible for conducting research and making recommendations for the prevention of work-related disease and injury. The institute is part of the Centers for Disease Control and Prevention (CDC). NIOSH is responsible for conducting research on the full scope of occupational disease and injury, ranging from lung disease in miners to carpal tunnel syndrome in computer users. NIOSH is a diverse organization made up of employees representing a wide range of disciplines including industrial hygiene, nursing, epidemiology, engineering, medicine, and statistics. NIOSH has developed an extensive agricultural safety and health program to address the high risks of injuries and illnesses experienced by workers and families in agriculture (USDHHS-NIOSH, April 1996, 1997).

At university centers in 20 states, prevention programs and research are conducted on pesticide exposure, pulmonary disease, musculoskeletal disorders, hearing loss, stress, and injuries associated with different farm operations. The University of California–Davis Center, an example of a university center, is a forum for agricultural health and safety communication. It provides electronic media, newsletters, conferences, focused talks and courses, as well as investigator meetings, advisory panels, and interactions among the agricultural community. The center is developing innovative and effective outreach programs to improve health among pesticide applicators, farmers, farm family members, and farm workers. An example is its agricultural engineering program that is designing safer and more ergonomic farm equipment to reduce traumatic and cumulative trauma injuries. Researchers in the School of Medicine are identifying risk factors for acute and chronic illnesses from toxic exposures so that effective prevention efforts can be targeted to those individuals at highest risk (Klassen, 1996).

The Migrant and Seasonal Agricultural Worker Protection Act

Migrant and seasonal farm workers have specific rights granted in the Migrant and Seasonal Agricultural Worker Protection Act through the U.S. Department of Labor (USDOL). This act was passed to help prevent employer abuse of migrant and seasonal agricultural workers. The act specifies that all labor contractors or "crew leaders" be registered by the USDOL. The act specifies that workers have the following rights:

- To receive accurate information in their language about wages and working conditions before beginning work.
- To have farm labor contractors show proof of their registration at the time workers are recruited.
- To be paid agreed-upon wages when due (at least minimum wage).
- To receive itemized, written statements of earnings and deductions for each pay period.
- To purchase goods such as household supplies and food from sources of their choice.
- To be transported in vehicles that are properly insured and operated by licensed drivers and that meet federal and state safety standards.
- For migrant farmworkers who are provided housing:
  — To be housed in a property that meets federal and state safety and health standards.
  — To have the housing information (including cost, if any) presented to them at the time of recruitment (Kurtz, 1997a).

OSHA regulations require that agricultural employers of 11 or more workers provide drinking water, handwashing facilities, and toilets for their employees working in the fields. Farmers with 10 or fewer employees are exempt from these requirements. When OSHA inspectors visit farms or other agricultural workplaces that employ migrant workers, the two standards most often cited by OSHA inspectors are the ones that cover housing conditions in temporary migrant worker labor camps and the field sanitation standard. In 1990 OSHA found field violations in 69% of its field inspections. In 1995 OSHA's federal database showed that there were 275 citations issued for violations of these two standards (Kurtz, 1997b; NCFH,

1997). Clearly, these violations of migrant worker rights are not only continuing but are on the increase.

The Office of Rural Health Policy (ORHP)

The Office of Rural Health Policy (ORHP), authorized by Congress in December 1987, promotes better health care service in rural America. ORHP activities are funded directly through Congress, which appropriated $39.5 million for 1997. The ORHP works both within government, at federal, state, and local levels, and with the private sector—with associations, foundations, providers, and community leaders—to seek solutions to rural health care problems. It is responsible for policy advocacy and information development.

ORHP responsibilities include the following:

- Express the views of rural constituencies within the federal government; advise the Secretary of Health and Human Services on the rural impact of the department's policies and regulations.
- Promote **rural health clinics**—clinics that are certified under a federal law to provide care in underserved areas, and therefore receive cost-based Medicare and Medicaid reimbursements. In part, because of these efforts, the rural health clinic program has grown dramatically in recent years: from 484 clinics in 1989 to some 2,500 in 1996.
- Provide staff support to the National Advisory Committee on Rural Health. This committee is an 18-member citizens' panel of nationally recognized rural health experts. It was chartered in 1987 to advise the Secretary of Health and Human Services on ways to address health care problems in rural America.
- Promote federal, state, and local cooperation by supporting and working with state offices of rural health. ORHP promotes state and local empowerment to meet rural health needs in several ways: by supporting state offices of rural health; by encouraging the formation of state rural health associations; and by working with a variety of state agencies to improve rural health.

Rural Information Center Health Service (RICHS)

The ORHP initiated a national Rural Information Center Health Service (RICHS) that provides a toll-free line accessible to rural residents throughout the nation. It provides customized assistance to individuals seeking rural health information, searches databases on requested topics, and distributes monographs available from other government offices and agencies to organizations and experts in the field. It posts on its Web site rural health information on funding resources, upcoming conferences, publications, full-text documents, and links to other relevant sites on the World Wide Web.

The National Rural Recruitment and Retention Network

The ORHP supported the development of the National Rural Recruitment and Retention Network to improve the recruitment and retention of health professionals in rural areas. It consists of 45 state-based organizations committed to assisting health professionals to locate suitable practices in rural and frontier areas throughout the country. They have information regarding rural practice sites in their respective states and will assist health professionals and their families to identify the resources necessary to meet their personal and professional needs (National Rural Recruitment and Retention Network [NRRRN], 1997).

ALTERNATIVES TO IMPROVE RURAL HEALTH CARE

Recent advances in technology and the restructuring of health care delivery have improved the outlook for rural health services.

Telecommunications

Telemedicine is the most recent addition in the available improvements for rural health. It is the practice of health care delivery, diagnosis, consultation, treatment, transfer of medical data, and education using interactive audio, video, and data communications. For example, a client may have an x-ray taken in the local rural health clinic and read by a radiologist at a medical center or home office. Clinical information is shared using available technologies including electronic mail, the transmission of still images via facsimile, or full interactive video conferencing. Community health nurses can use telehealth to monitor the health status of their clients, to transfer client electronic medical records, to assist in diagnosis for clients, and to consult with other professionals. It is a resource for community health nurses for interactive continuing education, and an electronic library (Rural Health Futures [RHF], 1997).

ᎧᏓ REFLECTIVE THINKING ᎧᏓ

Use of Telemedicine

How would you react to a diagnosis given to you by a practitioner reading an x-ray study that had been taken by you at the local rural clinic but read from a computer terminal an eight-hour drive away?

- Would you feel confident in the diagnosis?
- Would you feel that the process is impersonal?

An example of the use of telemedicine is the project at Hays Medical Center in northwestern Kansas. The Medical Center is creating a network of clinics linked by a medical information computer system. Thirty-six hospitals are linked with telemedicine and teleradiology. The specialists are available as resources to outlying clinics. Another system linked by telecommunications is the Kansas Primary Care Nurse Practitioner Program in Kansas City, Kansas. It is linked to classrooms in Garden City, Kansas, which is eight hours away by car. Using compressed video, the classroom at St. Catherine's Hospital in Garden City is linked to the University of Kansas School of Nursing in Kansas City. Educational programs allowing interaction between the receiver and the sender can be delivered to student nurses and practitioners. When the video is combined with the course work on the World Wide Web, nursing students can access a wide range of new material (Gorman, 1997, p. 61).

Emergency Medical Services (EMS)

Since the late 1960s when civilian emergency medical service (EMS) was first conceptualized and implemented, it has become institutionalized throughout the United States at the intersection of the public safety and the medical care systems. The EMS system is initiated by calling for emergency help or medical assistance, and most citizens expect to immediately receive life-saving medical advice from trained dispatchers, while paramedics and an ambulance race to their aid. EMS is particularly critical to rural and frontier residents because they experience disproportionate levels of serious injuries and their distance from traditional health resources increases the morbidity and mortality associated with trauma and medical emergencies. In many rural and frontier communities, however, these expectations are not met because of long distances, poor roads, difficult terrains, severe climate conditions, lack of or limited telephone service, inadequate public education, organizational instability, under-financing, inadequate access to training and medical direction, a lack of volunteers willing to commit to the considerable demands of emergency response, and insufficient infrastructure resources to support advanced emergency call systems or reliable radio communications systems between the field and base hospitals (NRHA, 1997).

All emergency personnel answering calls should have training in EMS techniques so that critical first-aid and medical advice can be given to callers before the emergency responders arrive. Dispatch centers should be considered as partners in implementing triage systems to direct clients to the appropriate level and source of health care service. In the traditional EMS system, clients in rural and frontier settings often are transported long distances to health care facilities that are not closely affiliated with local health care resources. In some cases, this practice is appropriate because some clients, particularly a severely injured trauma client, may require sophisticated tertiary care. However, far too often this long-distance transportation

simply reflects the traditional separation of the EMS service from local primary care providers, public health, and social service agencies that might be able to deal effectively with the needs of the client. It is essential to the health of rural and frontier communities that the EMS system be integrated into a health care system that is cooperative, shares limited health care resources, provides a broad education to the EMS providers, recognizes innovative methods of health care delivery, and is appropriately reimbursed (NRHA, 1997).

Rural Health Clinics

Passage of the federal Rural Health Clinic Services Act of 1977 (P.L. 95–120) provided for establishment of rural health clinics in underserved areas. It also established reimbursement of a fixed price per encounter to clinics. This law increased flexibility and allowed practitioners to see clients in clinics, homes, extended care facilities, or other settings. Individual states govern the scope of practice of the rural health clinic and its providers. State regulation allows the community to consider its needs and the needs of its diverse population.

THE NURSE'S ROLE IN RURAL COMMUNITY HEALTH NURSING PRACTICE

Bigbee (1993) defines **rural nursing** as the practice of professional nursing within the physical and sociocultural context of sparsely populated communities that involves continual interaction of the rural environment, the nurse, and her practice. It has a rich heritage, especially in rural community health and maternal child health (pp. 131–132).

Rural Nursing

The American Nurses Association (1996) cited the following characteristics of rural/frontier nurses:

- Their roles require them to be expert generalists because of the diverse skills they need to work with clients across the life span and with diverse health conditions.
- They need to be independent and self-reliant since they make on-site decisions in clinical settings (homes and rural health clinics) that can be at some distance from support.
- They have community ties and relationships that provide for close client contact and potential for continuity of care, unless they are a newcomer and then will have to gain the trust of the community.
- Social and professional roles intertwine so that inadvertent breaches of confidentiality are a concern.

- They have a positive community visibility that has been linked to professional pride, self-esteem, and a potential role in shaping health policy at the community health agency and community level (Turner & Gunn, 1991; ANA, 1996).

Rural community health nurses work in diverse communities that have clients with a variety of health care needs. They are an integral part of a community's health. They are resource persons and role models. Rural health nurses can assess the health needs of the client, family, and community by evaluating their health practices and providing primary care. They can provide counseling, health education, and advocacy services. They need electronic access to the latest nursing, medical, and psychiatric health information to keep up to date in their profession (ANA, 1996).

They need to be resourceful in meeting the preventive and treatment needs of the population, who are often geographically isolated, relatively older, poorer, and less insured. They need to be familiar with their community's resources, and work collaboratively with other health and social service professionals. They will need to prioritize their scarce health resources on the basis of the needs of the populations they serve. They need to be involved in planning, implementing, and coordinating community health programs and services.

They may find information from Table 28-4 useful as they begin their planning for the health needs of their communities (ANA, 1996; USDHHS-IHS, 1997).

Bushy (1992) identified rural nursing research priorities that are necessary to develop a body of knowledge for rural nursing. They include the need for research on the recruitment, retention, and training of health personnel; primary care; emergency medical service; the elderly and continuum of long-term care; maternal and child health; the poor and underinsured; and alternative rural delivery systems. Rural community health nurses are in an excellent position to contribute to this research agenda and to improve the quality of care for their clients and communities.

Professional–Community–Client Partnerships

The National Rural Health Association provides a set of principles, based on rural health services research and on the experiences of rural communities, that is correlated with community success in sustaining rural health care systems. The principles include:

- Well-informed community providers and residents who have access to relevant, practical information and successful rural models and who are knowledgeable

Perspectives...

Insights of a Rural Community Health Nurse

When I first began working in a rural community, it was easy to be so burdened with tasks and paperwork that I missed knowing the clients I was serving. As a rural community health nurse, I learned quickly that I needed to have insight into my own culture and the cultures of my clients. I assumed that clients had the same values and background that I had. As I gained more experience, I began to imagine that each client was surrounded by an invisible ring of light that reflected his inner life. The ring of light contains cultural practices, religious beliefs, habits, lifestyles, pride, dreams, and hopes. I realized that I could not fully assess clients without first recognizing that the halo exists and that I could not completely care for clients without incorporating it into my interventions. I also learned not to be judgmental and to be ex-

tremely careful not to breach client confidentiality, since I saw my clients in more than one role. The grocery clerk from the nearest supermarket was Friday night's alcohol poisoning admission and my referral for substance abuse counseling. The pitcher on my son's baseball team was admitted to the emergency room with bruises; the admitting nurse had to report the father for possible child abuse, and the case was referred to me for follow-up. Community health nurses need to learn as much as possible about their own cultures to understand the basis of their beliefs, to learn about the cultures of the clients they serve, to be nonjudgmental, and to be extremely confidential about their clients' problems. This knowledge will give them a basis for beginning to become compassionate community health nurses.

—*Anonymous*

about state and federal policies that affect rural health services.

- A bold vision of the desired local services and broad communitywide support for and participation in the work to sustain local health services and a willingness to take risks on behalf of their vision.
- Effective local health care leadership and system control of the elements of the delivery system—institutions such as hospitals and long-term care facilities, provider practices, and health care dollars.
- A high level of teamwork, respect, and collaboration among community providers and openness to partnerships and affiliations with other regional providers and with value-compatible urban providers (National Rural Health Association [NRHA], 1998).

Rural hospital closures, difficulty in recruiting physicians, and the ability to establish rural centers of health have stimulated thought on methods aimed at improving rural health. Partnership interventions among community agencies and health and social service professionals are a recent strategy to reduce health risks and to improve rural health services. Community assessment program planning and evaluation were discussed in Chapters 12 and 13 and provide foundational knowledge for community health nurses who wish to participate in partnership interventions for solving community problems. Leaders are needed who have these collaborative skills and who are able to work in partnership with others. Sensitivity to the rural community's values and lifestyles among the partners is essential to successful outcomes.

A community partnership begins with the identification of a problem area—immunization, cancer screening, or better nutrition, for example. Once an area of need has been identified, the community health nurses gather data to better assess the strengths and weaknesses of the com-

COMMUNITY NURSING VIEW

David, a 3-year old Native American, was brought to a tribal health center with symptoms of fever, malaise, nausea, abdominal discomfort, and loss of appetite. He appears jaundiced. He lives with his extended family on a large rural Native American reservation. He attends a tribal preschool during the day. David and his family attended the annual salmon festival one week prior to his clinic visit. He was diagnosed with hepatitis A.

Nursing Considerations

ASSESSMENT
- What other assessment data need to be obtained?
- What cultural beliefs would need to be considered?
- What issues need to be explored with David? With his family? With the community?

DIAGNOSIS
- What nursing diagnoses are appropriate to this client? Family? Community?
- What is the priority of his diagnoses?

OUTCOME IDENTIFICATION
- Are David and his contacts successfully identified and treated for hepatitis A?
- Do David, his family, and the community (preschool, etc.) understand the risks of hepatitis A and how to prevent it in the future?

- Are David, his family, and the community satisfied with the nursing services they received?

PLANNING/INTERVENTIONS
- How would a contract be developed with this family?
- How will the nurse explain the concept of communicable disease to the family?
- What teaching with the family would be initiated?
- How will the nurse explain to the family that this situation cannot be kept confidential?
- How will the nurse explain to the family the need to investigate possible contacts?
- What kind of plan would be developed to investigate possible contacts in a rural area?
- What referrals would be made to other agencies? Why?
- Is it a requirement to report this case to the local health authority? Why or why not?

EVALUATION
- What will the nurse do if the family or community is noncompliant or misunderstands how to care for David and themselves?
- How will the nurse know when to terminate visits with this family?

munity targeted. Analysis of the data in the community committee format allows sharing of the information and results in setting goals. A task force consisting of a community health officer, community health nurses, and members of the community must then decide what actions need to be taken.

A community partnership must be informed, flexible, and willing to change, if necessary. An informed partnership must recognize similarities and differences and must manage the challenges posed by differences, particularly those of culture, race, disease, and education. A consensus must be reached about the health practices by the community leaders and the health care providers. Once the program has been implemented, an evaluation must follow. The partnership must be negotiated whenever change occurs (Goeppinger, 1993, p. 2).

The Center for the Health Professions (UCSF, 1995) forecast that within a decade 80% to 90% of the insured U.S. population will receive care through an integrated care system that combines primary, specialty, and hospital services. The UCSF (1995) predicts that by the end of this century, the U.S. health care system will be:

- More managed, using fewer resources more effectively, with better integration of services and financing
- More accountable to and responsive to the needs of those who purchase and use health services
- More innovative and diverse in how it provides health care and more oriented to improving the health of the entire population
- More concerned with education, prevention, case management; less focused on treatment; and more reliant on outcome data and evidence

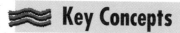 **Key Concepts**

- Rural health nursing has had a diverse history, with nurses working in the battlefields, small hospitals, clinics, and currently through telecommunications.
- Rurality is a complex concept that is defined by different standards by different federal agencies and researchers.
- Rural counties are diverse both economically and by policy types.
- Rural and urban residents' differences are due to demographic or socioeconomic composition of the areas in which they live, not necessarily their values.
- Rural minorities are at risk for health problems because of the nature of their work, lifestyles, and lack of adequate health care resources.
- Owing to the nature of their jobs, migrant and seasonal farm workers are exposed to many potential health problems and often only have intermittent follow-up care.
- Federal legislation affects the availability of health programs to rural residents.
- Regional health networks such as telemedicine and emergency medical services are an alternative for providing health care to rural communities.
- Rural community health nurses must be expert generalists, independent, and self-reliant.
- Rural community health nurses see clients in professional as well as social roles, so confidentiality must be closely guarded.

Health Care Delivery in the Global Community

Preparation for improving human health in the 21st century requires collaborative health care planning with a global perspective. Unit VII includes an overview of health status, in the United States and an examination of the major international health initiatives and a discussion of selected health care delivery systems around the world; the use of power, politics, and public policy in creating and maintaining new health care delivery systems and finally, a vision for the future of health care delivery systems and of community health nursing.

Health Status: National and International Perspectives

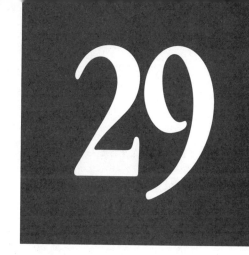

Sue A. Thomas, EdD, RN

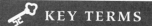
Historically, humans have found meaning in work, family, community, and shared faith. They have drawn upon collective resources to do what they could not do alone. United efforts—raising a barn, shoring a levee, rescuing earthquake victims, or singing a hymn—have brought people together, created enduring bonds, and exemplified the possibilities of collective spirit.

—Bollman & Deal (1995)

COMPETENCIES

Upon completion of this chapter, the reader should be able to:

- Discuss population health from national and international perspectives.
- Identify the determinants of population health, including the changes that have occurred in health professional perspectives.
- Identify the changes in the measurement of global health status from a public health perspective.
- Identify selected health problems from a population-based approach.
- Compare and contrast selected population changes with an international focus.
- Explain the community health nursing role in relation to caring for the health of communities from a national and international perspective.
- Discuss the implications for change in global health planning efforts.

Community health nurses provide care to clients in various communities throughout the world. The community health nurse functions within the multidisciplinary care model, a model that contributes to the comprehensive care of communities. When effective, the comprehensive holistic model exemplifies the collective spirit, the creation of caring communities in which human beings are respected, nurtured, and celebrated.

In order to function effectively in communities, community health nurses must examine the health of communities from national and international perspectives. Community health nurses must have knowledge of the various health problems that exist within the populations. Population characteristics need to be addressed in order to gain an understanding of changing population needs. It is also important to examine those factors that contribute to the health of populations, such as environmental and social determinants, as well as organizational efforts that are related to health status assessment, prevention, and control.

The purpose of this chapter is to examine the health of communities from national and international perspectives. Population health and selected characteristics will be discussed, in addition to those determinants that have an impact on health. The chapter will conclude with a discussion of the community health nursing role and community efforts to address community health.

POPULATION HEALTH

There are a variety of ways to describe the health of a population. There are different ways in which health and illness are defined and many different ways that people have thought about the relationship between the two.

In this chapter, a review of general and infant mortality estimates and life expectancy will provide a background for examining health progress. In addition, current thinking about approaches to measuring health status will be discussed. An initial examination of historical trends will demonstrate how the patterns of disease and life expectancy have changed dramatically over the course of this century.

Historical Perspectives

Since the 18th century, there has been a major shift in the health of populations, particularly in industrialized nations, and a significant decline in the death rate during the past 200 years (Lee & Estes, 1994). This decline reflects the decrease in the incidence of infectious diseases in industrialized nations that once claimed the lives of individuals in their early years. As McKeown (1978) pointed out, "over 90% of the reduction was due to a decrease of deaths from infectious diseases" (p. 6).

For example, in the 1800s, respiratory tuberculosis was the single largest cause of death (McKeown, 1978). There were remarkable changes in the course of the disease, however, as evidenced by the decline in British tuberculosis death rates from approximately 450 deaths per 100,000 people in 1810 to 180 per 100,000 in 1890 (Dubos & Dubos, 1952). This significant improvement could be linked to the sanitary reform movement, a reaction to the adverse impact of the Industrial Revolution. Even though the growth of industries brought about many benefits, the movement of workers and their families into cities not equipped to handle such influx resulted in very poor living conditions for many (Rosenberg, 1962).

In various cities throughout the world, pigs, dogs, and goats roamed the streets, serving as garbage disposal agents. In some cities, people had to get water from a pump in the street. Rooms were small, poorly lit and poorly ventilated, and often overcrowded. Infectious diseases such as tuberculosis, measles, diphtheria, and typhoid fever flourished. The inner city poor suffered the most; however, other social classes were also affected (Fee, 1987).

The development of the sulfonamides in the 1930s, penicillin in the 1940s, and broad-spectrum antibiotics in the 1940s and early 1950s played an important role in the declines in mortality from some of the infectious diseases; however, as the late British physician McKeown noted,

"the role of individual medical care in preventing sickness and premature death is secondary to that of other influences" (p. 12, as cited in Lee & Estes, 1994). McKeown argued that medical science and service are not the primary determinants of health; rather, environment and personal behavior play a significant role. Improved nutrition; a safer, cleaner environment; a change to fewer children in families; and changes in other personal health habits were more significant. The determinants of health will be explored further later in this chapter.

Today, the leading causes of death in many of the industrialized nations such as the United States are chronic diseases: for example, heart disease, cancer, and strokes. In industrialized nations, chronic diseases will remain the major causes of death in the future. In developing countries, infectious diseases will remain the leading causes of death. However, as their economies improve, noncommunicable diseases will become more prevalent (National Center for Health Statistics, 1992).

In the United States over the past 25 years, significant improvements have been made in reducing the mortality from heart disease and stroke: death rates for heart disease and stroke have declined by 49% and 58%, respectively. Much of this success has been attributed to a dual strategy that includes a high-risk and population approach. Improved high blood pressure control and high blood cholesterol control have been identified as the principal initiatives (U.S. Department of Health and Human Services [USDHHS], 1996). In the *Healthy People 2000,* 1995 midcourse review, however, major disparities and gaps were shown to exist among population groups and geographic regions, with a disproportionate burden of death and disability in minority and low-income groups (USDHHS, 1996).

Even though there has been a significant improvement in the mortality associated with certain chronic diseases in industrialized nations, the level of disability and handicap associated with chronic illness has increased. Many of the chronic illnesses are long term in nature, posing different types of problems in the community. As has been noted in Australia, for example, in its 1988 Survey of Disabled and Aged Persons, the Australian Bureau of Statistics (ABS) (1990) found that one or more disabilities were reported by almost 16% of the population. This percentage was significantly higher than the 13% reported in 1981 (ABS, 1991).

The Australian National Health Survey in 1989 and 1990, conducted by the ABS, found that, although most adults assessed their health status as excellent or good, 64% of the males and 68% of the females reported having one or more long-term or chronic health conditions (ABS, 1991).

Chronic disability conditions in the United States caused major activity limitations for 10.6% of the population in 1993, an increase from 9.4% in 1988. Many people, as many as 9 million, have functional limitations that are so severe they are unable to work, attend school, perform activities of daily living, or maintain a household. Chronicity has been identified as a priority area in the United

States. It was identified as a target area in the *Healthy People 2000* objectives, with a recognition of the need for prevention of disabilities, early diagnosis and treatment of chronic conditions, and the provision of information and support services to enable people to function as fully as possible in their communities (USDHHS, 1996). Chronic disability conditions in the United States and worldwide lead to physical, emotional, social, and economic costs to individuals, families, and nations.

The next two decades will see major changes in the health needs of all the world's populations. By the year 2020, noncommunicable diseases are expected to account for seven out of every 10 deaths in the developing nations of the world, compared with less than half in the latter part of the 20th century. These changes are expected because of the rapid aging of the populations in the developing countries worldwide. As the population ages, the major health problems become those of adults rather than children. The rapidity of change will present significant challenges to health care systems and will result in difficult decisions about the allocation of scarce resources (Murray & Lopez, 1996).

Determinants of Health

As mentioned previously in this text, in order for nurses to promote health in individuals, families, and groups, they must view health from a population perspective, as well as from a focus on individuals and families. It is important to examine the determinants of health in populations.

The health of a population is influenced by various factors: biology, lifestyle, environment, and the health care system. Determinants of health include not only health behaviors of clients and the influence of their family history but also social and environmental determinants. Lifestyles and environment are related to each country's level of development (Hunter, 1990) and position within the world division of labor (Elling, 1994).

An examination of the distribution of mortality and morbidity between social groups is necessary, as is an examination of the environmental determinants that affect health. As noted by Blane (1995), there is a definite consistency in the distribution of mortality and morbidity between social groups. The more-advantaged groups,

whether identified in terms of income, education, social class, or ethnicity, tend to have better health than the other members of society. The distribution is graded, not bipolar (advantaged versus others), so that a change in the level of advantage or disadvantage is associated with a change in health patterns, as measured by mortality and morbidity.

For most people, their cultural heritage, social roles, and economic situation have a profound influence on health behaviors and health outcomes. Blane (1995) states:

> This social patterning of health is important for a number of reasons. The size of the gap between the mortality rates of the most and least advantaged groups gives some indication of the potential for improvement in a nation's health. Identification of the groups who are at greatest risk of poor health can inform sound governance of medical services. . . . Understanding the causes of social variations in health should lead to intervention strategies which can reduce them (p. 903).

As clearly pointed out by Nijhius (1989), health is a complex phenomenon that is given form and meaning by the way it is perceived, but it is also definitely linked within the social context of living. Kickbusch (1989), from the World Health Organization (WHO), noted that "we need to re-think the understanding of health itself in view of changing lifestyles in our societies and the . . . more inner directed values emerging in the industrialized nations. New value orientations today look at human beings in the context of the ecological system which they are part of, they understand the individual to be part and parcel of a whole" (p. 58).

The environment is also critical in promoting the health of the population. Throughout history, citizens and leaders have made changes to improve their communities (Duhl & Drake, 1995). Whether making water available, removing sewage, or creating a market square, the ultimate goal has been to improve the quality of life. As Duhl and Drake (1995) have stated: "Before the scientific age of medicine, there was always an awareness of the interconnectedness of health and the environment" (p. 105).

When Florence Nightingale returned from the Crimean War in 1860, for example, she focused her energies on the health implications of broader issues. In the United States, Lillian Wald, Mary Brewster, and Lavinia Dock, among others, also recognized the linkage between health, the environment, and social determinants. They too focused on broader social and environmental issues related to health, as was noted in Chapter 2.

Although it is recognized that morbidity and mortality are affected by many interrelated factors, with the advent of the Industrial Age in the 18th century, a new intervention model emerged. A linear, rational, and reductionist model replaced the holistic perspective, which viewed health issues in a broader context. The new model suggested that successful intervention came from finding a causative agent associated with the problem and then removing it (Duhl & Drake, 1995).

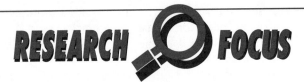

RESEARCH FOCUS

U.S. Mortality by Economic, Demographic, and Social Characteristics: The National Longitudinal Mortality Study

STUDY PROBLEM/PURPOSE

The purpose of the study was to measure the effects of race, employment status, income, education, occupation, marital status, and household size on mortality in the United States.

METHODS

There were 530,507 men and women, 25 years of age or more, identified from selected population surveys between 1979 and 1985. The population surveys involve a complex probability sample of households surveyed monthly to collect demographic, economic, and social information about the U.S. population. Surveys were conducted by personal and telephone interviews, with response rates close to 96%.

FINDINGS

African Americans less than 65 years of age had significantly higher age-adjusted mortality rates than Caucasians in the same age group. African Americans in the 25-to 44-year groups showed more than twice the rates of Caucasians, and those in the 45- to 64-year group showed 1.5-fold higher rates. Higher mortality rates were also found in persons not in the labor force, with lower incomes, with less education, and in service and other nonprofessional occupations, and in persons not married, living alone.

IMPLICATIONS

Employment status, income, education, occupation, race, and marital status have statistically significant associations with mortality. This study identified population target groups that need public health attention and demonstrated the importance of including these variables in morbidity and mortality studies.

SOURCE

From US Mortality by Economic, Demographic, and Social Characteristics: The National Longitudinal Mortality Study by P. D. Sorlie, E. Backlund, J. B. Keller, 1995, American Journal of Public Health, 85(7), pp. 949–956.

The reductionist model views the body as a machine that can be examined in terms of its parts, separate from the psychological, social, spiritual, and environmental aspects of illness. By focusing on the individual, this approach causes health professionals to ignore the complex interrelated web of relationships in a community and the interdependence of individual health and the social, ecological systems of which we are all a part.

As has been previously claimed, the medical model, with its focus on the individual, has resulted in life span improvement, a decrease in illness, and improvement in the well-being of people. McKeown explained with statistical detail, as noted by Kickbusch (1989), those factors that brought about the significant changes in the health of the population at the turn of the century. These factors were improved living conditions and better nutrition; in other words, changes in the standard of living.

Environmental Challenges—Global Perspectives

As discussed previously, the environment is a major determinant of population health. The health of the biosphere 1 significant impact on human health. Global atmos- ic change, ecotoxicity, and the depletion of natural resources pose serious environmentally based threats for the 21st century (Canadian Public Health Association, 1992).

Global atmospheric change has the potential to affect population health in a number of ways. The depletion of the ozone layer and the associated increase in ultraviolet radiation reaching the earth pose potentially serious problems: e.g., increased rates of cataracts and skin cancer, with possible immune system interference. Acid rain continues to be a serious problem because of its effects on ecosystems and association with respiratory diseases. Global warming is another major change with the potential to result in agricultural disruption, which could result in malnutrition and famine and an increase in tropical infectious diseases transmitted by insects (Hancock & Garrett, 1995).

Ecotoxicity, the effect of toxic chemical pollutants, is another major environmental health threat. The effects of air and water pollution, including pollution caused by seepage of toxic chemicals stored in the ground, have received a great deal of attention. Effects including detrimental genetic, hormonal, immunologic, and psychological consequences may pose very serious problems (Hancock & Garrett, 1995). Environmental toxification is a health threat that requires immediate attention and action.

Depletion of natural resources also has an impact on health, both directly and indirectly. The shrinking of pasturelands through desertification and erosion and the decline of harvestable terrestrial, marine, and freshwater species can lead to malnutrition and famine. Ground and surface water pollution threaten not only safe drinking water supplies but agricultural production as well. The development of safe and sustainable alternatives to dwindling fossil fuel resources is necessary to prevent energy supply problems, including heating of homes, transportation of agricultural products, and provision of basic services. As Hancock & Garrett (1995) point out:

> What is needed is a system of economic development that avoids harming the health of the ecosystem of which we are part and the global life support system upon which we depend for our health and survival. This will require a shift in the industrialized world toward a more environmentally sustainable form of economic development in the context of a consumer society (p. 940).

Achieving and maintaining health in the 21st century will require broad-based actions that address environmental health as well as the other major determinants of health at national and international levels. New policies and strategies have emerged to deal with these global challenges, strategies such as healthy public policy and investment in health through intersectoral collaboration.

The growth in the development and application of these strategies is occurring. They have the potential to continue to bring about changes in the 21st century, whereby people and communities can take part in defining and achieving progress in population health. The future of our health in the 21st century "involves much more than the future of medical care, since the major factors affecting health are environmental, social, and economic ones" (Hancock & Garrett, 1995, p. 935).

Measuring Health Status

A landmark publication, *The Global Burden of Disease and Injury Series,* published in 1996 with projections to the year 2020, is the result of a major study that began in 1992, a collaborative effort of the WHO, the World Bank, and the Harvard School of Public Health (Murray & Lopez, 1996). The researchers involved in this major effort developed a new approach to the measurement of health status, called the **global burden of disease (GBD).** The method quantifies not only the number of deaths but also the impact of premature death and disability on a population. These indicators are then combined into a single unit of measurement of the global burden of disease. As Jamison (as cited in Murray & Lopez, 1996, Content Introduction) states: "Publication of this Global Burden of Disease and Injury Series marks the transition to a new era—I firmly predict that by the turn of the century the official reporting of health outcomes in dozens of countries and globally will embody the approach and standards described in this series" (p. 2).

The GBD has three aims (Murray & Lopez, 1996):

1. To include nonfatal conditions, as well as mortality data, in assessments of health status. In many countries, the statistics on the health status of populations are limited, and the number of deaths from specific causes each year are difficult to obtain; thus only estimates can be made. Traditionally, mortality data have been widely used as indicators of health status; however, even in countries where the data are available, such as industrialized nations, they fail to identify the impact of nonfatal outcomes of disease and injury, such as blindness, dementia, or severe respiratory diseases on population health.

2. To produce "objective, independent, and demographically plausible assessments of the burdens of particular conditions and diseases" (p. 6).

3. To measure disease and injury burden in ways that can allow comparisons of the relative cost effectiveness of different interventions, in terms of cost per unit of disease burden averted: e.g., the treatment of long-term care for schizophrenia versus ischemic heart disease. Rational allocation of scarce resources requires this comparison.

The single measure of disease burden for the GBD is called the **disability-adjusted life year** (DALY), an internationally standardized measure. The DALY expresses years of life lost to premature death and years lived with a disability of specified severity and duration. One DALY is therefore one lost year of healthy life. In this measure, a premature death is defined as "one that occurs before the age to which the dying person could have expected to survive if [he or she] were a member of a standardized model population with a life expectancy at birth equal to that of the world's longest-surviving population, Japan" (Murray & Lopez, 1996, p. 7).

The inclusion of information about the GBD in this chapter is important for community health nurses to begin to understand because of the implications this landmark measurement has on examining the health status of nations. The reporting of health outcomes from a global perspective, using a different public health measure, is a true challenge for the future.

Global Mortality Estimates

Worldwide, one death in every three in 1990 was from the category Group I in the GBD—communicable, maternal, perinatal, and nutritional conditions. Most all of these deaths were in the developing regions. One death in 10 was from Group III causes (injuries) in the GBD, and just over half were from Group II causes (noncommunicable diseases) (Murray & Lopez, 1996). Figure 29-1 offers a listing of the different types of categories used in the Global Burden of Disease and Injury Series.

The developing regions of the world were estimated to have 47.4% of their deaths attributable to noncommunicable diseases and maternal, perinatal, and nutritional conditions and 10.7% to injuries. In the industrialized regions of the world, 86.2% of deaths were due to noncommunicable diseases, with 7.6% due to injuries, and 6.1% due to communicable, maternal, perinatal, and nutritional conditions. Only in India and sub-Saharan Africa do communicable diseases, maternal, perinatal, and nutritional conditions dominate as the major category for deaths, accounting for 51% and 65% of deaths, respectively. In Latin America and the Caribbean, there are almost twice as many deaths from noncommunicable disease as from those reported in the communicable disease category; whereas in China there are four and a half times as many deaths from noncommunicable diseases as from the communicable disease category (Murray & Lopez, 1996).

In the recent WHO World Health Report 1998, communicable diseases in Group I will continue to dominate in developing countries as the major cause of death. As the economies of the developing nations improve however, noncommunicable diseases from Group II will become more prevalent. This increase as noted in the report "will be due largely to the adoption of 'western' lifestyles and their accompanying risk factors—smoking, high-fat diet, obesity, and lack of exercise" (World Health Organization [WHO], 1998, p. 3).

Leading Causes of Death Worldwide

In 1990, just over 50 million people died worldwide, with ischemic heart disease (IHD) causing more deaths than any other disease or injury (Murray & Lopez, 1996). Only 2.7 million of the 6.3 million who died of IHD were in the industrialized nations, thus pointing to the need for greater recognition of the changing mortality patterns in the developing nations.

In 1997, there was a global total of 52.2 million deaths, with 15.3 due to circulatory diseases (WHO, 1998). Non-

communicable conditions are expected to climb from 28.1 million deaths in 1990 to 49.7 million in 2020 (an increase of 77% in absolute numbers), but deaths from Group I communicable diseases, maternal and perinatal conditions, and nutritional deficiencies continue to take a major toll even though control measures over the past 30 years have helped significantly. In 1990, 17.3 million deaths were due to Group I causes, with more than 16.5 million noted to be in developing regions, mainly India and sub-Saharan Africa. Of all deaths in the communicable disease category, four out of 10 were due to either pneumonia or diarrheal disease, accounting for more than 7 million deaths. Perinatal conditions accounted for more than 2.4 million reported deaths, and respiratory tuberculosis another 2.0 million (Murray & Lopez, 1996). In 1997, 17.3 million deaths worldwide were due to infectious and parasitic diseases, and 3.6 million were due to perinatal conditions. An estimate of 1.8 million adults died of AIDS in 1997 (WHO, 1998).

Health of Infants and Small Children

The significance of infant mortality as an indicator of a nation's health status and well-being has been well documented in the social and biomedical research literature. Since the early part of this century in the United States, for example, significant progress has been made in infant survival through improved sanitation and socioeconomic conditions, success against infectious diseases, improved nutrition and access to prenatal care, and the use of technology in neonatal intensive care units (Rice, 1994).

The overall mortality rates have improved significantly during this past century. One hundred years ago, one in two African American infants and one in four Caucasian infants in the United States died before reaching their first birthday. Today, fewer than two in 100 African American infants and one in 100 Caucasian infants die before their first birthday. Much of this improvement, as noted by Hogue and Hargraves (1993), resulted from the progressive child welfare movement inspired by Lillian Wald and other women of that time. Infant mortality was defined as a social problem, with multiple causes. The poverty paradigm was used by these socially conscious women, who collected empirical evidence, built community consensus, and harnessed political will to deal with the child welfare problem. Through the effectiveness of the child welfare movement—the reduction of poverty and the amelioration of the effects of poverty on the poor—the improvement of individual health occurred. The provision of safe milk supplies, improved housing and elimination of environmental hazards, elimination of exploitive child labor practices, as well as an increase in parenting education all provided a powerful means for public health action. As Hogue and Hargraves (1993) state: "We need broad-based policies to accelerate improvements in infant mortality, reduce social disparities, and reverse the ever increasing numbers of women and children in poverty" (p. 10).

Although the infant mortality rate in the United States has declined steadily since 1933, it is consistently higher

---

Figure 29-1   Global Burden of Disease and Injury Series Categories

Group I	Group II	Group III
Communicable diseases	Noncommunicable diseases	Injuries
Maternal conditions		
Perinatal conditions		
Nutritional conditions		

Adapted from Summary: The Global Burden of Disease, Global Burden of Disease and Injury Series *by C. J. Murray, A. D. Lopez, 1996, Cambridge, MA: Harvard School of Public Health on Behalf of the World Health Organization and the World Bank, Harvard University Press.*

than that found in many industrialized countries (Singh & Yu, 1995). The rate of decline in the United States has not equaled that of other industrialized countries. In 1960, the United States ranked 12th internationally in infant mortality. In 1988, the United States ranked 23rd in the world (MacDorman & Rosenberg, 1993). By 1991, compared with other industrialized nations, the United States ranked twenty-fourth in infant mortality (USDHHS, 1996).

Even though the past four decades in the United States have shown significant declines in the infant mortality rate, the United States has not made sufficient progress toward meeting several of the maternal–child health objectives identified in *Healthy People 2000* (USDHHS, 1996). The infant mortality rate in the United States is higher than in most other Western industrialized nations, as a result perhaps, as suggested by Singh and Yu (1995), of the excess mortality noted among certain minorities (African Americans, Native Americans, and Puerto Ricans) and low socioeconomic status groups.

In 1995, the infant mortality rate per 1,000 live births worldwide was 59 compared with 148 in 1955. It is projected to be 29 in 2025. The under-5-years of age mortality rates per 1,000 live births for 1955 was 210, 78 for 1995, and projected to be 37 in 2025. Significant progress has been made in reducing under-5 mortality since 1955, and it is projected to continue. Overall, there were about 10 million under-5 deaths in 1997 compared with 21 million in 1995 (WHO, 1998).

By 2025, it is projected that globally there will be approximately 5 million deaths among children under 5—97% of them in developing countries, with most of them due to infectious diseases such as pneumonia and diarrhea combined with nutritional deficiencies (Group I-GBD). There are approximately 24 million low birth weight babies born every year, with many likely to die early (WHO, 1998).

Health of Older Children and Adolescents

According to the recently released World Health Report 1998, one of the major 21st-century problems confronting children will be the continuing spread of HIV/AIDS. In 1997, 590,000 children 15 years of age became infected with HIV. This disease alone could reverse some of the major gains made in child health over the last 50 years. Other factors in the coming years will pose major risks in the transition from childhood to adulthood—such things as violence, delinquency, drug use, alcohol abuse, motor accidents, and sexual hazards such as HIV. Those most likely to be most at risk are children growing up in poor urban environments (WHO, 1998).

How various nations reduce the social disparities in infant mortality depends on how they identify and deal with such differences. Poverty is generally identified as the major cause of social class differences in infant mortality (Kessel et al., as cited in Hogue & Hargraves, 1993). In order to reduce infant mortality through reduction of poverty, health care workers must define the population at risk (the poor) and must determine why they are at risk

(factors such as environmental, social, and behavioral aspects) and how to reduce that risk (Hogue & Hargraves, 1993). Sweden, for example, has used this approach to reduce income differentials and to provide access to comprehensive health services. As Hogue and Hargraves (1993) suggest, "although the US public health community has used poverty to explain infant mortality differentials, we have not acted to eliminate poverty or ameliorate its effects as thoroughly or as consistently as has Sweden" (p. 9).

The Emergence and Reemergence of Infectious Diseases

Since 1986, a reemergence of concern about infectious diseases has occurred. As suggested by Khabbaz, Peters, and Berkelman from the U.S. National Center for Infectious Diseases, Centers for Disease Control and Prevention (CDC, 1995): "The claim of victory over infectious diseases made by prominent U.S. public health officials during the past two decades has unfortunately proven to be false" (p. 10). Infectious diseases continue to remain the cause of significant morbidity and mortality worldwide (WHO, 1992). In addition, emerging and reemerging infections continue to present themselves as problems. Many of the complex factors involved in disease emergence and reemergence are present, including transnational movement of people and goods, changes in the use of land and the environment, medical and technological changes, socioeconomic instability, and political unrest (Wilson, 1995).

As Wilson (1995) states:

Only a small fraction of the microbes that exist on the earth have been identified and characterized. As we probe the recesses of the earth we will continue to uncover microbial life as yet unknown. It is folly to think we have already discovered all existing microbes with pathogenic potential for humans. In addition, microbes mutate, recombine, and undergo genetic shift and drift. Because of their short generation time, microbes have the capacity for rapid adaptation through genetic change. Bacteria are enormously versatile, and have great metabolic diversity" (p. 93).

Wilson (1995) further points out that epidemiologic approaches will facilitate the detection and characterization of microbes, techniques such as constructing evolutionary trees, with the molecular mapping of the location and spread of a certain strain in different parts of the world. The focus on emerging diseases must integrate knowledge and skills from many disciplines in the social, biological, and physical sciences, because it is evident that the causes of various diseases and their prevention are multifactorial.

As has been noted previously in Chapter 20, one of the major infectious diseases to reemerge in the United States and other industrialized countries is tuberculosis (Jereb, Kelly, Dooley, et al., 1991; CDC, 1993b). Historically, respiratory tuberculosis (TBc) was the single largest cause of death in the mid-19th century, with mortality from the disease declining after 1938, when it was first registered in England and Wales as a cause of death (McKeown, 1978).

Tuberculosis and its control are related to social and economic determinants. During the Industrial Revolution, as noted by Friedan (1994), crowding and other factors contributed to the increase in the number of TBc cases. During this century, TBc rates fell steadily in most industrialized countries, except during periods of social stress such as war, with higher rates occurring among immigrants from countries with high prevalence rates (Dubos & Dubos, 1952).

With the discovery of antituberculosis medications and the development of early detection and follow-up programs, the decline in TBc rates was noted, bringing about the possibility of eliminating TBc from the United States, for example (CDC, 1988). Because TBc declined in the United States in the 1970s and 1980s, many of the follow-up programs that had been established for its control, often carried out by public health nurses in local health departments, were disbanded (Brodney & Dobkin, 1991). In 1980, many people incorrectly assumed that TBc in the United States had been controlled; therefore, the effective programs were no longer needed. Fueled by poverty, homelessness, and AIDS, as well as erosion of the public health infrastructure, the reemergence of TBc occurred (Hamburg, 1995). Because of this lack of foresight, as stated by Friedan (1994):

We have seen a dramatic increase in tuberculosis and drug resistance in recent years. In response, federal, state, and local efforts have begun to reestablish effective TBc control programs. As the disease once again begins to decline in the U.S. and leaves the front pages, our challenge will be to persevere. We must expand effective outreach programs . . . , provide services to underserved populations . . . , target services to groups identified by epidemiological studies . . . , conduct epidemiologic investigations . . . , and work to improve the social and economic environment that provides that substrate for the TBc epidemic in the U.S. and abroad" (pp. 1722–1723).

The decline in the number of TBc cases reported annually in the United States during 1992 to 1995 (14.5%) has been attributed to a variety of factors: (1) improved laboratory methods to allow for prompt identification of *Mycobacterium tuberculosis;* (2) broader use of drug-susceptibility testing; (3) increased use of preventive therapy in high-risk groups; (4) decreased transmission of the bacillus in congregated settings (e.g., correctional facilities and hospitals) through adherence to infection control guidelines; (5) improved follow-up of persons with TBc initially reported to the health department; and (6) increased federal resources for state and local TBc control efforts. Beginning in 1992, federal resources for assisting in TBc control efforts were increased (CDC, 1996a). Various activities demonstrated the recognition in the United

States that TBc, as a serious infectious disease, required continued and ongoing program efforts.

The recent national decreases in TBc morbidity in the United States can continue if efforts to promptly identify, treat, and follow those persons with TBc are sustained. In addition, TBc skin tests among high-risk persons, such as the homeless and near homeless, will enable the identification of those who could potentially benefit from preventive chemotherapy.

Worldwide, however, TBc continues to remain a major infectious disease, resulting in more deaths than any other infectious disease. In 1990, the TBc bacterium infected approximately 1.7 billion people, causing about 8 million cases and 2 to 3 million deaths annually worldwide (CDC, 1990). In 1997, TBc remained a leading cause of death, with 2.9 million dying from the disease (WHO, 1998). Friedan (1994) suggests that if we were as concerned about TBc in the developing world as we are about TBc in the United States, cases could be prevented here and abroad for decades to come. With nearly one in three U.S. TBc reported cases occurring in persons born outside the United States and its territories (i.e., foreign born), 31.3% in 1994, the U.S. policy of public health isolationism cannot afford to continue (CDC, 1996a).

Another major occurrence specific to infectious diseases is the emergence of acquired immunodeficiency syndrome (AIDS), which has become a leading cause of death in the United States, particularly among young adults. During the earliest years of the epidemic, from 1981 to 1982, nearly 80% of all reported AIDS cases were from six large metropolitan areas in five states—New York City, San Francisco, Los Angeles, Miami, Newark, and Houston. By 1991, 31 metropolitan areas in 25 states and the Commonwealth of Puerto Rico had reported 1,000 or more cumulative AIDS cases (CDC, 1993a). It was estimated in the early 1990s that 13 million people were infected worldwide (WHO, 1993). As was predicted, HIV disease continues to rise. In 1997, there were 2.3 million global deaths from HIV/AIDS (WHO, 1998). By 2020 it is projected that HIV could rank as high as tenth as a leading cause of global disease burden (see Figure 29-2).

As noted by the U.S. Centers for Disease Control and Prevention, HIV disease has a devastating impact on those who are already marginalized members of society. Growing numbers of HIV infection and AIDS cases occur among poor residents of inner cities. AIDS afflicts many people enduring social problems in the United States and other nations—poverty, drug use, prostitution, and discrimination, as well as limited access to health care. As pointed out by the National Commission on AIDS (CDC, 1993a), the association of poverty, homelessness, and disease is dramatized by the impact of the HIV epidemic on those who are disenfranchised, those in inner cities who are living at the margins of society. Without permanent addresses or steady incomes, the homeless and many of America's poor often are precluded from all but the most basic health care.

In addition to the limited access to health care, the issue of stigma attached to AIDS is a major problem. AIDS-

Figure 29-2 The 12 Leading Causes of Global Burden of Disease and Injury

1990	2020
Pneumonia	Ischemic heart disease
Diarrheal disease	Depression
Perinatal conditions	Road traffic accidents
Unipolar major depression	Cerebrovascular disease
Ischemic heart disease	Chronic obstructive pulmonary disease
Cerebrovascular disease	Lower respiratory infections
Tuberculosis	Tuberculosis
Measles	War
Road traffic accidents	Diarrheal diseases
Congenital anomalies	HIV
Malaria	Perinatal conditions
Chronic obstructive pulmonary disease	Violence

Adapted From Summary: The Global Burden of Disease, Global Burden of Disease and Injury Series *by C. J. Murray & A. D. Lopez, 1996, Cambridge, MA: Harvard School of Public Health on Behalf of the World Health Organization and the World Bank, Harvard University Press.*

related discrimination in the United States reflects the racism and homophobia that pervade U.S. society and, like poverty, limit people's access to care and compassion.

Global projections for HIV demonstrate that the death toll from AIDS may be even greater than expected in the future. In sub-Saharan Africa, for example, death rates from HIV/AIDS are expected to peak around 2005, with approximately 800,000 deaths per year. In India, death rates are expected to peak around 2010, at approximately half a million a year. During the year 2006, HIV deaths are anticipated to peak worldwide, with an estimate of 1.7 million deaths that year. It must be understood however that these projections are estimates only (Murray & Lopez, 1996).

Understanding and coping with infectious disease emergence requires a global perspective, geographically and conceptually. As Wilson (1995) suggests:

> We should anticipate increases in new and resurgent infectious diseases. The global movement and the evolution of microbes will continue. Introduction of new and old organisms into new areas and populations will continue. The persistence, amplification, and spread of microbes and the impact of infection on a population depend on environmental, social, behavioral, and economic factors. Only with a better understanding of the interactions among these factors and their relative contributions to disease emergence can we develop informed interventions (p. 94).

Injuries and Accidents

Although injuries are another major cause of morbidity and mortality worldwide, many countries lack adequate

data to routinely monitor these conditions. Injuries have not received the attention given to conditions of comparable or lesser public health importance (Murray & Lopez, 1996). Injuries, however, are important to examine, both fatal and nonfatal, as emphasized in *The Global Burden of Disease and Injury Series*.

Deaths from injuries (unintentional injuries) are among the most frequently recorded causes of death in populations for which mortality data are available and reasonably complete. Because of the availability of data, most injury research focuses on fatalities. As mentioned in the *Healthy People 2000 Midcourse Review and 1995 Revisions* (USDHHS, 1996), data are needed on the causes and outcomes of both fatal and nonfatal injuries to more clearly reflect the extent of the injury problem in the United States and elsewhere.

Unintentionally fatal injuries include motor vehicle accidents, falls, drownings, poisonings, and residential fire deaths, primarily. In 1993, the U.S. *Healthy People 2000*

⊚⊙ REFLECTIVE THINKING ⊙⊚

Infectious Diseases

• What contributions do you think you could make in the prevention of infectious diseases such as tuberculosis or AIDS?

• Why is it important to have a global understanding of the distribution and emergence of infectious diseases?

• What infectious diseases are prevalent in your community? Why would it be important to know the incidence and prevalence of these diseases?

target for reducing unintentional injury deaths was reached, with 29.2 deaths per 100,000 (USDHHS, 1996). These successes have occurred in declining motor vehicle crash-related deaths and the declining rates of injuries from falls, drowning, fires, and poisonings. Preventive program initiatives such as seatbelt use laws, use of helmets by motorcyclists and bicyclists, and safety prevention measures in the home have been introduced; however, they need to continue to be reinforced.

Worldwide, in 1990, approximately 5 million people died of injuries of all types; two-thirds of them were men, with most of the deaths being concentrated among young adults. Road traffic accidents, suicide, war, fire, and violence all were included within the 10 leading causes of death. Among adults aged 15 to 44 worldwide, road traffic accidents were the leading cause of death for men, fifth for women. Suicide was second only to TBc as a cause of death for women between age 15 and 44. In China, in 1990, more than 180,000 women killed themselves. In sub-Saharan Africa, the leading cause of fatal injuries was war (Murray & Lopez, 1996).

The global burden of injury in 1990 was highest in the formerly socialist economies of Europe, with almost 19% of all burden attributed to injury causes. China had the second highest injury burden; Latin America and the Caribbean third highest; and sub-Saharan Africa fourth (Murray & Lopez, 1996). In almost all regions of the world, except the Middle East crescent, unintentional injuries were a much bigger source of ill health in 1990 than injuries that were intentional, such as war and violence.

The challenge remains for health professionals to routinely inquire and counsel clients about their activities at home and in automobiles. Primary care providers can help to prevent injuries. In addition, there needs to be a greater emphasis on surveillance of injury morbidity, disability, and costs in order to identify risk factors and to evaluate injury prevention programs. Community health nurses have a very important role to play in the prevention efforts.

Chronic Diseases and Disability

As discussed earlier in this chapter, chronic diseases and disabilities pose serious problems for both developing and industrialized nations now and in the future.

In 1990, the three leading causes of global disease burden were pneumonia, diarrheal diseases, and perinatal conditions, in descending order. Projected to take their place by 2020 are ischemic heart disease, depression, and road traffic accidents. Figure 29-2 lists the top 12 leading causes of global disease burden from 1990 as compared with estimates for 2020.

Chronic, noncommunicable diseases are expected to increase worldwide as the population ages, augmented by the large numbers of people in developing regions who are now exposed to tobacco. By 2020, the burden of disease attributable to tobacco is projected to outweigh that caused by any single disease. Tobacco is expected to

increase its share to just under 9% of the total global burden of disease in 2020, compared with just under 6% for ischemic heart disease, the leading projected disease. In 1990, the level of 2.6% of all disease burden worldwide was attributed to tobacco use. As Murray & Lopez (1996) state: "This is a global emergency that many governments have yet to confront" (p. 38).

The burdens of mental illness, such as depression, alcohol dependence, and schizophrenia, for example, have been seriously underestimated by health status measures that do not take into account disability. Psychiatric conditions account for almost 11% of the disease burden worldwide (Murray & Lopez, 1996). Of the 10 leading causes of disability worldwide in 1990, measured in years lived with the disability, five were psychotic conditions: unipolar depression, alcohol use, bipolar affective disorder (manic depression), schizophrenia, and obsessive-compulsive disorder. The predominance of these conditions was not restricted to wealthy countries, although the burden is highest in the industrialized nations, such as the United States and Great Britain.

World Mental Health Perspectives

The past 50 years have seen significant improvements in the general level of physical public health in countries worldwide. Life expectancy has increased, infant mortality rates are reduced, and many of the common infectious diseases are less of a threat, although they still require concerted and ongoing surveillance, identification, treatment, and follow-up (Heggenhougen, 1995). Yet as Heggenhougen (1995) states: "Public health, in terms of mental and behavioral problems, including human rights abuses and social pathologies, is appalling throughout the world, requiring immediate attention and a new perspective" (p. 267).

The burden of psychiatric conditions has been seriously underestimated. Unipolar depression was the leading cause of disability worldwide in 1990, with an estimated 50.8 million people affected, constituting 10.7% of the total percentage of the leading causes of disability in the world (Murray & Lopez, 1996). As estimated by the World Bank in 1993, neuropsychiatric disorders in adults in developing countries contributed 12% to the global distribution. It was projected that by the year 2000, the number of cases of schizophrenia in developing countries will increase by 45% from the 1985 rate, to 24.4 million. Mental retardation and epilepsy rates are more than three times higher in developing nations than in industrialized countries. Seventy-five percent of the elderly with dementia will live in developing nations (approximately 80 million) by the year 2025 (World Bank, 1993).

A sizable portion, 5% to 10%, of the total world population is affected by alcohol-related diseases. Drug use and abuse are increasing at alarming rates and are often associated with violence. The World Bank (1993) also estimated that 34% of the global burden of disease is due to behavior-related problems, such as violence, AIDS, drug abuse, and injuries sustained in alcohol-related motor vehicle accidents. Violence will be discussed in more detail later in this chapter.

In the United States, an estimated 41.1 million adults have had a mental disorder at some time in their lives. An estimated 7.5 million children suffer from mental and emotional disturbances, such as autism, attention deficit disorder, and depression. In the United States, major depression accounts for more bed days than any impairment except for cardiovascular disease, as reported in the 1996 *Healthy People 2000* report (USDHHS, 1996).

Heggenhougen (1995) suggests that a new paradigm for understanding the processes contributing to the health of communities and societies is needed. The concern must be for human suffering in all of its various forms: social maladies, such as violence, mental and behavioral pathologies; human rights abuses; and the basic concern for physical health. The new public health lies at the intersection of these various forms.

Although there are major mental and social health problems worldwide, there is evidence of major efforts to respond. New pharmaceutical agents have enabled the effective treatment of many of the most severe mental illnesses. Community-based, integrated programs that focus on families have been shown to have great potential for improving lives (Heggenhougen, 1995). Creative public health initiatives focused on violence, abuse of women, and substance abuse are emerging in communities. New public health models have been introduced, including epidemiologic models for research and risk evaluation, with research focused on addressing the social and cultural context of particular behaviors. There is greater recognition of local strengths and resources, with community assets identified and reinforced.

Higher priority must be given to mental health, however, and to placing resources—human and material—into relevant programs and policies. As Heggenhougen (1995) states: "Mental health represents one of the great frontiers in the improvement of the human condition—mental health must be placed on the international agenda" (p. 269).

Violence

One of the major public health problems that has received a greater public health emphasis is violence, as discussed in Chapter 24. The recent public health focus on violence has helped to redefine the problem in measurable terms. One of the current definitions of violence is "the threatened or actual use of physical force or power against another person, against oneself, or against a group or community, that either results in or has a high likelihood of resulting in injury, death, or deprivation" (Mercy, Rosenberg, Powell, Broome, & Roper, as cited in Foege, Rosenberg, & Mercy, 1995, p. 2). The injuries may be psychological or physical. Violence includes suicide or attempted suicide, as well as interpersonal violence such as domestic and child abuse, rape, elder abuse, or assaults (Rosenberg & Fenley, 1990).

Violence and infectious diseases have both contributed to much of the world's premature mortality, yet two of the most devastating diseases, smallpox and polio, have responded to public health interventions. Violence can also be interrupted with interventions to break the cycle. The search for solutions must focus on the social and economic factors that contribute to violence, as well as individual factors (Foege et al., 1995).

Recently receiving attention is the connection between violence involving individuals or families and violence involving cultures, societies, and nations. Violence is a global problem, with interpersonal violence, ethnic violence, and national conflict being interrelated (Foege et al., 1995).

Violence must be considered a major public health problem because of the toll it takes on society. In the United States, for example, injuries from violence resulted in the loss of over 149,000 lives in 1991 and resulted in the loss of more years of potential life than heart disease, cancer, and stroke together (National Center for Health Statistics, 1992). In comparison with other industrialized countries, the United States experienced the highest homicide rates among males 15 to 24 years of age from 1988 to 1991 (WHO, 1991). Violence accounts for about 38% of all fatal injuries in the United States, with over 25,000 people dying from homicide and 30,000 from suicide (National Center for Health Statistics, 1992).

According to Foege, Rosenberg, and Mercy (1995), violence in the United States among young people is an epidemic out of control. Violence is a major problem of concern to public health; however, it is a problem of concern to other branches of government and other countries as well. Public health focuses on primary prevention and thus views the prevention of violence as critical. The public health and community health nursing approach to violence focuses on ways to break the cycle of violence, whatever the form, and stops a pattern that so often begins in infancy and childhood and carries over into young adulthood, middle age, and older age. The public health approach focuses on the bridging of many different disciplines, different parts of government, and outreach to the public and private sectors, as well as to community residents themselves.

Community health nurses are in vital positions to participate in collaborative multidisciplinary, community-based coalitions to work on developing multiple complementary activities that can assist in preventing violence effectively. As Foege, Rosenberg, and Mercy (1995) point out: "Communities that can effectively coordinate their diverse resources and perspectives will have a great advantage in addressing this problem" (p. 7).

Global Imbalances in the Burden of Disease

The people of sub-Saharan Africa and India together had more than four-tenths of the total global burden of disease in 1990, although they make up only 26% of the world population. The established market economies and the formerly socialist economies of Europe, with approximately a fifth of the world's population together, had less than 12% of the total disease burden. China was identified as the "healthiest" of the developing nations, with 15% of the global disease burden and a fifth of the world's population. Measured in DALYs per 1,000 population, approximately 579 years of health life were lost for every 1,000 people in sub-Saharan Africa, compared with just 124 for every 1,000 people in the established market economies. The rates of premature death varied sharply between regions, with the rates seven times higher in sub-Saharan Africa than in the established market economies.

These data clearly indicate the major differences and inequalities of world health at the end of the 20th century (Murray & Lopez, 1996). Such indicators point to the need for global collaboration to assist in dealing with the inequalities in health status. The findings pose definite challenges to public policy formation and health initiatives in the 21st century.

POPULATION CHARACTERISTICS— PROJECTED CHANGES

Population growth and changes have a significant impact on social and economic conditions. Population changes also have an influence on health and well-being and rank among the major determinants of health care needs.

One of the major changes in the population in many countries throughout the world, in both developing and industrialized nations, has been significant shifts in population age structures. These shifts have been characterized, to a great extent, by very low levels of fertility, declining mortality levels at older ages, and growth of the elderly populations (United Nations, 1992a, p. iii). These shifts are projected to result in important consequences and implications for various countries. It is necessary, therefore, to have an understanding of these changes and their projected results as the world moves into the 21st century. It is also necessary to examine the contributing factors that influence the population age structure.

In the following discussion, global changes in the age structure are reviewed. It is important to mention that the major source of the population estimates is the population census. Census data, as well as survey data, on age distribution in a number of developing countries may be significantly biased by misreporting of ages and age-selective undernumeration (Horiuchi, 1992). Results of the analysis should therefore be viewed with these factors in mind.

The population of the world in nine major areas will be presented initially, with long-range projections to the year 2150. These projections, presented by the United Nations in 1992, are based on possible scenarios of future levels of fertility and mortality, both central demographic determinants affecting population age structures. The projections are in no way to be viewed as a prevision of the future population trends in the world (United Nations, 1992a).

The population of the world is estimated to multiply by 4.6 between the years 1950 and 2150, growing from 2.5 billion to 11.5 billion (United Nations, 1992b). From 1950 to 1990, population growth was rapid, with an average increase of 1.9%, resulting in a multiplication by 2.1 of the initial population to 5.3 billion. The growth of the population is projected to slow gradually thereafter, with increases of 89% between 1990 and 2050 (to 10.0 billion), 12% between 2050 to 2100 (to 11.2 billion) and 3% between 2100 and 2150 (to 11.5 billion). On the basis of these estimates, the population of the world will ultimately reach 11.6 billion before stabilizing (United Nations, 1992b).

There are expected to be major changes in the age structure of the world's population. By the year 2150, the world population will have aged significantly. The median age will have risen to 42 years, from 24 years in 1990. In 2150, 18% of the world's population will be under age 15, having declined from 32% in 1990. One of the most dramatic changes projected is among the very old, those aged 80 and over. Their proportion is projected to increase ninefold, from 1% in 1990 to 9% in 2150 (United Nations, 1992b). These changes will have major implications for health care professionals in the years to come.

In developing nations, for example, declines in fertility rates and an increase in life expectancy are leading to a rapid rise in the age of their populations (Sepulveda, Lopez-Cervantes, Frenk, deLeon, et al., 1992). In the next three decades, many developing nations will witness a threefold or fourfold increase in their elderly population. As noted by Sepulveda et al. (1992), "the absolute numbers will be staggering" (p. 70). By the year 2020, China will have an increase of 200 million persons at least 55 years of age. India's older population will increase to 120 million by the same year. In addition, the number of older, disabled persons will also increase as the population ages. If the rates of disability among the elderly continue to rise (as has occurred in developed countries), the number of disabled persons will be enormous. The antic-

REFLECTIVE THINKING

Population Increases

• What impact do you think the changing population age structures will have on health care service needs?

• What recommendations do you have in relation to dealing with the projected population increases in older adults?

• How might you participate in community-based initiatives that focus on health-promotion activities for older adults?

ipated continued aging of populations will result in the need for substantially reorganized health services.

Tables 29-1, 29-2, and 29-3 show the percentage of the population projected for 2025 for those age groups under age 15, aged 15 to 24, and aged 65 and over (Horiuchi, 1992). In Table 29-4, estimates and projections are included for the median age distribution. Various regions in the world are identified in each of the tables. The tables also include data that are important to examine specific to population trends and projected estimates between 1950 and 2025.

COMMUNITY HEALTH NURSING ROLE

A focus on global population health, changing population characteristics, and factors that contribute to population health is necessary in community health nursing. Community health nurses have excellent opportunities to participate in communitywide health-care and will have even more in the future. Community health nurses have the ability to integrate concepts of health and disease, indi-

Table 29-1 Percentage of Population under Age 15, by Major Area and Region

MAJOR AREA AND REGION	1950	1970	1990	2025
World Total	34.6	37.5	32.3	24.5
More developed regions	27.8	26.6	21.3	17.8
Less developed regions	27.9	41.8	35.6	25.8
Least developed countries	41.0	44.1	44.5	33.3
Other developing countries	37.6	41.5	34.5	24.6
Africa	42.6	44.8	45.0	34.8
Eastern Africa	43.6	45.7	47.1	37.5
Middle Africa	41.2	43.0	45.4	38.5
Northern Africa	41.3	44.6	41.5	26.6
Southern Africa	39.0	41.5	38.3	28.6
Western Africa	44.1	45.6	46.8	36.0
Latin America	40.5	42.5	35.9	25.7
Caribbean	38.5	40.8	31.2	25.3
Central America	43.7	46.8	38.7	26.5
South America	39.8	41.2	35.3	25.4
North America	27.2	28.4	21.4	17.7
Asia	36.7	40.3	32.9	22.6
Eastern Asia	34.1	38.2	25.7	18.2
Southeastern Asia	39.3	43.4	36.7	23.4
Southern Asia	38.9	41.7	38.6	27.4
Western Asia	40.1	42.8	40.4	30.6
Europe	25.4	25.0	19.6	16.5
Eastern Europe	26.7	24.7	22.9	18.2
Northern Europe	23.5	24.2	19.1	17.1
Southern Europe	27.8	26.5	19.5	15.7
Western Europe	23.4	24.2	17.5	15.6
Oceania	29.7	32.2	26.5	20.8
Australia—New Zealand	27.0	29.4	22.2	18.0
Melanesia	40.5	42.6	40.4	27.8
Micronesia	39.1	42.5	37.8	23.8
Polynesia	44.1	47.4	42.8	26.4
Former U.S.S.R.	30.1	28.9	25.5	20.8

From United Nations (1992). Changing population age structures: Demographic and economic consequences and implications. Geneva: United Nations.

Table 29-2 Percentage of Population Aged 15–24, by Major Area and Region

MAJOR AREA AND REGION	1950	1970	1990	2025
World Total	18.3	18.0	19.1	16.0
More developed regions	17.2	16.7	14.8	12.3
Less developed regions	18.8	18.6	20.4	16.7
Least developed countries	18.6	18.3	19.5	20.4
Other developing countries	18.9	18.6	20.5	16.1
Africa	18.9	18.6	19.0	20.6
Eastern Africa	18.9	18.7	18.9	21.3
Middle Africa	18.7	18.5	18.9	21.1
Northern Africa	19.0	18.5	19.5	18.1
Southern Africa	18.5	18.8	19.1	18.3
Western Africa	19.1	18.6	18.8	21.5
Latin America	18.9	18.8	20.0	16.2
Caribbean	17.7	18.1	20.6	15.3
Central America	19.2	18.5	21.9	16.5
South America	19.0	19.0	19.1	16.1
North America	14.8	17.9	14.4	11.9
Asia	18.9	18.5	20.5	15.4
Eastern Asia	18.5	19.0	21.5	12.0
Southeastern Asia	19.4	18.2	20.8	15.5
Southern Asia	19.2	18.1	19.4	17.6
Western Asia	19.7	18.5	19.5	18.3
Europe	16.2	15.5	15.0	11.6
Eastern Europe	17.4	16.9	14.5	12.8
Northern Europe	13.7	15.2	14.8	11.5
Southern Europe	18.3	15.6	16.1	11.4
Western Europe	14.9	14.7	14.4	10.8
Oceania	15.5	17.7	17.5	14.1
Australia—New Zealand	14.6	17.5	16.5	12.4
Melanesia	19.2	18.7	20.6	18.3
Micronesia	19.9	18.7	19.6	16.8
Polynesia	18.8	18.4	21.5	17.7
Former U.S.S.R.	20.7	16.7	14.6	13.8

From United Nations (1992). Changing population age structures: Demographic and economic consequences and implications. Geneva: United Nations.

Table 29-3 Percentage of Population Aged 65 and over, by Major Area and Region

MAJOR AREA AND REGION	1950	1970	1990	2025
World Total	5.1	5.4	6.2	9.7
More developed regions	7.6	9.6	12.1	19.0
Less developed regions	3.8	3.7	4.5	8.0
Least developed countries	3.4	3.1	3.0	4.0
Other developing countries	3.9	3.8	4.6	8.7
Africa	3.2	3.1	3.0	4.1
Eastern Africa	3.1	2.8	2.7	3.3
Middle Africa	3.8	3.1	3.0	3.5
Northern Africa	3.5	3.9	3.6	6.4
Southern Africa	3.6	3.7	4.1	6.6
Western Africa	2.7	2.6	2.7	3.5
Latin America	3.3	3.9	4.8	8.6
Caribbean	4.4	5.2	6.5	10.0
Central America	3.2	3.3	3.8	7.5
South America	3.2	4.0	5.0	9.0
North America	8.1	9.6	12.5	19.9
Asia	4.0	4.0	5.0	9.6
Eastern Asia	4.5	4.5	6.3	13.7
Southeastern Asia	3.7	3.3	3.9	8.2
Southern Asia	3.6	3.6	4.1	7.2
Western Asia	3.6	4.0	3.6	6.0
Europe	8.7	11.4	13.4	20.1
Eastern Europe	7.0	10.4	11.3	17.6
Northern Europe	10.3	12.7	15.4	19.8
Southern Europe	7.4	9.9	12.8	20.0
Western Europe	10.1	12.8	14.5	22.3
Oceania	7.5	7.3	9.0	13.9
Australia—New Zealand	8.3	8.4	10.9	17.5
Melanesia	4.1	2.9	2.6	4.7
Micronesia	4.5	4.0	3.7	8.6
Polynesia	4.5	2.9	4.2	7.4
Former U.S.S.R.	6.1	7.4	9.6	14.8

From United Nations (1992). Changing population age structures: Demographic and economic consequences and implications. *Geneva: United Nations.*

Table 29-4 Median Age (in Years), by Major Area and Region

MAJOR AREA AND REGION	1950	1970	1990	2025
World Total	23.4	21.6	24.2	31.1
More developed regions	28.2	30.1	33.7	40.8
Less developed regions	21.2	18.9	22.0	29.6
Least developed countries	19.5	18.0	17.6	23.2
Other developing countries	21.4	19.0	22.5	30.8
Africa	18.6	17.5	17.4	22.2
Eastern Africa	18.1	17.1	16.4	20.6
Middle Africa	19.4	18.5	17.2	20.1
Northern Africa	19.3	17.6	19.1	28.1
Southern Africa	20.6	19.1	20.9	26.8
Western Africa	17.9	17.2	16.6	21.3
Latin America	19.7	18.6	21.9	30.3
Caribbean	21.3	19.7	24.1	31.5
Central America	18.1	16.5	19.8	29.4
South America	20.1	19.2	22.6	30.5
North America	30.0	27.7	33.1	41.1
Asia	21.9	19.7	23.3	32.5
Eastern Asia	23.5	20.6	36.5	38.4
Southeastern Asia	20.2	18.2	21.2	31.9
Southern Asia	20.5	19.2	20.6	29.4
Western Asia	19.6	18.5	19.6	25.6
Europe	30.5	32.2	35.0	42.9
Eastern Europe	28.7	31.4	33.7	40.0
Northern Europe	33.7	33.3	35.6	42.1
Southern Europe	27.4	31.0	34.3	44.4
Western Europe	33.9	33.1	36.4	44.7
Oceania	27.9	25.1	28.7	35.8
Australia—New Zealand	30.2	27.3	31.8	40.0
Melanesia	19.6	18.7	19.4	24.2
Micronesia	20.6	18.8	20.8	31.3
Polynesia	17.9	16.2	18.0	28.6
Former U.S.S.R.	24.7	28.9	31.1	36.4

From United Nations (1992). Changing population age structures: Demographic and economic consequences and implications. *Geneva: United Nations.*

vidual and aggregate approaches, public health and nursing, and health promotion and disease prevention. Nurses have the ability to demonstrate understanding of the relationships between the personal and environmental factors that affect health and thus are able to intervene at individual, family, and community levels.

Community health nurses can play a vital role in building partnerships with communities that can assist in addressing the current and projected health needs. Participating in partnerships with other health care profession-

als and members of the community—local, state, national, and international—will assist in the creation of healthier communities.

The international Healthy Cities/Communities movement, referred to in Chapter 1, focuses on mobilizing local resources and political, professional, and community members to improve the health of the community. It is a public health approach that examines the many interrelated factors that influence the health of a community. In order to participate in this movement and in the process

Perspectives...

Insights of a Community Health Nursing Instructor

It is critically important for community health nurses, and other nurses as well, to develop a knowledge of global health problems and issues. We live in a global society, and it is no longer sufficient for nurses to focus only on the population health needs in their respective countries. Nurses are in a vital position to assist in shaping public policy at national and international levels.

As a community health nursing faculty member in California, I have had the privilege of traveling to Australia each year since 1981 to participate in professional activities in a variety of ways: as curriculum consultant, a visiting fellow, presenter at research colloquia, international coordinator of an international research conference held in Melbourne in 1992, and as a professional colleague and friend of nurses in that country. These experiences, coupled with experiences as a board officer of the International Association for Human Caring and as a member of a collaborative research team that conducted a cross-national study in 1996 and 1997, have provided a rich tapestry of knowledge about nursing and health care issues in other countries. It has become evident that a global knowledge of health concerns and needs, as well knowledge of nursing's role in building caring, healthy communities, is imperative for our profession now and in the 21st century. Faculty members have a major responsibility to expand their focus on population health to include global perspectives. It is also an imperative to expand our knowledge in cultural care, on the cultural strategies that groups and communities use for negotiating our various health care systems. Listening to the perceptions of nurses, health care providers, and consumers from other countries share their knowledge with us is critical.

We are interconnected as nations; we do not exist in isolation. As nurses, we must become knowledgeable about global health problems and issues, cultural negotiation strategies, and the role that we can play in shaping public policy at local, state, national, and international levels. As Ramos (1997) so clearly states: "If the world is to be a healthier place, we cannot limit our caring to the interface with patients. There are huge steps to be taken in unifying health care professionals to design . . . care delivery systems that bring health to the people of the world. . . . If we care about the world we live in, if we translate our caring into a larger effort, we can make a difference" (p. 16).

Let us move forward with courage, commitment, compassion, excitement, and confidence that we, as nurses, can participate, personally and collectively, in building healthier communities worldwide in the next century.

—*Sue A. Thomas, EdD, RN*

of population health improvement, community health nurses must be prepared to function in multidisciplinary teams, to work with community residents and leaders, and to participate in changing health care delivery systems, given the projections in health status and population characteristics for the future.

Community health nurses can participate in policy making at local, state, national, and international levels to improve access to basic and preventive care, taking the initiative to work with community residents, leaders, and other health professionals to usher in the necessary changes. The nurse must place greater emphasis on participating in policy development aimed at quality-of-life issues, based on the caring concepts of mutual respect, trust, compassion, and courage. For example, by educating the public about population health problems and issues and eliciting their perspectives about their own community's health and population needs, the community health nurse is in a position to influence health outcomes and policy changes. The nurse can talk to policymakers about identified health needs and populations at risk and can serve on committees that address population health improvement strategies, such as educational programs, outreach services, and legislative action, among others. The nurse can also assist in identifying priorities and strategic planning for local, national, and international action, as well as participate in program evaluation research.

Participating with community leaders and citizens to establish a balanced approach to health improvement is another role for the nurse. Population health improvement efforts must balance an emphasis on personal responsibility with the social, structural, and environmental dimensions of health. Community health nurses are in pivotal positions to assist in this effort.

Because community health problems and issues transcend international borders, an international focus in community health nursing is also needed. Knowledge of the findings and projections from the Global Burden of Disease Study can provide the nurse with a much needed picture of global projections for the future as well as knowledge of the more current public health measures used to assess the health status of nations. International cooperation is required to deal with the challenges for the future. Basic to international collaborative efforts is the need for health care professionals to be culturally informed and cognizant of cultural differences.

Although disease, disability, injury, birth, death, and aging are universal, there are cultural differences in ways of defining health and illness, different systems for preventing and treating deviations from health, and different

DECISION MAKING

Culturally Congruent Care

A community health nurse is working in a multicultural urban neighborhood with families representing different racial and ethnic groups from different countries of origin. One of the major goals of the community health nurse is to provide services that are culturally congruent. Nursing interventions that are culturally relevant and sensitive to client and community needs decrease the possibility of conflict arising from cultural misunderstanding.

• What assessment domains should be included in order to understand the health needs of the selected populations in the neighborhood?

• What pertinent cultural factors should be included in a community nursing assessment?

• Why is cultural information important in the care of all clients?

COMMUNITY NURSING VIEW

A community health nurse is working in a community with a large population of at-risk and high-risk childbearing and childrearing Hispanic women, many of whom sought prenatal care late in their pregnancies. The infant mortality rate is higher in this community than in others surrounding it. Goals for this community are to reduce barriers to prenatal care and to provide care that is culturally relevant. The community health nurse is asked to serve as project director of a new program designed to reduce barriers to early prenatal care.

Nursing Considerations

ASSESSMENT
• What should the community health nurse include in the needs assessment process?
• What data should be collected regarding barriers to prenatal care? Who should collect the data?
• What factors need to be considered specific to data collection?

DIAGNOSIS
• Who should be involved in the formulation of community health diagnoses?

OUTCOME IDENTIFICATION
• What outcomes could be formulated specific to the prenatal care issue?
• What is the benefit to the community? To the mothers?

PLANNING/INTERVENTIONS
• Who should be involved in the planning with regard to the where, when, who, and how of program development?
• What factors should be considered when planning the program?
• What methods might be used to reduce barriers to prenatal care for the Hispanic women?

EVALUATION
• What indicators would suggest that the program has been effective?
• What might be suggested as the next course of action if the program is determined to be unsuccessful? Successful?

ways of coping with developmental and situational events (Dreher, 1996). Because of these differences, health care in the future will call for culturally informed health professionals. As the countries become even more interconnected, nurses as healers will be challenged to discover cultural meanings of health events, health beliefs, practices, and behaviors. Working with nurses and colleagues from both developing and industrialized nations will require cultural knowledge and sensitivity to culturally diverse ways of being. Appreciating cultural diversity will enhance nursing's contribution to building healthier communities.

The focus on healthy public policy and the concept of investing in health are emerging as important concepts, as evident in the Healthy Cities/Communities movement. The movement is a public health approach that encompasses the recognition that health and well-being are interconnected with social, cultural, physical, economic, and other factors and that community participation and collaboration are necessary to improve health and the quality of life. As Hancock and Garrett (1995) point out: "Primary advances in health during the 21st century are unlikely to be based mainly on medical care breakthroughs. They will be based instead on improvements in macro-environmental conditions—ecological, social, economic, political, and technological—that most influence health status" (p. 943). Because of this recognition, questions have been raised regarding the need for a new health economics. The European Regional Office of the WHO, for example, recently held a conference on the topic "investing in health." Questions posed by Dr. Ilona Kickbusch, director of WHO's Department of Health Promotion, Education, and Communications, were among those questions that were addressed at the conference, including: Where is health created? Which investment creates the largest health gain? Does the investment reduce inequity and respect human rights? (Hancock & Garrett, 1995). As Hancock and Garrett (1995) also noted, similar questions are beginning to receive serious consideration by other national and international agencies.

The growing worldwide movement for healthy cities and communities, which was initiated by the WHO in the 1980s, could result in new public health systems in the 21st century, ones that will be just as effective in improving health as their counterparts were in the 19th century (Hancock & Garrett, 1995). Community health nurses have the potential to play a vital role in the creation of healthier communities, as did nursing leaders such as Florence Nightingale, Lillian Wald, Mary Brewster, and Lavinia Dock, among others, over a century ago. Community health nurses are in a position to participate in the debates regarding changing priorities for public health in the decades ahead. The findings from the landmark Global Burden of Disease Study, which resulted in the production of a comprehensive and comparable set of current patterns of mortality, disease, disability, and injury for all regions of the world, with projections to the year 2020, pose challenges to nurses and policymakers throughout the world.

Key Concepts

- It is essential that community health nurses have a knowledge of population health problems from both national and international perspectives in order to function effectively in the global community as well as in their own community.

- Population health assessments must include knowledge not only of global mortality patterns but also of disease patterns, disabilities, and injuries in populations.

- Chronic diseases and disabilities are expected to increase as the population ages.

- The crusade against infectious disease must continue as long as diseases continue to exist.

- There needs to be greater emphasis on surveillance of injury morbidity, disability, and costs in order to identify risk factors and to evaluate injury-prevention programs.

- It is of vital importance to examine changing perspectives related to understanding the determinants of health.

- The global burden of disease (GBD) quantifies not only the number of deaths but also the impact of premature death and disability on a population.

- Changing global population growth patterns have a major impact on the nature of health care service needs.

- Knowledge of cultural factors is critical in the building of healthy communities.

- Community health nurses are in a vital position to contribute to the creation of community partnerships for the purpose of enhancing community health at local, state, national, and international levels.

Health Care Delivery Systems around the World

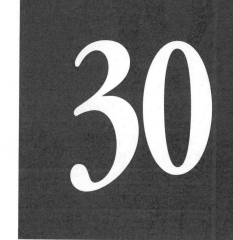

Sue A. Thomas, EdD, RN

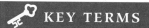 **KEY TERMS**

intergovernmental
   organizations
International Council of
   Nurses (ICN)
official international
   health organizations
Pan-American Health
   Organization (PAHO)
philanthropic
   foundations
private organizations
private voluntary
   organizations
Sigma Theta Tau,
   International (STT)
United Nations
   Children's Fund
   (UNICEF)

*By the year 2000, all people should have the opportunity to develop
and use their own health potential in order to lead socially,
economically, and mentally fulfilling lives.*

—*Target 2: Health and Quality of Life,*
World Health Organization, 1993

COMPETENCIES

Upon completion of this chapter, the reader should be able to:

- Discuss the major international health and health-promotion efforts from a global perspective.
- Discuss the role of primary health care in promoting the health of nations.
- Identify the major national and international health initiatives that affect public health.
- Describe major international health organizations and their contributions to promoting health.
- Discuss the nature of health sector reform from an international perspective.
- Discuss selected health care system trends in the United Kingdom, Australia, Canada, and Russia.
- Discuss cross-sectoral and cross-national collaboration as emerging strategies for the future.
- Discuss nursing's contribution to cross-sectoral collaboration efforts.

Because of the recognition of the global connectedness among nations and the increasing concern for international health and health care, community health nurses need to understand the organizational issues in health care delivery systems from an international perspective. Exploring the nature of the changes that are occurring in health care delivery can assist in the analysis of various approaches to international health care.

As Dreher (1997) states:

> It is clear that worldwide health cannot be achieved by a single nation. Indeed, even the health of a single nation cannot be achieved only through the efforts of that nation. Damage to the rain forest in Brazil affects the atmosphere that the whole world breathes, wars in Eastern Europe impact countless other nations, a virus originating in Africa has pandemic implications and television violence from the U.S. is broadcast throughout the world. Health is a dynamic and worldwide relationship between human societies and their environments. Like it or not, we live in a global society, and health is a global responsibility (p. 5).

This chapter provides a discussion of international health initiatives that have particular relevance for community health nursing. It also discusses the major international health organizations, including those in nursing. Changing perspectives in health care delivery systems are described, with a focus on selected health care systems. Last, implications for the future are explored.

INTERNATIONAL HEALTH AND HEALTH PROMOTION

As discussed in earlier chapters, the World Health Organization (WHO) initiative Health for All by the Year 2000 (HFA 2000) has resulted in significant growth of interest in world health and how best to achieve it. This interest is reflected in the recognition of the need to better understand health care issues and concerns on a global level.

All countries of the world have health problems and concerns. There is a difference in the nature of the problems and how to deal with them, however. Some countries experience higher infant and child mortality rates than others. Some countries have higher rates of certain infectious diseases, differences in environmental health hazards, chronic diseases, lifestyles, and mental health problems, among others. Examining the major problems and concerns of the world's health is of critical importance to community health nurses. One of the major ways the World Health Organization proposes to deal with various health problems and concerns is through a greater emphasis on health promotion and disease prevention efforts.

Health Promotion

Health promotion is central to the work of community health nurses, as well as all health professionals, whether in Australia, Canada, Russia, Finland, Brazil, the United Kingdom, the United States, or other countries. The emphasis on health promotion is an expanding one in nursing and health care generally, as discussed in Chapters 1 and 9.

Health promotion reflects a shift in focus toward care in community settings and an increased emphasis on the public's health. At the international level, health promotion efforts are enhanced through the process of countries working together, for the purpose of sharing knowledge, resources, and skills to promote world health. An integrated approach reflects the important position that health promotion increasingly occupies in nursing and in all of the various health care activities in many countries throughout the world. It is an approach that focuses on the premise that the basic conditions and resources for health are peace, shelter, food, income, education, a stable ecosystem, sustainable resources, social justice, and equity (World Health Organization, 1986). The integrated approach is based on the WHO health-promotion initiatives, which acknowledge the global nature of many of

today's health problems and the importance of the environment and ecological sustainability in promoting world health.

Health promotion is central to the whole view of health and caring, not marginal to mainstream care (Pike & Forster, 1995). It is a major challenge for the 21st century. Health promotion is not a new concept; however, it has historically been viewed primarily as the province of public health in Western industrialized nations. The crisis in health care costs, together with the demographic changes, changing patterns of health and disease, plus the recognition that prevention can reduce costs and illness, have led to a far greater emphasis on community health and on health promotion.

Health promotion in this chapter and book is viewed within the context of Ottawa's Charter for Health Promotion and the WHO targets for "Health for All" (WHO, 1993). The Ottawa Charter has become influential in promoting health and assisting the process to make it operational. This charter has integrated the concept of healthy public policy with the need for personal and individual involvement in health promotion. The Charter was based on principles of social justice, equity, and the achievement of "Health for All by the Year 2000" (Pike, 1995). The Ottawa strategy emphasizes both individual and community dimensions of health promotion, with the recognition that the two need to work together. It clearly points out that both the individual context and a public/community approach are vital to health promotion.

WHO recognized the significance of the Ottawa Charter and through the Healthy Cities/Communities movement has developed a far greater emphasis on public health and environmental issues. WHO has shifted from a major focus on individual and lifestyle behaviors to a far greater emphasis on public health and the environment, thus attempting to create and maintain a better balance between lifestyle, the environment, and health service issues (Pike, 1995).

The Role of Primary Health Care

Primary health care in international health is associated with the global conference held at Alma Ata in 1978, the conference that promoted the initiative Health for All by the Year 2000 (WHO, 1978). Primary health care (PHC), defined broadly at Alma Ata, emphasized universal health care access to all individuals and families, encouraged participation by community members in all aspects of health care planning and implementation, and promoted the delivery of care that would be "scientifically sound, technically effective, socially relevant and acceptable" (WHO, 1978, p. 2).

A major initiative produced in 1974, which had an influence at Alma Ata, was the LaLonde Report, called "A New Perspective on the Health of Canadians." This report stimulated discussion regarding the need for a new perspective on the health of the Canadian population. As the Canadian Minister of National Health and Welfare,

LaLonde recommended a more comprehensive approach to health care. LaLonde identified the major determinants of health as human biology, environment, lifestyle, and health care. Ashton and Seymour (1988) argued that this report was a major turning point in international policy with the reaffirmation of earlier public health strategies that focused on a broader approach to health rather than only a personal approach.

Thus, a major shift in perspective that emerged from the LaLonde Report, the Alma Ata Conference, and the Healthy Cities/Communities movement, referred to initially in Chapter 1, was the shift from an individual focus to one of community participation. The involvement of community members as participants in planning for health is viewed as a critical ingredient for effective public health practice for the 21st century. The commitment to shared values and common goals enables the group to deal with complex problems and issues more effectively than individuals alone. Thus, community health nurses are in a vital position to participate as leaders in the process.

Katz and Kreuter (1997) suggest that the justification for making community participation an essential aspect for public health practice can be summarized as follows:

• Nonmedical factors, such as social conditions and community values, have a major influence on health status.
• Planners and policymakers must actively involve the public in the development of solutions to health problems because medical interventions alone are not sufficient to result in health status improvements.
• Policy development requires the active involvement of people who are affected by public health programs.

MAJOR INTERNATIONAL ORGANIZATIONS

There are a variety of organizations concerned with international health. Because nursing is a global discipline and health is a global concern, nurses must be knowledgeable about international health organizations that work to improve the world's health.

Types of International Health Organizations

International health organizations can be classified as private voluntary agencies, philanthropic foundations, private organizations, and official (governmental, intergovernmental) agencies, as well as professional and technical organizations (Basch, 1990). **Private voluntary organizations** include both religious and secular groups that provide different health care assistance programs. Many of the religious institutions, such as the Maryknoll Missionaries from the Catholic Church, conduct health service projects worldwide. Secular groups, such as the International Council of Voluntary Agencies, assist in coordination activities. Other examples are Project HOPE and CARE.

Philanthropic foundations are those that use funds from private endowments to provide grants for health-related projects. Examples of the philanthropic organizations involved in health care globally include the Rockefeller Foundation, the W. K. Kellogg Foundation, and the Hewlett Foundation. The program goals and projects vary. **Private organizations** such as pharmaceutical companies (the Johnson and Johnson Company, for example) provide financial and technical assistance for health care, employment, and access to health care.

Official international health organizations are those agencies throughout the world that participate in collaborative arrangements via official governmental structures. Bilateral arrangements may occur between countries through various governmental organizations. Many of these arrangements are made between two countries with the focus on a single project. **Intergovernmental organizations** also exist. These organizations deal with health concerns on an ongoing basis and collaborate with governments, private foundations, and other efforts to improve health. Professional and technical organizations address specific professional as well as scientific goals and participate in the sharing of knowledge. An example is the International Council of Nurses.

The major intergovernmental organization that deals with health concerns at the international level is the World Health Organization (WHO). WHO was created in 1946 through the efforts of the League of Nations, which became the United Nations (UN). WHO was the outcome of a variety of global activities begun in the mid-1880s, directed by various countries to control cholera (Basch, 1990). The UN Charter resulted in formation of a special health agency that could deal with global health problems. The central office for WHO is in Geneva, Switzerland, with six regional offices in Copenhagen, Alexandria, Brazzaville, Manila, New Delhi, and Washington, D.C. The World Health Assembly, which meets yearly in May, is the policy formation arena for WHO. The scope of WHO's responsibilities is comprehensive and consists of many major functions, with over 100 subfunctions. It is responsible for monitoring global disease incidence and prevalence and for setting international health standards specific to sanitation, laboratory procedures, pharmaceutical manufacturing, and biological products. It also monitors environmental pollution, sponsors a variety of programs with emphasis on training medical personnel, health services development, primary health care, and disease control programs. As noted earlier in this chapter, the WHO is the major sponsor of the Healthy Cities/Communities movement that emerged in the 1980s as a way to implement the Health for All by the Year 2000 initiative.

At the fiftieth World Health Assembly held in May 1997 in Geneva, for example, more than 1,200 delegates from 191 member states attended the meeting of the WHO's governing body (American Public Health Association, 1997). One of the major global problems unanimously endorsed by the delegates was an international plan of action to deal with violence as a public health problem. The WHO plan on violence, prepared by a task force at the request of the assembly in 1996, asks for a description of the public health scope of violence in all of its various forms, which will require internationally accepted methodology. It is anticipated that quantifiable targets for violence prevention could be established by the year 2000.

Three other international organizations are also well known for their health-related efforts: the World Bank, the United Nations Children's Fund, and the Pan-American Health Organization. The World Bank places its major emphasis on assisting countries where economic development is needed. It provides financial assistance to governments and foundations to develop projects that address the health of those countries where economic development is limited. The bank assists with projects that focus on economic growth, affordable housing, safe and usable water, and sanitation systems, among others.

The **United Nations Children's Fund (UNICEF)** was formed after World War II to assist the children who lived in European war countries. Since that time, however, the UN Children's Fund expanded its focus worldwide. Health

projects have been developed throughout the world to control leprosy, tuberculosis, yaws, and other diseases. Maternal and child health programs are other global efforts supported by UNICEF.

The **Pan-American Health Organization (PAHO)**, founded in 1902, was developed to assist those countries of the Western Hemisphere. It focuses its efforts on the Americas, all of the countries of the Western Hemisphere, particularly those in Latin America. Two of its major functions are to identify public health hazards and to distribute public health data that include epidemiologic information, information about the health systems within the countries, and various environmental issues. The PAHO supports public health research efforts and professional education. The national profiles it creates provide significant assistance to health planning efforts.

Major International Nursing Organizations

In nursing, two major international organizations need to be discussed: the International Council of Nurses and Sigma Theta Tau, International. The **International Council of Nurses (ICN)** represents 112 national organizations (Ohlson & Styles, 1997) as members, with as many as 1 million nurses (Splane & Splane, 1994). The ICN, founded in 1899 (Bridges, 1965), was the first international organization for professional women in history and is the only organization that represents the nursing profession worldwide. The ICN is the primary organization for the advancement of international nursing. The purpose of the ICN is "to provide a medium through which the interests, needs, and concerns of member national nurses associations can be addressed to the advantage of the public and nurses" (Bridges, 1965). The ICN's program is based on the following objectives (Quinn, 1981):

1. To promote the development of strong national nursing associations (NNAs)
2. To assist NNAs in improving nursing standards and the competence of nurses—their education and practice
3. To assist NNAs in improving the status of nurses—their economic and social welfare
4. To serve as a unified voice for nurses and nursing internationally

Sigma Theta Tau, International (STT) is the international honor society of nursing. It was founded in 1922 at the Indiana University Training School for Nurses. In 1997, STT celebrated its seventy-fifth anniversary, with more than 200,000 members worldwide who live and work in 73 nations. There are 356 chapters located at colleges and universities in Australia, Canada, Puerto Rico, South Korea, Taiwan, and the United States. It is the second largest nursing organization in the United States and one of the five largest in the world.

DECISION MAKING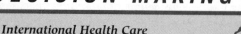

International Health Care

Select a country or area of the world outside the United States that interests you.

• How might you find out about the status of health care in that country, its major health problems, and which international health organizations are involved with health care delivery in that country?

• What types of questions would you need to ask in order to determine the role of primary health care in that country and the role of the community health nurse?

The purpose of STT is to recognize, encourage, and support nursing excellence in clinical practice, education, research, and leadership. The organization is dedicated to improving the health of people worldwide through increasing the scientific base of nursing practice.

HEALTH CARE SYSTEMS: CHANGING PERSPECTIVES

It is important that nurses recognize the significance of global sharing of knowledge about the provision of health services in different countries. Because nursing is a global enterprise and is committed to improving the health of citizens worldwide, a discussion of various health systems is included in this chapter. As Dreher (1997) points out, most of the major changes in disease prevention and control came not from medicine, as it is currently understood and practiced, but from public health practice, in which nurses have the primary responsibility for promoting healthy lifestyles, providing health education, and improving sanitation and hygiene. Thus, a focus on global knowledge related to health care systems is critical

DECISION MAKING

Global Levels of Health Care

It is most important that nurses develop knowledge of international health and those activities that contribute to the health of people worldwide. You have been asked to participate in a discussion focused on international health.

• What information do you think you would need to discuss international health issues? From what sources might you obtain information regarding the major international health problems?

• How do you think nurses should be prepared to think and act at both local and global levels?

because nurses can work together throughout the world to enhance care and caring in changing political climates.

As the world's people become more interdependent, it is imperative that nurses be prepared to deal with international health and that international health be integrated

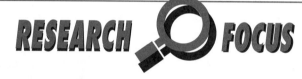

RESEARCH FOCUS

Nursing Education and International Health in the United States, Latin America, and the Caribbean

STUDY PROBLEM/PURPOSE

There is little research about the preparation and activities of nurses to assist them in dealing with international health and little information about the extent of international health activities in U.S. schools of nursing. The purpose of this study was to identify international health activities in schools of nursing in the United States, Latin America, and the Caribbean.

METHODS

A descriptive study design with a 16-item survey questionnaire was used to obtain information from a random sample of 100 U.S. university schools of nursing and 15 schools with known international activities (10 from the United States and five from Latin America and the Caribbean). Responses were received from 59 of the U.S. randomly sampled schools and from eight of those known to have international activities. All five schools from Latin America and the Caribbean responded.

FINDINGS

International health as a topic was found in one-third of the U.S. schools of nursing, but international

health was not integrated with other subjects. Of the U.S. respondents, 54 (84%) expressed interest in the field of international health. All five of the Latin American and Caribbean schools of nursing confirmed the Pan-American Health Organization's indications of international health activities. International health activities were usually individual initiatives with limited institutional support.

IMPLICATIONS

This study indicates a growing interest in international health among schools of nursing. However, they have contributed in a limited way to the development of the international health field. The study reveals a definite need for schools of nursing to include a nursing curriculum with international health, an interdisciplinary approach to the international health curriculum, and a vision of international health as a leadership responsibility for nurses.

SOURCE

From "Nursing Education and International Health in the United States, Latin America, and the Caribbean by M. M. Wright, C. Godue, M. Manfredi, & D. Korniewicz, 1998, Image: Journal of Nursing Scholarship, 30(1), pp. 31–36.

into the nursing curriculum. Wright, Godue, Manfredi, and Korniewicz (1998) conducted a study that focused on how nursing education and associated activities prepared nurses to develop a knowledge of international health. This study is particularly significant because it was the first known study that focused on the extent and nature of international health activities among U.S. schools of nursing and from schools in Latin America and the Caribbean. See the accompanying Research Focus for further exploration.

Health care systems in countries throughout the world vary in relation to their philosophies, structures, and functions. Several basic elements, however, are addressed in all the various systems (Basch, 1990): (1) the type of coverage a citizen or consumer could anticipate; (2) who can utilize the system; (3) the providers and the types of care they provide; (4) location of the health care services and nature of the facilities; and (5) who has the influence or power to determine access and availability. There is currently one additional major element that many are experiencing: rapidity of change. System changes are occurring throughout the world. The context of change and changes in government policy in various countries are occurring in all elements of services and in all types of services, including services for the elderly, child health and welfare, mental health, alcohol and drug services, and disability services.

Health Sector Reform: A Global Perspective

The emergence of health sector reform as a major international public health issue suggests that there is a widespread recognition of health sector problems and some solutions (Berman, 1996). Berman (1996) suggests that health sector reform may be defined as "sustained, purposeful, and fundamental change in the policies, programs, and institutions providing health care services" (p. 34). *Sustained change* refers to an effort over time—a process. It does not mean a single action. *Purposeful change* requires goals and implies that outcomes can be evaluated. *Fundamental change* differentiates the nature of health sector reform, with the inclusion of programs, institutions, and policies, from a specific programmatic change.

Health sector reform is needed in order to meet the current diverse health needs of populations and to incorporate rapid technological change. The goal of health sector reform is to provide health care that is affordable and manageable for future generations—to create systems that will be driven not by market forces alone but also by public policy and government.

Countries with different social and economic conditions are considering or developing programs to meet future needs. In the higher-income countries, a variety of concerns have resulted in reform efforts: (1) the rapid

increase in health care costs, (2) consumer dissatisfaction with access to and the quality of their health care, and (3) major disparities in access to health care for certain population groups (Berman, 1996). These factors are important in the examination of reform efforts in such countries as the United Kingdom, Sweden, and the Netherlands. In 1994 reform efforts were the major motivational factors for the unsuccessful health reform proposals in the United States.

In the formerly socialist countries, such as the former Soviet Union, Eastern Europe, Vietnam, and China, because of the major political and economic changes, government-financed and -operated health care services can no longer rely on adequate government support. There are current efforts to find new ways to satisfy the health care need. Many of these countries are struggling, however, with the issues of providing care to their populations, particularly those who are poor and vulnerable.

Middle-income and poorer countries have different pressures for reform. Countries such as Mexico, Colombia, and Thailand are experiencing shifts in disease patterns from high rates of infectious and communicable diseases to high rates of chronic diseases while, at the same time, trying to deal with the poor population groups who suffer from the conditions found in the poorest countries (Berman, 1996).

In many of the poorer countries such as those in Latin America and sub-Saharan Africa, declining incomes and public revenues have resulted in reduction in government health care expenditures. The most basic health care services have become more limited, as a result.

As Berman (1996) states:

> Although there is no single formula for health sector reform among such diverse countries, there are common themes. These include social solidarity in redistributing resources from the wealthier to the poorer and from the healthier to the sicker groups; increased use of regulated market-like forces to encourage efficiency and quality; focus of resources on more cost effective services; and increased recognition and wise use of pluralism in government and private participation in the health sector" (p. 36).

Countries have developed many different types of health care systems; however, the current predominant theme is one of change. Nursing varies from country to country, and nurses' roles are diverse given the nature of the different health care systems. Nursing is in a position to make a difference during this period of change. We need to assist each other through global sharing of knowledge, participating in healthy public policy development, and caring about one another with respect for our various cultures.

United Kingdom

The United Kingdom (UK) uses a government health system, the National Health Service. It began in 1946 for the purpose of providing everyone with health services and is supported by individual and corporate taxation. Services are administered through a system of health authorities. The services provided by the health authorities include general medicine, disability, surgery, and rehabilitation. Services are made available through private physicians, hospitals, nurses and allied health professionals, clinics, health outreach programs such as hospice, boroughs, district nursing, and environmental health services.

The British health care system still provides the majority of health care services (Pike, 1995), but it has undergone many changes. The changes have been particularly rapid since the mid-1980s, primarily in relation to the delivery process.

The health services are now operated in a climate that is influenced by business management principles (Pike, 1995). One of the major pressures to change health services has been to contain costs, and this has resulted in the movement toward a more businesslike climate. There is a greater emphasis on providing efficient and effective services. As a result, disease-prevention and health-promotion activities are receiving increased funding. Decision makers and health care providers are recognizing that it makes sense to try to curtail spending on high-technology hospital treatment (curative in nature) by preventing any need for it, and they are acknowledging the burden of preventable diseases. The shift of the balance of funding toward a greater emphasis on prevention and health promotion is also consistent with the WHO strategy and the focus on primary health care (Pike, 1995).

The shift in funding has resulted in the orientation toward a community basis for the delivery of care. This community focus is occurring in the health sector and in social work and social care. Large institutions, such as those that housed people with mental health problems, institutions for those with learning disabilities, large homes for older adults, and many of the larger hospitals that were a legacy from the last century are disappearing. Smaller units in the community are thought to be more appropriate. Larger institutions are often viewed as too expensive to manage. Community care is viewed as a more appropriate model because many of the conditions today are amenable to a caring approach rather than a primary focus on curing actions.

A number of conditions are bringing about the changes in the British health system plans for the future. The rise in the incidence of chronic diseases, degenerative conditions, and disability, along with the increase in the number of older adults in the population, has resulted in the recognition of the need for changes in health delivery. Mental health problems concerned with depression, stress, and substance abuse are also issues that require a community care focus.

Most people suffering from chronic diseases and disability are cared for in the community, not in institutions or hospitals. Thus, there is greater recognition in the United Kingdom than there is in the United States that health problems need to be prevented. Health promotion is viewed as a most important way to deal with current and future health problems.

Australia

Australia also uses a government system, a system of national health insurance for basic health care services—acute, subacute, and home care—for all persons in the population. Medicare, Australia's system of national health insurance, was instituted in 1984. Changes in government policy and in the role and structure of Australian families, the aging of the population, and the recognition of the need to control health care costs all began in the 1980s. Given these changes, significant shifts have occurred in the Australian health care system also. In Australia, as in the United States, there has been a major shift away from acute care institutions to home-based care in all service sectors, including services for the aging, child welfare, mental health, alcohol and drug abuse, and disability services (Zamurs, 1995). Thus, community-based care plays a major role in the health care system.

Community-based care in Australia now involves diverse providers and requires coordination of services. The major changes in the acute care system, based on technological changes, improved clinical practice, and further development of care management and nursing services at home have reduced the length of stay in hospitals. Because of this shift, improving the linkages between the hospital and community-based services has been increasingly emphasized in order to continue improvements in care management through effective discharge planning.

One of the results of earlier hospital discharges, coupled with the changing demographics and the resultant increase in the proportion of people with chronic health conditions, is the ever-increasing demand on family caregivers; these patterns are also identified in the United States. Complex care demands related to the increased acuity of family members being cared for at home have resulted in difficulty for the health and well-being of caregivers, particularly those without supportive families or community networks to share responsibilities (Zamurs, 1995).

In Australia, there is a great emphasis on shifting resources to the primary and continuing care system, because it is anticipated that the greatest demand and need will be for community-based services. With the shift to community-based services, health promotion and well-being receive greater emphasis.

The health services in Australia, similar to those in the United Kingdom and the United States, are operated in a climate influenced by privatization, economic considerations, and the culture of consumerism. There is a great emphasis on the need for efficient and effective services.

One of the health and community service provisions is the national health insurance system called Medicare, referred to earlier. The national health insurance system is popular with consumers, "playing a central role in making Australia a just society" (Duckett, 1995, p. 15). The five principles underpinning Medicare are universality, access, equity, efficiency, and simplicity (Commonwealth Department of Health, Housing, and Community Services, 1992). All residents are eligible for benefits, which include access to free inpatient and outpatient treatment in public hospitals and private medical services. Individuals who wish to use the services of a private medical practitioner of their choice will receive a benefit of 85% of the schedule fees (Commonwealth Department of Human Services and Health, 1995). Private insurance offers ancillary benefits only, hospital benefits only, or a combination of the two. Hospital benefits provide reimbursement for private hospital accommodation.

Although the national health insurance system is viewed as a strength, it has problems, such as lengthy hospital waiting lists, limited access to costly new technology, gaps in service provisions for people with chronic conditions, and difficulty in navigating the complexity of an array of programs and services. Because of the identified problems, changing community expectations, the changing care environment, and pressures on government to control costs, reform was viewed as necessary (Duckett, 1995).

The Council of Australian Governments (COAG) in 1994 identified reforms of health and community services that it viewed as necessary for the future (Duckett, 1995). The COAG approach to dealing with the identified problems was to conceptualize "streams of care as the basis for change." Three major categories of care were identified:

1. General care—Refers to primary health care, home and community care services, and selected outpatient services considered episodic in nature.

2. Acute care—Refers to care in day surgery centers and acute care hospitals. Viewed as all activities directly related to the services provided prior to the acute intervention, the acute care service itself, and any post-acute services directly related to the specific acute episode.

3. Coordinated care—Refers particularly to care and support that are long term and complex. This stream of care is viewed in Australia as one of the major areas needed for the future (Duckett, 1995). Coordinated care services, provided by a care coordinator, are believed to be particularly important for persons with chronic diseases—the frail elderly, disabled, those with long-term psychiatric problems, and those with long-term rehabilitation problems. Such care coordination has been identified as one way to prevent other health problems from arising and to address them early when they do, thus reducing the need for hospitalization or institutionalization. Nurses, particularly community health nurses, can play a vital role in this effort.

Duckett (1995) proposes that a focus on population health provides a way to measure how each of the care streams contributes to improving the community's health. Population health focuses on health promotion and improvements in the community's health as well as on the distribution of health conditions specific to particular populations, such as the indigenous population, non-English-speaking people, and others. Examining the different streams of care from a population perspective enhances outcome measurement, which has received great emphasis in Australia.

Canada

The Canadian health care system is based on a national health insurance program also. Federal legislation to institute national health insurance was enacted in 1957. The program provided for comprehensive in-hospital client care services with universal coverage for residents of participating provinces. This initial legislation created a program administered in the respective provinces. Currently, the provincial and federal governments provide funds through personal income taxes. Benefits cover primarily in-hospital and physician-centered care, the dominant features of the system that evolved since 1957. The high cost of these methods of providing care, however, has led to a search for more cost-effective and efficient, lower-cost services. Canadians believe that health insurance coverage is a right of citizenship (Ross Kerr, 1997). The tax-supported Medicare program is a valued initiative of the government.

The rationale for the evolution of the federal health legislation is based on five principles of health care (Ross Kerr, 1997):

1. Universality—Extending coverage to the entire population rather than to selected groups

2. Comprehensiveness—Coverage of all medically necessary services

3. Accessibility—Reasonable access to health care services

4. Portability—Coverage required for residents of one province when they move to another province and require services

5. Public administration—Nonprofit operation by an organization fiscally responsible to the provincial government

In the 1980s and 1990s the rising costs of health care, specifically hospital and physician services, served as a major impetus for change in the Canadian system. The aging of the population, increasing rates of health care utilization, and rising costs have raised issues that are being debated regarding payment for health services. These debates have given impetus to health system changes (Ross Kerr, 1997) that place greater emphasis on community-based care.

With the movement toward community-based care, major restructuring efforts are occurring in Canada. With the intent to increase the efficiency of service delivery and yet maintain quality of care, critical issues are being discussed in Canada, as in other countries. In addition to the increased emphasis on health promotion and cost efficiency, there is a greater recognition of the various determinants of health discussed in the landmark LaLonde Report, determinants such as income, education, and the environment. Health is being viewed more broadly than as being merely the absence of illness, and new approaches are being examined in relation to the meaning of health (Ross Kerr, 1997).

In a recent report commissioned by the provincial ministers of health, primary care organizations were promoted. Physicians are grouped together in large clinic settings where they practice with other health professionals. Physicians would be paid an annual fee for each person registered, thereby providing an incentive for health-promotion and disease-prevention efforts. Moving to a community-based model emphasizing disease prevention, health promotion, and multidisciplinary collaboration is viewed as holding the greatest potential for improving health (Ross Kerr, 1997).

Because of the changes occurring in Canada, providing accessible primary and community-based health care and linkages between hospitals and community services are challenges for the future. As Ross Kerr (1997) points out, although it is recognized that there are limits to the nature and amount of care that can be provided, measures need to be taken to ensure that universal availability and access to needed services are provided in a publicly funded, nonprofit, affordable system.

Russia

Health care in Russia is also in the midst of major changes. A discussion of health care must be viewed within the context of the political changes that occurred in Russia since 1991 and the significant changes that have occurred in nursing in that country. The Independent Republic of the Russian Federation, a reality since December 25, 1991, and its constitution set forth a health care system free of charge to all citizens (Smith, 1997).

Before 1991, health care was delivered by a centrally ordered, hierarchical system (Curtis, Petukhova, & Taket, 1995). Clients did not pay for care directly, and health care professionals were considered state employees. Health care concerns were given a lower priority than other governmental endeavors such as industrial and military activities. The gross domestic product for health care spending was approximately 2.4% (Curtis et al., 1995). Because of this lower priority rating, chronic underfunding and rationing occurred. Long waits for service and medicinal supply shortages were prevalent.

Since 1991, Russia has struggled to enact social reforms and a market-driven economy. Russia is a nation trying to overcome its history of oppression and human rights violations, as is evident in its new national charter. With this effort, problems have arisen. Inflation, poverty, crime, and concerns about the infrastructure are having a major impact on the people. The crumbling infrastructure and political changes are posing very serious problems for the health care system in Russia (Smith, 1997). Health care funding is not a priority of the government.

Hospitals are finding it difficult to operate, with shortages of food, supplies, and medicines in many areas. Each hospital has two parts; one part is designated for people without money or insurance. Their care is free, but they receive no or few medications and limited attention. The other part of the hospital is reserved for clients who pay for their care. These clients receive medications and more attention from staff. In addition, they are better fed because of their ability to pay for their care. Some hospitals provide little or no food on the free side because of severe funding shortages. Family members are expected to bring food, but clients who have no family have a very serious problem (Smith, 1997).

Picard and DiVitto (1997), describing a visit to Russia in 1995, gave an example of a health care center burn unit. The unit staff had one pair of gloves for each shift; the gloves were washed and reused. Nurses reported that the infection rate was 100%. Antibiotics and other medications were scarce, used in diluted doses, and given only for severe infections. Such shortages were reported to be present at other centers also.

Because nursing constitutes a major portion of the health professional work force, it is important to describe the historical context and the changes that have taken place in nursing in Russia. Historically, nursing was and still remains a physician-dominated, task-oriented profession. The status and income of nursing are low. Nurses' wages have been just above the poverty line (Perfiljeva, 1997). The working conditions are poor, and nurses are required to increase the workload which has resulted in work that is very demanding. As Perfiljeva states: "Most of them hold down two jobs to make ends meet" (p. 8).

Since 1991, however, physician dominance has been fading. Through the vision of Perfiljeva, who is the Dean of the School of Nursing at the Moscow Medical Academy, the academy initiated the first master's program in nursing in the country (Smith, 1997). In very difficult circumstances, progress has been made in nursing education in Russia, with curricula focused on both hospital nursing and community nursing at the baccalaureate level as well.

Perfiljeva (1997) comments: "It is recognized in the country that effectiveness, efficiency, and humanity—the cornerstones of a high quality service—depend to a large extent on the work of nurses. As the national debt rises and economic pressures continue to affect health care budgets, providing the most efficient and cost effective care is vital. Nurses can potentially save hospitals a great deal of money by working daily with patients in the community to prevent serious illnesses, or prevent people going into the hospital in the first place" (p. 8). Thus health promotion and disease prevention efforts will become a major role for nurses in the future. Perfiljeva also states: "We are very proud of our nursing students— They are the change agents in the health care delivery system and particularly, in their health care settings" (p. 9).

IMPLICATIONS FOR THE FUTURE

Many nations are engaged in health system reforms that imply substantial changes in policies, programs, and insti-

Perspectives...

Insights of a Community Health Nursing Instructor

Developing a knowledge of international perspectives about health and health care systems is an imperative for nursing today and in the future. The importance of sharing knowledge about the world's health problems and the nature of the health care delivery systems cannot be underestimated. We live in a global society, and as nurses we have knowledge to share, knowledge of the commonalities and differences in nursing and health care worldwide. We can assist each other, as colleagues and friends, in health promotion and disease prevention efforts. We must work together as nurses and with other health professionals to build healthy, caring communities.

One of the challenges for nursing in the next century is to incorporate into nursing curricula a much greater emphasis on international health perspectives. As a faculty member who has had the opportunity to teach and consult in a country outside the United States since the 1980s and the opportunity to participate in the development of an international association in nursing, I have found that there is a growing interest in international health in nursing. There is a need, however, to encourage the study of international health in schools of nursing and to conduct research that reflects cross-national collaborative efforts. Providing opportunities for faculty and students to

learn more about international health and international health issues in nursing will require formal commitments by schools and their universities to develop partnerships, student exchange programs, and faculty projects with universities in other countries. If we truly believe that we live in a global society, then we must expand our knowledge of international health and participate in international health efforts, such as the examples discussed in this chapter. As Picard and DeVitto (1997) so clearly point out: We must "think and act both locally and globally" (p. 6).

As community health nurses, with our understanding of the global public health and primary health care initiatives, we have a broad perspective of health care that incorporates a tradition in the international health field. We can assist others in this challenge for the future, developing knowledge about health and disease patterns throughout the world, coupled with the recognition of the cultural significance of health, disease, and illness. Throughout our journey of global sharing, our exchanges will need to be culturally sensitive, modified, and negotiated. As nurses we must view ourselves as part of the global community in which problems, resources, and opportunities for community action efforts are shared.

—Sue A. Thomas

tutions providing health care services. These changes require health professionals to reexamine their present and future roles. Given the nature of these changes, it is increasingly recognized that to improve the health of the community, address health problems, and respond to economic and performance pressures, interdisciplinary, cross-cultural collaboration is necessary. Collaboration within and between countries can provide powerful strategies for dealing with current and future health care delivery problems.

Health professionals are working in a rapidly changing world environment. These changes present a valuable opportunity to engage in collaborative endeavors for the purpose of learning from each other and taking a proactive approach to dealing with current and future health

care environments. These collaborative efforts can enhance not only the health of the individuals and populations that health professionals serve but also their own effectiveness and influence.

Cross-sectoral and cross-national partnerships provide the opportunity to bring together a broad range of health professionals, community leaders, and health organizations. International cooperation through international organizations, universities, and consulting firms has assisted national leaders to develop health sector information that can and does assist in health reform efforts (Berman, 1996). Continued exchange and transfer of knowledge, technology, and experience between and within countries will assist in dealing with problems in financing, organizing, and managing health care systems.

COMMUNITY NURSING VIEW

A community health nurse working in a city has been asked to be on a steering committee to identify and implement the process for assessing the health of the city, using the WHO Healthy Cities model. The ultimate purpose of the community assessment project is to provide a document that will assist in building a healthier city, through the formulation of community health diagnoses and proposed interventions. The community itself is multicultural, with varying socioeconomic levels represented. The community health nurse is well known for her knowledge of the community as well as for her knowledge of the community assessment process. She previously served on several other citywide committees whose purposes were to address special target population needs, such as high rates of family violence and of older adults with chronic disabling conditions, many of whom were identified as poor.

Nursing Considerations

ASSESSMENT
• What steps should be taken to begin the assessment process?

• Who should be involved in the community assessment process?
• What kind of structure, organization, and funding will be necessary?
• What data will be needed? From what sources?

DIAGNOSIS
• Who should participate in formulating the diagnoses? In setting priorities?
• What process would you recommend specific to the analysis?

OUTCOME IDENTIFICATION
• What outcome indicators would you use to evaluate the assessment?

PLANNING/INTERVENTIONS
• Who should participate in planning the interventions?
• What methods would you recommend?
• How should the priority problems and proposed interventions be determined?

EVALUATION
• Who should participate in the evaluation process?
• What methods would you suggest? Why?

An example of a cross-national collaborative effort is the partnership created between the Epsilon Beta Chapter, Sigma Theta Tau, International (Fitchburg State College, Massachusetts) and the School of Nursing at Moscow Medical Academy. Since 1990, with the effective leadership of Dr. Galina Perfiljeva, Dean of the Moscow Medical School of Nursing Academy, and Carol Picard, Associate Professor of Nursing at Fitchburg State College, a successful collaborative project was initiated. Because of the serious underfunding of health care and nursing education in Russia, journals and textbooks were needed. These were procured for use in Russia, and after the inception of the partnership, a successful fund-raising project was launched in 1995 that provided funds to purchase needed equipment for the School of Nursing in Russia. In addition to the above, collaborative conferences have been held in Russia, and joint scholarly projects have been negotiated. Perfiljeva (1997) commented recently: "I fully believe that what unites nurses in my country and the United States, indeed across the globe, is stronger than what divides us. We are grateful for our colleagues from the United States of America and other countries who have supported us over the past years" (p. 9).

As cross-sectoral collaboration within countries and cross-national collaborative efforts expand, it will be critical that community health nurses, as well as all nurses, develop knowledge and competencies in intersectoral and interdisciplinary collaboration, as well as knowledge of the major international health care system issues. Collaboration enhances each health sector's stature and sphere of influence (Lasker and the Committee on Medicine and Public Health, 1997). It requires competencies in negotiation, communication, and community development; a population focus; the ability to use information systems; and the ability to use culturally congruent care strategies to improve health care.

The collaborative paradigm was a framework used by leaders in public health and medicine in the 19th century when they worked together on health boards and sanitary reforms. Lillian Wald, the founder of public health nursing in the United States, demonstrated the value of collaborative efforts toward the beginning of the 20th century, as did Lavinia Dock and Mary Brewster, among others. Today, such a framework enhances the ability of community health nurses and other health professionals to achieve the powerful synergies of cross-sectoral collaboration.

As we think about the future, with the approach of the new millenium, it is important to emphasize that what each of us does contributes to tomorrow. Salmon (1998) so clearly states: "What is good about today reflects what we have done in the past. So, too, will the future be a mirror of what each of us cares about, is committed to, knows and does" (p. 3).

Working together to improve the health of our communities, nationally and internationally, is an example of caring in action. As Roach (1995) concludes: "Caring is the human mode of being" (p. 9). Thus, caring actions are critical, actions that include respect for others and compassion for those whose health care and life are compromised. Empowering community members, nurses, and other health professionals through interdisciplinary cross-national collaborative efforts will provide opportunities to demonstrate caring in action. Caring represents an ongoing commitment to work together to help meet the health care needs of the people throughout the world.

Key Concepts

- Health for all of the world's people is an international goal and is promoted by the major world health organizations.

- Primary health care is one of the key strategies for promoting the health of the world's populations.

- The major international health organizations that are involved in world health include (1) private voluntary agencies, (2) philanthropic foundations, (3) private organizations, (4) official (governmental and intergovernmental) agencies, and (5) professional and technical organizations.

- Health sector reform has emerged as a major international public health issue, with the recognition of health sector problems that need to be addressed.

- Cross-sectoral collaboration within countries is a framework that offers health professionals powerful strategies for dealing with current and future health care problems and challenges.

- Cross-national collaboration provides opportunities for health professionals to assist others in their endeavors to improve the health of their communities.

- Community health nurses, as well as other nurses, must develop a knowledge of international health and health care system issues.

Power, Politics, and Public Policy

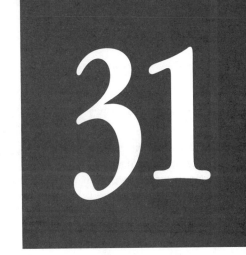

31

Laurel A. Freed, RN, MN, PNP

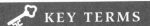
Genuine politics—politics worthy of the name, and the only politics I am willing to devote myself to—is simply a matter of serving those around us: serving the community, and serving those who will come after us.

—*Havel, 1992*

COMPETENCIES

Upon completion of this chapter, the reader should be able to:

- Discuss the concept of caring applied at the community level.
- Describe the concept of power, including the varied power bases.
- Explain the differences in the terms *politics* and *policy*.
- Discuss how a bill becomes a law in the United States.
- Discuss the differences between collective values and traditional values and how they affect policy development.
- Discuss the American Nurses Association (ANA) grassroots political nurse network.
- Discuss issues that will enhance nursing's political base.
- Describe specific political action strategies and how they can affect health policy.
- Identify several resources for participating in political activism.
- List and describe several nursing organizations involved in public policy formation.

Politics is about communities: the local, state, national, and international communities. The profession of nursing has had an interesting past in regard to political involvement and is now recognizing its unique contributions for the future.

It is important to revisit the efforts made by the nursing profession and some of its political pioneers. Early leaders in nursing, including Florence Nightingale and Lillian Wald, modeled political activism as an important role in nursing. Despite the involvement of these early leaders, widespread political involvement by nurses has not been realized. There are many reasons, including gender issues, the socialization process, and the obstacles that can be inherent in power, the political process, and the development of health policy. However, during the past two decades there has been a heightened awareness among nurses about the political process, political activism, and the building of nursing's political base.

This chapter will explore the above concepts and political processes. The chapter will focus on health policy development and how the community health nurse can be involved in shaping nursing practice and public policy by employing strategies of political activism. This chapter concludes with an overview of sources of information and organizations involved in health policy formation.

CARING AND THE POLITICAL ACTIVIST— HISTORICAL PERSPECTIVES

It is no accident that the founder of public health nursing in the United States was also an avid political activist. From the very inception of the Henry Street Settlement, Lillian Wald recognized the link between politics and the economic and social needs of the public. Like Florence Nightingale many years earlier, Wald astutely realized the connection between poor social, environmental, and economic living conditions and the poor health of the people living in those conditions. Like Nightingale, Wald conceptualized nursing not as a profession whose mission was limited to offering comfort and care in specified health care institutions but as one that encompassed the whole of people's lives. She chose to practice her nursing skills in the community and opened the Henry Street Settlement in one of the poorest neighborhoods of Manhattan to improve not just individuals' health but the health of the community as well.

Though the initial purpose of the Henry Street Settlement was to serve as a clinic for neighborhood residents, it gradually developed into a political power base for Wald's many social and political activities. Combining a fierce sense of justice with a social conscience, Wald quickly attracted like-minded women to the Settlement. Among the members of her inner circle was Lavinia Dock, a nurse, feminist, educator, and union organizer. Adelaide Nutting was an innovator in nursing education at Columbia Teachers College as well as a suffragist. Lina Rogers became the head of the first public school nursing service. Together, these women shared and supported each others' ideas and activities for social improvement. Included among the many political issues Lillian Wald participated in were the sanitation and health care problems in New York City's tenements, worker conditions, labor unions, children's rights and health issues, racial justice, and feminism and the suffrage movement.

Lillian Wald developed both a public and a private self that allowed her to accomplish major social reforms. "Through her public self she connected her caring with activism by initiating practice and policy changes via administrative and organizational skills, persuasiveness, coalitions, delivering testimony and political power" (Backer, 1993, p. 128). It is Wald's enduring conceptualization of the community health nurse as a health professional who both witnesses and seeks to improve the health, economic, and social conditions of those people with whom she works that laid the foundation for caring in the political arena.

Caring beyond the Individual and Family

Many people see nursing as a hands-on, one-to-one activity. The nurse is assumed to be the bedside practitioner,

the one health care professional who is accessible and constantly available for the client. Community health nursing, with its emphasis on the aggregate and its dedication to improving the health of communities, has long been seen as something of an outlier within the nursing profession and often requires a mental leap by nursing students as they are introduced to the concepts of aggregate nursing and population-focused practice. Similarly, the political activists among nurses are seen not as "real nurses," who by definition would remain at the bedside, but rather as people who have somehow lost touch with the basics of health care and health care recipients. Yet recent studies and news events reflect a gradual awareness by consumers about the linkages between a community's social and economic conditions and its health status. Consider recent news articles citing the rise in tuberculosis rates and its prevalence in homeless and immigrant populations. Consider the increasing American obsession with violent crime and teenage gangs, often associated with poor urban neighborhoods. Recall the poorly defined political campaign for "family values" in the 1996 presidential race, which attempted to link single-parent households to a variety of social ills including high rates of teen pregnancies. Yet few of these sensationalistic news stories examined and unraveled the many interlinked causes that contribute to the problems reported.

Clearly, the community health nurse is one of the few health professionals who directly observes many of the sources or causes of preventable health problems. The community health nurse visits the homes of families lacking the resources to adequately feed and clothe themselves. The community health nurse may participate in community clinics and identify children who have never had a visit with a primary care provider for routine health maintenance. The community health nurse may be the first to notice a number of similar cases of illness within the community and to identify environmental or toxic hazards affecting a community's health. Backer (1993) states:

Nurses today face social conditions similar to those confronted by Wald and her colleagues. These issues include inadequate or lack of health care for many Americans, as well as their lack of housing, employment, and education, and the threat of infectious diseases (p. 128).

The community health nurse may be the first to realize the presence or scope of health problems affecting large segments of the population, and this most certainly is a mandate to action for the caring professional.

Earlier in this textbook, the reader was exposed to the elements of caring applied to communities. Community health nurses demonstrate caring for populations by recognizing and accepting the multiple elements that make a community the place that it is: a place where people work, play, and live together. The nurse supports the growth and empowerment of communities as they seek new ways to improve their health status. But often problems that affect a community's well-being arise not from within the community but from outside the community.

Economic, social, environmental, and cultural factors may directly influence a community, and yet decisions about these factors may be occurring miles away from the community of concern. Often, decisions are made at the county, state, or federal level that directly affect communities. Consider the fierce political battles waged over the North American Free Trade Agreement (NAFTA), which opened trading between the United States and Mexico and with other nations. New public policies that mandate withholding medical services from immigrants are affecting western and southern border states in the United States and have a major impact on the health of populations in many near-border towns in California, Texas, and Arizona. Some health care programs continue to provide services to undocumented immigrants despite the policy. Off-shore oil drilling, lumber and land use regulations, hazardous materials disposal—all these are issues that are not only subject to heated national debate but also hold the potential for affecting the small communities to which they are adjacent. These issues, so clearly related to health, will be decided at the political and policymaking levels.

As the industrialized nations move forward, we are witnessing the end of the Industrial Revolution, which began at the start of this century. We are seeing the beginning of a new world whose economy depends less on labor and production and more on the gathering and exchange of information. The rapidly escalating use of computers and the international exchange of information and data have led some people to call this the beginning of the Information Age. Health care will be revolutionized as well by this explosion of information exchange. And at the center of the changing health care arena will be nurses, representing the largest number of health care workers. At a time when many see this new paradigm of health care delivery as increasingly computer and information based, it is important that nurses ensure that the human, caring aspects of health care be incorporated as well into the new system. Nurses need to become political players in health care reform. Not only do nurses need to be prepared to debate the issues; they need to step forward and define the issues as health care moves toward the 21st century.

CONCEPTS OF POWER, POLICY, AND POLITICS

The concepts of power, policy, and politics are important for the nurse to understand. Power has traditionally been viewed by many nurses as a negative concept. The discussion of the many dimensions of power and the various power bases will provide nurses with another way of viewing and applying the concept in their practice setting. The concepts of policy and politics are also often associated with negative images such as smoke-filled rooms, bribes, and payoffs, to mention only a few. Both terms are value laden and thus can be perceived as ethical or nonethical depending upon the situation. A detailed dis-

REFLECTIVE THINKING

Communities

• What types of communities do you know that are currently feeling threatened by pending governmental regulations?

• Why would communities dependent on only one main industry (such as tourism, lumber, coal mining) be most vulnerable to policy changes?

• How would the loss of a major industry affect the health status of a community?

cussion of all three concepts—power, policy, and politics—will provide the student with a framework for the rest of this chapter.

Power

Power is defined as the ability to influence others; the ability to do or act; achievement of the desired result. Nurses have not been socialized to the concept of power. To many, the concept carries with it a negative connotation. Many nurses view themselves as powerless, and, often, the public also perceives nurses as powerless. There are several reasons, most having to do with gender: (1) Nursing is a female-dominated profession; (2) power is related to the male gender; (3) power is not "feminine"; (4) the majority of nurses still work in male-dominated organizations (hospitals) with powerful males (physicians); (5) the profession is perceived as altruistic rather than power based.

Even though nurses are the largest professional group in the health care industry, they still have not fully appreciated their potential and used the power they could attain. As one nurse who participated in a political internship program stated: "The internship experience reemphasized to me the importance of one strong nursing voice. One in 44 female voters in America is a nurse. Though nurses are an extremely large segment of the population, they have not yet learned to harness the political power of their numbers" (Chaffee, 1996, p. 22).

In order to change the concept of power from negative to positive, we must remember that power is multidimensional and that there are many sources or bases of power. Understanding those facts can help in the analysis of the dynamics of power in specific situations. The more bases of power one incorporates, the more powerful she or he will become.

A typology of power bases has been established by various authorities (Mason, Talbott, & Leavitt, 1993, p. 120):

1. Coercive power is rooted in real or perceived fear of one person by another.

2. Reward power affects behavior as one person perceives the potential for rewards or favors by honoring the wishes of a powerful person.

3. Legitimate power derives from an organizational position or title rather than from a personal quality.

4. Expert power comes from knowledge, special talents, and skills; it is person power as contrasted with position power.

5. Referent power is apparent when a subordinate identifies with and follows the direction of a leader whom the subordinate admires and believes in.

6. Information power results when one individual has (or is perceived to have) special information that another individual desires.

7. Connection power is accorded to those who are thought to have a privileged connection with powerful individuals or organizations.

Policy

Policy is the governmental practice that guides and directs action in all spheres of social interaction such as national defense policy, environmental policy, economic policy, and health care policy. **Health care policy** is action taken by government to direct decisions and actions to safeguard and promote the health of the public and provide for health care services. "Policy encompasses the choices that a society, segment of society, or organization makes regarding its goals and priorities and how it will allocate its resources" (Mason et al., 1993, p. 5).

In the early stages of policy formation, the direction may not be completely clear, as in the current profusion of health care reform measures being proposed in various countries worldwide. Eventually, however, a number of measures that have been proposed, debated, and approved, will coalesce to show a picture of governmental purpose and direction. Though many people may speak of policy as if it were a plan or a single decision, governments often express one intent while enacting policy with differing or even opposite effect from the stated goal. It is important for nurses to distinguish between stated values or spoken goals and the actual direction dictated by public policy, for it is that actual direction rather than the stated values that will affect our lives.

Who determines policy? Although elected officials propose and participate in the development of policies, the public, including nurses, has a role in shaping public policy. Milio (1981), in her classic text, *Promoting Health through Public Policy,* writes about the importance of nursing's becoming involved and participating in shaping health policy. Nurses at all levels—at the bedside, in administration, and in the community—are affected on a daily basis by public policy. Individual nurses can influence policy decisions at all governmental levels. Organized nursing's unified efforts, such as those outlined in

Nursing's Agenda for Health Care Reform (Tri-Council for Nursing, 1991) is a good example of a **collective**, or group pursuing an agreed-upon goal, action or set of actions, and a **coalition**, which is a temporary alliance of diverse members who come together for joint action in support of a defined goal. It is important that nurses be proactive in the earliest stages of policy development so that they can exert nursing's influence early in the political process.

Although it might seem ideal to develop an idea and be able to enact it into law quickly, our government is structured to allow input from a variety of persons at many stages of policy development. It is these many opinions, and the resulting modifications to legislation or policy being developed, that determine what the final law looks like. Although this system of weighing various opinions, making compromises and modifications, eliminating controversial pieces of legislation, pressuring influential groups, and courting or opposing political parties can seem frustrating to some outside observers, many find it fascinating and exciting. The formation of policy involves the use of the political process.

Politics

Politics means "influencing." "It is defined as a process by which one influences the decisions of others and exerts control over situations and events. It is a means to an end" (Mason et al., 1993, p. 6). Frequently, politics is associated with conflicting values, and multiple interest groups compete for scarce resources. Being involved in politics and developing actions and strategies to influence the political process is known as **political action** or **political activism**.

Mason, Talbott, and Leavitt (1993) have advanced four spheres of political action. "Politics and policy are usually associated with government, but there are three other spheres for nurses' political action: the workplace, professional organizations, and the community" (p. 10). The community encompasses all three spheres of influence, which are an integral part of the community.

> The community is a social unit with a variety of special interest groups, community activities, health and social problems, and numerous resources for solving those problems. The community can be a neighborhood, or it can be international connections that will characterize the world into the twenty-first century (p. 10).

Nurses can effect change in all four spheres of political influence. The four spheres are interconnected and overlapping, and nurses' involvement in one sphere will affect the other spheres (Mason et al., 1993). See Figure 31-1.

How has nursing evolved as a body politic—that is, as the political arm of nursing? Cohen, Mason, Korner, Leavitt, and colleagues (1996) have advanced a framework that conceptualizes the political development of the nursing profession. They identify four stages of development

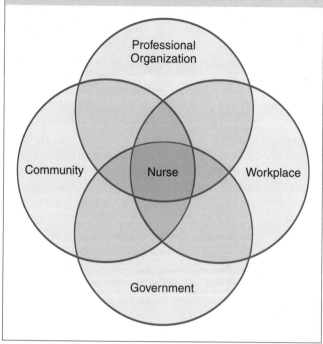

Figure 31-1 Nurses Opportunity to Effect Political Change in Four Spheres of Influence

Professional Organization

Community

Nurse

Workplace

Government

as election strategies and public relations techniques (Cohen et al., 1996).

The fourth and final stage in the profession's political development has not been realized and is termed "leading the way." Cohen et al. (1996) state:

> In this stage nurses become the initiators of crucial health policy ideas and innovations. Reaching this stage will require that nursing seek out, develop, and support its visionaries and risk-takers. The further the professional development, the more the public will benefit from nursing's expertise and advocacy (p. 263–264).

Now, during the period of reorganization of health care delivery in the United States and other countries, is a crucial time in transition toward stage four. Pursuit of stage four can be enhanced in the following ways:

- Build coalitions and constituencies.
- Enhance leadership development.
- Mobilize nurses to run for office.
- Integrate health policy into curricula.
- Develop public media expertise.
- Increase sophistication in policy analysis and related research (Cohen et al., 1996).

Because community health nursing focuses on the health of population groups, it is, by definition, political in nature. Community health nurses need to be advocates for aggregates with special needs and special concerns or problems. To be an advocate for special populations includes using a variety of political strategies and becoming sophisticated players in the political system.

POLITICAL PROCESSES: HOW LEGISLATION IS MADE

An important initial step in becoming a political activist is to have a basic grasp of the political system, to understand how laws are made, and to examine the finer points of the political process in a particular community, state, or nation. When nurses take time to study how laws and political decisions are made, they realize where they can effectively influence those decisions as health care professionals.

Think about some issues involving health that should be addressed in a community. Has there been a communicable disease outbreak recently in the community, and how would the community treat or prevent future outbreaks of this disease? Is there anything nurses can do to improve the health of children or to decrease the incidence of domestic violence? What can be done to facilitate healthier lifestyles for a particular population? Almost any health issue can be influenced by well-crafted legislation. Many health problems are negatively affected by legislation that either gives inadequate consideration to all the ramifications of the law (perhaps by not involving enough health care experts such as nurses) or is altered by people with differing economic or political motives.

to "analyze previous accomplishments and plan future actions that will enhance the political involvement of nursing as it seeks to improve the health care delivery system" (Cohen et al., 1996, p. 259).

The first stage of nurses' political activism, which began in the 1970s, sought to promote political awareness of nurses. At this time, the first of many books and articles were published that emphasized the importance of nurses' becoming politically active to advance the profession. The need for a power base among nurses' was emphasized by the American Nurses Association (ANA), the primary professional nursing association in the United States. These efforts began the identification of ways nurses could become involved in politics (Cohen et al., 1996).

The second stage highlighted the activities that enhance the profession's identity as a special interest in the political arena and began to develop its own sense of uniqueness. This stage was "characterized by a new sense of identity emanating from the development of nursing coalitions and the building of nursing's political base" (Cohen et al., 1996, p. 261). During this stage in the 1980s, the ANA's political activities expanded and a grassroots political network was developed and grew rapidly. There was a sudden increase in specialty organizations, many of which became politically active.

The third stage in the political development of the nursing profession, occurring in the 1990s, was marked by "political sophistication." The major achievements during this stage were (1) the development of Nursing's Agenda for Health Care Reform, discussed later in this chapter; (2) the appointment of nurses to federal panels and agencies; and (3) increasing savvy shown by nurses in areas such

The Legislative Process

The U.S. government has three levels of governance: federal, state, and local. Local government may include counties, cities, or different specified districts such as school districts, hospital districts, or other special-interest areas. Local politics may differ radically from one city or county to another. Major decisions may be made by city councils or county supervisors.

Federal and state governments are similar to each other. They both have three main branches: legislative, executive, and judicial.

The executive and legislative branches are intended to be open and accessible to the people and are able to be influenced by citizens in order to make laws that serve everyone equally. However, the way in which citizens may wield their influence differs for each branch.

The Legislative Branch

The legislative branch is the law-making body of government. On the federal level, the legislative branch, Congress, is made up of two bodies: the U.S. Senate and the U.S. House of Representatives.

A single bill may be considered by several different committees. Once it has been passed by the committee(s), it is returned to the **house of origin**. The house of origin is the governing body of which the bill's **author**, the legislator who submits the bill, is a member (i.e., either the House or the Senate). The bill is presented in its **amended** (i.e., including any changes made to the printed bill) form for a full vote by all the members of the house of origin. The members vote, and the bill is either passed or defeated, or **killed**. Once a bill has passed through its house of origin, it is then sent to the other house and the process is repeated. It may go through committees and then be voted upon by the full membership of that house. Only after a bill has been passed by both houses of the legislature is it sent to the executive branch of government and signed into law or vetoed by the chief of the executive branch. On the federal level this is the president, and on the state level it is the state's governor. See Figure 31-2.

꧁ REFLECTIVE THINKING ꧂

Community Political Structure

- How is your local city or county structured?

- Who are the major decision makers in your city or county?

- Who are the official (i.e., elected or appointed) leaders in your community? Who are the unofficial leaders? Consider church, cultural, and business leaders and the roles they play in your town.

- Who do you know who has participated in local or state politics?

There are many ways that nurses can influence the legislative process. At the state level, nurses may serve as the **sponsor** of a bill: that is, the originator of the idea for the bill. An individual nurse may contact her or his representative to meet and suggest an idea, or, more commonly the state nurses' association will propose an idea to a legislator. The legislator who first introduces a bill to the legislature is then known as the bill's author. Once the bill is introduced, nurses may augment its progress by garnering support for the bill from lobbyist groups within the state. Many health care groups actively follow and **lobby**, (take actions to influence legislators to take a certain position on prospective bills or issues) a number of bills as they progress through the legislative process. Several health-related associations may align with each other in order to stimulate legislators to pass legislation that may benefit them all.

Joining with special-interest groups to lobby politicians is one of the most effective means of supporting legislation because legislators recognize that such groups represent large numbers of potential voters. Seeking the support of influential groups is the business of politicians. Politicians want to serve and please the people who voted them into office because these constituents represent future votes the next time they run for office.

Aside from joining lobbying groups, nurses have a unique and perhaps more powerful lever for influencing health legislation: their experience within the health care system. Every nurse who has held a job in nursing has seen the health care system in action and the effect it has on clients. Each nurse has a story to tell. Often a story well-told will influence a politician to support or oppose a piece of legislation. Providing **testimony**, or evidence in support of a bill, at legislative committee hearings, keeping track of pieces of legislation, and calling or writing a legislator may have a significant impact on a proposed bill. In order to track and affect legislation at key times in the life of a bill, interested parties must contact committees and key players at the appropriate state and federal levels. Figure 31-2 depicts the typical progress of a bill at the federal level. The left side of the figure indicates points in the process at which community health nurses might become involved and influence legislation.

The Executive Branch

The executive branch of government is responsible for carrying out the laws passed by the legislative branch. At the federal level, the chief executive is the President of the United States. At the state level it is the state's governor. Among the responsibilities of the executive branch are signing bills passed by the legislative branch and making them into laws. The chief executive has the power to **veto,** or reject, bills passed by the legislature. If the legislative branch wishes to override an executive veto, a second vote on the bill is taken in both houses and a two-thirds vote is required to effect an override.

At the federal level, another responsibility of the executive branch includes appointing persons to key positions

Figure 31-2   How a Bill Becomes a Law at the Federal Level in the United States

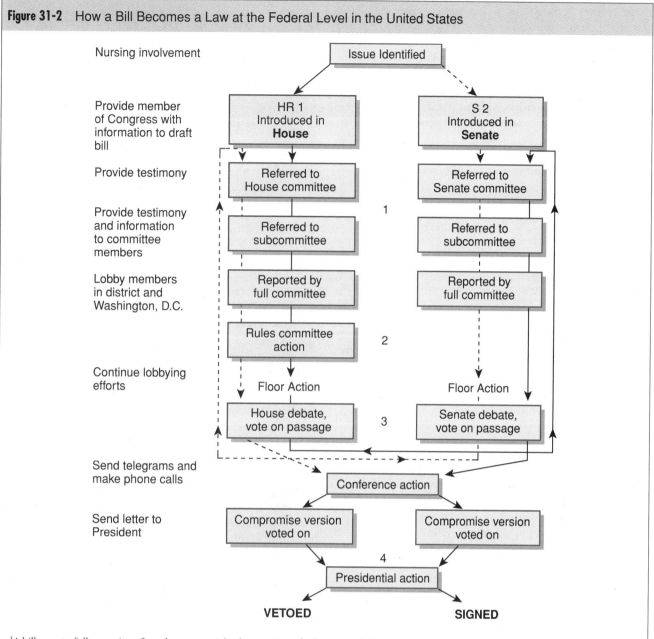

Nursing involvement

Provide member of Congress with information to draft bill

Provide testimony

Provide testimony and information to committee members

Lobby members in district and Washington, D.C.

Continue lobbying efforts

Send telegrams and make phone calls

Send letter to President

[1]A bill goes to full committee first, then to special subcommittees for hearings, debate, revisions, and approval. The same process occurs when it goes to full committee. It either dies in commitee or proceeds to the next step.

[2]Only the House has a Rules Committee to set the "rule" for floor action and conditions for debate and amendments. In the Senate, the leadership schedules action.

[3]The bill is debated, amended, and passed or defeated. If passed, it goes to the other chamber and follows the same path. If the two chambers pass a similar bill, both versions go to conference.

[4]The President may sign the bill into law, allow it to become law without his signature, or veto it and return it to Congress. To override the veto, both houses must approve the bill by a 2/3 majority vote.

From Policy and Politics for Nurses: Action and Change in the Workplace, Government, Organization and Community *(2nd ed.) by D. J. Mason, S. W. Talbott, & J. K. Leavitt, (Eds.), 1993, Philadelphia, PA: W. B. Saunders. Reprinted with permission.*

such as cabinet members, ambassadors, and federal judges. Nursing organizations can support the appointment of persons with knowledge of health care issues to key posts. Kristine Gebbie, a nurse and former Secretary of Health in the state of Washington, was appointed to chair the President's AIDS Commission by President Clinton in 1993. Other executive duties include making treaties with other nations and, most important, reporting on the state of the nation to the legislative branch. The President makes a yearly State of the Union address to Congress in January.

At the state level, many of the laws passed by the legislature are then sent to regulatory agencies that transform the laws into enforceable regulations. The regulatory agencies are considered to be part of the executive branch, and the directors of these powerful agencies are appointed by the governor.

Nurses should feel comfortable writing or calling either the White House or their state governor's office to offer comments on pending legislation or upcoming appointments. Comments by citizens are tallied by staff, and opinion trends can significantly affect executive decisions. In addition, a brief well-told anecdote of some personal encounter that illustrates an opinion may be utilized by a leader to make a point in a political debate.

The Judicial Branch

The third branch of government is the judicial branch. This branch is the court system of the federal government. The judicial branch is divided into three levels: Federal District Court, Appellate Courts, and the Supreme Court. Most federal cases originate in District Courts, whose decisions may be appealed to the Appellate Courts and, finally, the Supreme Court of the United States. The judicial branch is responsible for interpreting federal law, and it has the power to resolve disputes over the Constitution that might arise from the legislative and executive branches.

Regulation

Regulations are intended to promote individual accountability for actions and to protect the public health and welfare. Regulations specify how policies are to be realized; they fill out the details of new or amended laws.

At the federal level, proposed regulations are published in the *Federal Register*, after which concerned parties may comment on the proposed regulations and suggest changes. Community health nurses can have input into regulations that affect their professional practice as well as legislation that shapes public health policy.

PARTICIPATION IN HEALTH POLICY FORMATION

Whereas the concept of politics may seem overwhelmingly broad and intimidating to many Americans, the concept of public policy is even less clearly delineated. What is public policy, and how does it affect us? Why would a person in a caring profession, whose expertise involves working with people around health issues, be interested in policy? If you find yourself asking these questions, consider the following effects of policies today:

- Both prescription and nonprescription drugs in the United States are tightly regulated by the Food and Drug Administration. Yet tobacco containing nicotine, one of the most harmful drugs known to humans, remains unregulated. Approximately 390,000 people die from cigarette smoking each year in this country alone.

DECISION MAKING

Political Influence

A federal bill related to early intervention for pregnant women is at the committee level. As a community health nurse you are aware of how important the passage of this bill would be to your practice.

- What could you and other community health nurses do to influence this legislation?

- Statistics indicate a strong link between the number of handguns in a given society and the number of gunshot-related injuries and deaths. Yet the U.S. government has yet to ban personal weapons.
- Attempts to hold down Medicare costs in this country in the early 1980s caused the initiation of measures limiting days in the hospital for the elderly. Yet, health care professionals have increasingly warned of the increased potential of incomplete recovery for persons released prematurely to their homes.

All of these issues represent different aspects of public policy. Clearly, they are connected to the health of the people in communities where community health nurses work. Nurses are in a unique position to address many health problems that can be modified by public policy. Because community health nurses share common goals with clients and because they recognize that individuals are embedded in family and community systems, they are prepared to play a vital role in policy and population-based efforts to enhance care. In the next sections, public policy and specific strategies nurses can use to help shape it will be explored in more depth.

Policy Formation

Public policy is the action taken by the government of a country to guide its direction and produce outcomes. From a global perspective, one approach to policy formation has been the "Healthy Cities" movement. Healthy Cities is an innovative grassroots approach to health promotion and disease prevention. Originating in Europe in 1986, Healthy Cities has been a successful model to ensure that the local community is involved and participates in the treatment of its health problems. This model was discussed in Chapters 1 and 29. "Aimed at developing healthy public policy, Healthy Cities ensures diversity and collaboration by involving persons from all walks of life to improve the community's health" (Flynn, 1995, p. 7).

Occasionally, ambitious proposals seem to radically change the course of a country's public policies. In the United States, for example, much of the criticism of President Clinton has revolved around his overly ambitious attempts to make major policy changes. His proposals for health care reform and for reform of the criminal justice system via a major crime bill were at odds with the current direction of policies in those areas. Rarely has a president tackled a major restructuring of national policy, however, historians can quickly cite the few instances. One example is the New Deal by President Franklin Roosevelt during the 1930s. The New Deal was a term applied to a number of economic and social measures initiated to bolster the national economy and productivity. Social Security was one government program that emerged as part of the New Deal. Other examples are President Johnson's Medicare and President Clinton's welfare reform.

Although it is easier to visualize public policy by imagining the larger sweeping reforms mentioned above, most public policy is in fact created in small, individual steps. Individual laws, enacted piece by piece, relating to a common concept such as welfare, health access, or education come together to form a direction that is, if not mutually decided upon, at least silently condoned.

Policy, then, is rarely developed with a broad vision in sweeping reforms. It is an incremental process in which pieces are added and refined as policymakers see fit. The ultimate goal of nursing involvement in politics is not to become overly concerned with the political process but rather to use that process as a tool to influence public policy.

In policy formation, there is often a conflict in values. When nurses begin a study of public policy, and specifically health policy, it is necessary to examine the values of the society that has developed the policies. MacPherson's (1987) article examining health care policy and values lists three areas in which U.S. culture differs significantly from nursing values. The opposing values include individualism versus collectivism, competition versus cooperation, and inequality versus equality. She points out that the fierce individualism that has created self-reliant heroes like explorers and cowboys also has undermined the capacity of Americans for commitment to one another. It is natural then, in a country such as the United States, which stresses individualism, pursuit of self-interest, and competitiveness, that health care policies tend to promote structured inequalities (p. 3).

Traditional U.S. ideals of individualism and the free market are in conflict with nursing values and especially with the work and concepts inherent in community health nursing. Community health nurses work to promote a collective identity among the aggregates they work with in order to empower the community to resolve health-related problems. They see the strength of communities as residing in an increasing ability to plan and work together toward common goals. Cooperation and collaboration rather than competition yield a strong base from which to identify and deal with community problems.

Emerging values emphasizing collectivist or community-oriented solutions are challenging traditional values. Collective orientation emphasizes society's responsibility to solve social problems. Debates regarding collective versus individual rights have been increasing in U.S. politics;

examples include struggles to enact legislation on the wearing of seatbelts, use of motorcycle helmets, gun control, and health care reforms (Weis, 1995).

Americans will not be able to solve the problems of the health care system unless the country shifts priorities and biases away from an individual-centered view of health and human welfare toward a more community-centered approach (p. 26).

Collectivism strives for collaborative efforts or partnerships throughout society.

Nursing and the Political Network

Although some specialty groups follow legislation pertinent to their particular group, the vehicle for collective action or political action is nursing's primary professional organization in various nations throughout the world. Worldwide, the major international organization is the International Council for Nurses (ICN), discussed previously in Chapter 29. In the United States, for example, the American Nurses Association (ANA) is the major organization. The ANA has a long history and has been the major voice for nursing at the federal level. The ANA began in the early part of the century and formed a special committee on legislation in 1923. "Throughout its history, ANA has demonstrated its commitment to the delivery of quality, cost-effective health care services to the public by fostering high standards of nursing practice and by lobbying the U.S. Congress on health issues affecting the public" (Mason et al., 1993, p. 582).

In 1951, ANA opened its Washington, D.C. office in order to have access to legislators and to lobby Congress on issues important to the nursing profession. In 1992, the ANA launched an effective "Nursing on the Move Campaign." The ANA moved its entire headquarters from Kansas City to Washington, D.C., Capitol Hill, to be more visible to policymakers in Congress. The primary departments involved in legislative activities at ANA headquarters are Government Relations, American Nurses Association Political Action Committee (ANA-PAC), and Political Education, hub of the political network grassroots program.

The Government Relations Department at ANA headquarters includes a cadre of lobbyists and political staff who ensure that nursing is visible and active during key policy debates. The primary purpose of the Government Relations Department is to lobby and network with legislators. This department is concerned with a myriad of issues and concerns about which lobbyists and staff must become knowledgeable and gain expertise in order to move key and important legislation for nursing and health care.

In 1971, a small group of nurses in New York State organized the "political arm of ANA." The name of the group was Nurses for Political Action (NPA). "A political action committee increases member participation, empowers its members to play a greater role in the development of public policy, raises money to contribute to candidates running for political office and better positions the profession in the legislative arena" (ANA, 1996, p. 5).

In 1974, under the auspices of the ANA, the political action arm became Nurses' Coalition for Action in Politics (N-CAP). Its focus was on education, stimulating participation, and political education of nurses as well as nonpartisan fund raising. In 1986, N-CAP was renamed the ANA-PAC.

By 1994, ANA-PAC ranked the third largest health care political action committee in the United States, surpassed only by the American Medical Association (AMA) and the American Dental Association (ADA). Owing to thousands of nurses who contributed to ANA-PAC, it became the fastest-growing PAC association from the 1991–1992 election cycle to the 1993–1994 election cycle. In the booklet *Successes and Challenges in the Federal Legislative Arena,* the ANA (1996) states: "Political action committees increase citizen participation in our nation's political and legislative processes. Involvement in ANA-PAC is one way that nurses are speaking with one strong voice about the critical health care concerns facing our nation" (p. 9).

The development of nursing as a special interest included the growth of ANA's political activities. In 1981, the ANA established its political nurse network. The ANA legislative network is coordinated by the ANA's Department of Political Education in Washington, D.C. The goal of this legislative network is to have a grassroots structure of nurses established in every one of the 435 congressional districts in the United States. District activities are coordinated under the leadership of a nurse residing in that particular district, who assumes the role and title of "Congressional District Coordinator," or CDC. This nurse acts as a liaison between Washington and her or his district. In the late 1980s, the ANA legislative network also established Senate coordinators (SCs), accomplishing the ANA's goal to have one nurse as primary contact to all senators and congresspersons across the nation. The ANA's political network proliferated across the United States and enabled nurses to organize within their congressional districts and states, thereby increasing their visibility, access to legislators, and influence in the political process.

Congressional district coordinators and Senate coordinators work with the ANA's political and legislative departments to keep abreast of issues and serve as the ANA's link educating nurses on the political issues and process and educating members of Congress on nursing's issues. These nurses gather information on the local "political scene" for ANA and ANA-PAC, work on the campaigns of ANA-PAC–endorsed candidates, provide information on federal legislation, and encourage nurses to lobby. As the CDC for the First Congressional District of California, this writer can attest to the influence this network has on nursing's political machine.

In 1993, during the health care reform debate, the ANA coordinated an action team, Nurses Strategic Action Team (N-STAT). This grassroots program established communication links and mobilized nurses to respond quickly to congressional decisions in order to influence the health care reform debate. The former CDCs and SCs, which

were established in the early 1980s, became known as the N-STAT Leadership Team during the period of the Clinton administration's health care reform debates during the 1990s. The N-STAT Team continued to establish effective working relationships with their senators and representatives in Congress through political and grassroots activities. The other arm of N-STAT is the Rapid Response Team. The Rapid Response Team is basically a communication network; its members provide thousands of voices speaking to public policy makers on nursing issues. Nurses may become members of the team if they belong to their State Nurses Association (SNA). Today, approximately 40,000 nurses are members of N-STAT. "The heart of nursing's power on Capitol Hill lies in the participation of thousands of nurses at the grassroots level; as that participation increases, so will the voice and victories of nursing in the legislative arena" (ANA, 1996, p. 4).

Recognizing and Prioritizing the Issues

One unique purpose of the ANA is to shape public policy about health care to be consonant with the goals of nurses, nursing, and the public health. The ANA establishes policies and goals for the profession that form the basis for nursing's contribution to the advancement of health care policy.

These goals serve as the foundation for a variety of ANA program activities. One of these activities is the ANA's legislative and political effort. The ANA seeks enactment and implementation of legislation that will benefit the health and welfare of the nation's citizens. It also participates in the election of candidates to public office who are knowledgeable about and supportive of the profession's policies.

In addition to political and legislative activities, the ANA is involved in other nursing activities and health care issues such as access to quality health care services, financing of health care, funding for nursing education and nursing research, human rights, and the economic and general welfare of nurses.

As indicated above, the ANA has many categories for prioritizing their political efforts. In the formulation of health policy, it is important to identify the issues and prioritize them. In this section, nursing issues on a national and international level will be identified and issues that will enhance the political development of nursing will be explored.

On the national level, the following list of nursing issues is by no means exhaustive. However, it will provide the reader with an overview of current nursing concerns. It is important to remember that policy formation is often a lengthy process; an issue may carry over for several sessions of Congress before legislation is passed.

ANA nursing issues are as follows:

• Health care reform: the next step
• Medicaid reform and Medicare restructuring

- Reimbursement for advanced practice nurses
- Community nursing organizations (CNOs)
- Workforce and quality issues
- Patient safety
- Long-term care

In the international community, nursing's basic problems and issues are very similar to national issues. Mason, Talbott, and Leavitt (1993) state, "What creates the differences among countries and regions is the degree to which a problem exists in relationship to geography, history, culture (including the role of women) and, increasingly, economics" (p. 636). In the 1990s, a number of major policy issues are facing nurses and nursing in all parts of the world:

- Decreasing resources for health services and a concomitant demand by policymakers for measures for proving the effectiveness of care.
- Increasing longevity
- Employment of general managers, rather than health professionals, to manage health services
- Health for all through primary health care availability and accessibility
- The impact of HIV/AIDS on society and health systems
- Inadequate numbers of effective nurse leaders in many countries (Mason et al., 1993, p. 636)

There are specific issues that will enhance the political development of nursing. These issues cannot be prioritized because it is important to remember that (1) the stages of nursing's political development are not time bound; (2) depending on the issues, there may be movement back and forth among stages; and (3) the events that categorize each stage of nursing's political development are ongoing and are not intended to end or be replaced by those of other stages (Cohen et al., 1996).

Some of the issues that will enhance nursing's body politic are:

- **Development of nursing as a special interest**
  The development of nursing as a special interest has not been a hasty process. It was necessary to grow as a profession—to move schools of nursing into academia, develop nursing's unique theory base, and increase research in nursing. The profession strived to develop its own identity. Attainment of nursing as a special interest will always be advantageous to nursing as well as the public. In the later stages of political development, nursing can advocate for groups in society or a community to improve the well-being of others.
- **Formation and growth of the Political Action Committee for Nurses**
  In 1997, ANA-PAC celebrated its twenty-fifth anniversary (personal communication, ANA-PAC director, May 1997). In the future ANA-PAC must continue to grow. Largely as a result of telemarketing, by 1994, ANA-PAC ranked third among health-related PACs in contributions made to federal candidates. This achievement marked a new type of political sophistication for the ANA and its members (Cohen et al., 1993).

- **Building coalitions**
  The formation of nursing coalitions in the legislative arena is very important for nursing. One powerful coalition, the Tri-Council of Nursing—consisting of the ANA, American Association of Colleges of Nursing (AACN), National League for Nursing (NLN), and American Organization of Nurse Executives (AONE)—was very significant in the development of a plan for nursing's agenda for health care reform. There are three reasons to enter into coalitions: to "borrow" power, to build a base of support, and to prevent another group from challenging a plan (Mason et al., 1993, p. 169). Perhaps all of those reasons were influential in the success of the agenda.

  The ability to forge coalitions and compromises symbolized a new level of maturity for the profession. In the future, the profession will need to build coalitions beyond nursing for broad health policy concerns. "Nursing will have to form political and economic coalitions, not only with consumer groups, but with the other economic and political players in ways which will associate nurses with these groups" (Porter-O'Grady, 1994, p. 36).
- **Fostering nurse appointments and campaigns**
  Appointments of nurses to federal panels and agencies, ranging from the Prospective Payment Assessment Commission to the Agency for Health Care Policy and Research (AHCPR), have increased over the years. Also, there has been a proliferation of nurses elected or appointed to positions at the federal and state levels of government. By 1996, 71 nurses held elected positions in state legislatures, and many more were members of legislative staffs in Congress or state governments. In the future, the profession needs to mobilize nurses for campaigns to promote the election of nurses to public offices. Until nurses can be more a part of the legislative arena, it will be difficult to influence "healthy policy."
- **Increasing research and policy analysis**
  Congress established the National Center for Nursing Research in 1985, which Congress upgraded to the National Institute of Nursing Research in 1993. In the last several decades, nursing research has grown immensely, but policy research has not. Research on nursing's political socialization is still in its infancy. "Actual policy studies in nursing have minimally increased since Milio's (1981) comprehensive literature review in nursing and no nursing policy analysis research has been done by nurses" (Hall-Long, 1995, p. 27). In the future, nursing needs to increase research related to nursing's political socialization, education, and participation. In addition, "nursing needs to develop sophistication in conducting policy analysis, policy research, and nursing research with policy implications" (Cohen et al., 1993, p. 265).
- **Increasing education in relation to policy formation and participation**
  During the first stage of nursing's political development, the importance of including health policy in nursing curricula was recognized. This importance was

espoused by nursing leaders in the mid-1980s and into the 1990s. "Nurses must incorporate a political component into their professional role identity. A political thread must be woven through the nursing curricula" (Brown, 1996, p. 3).

In her article "Community Health Learning Experiences and Political Activism: A Model for Baccalaureate Curriculum Revolution Content," Williams (1993) suggests that political activism content, theory, and practice be a part of community health nursing curricula. She states that with their "emphasis on public health programs and services, legislative influences on health care, and health policy issues, community health nursing content and practice are the logical areas of the baccalaureate curriculum for political activism education" (p. 353). She advocates that nursing faculty be involved in political issues and activities so that they can serve as role models and mentors for students. Students are constantly hearing about and are interested in health-related political issues: health care reform, America's aging population, motorcycle safety, right-to-life and living-will concerns, to mention just a few. "Unless students see faculty members involved in such concerns, it may be difficult for them to integrate activism into the nursing role" (p. 354).

In its 1990 document *Essentials of Baccalaureate Nursing Education for Entry Level Community Health Nursing Practice*, the Association of Community Health Nurse Educators (ACHNE) recommended that the theoretical content of baccalaureate programs should include "health policy, and political and legislative concepts and processes including nursing's role in affecting policy" (ACHNE, 1990, p. 3). The National League for Nursing (NLN) (1988) document *Curriculum Revolution: Mandate for Change* advocates a curriculum revolution that incorporates political activism. Unfortunately, although these documents bow to the concept, implementation has not been accomplished.

In the future, nursing educators can make sure that political content is included at the baccalaureate level. To hasten this action, the NLN Council of Baccalaureate and Higher Degree Programs in Nursing could include the requirement of political action content as one of the criteria for the accreditation of baccalaureate programs in nursing.

• **Reaffirm nursing's agenda for health care reform**

Nursing's Agenda for Health Care Reform (Tri-Council for Nursing, 1991) was a milestone for the profession in terms of consensus building and collaboration among organizations. For the first time, the entire profession had a document that depicted the values that nursing stands for in terms of health policy and quality client care. This document enhances the ability of nurses to represent themselves to legislators and others during deliberations of health care reform (Cohen et al., 1996). The development of the agenda reflected a new level of maturity for the nursing profession. In the future, there must be a reaffirmation of nursing's agenda for health care reform and

DECISION MAKING

The Future

Nursing has come a long way in its political development. What particular ideas or strategies would be important to enhance nursing's future development?

a commitment to be diligent in all efforts to create meaningful reform.

• **Participation in health care reform and health care delivery**

Evaluating the effectiveness of the nation's health care system continued at a rapid rate during the 1990s. The issues are complex and have profound implications for nursing in an evolving health care delivery system. To date, there have been many problems in health care reform because of the current "erosion" of care. In the future, there will be reorganization of health care delivery and new opportunities for true health care reform. "Nursing offers just what the American health consumer hopes for. This is the time to take the lead and aggressively persevere in negotiating a truly reformed and effective health-based system (Porter-O'Grady, 1994, p. 38).

There is a fit between the values of the community health nurse and the values of the community. The more the profession pursues its political development and participates in policy making, the more the public will benefit from nursing expertise and the advocacy that nurses can provide on behalf of the public.

Nursing's Role in Shaping Health Policy

Nurses are becoming more political in their workplace and community and on state, national and international

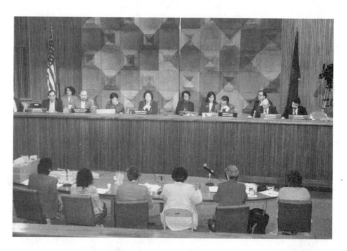

Nurses making a presentation before a state legislature.
Photo courtesy of the New York State Nurses Association.

levels. In the workplace, collective bargaining unions are becoming prevalent. Nurses participating in such unions must know the political structure of an organization and the negotiating process. The State Nurses Associations (SNAs) and the ANA in the United States have legislative networks in place. Nurses in increasing numbers are participating and taking leadership in these networks. Knowledge of politics and political action is needed if nurses are to participate in decisions about the health care system of which they are so essential a part.

Community health nurses need to be politically active in the community because of shared values and because of the pervasive role the government has on health care. The local level delivers direct services to combat risk factors for disease and injury and seeks to improve health levels through government-funded clinics and other programs. Community health nurses need to educate policymakers regarding the needs of the public. Policymakers rarely have backgrounds related to health and may be unaware of health issues or lack understanding of the implications for the health of the public. Policymakers at all levels need input from nurses.

Communicating with legislators or other policy makers is necessary for effective political action. Communicating with a legislator may be accomplished by writing letters, telephoning, attending meetings, and participating in events featuring legislators.

Each of the above methods is effective in a particular situation. Constituent letters, if well written, can be a powerful vehicle for ensuring that multiple voices are heard. Use of the telephone in contacting your legislator can save time; also, it often provides a more direct and rapid means of delivering your message. Scheduled meetings with legislators in their district or legislative offices are an important activity for nurse leaders. As the role of the state and federal legislature in determining health issues continues to escalate, personal communication with individual legislators becomes increasingly important. Visits by nurses as health care professionals provide for face-to-face dialogue on pertinent health issues and allow for personalization of an organizational relationship with the legislator and the legislator's staff. Finally, attending candidate campaign events is very important. Endorsing candidates and contributing to (and/or working in) their campaigns ensure our influence as nurses with elected officials. Refer to Tables 31-1 through 31-4 for specific guidelines on communicating with legislators and other policymakers.

To help shape health policy, one must know and use the strategies of political action. Communicating with a policymaker is only one example of political action; there are many other strategies nurses can learn and use to affect health policy. Many of these strategies were discussed in the previous section as the issues pertinent to nursing's political development were explored. Political action strategies may be categorized into levels of sophistication from the least to the most sophisticated: basic political participation, political awareness, political activism, and political sophistication. These levels and strategies are summarized in Table 31-5. By reviewing this table, the nurse should be able to recognize her or his personal level of sophistication. This table will also provide the nurse with information about how she or he can use additional political action strategies in order to reach a new level of sophistication.

It is important for community health nurses to focus on health policy issues that concern the public, because nursing values can improve the health and health care of people. Emerging values may remain on a collision course with dominant or traditional value systems in our country. Nursing's long-held belief in a more collective approach to health care should continually be voiced. Nurses can help shape the values debate to seek support for increased access to quality, cost-effective health care for all Americans. "Nurses are in a unique position to take the heartbeat of their clients and translate it into caring health policy. The time is now for us to capture our legislators' attention and make our concerns known" (Jennings, 1995).

Table 31-1   Writing to Your Legislator

DO	DO NOT
1. Use plain or personal stationery when you write as an individual. If you are writing as the representative of a group, use the organization's stationery.	1. Make threats or personal attacks.
2. Identify the bill with which you are concerned, using title and number when possible.	2. Berate your legislator. If you disagree with him or her, give reasons for your position.
3. If you belong to an association that evaluates legislation, know its position. You have maximum impact when you back up your association's position.	3. Overstate or exaggerate your position.
4. Be concise and factual.	4. Use mimeographed letters, printed postal cards, or form letters.
5. Let the legislator know how the particular measure will affect his or her district.	5. Write only letters of criticism.
6. Include enough pertinent facts and reasons to substantiate your position.	

From Political Action Handbook for Nurses *by L. Freed, 1996, Santa Rosa, CA: Professor Publishing.*

Table 31-2 Telephoning Your Legislator

Preparation

1. Decide the purpose of your call, and list the points you wish to make in the course of the telephone conversation.
2. Know the number of the bill you want to discuss, its author, its general purpose and contents.
3. If possible, find out when and where the next action is scheduled on that bill.
4. If you are representing an organization, know approximately how many organization members live or work in the legislator's district.
5. Make sure you understand and can explain simply your rationale for support of or position on the legislation.

Suggestions for Conversation

1. Make the reason for your call clear at the beginning of the conversation.
2. State your name and what county you work in, the association position you hold (if any), and the legislative district in which you live (if applicable).
3. If you are calling about a bill and the legislator is not available, ask to speak to a legislative aide.
4. Ask for the appointment secretary or personal secretary if you are calling to make an appointment with the legislator.
5. As briefly as possible, state the state nurses association's position on the bill or issue and clearly stress the local support of that position.
6. Try to determine the position held by the legislator on the bill or issue.
7. If you spoke with a legislative staff person, make a note of the name.
8. Thank the legislator or legislative staff person for his or her time and assistance.
9. Make a brief report, verbally or in writing, to the state nurses association legislative chairperson or other appropriate person.

From Political Action Handbook for Nurses *by L. Freed, 1996, Santa Rosa, CA: Professor Publishing.*

Table 31-3 Meeting with Your Legislator

Contacting the District Office

1. Contact the district office during legislative recess or make arrangements to visit your state capital or Washington, D.C.
2. Write or call in advance for an appointment.
3. Make your appointment for a specific time period; usually half an hour to an hour in length is appropriate.
4. If the meeting is going to focus on a specific legislative topic, let the legislator's staff know this at the time the meeting is arranged.
5. When a legislator is not available, make an appointment with the legislator's staff person.

Preparing for the Meeting

1. Select a small group of knowledgeable nurses to attend meetings.
2. Meet as a group in advance of the meeting with the legislator to:
   a. Determine the primary goal of the meeting.
   b. Identify which issues or legislation need to be discussed to meet that goal.
   c. Review the rationale for positions on issues or legislation.
   d. Determine the roles and responsibilities of individual members for the conduct of the meeting.

During the Meeting

1. Be prepared to be brief and speak to the point.
2. Stick to the topic(s) you planned to discuss.
3. Supply a fact sheet or other information on the topic or issue being addressed.
4. Leave on time unless the legislator clearly wishes to continue.
5. Thank the legislator (or staff person) for his or her time.

After the Meeting

1. Take time to debrief and to summarize impressions of the meeting and the legislator's positions.
2. Write a brief summary of the meeting and forward it to the legislative chairperson of the state nursing association.
3. Discuss and plan strategy for follow-up.

From Political Action Handbook for Nurses *by L. Freed, 1996, Santa Rosa, CA: Professor Publishing.*

Table 31-4 Reasons for Participating in Events Featuring Legislators

1. To get better acquainted with legislators.
2. To listen to legislators' concerns.
3. To question legislators about issues and bills in your state capital and Washington.
4. To make a statement to your legislators about the viewpoint of your state nursing association.
5. To showcase your clout as an organization.

From Political Action Handbook for Nurses *by L. Freed, 1996, Santa Rosa, CA: Professor Publishing.*

Table 31-5   Levels of Political Sophistication and Political Action Strategies

LEVEL	POLITICAL ACTION STRATEGIES
Basic	• Voting • Reading newspapers, magazines, and journals • Understanding the political process
Political awareness	• Learning about politics, policy, and political action committees (PACs) • Lobbying: writing a legislator, telephoning a legislator • Participating in a grassroots political network—local or state level • Participating in voter registration programs • Campaigning • Supporting nursing organizations
Political activism	• Lobbying: meeting with a legislator, participating in events featuring legislators • Participating in a grassroots political nurse network—federal level • Leading a grassroots political nurse network • Participating in coalition building • Participating in campaigns • Contributing to PACs • Electioneering • Attending conferences and workshops and completing internships related to policy making • Supporting nursing organizations and lobbying for their interests • Presenting testimony—local level • Participating in community partnerships
Political sophistication	• Forming coalitions • Presenting testimony—state or federal level • Becoming appointed to federal panels or agencies • Conducting public policy research • Running for public office

SOURCES OF INFORMATION

There are many sources of information and resources for nurses who are interested and wish to participate in political activism. The most important first step in the decision to take a political stance and attempt to influence the political process is to become an informed student of politics. To become informed, one must read, listen, and watch. Local newspapers, magazines, and even professional journals are filled with reports of policy decisions. Radio and television news reports are both excellent sources of information and a gauge of public opinion.

When an issue or a piece of legislation is of particular interest or concern, be sure to know the topic well. The nurse should become knowledgeable about the issue or bill so that when it is debated he or she will be able to answer any questions that may be posed by lawmakers, voters, or others. Nurses should study the political process to ensure they can anticipate the paths the legislation or politician needs to travel. Nurses should form coalitions with organizations that are similarly interested in the issue and should identify the point in the political process where they are most likely to have the most influence; this point will depend on the resources, alliances, and strategies developed. With persistence, political activism can be the most rewarding way of demonstrating community health nursing's strength in caring for the people community health nurses serve.

The following sections include selected resource information. This list is not exhaustive. Refer to Appendix B for more resources.

Books

Policy and Politics for Nurses: Action and Change in the Workplace, Government, Organization and Community, 2nd ed. by Mason, Talbott and Leavitt (1993) is an excellent book suitable for a reference in nursing and politics.

Healthy People 2000 by the U.S. Department of Health and Human Services (1995) includes the current U.S. health priorities for disease treatment and prevention and serves as a logical starting point for nurse activists. Familiarity with the *Healthy People 2000* Priority Areas provides both a priority list for nurses and an insight into the discrepancies between the country's stated agenda and the actual actions taken on that agenda. Accessing the Internet for updates on the development of the Healthy People 2000 initiative is also important. An examination of similar initiatives in other countries will enhance nursing's knowledge of global actions to improve health.

Perspectives...

Insights of a Nursing Activist

In 1983, during a sabbatical leave from teaching, I served as a legislative intern for the ANA in Washington, D.C. An exciting piece of legislation that had been introduced in the Senate sparked my interest because it was directly related to community health nursing—one of my practice areas in nursing. The legislation provided for a demonstration project for four community nursing organizations (CNOs). A CNO is a nurse-run, nurse-managed center serving Medicare beneficiaries in home- and community-based settings under contracts that provide a fixed monthly capitation payment for each enrollee. The benefits include an array of services including Medicare-covered home care, physical, occupational and speech therapies, and medical equipment and supplies. In addition, the CNO would offer other services such as case management and health education. How exciting for nursing! If this legislation passed, it would be the first time in history that nurses would obtain direct reimbursement for their services. I thought a great deal about the implications that this legislation could have for the profession of nursing.

After my return to California, my interest in this legislation did not wane. I taught about the legislation in one of my nursing courses: "Nursing in a Socio-Political Environment." I continued my involvement and communication with the ANA and their lobbyists in government relations in order to maintain currency on the status of this legislation. I apprised nursing leaders in the community about the legislation, and a committee was formed (CNO Sonoma) to track this and other nursing legislation. Our committee met bimonthly for years with a goal to apply as one of the demonstration sites after passage of the bill. In 1987, the CNO project was authorized under the Omnibus Reconciliation Act (OBRA) of 1987; the legislation became Public Law (PL) 100-203. The Health Care Financing Administration (HCFA) established guidelines for the demonstration sites, and in 1992 CNO Sonoma submitted a grant proposal to become a demonstration site. However it was not funded.

The four sites selected and operating today are: the Living at Home Block Nurse Program in St. Paul, Minnesota; Carle Clinic in Urbana, Illinois; Carondelet Health Care in Tucson, Arizona; and the Visiting Nurse Service of New York in Long Island City, New York. Recent evaluation studies indicate improved access and quality, cost savings, and high levels of client satisfaction with this model of health care delivery. Because of the need for continued evaluation studies, there is a bill in the House of Representatives (HR 686) to reauthorize the demonstration project for an additional three years. CNO Sonoma plans to reconvene their meetings and to continue political action for this and other important nursing legislation. I will continue to advocate for the CNO model, because I believe it will well serve the profession and the public.

—Laurel Freed

Magazines and Newsletters

The American Nurse is the official publication of the American Nurses Association. This monthly news magazine is distributed to state nurses association and ANA members and includes invaluable information on policy issues and political action.

Capitol Update is the legislative newsletter for nurses. This bimonthly newsletter is compiled by the Departments of Federal Government Relations and Political and Grassroots Programs at ANA Headquarters, Washington, D.C. Each issue usually includes "Legislative Update," "In the Agencies," "Political Update," and announcements. This newsletter is a must for the political activist.

Specialty Organizations

Many specialty nursing organizations such as the American Association of Critical Care Nurses (AACN), the Organization for Obstetric, Gynecologic, and Neonatal Nurses (NAACOG), and the Association of Operating Room Nurses (AORN), to name just a few, are active in politics and distribute legislative newsletters. Nurses who belong to a specialty organization and wish to increase their political involvement should request specific newsletters from their organization.

Political Internships

Nurse in Washington Internship (NIWI) is an internship program sponsored by the National Federation for Specialty Nursing Organizations (NFSNO). This program is for nurses who wish to develop legislative knowledge and skills of political activism. This annual intensive four-day program educates nurses throughout the United States about the policy process in the nation's capital. Since its inception in 1985, 1,129 nurses have completed the internship and have developed the ability to become participants in nursing political activities. Mary Wakefield, nurse and Chief Staff to U.S. Senator Kent Conrad (D-ND) stated, "There is a direct link between what happens in D.C. and how we practice, what we teach, and what we research" (Chaffee, 1996, p. 21).

ORGANIZATIONS INVOLVED IN POLITICS AND POLICY

Nursing and health care organizations provide an opportunity for nurses to influence health and public policy through collective action. Perhaps one of the best examples of collective action in the United States was Nursing's Agenda for Health Care Reform, a policy statement on national health care. More than 60 organizations supported the agenda. Many nursing organizations have recognized the importance of political action for their members. And some specialty nursing organizations have enhanced their specialty by intense political involvement. It is also important for nurses to be active participants in multidisciplinary organizations such as the American Public Health Association (APHA), because their participation can lead to coalition building. Representation in multidisciplinary groups strengthens political efforts.

These nursing organizations have been involved in politics and political activism longer than other nursing organizations: American Nurses Association (ANA), state nurses associations (SNAs), National League for Nursing (NLN), and the Tri-Council for Nursing. By the mid-1980s, owing to the growth of specialty groups, there was also a proliferation of specialty organizations.

The American Nurses Association (ANA) began in the early part of the century and formed a Special Committee on Legislation in 1923. The departments that have to do with politics and policy are:

Government Relations—lobbies legislators and follows legislation in Congress

ANA-PAC—a powerful political action committee

Political Grassroots Program—a political grassroots network for nurses

The state nurses associations (SNAs) determine preferred state policy and lobby on most issues of concern to nursing. They also have their own PACs. Each state has an affiliated association with the ANA.

The National League for Nursing (NLN) was formed in the early 1950s and has joined with the ANA on many issues of concern to nursing. This organization is one arm of the Tri-Council for Nursing, which developed Nursing's Agenda for Health Care Reform. Although the focus of the League is on nursing education and the accreditation of schools of nursing, the NLN has participated in policy and political debates at all levels of government.

The Tri-Council for Nursing originated in 1981 and is composed of the American Nurses Association (ANA), National League for Nursing (NLN), American Colleges of Nursing (AACN), and the American Organization of Nurse Executives (AONE). (AONE joined the alliance in 1985 without any change in the title.) Its purpose is to facilitate coordination and communication on key professional issues and to promote federal legislation of mutual concern. The alliance has played a major role in advancing the profession and the nation's health in the policy arena (Hall-Long, 1995).

The National Federation of Specialty Nursing Organizations (NFSNO) is a loosely structured alliance of large and small nursing specialty organizations whose purpose is to coordinate efforts of practice, education, and other areas of mutual concern among nursing organizations" (Hall-Long, 1995, p. 26).

The National Organization Liaison Forum (NOLF) was formulated in the early 1980s. It is a diverse forum within the ANA made up of a coalition of nursing organizations. Its purpose is to "provide a unified approach to national policy issues and nursing interests" (Hall-Long, 1995, p. 26).

The American Association of Critical Care Nurses (AACN) Certification Corporation certifies critical care nurses and promotes critical care nursing practice that contributes to desired client outcomes through the CCRN certification program in adult, pediatric, and neonatal critical care nursing. This corporation is a separate affiliate of the American Association of Critical Care Nurses, the world's largest specialty nursing organization. In an article titled "AACN Perspective, Redefining Nursing in the Midst of Health Care Reform," Caterinicchio (1995) states: "Nurses are constants in every phase of health care delivery—and reform. Through a shared and mutual commitment to promote a health care system driven by the needs of patients and their families, nurses have the power to set the tone for change across the entire nation" (p. 9).

The American Organization of Nurse Executives (AONE) is an association dedicated to advancing the practice of nurses who facilitate, design, and manage care. The organization focuses on resources that promote education, advocacy, research, information sharing, networking, and career advancement opportunities. Since 1994, the AONE has strengthened its linkages between the national organization and the Organization of Nurse Executives (ONE) at the state and local levels. It strengthened its linkages because the AONE recognized that both leadership and policy development begin at the local level, where real health care reform is taking shape (Swan, 1995).

The American Academy of Nurse Practitioners (AANP) is an organization that includes all nurse practitioner specialties. Its purposes are to promote high standards of health care delivered by nurse practitioners and to act as a forum to enhance the identity and continuity of nurse practitioners at a national and international level. The organization actively promotes health policy through its governmental affairs activities in Washington, D.C. Participating in the development of health policy has become an important part of the role of the nurse practitioner (Towers, 1995).

The American Association of Occupational Health Nurses, Inc. (AAOHN) is the national professional association for registered nurses who provide on-the-job health care for the nation's workers. As the largest group of providers of health care at the worksite, occupational health nurses are key players in directing public policy. After many years of working with the Occupational Safety and Health Administration (OSHA), in 1993 the OSHA of Occupational Health Nursing was established. In an article about AAOHN, Livsey (1995) states, "In today's work environment, it is imperative that nurses take a proactive position in influencing health policy at national, state, and local levels" (p. 14).

There are other specialty nursing organizations involved in politics. Some have their own lobbyists on Capitol Hill; others do not. It is important to remember not to work alone on a policy or issue and thus fragment nursing. The more one specialty organization can work with other orga-

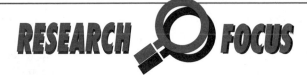

Long-Term Effects of Home Visitation on Maternal Life Course and Child Abuse and Neglect: Fifteen-Year Follow-up of a Randomized Trial

STUDY PROBLEM/PURPOSE

Home visitation services have been promoted as a means of improving maternal and child health and functioning. Long-term effects had not been examined, however.

The study was conducted to examine the long term effects of a program of prenatal and early childhood home visitation by nurses and to determine if the program, instituted early in the life cycle, would alter life outcomes of the mothers through the child's fifteenth birthday. Two domains of maternal functioning were examined: (1) subsequent pregnancy, use of Aid to Families with Dependent Children (AFDC), employment, substance abuse, encounters with the criminal justice system and (2) perpetration of child abuse and neglect.

METHODS

The study was conducted in a semirural community in New York State. Pregnant women were recruited from the county health department and the offices of private obstetricians if they had had no previous live births and could participate before the twenty-fifth week of gestation. Having at least one of three of the following sociodemographic risk characteristics was preferred but not required: young age (under 19 years at registration), unmarried, or low socioeconomic status. Of 500 eligible clients, 100 refused participation. The 400 participants were randomized according to treatment conditions: treatments one and two were combined to form a

comparison group; treatment three was nurse visitation during pregnancy and through the child's second birthday. Three hundred and twenty-four families participated in a follow-up study when their children were 15 years old.

In the home visits, the nurses promoted three aspects of maternal functioning: health-related behaviors during pregnancy and parenting, parental role behaviors, and personal life planning.

The nurses used detailed assessments and protocols to guide their work with families.

The nurses completed an average of nine home visits during the pregnancy and 23 visits from the child's birth to second birthday.

FINDINGS

Findings from this study indicated that early childhood home visitation by nurses resulted in positive outcomes. The number of subsequent pregnancies was reduced; child abuse and neglect were reduced. There was increased participation in the labor force, and there was reduced government spending for low-income unmarried women for up to 15 years after the birth of the first child.

IMPLICATIONS

Prenatal and early childhood home visitation was effective in improving the quality of life for disadvantaged women.

SOURCE

Long-Term Effects of Home Visitation on Maternal Life Course and Child Abuse and Neglect: Fifteen Year Follow-up of a Randomized Trial *by D. L. Olds, J. Eckenrode, C. Henderson, H. Kitzman, J. Powers, R. Cole, K. Sidora, P. Morris, L. Pettit, & D. Luckey, 1997, Journal of the American Medical Association, 278, pp. 637–643.*

COMMUNITY NURSING VIEW

The Olds study of prenatal and early home visitation (see this chapter's Research Focus) is well known among community health nurses for demonstrating primary prevention in home visitation by nurses. This highly acclaimed and tested model improves the social functioning of low-income first-time mothers and their babies. To date, there have been two randomized clinical trials: one in Elmira, New York, and the other in Memphis, Tennessee. Other replication sites are in place, and there are plans to expand to 20 replication sites across the nation. The trials produced the following results:

- 25% reduction in cigarette smoking during pregnancy among women who smoked cigarettes at registration
- 80% reduction in rates of child maltreatment among at-risk families from birth through child's second birthday
- 56% reduction in the rates of children's health care encounters for injuries and ingestions, from birth through child's second birthday
- 43% reduction in subsequent pregnancy among low-income, unmarried women by first child's birthday
- 83% increase in the rates of mother's labor force participation by first child's fourth birthday

In 1997, an Assembly bill was presented in the California legislature that provides for a home visitation program for low-income mothers to aid in the prevention of maternal and child health problems and to improve outcomes of mothers and children.

Nursing Considerations

ASSESSMENT
- This piece of legislation is very important for community health nurses; what initial data would be important to collect in order to effectively lobby for the bill?
- What data would be necessary to begin planning and intervention strategies?

DIAGNOSIS
- How would you state a community diagnosis in this situation?

OUTCOME IDENTIFICATION
- What are the expected outcomes of this legislation?

PLANNING/INTERVENTIONS
- This legislation is at the committee level. According to knowledge about "how a bill becomes law," how should the community health nurse proceed?
- What other information is needed?
- What should the community health nurse specifically do to affect this piece of legislation?
- What strategies are necessary to "track," or follow, this legislation?
- How can the community health nurse involve other nurses to influence this piece of legislation?

EVALUATION
- How might the community health nurse have developed a stronger power base to influence this legislation?

nizations to form coalitions, the more influence the profession will have on legislators and other policymakers. The following is only a partial listing of other specialty nursing organizations involved in the policy arena:

- American Nephrology Nurses' Association
- Association of Operating Room Nurses
- Organization for Obstetric, Gynecologic and Neonatal Nurses (NAACOG)
- Oncology Nursing Society

Other national and international organizations include the American Public Health Association (APHA), which was founded in 1882 and represents approximately 50,000 public health workers. It is a multidisciplinary organiza-

tion representing varied health professionals and health organizations. The APHA has numerous special-interest sections, including a Public Health Nursing Section. The association is nationally and internationally recognized for its expertise and leadership in public health. The APHA frequently provides testimony to Congress and is involved with both public policy and regulatory issues. The APHA is a member of the World Federation of Public Health Associations and serves as that organization's secretariat.

The Agency for Health Care Policy and Research (AHCPR) is one of eight agencies of the U.S. Public Health Service. This agency was established by Congress in 1990 and is the nation's focal point of health services research. The AHCPR seeks answers to some of the most pressing health concerns facing the population and serves as a bridge between researchers, clinicians, and policymakers. Participation by nurses from all backgrounds is welcomed and encouraged by the agency (Bavier, 1995).

The International Council of Nurses (ICN) was formed by a group of British nurses at the turn of the century. It is composed of over 90 nursing associations (only one from each country may belong). The American Nurses Association is the member from the United States. The organization provides a medium through which national nurses' associations share their common interests and goals and work together for the health of their nations.

The World Health Organization (WHO) was established in 1946 and is related to the United Nations (UN). The World Health Assembly, one of the three branches of the WHO, meets annually with all UN members and is the policy-making body of the WHO. The WHO's main goal is to attain the highest possible level of health for all. The headquarters for the WHO is in Geneva, Switzerland, and it has six regional headquarters.

Key Concepts

- Early community health nurses were involved in influencing health-related policy decisions. However, only in the last two decades has nursing become visible in the political arena.

- The community health nurse is one of the few health professionals to realize the scope of health problems affecting large segments of the population; this knowledge is a mandate to action for the caring professional.

- By learning the various power bases, the nurse can understand and use power in a positive and productive way.

- Policy represents the actions of a government and develops incrementally over time.

- Politics is associated with conflicting values, and often multiple interest groups compete for scarce resources.

- Four stages of political development in the nursing profession have been identified in order to analyze previous accomplishments and plan future actions.

- Local politics may differ radically from one city or county to another; federal and state governments are similar to each other.

- The private sector, including nurses, can influence legislation in many ways, especially through influencing the process of writing regulations.

- The community health nurse should use the political process as a tool to influence health care policy.

- Nursing values, although different from the public's traditional values, are useful for focusing the policy debate on issues of human rights, individual worth, and caring.

- Nursing's political network encompasses the professional associations with their myriad activities including lobbying, electioneering, and grassroots political action.

- In the international community, nursing's basic problems and issues are very similar to national issues.

- Community health nurses need to be politically active in the community because of community and professional shared values and because of the pervasive role the government has on the impact of health care.

- Major strategies for political action include lobbying, electioneering, coalition building, and participating in political networks.

- Nurses can access a variety of specialty organizations with expertise in political activism to ensure that nursing's voice is heard at all levels of government.

- The primary goal of the World Health Organization is to attain the highest possible level of health for all people.

Visions for the Future

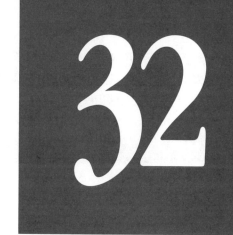

Phyllis Schubert, DNSc, RN, MA
Janice Hitchcock, DNSc, RN
Sue A. Thomas, RN, EdD

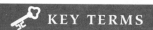
It's as if the milestone of the millennium acts like a deadline, encouraging us to confront and resolve our problems so we can meet the next century with a clean slate. Will it be Apocalypse or Golden Age? The choice is clearly ours.

—*John Naisbitt*

COMPETENCIES

Upon completion of this chapter, the reader should be able to:

- Discuss concerns and possibilities recommended by health and health care futurists.
- Describe current efforts of global, regional, and local leaders to transform a disease-oriented sick care system to a wellness-oriented health care system for the 21st century.
- Discuss efforts to include environmental, social, health, and economic intersectoral factors while working to meet *Healthy People 2000* goals.
- Describe socioeconomic, environmental, and epidemiologic factors driving the need for community health nursing knowledge and skills.
- Discuss efforts to form nursing and interdisciplinary partnerships to promote health and prevent disease.
- Explain conceptual frameworks for clinical nursing practice that serve as guides for community nursing in the future.
- Discuss images of nursing theory-based community health centers and interdisciplinary settings established to promote health and healing and to serve people of diverse cultures.
- Describe contemporary and futuristic visions of community health nursing practice, research, and education in the 21st century.

Health for all is a global vision that will continue to direct our energies as we move into the 21st century. Our images and beliefs about the future are relevant because they determine what we do and how we live today. In general, those who study the future take a proactive stance, believing the future can be shaped and guided by human decisions and actions (Hancock & Bezold, 1994). This chapter includes a look at work by futurists about health in the next century, major risk factors related to changing human–environment processes, current international and national efforts to move health care delivery systems from a disease-oriented system to one of health promotion and disease prevention, the impact of these changing social forces on community health nursing, and proposed innovations for nursing theory-based practice, research, and education that use conceptual models and theories of nurse theorists that define nursing in terms of the nursing metaparadigm—health, person, environment, and nursing.

FUTURISTS LOOK AT POSSIBILITIES

Futurists, according to Hancock & Bezold (1994), think about the future in four ways. They consider all the imaginable possibilities and then select and examine those that are most plausible. Various scenarios are then created from the most plausible known at the time. A probable future scenario is seen as an extension of the present without significant change. This probable scenario is often undesirable. The futurist then selects a preferable scenario by envisioning one that is desirable. The immediate future (one to five years) is shaped by decisions previously made. The medium-term (six to 20 years) and the long-term (20 to 50 years) futures are shaped by decisions made today and in the years ahead (see Figure 32-1). Thinking beyond 50 years is difficult and requires imagination and creativity.

Concerns for the Future of Health

Futuristic study of health and health care is very different from the study of medical care. Health care also involves environmental, social, economic, and political determinants. To a lesser extent biophysiological, genetic, and medical care factors affect future health. According to Hancock and Garrett (1995), health has generally improved during the last century. However, population growth, urbanization, environmental changes, poverty, inequity, war, and existing and possible new communicable and chronic diseases put the health of future generations in grave danger.

Chronic diseases such as cancer, heart disease, musculoskeletal conditions, and neuropsychiatric disorders are expected to remain prevalent in more developed countries; and communicable, maternal, and childhood diseases in lesser developed countries. One ray of hope arises from indications that people in more developed countries may be reversing the trend of chronic disease by leading healthier lifestyles. Increasing population growth, however, is causing rapid urbanization and environmental deterioration, which in turn lead to poor housing and sanitary conditions, disease, social disintegration, and violence (Hancock & Garrett, 1995).

In addition, increasing stress on the planet's resources and ecology is expected to take a toll on human health. This stress includes: (a) global atmospheric changes (depletion of the ozone layer leading to skin cancer, cataracts, and interference with immune functioning); (b) depletion of natural resources (desertification leading to malnutrition and famine); and (c) **ecotoxicity** (contamination of the planet with toxic chemicals that poison and have genetic, hormonal, immunologic, and psychological consequences). Equity, a major issue in health concerns, addresses more than distribution of wealth. It involves education, living and working conditions, social status, and power. War and conflict carry unspeakable possibilities that very few people are even willing to consider.

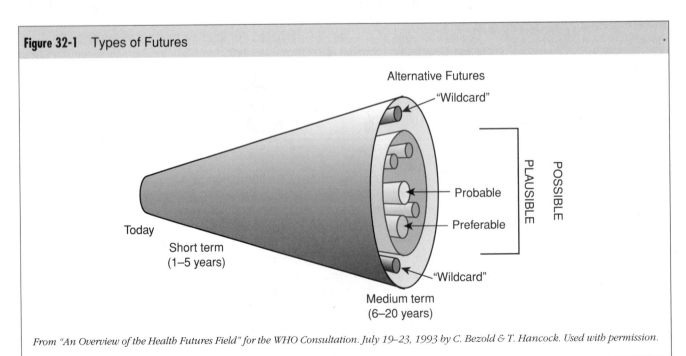

Figure 32-1 Types of Futures

From "An Overview of the Health Futures Field" for the WHO Consultation. July 19–23, 1993 by C. Bezold & T. Hancock. Used with permission.

Create Your Image of a Healthy Community or City

Let yourself relax with a small group of peers, and draw your attention inward. Allow an image to form of yourself touring a community or city of the future that, by your standards, reflects health. When you have completed your tour, use colored pencils or crayons to draw what you saw. Share with each other what you saw—people involved in various activities, stores, workplaces, residences, recreational settings, cars, plants, trees, street life, social centers, water, and sky. Share any strategies you could use to make your community of the present more like the one you imagined.

Futurists Make Suggestions

Hancock and Garrett (1995) have summarized suggestions made by futurists to improve health for the 21st century. These include:

- Continue evolution of community-based, integrated, primary care systems that use fewer physicians and more nurses and allied health professionals.
- Increase psychoneuroimmunology research and development of noninvasive alternative and complementary care therapies which are used to integrate body, mind, and spirit.
- Continue biomedical developments in diagnostic and treatment technology even though proportionate impact on health status of the world population will be limited.
- Make improvements in macro-environmental conditions—ecological, social, economic, political, and technologic—that most influence health status.

The last suggestion includes goals related to: (a) education and empowerment of women, (b) effective management of urbanization, (c) protection of environmental quality, (d) equitable distribution of wealth and power, and (e) encouragement of healthy lifestyles, including education and anti-tobacco campaigns.

Formulation of public policy that focuses on health care must be a priority. A new approach to health economics that emphasizes the largest health gain rather than monetary profit as investment outcome is also needed. Last, establishment of innovative partnerships is needed to develop integrated structures that recognize the interdependent and ecological nature of the problems being faced. Such structures would encourage the societal participation in governance considered necessary to meet these goals (Hancock & Garrett, 1995).

Hancock (1993a) suggests a bottom-down health system as an ideal for health care delivery (see Figure 32-2).

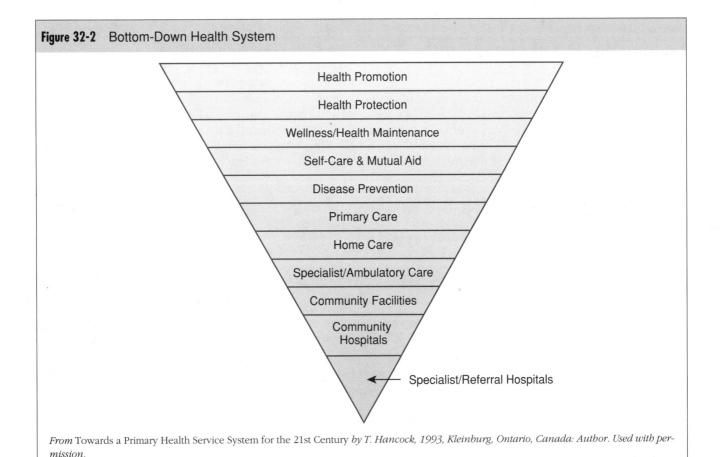

Figure 32-2 Bottom-Down Health System

Health Promotion

Health Protection

Wellness/Health Maintenance

Self-Care & Mutual Aid

Disease Prevention

Primary Care

Home Care

Specialist/Ambulatory Care

Community Facilities

Community Hospitals

← Specialist/Referral Hospitals

From Towards a Primary Health Service System for the 21st Century *by T. Hancock, 1993, Kleinburg, Ontario, Canada: Author. Used with permission.*

In this system the main emphasis is on health promotion, protection, and maintenance. Various sectors of the community come together to develop healthy public policy. Teams of health care workers include community health nurses, nurse practitioners, midwives, physicians, and other primary care providers. Services occur in a wide variety of settings, such as community health centers, schools, the workplace, malls, and senior housing.

Health and health care futurists help us look ahead, plan for, and develop skills needed to anticipate challenges and avert disaster. Five scenarios for health care delivery in the United States early in the 21st century were created by five futurists (Healthcare Forum, 1992). The scenarios, listed in Table 32-1, indicate several possible directions the health care movement might take.

Leadership Development and Future Health

Leadership development was an initial and major focus of the Kellogg Foundation when it funded the Healthy Cities Indiana project—an ongoing collaborative effort between the Indiana University School of Nursing, the Institute of Action Research for Community Health, the Indiana Pub-

lic Health Association, and six Indiana cities. Preparation of community leaders in this movement to build healthy cities and communities was seen as essential. The leadership skills found necessary for the success of this project were: (a) ability to gather and interpret information, (b) interpersonal skills in working with each other and the broader community, and (c) decision-making skills that would serve the broader community rather than a smaller segment of the population (Flynn, 1992).

Intersectoral Partnerships

Solutions to complex issues require networking and partnership. Persons concerned about future health and health-related issues have addressed the need for partnerships in all arenas. Visions linking nurses, consumers of health care, and health care disciplines are addressed later in this chapter. But first, the need for **intersectoral partnerships,** or working relationships between different sectors of the community or of society, such as education, business, and government, are addressed.

It is clear from the WHO perspective that a comprehensive health system emphasizing primary and secondary prevention must include coordination with and cooperation from all sectors of society, not just the health sector. An intersectoral approach to health care focuses on creating community partnerships in health care planning, implementation, and evaluation. With this approach, power is manifest through influence rather than authority (Hudson-Rodd, 1994).

The Healthy Cities/Healthy Communities model challenges citizens and local leaders in all sectors to "develop a broad range of strategies to address the broad social, environmental and economic determinants of health, and ultimately to change the corporate and community culture by incorporating health" (Hancock, 1993b, p. 8).

Like Health for All (HFA) programs, the Healthy Cities/Healthy Communities model focuses on intersectoral partnerships in addressing the health needs of the community.

Table 32-1   Five Scenarios for Future Health Care Delivery

SCENARIO	EXPECTATION
1. Continued growth/high tech	Major biomedical advances, but continuing toward unequal access to care.
2. Hard times/government leadership	Continued economic difficulties and a revolt against the healthcare system. Replacement with a more frugal and universal system.
3. The buyer's market	Providers compete on the basis of outcomes. Consumer tax deductions for care removed.
4. A new civilization	Western civilization in process of rebirth as paradigms in science, technology, society, and government change dramatically. Health care becoming more sophisticated, focused, and directed by the individual and concerned with community health.
5. Healing and health care	Assumes an emerging new civilization, as does the previous scenario, but focused more on greater use of our mental, emotional, and spiritual capacities in healing.

Adapted from "Possible Futures, Preferable Futures" by T. Hancock and C. Bezold, 1994, Healthcare Forum Journal, *March/April.*

Areas addressed include employment, schooling, agriculture, pollution, energy use and transport, ecology, and other issues common around the world. Other concerns include community and family violence, effects of substance abuse on the community, reemergence of infectious disease in the Western world, and media effects on all of these issues. Threats to the community's health also include the focus on illness care, the impact of poverty, the widening gap between rich and poor, community overdevelopment, and environmental degradation.

EFFORTS BY CURRENT LEADERS—INTERNATIONAL AND NATIONAL

Global efforts to achieve a goal of health for all began with the Declaration of Alma Ata in 1978. Delegates from 134 countries plus representatives from the World Health Organization (WHO) met in what was then Alma Ata, USSR (now Almatay, Kazakhstan). That meeting brought the first international recognition that shifting the focus of care from illness to health was imperative (WHO, 1981; Anderson & McFarlane, 1996).

The Alma-Ata document (WHO, 1978) emphasized that "health development is essential for social and economic development, that the means for attaining them are intimately linked, and that actions to improve the health and socioeconomic situation should be regarded as mutually supportive rather than competitive" (pp. 15–16). Global Strategies for Health for All by the Year 2000, which arose from this Declaration, asserts that delivery of programs and services that promote health and prevent disease to the whole population must start with primary health care (WHO, 1981; Ashton, 1991).

According to Anderson and McFarlane (1996), confusion of the terms primary health care and primary care inhibits efforts of developed countries such as the United States. In the United States, *primary care* represents entry into the health care delivery system. Linkage with a primary care provider enhances accessibility, comprehensiveness, coordination of services, and continuity. *Primary health care*, as implied in the Alma-Ata mandate, includes public health efforts such as community participation, occupational health, and environmental health issues.

Primary health care includes: (a) education for identification and prevention of prevailing health problems for the community involved; (b) proper food supplies and nutrition; (c) safe water and basic sanitation; (d) maternal and child care and family planning; (e) immunization against major infectious diseases; (f) prevention and control of endemic diseases; (g) appropriate treatment of common diseases; (h) promotion of mental health; and (i) provision of essential drugs (WHO, 1978). Although it has been assumed that the United States led the world in these areas, morbidity and mortality statistics indicate poor standing compared with other developed countries. Bryant,

Zuberi, and Thaver (1991) note that in this time of constrained economics, primary health care is essential to achieving **equity in health care,** which is the goal of equal access to medical or illness care, but may also refer to equal access to health and wellness care, education, a clean and caring environment, and opportunity to fulfill one's fullest life potential.

Health care delivery systems within the United States are undergoing change as creative efforts are made to solve certain problems. Some current efforts within the health care system are addressed here.

Managed Care

Attempts to reform health care also affect community health nursing. Major changes are under way in the U.S. health care system to decrease the cost of health care delivery. Restructuring, downsizing, and mergers have changed health care delivery models. Managed care delivery systems, in which one health professional oversees and coordinates health care services of the individual, integrated networking systems, community health nursing organizations, school-based family health centers, and health ministries, in which the clients or consumers, clergy, and health care professionals work together to preserve and promote the health of people within communities, have changed the way care is delivered. As discussed in previous chapters, these changes will continue to have a major impact on the delivery of community health nursing services.

Managed care is currently a major force in the changing structure of health care delivery in the United States, reshaping the financing and delivery of health care services. Health care networks or systems are encouraged to provide comprehensive services, such as disease prevention, health promotion, and care for sickness within the community. Health maintenance organizations (HMOs) emphasize prevention; wellness, which is the fulfillment of one's potential physically, emotionally, mentally, and spiritually; and coordination of primary care, with financial incentives to decrease utilization of high-cost, high-tech acute care services. Low-tech health care services are provided in community agencies such as libraries and schools (Gray, 1994). These services include such activities as health teaching, counseling, the provision of complementary therapies, and immunizations. Integrated computerized communication systems link all the components of the system so that client data is accessible and available as needed.

Integrated health care systems, which offer networks and linkages of services to ensure continuity of care, discussed in Chapters 3 and 4, are being created to deliver seamless care (effective and efficient, without gaps) to managed care enrollees. Case management, the process in which a care provider serves to assess, plan, intervene, and evaluate according to the needs of the client, now holds a major role in managed care systems. Nurses are in a pivotal position to serve in that role, helping clients and families to move across various developmental phases and community settings (Sims, 1994).

In many states public health departments are moving into managed care with the Medicaid population, those individuals who are receiving state and federal funds to pay for medical services. Public health nurses are functioning as case managers, focusing on health promotion and disease prevention. Nurses also serve as case managers in other managed care systems. The process commonly spans the continuum of care—home-based care, ambulatory services, emergency, inpatient, board and care, and skilled nursing facility care.

These changes seem like small steps in the overall system, but efforts to create major reform are difficult in the United States. Political differences and powerful special interest groups impede efforts to meet HFA goals. Debate persists concerning whether individual states or the federal government should make health care and environmental decisions. The balance between individual freedom and responsibility is at issue. That balance is perhaps skewed somewhat toward freedom but will most likely always be moving one way or the other in an attempt to achieve balance or maintain equilibrium.

New forms of nationalism, ethnic identity, religious fundamentalism, and fascism present divisive threats to peaceful solutions in the United States and many other countries (Anderson & McFarlane, 1996). Counterefforts by many make the movement toward a healthier world difficult. Yet, community health nurses and those of many other disciplines hold great potential to serve communities in ways they have never before used. Many nurses have knowledge and skills to promote and participate in healing dialogue in communities of all kinds.

COMMUNITY HEALTH NURSING AND THE FORCES FOR CHANGE

Changing social and environmental forces will influence the evolution of community health nursing greatly during the next several years. The work of health care futurists provides only part of the backdrop. Another aspect is provided by the mandates cited in the previous section, those related to broader socioeconomic and global contexts.

The forces of change in health care are driven by the need to achieve some combination of cost reduction, enhanced client and consumer satisfaction, and improvement of health care outcomes. A Pew Health Professions Commission Report (1995) states: "A trillion dollar health care industry in the U.S. is undergoing enormous changes as it anticipates the move from a disease care emphasis to one of health promotion and disease prevention." A few of the recommendations made by the Pew Commission (the commission responsible for guiding and making recommendations for education and practice in the health professions) directly affecting community health nursing are as follows (Pew Health Professions Commission, 1995):

> ### REFLECTIVE THINKING
> **Changing Health Care Delivery Systems**
>
> • What aspects of the health care delivery system in your nation would you choose to retain to benefit society as a whole? To benefit families? Individuals?
>
> • What aspects would you change because of detrimental effects to society? To families? To individuals?

- Education of health professional schools must increase content related to psycho-social-behavioral sciences and population and health management.
- Clinicians of the future must have skills in the use of sophisticated information and communications technology to promote health and prevent disease; to use the political process to help create a more consumer-focused system; and to strike a more equitable balance between resources and needs.
- Clinicians must be prepared to serve consumers within the consumers' own cultural context.
- Nursing must recover its clinical management role and recognize management as an important aspect of professional practice.
- Nursing must decrease the number of associate degree and diploma programs and increase the number of master's-level nurse practitioner training programs.

The move from disease-oriented health care to health promotion and disease prevention is expected by the Pew Commission to affect health care workers in many ways. It is expected that about half of the nation's hospitals will close. There will be massive expansion of primary care in ambulatory and community settings. A surplus of physicians, nurses, and pharmacists will occur as hospitals close and dispensing of drugs is automated and centralized. Demands for public health professionals will increase greatly to meet the needs of the market-driven system. Educational programs and curricula for health professionals must undergo fundamental alterations to prepare for changes in practice, research, and education (Pew Health Professions Commission, 1995).

The strength of community health nursing has traditionally been providing primary health care services. Primary health care shifts the emphasis from aggregates to individuals and families in their homes, schools, workplace, and back to aggregates. The philosophy of primary health care focuses on social justice, equity, and self-reliance. Because of their services, nurses are increasingly acknowledged as necessary for healthy communities throughout the world. Shalala (1993) asserts that

nurses are the agents and leaders for health in our society. That means they also are among the primary agents for educational success, job capability, social productivity, and able parenting—because all these things are by-products of a healthy life beginning at birth (p. 289).

Because nursing theory links the concepts of person, environment, health, and nursing, increasing knowledge and understanding of health as the interrelationship of person and environment has great impact. One example involves the growing knowledge of epidemiology. Epidemiologic skills—traditionally of great importance to the community health nurse—are becoming increasingly complex in the modern world. Environmental conditions, changing lifestyles, and health-promotion strategies have expanded a system in which the view of agent as an infectious organism, environment as physical surroundings, and host as a person was very narrow.

Now, the agent may be prematurity, low birth weight, birth injury, congenital malformation, sudden infant death syndrome, or accidents. The environment may include maternal age, ethnicity, parity, prenatal care, education, socioeconomic status, migration, adult mortality and morbidity, changes in health services, policies, personnel, or funding policy and procedure. The host may be identified as the infant population or as birth and death patterns related to age, ethnicity, sex, or birth weight, for example. Also, screening not only identifies problems; it also implies ethical commitment for diagnosis and treatment.

The national and international mandates discussed earlier focus on primary prevention and emerge from a vision that emphasizes wellness, not illness, as the true key to improved health care. During the past 20 to 30 years, the working definition of health has shifted from absence of death, disease, and disability to a current understanding that health involves broader holistic concerns related to social, economic, and political issues. Considering nursing's concern with human health, this shift is of great consequence to the discipline.

Major changes are occurring in health care at all levels. Emerging models require community health nurses to be flexible and proactive, to reaffirm their social mission, and to collaborate with others in the assessment, planning, implementation, and evaluation of health care services. Six issues associated with HFA strategies and creation of healthy communities will be of central concern for the nurse of the future. They are equity, health promotion, community involvement, intersectoral partic-

ipation, primary health care, and international cooperation (Rathwell, 1992).

Coupled with this worldwide recognition of a need to create different models of health care are reemergence of infectious diseases, many of them drug resistant; disenfranchisement of significant parts of the population; a problematic economic environment; and unmet health care needs of vulnerable populations (Buhler-Wilkerson, 1993).

COMMUNITY HEALTH NURSING LEADERS AND VISIONS OF PARTNERSHIP

Community health nurses are helping to shift the focus from medical/curative factors to disease prevention and health promotion. This change of focus requires increased activity by nurses in policy arenas, forming partnerships with communities and organizations at local, regional, and national levels (Mason, Talbott & Leavitt, 1993).

Nurse-managed centers guided by community members and professionals provide opportunity for engagement in the community (Anderson & McFarlane, 1996). Social, cultural, and environmental determinants of health are major considerations in such settings.

Nurses and Consumers in Partnership

Community health nurses are favorably positioned to provide leadership in coalition and community building efforts. Pioneer community health nurses have viewed nursing's role as a crucial social mission and have envisioned nurses as creating "a public sphere that (draws) upon the diversity of cultural beliefs and societal demands of the populace" (Reverby, 1993, p. 1662). The concepts of partnerships and community building, similar to the ideas advocated by the HFA initiative and Healthy Communities model, are central to the mission of early nursing leaders. More than 100 years ago, they focused on collaborating with city leaders, philanthropists, and neighborhood and community leaders to create models of care that would help people improve their health and would enhance healing—at the individual and family level as well as at the public policy level. These models of care remain relevant today.

Community health nurses and other health care workers are challenged to form **community partnerships** with community leaders to work for better health by participating in assessing, planning, building programs, implementing, and constantly evaluating. Hudson-Rodd (1994) encourages shifting the emphasis from discipline-specific public health workers to community members working together. She sees local, state, national, and global activities as necessary to create viable, sustainable, healthy places in which people can live.

☙ REFLECTIVE THINKING ☙

Building Partnerships for Community Health

• How do you think community health nurses could participate in creating partnership models in the community?

• What skills do you think are needed for community health nurses to establish linkages with community residents for the purpose of participating in health planning efforts?

• What does the concept of partnership mean to you in relation to community building?

Reaching out to people in their communities—a basic community health nursing practice—includes creating partnerships for the purpose of community building. Creation of partnerships between the various sectors—providers and consumers—has been, and will be, a crucial determinant in improving the health of our communities at all levels. Alliances formed with consumers will aid in developing coalitions to improve access to health care for all (Tietebaum and Bieg, 1994).

Anderson and McFarlane (1996) suggest that nursing ethics should address advocacy as a moral position of the nurse in the community-as-partner model. The concept of advocacy represents commitment to nurturing client autonomy, honoring client choices, and engaging with clients in a manner that encourages expression of values, as well as serving to communicate the needs of the clients to relevant persons or agencies.

Interdisciplinary Partnerships

As the nursing profession enters the 21st century, a major role transition is occurring throughout the world. Nursing is moving toward more independent functioning, interdependence with flexible role boundaries, and a focus on health promotion. Nurses are expected to take part in interactive, interdisciplinary teams focusing on issues within a political, social, cultural, policy, and economic context (Lewis & Farrell, 1995). Negotiation and conflict resolution and management skills are increasingly important as participation in health care delivery systems addresses and heightens cultural and political awareness.

Partnerships among consumers, universities, community health centers, health departments, faith communities, schools, and hospitals are helping to create seamless health care systems (Meservey, 1995). Community health nurses will increasingly work in such systems, assist in facilitating their development, and function in teams with shared ownership and shared responsibilities. Flexibility and readiness to respond to emerging needs are required.

The current disease-oriented medical system is technologically sophisticated and complex but very costly in both economic and human terms. Although it achieves excellent results in many situations, it often leaves a trail of chronic health problems that are of little interest to acute care professionals. The challenge is for community nursing to assert distinctive knowledge and skills to tackle these problems in partnership with medicine and other professions. Nurses will apply the rich heritage of nursing's conceptual models in the process of building collaborative, cooperative relationships and functioning as full and equal partners with those from different professional perspectives, all being committed to the health and well-being of consumers.

Nurses have historically provided a unique and significant community service throughout the world. Grace (1995) notes that she has seen nurses seize the opportunity to work with communities in Brazil, townships of South Africa, rural areas in Zimbabwe, barrios in Mexico, and inner cities and rural areas in the United States among others to create projects and models that address health needs

and problems. As we enter the 21st century, nurses will be in a pivotal position to help reconfigure health care delivery and to create health care systems that are more community responsive and consumer friendly (Smith, 1995).

Even more, nurses will need to recognize and support the role of the consumer as an "informed participant in decisions that affect . . . care" (National League for Nursing, 1993, p. 6). The W. K. Kellogg Foundation currently funds projects specified for and about community partnerships. There are hundreds of these projects around the world; the Healthy Cities Indiana project mentioned earlier in this chapter is the first in the United States. In response to these projects, Smith (1995) stated:

> We are seeing communities in many parts of the world engage in redefining health and designing new approaches to organizing health care services. Comprehensive community-based care and primary care are ascending in importance. We are seeing nursing strive to develop partnerships with consumers and communities (p. 189).

Nurses will need new knowledge and skills to function in redesigned health care systems of the future—systems that utilize community development models to meet health needs. Nursing leaders must look at nursing practice in a broader context of health care and commit to work with policymakers in government, education, and health care service systems to improve health care delivery locally, nationally, and globally.

NURSING THEORY–BASED HEALTH CENTERS FOR THE 21ST CENTURY

If nursing theory should become the guide for the discipline in the 21st century, community health nursing practice would look very different than it does today. Nursing theories, and conceptual models of nursing in general, could be categorized as visionary, because nursing, in general, has not been practiced as a unique and autonomous profession, even though community health nurses have enjoyed some degree of autonomy in their nursing practice. And if nursing theory guided the discipline of nursing, nursing research and education would also be based in the theories and conceptual models of nursing. The field of nursing would fit well in the present world, which is concerned with the nature of the person–environment relationship and health. This section outlines visions for the future of community health nursing practice, research, and education beyond the year 2000. These **theory-based nursing practice** visions for the future are derived from the ideas of nurse theorists and leaders.

Nurse Visionaries

Recognized nurse theorists whose work is relevant to community theory–based practice include Imogene King

(1981), Madeleine Leininger (1988), Betty Neuman (1982), Margaret Newman (1994), Dorothea Orem (1985), Rosemarie Parse (1987), Martha Rogers (Madrid & Barrett, 1994), Callista Roy (1982), and Jean Watson (1985). The models represented by these theorists have been discussed throughout this book. Martha Rogers and Madeleine Leininger are discussed here because they have spoken as visionaries for the future practice of nursing. Margaret Newman addresses professional responsibility, and Betty Neuman focused on community health nursing in particular. Although not a theorist, Lillian Wald is included here because of her visionary perspective on community health nursing.

Martha Rogers

Martha Rogers (1914–1994) perceived herself as a visionary for the future of nursing, and many others have agreed. The Rogerian Model for Science-Based Nursing has been discussed frequently throughout this book; the significance of her thought as a futurist is addressed here. Rogers' work speaks eloquently of the essential need for autonomous community-based nursing practice. She was particularly concerned that nursing develop and practice its own discipline rather than that of medicine. Barrett (1994) identified Rogerian themes that have set the stage for increasing professional responsibility to society. These themes, which support visions for nursing practice, education, and research addressed in this section, include: (1) nursing as a basic science of person-environment interrelationship, (2) baccalaureate education as preparation for beginning professional autonomous nursing practice, (3) increased collaborative relationships between the nurse and other health professionals, and (4) nursing services available in differing degrees of complexity to people in various life situations.

Rogers encouraged nurses to help shape the future by participating in its creation. She identified potentials for nursing and suggested possibilities from her own optimistic perspective, thus helping to shape visions for nursing and for the world. She insisted that the future demands "new visions, flexibility, curiosity, imagination, courage, risk-taking, compassion, and an excellent sense of humor" (Rogers, 1988, p. 102). Space nursing was an area of concern for her, and she encouraged nurse involvement in planning for health promotion and disease prevention as people begin to move away from the earth toward other worlds. Her futuristic ideas will undoubtedly influence nursing and nurses for many years to come.

Madeleine Leininger

Futurists predict that by the middle of the 21st century people of European descent will be a minority in the United States (Congress & Lyons, 1992). Madeleine Leininger (1991) optimistically suggests that by the year 2010, nursing will have changed from a **unicultural** (all parties sharing the same cultural beliefs, values, and health care practices) to a **multicultural** (many and diverse cultures) perspective. **Transcultural** nursing, in which more than one belief system is at work, will be highly valued as a philosophy and mode of education, research, and practice. All nurses will be expected to be transculturally focused in their work as clinicians, educators, and researchers.

Leininger anticipates a transculturally transformed nursing practice that values **human diversity,** the myriad of differences reflected in and among human beings and the human experience, as well as **universality,** the commonalities of all human beings. She encourages development of a classification system for nursing diagnosis suited to meet the needs of diverse cultural groups and useful in collaborative interdisciplinary partnerships.

Leininger insists that nursing organizations move beyond the present focus on **cultural sensitivity,** the awareness of cultural influences on health care and being respectful of differences in cultural belief systems, to in-depth cultural knowledge and competency. She expects formation of various cultural groups and institutions with particular values, beliefs, and customs. These groups will regulate and control the quality of care as governing councils provide policy. In her view, increased funding for transcultural nursing and worldwide cooperative nursing care research will become available as practice expands globally.

Margaret Newman

Margaret Newman (1994) concluded that professional responsibility within any autonomous and independent practice includes building a relationship with the client to identify health care needs and facilitate client action potential and decision-making ability. In addition, the responsibility includes communicating and collaborating with other nurses and associates in various settings. The emerging whole-person perspective of nursing requires high-level communication, cooperation, and collaboration skills. Differentiation of practice roles based on levels of preparation is required to make the most efficient use of nursing knowledge and skills.

One of many concerns regarding practice has been the wide variation in education and skills, with some nurses overextended and others underutilized. This situation exists because when hiring, health care agencies often fail to consider how levels of education affect job skills. Newman (1994) forecasts that nurses with various levels of education will be integrated in interdisciplinary settings, practicing according to their abilities and moving about the community serving their clients.

Newman sees "the nurse coming together with clients at critical choice points in their lives and participating with them in the process of expanding consciousness" (1994, p. 129). The nurse's stance in the relationship is characterized by compassion, continuity, and respect for client choice. Newman recognizes New Zealand nurse leaders who, during health care reform efforts there, introduced the concept of family nurse (FN). Family nurse practice in that country involves a professional partnership with families in crisis who do not know how to handle their situations. The FN gives support while the family assumes control over health circumstances and begins to seek and use available services.

Betty Neuman

The Neuman Systems Model was developed primarily for community health nursing and is used internationally. Primary, secondary, and tertiary levels of prevention are addressed in ways that are especially helpful to community health nursing and other health-related disciplines. The model provides a systems perspective to the understanding of person, environment, health, and nursing and addresses numerous factors related to health. Application is appropriate whether persons are sick or well and includes environmental issues and concerns (Fawcett, 1984).

Anderson and McFarlane (1996) have adapted the Neuman model to specifically guide application of the nursing process to communities in a community-as-partner model. This model guides the nursing process of community assessment, analysis, and diagnosis; community planning for primary, secondary, and tertiary prevention programs; and program evaluation. Lines of resistance and defense within the community structure reflect the community's ability to deal with stress.

The focus of this model is the aggregate, and the actual or potential ability of the community to function. The role of the nurse is to promote and protect health and act as a facilitator, catalyst, and advocate for health so that the community as a whole is able to control its response to stress. The intervention may be primary, secondary, and tertiary prevention. The intended consequences are a strengthened normal line of defense, increased resistance to stressors, and a diminished degree of reaction to stressors by the community.

Lillian Wald

Lillian Wald (Buhler-Wilkerson, 1993) was an early 20th century nurse visionary. Her stated mission for public health nursing continues to be relevant in the atmosphere of *Health for All 2000* and *Healthy People 2000*. Wald's vision of nursing practice went beyond sickness care, health education, and caring for families in their homes. It included an agenda of reform in health, industry, education, recreation, and housing in the community. She addressed individual ills within a broader context of social concern—the same vision held by today's futurists. The nursing profession has the potential to meet this vision more powerfully than ever before, but currently it has been diverted from its ideal of primary prevention to provide damage control for individuals and families already suffering from medical, psychological, and social problems (Zerwekh, 1993, p. 1676). The challenge is to address both issues at once.

Other Nurse Visionaries

Current nurse leaders with 21st-century visions of community health nursing practice, research, and education include Margretta Styles (1994), Karen Buhler-Wilkerson (1993), and Marlo Salmon (1993).

Styles (1994) points out the many efforts of nurses who are planning for the future of community health nursing in international settings. These efforts include nutrition and disease-prevention education in Mexico; counseling and teaching care and prevention to HIV/AIDS clients and families in Africa; and managing nursing employment agencies for families and institutions in Italy. In Korea, 2,000 community health posts are being staffed and managed by specially trained nurses, and in Tokyo a school of nursing has established a comprehensive system of care for the elderly. In New Zealand, hospitals are being replaced by community services where the emphasis is on primary care. In many countries throughout the world, nurses are also finding ways to provide independent and autonomous care for their clients.

Buhler-Wilkerson (1993) identifies the most successful responses by public health nurses to both public sentiment and community need:

1. Invent a diverse mix of public and private programs that respect local custom, link effectively with mainstream health care institutions, and are substitutive, additive, or complementary to community needs.

2. Counterbalance perceived costliness of community-based care by documenting cost effectiveness, benefits valued by society, patient satisfaction, and responsiveness to sponsors' pluralistic agendas.

3. Gain sufficient control over the structure and process of practice to produce the desired outcomes.

4. Place practice within systems of reimbursement that provide payment appropriate to service costs.

5. Articulate clearly the concept of comprehensive community-based nursing care, a concept that cuts across race and class and occurs at home, as an innovative and practical solution to the complex needs of vulnerable individuals and families.

6. Produce practitioners with enough training and ability to manage all the complexities of community-based care.

7. Couple preventive services with immediate health and social needs, rather than offering them in isolation.

8. Provide culturally relevant services according to local custom and linguistic preference (pp. 1784–1785).

Marlo Salmon, speaking from the Division of Nursing, U.S. Public Health Services (1993), encouraged use of nursing as the centerpiece in health departments and stated that public health nurses are generalists who build bridges between science, policy, and the people. According to Salmon, public health nurses are able to assess environmental hazards, networking with communities concerning information about hazards and health risks.

Their "assessment, communication, and management skills allow them to expand or contract their roles as needed. Nurses move easily across settings and roles; they are translators among disciplines and interpreters of and for communities" (p. 1675).

There is a great deal that nurses can do to advance the public health mission, but the broader public health community as well as the public must come to recognize that what nursing has to offer in terms of culturally appropriate preventive and primary health care is of value to society. Nursing visionaries have spoken up repeatedly but have found it difficult to mobilize institutional support in the face of a competitive medical world, disagreements over what kind of education a nurse really needs, the belief that access to more medical care will create health, prevention programs, and weakness in collective political power.

Models of Nursing Practice for the 21st Century

Several models of future community health practice have been developed. They include community-, school-, church-, and neighborhood-based centers.

Community-Based Nursing Centers

Jenkins and Sullivan-Marx (1994) suggest a model that emphasizes primary care and a partnership between nurse practitioners and community health nurses. In their model, shown in Figure 32-3 as a pyramid, consumer access to primary care nursing services in community-based settings is enhanced. Such a plan would increase community health access and provide continuity of care between levels.

The foundation of the pyramid includes basic public health functions including nursing functions. On the next level are the nursing centers, the heart of primary care delivery. Home care, partial hospitalization, and nursing home care form the next level. Medical management and acute and critical care are at the apex of the pyramid. This model joins primary care nurse practitioners and community health nurses in a partnership that forms the foundation of a coordinated, community-based health care system focused on both primary and secondary prevention.

School-Based Family Health Centers

Partnership between education and health in school-based health centers has improved children's access to health care (Biester, 1994; Passarelli, 1994; Salmon, 1994).

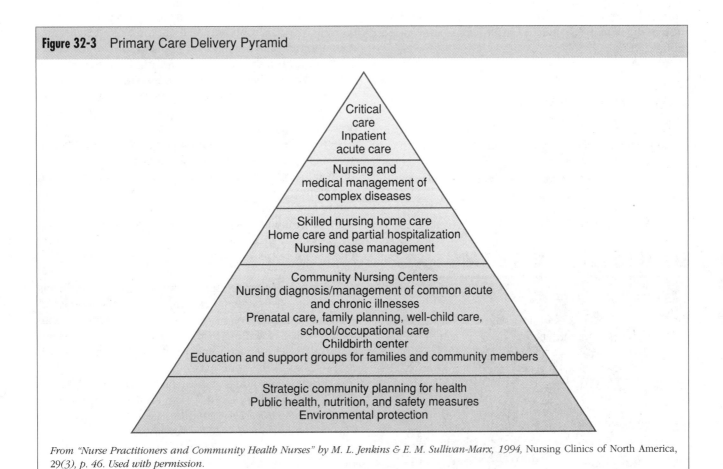

Figure 32-3 Primary Care Delivery Pyramid

Critical care
Inpatient
acute care

Nursing and
medical management of
complex diseases

Skilled nursing home care
Home care and partial hospitalization
Nursing case management

Community Nursing Centers
Nursing diagnosis/management of common acute
and chronic illnesses
Prenatal care, family planning, well-child care,
school/occupational care
Childbirth center
Education and support groups for families and community members

Strategic community planning for health
Public health, nutrition, and safety measures
Environmental protection

From "Nurse Practitioners and Community Health Nurses" by M. L. Jenkins & E. M. Sullivan-Marx, 1994, Nursing Clinics of North America, *29(3), p. 46. Used with permission.*

One model still in the early stages of development is the family health center, located at or near schools. This model is designed to deliver easily accessible, family-focused, primary health care that is linked with other community health care delivery systems (Passarelli, 1994).

Health Ministries

With the shift toward community-based care, one important recent trend is the development of health ministries and **parish nursing,** in which a nurse provides services to the members of church or religious group, in partnership with health care systems. In the late 1970s, the Rev. Granger Westberg, a Lutheran clergyman and medical school professor at the University of Illinois, founded the health ministries model, seeking to develop partnerships between consumers, clergy, and health care professionals. Since the early 1980s, nurses and religious congregations throughout the United States have begun using health ministries to bring health care to communities. In 1996 it was estimated that there were 4,000 parish nurse programs in the United States. Canada and Australia are also developing such programs (Peacock, 1996).

The purpose of health ministries is to promote health and wellness, with a focus on expanding knowledge about whole-person wellness and increasing access to health resources. As the U.S. government reduces its role in public health and social services, health ministries address health education, health assessment, and health promotion activities, such as health fairs and support groups.

Neighborhood Nursing

Zerwekh (1993) proposes neighborhood-oriented nursing as the practice structure for the future. Present health care delivery problems include failure to manage a person's safe passage through the system. Neighborhood-oriented

nursing would provide broad-based case management and care coordination within neighborhoods or rural regions. In such a setting, care of the individual would be determined by knowledge of community needs, and care of the community by knowledge of the people as individuals. The neighborhood nurse would be a generalist responsible for a neighborhood or region. Trusting relationships would be developed so that the nurse, as the ultimate case manager, would know both the people needing services and the community resources available. This neighborhood nurse would work in partnership with social agencies and health professionals as well as community health assistants who could do a variety of tasks, according to their skill levels. Tasks would range from cooking, cleaning, and personal care to advocacy and health education.

Provision of these personal services would promote family self-care and offer a humane approach to prevention of the problems that result in extraordinary social and economic costs for emergency care, intensive care, lifelong special education, and penitentiaries for people who could have been helped by early intervention (Zerwekh, 1993, p. 1678).

Issues for Community Health Nursing in the 21st Century

Hopes were high in 1993 when national health care reform seemed to be a strong possibility in the United States and community health nursing had so much to offer the country. Political forces against such reform however, proved to be stronger than the efforts being made to support changes. Health care reform continues to occur, though in small increments without overall planning for what would best serve the populace.

Regardless of the disappointments, community health nursing continues to evolve. In response to expanding knowledge related to health and healing, changing health care delivery systems, and changing gender roles and influences, nursing in general is being transformed in some fundamental ways. Expansion of knowledge related to health and healing is not only advancing biomedical technology but is also clarifying the value of alternative and complementary therapies that enhance natural healing processes. Another area of knowledge expansion is the human-environment relationship and the impact of environmental disruption on human health. The emphasis in nursing is shifting from highly technical acute care in hospital settings to home health and primary health care settings in the community.

Although community health nursing currently serves individuals, families, groups, communities, and populations, the health nurse of the future will work in partnership with other nurse specialists who may also work in a variety of community settings, focusing their work on individuals and families according to the expertise needed in a particular situation.

DECISION MAKING

Community-Based Nursing Centers

• Imagine that you are participating in the development of a community-based nursing center. What would you need to consider in relation to planning for the creation of such a center?

• What approaches would you use to encourage community residents and leaders to participate in the planning process?

• How would you evaluate the effectiveness of your planning process and the effectiveness of the center?

The Ethics of Individual Responsibility versus Social Responsibility

Increasing knowledge of the relationship between health behavior and health status is beginning to present ethical questions related to funding for care of persons whose behaviors, contributed to their illness. Some maintain that it is appropriate to hold each person or family (depending on the culture) responsible for causing their own illness by practicing certain destructive behaviors. Others take the position that the environment and those who make decisions about the environment are responsible.

The position stressing individual responsibility is consistent with the position taken in Chapter 5 that, as individual consciousness expands, there is an increased sense of responsibility not only for oneself but also for the total environment. Individuals vary in their ability to create or contribute to the creation of healthy environments. Many environmental qualities can be changed by a group effort, but a group is made up of individuals, each taking social responsibility to prevent or solve a problem.

Alternative and Complementary Care Therapies in Nursing

In 1983, Rogers addressed the public demand for freedom of choice, informed consent, and health provider and health service alternatives. She anticipated the creation of independent nursing practice, autonomous nursing, and autonomous birthing centers, because she believed that such nursing services would accommodate a strong societal emphasis on health promotion. She also expected that the future would bring a predominance of noninvasive and meditative modalities. One example of these modalities is Therapeutic Touch, which is a holistic therapy involving consciously directed manipulation of energy in which the

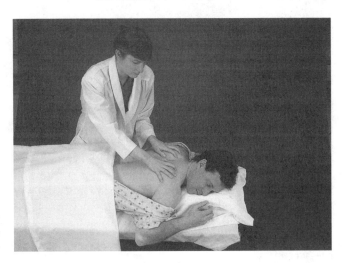

Therapeutic massage is an example of a noninvasive modality.

practitioner uses the hands to facilitate the healing process. Another example is interactive guided imagery, a technique in which the health care provider gives support and structure while the client explores images and their meanings arising from within (see Chapter 6).

New types of interventions to promote health and healing are emerging in the Western world. Many have come from other cultures in which these therapies have been used for centuries to balance and harmonize energy patterns (see Chapter 6). Increasing the routine use of non-invasive alternative and complementary care therapies supported by research is anticipated (Belmont Vision Project, 1995; Hancock & Garrett, 1995). With increasing knowledge of psychoneuroimmunology, there may be a greater emphasis in nursing on helping people alter personal health behaviors, especially those related to sleeping, eating, exercise, addiction, and coping with stress. Health counseling and education for individuals, families, and groups will be a major role for nurses in the delivery of primary health care services.

Bulechek and McCloskey (1992) used Rogerian theory to support using specific interventions as treatment for identified nursing diagnoses. For example, interventions listed with the diagnosis of anxiety are "active listening, assertiveness training, discharge planning, music therapy, presence, relaxation training . . . , support groups, truth telling and Therapeutic Touch" (p. 402). These therapies may now be used in autonomous nursing practice to promote health and healing by nurses with training in specific modalities.

The Mutual Connectedness Model was an outcome of the study presented as the Research Focus (see also Chapter 8). A nonprofit organization was created to implement and test Schubert and Lionberger's Mutual Connectedness model. An educational program offers university extension units and continuing education units for nurses. Nursing students at a nearby university are invited to participate in activities and internships. Graduate students' research projects concerning healing are supported and

---

⊘⊘ REFLECTIVE THINKING ⊘⊘

Who Is Responsible?

You are 45 years of age and have been diagnosed with cancer of the lung. You have smoked a pack of cigarettes a day for many years and started smoking at 13 years of age. What is the responsibility of society at large for this problem? Of the government? The tobacco companies? Your parents? Your children? You?

Now assume that you are a person who is strong and healthy. You may or may not be a health professional. You become aware of the high incidence of breast cancer in your area. What is your responsibility as part of society for this problem? What is the responsibility of the government? Of companies that feel threatened by environmentalist attacks concerning the release of carcinogens in the environment? Of your children?

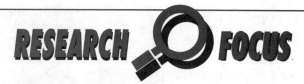

Mutual Connectedness: A Study of Client–Nurse Interaction Using the Grounded Theory Method

STUDY PROBLEM/PURPOSE

To examine theory-based nursing practice in a private community nursing practice setting. To gain knowledge of the client experience in such a relationship (presented in Chapter 8).

METHODS

Twelve nurses in private practice within the greater San Francisco Bay Area were interviewed one time each to determine the nature of their practices and their beliefs about human beings, environment, health, and nursing. Eighteen of the nurses' clients were then interviewed three times each over the course of the first three months of their experiences with the nurses. The clients received all their medical care from physicians in addition to the nursing therapy.

Interview data were analyzed using the Grounded Theory Method. The nurses used touch therapies (Therapeutic Touch, Jin Shin Jyutsu®; acupressure, a system of applying pressure with the thumbs to acupoints along the meridians; and massage), interactive guided imagery, counseling (listening), and teaching (sharing of knowledge).

FINDINGS

Both nurses and clients described relationships of caring experienced as connecting and bonding. Nursing therapies were carried out within the relationship bond. The data yielded the Mutual Connectedness Model of client–nurse interaction presented in Chapter 8.

A picture of theory-based nursing practice in private settings emerged as follows. The nurses ranged in age from 31 to 65 years and had 10 to 43 years of nursing experience. Most had worked in a variety of hospital and community settings. They had been or were currently administrators or instructors in universities, colleges, or continuing education programs. Two were working in hospitals as staff nurses.

The nurses assumed a variety of roles in their practices ranging from using touch therapies and guided imagery with individuals; teaching family members self-help interventions; counseling individuals, families, and groups; teaching individuals and groups in various settings; holding neighborhood social events; and serving on various community health planning boards. Some of these nurses saw their homes or businesses as neighborhood health centers within their communities.

The nurses' beliefs about health, person, and environment were synchronistic with those expressed by Martha Rogers and Margaret Newman. Figure 32-4 depicts the configuration of the nurse–client relationship as derived from the data from study participants. The nurses expressed their commitment to this type of practice, saying it was consistent with their beliefs about nursing and about themselves as nurses. Several nurses identified having had a serious health problem that influenced their search for a better way to work with their own health and that of others.

IMPLICATIONS

These nurses and their neighborhood centers served as exemplars for nursing-theory–based practice: autonomous and independent clinical practice based on caring relationships and the use of nursing therapies to promote health and facilitate healing. Clients reported, in addition to relief of symptoms, an increasing sense of wholeness, harmony, and balance in their lives. These feelings were experienced as transformational in their lives.

SOURCE

"Mutual Connectedness: A Study of Client–Nurse Interaction Using the Grounded Theory Method" by P. Schubert & H. Lionberger, 1995, Journal of Holistic Nursing, 13(2), pp. 102–116.

encouraged. Weekly free Therapeutic Touch and Jin Shin Jyutsu® clinics are open to the community.

The activities at the non-profit organization occur at a facility where nurse entrepreneurs as sole proprietors also provide services for a set fee or on a sliding scale. Clients from all walks of life utilize health promotion, health maintenance, and disease prevention services. Most come for healing of long-standing chronic conditions. Interventions include health counseling and teaching, touch therapies, and imagery for individuals, couples, families, and groups. This organization represents efforts by nurses to build partnerships with a community and to test a nursing practice model using therapies that promote health and healing.

Research in Community Health Nursing for the 21st Century

For Schoenhofer (1993) the question of what constitutes **nursing research,** or the development of nursing scien-

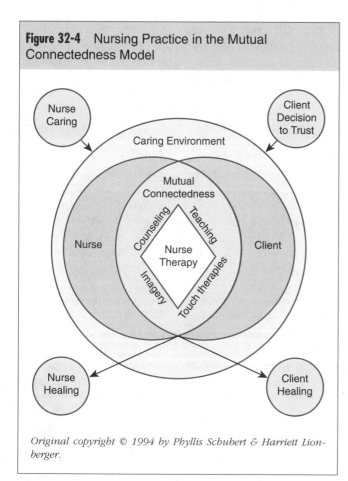

Figure 32-4 Nursing Practice in the Mutual Connectedness Model

Original copyright © 1994 by Phyllis Schubert & Harriett Lionberger.

environment interrelationship and health. This paradigm assumes the metaphor of the living organism interconnected with its environment; that human beings are unpredictable, diverse, and complex in nature; that nature is holistic and evolutionary, so that the whole is the focus for study and that development is both **qualitative,** in which data consist of words and observations, and **quantitative,** in which the data are based on numbers (Fawcett, 1993).

Community health nursing research must address application of the nursing process to aggregates. Research must aid in the acquisition of knowledge needed for health policy development, implementation, and evaluation to improve the health of aggregates if nursing is to assume leadership in health care delivery in the 21st century. And finally, it will include ecological connections such as carcinogenic potential of pollutants in the air, water, and solid waste and interdependence of humans and the environment as a major determinant of health.

tific knowledge by conducting research studies to test theory used in nursing practice, is a core issue in nursing. The answer for Schoenhofer is that nursing research occurs when questions arise from a particular conception of nursing embedded in one of the formal general frameworks of nursing. If nursing is the promotion of health and facilitation of the healing process by providing and supporting healthy/healing environments as proposed in this text, then nursing research is the study of client experience and public health efforts related to these phenomena.

The question then arises: How does one conduct research that addresses health, healing, caring, wholeness, pattern, organization, interconnectedness, interrelatedness, and mutual process? Philosophically, the assumptions that underlie the study question must match assumptions implied in the research method. Assumptions of the traditional Western **mechanistic view,** which is the perspective that the universe is made up of parts and together these parts create a whole, are different from those of the **holistic worldview,** which is the perspective that everything in the universe is interconnected and that everything affects everything else. The holistic view, however, can be seen to transcend and include the mechanistic view as one of its parts (Wilber, 1996), clearing the way for studies combining the two.

The holistic **paradigm,** or way of perceiving the world, is more apt to lead to understanding of the person–

Methods for Nursing Research

Phillips (1994) encourages the use of methods that study wholeness in the human experience. **Basic research,** which is intended to extend the base of knowledge in a discipline for the sake of knowledge production or theory construction, related to the nature of health and healing and supportive of community nursing practice is needed. This would include creative studies of nursing interventions and health outcomes in community health nursing, health promotion, and healing. When these studies emphasize partnerships with community and other disciplines they will be particularly powerful.

Increasingly, community health nurses will be called upon to participate in collaborative research with other disciplines. Creativity is an essential need as nursing enters the new millennium and participates in a **paradigm shift,** a change of perception or worldview about the nature of reality, from a focus on disease to a view of health and wellness as wholeness, harmony, and balance. Because qualitative methods are philosophically congruent with the study of wholeness, **pattern** (ways of behaving, feeling, believing, choosing, valuing, and perceiving that form a picture of the person–environment interrelationship), and organization, new methods using qualitative data are being developed and used.

Rogers has consistently encouraged creativity in developing and using research methods. A major issue involved is attaining dynamic knowledge that evolves in relationship with environment and consciousness. Newman (1990) suggested involving practice and research in the same study. The proposed method is rooted in the mutuality of the nurse–person/researcher–participant relationship and focuses on meanings of relationship and events in the person's life. The researcher identifies patterns in the person's life and shares these in narrative form while seeking revision or confirmation. During this process both gain insight into their own patterns. Newman calls this process research-as-praxis; meanings shift, and interpretation of meanings provides the working process for both practice and research.

Leininger (1988) recommended an **ethno-nursing research** method in which the researcher obtains *meanings-in-context data* by entering the world of the people under study, gaining access to "*back-stage reality*" and becoming *a trusted friend*. Entry into the world of relationship, and resulting collections of healing stories as case studies, may enrich and strengthen the science of nursing as caring.

Watson (1985) has also stated that a variety of qualitative methods are suitable for testing her theory of human caring and for exploring meanings related to the human experience of health and healing. Research in caring involves meanings of both the person receiving care and the nurse, with the meaning of the nurse to the person a focal interest.

Community health nurses will also be expected to participate in public health outcome measurement projects. Program evaluation skills will become even more important in the future as community health nurses work in collaborative teams to determine program effectiveness.

Education for the 21st Century

The nursing leaders 20 years hence are being educated now. The need is clear for creative, caring, critical thinkers who are committed to excellence in nursing and health care.

Changes in nursing practice to meet the demands of society for the next century call for fundamental changes in education. A major challenge is the wide variance in practice roles. Systematic planning may lead to improved utilization of the various educational levels. The existence of many levels of education in the United States is a problem when there is little differentiation in the role of the nurse in different practice settings, yet it is a strength when nurses are used in a wide variety of ways in a broad range of settings (Anderson & McFarlane, 1996).

Schools of nursing and institutes are expected to become identified with cultural areas or regions serving different cultural groups. Nursing curricula will be developed by faculty with cultural expertise and community representatives who support cultural health practices.

With the trend for nurses to practice in community-based settings, nursing education is preparing nurses for community practice. Knollmueller (1994) anticipates that the student of the future will spend only one or two terms in an acute care facility for clinical practice and the rest will be in community-based settings. New graduates will be hired by community agencies because students have been prepared for that role.

Skills needed for community health nursing of the future are changing. Educators are constantly revising and updating their curricula in an attempt to meet the demands of society. Styles (1994) observed the need for courses in economics in health care to provide nurses with the tools necessary to create cost-effective care. Students must be prepared for decision making for health policy and planning responsibilities. Knollmueller (1994) argued that the skills most needed for the future are problem identification, problem solving, and the ability to connect those who can identify problems with those who can solve them. The ability to resolve conflicts and to mediate through effective communication is essential for interdisciplinary teamwork. **Critical thinking** involves consideration of all factors, such as examination of beliefs, values, and action, before decision making and is a must for nurses of the future.

Nurses in the future will also need to be knowledgeable about international health and nursings' role in global health efforts. Thinking and acting both locally and globally will be necessary in order for nurses to participate effectively in the future. Educators must be prepared to expand their knowledge of global health as well as nursings' role in international public health efforts.

Technologic Influence on Practice, Research, and Education

Technology is influenced by and, in turn, influences social change. A major change began to occur in the U.S. in the

---

ॐ REFLECTIVE THINKING ॐ

Sky Diving and the Nursing Profession

Margretta Styles, former president of the American Nurses Association and executive director of the International Council of Nurses, told a class of students that she had taken sky diving lessons the previous summer. As she was hanging onto the wing girders of the plane and deciding whether to let go or crawl back in the plane, the thought crossed her mind: "This is where nursing is—we must either jump or crawl back inside." And with that she let go.

• What do you think she meant when she said that nursing has to either "jump" or "crawl back inside"?

• What qualities do you think might be required of you to "jump" with the profession? What support might you need and from whom?

Perspectives...

Insights of a Community Health Professional

We live in an era of rapid change; an era in which change is so profound, the past is of little help in dealing with the future. Phrases used to describe this era are "continuous paradigm shifts," "the absence era, i.e., the absence of certainty, of understanding, and of predictability," "living in constant whitewater," and "non-linear dynamic systems."

In this context, there are four major change drivers that are altering the nature of health care delivery:

- Market-driven economic policy
- Technology
- Demographics
- Science

For most of the 20th century, people in the United States believed in government as a vehicle for improving the lives of citizens. For example, public schools were funded with the dream of making 12 to 14 years of education available to all. Health care programs funded with tax dollars and cost shifting from those without insurance to those with insurance were strategies accepted in an effort to make health care available to all. The government built roads and subsidized transportation. We, the public, trusted government. However, since the 1960s, values and beliefs have shifted. A new generation of leaders is influencing national and local policy. The predominant theme is that government is too large and is not to be trusted. What has emerged is a belief in the marketplace. As a consequence, the delivery of health care is influenced more by stockholders than by health care providers. The marketplace is now expected to find ways to control costs, determine utilization of health care resources, and set the standards for quality.

Technology, another change driver, is making the impossible possible. First it made it possible to save lives that otherwise would not have been saved. Then it enabled health care providers to work more effectively and efficiently. For example, using the computer to determine potential drug interactions is more effective and efficient than trying to determine the potential by reading about each individual drug. As one looks to the future, it is clear that technology will continue to transform the "what" and "how" of clinical care. Self-diagnostic tests and monitoring devices will enable individuals to have greater control over their care. Computerized databases will be used to direct care with or without the involvement of a health care provider. Hospitalization will be rare and used only when an acute episode of a curable condition has occurred. People will die under hospice care. People will live with community-based preventive services.

The population of the United States is becoming more and more heterogeneous in terms of race, culture, and ethnicity. Changing demographics is a major change driver for health care because the impact influences all of our social institutions. The population of the oldest old, those over 85, will increase most dramatically. Currently, Hawaii is the only state where non-Hispanic Caucasians are in the minority. In the near future, non-Hispanic Caucasians will also be in the majority in New Mexico, Texas, California, and possibly Florida. Between 1980 and 1992, the total U.S. population grew by 13%, but the Hispanic population increased by 65% and the Asian and Pacific Islander population doubled. The average household size is decreasing, and the number of husband–wife households is also decreasing. The impact of these changing demographics is seen in many ways, from the development of retirement communities, to specialized grocery stores, to the demand for alternatives to Western medicine. Health care providers can no longer assume there is a dominant set of values and beliefs about health care. Scientific developments are occurring so rapidly they are taken as normal. But even 10 years ago, who would have thought that cloning was on the horizon? In the near future, scientific advances in genetics will have a great impact on health care. Individuals will be able to know the likelihood of developing a genetically based disease. Treatment programs can be based on an analysis of an individual's genetic makeup. The origin of currently poorly understood diseases will be discovered. As a result, morbidity will be compressed; that is, chronic illnesses will occur later in life and quality of living will be improved.

For community-based health care providers the future offers unlimited possibilities. The key to success is the willingness to give up notions of control and predictability and enjoy change and ambiguity. It is indeed a new world.

—*Carol A. Lindeman, PhD, RN, FAAN*

COMMUNITY NURSING VIEW

A Contemporary and Visionary Approach to Community Health Nursing

Currently, nurses are experimenting with various visionary approaches to community health nursing services. One example may be found in a nonprofit urban community health center in Portland, Oregon, run by and for Native Americans. The purpose of this health patterning center is to empower people to achieve maximum well-being and harmony in their lives. The identified goal for the center is to "create a diverse and evolving healing environment that helps individuals, families, and the community repattern their lives in healthy ways" (Barrington, 1995). Assumptions from conceptual frameworks of nursing, specifically those of Rogers (1994), Newman (1994), Roach (1991), and Leininger (1991), provide the foundation for the focus of clinic structure and activities. Theoretical assumptions from the work of the mentioned theorists provide the framework for the services offered (Barrington, 1995):

- People are irreducible wholes of open, resonating energy fields, engaging in continuous mutual process with environmental energy fields, with integration and evolution of the person–environment relationship.
- Health, as a process of wholeness, is personally, culturally, spiritually, and socially defined.
- Nurses engage in conscious therapeutic use of self, mobilizing client healing patterns to facilitate achievement of the greatest health potential.
- Caring is a dominant theme of nursing practice, expressed as the nurse's commitment, competence, confidence, conscious intention, and compassion.
- Nursing is engaged in the care of people within environments where there is increasing diversity and complexity, while using nursing arts and science based on nursing theory and research.

These basic assumptions of nursing resonate with traditional Native American spiritual and cultural beliefs.

The community center is staffed by two nurses (a master's-prepared adult nurse practitioner, who serves as director and a community health nurse), a part-time psychiatrist, a family practice physician, a social worker, and office staff. Although the health center is 70% funded by the Indian Health Service, a governmental agency, the nurse practitioner position is funded by the Center for Substance Abuse Treatment to link primary care and treatment of addiction. A program based in concepts of primary and secondary prevention activities designed to prevent addiction or relapse in this high-risk population is provided.

Prior to the hiring of the nurse practitioner, the clinic had functioned as a medically oriented, disease-focused center for urgent care, with diagnosis, treatment, and referral services for the population. The physical environment was described by the nurses as lifeless, stark, and dingy. Attendance was poor, and people tended not to follow through with recommended return visits or to show up for appointments. Word of mouth in the Native American community was that services at the clinic were poor and did not reflect caring. It was considered a place of last resort by much of the community.

The nurses and clients repatterned the environment by making it beautiful. They redecorated and furnished the center in ways that reflect the spiritual and cultural beliefs and the heritage of the people by using Native American art, music, love of nature, and crystals used in traditional healing practices.

The organizational structure of the center has also been repatterned. The top-down management style has been replaced with a leadership circle in keeping with Native tradition and belief. The belief is that each person's input is necessary for building the organization. All people of the tribe are seen as valuable to the whole. The staff has been retrained to work in cooperation and mutual processing styles with each other. Workers are selected whose concepts of spirituality and healing, health, and harmony are consistent with the beliefs of the population served and are reflected in the tenets of the community health center.

Job descriptions for the nurses include health education for groups, schools, families, and individuals and immunizations outreach into the community. Responsibilities of the

Continued

COMMUNITY NURSING VIEW

(Continued)

nurses include triage, phone and walk-in health advising, teaching, crisis counseling, direct primary care, independent RN practices, administrative duties, program development and implementation, community education, speaking to community groups, networking and teaching in the medical/health care community, and writing newspaper articles. The master's-prepared nurse has additional responsibilities as an independent nurse practitioner, leader, and mentor.

The health education program is based in culturally specific content and traditional practices such as healing circles and cradleboard-making classes. The nurse practitioner provides healing therapies, such as Therapeutic Touch, and also medically related services of diagnosis and prescriptive drug treatment. (In Oregon, nurse practitioners have independent practice and prescriptive drug privileges.)

There has also been a repatterning of services to include Native American cultural healing practices used at the health center by the **multidisciplinary** team, which consists of people from many different professional disciplines, or branches of learning. For example, the social worker now uses guided imagery and dream work; the nurse educator incorporates traditional Native American foods into her dietary counseling; and the nurses use Therapeutic Touch, which is considered a primary therapy for the clients. The time allotted for health care visits has been extended; the nurses believe that a visit with one person affects at least 50 other family and community members.

The culture-specific program planning led to creation of weekly healing circles for women of all ages. The purpose of the groups is to promote individual health of the women as well as the families and communities they represent and serve. Mutually agreed upon topics are discussed by participants in the nurse-guided healing circles. The women share stories, prose, and poetry while reminiscing about days on the reservations.

The "seven generation prenatal linkage program" designed by Barrington (1995) uses contemporary Rogerian nursing theory as implemented in Barrett's (1990) Power Model for Practice. In this model, power is reflected in awareness, choices, freedom to act intentionally, and involvement in creating changes. The seven-generation concept is presented through the cradleboard-making class for women of all ages, which is taught by an elder. In this class, the nurse practitioner provides contemporary prenatal and infant care education, while the native elder brings forth the wisdom of the grandmother in child-rearing through story and song. Thus, cultural belief systems and practices are used to strengthen personal power, a powerful determinant of health status. Clients are taught the pride of seven generations in the past and seven generations into the future. Adoption and foster parenting often alter the concept of seven generations past, but the nurse asks that mothers commit not only to the children they are carrying in their wombs but also to the children born to those children, and all children born for seven generations in the future. The commitment requested is that all will know who they are, what they stand for, and that all will be proud and strong. This program includes the idea that prenatal care begins at puberty, with preconception education for both boys and girls.

Home visits are not a part of the program, although some are made when deemed appropriate or necessary. The nurses schedule family visits at the health center, and families are invited to attend the healing circles, cradleboard classes, and health talks. Attendance at powwows, spiritual gatherings, and funerals is an ongoing part of the work with families.

Linkage of services is a major focus of the nurse practitioner's work in this health center. A community partnership network serving on behalf of the client population includes the following organizations: Northwest Portland Indian Health Board, Women's Wellness Coalition (40 tribes in the Northwest), Oregon Breast and Cervical Cancer Coalition, Indian Health Service/University of Oklahoma Wellness Programs, county drug and alcohol rehabilitation programs, city and county family violence network, University of Portland (nursing preceptor), all major hospitals, physician groups, childbirth educators, nurse

Continued

COMMUNITY NURSING VIEW

(Continued)

practitioner and midwife groups, and the American Cancer Society.

Evaluation outcomes have indicated: (a) decreased hospital utilization for crisis care, (b) decreased prescription budget expenditures, (c) increased utilization of preventive health care, (d) prolonged abstinence in recovering addicts, (e) client expression of improved well-being, expanded support systems, and empowerment, and (f) increased trust of health care providers and practices reflected in self-disclosure with care providers, increased follow-up after treatment, and increased attendance at the center and participation in activities.

The community health center has become highly visible in the community and is known for:

- Culturally specific primary care providers
- Excellence in women's health care
- Co-management of prenatal care with obstetric-gynecologic services
- Incorporating Therapeutic Touch with primary care
- Offering a practice opportunity for BSN and nurse practitioner students
- Application of Rogerian Science in grassroots nursing practice

Nursing Considerations

Consider the nursing process as you address the following questions with fellow student or colleague:

ASSESSMENT
- What methods for pattern appraisal could be used in this setting?

DIAGNOSIS
- How would you address nursing diagnoses in this setting?

OUTCOME IDENTIFICATION
- In what way would you carry out the task of outcome identification, so that the process would harmonize with the philosophical perspective of Rogerian theory?

PLANNING/INTERVENTIONS
- What approach would you use for planning with individuals, families, health care workers in the community, staff, and community groups?
- What interventions would you support in a health center for those of a culture different from your own?

EVALUATION
- How would you evaluate health outcomes for clients? For the community? For the health center?

1980s when advanced biomedical technology was introduced in the care of clients in the home. Nurses from home health care agencies were expected to provide services to clients who required intravenous therapy, total parenteral nutrition, ventilator care, and intensive wound care. These skills are technical in nature and require expert clinical judgment in a complex environment. In addition to changing biomedical technological skills, technology is advancing rapidly in all areas of nursing—practice, research, and education. Styles (1994) anticipates significant changes in nursing practice as computer-based client records provide data about persons from birth to death. With these technologies and the focus moving from illness to wellness, nurses will be expected to be increasingly productive, responsible, and accountable for care.

Creativity in the development of technological tools is rapidly increasing the diversity and complexity of research methods, both qualitative and quantitative. Efficiency and creativity in the use of computer systems increase the possibility of combining research and practice in building nursing science.

Computers and telecommunications systems are increasing the possibilities for basic and continuing education in nursing as well as the means for providing health education through media in the home and community. Advancement of technology also requires that the nurse keep abreast of new technologies as they develop (Styles, 1994). The complexity of these changes forces the nurse to expand in global consciousness yet stay focused in the present situation (see Chapter 5).

SHARED VISIONS OF THE FUTURE

Nursing is challenged to form a wide variety of partnerships to meet the health care needs of people—regionally, nationally, and globally. As Grace (1995) points out, "the challenge is not only that of building infrastructures to support appropriate and quality nursing education and practice, but to provide leadership to other health professionals, including medicine, and to a wide array of workers at the community level" (p. 172).

If nurses step forward to meet the challenge of bringing about *Health for All* and work together with consumers and others to have their voices heard, improvement of the health of peoples around the world can become a reality. Changing the ways in which we deliver health care is a long-term process and certainly will not be fully realized by the year 2000. As we strive to achieve these visions, however, we are participating in the global movement to improve quality of life for the world.

≋ Key Concepts

- Future health studies encourage proactive efforts to shape a stronger health-promotion and disease-prevention focus to achieve health for the world.
- International, national, and community health care planning and strategy are moving the focus in health care from disease to health promotion and disease prevention.
- Intersectoral partnerships among leaders of environmental, social, economic, and health disciplines are required if there is to be health for all.
- Socioeconomic realities and increasing knowledge related to the human-environment interrelationship and health are among the forces of change driving the need for increased community health nursing knowledge and skills.
- Nursing and interdisciplinary partnerships in community-based services are being planned to increase utilization of nursing knowledge, skills, and resources.
- Nurse theorists and visionaries encourage that nursing centers be based on nursing's theoretical frameworks rather than on the medical model.
- Nursing theory–based community centers are being developed in which community health nurses can serve their communities in ways long imagined by visionary nurse clinicians, theorists, and educators.

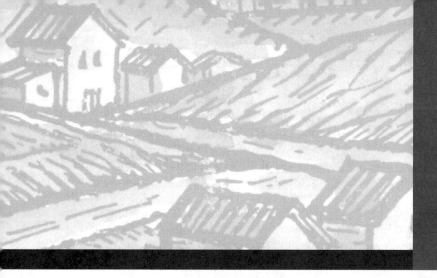

APPENDIX A
Healthy People 2000: Priorities and Objectives (1995)*

The Healthy People 2000 project identifies 22 priority areas to meet the goals of health promotion, health protection, and preventive services. Specific objectives for each priority area are listed here along with quantitative indicators that were determined for the mid-1990s. These percentages reflect movement toward or away from predetermined goals set at the beginning of the 1990s for the year 2000. Baseline data for these objectives are not included here but are included in the *Healthy People 2000: Midcourse Review and 1995 Revisions*, which is the source of this material. Graphs accompany the discussion of the 22 priorities to illustrate the status of the objectives.

PHYSICAL ACTIVITY AND FITNESS

Physical activity and fitness constitute one of 22 priority areas in Healthy People 2000: National Health Promotion and Disease Prevention Objectives. The lead agency for coordinating achievement of the 12 health-promotion objectives in this priority is the President's Council on Physical Fitness and Sports.

Health Status Objectives

1.1 Reduce coronary heart disease deaths to no more than 100 per 100,000 people.

1.2 Reduce overweight to a prevalence of no more than 20 percent among people aged 20 and older and no more than 15 percent among adolescents aged 12 to 19.

*From *Healthy People 2000: Midcourse Review and 1995 Revisions* by U.S. Department of Health and Human Services, 1996, Sudbury, MA: Jones & Bartlett. Copyright 1996 by Jones & Bartlett. Reprinted with permission.

Risk Reduction Objectives

1.3 Increase to at least 30 percent the proportion of people aged 6 and older who engage regularly, preferably daily, in light to moderate physical activity for at least 30 minutes per day.

1.4 Increase to at least 20 percent the proportion of people aged 18 and older and to at least 75 percent the proportion of children and adolescents aged 6 to 17 who engage in vigorous physical activity that promotes the development and maintenance of cardiorespiratory fitness 3 or more days per week for 20 or more minutes per occasion.

1.5 Reduce to no more than 15 percent the proportion of people aged 6 or older who engage in no leisure-time physical activity.

1.6 Increase to at least 40 percent the proportion of people aged 6 and older who regularly perform physical activities that enhance and maintain muscular strength, muscular endurance, and flexibility.

1.7 Increase to at least 50 percent the proportion of overweight people aged 12 and older who have adopted sound dietary practices combined with regular physical activity to attain an appropriate body weight.

Services and Protection Objectives

1.8 Increase to at least 50 percent the proportion of children and adolescents in 1st to 12th grades who participate in daily school physical education.

1.9 Increase to at least 50 percent the proportion of school physical education class time that students spend being physically active, preferably engaged in lifetime physical activities.

1.10 Increase the proportion of worksites offering employer-sponsored physical activity and fitness programs.

1.11 Increase community availability and accessibility of physical activity and fitness facilities.

1.12 Increase to at least 50 percent the proportion of primary care providers who routinely assess and counsel their patients regarding the frequency, duration, type, and intensity of each patient's physical activity practices.

Health Status Objective (*Added in 1995*)

1.13 Reduce to no more than 90 per 1,000 people the proportion of all people aged 65 and older who have difficulty in performing two or more personal care activities, thereby preserving independence.

NUTRITION

The lead agencies for coordinating achievement of the 27 nutrition objectives are the Food and Drug Administration and the National Institutes of Health.

Health Status Objectives

2.1 Reduce coronary heart disease deaths to no more than 100 per 100,000 people.

2.2 Reverse the rise in cancer deaths to achieve a rate of no more than 130 per 100,000 people.

2.3 Reduce overweight to a prevalence of no more than 20 percent among people aged 20 and older and no more than 15 percent among adolescents aged 12 to 19.

2.4 Reduce growth retardation among low-income children aged 5 and younger to less than 10 percent.

Risk Reduction Objectives

2.5 Reduce dietary fat intake to an average of 30 percent of calories or less and average saturated fat intake to less than 10 percent of calories among people aged 2 and older. In addition, increase to at least 50 percent the proportion of people aged 2 and older who meet the *Dietary Guidelines'* average daily goal of no more than 30 percent of calories from fat, and increase to at least 50 percent the proportion of people aged 2 and older who meet the average daily goal of less than 10 percent of calories from saturated fat.

2.6 Increase complex carbohydrate and fiber-containing foods in the diets of people aged 2 and older to an average of five or more daily servings for vegetables (including legumes) and fruits and to an average of six or more daily servings for grain products. In addition, increase to at least 50 percent the proportion of people aged 2 and older who meet the *Dietary Guidelines'* average daily goal of 5 or more servings of vegetables and fruits, and increase to at least 50 percent the proportion who meet the goal of six or more servings of grain products.

2.7 Increase to at least 50 percent the proportion of overweight people aged 12 and older who have adopted sound dietary practices combined with regular physical activity to attain an appropriate body weight.

2.8 Increase calcium intake so at least 50 percent of people aged 11 to 24 and 50 percent of pregnant and lactating women consume an average of three

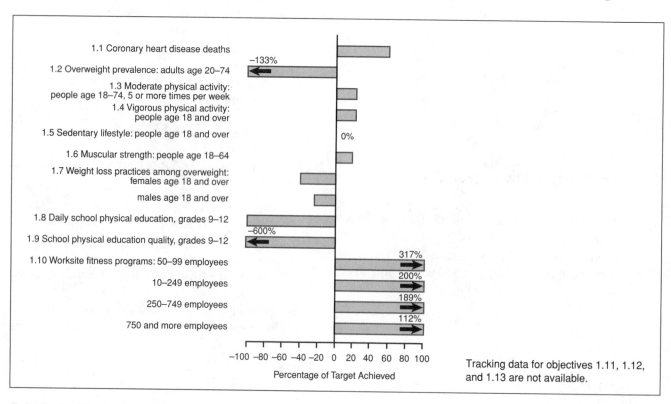

Tracking data for objectives 1.11, 1.12, and 1.13 are not available.

Priority 1—Physical Activity and Fitness; Lead Agency: President's Council on Physical Fitness and Sports

or more daily servings of foods rich in calcium, and at least 75 percent of children aged 2 to 10 and 50 percent of people aged 25 and older consume an average of two or more servings daily.

2.9 Decrease salt and sodium intake so at least 65 percent of home meal preparers prepare foods without adding salt, at least 80 percent of people avoid using salt at the table, and at least 40 percent of adults regularly purchase foods modified or lower in sodium.

2.10 Reduce iron deficiency to less than 3 percent among children aged 1 to 4 and among women of childbearing age.

2.11 Increase to at least 75 percent the proportion of mothers who breastfeed their babies in the early postpartum period and to at least 50 percent the proportion who continue breastfeeding until their babies are 5 to 6 months old.

2.12 Increase to at least 75 percent the proportion of parents and caregivers who use feeding practices that prevent baby bottle tooth decay.

2.13 Increase to at least 85 percent the proportion of

people aged 18 and older who use food labels to make nutritious food selections.

Services and Protection Objectives

2.14 Achieve useful and informative nutrition labeling for virtually all processed foods and at least 40 percent of ready-to-eat carry-away foods. Achieve compliance by at least 90 percent of retailers with the voluntary labeling of fresh meats, poultry, seafood, fruits, and vegetables.

2.15 Increase to at least 5,000 brand items the availability of processed food products that are reduced in fat and saturated fat.

2.16 Increase to at least 90 percent the proportion of restaurants and institutional food service operations that offer identifiable low-fat, low-calorie food choices consistent with the *Dietary Guidelines for Americans*.

2.17 Increase to at least 90 percent the proportion of school lunch and breakfast services and child care

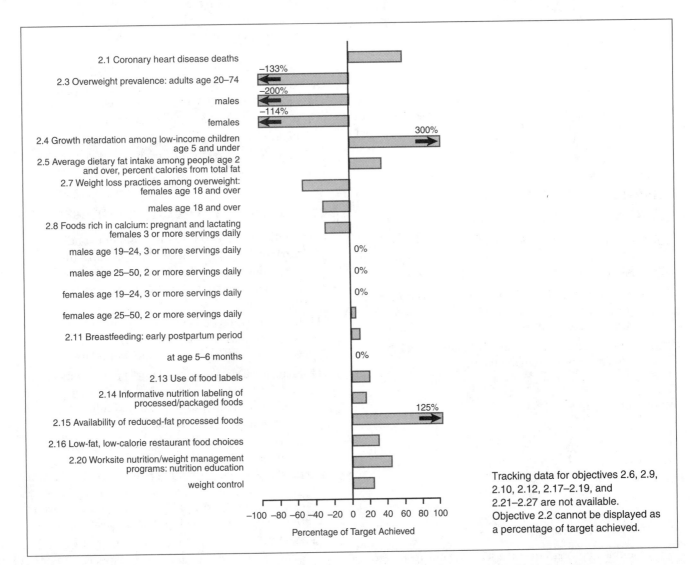

Tracking data for objectives 2.6, 2.9, 2.10, 2.12, 2.17–2.19, and 2.21–2.27 are not available. Objective 2.2 cannot be displayed as a percentage of target achieved.

Priority 2—Nutrition; Lead Agencies: National Institutes of Health and Food and Drug Administration

food services with menus that are consistent with the nutrition principles in the *Dietary Guidelines for Americans*.

2.18 Increase to at least 80 percent the receipt of home food services for people aged 65 and older who have difficulty in preparing their own meals or are otherwise in need of home-delivered meals.

2.19 Increase to at least 75 percent the proportion of the nation's schools that provide nutrition education from preschool to 12th grade, preferably as part of comprehensive school health education.

2.20 Increase to at least 50 percent the proportion of worksites with 50 or more employees that offer nutrition education and/or weight management programs for employees.

2.21 Increase to at least 75 percent the proportion of primary care providers who provide nutrition assessment and counseling and/or referral to qualified nutritionists or dietitians.

Health Status Objectives (*Added in 1995*)

2.22 Reduce stroke deaths to no more than 20 per 100,000 people.

2.23 Reduce colorectal cancer deaths to no more than 13.2 per 100,000 people.

2.24 Reduce diabetes to an incidence of no more than 2.5 per 1,000 people and a prevalence of 25 per 1,000 people.

Risk Reduction Objectives (*Added in 1995*)

2.25 Reduce the prevalence of blood cholesterol levels of 240 mg/dl or greater to no more than 20 percent among adults.

2.26 Increase to at least 50 percent the proportion of people with high blood pressure whose blood pressure is under control.

2.27 Reduce the mean serum cholesterol level among adults to no more than 200 mg/dl.

TOBACCO

The lead agency guiding the nation toward meeting the 26 tobacco objectives is the Centers for Disease Control and Prevention.

Health Status Objectives

3.1 Reduce coronary heart disease deaths to no more than 100 per 100,000 people.

3.2 Slow the rise in lung cancer deaths to achieve a rate of no more than 42 per 100,000 people.

3.3 Slow the rise in deaths for the total population from chronic obstructive pulmonary disease to achieve a rate of no more than 25 per 100,000 people.

3.4 Reduce cigarette smoking to a prevalence of no more than 15 percent among people aged 18 and older.

Risk Reduction Objectives

3.5 Reduce the initiation of cigarette smoking by children and youth so that no more than 15 percent have become regular cigarette smokers by age 20. (Baseline: 30 percent of youth had become regular cigarette smokers by ages 20 to 24 in 1987.)

3.6 Increase to at least 50 percent the proportion of cigarette smokers aged 18 and older who stopped smoking cigarettes for at least one day during the preceding year.

3.7 Increase smoking cessation during pregnancy so that at least 60 percent of women who are cigarette smokers at the time they become pregnant quit smoking early in pregnancy and maintain abstinence for the remainder of their pregnancy.

3.8 Reduce to no more than 20 percent the proportion of children aged 6 and younger who are regularly exposed to tobacco smoke at home.

3.9 Reduce smokeless tobacco use by males aged 12 to 24 to a prevalence of no more than 4 percent.

Services and Protection Objectives

3.10 Establish tobacco-free environments and include tobacco use prevention in the curricula of all elementary, middle, and secondary schools, preferably as part of comprehensive school health education.

3.11 Increase to 100 percent the proportion of worksites with a formal smoking policy that prohibits or severely restricts smoking at the workplace.

3.12 Enact in 50 states and the District of Columbia comprehensive laws on clean indoor air that prohibit smoking or limit it to separately ventilated areas in the workplace and enclosed public places.

3.13 Enact in 50 states and the District of Columbia laws prohibiting the sale and distribution of tobacco products to youth younger than age 18. Enforce these laws so that the buy rate in compliance checks conducted in all 50 states and the District of Columbia is no higher than 20 percent.

3.14 Establish in 50 states and the District of Columbia plans to reduce tobacco use, especially among youth.

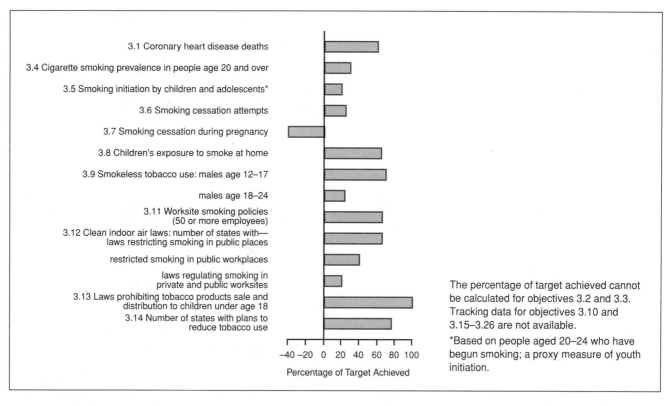

3.1 Coronary heart disease deaths
3.4 Cigarette smoking prevalence in people age 20 and over
3.5 Smoking initiation by children and adolescents*
3.6 Smoking cessation attempts
3.7 Smoking cessation during pregnancy
3.8 Children's exposure to smoke at home
3.9 Smokeless tobacco use: males age 12–17
males age 18–24
3.11 Worksite smoking policies (50 or more employees)
3.12 Clean indoor air laws: number of states with— laws restricting smoking in public places
restricted smoking in public workplaces
laws regulating smoking in private and public worksites
3.13 Laws prohibiting tobacco products sale and distribution to children under age 18
3.14 Number of states with plans to reduce tobacco use

−40 −20 0 20 40 60 80 100
Percentage of Target Achieved

The percentage of target achieved cannot be calculated for objectives 3.2 and 3.3. Tracking data for objectives 3.10 and 3.15–3.26 are not available.

*Based on people aged 20–24 who have begun smoking; a proxy measure of youth initiation.

Priority 3—Tobacco; Lead Agency: Centers for Disease Control and Prevention

3.15 Eliminate or severely restrict all forms of tobacco product advertising and promotion to which youth younger than age 18 are likely to be exposed.

3.16 Increase to at least 75 percent the proportion of primary care and oral health care providers who routinely advise cessation and provide assistance and follow-up for all of their tobacco-using patients.

Health Status Objectives (*Added in 1995*)

3.17 Reduce deaths due to cancer of the oral cavity and pharynx to no more than 10.5 per 100,000 men aged 45 to 74 and 4.1 per 100,000 women aged 45 to 74.

3.18 Reduce stroke deaths to no more than 20 per 100,000 people.

Risk Reduction Objectives (*Added in 1995*)

3.19 Increase by at least 1 year the average age of first use of cigarettes, alcohol, and marijuana by adolescents aged 12 to 17.

3.20 Reduce the proportion of young people who have used alcohol, marijuana, cocaine, or cigarettes in the past month. (Target percentages vary with age and substance.)

3.21 Increase the proportion of high school seniors who perceive social disapproval of heavy use of alcohol (70%), occasional use of marijuana (85%), and experimentation with cocaine (95%), or regular use of cigarettes (95%).

3.22 Increase the proportion of high school seniors who associate physical or psychological harm with heavy use of alcohol (70%), occasional use of marijuana (90%), and experimentation with cocaine (80%), or regular use of tobacco (95%).

Services and Protection Objectives

3.23 Increase the average (state and federal combined) tobacco excise tax to at least 50 percent of the average retail price of all cigarettes and smokeless tobacco.

3.24 Increase to 100 percent the proportion of health plans that offer treatment of nicotine addiction (e.g., tobacco use cessation counseling by health care providers, tobacco use cessation classes, prescriptions for nicotine replacement therapies, and/or other cessation services).

3.25 Reduce to zero the number of states that have clean indoor air laws preempting stronger clean indoor air laws on the local level.

3.26 Enact in 50 states and the District of Columbia laws banning cigarette vending machines except in places inaccessible to minors.

SUBSTANCE ABUSE: ALCOHOL AND OTHER DRUGS

The Substance Abuse and Mental Health Services Administration is the agency identified to lead the nation in meeting the 20 objectives related to substance abuse.

Health Status Objectives

4.1   Reduce deaths caused by alcohol-related motor vehicle crashes to no more than 5.5 per 100,000 people.

4.2   Reduce cirrhosis deaths to no more than 6 per 100,000 people.

4.3   Reduce drug-related deaths to no more than 3 per 100,000 people.

4.4   Reduce drug abuse-related hospital emergency department visits by at least 20 percent.

Risk Reduction Objectives

4.5   Increase by at least 1 year the average age of first use of cigarettes, alcohol, and marijuana by adolescents aged 12 to 17.

4.6   Reduce the proportion of young people who have used alcohol, marijuana, cocaine, or cigarettes in the past month. (Target percentages by age group and by substance.)

4.7   Reduce the proportion of high school seniors and college students engaging in recent occasions of heavy drinking of alcoholic beverages to no more

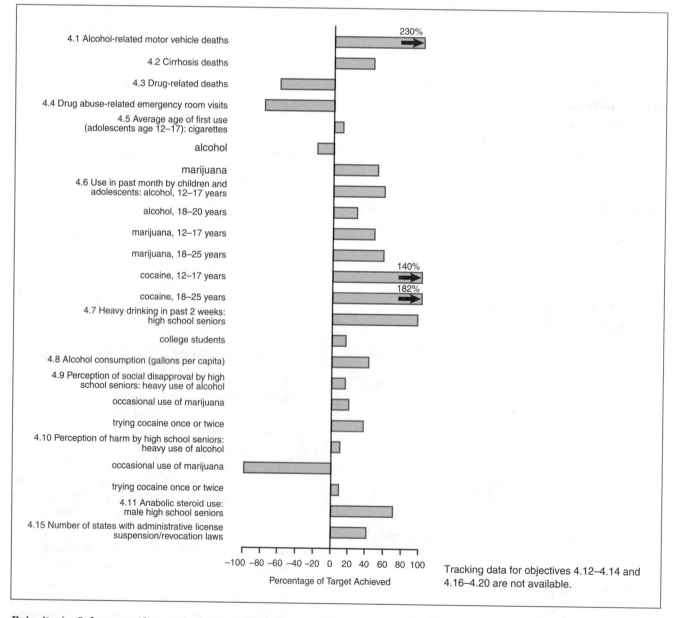

Priority 4—Substance Abuse: Alcohol and Other Drugs; Lead Agency: Substance Abuse and Mental Health Services Administration

than 28 percent of high school seniors and 32 percent of college students.

4.8   Reduce alcohol consumption by people aged 14 and older to an annual average of no more than 2 gallons of ethanol per person.

4.9   Increase the proportion of high school seniors who perceive social disapproval of heavy use of alcohol (70%), occasional use of marijuana (85%), and experimentation with cocaine (95%), or regular use of tobacco (95%).

4.10   Increase the proportion of high school seniors who associate physical or psychological harm with heavy use of alcohol (70%), occasional use of marijuana (90%), and experimentation with cocaine (80%), or regular use of cigarettes (95%).

4.11   Reduce to no more than 3 percent the proportion of male high school seniors who use anabolic steroids.

Services and Protection Objectives

4.12   Establish and monitor in 50 states comprehensive plans to ensure access to alcohol and drug treatment programs for traditionally underserved people.

4.13   Provide to children in all school districts and private schools primary and secondary school educational programs on alcohol and other drugs, preferably as part of comprehensive school health education.

4.14   Extend adoption of alcohol and drug policies for the work environment to at least 60 percent of worksites with 50 or more employees.

4.15   Extend to 50 states administrative driver's license suspension/revocation laws or programs of equal effectiveness for people determined to have been driving under the influence of intoxicants.

4.16   Increase to 50 the number of states that have enacted and enforce policies, beyond those in existence in 1989, to reduce access to alcoholic beverages by minors.

4.17   Increase to at least 20 the number of states that have enacted statutes to restrict promotion of alcoholic beverages that is focused principally on young audiences.

4.18   Extend to 50 states legal blood alcohol concentration tolerance levels of 0.08 percent for motor vehicle drivers aged 21 and older and zero tolerance (0.02 percent and lower) for those younger than age 21.

4.19   Increase to at least 75 percent the proportion of primary care providers who screen for alcohol and other drug use problems and provide counseling and referral as needed.

Services and Protection Objective (*Added in 1995*)

4.20   Increase to 30 the number of states with hospitality resource panels (including representatives from state regulatory, public health, and highway safety agencies; law enforcement; insurance associations; and alcohol retail and licensed beverage associations) to ensure a process of management and server training and define standards of responsible hospitality.

FAMILY PLANNING

The Office of Population Affairs is the lead agency in meeting the 12 family planning objectives.

Health Status Objectives

5.1   Reduce pregnancies among females aged 15 to 17 to no more than 50 per 1,000 adolescents.

5.2   Reduce to no more than 30 percent the proportion of all pregnancies that are unintended.

5.3   Reduce the prevalence of infertility to no more than 6.5 percent.

Risk Reduction Objectives

5.4   Reduce the proportion of adolescents who have engaged in sexual intercourse to no more than 15 percent by age 15 and no more than 40 percent by age 17.

5.5   Increase to at least 40 percent the proportion of ever sexually active adolescents aged 17 and younger who have not had sexual intercourse during the previous 3 months.

5.6   Increase to at least 90 percent the proportion of sexually active, unmarried people aged 15 to 24 who use contraception, especially combined method contraception that both effectively prevents pregnancy and provides barrier protection against disease.

5.7   Increase the effectiveness with which family planning methods are used, as measured by a decrease to no more than 7 percent in the proportion of women experiencing pregnancy despite use of a contraceptive method.

Services and Protection Objectives

5.8   Increase to at least 85 percent the proportion of people aged 10 to 18 who have discussed human sexuality, including correct anatomical names, sexual abuse, and values surrounding sexuality, with

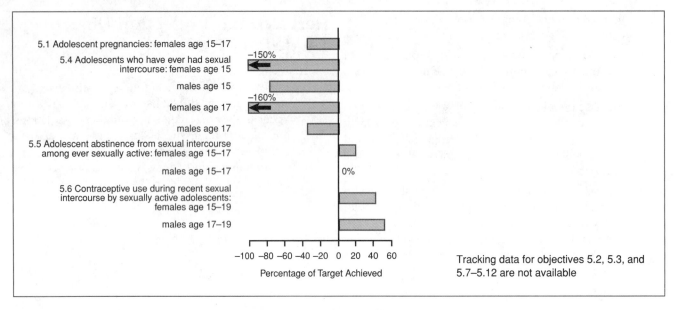

5.1 Adolescent pregnancies: females age 15–17

5.4 Adolescents who have ever had sexual intercourse: females age 15   −150%

males age 15

females age 17   −160%

males age 17

5.5 Adolescent abstinence from sexual intercourse among ever sexually active: females age 15–17

males age 15–17   0%

5.6 Contraceptive use during recent sexual intercourse by sexually active adolescents: females age 15–19

males age 17–19

−100 −80 −60 −40 −20 0 20 40 60
Percentage of Target Achieved

Tracking data for objectives 5.2, 5.3, and 5.7–5.12 are not available

Priority 5—Family Planning; Lead Agency: Office of Population Affairs

their parents and/or have received information through another parentally endorsed source, such as youth, school, or religious programs.

5.9   Increase to at least 90 percent the proportion of family planning counselors who offer accurate information about all options, including prenatal care and delivery, infant care, foster care, or adoption and pregnancy termination to their patients with unintended pregnancies.

5.10   Increase to at least 60 percent the proportion of primary care providers who provide age-appropriate preconception care and counseling.

5.11   Increase to at least 50 percent the proportion of family planning clinics, maternal and child health clinics, sexually transmitted disease clinics, tuberculosis clinics, drug treatment centers, and primary care clinics that provide on-site primary prevention and provide or refer for secondary prevention services for HIV infection and bacterial sexually transmitted diseases (gonorrhea, syphilis, and chlamydia) to high-risk individuals and their sex or needle-sharing partners.

Risk Reduction Objective

5.12   Increase to at least 95 percent the proportion of all females aged 15 to 44 at risk of unintended pregnancy who use contraception.

MENTAL HEALTH AND MENTAL DISORDERS

The Substance Abuse and Mental Health Services Administration and the National Institutes of Health are the lead agencies in meeting the 15 mental health and mental disorders objectives.

Health Status Objectives

6.1   Reduce suicides to no more than 10.5 per 100,000 people. (Target percentages vary with age and race.)

6.2   Reduce to 1.8 percent the incidence of injurious suicide attempts among adolescents aged 14 to 17.

6.3   Reduce to less than 17 percent the prevalence of mental disorders among children and adolescents.

6.4   Reduce the prevalence of mental disorders (exclusive of substance abuse) among adults living in the community to less than 10.7 percent.

6.5   Reduce to less than 35 percent the proportion of people aged 18 and older who report adverse health effects from stress within the past year.

Risk Reduction Objectives

6.6   Increase to at least 30 percent the proportion of people aged 18 and older with severe, persistent mental disorders who use community support programs.

6.7   Increase to at least 54 percent the proportion of people with major depressive disorders who obtain treatment.

6.8   Increase to at least 20 percent the proportion of people aged 18 and older who seek help in coping with personal and emotional problems.

6.9   Decrease to no more than 5 percent the proportion of people aged 18 and older who report experiencing significant levels of stress who do not take steps to reduce or control their stress.

Services and Protection Objectives

6.10   Increase to 50 the number of states with officially established protocols that engage mental health, al-

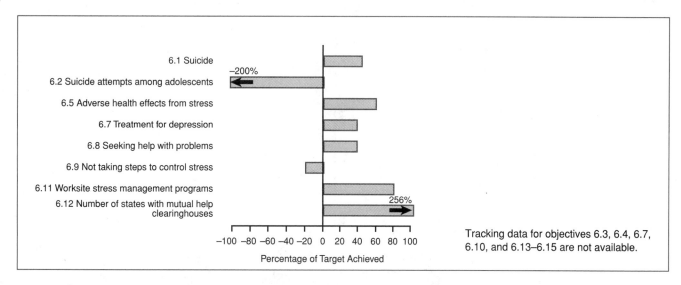

Priority 6—Mental Health and Mental Disorders; Lead Agencies: Substance Abuse and Mental Health Services Administration and National Institutes of Health

cohol and drug, and public health authorities with corrections authorities to facilitate identification and appropriate intervention to prevent suicide by jail inmates.

6.11 Increase to at least 40 percent the proportion of worksites employing 50 or more people that provide programs to reduce employee stress.

6.12 Establish a network to facilitate access to mutual self-help activities, resources, and information by people and their family members who are experiencing emotional distress resulting from mental or physical illness.

6.13 Increase to at least 60 percent the proportion of primary care providers who routinely review with patients their patients' cognitive, emotional, and behavioral functioning and the resources available to deal with any problems that are identified.

6.14 Increase to at least 75 percent the proportion of providers of primary care for children who include assessment of cognitive, emotional, and parent–child functioning, with appropriate counseling, referral, and follow-up, in their clinical practices.

Health Status Objective (*Added in 1995*)

6.15 Reduce the prevalence of depressive (affective) disorders among adults living in the community to less than 4.3 percent.

VIOLENT AND ABUSIVE BEHAVIOR

The lead agency for coordinating achievement of the 19 violent and abusive behavior objectives is the Centers for Disease Control and Prevention.

Health Status Objectives

7.1 Reduce homicides to no more than 7.2 per 100,000 people.

7.2 Reduce suicides to no more than 10.5 per 100,000 people.

7.3 Reduce firearm-related deaths to no more than 11.6 per 100,000 people from major causes.

7.4 Reverse to less than 22.6 per 1,000 children the rising incidence of maltreatment of children younger than age 18.

7.5 Reduce physical abuse directed at women by male partners to no more than 27 per 1,000 couples.

7.6 Reduce assault injuries among people aged 12 and older to no more than 8.7 per 1,000 people.

7.7 Reduce rape and attempted rape of women aged 12 and older to no more than 108 per 100,00 women.

7.8 Reduce by 15 percent the incidence of injurious suicide attempts among adolescents aged 14 to 17.

Risk Reduction Objectives

7.9 Reduce to 110 per 1,000 the incidence of physical fighting among adolescents aged 14 to 17.

7.10 Reduce to 86 per 1,000 the incidence of weapon carrying by adolescents aged 14 to 17.

7.11 Reduce by 20 percent the proportion of people who possess weapons that are inappropriately stored and therefore dangerously available.

Services and Protection Objectives

7.12 Extend protocols for routinely identifying, treating, and properly referring suicide attempters, victims of sexual assault, and victims of spouse, elder, and

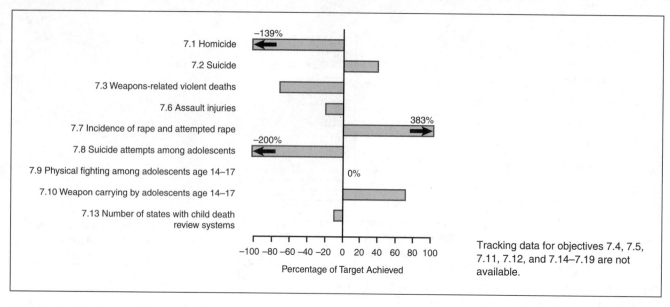

Priority 7—Violent and Abusive Behavior; Lead Agency: Centers for Disease Control and Prevention

child abuse to at least 90 percent of hospital emergency departments.

7.13 Extend to at least 45 states implementation of unexplained child death review systems.

7.14 Increase to at least 30 the number of states in which at least 50 percent of children identified as neglected or physically or sexually abused receive physical and mental evaluation with appropriate follow-up as a means of breaking the intergenerational cycle of abuse.

7.15 Reduce to less than 10 percent the proportion of battered women and their children turned away from emergency housing because of lack of space.

7.16 Increase to at least 50 percent the proportion of elementary and secondary schools that teach nonviolent conflict-resolution skills, preferably as a part of comprehensive school health education.

7.17 Extend coordinated, comprehensive violence prevention programs to at least 80 percent of local jurisdictions with populations over 100,000.

7.18 Increase to 50 the number of states with officially established protocols that engage mental health, alcohol and drug, and public health authorities with corrections authorities to facilitate identification and appropriate intervention to prevent suicide by jail inmates.

Services and Protection Objective (*Added in 1995*)

7.19 Enact in 50 states and the District of Columbia laws requiring that firearms be properly stored to minimize access and the likelihood of discharge by minors.

EDUCATIONAL AND COMMUNITY-BASED PROGRAMS

The lead agencies for coordinating achievement of the 14 objectives developed in the priority area of educational and community-based programs are the Centers for Disease Control and Prevention and the Health Resources and Services Administration.

Health Status Objective

8.1   Increase years of healthy life to at least 65.

Risk Reduction Objective

8.2   Increase the high school completion rate to at least 90 percent, thereby reducing risks for multiple problem behaviors and poor mental and physical health.

Services and Protection Objectives

8.3   Achieve for all disadvantaged children and children with disabilities access to high-quality and developmentally appropriate preschool programs that help prepare children for school, thereby improving their prospects with regard to school performance, problem behaviors, and mental and physical health.

8.4   Increase to at least 75 percent the proportion of the nation's elementary and secondary schools that provide planned and sequential kindergarten to 12th grade comprehensive school health education.

8.5   Increase to at least 50 percent the proportion of postsecondary institutions with institutionwide

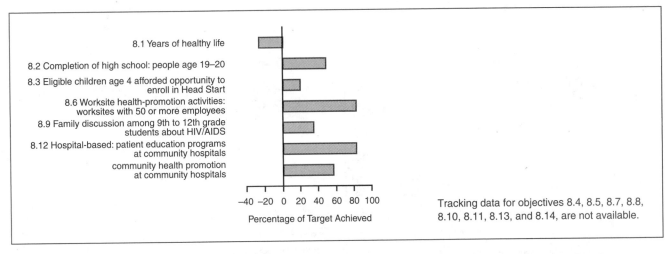

Priority 8—Educational and Community-Based Programs; Lead Agencies: Centers for Disease Control and Prevention and Health Resources and Services Administration.

health-promotion programs for students, faculty, and staff.

8.6   Increase to at least 85 percent the proportion of workplaces with 50 or more employees that offer health-promotion activities for their employees, preferably as part of a comprehensive employee health-promotion program.

8.7   Increase to at least 20 percent the proportion of hourly workers who participate regularly in employer-sponsored health-promotion activities.

8.8   Increase to at least 90 percent the proportion of people aged 65 and older who had the opportunity to participate during the preceding year in a least one organized health-promotion program through a senior center, lifecare facility, or other community-based setting that serves older adults.

8.9   Increase to at least 75 percent the proportion of people aged 10 and older who have discussed issues related to nutrition, physical activity, sexual behavior, tobacco, alcohol, other drugs, or safety with family members on at least one occasion during the preceding month.

8.10 Establish community health-promotion programs that separately or together address at least three of the Healthy People 2000 priorities and reach at least 40 percent of each state's population.

8.11 Increase to at least 50 percent the proportion of counties that have established culturally and linguistically appropriate community health-promotion programs for racial and ethnic minority populations.

8.12 Increase to at least 90 percent the proportion of hospitals, health maintenance organizations, and large group practices that provide patient education programs and to at least 90 percent the proportion of community hospitals that offer community health-promotion programs addressing the priority health needs of their communities.

8.13 Increase to at least 75 percent the proportion of local television network affiliates in the top 20 television markets that have become partners with one or more community organizations around one of the health problems addressed by the Healthy People 2000 objectives.

8.14 Increase to at least 90 percent the proportion of people who are served by a local health department that is effectively carrying out the core functions of public health.

UNINTENTIONAL INJURIES

The lead agency for coordinating achievement of the 26 objectives related to unintentional injury is the Centers for Disease Control and Prevention.

Health Status Objectives

9.1   Reduce deaths caused by unintentional injuries to no more than 29.3 per 100,000 people.

9.2   Reduce nonfatal unintentional injuries so that hospitalizations for this condition are no more than 754 per 100,000 people.

9.3   Reduce deaths caused by motor vehicle crashes to no more than 1.5 per 100 million vehicle miles traveled (VMT) and 14.2 per 100,000 people.

9.4   Reduce deaths from falls and fall-related injuries to no more than 2.3 per 100,000 people.

9.5   Reduce drowning deaths to no more than 1.3 per 100,000 people.

9.6   Reduce residential fire deaths to no more than 1.2 per 100,000 people.

9.7   Reduce hip fractures among people aged 65 and older so that hospitalizations for this condition are no more than 607 per 100,000.

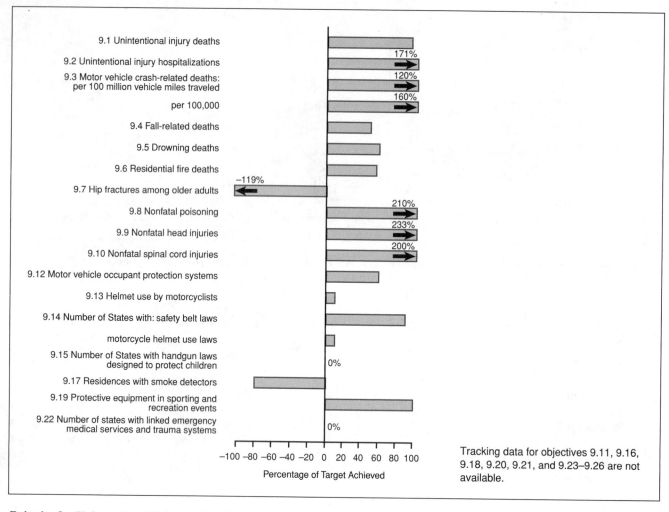

9.1 Unintentional injury deaths
9.2 Unintentional injury hospitalizations — 171%
9.3 Motor vehicle crash-related deaths: per 100 million vehicle miles traveled — 120%
    per 100,000 — 160%
9.4 Fall-related deaths
9.5 Drowning deaths
9.6 Residential fire deaths
9.7 Hip fractures among older adults — −119%
9.8 Nonfatal poisoning — 210%
9.9 Nonfatal head injuries — 233%
9.10 Nonfatal spinal cord injuries — 200%
9.12 Motor vehicle occupant protection systems
9.13 Helmet use by motorcyclists
9.14 Number of States with: safety belt laws
    motorcycle helmet use laws
9.15 Number of States with handgun laws designed to protect children — 0%
9.17 Residences with smoke detectors
9.19 Protective equipment in sporting and recreation events
9.22 Number of states with linked emergency medical services and trauma systems — 0%

−100 −80 −60 −40 −20 0 20 40 60 80 100
Percentage of Target Achieved

Tracking data for objectives 9.11, 9.16, 9.18, 9.20, 9.21, and 9.23–9.26 are not available.

Priority 9—Unintentional Injuries; Lead Agency: Centers for Disease Control and Prevention

9.8 Reduce nonfatal poisoning to no more than 88 emergency department treatments per 100,000 people.

9.9 Reduce nonfatal head injuries so that hospitalizations for this condition are no more than 106 per 100,000 people.

9.10 Reduce nonfatal spinal cord injuries so that hospitalizations for this condition are no more than 5 per 100,000 people.

Risk Reduction Objectives

9.11 Reduce by 20 percent the incidence of secondary conditions (e.g., pressure sores) associated with traumatic spinal cord injuries.

9.12 Increase use of safety belts and child safety seats to at least 85 percent of motor vehicle occupants.

9.13 Increase use of helmets to at least 80 percent of motorcyclists and at least 50 percent of bicyclists.

Services and Protection Objectives

9.14 Extend to 50 states laws requiring safety belt and motorcycle helmet use for all ages.

9.15 Enact in 50 states laws requiring that new handguns be designed to minimize the likelihood of discharge by children.

9.16 Extend to 2,000 local jurisdictions the number whose codes address the installation of fire suppression sprinkler systems in those residences at highest risk for fires.

9.17 Increase the presence of functional smoke detectors to at least one on each habitable floor of all inhabited residential dwellings.

9.18 Provide academic instruction on injury prevention and control, preferably as part of comprehensive school health education, in at least 50 percent of public school systems (grades K–12).

9.19 Extend requirement of the use of effective head, face, eye, and mouth protection to all organizations, agencies, and institutions sponsoring sporting and recreation events that pose risks of injury.

9.20 Increase to 50 the number of states that have design standards for markings, signs, and other characteristics of the roadway environment to improve the visual stimuli and protect the safety of older drivers and pedestrians.

9.21 Increase to at least 50 percent the proportion of primary care providers who routinely provide age-appropriate counseling on safety precautions to prevent unintentional injury.

9.22 Extend to 20 states the capability to link emergency medical services, trauma systems, and hospital data.

Health Status Objective (*Added in 1995*)

9.23 Reduce deaths caused by alcohol-related motor vehicle crashes to no more than 5.5 per 100,000 people.

Services and Protection Objectives (*Added in 1995*)

9.24 Extend to 50 states laws requiring helmets for bicycle riders.

9.25 Enact in 50 states laws requiring that firearms be properly stored to minimize access and the likelihood of discharge by minors.

9.26 Increase to 35 the number of states having a graduated driver licensing system for novice drivers and riders under the age of 18.

OCCUPATIONAL SAFETY AND HEALTH

The Centers for Disease Control and Prevention is the lead agency for meeting the 20 occupational safety and health objectives.

Health Status Objectives

10.1 Reduce deaths from work-related injuries to no more than 4 per 100,000 full-time workers.

10.2 Reduce work-related injuries resulting in medical treatment, lost time from work, or restricted work activity to no more than 6 cases per 100 full-time workers.

10.3 Reduce cumulative trauma disorders to an incidence of no more than 60 cases per 100,000 full-time workers.

10.4 Reduce occupational skin disorders or diseases to an incidence of no more than 55 per 100,000 full-time workers.

Risk Reduction Objectives

10.5 Reduce hepatitis B among occupationally exposed workers to an incidence of no more than 623 clinical cases.

10.6 Increase to at least 95 percent the proportion of worksites with 50 or more employees that mandate employee use of occupant protection systems, such as seatbelts, during all work-related motor vehicle travel.

10.7 Reduce to no more than 15 percent the proportion of workers exposed to average daily noise levels that exceed 85 dBA.

10.8 Eliminate exposures that result in workers' having blood lead concentrations greater than 25 µg/dl of whole blood.

10.9 Increase hepatitis B immunization levels to 90 percent among occupationally exposed workers.

Services and Protection Objectives

10.10 Implement occupational safety and health plans in 50 states for the identification, management, and prevention of leading work-related diseases and injuries within each state.

10.11 Establish in 50 states exposure standards adequate to prevent the major occupational lung diseases to which their worker populations are exposed (byssinosis, asbestosis, coal workers' pneumoconiosis, and silicosis).

10.12 Increase to at least 70 percent the proportion of worksites with 50 or more employees that have implemented programs on worker health and safety.

10.13 Increase to at least 50 percent the proportion of worksites with 50 or more employees that offer back injury prevention and rehabilitation programs.

10.14 Establish in 50 states either public health or labor department programs that provide consultation and assistance to small businesses to implement safety and health programs for their employees.

10.15 Increase to at least 75 percent the proportion of primary care providers who routinely elicit occupational health exposures as a part of patient history and provide relevant counseling.

Health Status Objectives (*Added in 1995*)

10.16 Reduce deaths from work-related homicides to no more than 0.5 per 100,000 full-time workers.

10.17 Reduce the overall age-adjusted mortality rate for four major preventable occupational lung diseases (byssinosis, asbestosis, coal workers' pneumoconiosis, and silicosis).

Services and Protection Objectives (*Added in 1995*)

10.18 Increase to 100 percent the proportion of worksites with a formal smoking policy that prohibits or severely restricts smoking at the workplace.

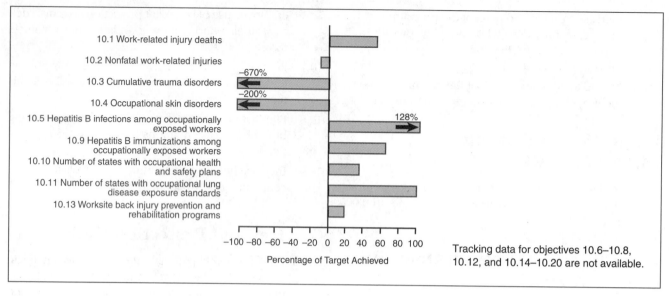

Priority 10—Occupational Safety and Health; Lead Agency: Centers for Disease Control and Prevention

10.19 Enact in 50 states and the District of Columbia comprehensive laws on clean indoor air that prohibit smoking or limit it to separately ventilated areas in the workplace and enclosed public places.

10.20 Reduce to zero the number of states that have clean indoor air laws preempting stronger clean indoor air laws on the local level.

ENVIRONMENTAL HEALTH

The lead agencies responsible for achievement of the 17 environmental health objectives are the National Institutes of Health and the Centers for Disease Control and Prevention.

Health Status Objectives

11.1 Reduce asthma morbidity, as measured by a reduction in asthma hospitalizations, to no more than 160 per 100,000 people.

11.2 reduce the prevalence of serious mental retardation among school-aged children to no more than 2 per 1,000 children.

11.3 Reduce outbreaks of waterborne disease from infectious agents and chemical poisoning to no more than 11 per year.

11.4 Reduce the prevalence of blood lead levels exceeding 15 μg/dl and 25 μg/dl among children aged 6 months to 5 years to no more than 300,000 and zero, respectively.

Risk Reduction Objectives

11.5 Reduce human exposure to criteria air pollutants, as measured by an increase to at least 85 percent in the proportion of people who live in counties that have not exceeded any Environmental Protection Agency standard for air quality in the previous 12 months.

11.6 Increase to at least 40 percent the proportion of homes in which homeowners or occupants have tested for radon concentrations and that have either been found to pose minimal risk or have been modified to reduce risk to health.

11.7 Reduce human exposure to toxic agents by decreasing the release of hazardous substances from industrial facilities: a 65 percent decrease in the substances on the Department of Health and Human Services list of carcinogens and a 50 percent reduction in the substances on the Agency for Toxic Substances and Disease Registry (ATSDR) priority list of the most toxic chemicals.

11.8 Reduce human exposure to solid waste–related water, air, and soil contamination, as measured by a reduction in average pounds of municipal solid waste produced per person each day to no more than 4.3 pounds before recovery and 3.2 pounds after recovery.

11.9 Increase to at least 85 percent the proportion of people who receive a supply of drinking water that meets the safe drinking water standards established by the Environmental Protection Agency.

11.10 Reduce potential risks to human health from surface water, as measured by an increase in the proportion of assessed rivers, lakes, and estuaries that support beneficial uses such as consumable fish and recreational activities.

Services and Protection Objectives

11.11 Perform testing for lead-based paint in at least 50 percent of homes built before 1950.

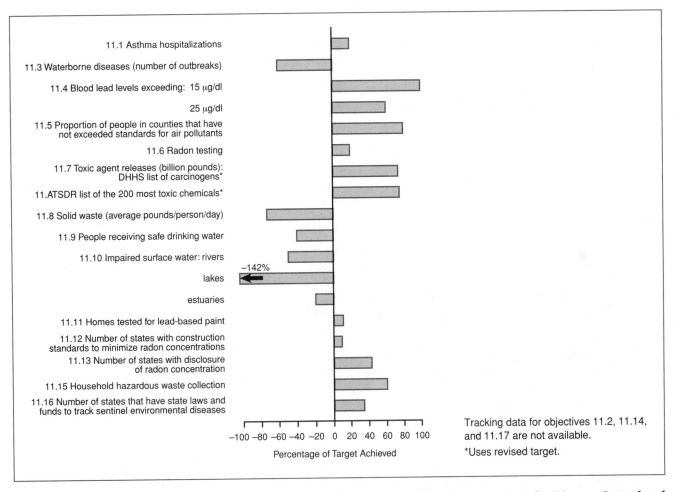

Priority 11—Environmental Health; Lead Agencies: National Institutes of Health and Centers for Disease Control and Prevention

11.12 Expand to at least 35 the number of states in which at least 75 percent of local jurisdictions have adopted construction standards and techniques that minimize elevated indoor radon levels in those new building areas locally determined to have elevated radon levels.

11.13 Increase to at least 30 the number of states requiring that prospective buyers be informed of the presence of lead-based paint and radon concentrations in all buildings offered for sale.

11.14 Eliminate significant health risks from National Priority List hazardous waste sites, as measured by performance of cleanup at these sites sufficient to eliminate immediate and significant health threats as specified in health assessments completed at all sites.

11.15 Establish curbside recycling programs that serve at least 50 percent of the U.S. population and continue to increase household hazardous waste collection programs.

11.16 Establish and monitor in at least 35 states plans to define and track sentinel environmental diseases.

Risk Reduction Objective (*Added in 1995*)

11.17 Reduce to no more than 20 percent the proportion of children aged 6 and younger who are regularly exposed to tobacco smoke at home.

FOOD AND DRUG SAFETY

The Food and Drug Administration (FDA) is the lead agency in meeting the 8 food and drug safety objectives.

Health Status Objectives

12.1 Reduce infections caused by key foodborne pathogens to no more than 16 cases of *Salmonella* per 100,000 people; 25 cases of *Campylobacter jejuni*; 4 cases of *Eschericia coli* O157:H7; and 0.5 cases of *Listeria monocytogenes*.

12.2 Reduce outbreaks of infections due to *Salmonella enteritidis* to fewer than 25 outbreaks yearly.

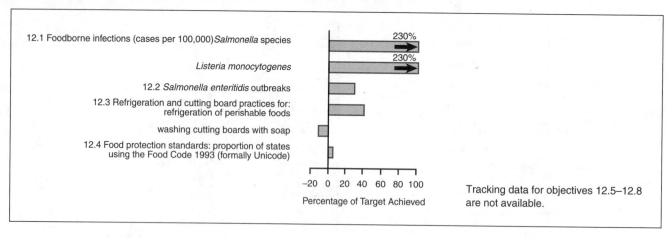

12.1 Foodborne infections (cases per 100,000) *Salmonella* species — 230%
Listeria monocytogenes — 230%
12.2 *Salmonella enteritidis* outbreaks
12.3 Refrigeration and cutting board practices for:
refrigeration of perishable foods
washing cutting boards with soap
12.4 Food protection standards: proportion of states
using the Food Code 1993 (formally Unicode)

-20 0 20 40 60 80 100
Percentage of Target Achieved

Tracking data for objectives 12.5–12.8
are not available.

Priority 12—Food and Drug Safety; Lead Agency: Food and Drug Administration

Risk Reduction Objective

12.3 Increase to at least 75 percent the proportion of households in which principal food preparers routinely refrain from leaving perishable food out of the refrigerator for over 2 hours and wash cutting boards and utensils with soap after contact with raw meat and poultry.

Services and Protection Objectives

12.4 Extend to at least 70 percent the proportion of states and territories that have implemented Food Code 1993 for institutional food operations and to at least 70 percent the proportion that have adopted the new uniform food protection code that sets recommended standards for regulation of all food operations.

12.5 Increase to at least 75 percent the proportion of pharmacies and other dispensers of prescription medications that use linked systems to provide alerts to potential adverse drug reactions among medications dispensed by different sources to individual patients.

12.6 Increase to at least 75 percent the proportion of primary care providers and other dispensers of medicine who routinely review with their patients aged 65 and older all prescribed and over-the-counter medicines taken by their patients each time a new medication is prescribed or dispensed.

Services and Protection Objectives (*Added in 1995*)

12.7 Increase to at least 75 percent the proportion of the total number of adverse event reports voluntarily sent directly to the FDA that are regarded as serious.

12.8 Increase to at least 75 percent the proportion of people who receive useful information verbally and in writing for new prescriptions from prescribers or dispensers.

ORAL HEALTH

The National Institutes of Health and the Centers for Disease Control and Prevention are the lead agencies responsible for achievement of the 17 oral health objectives.

Health Status Objectives

13.1 Reduce dental caries (cavities) so that the proportion of children with one or more caries (in permanent or primary teeth) is no more than 35 percent among children aged 6 to 8 and no more than 60 percent among adolescents aged 15.

13.2 Reduce untreated dental caries so that the proportion of children with untreated caries (in permanent or primary teeth) is no more than 20 percent among children aged 6 to 8 and no more than 15 percent among adolescents aged 15.

13.3 Increase to at least 45 percent the proportion of people aged 35 to 44 who have never lost a permanent tooth due to dental caries or periodontal disease.

13.4 Reduce to no more than 20 percent the proportion of people aged 65 and older who have lost all of their natural teeth.

13.5 Reduce the prevalence of gingivitis among people aged 35 to 44 to no more than 30 percent.

13.6 Reduce destructive periodontal diseases to a prevalence of no more than 15 percent among people aged 35 to 44.

13.7 Reduce deaths due to cancer of the oral cavity and pharynx to no more than 10.5 per 100,000 men aged 45 to 74 and 4.1 per 100,000 women aged 45 to 74.

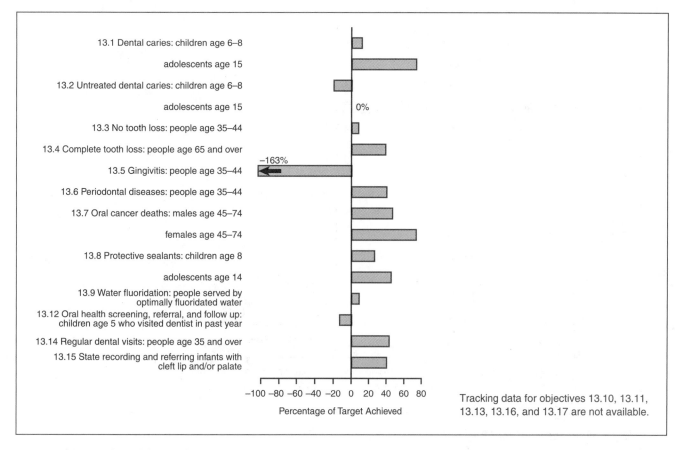

Priority 13—Oral Health; Lead Agencies: National Institutes of Health and Centers for Disease Control and Prevention

Risk Reduction Objectives

13.8   Increase to at least 50 percent the proportion of children who have received protective sealants on the occlusal (chewing) surfaces of permanent molar teeth.

13.9   Increase to at least 75 percent the proportion of people served by community water systems providing optimal levels of fluoride.

13.10   Increase use of professionally or self-administered topical or systemic (dietary) fluorides to at least 85 percent of people not receiving optimally fluoridated public water.

13.11   Increase to at least 75 percent the proportion of parents and caregivers who use feeding practices that prevent baby bottle tooth decay.

Services and Protection Objectives

13.12   Increase to at least 90 percent the proportion of all children entering school programs for the first time who have received an oral health screening, referral, and follow-up for necessary diagnostic, preventive, and treatment services.

13.13   Extend to all long-term institutional facilities the requirement that oral examinations and services be provided no later than 90 days after entry into these facilities.

13.14   Increase to at least 70 percent the proportion of people aged 35 and older using the oral health care system during each year.

13.15   Increase to at least 40 the number of states that have an effective system for recording and referring infants with cleft lip and/or palate to craniofacial anomaly teams.

13.16   Extend requirement of the use of effective head, face, eye, and mouth protection to all organizations, agencies, and institutions sponsoring sporting and recreation events that pose risks of injury.

Risk Reduction Objective (*Added in 1995*)

13.17   Reduce smokeless tobacco use by males aged 12 to 24 to a prevalence of no more than 4 percent.

MATERNAL AND INFANT HEALTH

The Health Resources and Services Administration is the lead agency in meeting the 17 maternal and infant health objectives.

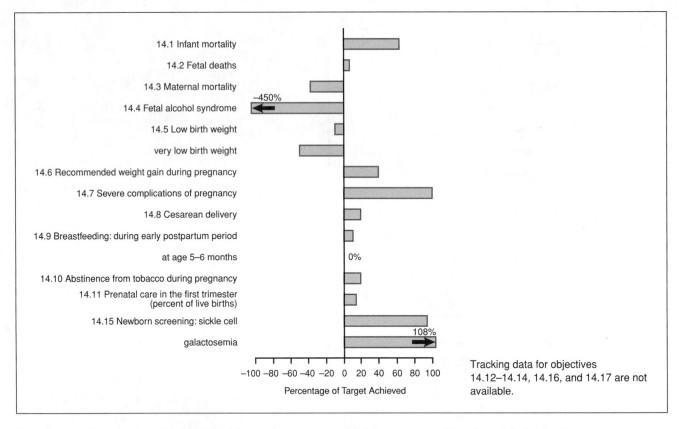

Priority 14—Maternal and Infant Health; Lead Agency: Health Resources and Services Administration

Health Status Objectives

14.1   Reduce the infant mortality rate to no more than 7 per 1,000 live births.

14.2   Reduce the fetal death rate (20 or more weeks of gestation) to no more than 5 per 1,000 live births plus fetal deaths.

14.3   Reduce the maternal mortality rate to no more than 3.3 per 100,000 live births.

14.4   Reduce the incidence of fetal alcohol syndrome to no more than 0.12 per 1,000 live births.

Risk Reduction Objectives

14.5   Reduce low birth weight to an incidence of no more than 5 percent of live births and very low birth weight to no more than 1 percent of live births.

14.6   Increase to at least 85 percent the proportion of mothers who achieve the minimum recommended weight gain during their pregnancy.

14.7   Reduce severe complications of pregnancy to no more than 15 per 100 deliveries.

14.8   Reduce the cesarean delivery rate to no more than 15 per 100 deliveries.

14.9   Increase to at least 7.5 percent the proportion of mothers who breastfeed their babies in the early postpartum period and to at least 50 percent the proportion who continue breastfeeding until their babies are 5 to 6 months old.

14.10   Increase abstinence from tobacco use by pregnant women to at least 90 percent and increase abstinence from alcohol, cocaine, and marijuana by pregnant women by at least 20 percent.

Services and Protection Objectives

14.11   Increase to at least 90 percent the proportion of all pregnant women who receive prenatal care in the first trimester of pregnancy.

14.12   Increase to at least 60 percent the proportion of primary care providers who provide age-appropriate preconception care and counseling.

14.13   Increase to at least 90 percent the proportion of women enrolled in prenatal care who are offered screening and counseling on prenatal detection of fetal abnormalities.

14.14   Increase to at least 90 percent the proportion of pregnant women and infants who receive risk-appropriate care.

14.15   Increase to at least 95 percent the proportion of newborns screened by state-sponsored programs for genetic disorders and other disabling conditions and to 90 percent the proportion of newborns testing positive for disease who receive appropriate treatment.

14.16   Increase to at least 90 percent the proportion of babies aged 18 months and younger who receive recommended primary care services at the appropriate intervals.

Health Status Objective (*Added in 1995*)

14.17 Reduce the incidence of spina bifida and other neural tube defects to 3 per 10,000 live births.

HEART DISEASE AND STROKE

The National Institutes of Health is the lead agency in guiding achievement of the 17 objectives related to heart disease and stroke.

Health Status Objectives

15.1 Reduce coronary heart disease deaths to no more than 100 per 100,000 people.

15.2 Reduce stroke deaths to no more than 20 per 100,000 people.

15.3 Reverse the increase in end-stage renal disease (requiring maintenance dialysis or transplantation) to attain an incidence of no more than 13 per 100,000.

Risk Reduction Objectives

15.4 Increase to at least 50 percent the proportion of people with high blood pressure whose blood pressure is under control.

15.5 Increase to at least 90 percent the proportion of people with high blood pressure who are taking action to help control their blood pressure.

15.6 Reduce the mean serum cholesterol level among adults to no more than 200 mg/dl.

15.7 Reduce the prevalence of blood cholesterol levels of 240 mg/dl or greater to no more than 20 percent among adults.

15.8 Increase to at least 60 percent the proportion of adults with high blood cholesterol who are aware of their condition and are taking action to reduce their blood cholesterol to recommended levels.

15.9 Reduce dietary fat intake to an average of 30 percent of calories or less and average saturated fat intake to less than 10 percent of calories among people aged 2 and older. In addition, increase to at least 50 percent the proportion of people aged 2 and older who meet the *Dietary Guidelines'* average daily goal of no more than 30 percent of calo-

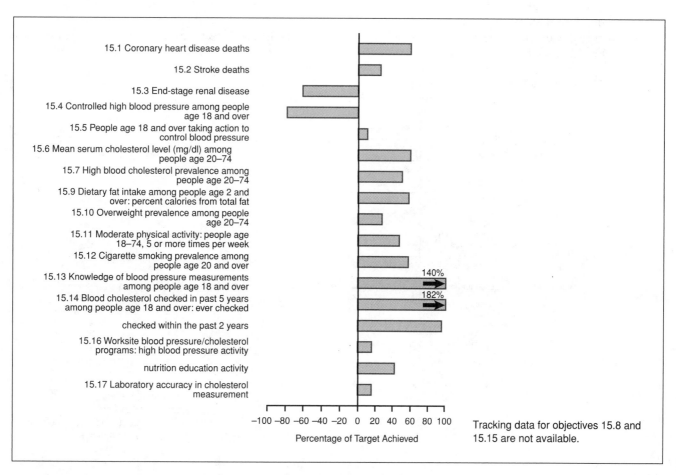

Tracking data for objectives 15.8 and 15.15 are not available.

Priority 15—Heart Disease and Stroke; Lead Agency: National Institutes of Health ries from fat, and increase to at least 50 percent the proportion of people aged 2 and older who meet the average daily goal of less than 10 percent of calories from saturated fat.

15.10   Reduce overweight to a prevalence of no more than 20 percent among people aged 20 and older and no more than 15 percent among adolescents aged 12 to 19.

15.11   Increase to at least 30 percent the proportion of people aged 6 and older who engage regularly, preferably daily, in light to moderate physical activity for at least 30 minutes per day.

15.12   Reduce cigarette smoking to a prevalence of no more than 15 percent among people aged 18 and older.

Services and Protection Objectives

15.13   Increase to at least 90 percent the proportion of adults who have had their blood pressure measured within the preceding 2 years and can state whether their blood pressure was normal or high.

15.14   Increase to at least 75 percent the proportion of adults who have had their blood cholesterol checked within the preceding 5 years.

15.15   Increase to at least 75 percent the proportion of primary care providers who initiate diet and, if necessary, drug therapy at levels of blood cholesterol consistent with current management guidelines for patients with high blood cholesterol.

15.16   Increase to at least 50 percent the proportion of worksites with 50 or more employees that offer high blood pressure and/or cholesterol education and control activities to their employees.

15.17   Increase to at least 90 percent the proportion of clinical laboratories that meet the recommended accuracy standard for cholesterol measurement.

CANCER

The National Institutes of Health is the lead agency in directing achievement of the 17 objectives related to cancer.

Health Status Objectives

16.1   Reverse the rise in cancer deaths to achieve a rate of no more than 130 per 100,000 people.

16.2   Slow the rise in lung cancer deaths to achieve a rate of no more than 42 per 100,000 people.

16.3   Reduce breast cancer deaths to no more than 20.6 per 100,000 women.

16.4   Reduce deaths from cancer of the uterine cervix to no more than 1.3 per 100,000 women.

16.5   Reduce colorectal cancer deaths to no more than 13.2 per 100,000 people.

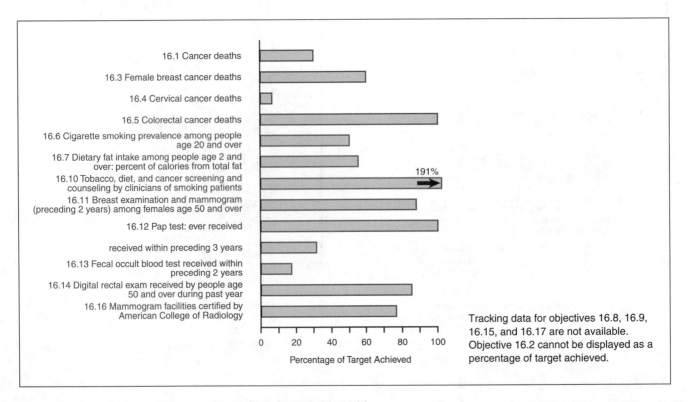

Tracking data for objectives 16.8, 16.9, 16.15, and 16.17 are not available. Objective 16.2 cannot be displayed as a percentage of target achieved.

Priority 16—Cancer; Lead Agency: National Institutes of Health

Risk Reduction Objectives

16.6   Reduce cigarette smoking to a prevalence of no more than 15 percent among people aged 18 and older.

16.7   Reduce dietary fat intake to an average of 30 percent of calories or less and average saturated fat intake to less than 10 percent of calories among people aged 2 and older. In addition, increase to at least 50 percent the proportion of people aged 2 and older who meet the *Dietary Guidelines'* average daily goal of no more than 30 percent of calories from fat, and increase to at least 50 percent the proportion of people aged 2 and older who meet the average daily goal of less than 10 percent of calories from saturated fat.

16.8   Increase complex carbohydrate and fiber-containing foods in the diets of people aged 2 and older to an average of five or more daily servings for vegetables (including legumes) and fruits and to an average of six or more daily servings for grain products. In addition, increase to at least 50 percent the proportion of people aged 2 and older who meet the *Dietary Guidelines'* average daily goal of 5 or more servings of vegetables and fruits and increase to at least 50 percent the proportion who meet the goal of six or more servings of grain products.

Services and Protection Objectives

16.9   Increase to at least 60 percent the proportion of people of all ages who limit sun exposure, use sunscreens and protective clothing when exposed to sunlight, and avoid artificial sources of ultraviolet light (e.g., sun lamps, tanning booths).

16.10   Increase to at least 75 percent the proportion of primary care providers who routinely counsel patients about the following: tobacco use cessation, diet modification, and cancer screening recommendations, which includes providing information on the potential benefit or harm attributed to the various screening modalities and discussion of risk factors associated with breast, prostate, cervical, colorectal, and lung cancers.

16.11   Increase to at least 60 percent those women aged 50 and older who have received a clinical breast examination and a mammogram within the preceding 1 to 2 years.

16.12   Increase to at least 95 percent the proportion of women aged 18 and older who have ever received a Pap test and to at least 85 percent those who received a Pap test within the preceding 1 to 3 years.

16.13   Increase to at least 50 percent the proportion of people aged 50 and older who have received fecal occult blood testing within the preceding 1 to 2

years and to at least 40 percent those who have ever received proctosigmoidoscopy.

16.14   Increase to at least 40 percent the proportion of people aged 50 and older visiting a primary care provider in the preceding year who have received oral, skin, and digital rectal examinations during one such visit.

16.15   Ensure that Pap tests meet quality standards by monitoring and certifying all cytology laboratories.

16.16   Ensure that mammograms meet quality standards by inspecting and certifying 100 percent according to the requirements of the Mammography Quality Standards Act.

Health Status Objective (*Added in 1995*)

16.17   Reduce deaths due to cancer of the oral cavity and pharynx to no more than 10.5 per 100,000 men aged 45 to 74 and 4.1 per 100,000 women aged 45 to 74.

DIABETES AND CHRONIC DISABLING CONDITIONS

The lead agencies for coordinating achievement of the 23 objectives in the priority area of diabetes and chronic disabling conditions are the Centers for Disease Control and Prevention and the National Institutes of Health.

Health Status Objectives

17.1   Increase years of healthy life to at least 65.

17.2   Reduce to no more than 8 percent the proportion of people who experience a limitation in major activity due to chronic conditions.

17.3   Reduce to no more than 90 per 1,000 people the proportion of all people aged 65 and older who have difficulty in performing two or more personal care activities, thereby preserving independence.

17.4   Reduce to no more than 10 percent the proportion of people with asthma who experience activity limitation.

17.5   Reduce activity limitation due to chronic back conditions to a prevalence of no more than 19 per 1,000 people.

17.6   Reduce significant hearing impairment to a prevalence of no more than 82 per 1,000 people.

17.7   Reduce significant visual impairment to a prevalence of no more than 30 per 1,000 people.

17.8 Reduce the prevalence of serious mental retardation among school-age children to no more than 2 per 1,000 children.

17.9 Reduce diabetes-related deaths to no more than 34 per 100,000 people.

17.10 Reduce the most severe complications of diabetes: end-stage renal disease to 1.4/1,000; blindness to 1.4/1,000; lower extremity amputation to 4.9/1,000; perinatal mortality to 2%; and major congenital malformations to 4%.

17.11 Reduce diabetes to an incidence of no more than 2.5 per 1,000 people and a prevalence of no more than 25 per 1,000 people.

Risk Reduction Objectives

17.12 Reduce overweight to a prevalence of no more than 20 percent among people aged 20 and older and no more than 15 percent among adolescents aged 12 to 19.

17.13 Increase to at least 30 percent the proportion of people aged 6 and older who engage regularly, preferably daily, in light to moderate physical activity for at least 30 minutes per day.

Services and Protection Objectives

17.14 Increase to at least 40 percent the proportion of people with chronic and disabling conditions who receive formal patient education including information about community and self-help resources as an integral part of the management of their condition.

17.15 Increase to at least 80 percent the proportion of providers of primary care for children who routinely refer or screen infants and children for impairments of vision, hearing, and speech and language and who assess other developmental milestones as part of well-child care.

17.16 Reduce the average age at which children with significant hearing impairment are identified to no more than 12 months.

17.17 Increase to at least 60 percent the proportion of providers of primary care for older adults who routinely evaluate people aged 65 and older for urinary incontinence and impairments of vision, hearing, cognition, and functional status.

17.18 Increase to at least 90 percent the proportion of perimenopausal women who have been counseled about the benefits and risks of estrogen replace-

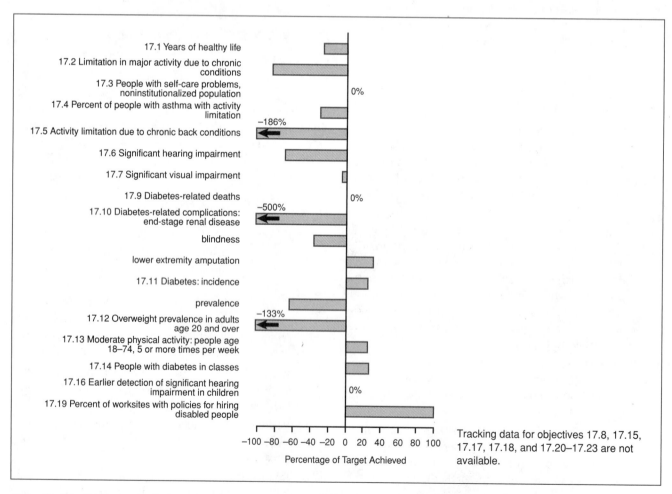

Priority 17—Diabetes and Chronic Disabling Conditions; Lead Agencies: National Institutes of Health and Centers for Disease Control and Prevention

ment therapy (combined with progestin, when appropriate) for prevention of osteoporosis.

17.19 Increase to at least 75 percent the proportion of worksites with 50 or more employees that have a policy or program for the hiring of people with disabilities.

17.20 Increase to 50 the number of states that have service systems for children with or at risk of chronic and disabling conditions, as required by Public Law 101-239.

Health Status Objectives (*Added in 1995*)

17.21 Reduce the prevalence of peptic ulcer disease to no more than 18 per 1,000 people aged 18 and older by preventing its recurrence.

17.22 Develop and implement a national process to identify significant gaps in the nation's disease-prevention and health-promotion data, including data for racial and ethnic minorities, people with low incomes, and people with disabilities, and establish mechanisms to meet these needs.

Services and Protection Objective (*Added in 1995*)

17.23 Increase to 70 percent the proportion of people with diabetes who have an annual dilated eye exam.

HIV INFECTION

The Office of HIV/AIDS Policy serves as lead agency for meeting the 17 HIV infection objectives.

Health Status Objectives

18.1 Confine annual incidence of diagnosed AIDS cases to no more than 43 per 100,000 population.

18.2 Confine the prevalence of HIV infection to no more than 400 per 100,000 people.

Risk Reduction Objectives

18.3 Reduce the proportion of adolescents who have engaged in sexual intercourse to no more than 15 percent by age 15 and no more than 40 percent by age 17.

18.4 Increase to at least 50 percent the proportion of sexually active, unmarried people who used a condom at last sexual intercourse.

18.5 Increase to at least 50 percent the estimated proportion of all injecting drug users who are in drug abuse treatment programs.

18.6 Increase to at least 75 percent the proportion of active injecting drug users who use only new or properly decontaminated syringes, needles, and other drug paraphernalia ("works").

18.7 Reduce to no more than 1 per 250,000 units of blood and blood components the risk of transfusion-transmitted HIV infection.

Services and Protection Objectives

18.8 Increase to at least 80 percent the proportion of HIV-infected people who know their serostatus.

18.9 Increase to at least 75 percent the proportion of primary care and mental health care providers who provide appropriate counseling on the prevention of HIV and other sexually transmitted diseases.

18.10 Increase to at least 95 percent the proportion of schools that provide appropriate HIV and other STD education curricula for students in 4th–12th grades, preferably as part of comprehensive school health education, based upon scientific information that includes the way HIV and other STDs are prevented and transmitted.

18.11 Increase to at least 90 percent the proportion of students who received HIV and other STD information, education, or counseling on their college or university campus.

18.12 Increase to at least 90 percent the proportion of cities with populations over 100,000 that have outreach programs to contact injecting drug users (particularly injecting drug users) to deliver HIV risk reduction messages.

18.13 Increase to at least 50 percent the proportion of family planning clinics, maternal and child health clinics, sexually transmitted disease clinics, tuberculosis clinics, drug treatment centers, and primary care clinics that provide onsite primary prevention and provide or refer for secondary prevention services for HIV infection and bacterial sexually transmitted diseases (gonorrhea, syphilis, and chlamydia) to high-risk individuals and their sex or needle-sharing partners.

18.14 Extend to all facilities where workers are at risk for occupational transmission of HIV regulations to protect workers from exposure to bloodborne infections, including HIV infection.

Risk Reduction Objectives (*Added in 1995*)

18.15 Increase to at least 40 percent the proportion of ever sexually active adolescents aged 17 and

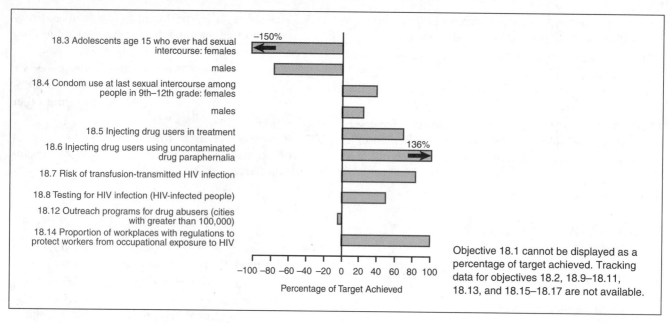

Priority 18—HIV Infection; Lead Agency: Office of HIV/AIDS Policy

younger who have not had sexual intercourse for the previous 3 months.

18.16 Increase to at least 50 percent the proportion of large businesses and to 10 percent the proportion of small businesses that implemented a comprehensive HIV/AIDS workplace program.

18.17 Increase to at least 40 percent the number of federally funded primary care clinics that have formal established linkages with substance abuse treatment programs and increase to at least 40 percent the number of federally funded substance abuse treatment programs that have formal established linkages with primary care clinics.

SEXUALLY TRANSMITTED DISEASES

The Centers for Disease Control and Prevention is the lead agency in guiding achievement of the 17 objectives related to sexually transmitted diseases.

Health Status Objectives

19.1 Reduce gonorrhea to an incidence of no more than 100 cases per 100,000 people.

19.2 Reduce the prevalence of *Chlamydia trachomatis* infection among young women (under the age of 25 years) to no more than 5 percent.

19.3 Reduce primary and secondary syphilis to an incidence of no more than 4 cases per 100,000 people.

19.4 Reduce congenital syphilis to an incidence of no more than 40 cases per 100,000 live births.

19.5 Reduce genital herpes and genital warts, as measured by a reduction to 138,500 and 246,500, re-

spectively, in the annual number of first-time consultations with a physician for the conditions.

19.6 Reduce the incidence of pelvic inflammatory disease, as measured by a reduction in hospitalizations for pelvic inflammatory disease, to no more than 100 per 100,000 women aged 15 to 44 and a reduction in the number of initial visits to physicians for pelvic inflammatory disease to no more than 290,000.

19.7 Reduce sexually transmitted hepatitis B infection to no more than 30,500 cases.

19.8 Reduce the rate of repeat gonorrhea infection to no more than 15 percent within the previous year.

Risk Reduction Objectives

19.9 Reduce the proportion of adolescents who have engaged in sexual intercourse to no more than 15 percent by age 15 and no more than 40 percent by age 17.

19.10 Increase to at least 50 percent the proportion of sexually active, unmarried people who used a condom at last sexual intercourse.

Services and Protection Objectives

19.11 Increase to at least 50 percent the proportion of family planning clinics, maternal and child health clinics, sexually transmitted disease clinics, tuberculosis clinics, drug treatment centers, and primary care clinics that provide onsite primary and secondary prevention services for HIV infection and bacterial sexually transmitted diseases (gonorrhea, syphilis, and chlamydia) to high-risk individuals and their sex or needle-sharing partners.

19.12 Increase to at least 95 percent the proportion of schools that provide appropriate HIV and STD ed-

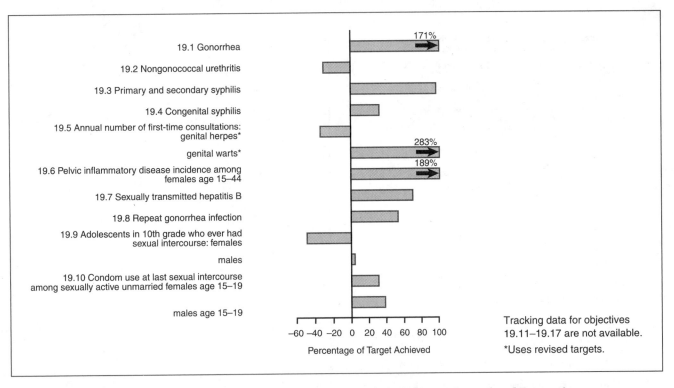

19.1 Gonorrhea — 171%

19.2 Nongonococcal urethritis

19.3 Primary and secondary syphilis

19.4 Congenital syphilis

19.5 Annual number of first-time consultations: genital herpes*

genital warts* — 283%

19.6 Pelvic inflammatory disease incidence among females age 15–44 — 189%

19.7 Sexually transmitted hepatitis B

19.8 Repeat gonorrhea infection

19.9 Adolescents in 10th grade who ever had sexual intercourse: females

males

19.10 Condom use at last sexual intercourse among sexually active unmarried females age 15–19

males age 15–19

−60 −40 −20 0 20 40 60 80 100
Percentage of Target Achieved

Tracking data for objectives 19.11–19.17 are not available.
*Uses revised targets.

Priority 19—Sexually Transmitted Diseases; Lead Agency: Centers for Disease Control and Prevention

ucation curricula for students in 4th–12th grades, preferably as part of comprehensive school health education, based upon scientific information that includes the way HIV infection and other STDs are prevented and transmitted.

19.13 Increase to at least 90 percent the proportion of primary care providers treating patients with sexually transmitted diseases who correctly manage cases, as measured by their use of appropriate types and amounts of therapy.

19.14 Increase to at least 75 percent the proportion of primary care and mental health care providers who provide appropriate counseling on the prevention of HIV and other sexually transmitted diseases.

19.15 Increase to at least 50 percent the proportion of all patients with bacterial sexually transmitted diseases (gonorrhea, syphilis, and chlamydia) who are offered provider referral services.

Risk Reduction Objective (*Added in 1995*)

19.16 Increase to at least 40 percent the proportion of ever sexually active adolescents aged 17 and younger who have not had sexual intercourse for the previous 3 months.

Services and Protection Objective (*Added in 1995*)

19.17 Increase to at least 90 percent the proportion of students who received HIV and other STD informa-

tion, education, or counseling on their college or university campus.

IMMUNIZATION AND INFECTIOUS DISEASES

The Centers for Disease Control and Prevention is the lead agency in coordinating the achievement of the 19 objectives related to immunization and infectious diseases.

Health Status Objectives

20.1 Reduce indigenous cases of vaccine-preventable diseases to 0% for diptheria, tetanus, polio, measles, rubella, and congenital rubella syndrome. Mumps will be reduced to 500 cases and pertussis to 1,000.

20.2 Reduce epidemic-related pneumonia and influenza deaths among people aged 65 and older to no more than 15.9 per 100,000.

20.3 Reduce viral hepatitis as follows: hepatitis B to 40 per 100,000; hepatitis A to 16 per 100,000; and hepatitis C to 13.7 per 100,000.

20.4 Reduce tuberculosis to an incidence of no more than 3.5 cases per 100,000 people.

20.5 Reduce by at least 10 percent the incidence of surgical wound infections and nosocomial infections in intensive care patients.

20.6 Reduce selected illness among international travelers as follows: typhoid fever to 140 cases; hepatitis A to 1,119 cases; and malaria to 750 cases.

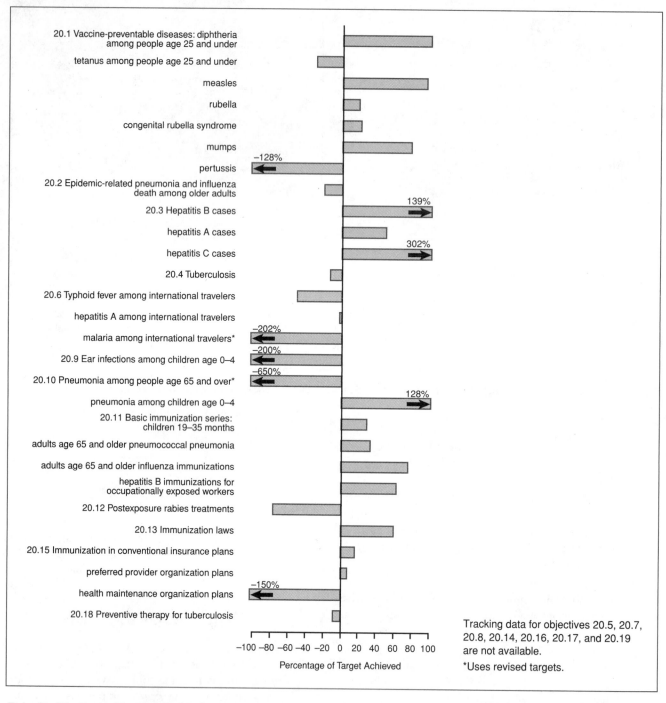

Priority 20—Immunization and Infectious Diseases; Lead Agency: Centers for Disease Control and Prevention

20.7   Reduce bacterial meningitis to no more than 4.7 cases per 100,000 people.

20.8   Reduce infectious diarrhea by at least 25 percent among children in licensed child care centers and children in programs that provide an Individualized Education Program (IEP) or Individualized Health Plan (IHP).

20.9   Reduce acute middle ear infections among children aged 4 and younger, as measured by days of restricted activity or school absenteeism, to no more than 105 days per 100 children.

20.10   Reduce pneumonia-related days of restricted activ-

ity as follows: 15.1 days for people 65 and older per 100 people; and 24 days for children aged 4 and younger per 100 people.

Risk Reduction Objectives

20.11   Increase immunization levels as follows: basic immunization series among children through age 2, at least 90%.

20.12   Reduce postexposure rabies treatments to no more than 9,000 per year.

Services and Protection Objectives

20.13 Expand immunization laws for schools, preschools, and day care settings to all states for all antigens.

20.14 Increase to at least 90 percent the proportion of primary care providers who provide information and counseling about immunizations and offer immunizations as appropriate for their patients.

20.15 Improve the financing and delivery of immunizations for children and adults so that virtually no American has a financial barrier to receiving recommended immunizations.

20.16 Increase to at least 90 percent the proportion of public health departments that provide adult immunization for influenza, pneumococcal disease, hepatitis B, tetanus, and diphtheria.

20.17 Increase to at least 90 percent the proportion of local health departments that have ongoing programs for actively identifying cases of tuberculosis and latent infection in populations at high risk for tuberculosis.

20.18 Increase to at least 85 percent the proportion of people found to have tuberculosis infection who completed courses of preventive therapy.

20.19 Increase to at least 85 percent the proportion of tertiary care hospital laboratories and to at least 50 percent the proportion of secondary care hospital and health maintenance organization laboratories possessing technologies for rapid viral diagnosis of influenza.

CLINICAL PREVENTIVE SERVICES

The lead agencies for achievement of the eight objectives related to clinical preventive services are the Centers for Disease Control and Prevention and the Health Resources and Services Administration.

Health Status Objective

21.1 Increase years of healthy life to at least 65.

Risk Reduction Objective

21.2 Increase the proportion of people who have received selected clinical preventive screening and immunization services and at least one of the counseling services appropriate for their age and gender as recommended by the U.S. Preventive Services Task Force. Objectives stipulate the following targets for preventive care by the year 2000.

Basic immunization series	90%
Routine check-up (over 65 years)	91%
Cholesterol checked in last 5 years	75%
Cholesterol ever checked	75%
Cholesterol checked in last 2 years	75%
Tetanus booster last 10 years	62%
Pneumococcal vaccine in lifetime (over 65)	60%
Influenza vaccine in last year (over 65)	60%
Pap test in last 3 years	85%
Breast exam and mammogram past 2 years	60%
Counseling services	80%

Services and Protection Objectives

21.3 Increase to at least 95 percent the proportion of people who have a specific source of ongoing primary care for coordination of their preventive and episodic health care.

21.4 Improve financing and delivery of clinical preventive services so that virtually no American has a financial barrier to receiving, at a minimum, the screening, counseling, and immunization services recommended by the U.S. Preventive Services Task Force.

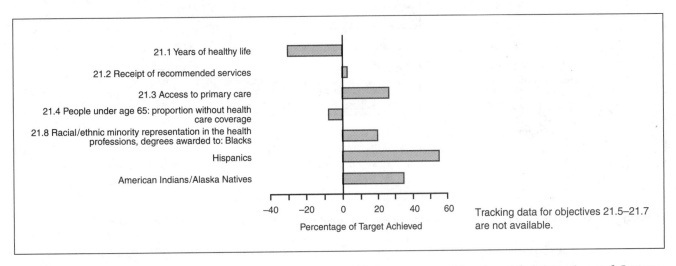

Priority 21—Clinical Preventive Services; Lead Agencies: Health Resources and Services Administration and Centers for Disease Control and Prevention

21.5 Ensure that at least 90 percent of people for whom primary care services are provided directly by publicly funded programs are offered, at a minimum, the screening, counseling, and immunization services recommended by the U.S. Preventive Services Task Force.

21.6 Increase to at least 50 percent the proportion of primary care providers who provide their patients with the screening, counseling, and immunization services recommended by the U.S. Preventive Services Task Force.

21.7 Increase to at least 90 percent the proportion of people who are served by a local health department that assesses and ensures access to essential clinical preventive services.

21.8 Increase the proportion of all degrees in the health professions and allied and associated health profession fields awarded to members of underrepresented racial and ethnic minority groups as follows: Blacks, 8% increase; Hispanics, 6.4%; and American Indians/Alaska Natives, 0.6%.

SURVEILLANCE AND DATA SYSTEMS

The Centers for Disease Control and Prevention is the lead agency in seeing that the seven surveillance and data systems objectives are met.

Health Status Objectives

22.1 Develop a set of health status indicators appropriate for federal, state, and local health agencies and establish use of the set in at least 40 states.

22.2 Identify, and create where necessary, national data sources to measure progress toward each of the year 2000 national health objectives.

22.3 Develop and disseminate among federal, state, and local agencies procedures for collecting comparable data for each of the year 2000 national health objectives and incorporate these into Public Health Service data collection systems.

22.4 Develop and implement a national process to identify significant gaps in the nation's disease prevention and health promotion data, including data for racial and ethnic minorities, people with low incomes, and people with disabilities, and establish mechanisms to meet these needs.

22.5 Implement in all states periodic analysis and publication of data needed to measure progress toward objectives for at least 10 of the priority areas of the national health objectives.

22.6 Expand in all states systems for the transfer of health information related to the national health objectives among federal, state, and local agencies.

22.7 Achieve timely release of national surveillance and survey data needed by health professionals and agencies to measure progress toward the national health objectives.

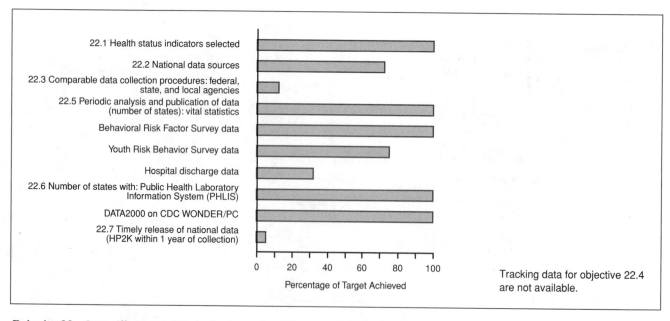

Priority 22—Surveillance and Data Systems; Lead Agency: Centers for Disease Control and Prevention

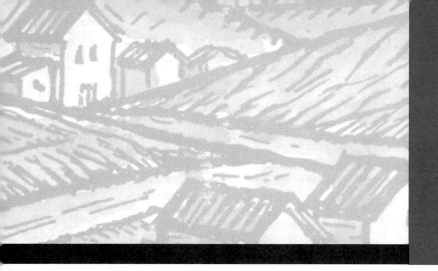

Community Resources

U.S. HEALTH-RELATED ORGANIZATIONS—GENERAL

American Health Care Association (AHCA)
  1200 15th Street, NW, Washington, DC 20005
American Health Foundation
  320 East 43rd Street, New York, NY 10018
American Public Health Association (APHA)
  1015 15th Street, NW, Suite 300, Washington, DC
  20005
  Telephone: (202) 789-5600
Association for Vital Records and Health Statistics
  c/o George van Amburg, Michigan Department of
  Public Health, 3423 Logan Street, North, P.O. Box
  30195, Lansing, MI 48909
Department of Health and Human Services
  200 Independence Avenue, SW, Washington, DC
  20201
  Telephone: (202) 679-0257
Food and Drug Administration (FDA)
  200 C Street, SW, Washington, DC 20204
  Telephone: (301) 443-2410
Health America
  315 West 105th Street, #1F, New York, NY 10025
W. K. Kellogg Foundation
  400 North Avenue, Battle Creek, MI 49017
National Health Council
  622 Third Avenue, 34th Floor, New York, NY 10017
Rockefeller Foundation
  420 Fifth Avenue, New York, NY 10018-2702

U.S. HEALTH-RELATED ORGANIZATIONS—SPECIFIC

Aging

American Association of Homes for the Aging
  901 East Street, NW, Suite 500, Washington, DC
  20004-2037
American Association of Retired Persons (AARP)
  601 East Street NW, Washington, DC, 20049

American Geriatrics Society
  770 Lexington Avenue, Suite 400, New York, NY
  10021
American Society on Aging
  833 Market Street, Suite 4511, San Francisco, CA
  94103
Gray Panthers
  2025 Pennsylvania Avenue, NW, Suite 831,
  Washington, DC 20006
National Center for Health Promotion and Aging
  c/o National Council on Aging, 409 Third Street, SW,
  2nd Floor, Washington, DC 20024
National Council on the Aging
  409 3rd Street, SW, Washington, DC 20024
National Council of Senior Citizens
  1331 F Street NW, Washington, DC 20004
National Support Center for Families of Aging
  P.O. Box 245, Swarthmore, PA 19081

Child Health

American School Health Association
  P.O. Box 708, Kent, OH 44240
Association for the Care of Children's Health
  3615 Wisconsin Avenue, NW, Washington, DC 20016
Children's Foundation
  815 15th Street, NW, Suite 928, Washington, DC
  20005
National Information Center for Children and Youth
  with Disabilities
  P.O. Box 1492, Washington, DC 20013-1492
(Toy) Guide for Differently-Abled Kids (free)
  P.O. Box 8501, Nevada, IA 50201-9968

Death and Dying

Children's Hospice International
  901 North Washington Avenue, Suite 700, Alexandria,
  VA 22314
Hospice Education Institute
  190 Westbrook Road, Essex, CT 06426

National Hospice Organization
  1901 North Moore Street, Suite 901, Arlington, VA
  22209

Dental Health and Treatment

American Dental Association
  211 East Chicago Avenue, Chicago, IL 60611

Disabilities (General)

March of Dimes Birth Defects Foundation
  1275 Mamaroneck Avenue, White Plains, NY 10605
National Genetics Foundation
  P.O. Box 1374, New York, NY 10101
National Organization on Disability
  910 16th Street, NW, Room 600, Washington, DC
  20006
National Parent Network on Disabilities
  1600 Prince Street, #115, Alexandria, VA 22314
Society for the Advancement of Travel for the
  Handicapped
  327 Fifth Avenue, Suite 610, New York, NY 10016

Disabilities (Mental)

Association for Children and Adults with Learning
  Disabilities
  4156 Library Road, Pittsburgh, PA 15234
Association for Retarded Citizens
  500 East Border Street, Suite 300, Arlington, TX 76010
Autism Society for America
  1234 Massachusetts Avenue, NW, Suite C-1017,
  Washington, DC 20005
National Association for Down's Syndrome
  P.O. Box 4542, Oak Park, IL 60522
National Center for Learning Disabilities
  99 Park Avenue, 6th Floor, New York, NY 10016
Stuttering Foundation of America
  P.O. Box 11749, 3100 Walnut Grove Road, #603,
  Memphis, TN 38111
  Telephone: (800) 992-9392

Disabilities (Physical)

Alexander Graham Bell Association for the Deaf
  3417 Volta Place, NW, Washington, DC 20007-2778
American Foundation for the Blind
  15 West 16th Street, New York, NY 10011
Association for Education and Rehabilitation of the Blind
  and Visually Impaired
  206 North Washington Street, Suite 320, Alexandria,
  VA 22314
Braille Institute
  741 North Vermont Avenue, Los Angeles, CA 90029
National Association of the Physically Handicapped
  76 Elm Street, London, OH 43140

Winners on Wheels
  2842 Business Park Avenue, Fresno, CA 93727

Disaster Care

American Red Cross
  17th and D Streets, NW, Washington, DC 20006
Salvation Army World Service Office
  P.O. Box 269, Alexandria, VA 22313
  Telephone: (703) 684-5528

Disease/Disorder Prevention and Research

Alzheimer's Disease and Related Disorders Association
  919 North Michigan Avenue, Suite 1000, Chicago, IL
  60611
American Cancer Society's Cancer Response System
  1599 Clifton Road, NE, Atlanta, GA 30329
  Telephone: (800) ACS-2345
American Diabetes Association National Service Center
  P.O. Box 25757, 1660 Duke Street, Alexandria, VA
  22313
American Epilepsy Society
  c/o Priscilla S. Bourgeois, 179 Allyn Street, #304,
  Hartford, CT 06103
American Heart Association
  7272 Greenville Avenue, Dallas, TX 75231-4596
American Hepatitis Association (AHA)
  30 East 40th Street, Room 305, New York, NY 10016
American Liver Foundation
  998 Pomptom Avenue, Cedar Grove, NJ 07009
American Lung Association
  1740 Broadway, New York, NY 10019
  Telephone: (212) 315-8700
American Lupus Society Information
  260 Maple Court, Suite 123, Ventura, CA 93003
American Parkinson Disease Association
  116 John Street, Suite 417, New York, NY 10038
Arthritis Foundation
  1314 Spring Street, NW, Atlanta, GA 30309
Asthma and Allergy Foundation of America
  1717 Massachusetts Avenue, Suite 305, Washington,
  DC 20036
Centers for Disease Control and Prevention (CDC)
  1600 Clifton Road, NE, Atlanta, GA 30333
Huntington's Disease Society of America
  140 West 22nd Street, 6th Floor, New York, NY
  10011-2420
International Association of Cancer Victims and Friends
  7740 W. Manchester Avenue, Suite 110, Playa del
  Rey, CA 90293
Juvenile Diabetes Foundation International
  432 Park Avenue, South, New York, NY 10016
Leukemia Society of America
  733 Third Avenue, New York, NY 10017
Living Bank
  P.O. Box 6725, Houston, TX 77625

Lupus Foundation of America
  1717 Massachusetts Avenue, NW, Suite 203,
  Washington, DC 20036
Mended Hearts
  c/o American Heart Association, 7320 Greenville
  Avenue, Dallas, TX 75231
Multiple Sclerosis Association of America
  601 White Horse Pike, Oaklyn, NJ 08107
Muscular Dystrophy Association
  810 Seventh Avenue, New York, NY 10019
Myasthenia Gravis Foundation
  53 West Jackson Boulevard, Suite 909, Chicago, IL
  60604
National Cancer Institute
  NIOH, 900 Rockville Pike, Bethesda, MD 20892
National Hemophilia Foundation
  110 Green Street, Room 406, New York, NY 10012
National Institute of Neuro Disorders and Stroke
  Building 31, Room 8AOy, 31 Center Drive, MSC 2540,
  Bethesda, MD 20892-2540
National Kidney Foundation
  2 Park Avenue, New York, NY 10003
National Lupus Erythematosus Foundation
  5430 Van Nuys Boulevard, Suite 206, Van Nuys, CA
  91401
National Organization for Rare Disorders
  P.O. Box 8923, New Fairfield, CT 06812-8923
National Osteoporosis Foundation
  1150 17th Street, Suite 500, NW, Washington, DC
  20036-4603
National Tay-Sachs and Allied Diseases Association
  385 Elliot Street, Newton, MA 02164
United Cerebral Palsy Association
  66 East 34th Street, New York, NY 10016

Ethnic Health

American Indian Health Care Association
  245 East 6th Street, Suite 499, Saint Paul, MN 55101
Asian American Health Forum, Inc.
  116 New Montgomery Street, Suite 531, San
  Francisco, CA 94105

Fitness

American Physical Fitness Research Institute
  654 North Sepulveda Boulevard, Los Angeles, CA
  90049

Health Care Delivery

Agency for Health Care Policy and Research
  Executive Office Center, Suite 603, 2101 East Jefferson
  Street, Rockville, MD 20852
American Association for Continuity of Care
  1730 North Lynn Street, Arlington, VA 22209
American Federation of Home Health Agencies
  1320 Fenwick Lane, Suite 100, Silver Spring, MD 20910

Center for Home Care Policy and Research
  107 East 70th Street, New York, NY 10021
Health Care Financing Administration (HCFA)
  6325 Security Boulevard, Baltimore, MD 21207
National Association for Home Care
  228 Seventh Street, SE, Washington DC 20003
  Telephone: (202) 547-7424

Injury Treatment and Prevention

Agency for Toxic Substances and Disease Registry
  (ATSDR)
  1600 Clifton Road, NE, Mail Stop E-28, Atlanta, GA
  30333
  Telephone: (404) 639-0501
American Association of Poison Control Centers
  3800 Reservoir Road, NW, Washington, DC 20007
  Telephone: (202) 784-4666; FAX: (202) 784-2530
American Burn Association
  c/o Shriners Burn Institute, 202 Goodman Street,
  Cincinnati, OH 45219
Consumer Product Safety Commission
  East West Towers, 4340 East West Highway,
  Bethesda, MD 20814
National Safety Council
  1121 Spring Lake Drive, Itasca, IL 60143-3201
  Telephone: (630) 285-1121

Maternal/Child Health

American Fertility Society
  2140 Eleventh Avenue, South, Suite 200, Birmingham,
  AL 35205
American Foundation for Maternal and Child Health
  (AFMC)
  439 East 51st Street, New York, NY 10022
International Childbirth Education Association
  P.O. Box 20048, Minneapolis, MN 55420
La Leche League International
  9616 Minneapolis Avenue, P.O. Box 1209, Franklin
  Park, IL 60131
National Association of Childbearing Centers
  3123 Gottschall Road, Perkiomenville, PA 18074-
  9546
National Sudden Infant Death Syndrome Foundation
  8200 Professional Plaza, Suite 104, Landover, MD
  20785
Planned Parenthood Federation of America
  810 Seventh Avenue, New York, NY 10019

Mental Illness

American Association of Suicidology
  Suite 310, 4201 Connecticut Avenue, NW,
  Washington, DC 20008
  Telephone: (202) 237-2280

American Mental Health Foundation
   2 East 86th Street, New York, NY 10028
National Alliance for the Mentally Ill (NAMI)
   200 North Glebe Road, Suite 1015, Arlington, VA
   22203-3754
   Telephone: (800) 950-6264
National Mental Health Association
   1021 Prince Street, Alexandria, VA 22314

Migrant Health

Migrant Clinicians Network
   2512 South Interstate Highway 35, Suite 220, Austin,
   TX 78704
National Migrant Resource Program
   2512 South Interstate Highway 35, Suite 220, Austin,
   TX 78704

Nursing Organizations

American Association of Occupational Health Nurses
   (AAOHN)
   50 Lenox Pointe, Atlanta, GA 30324
   Telephone: (800) 241-8014, (404) 262-1162
American Nurses Association (ANA)
   600 Maryland Avenue, SW, Suite 100 W, Washington,
   DC 20024-2571
   Telephone: (202) 554-4444
Hospice Nurses' Association
   P.O. Box 8166, Van Nuys, CA 91409-8166
International Association for Human Caring (IAHC)
   School of Nursing, La Salle University, Philadelphia,
   PA 19141
National Association of School Nurses
   Lamplighter Lane, P.O. Box 1300, Scarborough, ME
   04074
   Telephone: (207) 883-2117
National Nurses' Society on Addictions (NNSA)
   4101 Lake Boone Trail, Suite 201, Raleigh, NC 27607-
   6518
Nurse Healers—Professional Associates, Inc. (NH–PA)
   1211 Locust Street, Philadelphia, PA 19107
Visiting Nurse Associations of America
   3801 East Florida Street, Suite 900, Denver, CO
   80210

Nutritional Health

National Center for Nutrition and Dietetics Consumer
   Hotline
   Telephone: (800) 366-1655
National Dairy Council
   6300 North River Road, Rosemont, IL 60018-4289
Society for Nutrition Education
   2001 Killebrew Drive, Suite 340, Minneapolis, MN
   55425-1882

Occupational and Environmental Health

Association of Occupational and Environmental Clinics
   (AOEC)
   1010 Vermont Avenue, Suite 513, Washington, DC
   20005
The EnviroLink Network
   4618 Henry Street, Pittsburgh, PA 15213
   Telephone: (412) 683-6400
Environmental Protection Agency (EPA)
   401 M Street, SW, Washington, DC 20460
Extension Toxicology Network (EXTOXNET)
   University of Davis, Davis, CA 95616-8588
   Telephone: (916) 752-2936; FAX: (916) 752-0903
Job Accommodation Network
   West Virginia University, P.O. Box 6080,
   Morgantown, WV 26506-6080
National Coalition Against the Misuse of Pesticides
   (NCAMP)
   701 E Street, SE, Suite 200, Washington, DC 20003
National Environment Health Association
   720 South Colorado Boulevard, Suite 970, South
   Tower, Denver, CO 80222
   Telephone: (301) 756-9090
National Institute for Occupational Safety and Health
   (NIOSH)
   Hubert Humphrey Building, 200 Independence
   Avenue, SW, Room 715H, Washington, DC 20201
   Telephone: (202) 260-0901
Occupational Safety and Health Administration (OSHA)
   U.S. Department of Labor, 200 Constitution Avenue,
   NW, Washington, DC 20210
   Office of Information and Consumer Affairs
   telephone: (202) 219-8151
   Office of Statistics telephone: (202) 219-6463
Pesticide Education Center
   P.O. Box 420870, San Francisco, CA 94142-0870
   Telephone: (415) 391-8511
Society for Occupational and Environmental Health
   6728 Old McLean Village Drive, McLean, VA 22101
   Telephone: (703) 556-9222

Rural Health

National Association of Rural Health Clinics
   426 C Street, NE, Washington, DC 20002
   Telephone: (202) 543-0348; FAX: (202) 543-2565
National Association for Rural Mental Health
   P.O. Box 570, Wood River, IL 62095
   Telephone: (618) 251-0589
National Organization of State Offices of Rural Health
   Office of Rural Health, 1000 N.E. 10th Street, Fifth
   Floor, Oklahoma City, OK 73117-1299
   Telephone: (405) 271-8750; FAX: (405) 271-8877
National Rural Health Association (NRHA)
   1 West Armdour Boulevard, Suite 301, Kansas City,
   MO 64111
   Telephone: (816) 756-3140; FAX: (816) 756-3144

Rural Information Center Health Services (RICHS)
Rural Information Center Health Service, National Agricultural Library
Room 304, 10301 Baltimore Avenue, Beltsville, MD 20705-2351
Telephone: (800) 633-7701, (301) 504-5547
Online: http://www.nal.usda.gov/ric/richs
key words: Rural Health

Self-Help

National Council on Self-Help and Public Health
515 North State Street, Chicago, IL 60610

Sexual Health

American Association of Sex Educators, Counselors and Therapists (AASECT)
11 Dupont Circle, NW, Suite 220, Washington, DC 20036
State offices listed on the Internet
National Coalition Against Sexual Assault
912 North 2nd Street, Harrisburg, PA 17102-3119
Telephone: (717) 232-7460
National Lesbian and Gay Health Foundation
1407 S Street, NW, Washington, DC 20009
Telephone: (202) 939-7880

Substance Abuse/Addictions

AL-ANON Family Group Headquarters, Inc.
1372 Broadway, New York, NY 10018
Alcoholics Anonymous World Services
P.O. Box 459, Grand Central Station, New York, NY 10163
Alcohol and Drug Problems Association of North America, Inc.
444 North Capitol Street, NW, Suite 181, Washington, DC 20001
National Committee for the Prevention of Alcoholism and Drug Dependency
RR 1, Box 635, Appomattox, VA 24522
National Council on Alcoholism
12 West 21st Street, New York, NY 10010

Wellness

National Wellness Institute
1300 College Court, P.O. Box 827, Stevens Point, WI 54481-0827
Telephone: (715) 342-2969
Wellness Councils of America
555 Thirteenth Street, NW, Suite 1220 E, Washington, DC 20004-1109
Telephone: (202) 637-6841

Women's Health

National Women's Health Resource Center
5255 Loughboro Road, NW, Washington, DC 20016
Telephone: (202) 537-4015
Nursing Network on Violence Against Women
c/o Mary Jo Betler, 3110 McCorkle Avenue, SE, Charleston, WV 25304-1299

CANADIAN HEALTH-RELATED ORGANIZATIONS—GENERAL

(List compiled by Tania Nahulak, Judy Seguin, Cindy Zachow, and Chantelle Grahma, Nursing Students at Okanagan University College, Kelowna, British Columbia.)
The Canadian Health Network
Inquiries—13th Floor, Brooke Claxton Building, Ottawa, Ontario K1A 0K9
Telephone: (613) 957-2991
Canadian Medical Association
1867 Alta Vista Drive, Ottawa, Ontario K1G 3Y6
Telephone: (613) 731-9331
Canadian Public Health Association
1565 Carling Avenue, Suite 400, Ottawa, Ontario K1Z 8R1
Telephone: (613) 725-9826
David Foster Foundation Society
3795 Carey Road, Victoria, British Columbia V8T 6T8
Telephone: (250) 475-1223
Health Canada (General Inquiries)
13th Floor, Brooke Claxton Building, Tunney's, Ottawa, Ontario K1A 0K9
Telephone: (613) 957-2991
Statistics Canada
National Capital Region Statistics Canada, Ottawa, Ontario K1A 0T6
Telephone: (613) 951-8116
Vital Statistics
818 Fort Street, Victoria, British Columbia V8W 1H8

CANADIAN HEALTH-RELATED ORGANIZATIONS—SPECIFIC

Aging

Canadian Association on Gerontology
1306 Wellington Street, Suite 500, Ottawa, Ontario K1Y 3B2
Telephone: (613) 728-9347
Health Canada's Division of Aging and Seniors
473 Albert Street, 3rd Floor-4203A, Ottawa, Ontario K1A 0K9
Telephone: (613) 952-7606

Alternative Medicine

Acupuncture Foundation of Canada Institute
   2131 Lawrence Avenue, East, Suite 204, Scarborough,
   Ontario M1R 5G4
   Telephone: (416) 752-3988
Canadian Association for Music Therapy
   Wilfred Laurier University, Waterloo, Ontario, N2L 3C5
   Telephone: (519) 884-2970
Canadian Medical Acupuncture Society
   9904-106 Street, NW, Edmonton, Alberta, T5K 1C4
   Telephone: (403) 426-2760

Child Health

Canadian Child Care Federation
   30 Rosemount Avenue, Suite 100, Ottawa, Ontario
   K1Y 1P4
   Telephone: (613) 729-5289
Canadian Foundation for the Study of Infant Deaths
   586 Eglinton Avenue, East, Suite 308, Toronto,
   Ontario, N4P 2P2
   Telephone: (416) 488-3260
Canadian Institute of Child Health
   885 Prom. Meadowlands Drive, Suite 512, Ottawa,
   Ontario, K2C 3N2
   Telephone: (613) 224-4144
Kids Help Phone/Jeunesse J'Ecoute
   439 University Avenue, Suite 300, Toronto, Ontario
   M5G 1Y8
   Telephone: (416) 586-0100

Community Care

Canadian Association for Community Care
   45 Rideau Street, Suite 701, Ottawa, Ontario,
   K1N 5W8
   Telephone: (613) 241-7510

Death and Dying

Canadian Palliative Care
   Royal Victoria Hospital, R6, 687 Pine Avenue,
   Montreal, Quebec H3A 1A1
   Telephone: (613) 241-3663
Dying with Dignity
   188 Eglinton Avenue, East, Suite 706, Toronto,
   Ontario M4P 1P3
   Telephone: (416) 486-3998

Dental Health and Treatment

Canadian Dental Association
   1815 Alta Vista Drive, Ottawa, Ontario K1G 3Y6
   Telephone: (613) 532-1770

Disabilities (General)

Active Living Alliance for Canadians with a Disability
   1600 James Naismith Drive, Gloucester, Ontario
   K1B 5N4
   Telephone: (613) 748-5747
Canadian Abilities Foundation
   489 College Street, Suite 501, Toronto, Ontario
   M6G 1A5
   Telephone: (416) 923-1885
Neil Squire Foundation—National Office
   2250 Boundary Road, Suite 202, Burnaby, British
   Columbia V5M 4L9
   Telephone: (604) 473-9363

Disabilities (Physical)

Association for the Neurologically Disabled of Canada
   (ANDC)
   59 Clement Road, Etobicoke, Ontario M9R 1Y5
Canadian Association for the Deaf
   205-2435 Holly Lane, Ottawa, Ontario K1V 7P2
   Telephone: (613) 565-2882
Canadian Association for People Who Stutter (CAPS)
   P.O. Box 2274, Square One, 100 City Ce, Mississauga,
   Ontario L5B 3C8
Canadian Down's Syndrome Society
   811 14 Street, NW, Calgary, Alberta T2N 2A4
   Telephone: (403) 270-8500
Canadian Foundation for Physically Disabled Persons
   731 Runnymeade Road, Toronto, Ontario M6N 3V7
   Telephone: (416) 760-7351
Canadian Hard of Hearing Association
   2435 Holly Lane, Suite 205, Ottawa, Ontario K1V 7P2
   Telephone: (613) 526-1584
Canadian National Institute for the Blind—Toronto
   1929 Bayview Avenue, Toronto, Ontario M4G 3E8
   Telephone: (416) 480-7415
Canadian Paraplegic Association—National
   1101 Prince of Wales Drive, Suite 320, Ottawa,
   Ontario K2C 3W7
   Telephone: (613) 723-1033
Canadian Spinal Research Organization
   120 Newkirk Road, Unit 32, Richmond Hill, Ontario
   L4C 9S3
   Telephone: (905) 508-4000
Easter Seals/March of Dimes National Council
   45 Sheppard Avenue East, Toronto, Ontario
   M2N 5W9
   Telephone: (416) 250-7490
Learning Disabilities Association of Canada
   323 Chapel Street, Suite 200, Ottawa, Ontario K1N 7Z2
   Telephone: (613) 238-5721

Disaster Care

Canadian Red Cross Society
   1800 Alta Vista Drive, Ottawa, Ontario K1G 4S5
   Telephone: (613) 739-3000

Disease/Disorder Prevention and Research

Allergy Foundation of Canada
 Box 1904, Saskatoon, Saskatchewan S7K 2S5
 Telephone: (306) 652-1608

Arthritis Society—National
 393 University Avenue, Suite 1700, Toronto, Ontario
 M5G 1E6
 Telephone: (416) 979-7228

Asthma Society of Canada
 130 Bridgeland Avenue, Suite 425, Toronto, Ontario
 M6A 1Z4
 Telephone: (416) 787-4050

Autism Society of Canada
 Suite 202, 129 Yorkville Avenue, Toronto, Ontario
 M5C 4C4
 Telephone: (416) 922-0302

Autism Treatment Services of Canada
 404-94 Avenue, SE, Calgary, Alberta T2J 0E8
 Telephone: (403) 253-6961

Breast Cancer Society of Canada
 401 St. Clair Street, Point Edwards, Ontario N7V 1P2
 Telephone: (519) 336-0746

Canadian AIDS Society
 400-100 Sparks Street, Ottawa, Ontario K1P 5B7
 Telephone: (613) 230-3580

Canadian Cancer Society
 10 Alcorn Avenue, Suite 200, Toronto, Ontario
 M4V 3B1
 Telephone: (416) 961-7223

Canadian Cardiovascular Society
 222 Queen Street, Suite 1403, Ottawa, Ontario K1P 5V9
 Telephone: (613) 569-3407

Canadian Celiac Association—National
 6519B Mississauga Road, Mississauga, Ontario
 L5N 1A6
 Telephone: (905) 567-7195

Canadian Cystic Fibrosis Foundation
 2221 Yonge Street, Suite 601, Toronto, Ontario
 M45 ZB4
 Telephone: (416) 485-9149

Canadian Diabetes Association—National
 15 Toronto Street, Suite 800, Toronto, Ontario M5C 2E3
 Telephone: (416) 363-3393

Canadian Hemophilia Society
 625 President Kennedy Avenue, Montreal, Quebec
 H3A 1K2

Canadian Infectious Diseases Society, Ontario
 441 MacLaren, Suite 260, Ottawa, Ontario K2P 2H3
 Telephone: (613) 234-4387

Canadian Infectious Diseases Society, Quebec
 c/o Hospital Saint-Luc, 1057 rue Saint-D, Montreal,
 Quebec H2X 3J4
 Telephone: (514) 281-2100

Canadian Liver Foundation
 365 Bloor Street, East, Suite 200, Toronto, Ontario
 M4W 3L4
 Telephone: (416) 964-1953

Canadian Lung Association
 1900 City Park Drive, Suite 508, Gloucester, Ontario
 K1J 1A3
 Telephone: (613) 747-6776

Canadian Organization for Rare Disorders (CORD)
 P.O. Box 814, Coaldale, Alberta T1M 1M7
 Telephone: (403) 345-4544

Canadian Psoriasis Foundation—National
 1306 Wellington Street, Suite 500A, Ottawa, Ontario
 K1Y 3B2
 Telephone: (613) 728-4000

Candlelighters Childhood Cancer Foundation Canada
 55 Eglinton Avenue, East, Suite 401, Toronto, Ontario
 M4P 1G8
 Telephone: (416) 489-6440

CANFAR
 165 University Avenue, Suite 901, Toronto, Ontario
 M5H 3B8
 Telephone: (416) 361-6281

Crohn's and Colitis Foundation of Canada
 21 St. Clair Avenue, East, Toronto, Ontario M4T 1L9
 Telephone: (416) 920-5035

Environmental Illness Society of Canada
 536 Dovercourt Avenue, Ottawa, Ontario K2A 0T9
 Telephone: (613) 728-9493

Epilepsy Canada/Epilepsie Canada
 1470 Peel Street, Suite 745, Montreal, Quebec H3A 1T1
 Telephone: (514) 845-7855

Heart and Stroke Foundation of Canada—National
 Office
 160 George Street, Suite 200, Ottawa, Ontario K1N 9M2
 Telephone: (613) 241-4361

Huntington Society of Canada
 P.O. Box 1269, Cambridge, Ontario N1R 7G6
 Telephone: (519) 622-1002

Kidney Foundation of Canada—National Office
 5165, rue Sherbrooke Quest, Suite 300, Montreal,
 Quebec H4A 1T6

Lupus Canada
 P.O. Box 64034, 5512 Four Street, NW, Calgary, Alberta
 Telephone: (403) 274-5599

Migraine Association of Canada
 365 Bloor Street, East, Suite 1912, Toronto, Ontario
 M4W 3L4
 Telephone: (416) 920-4916

Multiple Sclerosis Society of Canada
 250 Bloor Street, East, Suite 1000, Toronto, Ontario
 M4W 3P9
 Telephone: (416) 922-6065

Muscular Dystrophy Association of Canada
 2345 Yonge Street, Suite 900, Toronto, Ontario M4P 2E5
 Telephone: (416) 488-0030

National ME/FM (Myalgic Encephalomyelitis/Chronic
 Fatigue Syndrome)
 3836 Carling Avenue, Nepean, Ontario K2K 2Y6
 Telephone: (613) 829-6667

National Tay-Sachs and Allied Disease of Ontario
 512 Wicklow Road, Burlington, Ontario L7L 2H8
 Telephone: (905) 634-4101

North American Chronic Pain Association of Canada
150 Central Park Drive, Unit 105, Brampton, Ontario L6T 1T9
Telephone: (905) 793-5230

Osteoporosis Society of Canada
33 Laird Drive, Toronto, Ontario M4G 3S9
Telephone: (416) 696-2663

Parkinson Foundation of Canada
390 Bay Street, Suite 710, Toronto, Ontario M5H 2Y2
Telephone: (416) 366-0099

Pediatric AIDS Canada
269 Juniper Avenue, Burlington, Ontario L7L 2T5
Telephone: (905) 631-8818

Sleep Disorders of Canada
3080 Yonge Street, Suite 5055, Toronto, Ontario M4N 3N1
Telephone: (416) 483-9654

Spina Bifida and Hydrocephalus Association of Canada
220-388 Donald Street, Winnipeg, Manitoba R3B 2J4
Telephone: (204) 957-1784

Terry Fox Foundation
60 St. Clair Avenue, East, Suite 605, Toronto, Ontario M4T 1N5
Telephone: (416) 962-7866

Thyroid Foundation of Canada
1040 Gardeiners Road, Suite C, Kingston, Ontario K7P 1R7
Telephone: (613) 634-3426

Turners Syndrome Society
7777 Keele Street, Floor 2, Concord, Ontario L4K 1Y7
Telephone: (905) 660-7766

Family Health

Canadian Association of Family Resource Programs
101-30 Rosemount Avenue, Ottawa, Ontario K1Y 1P4
Telephone: (613) 728-3307

Nobody's Perfect, Family and Child Health Unit—Health Canada
Health Promotion Directorate, 4th Floor, Je, Ottawa, Ontario K1A 1B4
Telephone: (613) 957-7804

One Parent Families Association of Canada
6979 Yonge Street, Suite 203, Willowdale, Ontario M2M 3X9
Telephone: (416) 226-0062

Fitness

Canadian Fitness and Lifestyle Research Institute
201-185 Somerset Street, West, Ottawa, Ontario K2P 0J2
Telephone: (613) 233-5528

Health Care Delivery

Canadian Institute for Health Information and Canadian Institute for Health Promotion
377 Dalhousie Street, Suite 200, Ottawa, Ontario K1N 9N8
Telephone: (613) 241-7860

Injury Treatment and Prevention

Canadian Association of Poison Control Centers
Health Sciences Center, 840 Sherbook, Winnipeg, Manitoba R3A 1S1
Telephone: (204) 787-2445

Canadian Injury Prevention Foundation
20 Queen Street, West, Suite 200, Toronto, Ontario M5H 3V7
Telephone: (416) 979-4012

MADD Canada
141-6200 McKay Avenue, Suite 524, Burnaby, British Columbia V5H 4M9
Telephone: (604) 515-9212

War Amps of Canada
530-140 Merton Street, Toronto, Ontario M4S 1A5
Telephone: (416) 488-0600

Maternal/Child Health

Infertility Awareness Association of Canada
Suite 104-1785 Alta Vista Drive, Ottawa, Ontario K1G 3Y6
Telephone: (613) 738-8968

Mother Risk Program
555 University Avenue, Toronto, Ontario M5G 1X8
Telephone: (613) 813-6780

Planned Parenthood Federation of Canada
1 Nicholas Street, Suite 430, Ottawa, Ontario K7B 7B7
Telephone: (613) 238-4474

Mental Illness

Alzheimer Society of Canada
20 Eglinton Avenue, West, Suite 1200, Toronto, Ontario M4R 1K8
Telephone: (416) 488-8772

Anorexia Nervosa and Bulimia Association
767 Bayridge Drive, P.O. Box 20058, Kingston, Ontario K7P 1C0
Telephone: (613) 547-3684

Canadian Association for Suicide Prevention
Suite 201, 1615 Tenth Avenue, SW, Calgary, Alberta T3C 0J7
Telephone: (403) 245-3900

Canadian Mental Health Association—National
2160 Yonge Street, 3rd Floor, Toronto, Ontario M4S 2Z3
Telephone: (416) 484-7750

National Clearinghouse on Family Violence—Health Canada
Health Promotion and Programs Branch, Ottawa, Ontario K1A 1B4
Telephone: (613) 957-2938

Schizophrenia Society of Canada
75 The Donway West, Suite 814, Don Mills, Ontario M3C 2E9
Telephone: (416) 445-8204

Nursing Organizations

Canadian Nurses Association
    50 The Driveway, Ottawa, Ontario K2P 1E2
    Telephone: (613) 237-2133
Canadian Nursing Students' Association (CNSA)
    325-350 Albert Street, Ottawa, Ontario K1R 1B1
    Telephone: (613) 563-1236

Nutritional Health

Dietitians of Canada
    480 University Avenue, Suite 604, Toronto, Ontario
    M5G 1V2
    Telephone: (416) 596-0857

Occupational and Environmental Health

Canada Safety Council
    1020 Thomas Spratt Place, Ottawa, Ontario K1G 5L5
    Telephone: (613) 739-1535
Canadian Centre for Occupational Health and Safety
    250 Main Street, East, Hamilton, Ontario L8N 1H6
    Telephone: (905) 572-4400
Canadian Standards Association
    178 Rexdale Boulevard, Etobicoke, Ontario M9W 1R3
    Telephone: (416) 747-4000

Sexual Health

Sex Information and Education Council of Canada
    850 Coxwell Avenue, East York, Ontario M4C 5R1
    Telephone: (416) 466-5304

Substance Abuse/Addictions

Al-Anon Family Group Headquarters
    P.O. Box 6433, Station J, Ottawa, Ontario K2A 3Y6
    Telephone: (613) 722-1783
Canadian Centre on Substance Abuse—FAS/FAE
    Information
    75 Albert Street, Suite 300, Ottawa, Ontario K1P 5E7
    Telephone: (613) 235-4048

Canadian Foundation on Compulsive Gambling
    505 Consumers Road, Suite 605, Willowdale, Ontario
    M2J 4V8
    Telephone: (416) 499-9800
Canadian Foundation for Drug Policy
    70 MacDonald Street, Ottawa, Ontario K2P 1H6
    Telephone: (613) 236-1027

Women's Health

Elizabeth Fry Society
    195A Bank Street, Ottawa, Ontario K2P 1W7
    Telephone: (613) 238-1171

List compiled by Tania Nahulak, Judy Seguin, Cindy
Zachow, and Chantelle Grahma, Nursing Students at
Okanagan University College, Kelowna, British
Columbia.

AUSTRALIAN HEALTH-RELATED ORGANIZATION

Disability Information and Communication Exchange
    (DICE)
    P.O. Box 407, Curtain ACT 2605, Australia
    Telephone: (06) 285-3713; FAX: (06) 285-3714

INTERNATIONAL HEALTH-RELATED ORGANIZATIONS

Global Health Network
    University of Pittsburgh, Pittsburgh, PA 15260
International Council of Nursing (ICN)
    1 place Jean-Marteau, CH-12101 Geneva, Switzerland
    Telephone: (22) 731-2960
International Healthy Cities Foundation
    One Kaiser Plaza, Suite 1930, Oakland, CA 94612
La Leche League International
    P.O. Box 4079, Schaumburg, IL 60173-4048
    Telephone: (847) 519-7730
National Council for International Health
    1701 K. Street, NW, Suite 600, Washington, DC 20006
World Health Organization (WHO)
    1211 Geneva, Switzerland

APPENDIX C
Lifestyle Assessment Questionnaire*

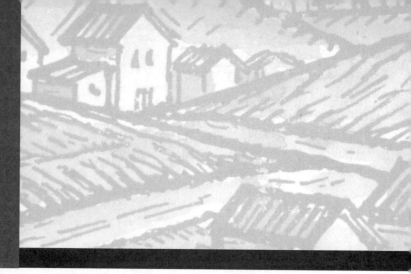

PURPOSE

This assessment tool and the analysis it provides are designed to help you discover how the choices you make each day affect your overall health.

By participating in this assessment process, you will also learn how you can make positive changes in your lifestyle, enabling you to reach a higher level of wellness.

Some of the questions are personal. While you may have leave them blank, the more information you provide about your current lifestyle, the more accurately the LAQ can assess your current level of wellness and risk areas.

CONFIDENTIALITY

The National Wellness Institute, Inc. subscribes to the guidelines established by the Society of Prospective Medicine concerning confidentiality in the use of health risk appraisals and risk reduction systems. These guidelines specifically state that only the participant and health professionals authorized by the participant should receive copies of his/her own health risk appraisal results.

The National Wellness Institute, Inc. strongly encourages all users of the LAQ to strictly follow these guidelines and maintain the confidentiality of all answers.

WHAT IS WELLNESS?

Wellness is an active process of becoming aware of and making choices toward a higher level of well-being. **Remember, leading a wellness lifestyle requires your active involvement.** As you gain more knowledge about what enhances your well-being, you are encouraged to use this information to make informed choices which lead to a healthier life.

The Lifestyle Assessment Questionnaire was written by the National Wellness Institute, Inc.'s Cofounders; Dennis Elsenrath, Ed.D., Bill Hettler, M.D., and Fred Leafgren, Ph.D.

*1997. Reprinted with permission. Copyright 1992 by the National Wellness Institute, Inc.

Section 1: PERSONAL DATA

INSTRUCTIONS:

Please complete the following general information about yourself. Please take your time and read each question carefully.

1. Sex
   a) male
   b) female
2. Race
   a) White
   b) Black
   c) Hispanic
   d) Asian
   e) American Indian
   f) other
3. Age
4. Height (feet and inches)
5. Weight (pounds)
6. Body frame size
   a) small
   b) medium
   c) large
7. Marital Status
   a) married
   b) widowed
   c) separated
   d) divorced
   e) single
   f) cohabiting
8. What was the total gross income of your household last year?
   a) under $12,000
   b) $12,000–$20,000
   c) $20,001–$30,000
   d) $30,001–$40,000
   e) $40,001–$50,000
   f) $50,001–$60,000
   g) over $60,000
9. What is the highest level of education you have completed?
   a) grade school or less
   b) some high school
   c) high school graduate
   d) some college or technical school
   e) college graduate
   f) postgraduate or professional degree
10. On the average day, how many hours do you watch television?
    a) 0 hours
    b) 1–3 hours
    c) 4–7 hours
    d) more than 8 hours
11. Where do you live?
    a) in the country
    b) in a city
    c) suburb
    d) small town
12. If you live in a city, suburb, or small town, what is the population?
    a) under 20,000
    b) 20,000–50,000
    c) 50,001–100,000
    d) 100,001–500,000
    e) over 500,000

Section 2: LIFESTYLE

INSTRUCTIONS:

This section will help determine your level of wellness. It will also give you ideas for areas in which you might improve. Some questions touch on very personal subjects. Therefore, if you prefer to skip certain questions, you may. However, the more questions you answer, the more you will learn about your health and how to improve it.

Please respond to these statements using the following responses. If an item does not apply to you, do not mark it.

   A. Almost always (90% or more of the time)
   B. Very often (approximately 75% of the time)
   C. Often (approximately 50% of the time)
   D. Occasionally (approximately 25% of the time)
   E. Almost never (less than 10% of the time)

PHYSICAL EXERCISE

Measures one's commitment to maintaining physical fitness.

1. I exercise vigorously for at least 20 minutes three or more times per week.
2. I determine my activity level by monitoring my heart rate.
3. I stop exercising before I feel exhausted.
4. I exercise in a relaxed, calm, and joyful manner.
5. I stretch before exercising.
6. I stretch after exercising.
7. I walk or bike whenever possible.
8. I participate in a strenuous activity (tennis, running, brisk walking, water exercise, swimming, handball, basketball, etc.).
9. If I am not in shape, I avoid sporadic (once a week or less often), strenuous exercise.
10. After vigorous exercise, I "cool down" (very light exercise such as walking) for at least five minutes before sitting or lying down.

NUTRITION

Measures the degree to which one chooses foods that are consistent with the dietary goals of the United States as published by the Senate Select Committee on Nutrition and Human Needs.

11. When choosing non-vegetable protein, I select lean cuts of meat, poultry, fish, and low-fat dairy products.
12. I maintain an appropriate weight for my height and frame.
13. I minimize salt intake.
14. I eat fruits and vegetables, fresh and uncooked.
15. I eat breakfast.
16. I intentionally include fiber in my diet on a daily basis.
17. I drink enough fluid to keep my urine light yellow.
18. I plan my diet to ensure an adequate amount of vitamins and minerals.
19. I minimize foods in my diet that contain large amounts of refined flour (bleached white flour, typical store bread, cakes, etc.).
20. I minimize my intake of fats and oils including margarine and animal fats.

21. I include items from all four basic food groups in my diet each day (fruits and vegetables; milk group; breads and cereals; meat, fowl, fish or vegetable proteins).
22. To avoid unnecessary calories, I choose water as one of the beverages I drink.
23. I avoid adding sugar to my foods. I minimize my intake of pre-sweetened foods (sugarcoated cereals, syrups, chocolate milk, and most processed and fast foods).

SELF-CARE

Measures the behaviors which help one prevent or detect early illnesses.

24. I use footgear of good quality designed for the activity or the job in which I participate.
25. I record immunizations to maintain up-to-date immunization records.
26. I examine my breasts or testes on a monthly basis.
27. I have my breasts or testes examined yearly by a physician.
28. I balance the type and amount of food I eat with exercise to maintain a healthy percent body fat.
29. I take action to minimize my exposure to tobacco smoke.
30. When I experience illness or injury, I take necessary steps to correct the problem.
31. I engage in activities which keep my blood pressure in a range which minimizes my chances of disease (e.g., stroke, heart attack, and kidney disease).
32. I brush my teeth after eating.
33. I floss my teeth after eating.
34. My resting pulse is 60 or less.
35. I get an adequate amount of sleep.
36. If I were to have sex, I would take action to prevent unplanned pregnancy.
37. If I were to have sex, I would take action to prevent giving and/or getting sexually transmitted disease.

VEHICLE SAFETY

Measures one's ability to minimize chances of injury or death in a vehicle accident.

38. I do not operate vehicles while I am under the influence of alcohol or other drugs.
39. I do not ride with drivers who under the influence of alcohol or other drugs.
40. I stay within the speed limit.
41. I practice defensive driving techniques.
42. When traffic lights change from green to yellow, I prepare to stop.
43. I maintain a safe driving distance between cars based on speed and road conditions.
44. Vehicles which I drive are maintained to assure safety.
45. Because they are safer, I use radial tires on cars that I drive.
46. When I ride a bicycle or motorcycle, I wear a helmet and have adequate lights/reflectors.
47. Children riding in my car are secured in an approved car seat or seat belt.
48. I use my seat belt while driving or riding in a vehicle.

DRUG USAGE AND AWARENESS

Measures the degree to which one functions without the unnecessary use of chemicals.

49. I use prescription drugs and over-the-counter medications only when necessary.
50. If I consume alcohol, I limit my consumption to not more than one drink per hour and no more than two drinks per day.
51. I avoid the use of tobacco.
52. Because of the potentially harmful effects of caffeine (e.g., coffee, tea, cola, etc.), I limit my consumption.
53. I avoid the use of marijuana.
54. I avoid the use of hallucinogens (LSD, PCP, MDA, etc.).
55. I avoid the use of stimulants ("uppers"—e.g., cocaine, amphetamines, "pep pills," etc.).
56. I avoid the use of nonmedically prescribed depressants ("downers"—e.g., barbiturates, quaaludes, minor tranquilizers, etc.).
57. I avoid using a combination of drugs unless under medical supervision.
58. I follow the instructions provided with any drug I take.
59. I avoid using drugs obtained from illegal sources.
60. I understand the expected effect of drugs I take.
61. I consider alternatives to drugs.
62. If I experience discomfort from stress or tension, I use relaxation techniques, exercise, and meditation instead of taking drugs.
63. I get clear directions for taking my medicine from my doctor or pharmacist.

SOCIAL/ENVIRONMENTAL

Measures the degree to which one contributes to the common welfare of the community. This emphasizes interdependence with others and nature.

64. I conserve energy at home.
65. I consider energy conservation when choosing a mode of transportation.
66. My social ties with family are strong.
67. I contribute to the feeling of acceptance within my family.
68. I develop and maintain strong friendships.
69. I do my part to promote a clean environment (i.e., air, water, noise, etc.).
70. When I see a safety hazard, I take action (warn others or correct the problem).
71. I avoid unnecessary radiation.
72. I report criminal acts I observe.
73. I contribute time and/or money to community projects.
74. I actively seek to become acquainted with individuals in my community.
75. I use my creativity in constructive ways.
76. My behavior reflects fairness and justice.
77. When possible, I choose an environment which is free of noise pollution.
78. When possible, I choose an environment which is free of air pollution.
79. I participate in volunteer activities benefiting others.
80. I help others in need.
81. I beautify those parts of my environment under my control.

82. Because of limited resources, I do my part to conserve.
83. I recycle aluminum, glass, and paper products.
84. I involve myself with people who support a positive lifestyle.

EMOTIONAL AWARENESS AND ACCEPTANCE

Measures the degree to which one has an awareness and acceptance of one's feelings. This includes the degree to which one feels positive and enthusiastic about oneself and life.

85. I have a good sense of humor.
86. I feel positive about myself.
87. I feel there is a satisfying amount of excitement in my life.
88. My emotional life is stable.
89. I am aware of my needs.
90. I trust and value my own judgment.
91. When I make mistakes, I learn from them.
92. I feel comfortable when complimented for jobs well done.
93. It is okay for me to cry.
94. I have feelings of sensitivity for others.
95. I feel enthusiastic about life.
96. I find it easy to laugh.
97. I am able to give love.
98. I am able to receive love.
99. I enjoy my life.
100. I have plenty of energy.
101. My sleep is restful.
102. I trust others.
103. I feel others trust me.
104. I accept my sexual desires.
105. I understand how I create my feelings.
106. At times, I can be both strong and sensitive.
107. I am aware when I feel angry.
108. I accept my anger.
109. I am aware when I feel sad.
110. I accept my sadness.
111. I am aware when I feel happy.
112. I accept my happiness.
113. I am aware when I feel frightened.
114. I accept my feelings of fear.
115. I am aware of my feelings about death.
116. I accept my feelings about death.

EMOTIONAL MANAGEMENT

Measures the degree to which one controls and expresses feelings, and engages in effective, related behaviors.

117. I share my feelings with those with whom I am close.
118. I express my feelings of anger in appropriate ways.
119. I express my feelings of sadness in healthy ways.
120. I express my feelings of happiness in desirable ways.
121. I express my feelings of fear in appropriate ways.
122. I compliment myself for a job well done.
123. I accept constructive criticism without reacting defensively.
124. I set appropriate limits for myself.
125. I stay within the limits that I have set.
126. I recognize that I can have wide variations of feelings about the same person (such as loving someone even though you are angry with her/him at the moment).
127. I am able to develop close, intimate relationships.
128. I say "no" without feeling guilty.
129. I would feel comfortable seeking professional help to better understand and cope with my feelings.
130. I reduce feelings of failure by setting achievable goals.
131. I relax my body and mind without using drugs.
132. I can be alone without feeling lonely.
133. I am able to be spontaneous in expressing my feelings.
134. I accept responsibility for my actions.
135. I am willing to take the risks that come with making change.
136. I manage my feelings to avoid unnecessary suffering.
137. I make decisions with a minimum of stress and worry.
138. I accept the responsibility for creating my own feelings.
139. I can express my feelings about death.
140. I recognize grieving as a healthy response to loss.

INTELLECTUAL

Measures the degree to which one engages her/his mind in creative, stimulating mental activities, expanding knowledge, and improving skills.

141. I read a newspaper daily.
142. I read twelve or more books yearly.
143. On the average, I read one or more national magazines per week.
144. When I watch TV, I choose programs with informational/educational value.
145. I visit a museum or art show at least three times yearly.
146. I attend lectures, workshops, and demonstrations at least three times yearly.
147. I regularly use some of my time participating in hobbies such as photography, gardening, woodworking, sewing, painting, baking, art, music, writing, pottery, etc.
148. I read about local, state, national, and international political/public issues.
149. I learn the meaning of new words.
150. I engage in some type of writing activity such as a regular journal, letter writing, preparation of papers or manuscripts, etc.
151. I am interested in understanding the views of others.
152. I share ideas, concepts, thoughts, or procedures with others.
153. I gather information to enable me to make decisions.
154. I listen to radio and/or TV news.
155. I think about ideas different than my own.

OCCUPATIONAL

Measures the satisfaction gained from one's work and the degree to which one is enriched by that work. Please answer these items from your primary frame of reference (e.g., your job, student, homemaker, etc.).

156. I enjoy my work.
157. My work contributes to my personal needs.
158. I feel that my job in some way contributes to my well-being.
159. I cooperate with others in my work.
160. I take advantage of opportunities to learn new work-related skills.
161. My work is challenging.
162. I feel my job responsibilities are consistent with my values.
163. I find satisfaction from the work I do.
164. I find healthy ways of reducing excessive job-related stress.
165. I use recommended health and safety precautions.
166. I make recommendations for improving worksite health and safety.
167. I am satisfied with the degree of freedom I have in my job to exercise independent judgments.
168. I am satisfied with the amount of variety in my work.
169. I believe I am competent in my job.
170. My co-workers and supervisors respect me as a competent individual.
171. My communication with others in my workplace is enriching for me.

SPIRITUAL

Measures one's ongoing involvement in seeking meaning and purpose in human existence. It includes an appreciation for the depth and expanse of life and natural forces that exist in the universe.

172. I feel good about my spiritual life.
173. Prayer, mediation, and/or quiet personal reflection is/are important part(s) of my life.
174. I contemplate my purpose in life.
175. I reflect on the meaning of events in my life.
176. My values guide my daily life.
177. My values and beliefs help me to meet daily challenges.
178. I recognize that my spiritual growth is a lifelong process.
179. I am concerned about humanitarian issues.
180. I enjoy participating in discussions about spiritual values.
181. I feel a sense of compassion for others in need.
182. I seek spiritual knowledge.
183. My spiritual awareness occurs other than at times of crisis.
184. I believe in something greater or that I am part of something greater than myself.
185. I share my spiritual values.

Section 3: HEALTH RISK APPRAISAL

INSTRUCTIONS:

This section is intended to help you identify the problems most likely to interfere with the quality of your life. It will also show you choices you can make to stay healthy and avoid the most common causes of death for a person your age and sex.

This Health Risk Appraisal is not a substitute for a checkup or physical exam that you get from a doctor or nurse. It only gives you some ideas for lowering your risk of getting sick or injured in the future. It is NOT designed for people who already have HEART DISEASE, CANCER, KIDNEY DISEASE, OR OTHER SERIOUS CONDITIONS. If you have any of these problems and you want a Health Risk Appraisal anyway, ask your doctor or nurse to read this section with you.

If you don't know or are unsure of an answer, please leave that item blank.

1. Have you ever been told that you have diabetes (or sugar diabetes)?
   a. yes
   b. no
2. Does your natural mother, father, sister or brother have diabetes?
   a. yes
   b. no
   c. not sure
3. Did either of your natural parents die of a heart attack before age 60? (If your parents are younger than 60, mark no).
   a. yes, one of them
   b. yes, both of them
   c. no
   d. not sure
4. Are you now taking medicine for high blood pressure?
   a. yes
   b. no
5. What is your blood pressure now?
   a. ____ systolic (high number)
   b. ____ diastolic (low number)
6. If you *do not* know the number, select the answer that describes your blood pressure.
   a. high
   b. normal or low
   c. don't know
7. What is your TOTAL cholesterol level (based on a blood test)?
   ____ (mg/dl)
8. What is your High Density Lipoprotein (HDL) cholesterol level (based on a blood test)?
   ____ (mg/dl)
9. How many cigars do you usually smoke per day?
   ____
10. How many pipes of tobacco do you usually smoke per day? ____
11. How many times per day do you usually use smokeless tobacco (chewing tobacco, snuff, pouches, etc.)? ____
12. How would you describe your cigarette smoking habits?
    a. never smoked **Go to 15**
    b. used to smoke **Go to 14**
    c. still smoke **Go to 13**

13. How many cigarettes a day do you smoke?
    ____ cigarettes per day **Go to 15**
14. a. How many years has it been since you smoked cigarettes regularly?
    ____ years
    b. What was the average number of cigarettes per day that you smoked in the 2 years before you quit?
    ____ cigarettes per day
15. In the next 12 months, how many thousands of miles will you probably travel by each of the following? (NOTE: U.S. averages = 10,000 miles)
    a. car, truck, or van: ____,000 miles
    b. motorcycle: ____,000 miles
16. On a typical day how do you USUALLY travel? (Check one only)
    a. walk
    b. bicycle
    c. motorcycle
    d. sub-compact or compact car
    e. mid-size or full-size car
    f. truck or van
    g. bus, subway, or train
    h. mostly stay home
17. What percent of the time do you usually buckle your safety belt when driving or riding?
    ____%
18. On the average, how close to the speed limit do you usually drive?
    a. within 5 mph of limit
    b. 6–10 mph over limit
    c. 11–15 mph over limit
    d. more than 15 mph over limit
19. How many times in the last month did you drive or ride when the driver had perhaps too much alcohol to drink?
    ____ times last month
20. When you drink alcoholic beverages, how many drinks do you consume in an average day? (If you *never* drink alcoholic beverages, write 0.)
    ____ alcoholic beverages/average day
21. On the average, how many days per week do you consume alcohol?
    ____ days/week

(MEN GO TO QUESTION 31)

WOMEN ONLY (QUESTIONS 22–30)

22. At what age did you have your first menstrual period?
    ____ years old
23. How old were you when your first child was born (if no children, write 0)?
    ____ years old
24. How long has it been since your last breast x-ray (mammogram)?
    a. less than 1 year ago
    b. 1 year ago
    c. 2 years ago
    d. 3 or more years ago
    e. never
25. How many women in your natural family (mother and sisters only) have had breast cancer?
    ____ women

26. Have you had a hysterectomy?
    a. yes
    b. no
    c. not sure
27. How long has it been since you had a Pap smear test?
    a. less than 1 year ago
    b. 1 year ago
    c. 2 years ago
    d. 3 or more years ago
    e. never
28. How often do you examine your breasts for lumps?
    a. monthly
    b. once every few months
    c. rarely or never
29. About how long has it been since you had your breasts examined by a physician or nurse?
    a. less than 1 year ago
    b. 1 year ago
    c. 2 years ago
    d. 3 or more years ago
    e. never
30. About how long has it been since you had a rectal exam?
    a. less than 1 year ago
    b. 1 year ago
    c. 2 years ago
    d. 3 or more years ago
    e. never

(WOMEN GO TO QUESTION 35)

MEN ONLY (QUESTIONS 31–34)

31. About how long has it been since you had a rectal or prostate exam?
    a. less than 1 year ago
    b. 1 year ago
    c. 2 years ago
    d. 3 or more years ago
    e. never
32. Do you know how to properly examine your testes for lumps?
    a. yes
    b. no
    c. not sure
33. How often do you examine your testes for lumps?
    a. monthly
    b. once every few months
    c. rarely or never
34. About how long has it been since you had your testes examined by a physician or nurse?
    a. less than one year ago
    b. 1 year ago
    c. 2 years ago
    d. 3 or more years ago
    e. never

35. How many times in the last year did you witness or become involved in a violent fight or attack where there was a good chance of a serious injury to someone?
    a. 4 or more times
    b. 2 or 3 times
    c. 1 time or never
    d. not sure

36. Considering your age, how would you describe your overall physical health?
    a. excellent
    b. good
    c. fair
    d. poor
37. In an average week, how many times do you engage in physical activity (exercise or work which lasts at least 20 minutes without stopping and which is hard enough to make you breathe heavier and your heart beat faster)?
    a. less than 1 time per week
    b. 1 or 2 times per week
    c. at least 3 times per week
38. If you ride a motorcycle or all-terrain vehicle (ATV), what percent of the time do you wear a helmet?
    a. 75% to 100%
    b. 25% to 74%
    c. less than 25%
    d. does not apply to me

39. Do you eat some food every day that is high in fiber, such as whole grain bread, cereal, fresh fruits, or vegetables?
    a. yes
    b. no
40. Do you eat foods every day that are high in cholesterol or fat, such as fatty meat, cheese, fried foods, or eggs?
    a. yes
    b. no
41. In general, how satisfied are you with your life?
    a. mostly satisfied
    b. partly satisfied
    c. not satisfied
42. Have you suffered a personal loss or misfortune in the past year that had a serious impact on your life? (For example, a job loss, disability, separation, jail term, or the death of someone close to you.)
    a. yes, 1 serious loss or misfortune
    b. yes, 2 or more
    c. no

Section 4: TOPICS FOR PERSONAL GROWTH

This section will help you identify areas in which you would like more information. In response to your selection from the following topics, we will provide you with resources or services to meet your requests.

Select topics on which you would like information. (Maximum of 4 topics.)

1. Responsible alcohol use
2. Stop-smoking programs
3. Sexuality
4. Gay issues
5. Depression
6. Loneliness
7. Exercise programs
8. Weight reduction
9. Self-breast exam
10. Medical emergencies
11. Nutrition
12. Relaxation
13. Stress reduction
14. Parenting skills
15. Marital or couples problems
16. Assertiveness training (how to say "no" without feeling guilty)
17. Biofeedback for tension headache and pain
18. Overcoming fears (e.g., high places, crowded rooms, etc.)
19. Educational or career goal setting/planning
20. Spiritual or philosophical values
21. Communication skills
22. Automobile safety
23. Suicide thoughts or attempts
24. Substance abuse
25. Anxiety associated with public speaking, tests, writing, etc.
26. Enhancing relationships
27. Time-management skills
28. Death and dying
29. Learning skills (e.g., speed-reading, comprehension, etc.)
30. Financial management
31. Divorce
32. Alcoholism
33. Men's issues
34. Women's issues
35. Medical self-care
36. Dental self-care
37. Self-testes exam
38. Aging
39. Self-esteem
40. Premenstrual syndrome (PMS)
41. Osteoporosis
42. Recreation and leisure
43. Environmental issues

IMPORTANT—If you have finished completing all sections of the LAQ, please make sure you have answered the questions in Section 1 requesting your sex, race, age, height and weight. Results cannot be generated for the Health Risk Appraisal section without this information.

YOU AND YOUR LIFESTYLE ARE THE MAJOR DETERMINANTS FOR JOYFUL LIVING

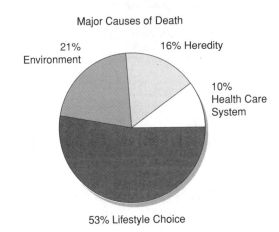

Major Causes of Death

21% Environment

16% Heredity

10% Health Care System

53% Lifestyle Choice

The circle graph to the left indicates the factors which contribute to your enjoyment and quality of life. While medical professionals contribute to the quality of your life, this graph clearly shows that the majority of those factors which contribute to your well-being are controlled by you. As you make responsible, informed choices, your chances of improving your health and well-being increase.

THE LAQ's ROLE . . .

We believe this instrument is useful in helping individuals identify the most likely causes of death and disability. More importantly, it identifies those areas of self-improvement which will lead to higher levels of health and well-being.

　　The areas assessed in the LAQ emphasize the importance of creating a balance among the many different aspects of your lifestyle. Each of these areas affects the others and determines your overall wellness status. Also, each provides an opportunity for learning, making responsible decisions, and personal growth.

　　We invite you to use the information provided by the LAQ to your best advantage to increase your level of wellness.

WORDS FROM THE PAST

Wellness is a term that has enjoyed growing popularity during the past several decades. Although the term was introduced relatively recently, the concept of prevention has been present for centuries. The following passages provide a brief glimpse of the wellness philosophy through the years. Wellness is a movement which has become a major part of modern culture and is the most important weapon available to combat lifestyle illnesses.

"For many years, while engaged in the practice of medicine, the author of this volume has been more and more impressed with the idea that the causes of suffering, diseases, and premature deaths, which we witness around us on every hand, lie near our own doors . . . and that the men and women of today, are, at least, equally as responsible for existing suffering, as those who have gone before them, and often much more so. In fact, he feels satisfied that by far the greatest portion of all the suffering, disease, deformity, and premature deaths which occur are the direct result of either the violation of or the want of compliance with the laws of our being; calamities, which, were the requisite knowledge possessed by the community, can and should be avoided."

—JOHN ELLIS, M.D., 1859

"It is universally admitted at the present time that preventive medicine is of far greater importance than curative medication, and many of the most eminent members of the profession are devoting themselves exclusively to this branch."

—J. H. KELLOGG, M.D., 1902

"To ward off disease or recover health, men as a rule find it easier to depend on the healers than to attempt the more difficult task of living wisely."

—RENE DUBOS, Ph.D., 1959

"It's what you do hour by hour, day by day, that largely determines the state of your health; whether you get sick, what you get sick with, and perhaps when you die."

—LESTER BRESLOW, M.D., 1969

APPENDIX D

The Friedman Family Assessment Model (Short Form)

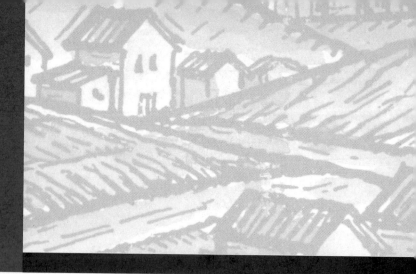

Before using the following guidelines in completing family assessments, two words of caution: First, not all areas included will be germane for each of the families visited. The guidelines are comprehensive and allow depth when probing is necessary. The student should not feel that every subarea needs be covered when the broad area of inquiry poses no problems to the family or concern to the health worker. Second, by virtue of the interdependence of the family system, one will find unavoidable redundancy. For the sake of efficiency, the assessor should try not to repeat data, but to refer the reader back to sections where this information has already been described.

IDENTIFYING DATA

1. **Family Name**
2. **Address and Phone**
3. **Family Composition**
   See Table D-1.
4. **Type of Family Form**
5. **Cultural (Ethnic) Background**
6. **Religious Identification**
7. **Social Class Status**
8. **Family's Recreational or Leisuretime Activities**

DEVELOPMENTAL STAGE AND HISTORY OF FAMILY

9. **Family's Present Developmental Stage**
10. **Extent of Family Developmental Tasks Fulfillment**
11. **Nuclear Family History**
12. **History of Family of Origin of Both Parents**

ENVIRONMENTAL DATA

13. **Characteristics of Home**
14. **Characteristics of Neighborhood and Larger Community**
15. **Family's Geographical Mobility**
16. **Family's Associations and Transactions with Community**
17. **Family's Social Support System or Network**
    Ecomap
    Family genogram

FAMILY STRUCTURE

18. **Communication Patterns**
    Extent of Functional and Dysfunctional Communication (types of recurring patterns)
    Extent of Emotional (Affective) Messages and How Expressed
    Characteristics of Communication within Family Subsystems
    Extent of Congruent and Incongruent Messages
    Types of Dysfunctional Communication Processes Seen in Family
    Areas of Open and Closed Communication
    Familial and Contextual Variables Affecting Communication

19. **Power Structure**
    Power Outcomes
    Decision-Making Process
    Power Bases
    Variables Affecting Family Power
    Overall Family System and Subsystem Power (family power continuum placement)

Table D-1   Family Composition Form

NAME (LAST, FIRST)	GENDER	RELATIONSHIP	DATE/PLACE OF BIRTH	OCCUPATION	EDUCATION
1. (Father)					
2. (Mother)					
3. (Oldest child)					
4.					
5.					
6.					
7.					
8.					

20. **Role Structure**

Formal Role Structure .
Informal Role Structure
Analysis of Role Models (optional)
Variables Affecting Role Structure

21. **Family Values**

Compare the family with American or family's reference group values and/or identify important family values and their importance (priority) in family.

Congruence between the Family's Values and Values of the Family's Reference Group or Wider Community
Congruence between the Family's Values and Family Members' Values
Variables Influencing Family Values
Values Consciously or Unconsciously Held
Presence of Value Conflicts in Family
Effect of the Above Values and Value Conflicts on Health Status of Family

FAMILY FUNCTIONS

22. **Affective Function**

Family Need–Response Patterns
Mutual Nurturance, Closeness, and Identification
Family attachment diagram
Separateness and Connectedness

23. **Socialization Function**

Family Child-Rearing Practices
Adaptability of Child-Rearing Practices for Family Form and Family's Situation
Who Is (are) Socializing Agent(s) for Child(ren)?
Value of Children in Family
Cultural Beliefs That Influence Family's Child-Rearing Patterns

Social Class Influence on Child-Rearing Patterns
Estimation about Whether Family Is at Risk for Child-Rearing Problems and If So, Indication of High-Risk Factors
Adequacy of Home Environment for Children's Needs to Play

24. **Health Care Function**

Family's Health Beliefs, Values, and Behaviors
Family's Definitions of Health–Illness and Their Level of Knowledge
Family's Perceived Health Status and Illness Susceptibility
Family's Dietary Practices
   Adequacy of family diet (recommended three-day food history record)
   Function of mealtimes and attitudes toward food and mealtimes
   Shopping (and its planning) practices
   Person(s) responsible for planning, shopping, and preparation of meals

Sleep and Rest Habits
Physical Activity and Recreation Practices (not covered earlier)
Family's Drug Habits
Family's Role in Self-Care Practices
Medically Based Preventive Measures (physicals, eye and hearing tests, and immunizations)
Dental Health Practices
Family Health History (both general and specific diseases—environmentally and genetically related)
Health Care Services Received
Feelings and Perceptions Regarding Health Services
Emergency Health Services
Source of Payments for Health and Other Services
Logistics of Receiving Care

FAMILY STRESS AND COPING

25. **Short- and Long-Term Familial Stressors and Strengths**

26. **Extent of Family's Ability to Respond, Based on Objective Appraisal of Stress-Producing Situations**

27. **Coping Strategies Utilized (present/past)**
    Differences in Family Members' Ways of Coping
    Family's Inner Coping Strategies
    Family's External Coping Strategies

28. **Dysfunctional Adaptive Strategies Utilized (present/past; extent of usage)**

This appendix lists the broad content areas recommended for family assessment. In-depth discussion of each of these content areas and related theoretical and research foundations, as well as relevant diagnoses and intervention guidelines, are included in the original source.

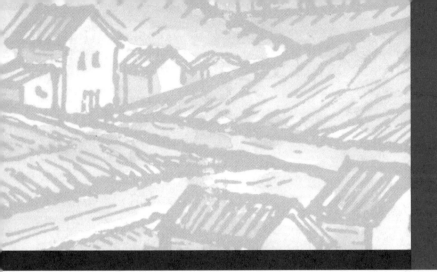

APPENDIX E
Mini Mental-Status Examination

The "mini" mental-status examination is a quick way to evaluate cognitive function. It is often used to screen for dementia or to monitor its progression.

Folstein Mini Mental-Status Examination

TASK	INSTRUCTIONS	SCORING	MAXIMUM SCORING POINTS
Date orientation	"Tell me the date." Ask for omitted items.	One point each for year, season, date, day of week, and month	5
Place orientation	"Where are you?" Ask for omitted items.	One point each for state, county, town, building, and floor or room	5
Register three objects	Name three objects slowly and clearly. Ask the client to repeat them.	One point for each item correctly repeated	3
Serial sevens	Ask the client to count backward from 100 by 7. Stop after five answers. (Or ask the client to spell "world" backwards.)	One point for each correct answer (or letter)	5
Recall three objects	Ask the patient to recall the objects mentioned previously.	One point for each item correctly remembered	3
Naming	Point to your watch and ask the client, "What is this?" Repeat with a pencil.	One point for each correct answer	2
Repeating a phrase	Ask the client to say, "No ifs, ands, or buts."	One point if successful on first try	1
Verbal commands	Give the client a plain piece of paper and say, "Take this paper in your right hand, fold it in half, and put it on the floor."	One point for each correct action	3
Written commands	Show the client a piece of paper with "CLOSE YOUR EYES" printed on it, and tell the client to read it and do what it says.	One point if the client's eyes close	1
Writing	Ask the client to write a sentence.	One point if sentence has a subject, a verb, and makes sense	1
Drawing	Ask the client to copy a pair of intersecting pentagons onto a piece of paper.	One point if the figure has 10 corners and two intersecting lines	1
Scoring	A score of 24 or above is considered normal.		30

Adapted from Folstein, M. F., Folstein, S. E., McHugh, P. R., Mini Mental State, 1975, Journal of Psychiatric Research, *12, pp. 196–198. Copyright 1975 by Pergamon Press. Adapted with permission.*

APPENDIX F
Functional Assessments:
Instrumental Activities of Daily Living (IADLs) and Physical Self-Maintenance Activities

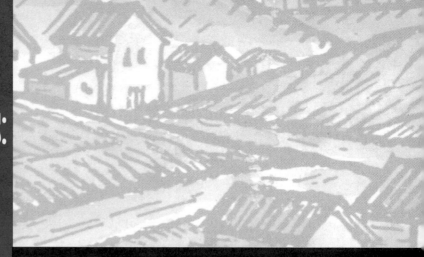

I. Instrumental Activities of Daily Living

A. Ability to use telephone
1. Operates telephone independently—looks up and dials numbers
2. Dials a few well-known numbers
3. Answers phone but does not dial or use touch tone
4. Does not use telephone at all

B. Housekeeping
1. Maintains house independently or with occasional assistance for "heavy work"
2. Performs light tasks such as bedmaking and dishwashing
3. Performs light daily tasks but cannot maintain adequate level of cleanliness
4. Needs assistance with all home maintenance tasks
5. Does not participate in any tasks

C. Laundry
1. Does personal laundry completely
2. Launders small items such as socks and stockings
3. All laundry must be done by others

D. Mode of transportation
1. Independently drives own car or uses public transportation
2. Arranges own travel via taxi or special transportation services, but does not use public transportation and does not drive
3. Travels on public transportation when assisted or with others
4. Travel limited to taxi or auto with assistance
5. Does not travel at all

E. Responsibility for medications
1. Takes medication in correct dosages at correct time independently
2. Takes medication if medication is prepared in advance in separate doses
3. Not capable of dispensing own medications

F. Ability to handle finances
1. Independently manages finances—writes checks, pays bills, keeps track of income
2. Manages own finances with assistance
3. Not capable of managing own finances

G. Shopping
1. Does all of the shopping independently
2. Shops for small purchases independently
3. Not able to go shopping without assistance
4. Unable to shop for any purchase

H. Food preparation
1. Able to prepare and serve food without assistance
2. Prepares adequate meals if supplied with food
3. Able to heat and serve prepared meals
4. Unable to prepare and serve meals

Adapted from "Assessment of Older People: Self-Maintaining and Instrumental Activities of Daily Living" by M. Lawton and E. Brody, 1969, The Gerontologist, 9, pp. 179–186. Adapted with permission.

II. Physical Self-Maintenance Activities

A. Feeding
1. Eats without assistance
2. Eats with minor assistance at meal times and helps in cleaning up
3. Feeds self with moderate assistance
4. Requires extensive assistance—all meals
5. Does not feed self at all and resists efforts of others to feed him/her

B. Toilet
1. Cares for self completely, no incontinence
2. Needs to be reminded or needs help in cleaning self
3. Soils the bed while asleep—more than once a week
4. Soils clothing while awake—more than once a week
5. No control of bladder/bowel

C. Grooming (hairs, nails, hands, face)
1. Able to care for self
2. Occasional minor assistance needed (e.g., with shaving)
3. Moderate and regular assistance needed

4. Needs total grooming care, but accepts some
5. Actively negates efforts of others to maintain grooming

D. Bathing
1. Bathes self without help
2. Bathes self with help into and out of tub or shower
3. Can wash face and hands only
4. Does not wash self but is cooperative
5. Does not try to wash self and resists efforts of others to help

E. Dressing
1. Dresses, undresses, and selects clothes from wardrobe
2. Dresses and undresses with minor assistance
3. Needs moderate assistance in dressing or selection of clothes
4. Needs major assistance
5. Completely unable to dress self and resists efforts of others to help

F. Ambulation
1. Ambulates about grounds or city without assistance
2. Ambulates within residence or nearby
3. Ambulates with assistance of
   a. another person
   b. a railing
   c. cane
   d. walker
   e. wheelchair
4. Sits unsupported in chair or wheelchair but cannot propel self
5. Bedridden more than half the time

APPENDIX G
Community Assessment Guide:
The Place, the People, and the Social System

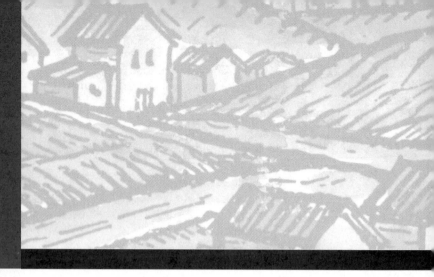

The community health assessment guide is a tool that guides the community health nurse in the systematic collection of data about the characteristics of an identified community and the formulation of community health diagnoses about the community's assets and health problems and concerns. The guide provides a method for assessing relevant community parameters and identifies categories and subcategories that provide direction for the organization of data in a meaningful way.

Community _____   Date _____

I. Overview
   A. Description of the community
      1. History
      2. Type of community: urban, suburban, rural
II. The Community As a Place
   A. Description: general identifying data
      1. Location
      2. Topography
      3. Climate
   B. Boundaries, area in square miles
   C. Environment
      1. Sanitation: water supply, sewage, garbage, trash
      2. Pollutants, toxic substances, animal reservoirs or vectors, flora and fauna
      3. Air quality: color, odor, particulates
      4. Food supply: sources, preparation
   D. Housing
      1. Types of housing (public and private)
      2. Condition of housing
      3. Percent owned, rented
      4. Housing for special populations
         a. Near homeless
         b. Homeless
         c. Frail elders
   E. Leading industries and occupations
III. The People of the Community
   A. Population profile
      1. Total population for ____ (year of last census)
      2. Population density
      3. Population changes in past 10 years
      4. Population per square mile
      5. Mobility

      6. Types of families
   B. Vital and demographic population characteriscs
      1. Age distribution
      2. Sex distribution
      3. Race distribution
      4. Ethnic group composition and distribution
      5. Socioeconomic status
         a. Income of family
         b. Major occupations
         c. Estimated level of unemployment
         d. Percent below poverty level
         e. Percent retired
      6. Educational level
      7. Religious distribution
      8. Marriage and divorce rates
      9. Birth and death rates
   C. Leading causes of morbidity
      1. Incidence rates (specific diseases)
      2. Prevalence rates (specific diseases)
   D. Mortality characteristics
      1. Crude death rate
      2. Age-specific death rate
      3. Infant mortality rate
      4. Maternal mortality rate
      5. Leading causes of death
IV. The Community As a Social System
   A. Government and leadership
      1. Type of government (mayor, city manager, board of supervisors)
      2. City offices (location, hours, services, access)
   B. Education
      1. Public educational facilities
      2. Private educational facilities

3. Libraries
4. Services for special populations
   a. Pregnant teens
   b. Adults with special problems
   c. Children and adults who are developmentally disabled
   d. Children and adults who are blind and/or deaf
C. Transportation
   1. Transport systems: bus, suburban train, private auto, air, streetcar, other
   2. Transportation provisions for special populations
      a. Elders
      b. Homeless/near homeless
      c. Adults with disabilities
D. Communication resources
   1. Newspapers
   2. Radio stations
   3. Television
   4. Key community leaders and/or decision makers
   5. Internet Web sites
   6. Other
E. Religious resources
   1. Churches and other religious facilities
   2. Community programs and services (e.g., health ministries, parish nursing)
   3. Major religious leaders
F. Recreation resources
   1. Public and private facilities
   2. Programs for special population groups
      a. People with disabilities
      b. Elders
      c. Blind and deaf
      d. Other
G. Community safety (protection)
   1. Fire protection (describe)
   2. Police protection, including county detention facilities (describe)
   3. Disaster preparation
H. Stores and shops
   1. Types and location
   2. Access
I. Community health facilities and resources (see Section V)

V. Community Health Facilities and Resources
(Resource access, availability, eligibility)
A. Health systems
   1. Hospitals (type and services rendered): acute care facilities—emergency medical, surgical, intensive care, psychiatric
   2. Rehabilitation health care facilities: physical conditions, alcoholism, and substance abuse
   3. Home health services: hospice and home health agencies
   4. Long-term care facilities (e.g., skilled nursing facilities)

5. Respite care services for special population groups
6. Ambulatory services
   a. Hospital ambulatory clinics
   b. Public health service clinics
   c. Nursing centers
   d. Community mental health centers
   e. Crisis clinics
   f. Community health centers
7. Special health services for targeted populations
   a. Preschool
   b. School age
   c. Adult or young adult
   d. Adults and children with handicaps (e.g., regional centers for developmentally disabled)
8. Other
   a. School health services
   b. Occupational health services
B. Public health and social services
   1. Health departments (various programs)
   2. Social services
      a. Department of social services
         (1) County level—location of suboffices
         (2) Official (public) social services, major programs (e.g., adult services, children's services, Welfare to Work)—eligibility, services rendered, location
      b. Social Security (USA)
         (1) Location and program availability
         (2) Eligibility
C. Voluntary health organizations
   1. Cancer Society
   2. Heart Association
   3. Red Cross
   4. Women's shelter
   5. Suicide prevention
   6. Rape crisis centers
   7. Family service agency
   8. Catholic Charities
   9. Alzheimer's Association
   10. Lung Association
   11. Diabetes Association
D. Health-related planning groups
   1. Area agency on aging
   2. Senior coordinating councils
   3. High-risk infant coordinating councils
   4. Healthy Communities Coordinating Teams
   5. Multipurpose agencies
   6. Teen violence prevention planning teams

VI. Summary
A. What are the major assets of the community and from whose perspective—health care provider's, community members', etc.?
   1. The place
   2. The people

3. The resources (availability, accessibility, acceptability; public and private)

B. What are the major health problems/needs?
   1. The place
   2. The people
   3. The resources (availability, accessibility, acceptability; public and private)

C. Identify and propose the contributions of nurses, other health care providers, community leaders, community residents, etc., to the solutions

D. Which of the health problems/needs should be given priority—first, second, and third? Why?

The Environmental Assessment guide is a tool that assists the community health nurse in the systematic collection of data about the home safety of diabled or older adults. It provides a way to assess the home for actual or potential safety hazards.

I. Entrance and Exit Areas

A. Is the housing on the ground level?   ____ Yes ____ No

    1. If **no,** is there an elevator?   ____ Yes ____ No

       Stairs?   ____ Yes ____ No

    2. If there are stairs, how many?   _____

B. Can the client get to and from the entrance easily?   ____ Yes ____ No

C. Are there any problems outside the house/apartment (e.g., steep path, lack of handrails on stairs)?   ____ Yes ____ No

    1. If **yes,** please describe _____

_____

_____

II. Living Area

A. What type of heating is there? (Circle all that apply.)

    1. Gas

    2. Electric

    3. Wood

    4. Central heating

    5. Space heater(s)

B. Is the heating system clean and operable?   ____ Yes ____ No

C. Are electrical cords well away from rugs and out of walkways?   ____ Yes ____ No

D. Are there any scatter (throw) rugs on the floor?   ____ Yes ____ No

E. If there are stairs, are they well lit?   ____ Yes ____ No

F. Are all chairs and sofas at a safe height for getting up and down?   ____ Yes ____ No

G. Is lighting adequate for walking?   ____ Yes ____ No

H. Is the furniture arranged for safety?   ____ Yes ____ No

I. Do the windows close completely?   ____ Yes ____ No

III. Kitchen Area

A. Is the kitchen easy to get to for the person?   ____ Yes ____ No

B. Are the appliances in good operating condition?   ____ Yes ____ No

C. Are sharp items placed safely in storage areas?   ____ Yes ____ No

D. Are poisonous and toxic items stored safely?   ____ Yes ____ No

E. Are the stove and cooking area free from grease and dust?   ____ Yes ____ No

F. Are the foods stored properly?   ____ Yes ____ No

G. Are the following facilities accessible?

     1. Refrigerator   ____ Yes ____ No

     2. Sink   ____ Yes ____ No

     3. Kitchen faucets   ____ Yes ____ No

     4. Stove   ____ Yes ____ No

     5. Cupboard   ____ Yes ____ No

     6. Kitchen counters   ____ Yes ____ No

IV. Bathroom Area

A. Is the toilet easily accessible?   ____ Yes ____ No

B. Are bathing facilities easily accessible?   ____ Yes ____ No

C. Are the bathing facilities safe?   ____ Yes ____ No

D. Are there railings or grab bars in the tub or shower area?   ____ Yes ____ No

     1. If there are railings or bars, are they secure and strong?   ____ Yes ____ No

E. Are there any visible electrical cords?   ____ Yes ____ No

     a. If **yes,** are they a safe distance from water?   ____ Yes ____ No

F. Is the floor nonskid?   ____ Yes ____ No

G. Is the bathtub or shower nonskid?   ____ Yes ____ No

V. Other Areas

A. Are there fire escape plans?   ____ Yes ____ No

B. Is there a fire alarm that can be heard by the person?   ____ Yes ____ No

C. Does the person know where the nearest fire alarm is?   ____ Yes ____ No

D. Are all flammable items stored safely away from the heat?   ____ Yes ____ No

E. Can the phone(s) be easily reached in an emergency?   ____ Yes ____ No

F. Are emergency numbers visible and easily accessible?   ____ Yes ____ No

SAFETY CHECKLIST

1. Insufficient heating/cooking   ____ Yes ____ No ____ Needs Action

2. Improper storage of poisonous and toxic items   ____ Yes ____ No ____ Needs Action

3. Improper food storage   ____ Yes ____ No ____ Needs Action

4. Insufficient/improper cooking facilities   ____ Yes ____ No ____ Needs Action

5. Railings or grab bars absent   ____ Yes ____ No ____ Needs Action

6. Elevators broken   ____ Yes ____ No ____ Needs Action

7. Unsafe toilets   ____ Yes ____ No ____ Needs Action

Environmental Summary: _____

_____

_____

_____

The Service Satisfaction Questionnaire is a tool that can be used to collect data regarding client perceptions of the nursing care received. The collection of this information is an important part of the outcomes measurement process. Service satisfaction questionnaires should be administered to clients on a regular basis, with response data analyzed in order to provide information that will assist in quality improvement.

Introduction

We would like your opinion on the nature of our community health nursing services. Your opinions are very important to us, and we thank you for your help. We want to provide our clients with the best community health nursing services possible. We ask these questions so that we may develop services that will be helpful to all of our clients. The information you provide is considered confidential. Your decision whether to complete this questionnaire will not affect your future relations with our nursing program. Your completion of this questionnaire indicates that you have given your consent to do so, having read the information provided above. Thank you.

Instructions: Please check your response to each of the questions below.

1. **When you first met the nurse, how well did she/he explain the reason for the visits with you?**
   - ____ Very well
   - ____ Well
   - ____ Moderately
   - ____ Poorly
   - ____ Very poorly

2. **Did the nurse involve you in planning for your health care?**
   - ____ Yes
   - ____ No

3. **How would you evaluate the nursing care and services you receive/have received?**
   - ____ Excellent
   - ____ Good
   - ____ Average
   - ____ Poor
   - ____ Very poor

4. **Did you feel that you could talk to the nurse about concerns or questions you had regarding your health and health care?**
   - ____ Yes
   - ____ No

5. **Did the nurse encourage you to ask questions about your health conditions and concerns?**
   - ____ Yes
   - ____ No

6. **Overall, how satisfied were you with the way information about your health condition was discussed with you?**
   - ____ Very satisfied
   - ____ Satisfied
   - ____ Neutral
   - ____ Dissatisfied
   - ____ Very dissatisfied

7. **Overall, how would you rate the respect and courtesy the nurse from (the agency's name) has shown to you?**

_____ Excellent

_____ Good

_____ Average

_____ Poor

_____ Very poor

8. **How much do you think you have been assisted by your visit(s) with the nurse?**

_____ A great deal

_____ Quite a bit

_____ Somewhat

_____ A little

_____ Not at all

_____ Not sure

9. **Do you think that additional health-related services should be provided by the nurse?**

_____ Yes

_____ No

_____ Not sure

If you answered **yes** to question 9, what services would you recommend? _____

_____

10. **Do you have any suggestions for ways that we could improve our nursing service to you? If yes, please comment.** _____

_____

_____

BACKGROUND INFORMATION

1. **What is your age?**

_____ 19 or younger

_____ 20–29

_____ 30–39

_____ 40–49

_____ 50–59

_____ 60–69

_____ 70–79

_____ 80+

2. **What is your gender?**

_____ Male

_____ Female

3. **What is your marital status?**

_____ Married

_____ Single

_____ Divorced

_____ Widowed

_____ Separated

4. **What is your ethnic origin?**

_____ Asian/Pacific Islander

_____ African American

_____ Latino

_____ Mixed race

Please indicate origins _____

_____ Native American/Alaskan

_____ Caucasian

_____ Other

Please indicate _____

_____ Decline to state

5. **What is your current family composition?**

_____ Single-parent/female

_____ Single-parent/male

_____ Two parents with children

_____ Single person

_____ Two adults with no children

_____ Extended family (e.g., aunt, grandmother living with you)

_____ Other (please specify: _____)

Thank you for taking the time to complete this questionnaire. We appreciate your assistance.

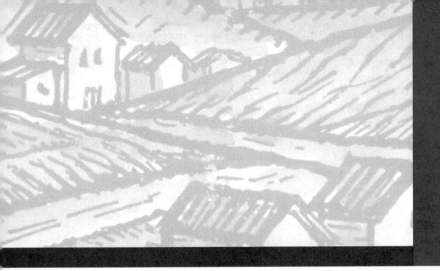

APPENDIX J
Recommended Childhood Immunization Schedule, United States, January–December 1998

Vaccines[1] are listed under the routinely recommended ages. ‭Bars‬ indicate range of acceptable ages for immunization. Catch-up immunization should be done during any visit when feasible. Shaded ‭ovals‬ indicate vaccines to be assessed and given if necessary during the early adolescent visit.

AGE VACCINE	BIRTH	1 MO	2 MOS	4 MOS	6 MOS	12 MOS	15 MOS	18 MOS	4–6 YRS	11–12 YRS	14–16 YRS
Hepatitis B[2,3]	Hep B-1										
			Hep B-2			Hep B-3				Hep B[2]	
Diphtheria, tetanus, pertussis[4]			DTaP or DTP	DTaP or DTP	DTaP or DTP		DTaP or DTP[4]		DTaP or DTP		Td
Haemophilus influenzae type b[5]			Hib	Hib	Hib	Hib					
Polio[6]			Polio[6]	Polio	Polio[6]				Polio		
Measles, mumps, rubella[7]						MMR			MMR[7]	MMR[7]	
Varicella[8]						Var				Var[8]	

Approved by the Advisory Committee on Immunization Practices (ACIP), the American Academy of Pediatrics (AAP), and the American Academy of Family Physicians (AAFP), and Centers for Disease Control and Prevention.

[1]This schedule indicates the recommended age for routine administration of currently licensed childhood vaccines. Some combination vaccines are available and may be used whenever administration of all components of the vaccine is indicated. Providers should consult the manufacturers' package inserts for detailed recommendations.

*[2]**Infants born to HBs Ag-negative mothers** should receive 2.5 μg of Merck vaccine (Recombivax HB®) or 10 μg of SmithKline Beecham (SB) vaccine (Engerix-B®). The 2nd dose should be administered at least 1 mo after the 1st dose. The 3rd dose should be given at least 2 mos after the second, but not before 6 mos of age.*

***Infants born to HBs Ag-positive mothers** should receive 0.5 ml hepatitis B immune globulin (HBIG) within 12 hrs of birth, and either 5 μg of Merck vaccine (Recombivax HB®) or 10 μg of SB vaccine (Engerix-B®) at a separate site. The 2nd dose is recommended at 1–2 mos of age and the 3rd dose at 6 mos of age.*

***Infants born to mothers whose HBs Ag status is unknown** should receive either 5 μg of Merck vaccine (Recombivax HB®) or 10 μg of SB vaccine (Engerix-B®) within 12 hrs of birth. The 2nd dose of vaccine is recommended at 1 mo of age and the 3rd dose at 6 mos of age. Blood should be drawn at the time of delivery to determine the mother's HBs Ag status. If it is positive, the infant should receive HBIG as soon as possible (no later than 1 wk of age). The dosage and timing of subsequent vaccines should be based upon the mother's HBs Ag status.*

[3]Children and adolescents who have not been vaccinated against hepatitis B in infancy may begin the series during any visit. Those who have not previously received 3 doses of hepatitis B vaccine should initiate or complete the series during the 11–12 year-old visit, and unvaccinated older adolescents should be vaccinated whenever possible. The 2nd dose should be administered at least 1 mo after the 1st dose, and the 3rd dose should be administered at least 4 mos after the 1st dose and at least 2 mos after the 2nd dose.

[4]DTaP (diphtheria and tetanus toxoids and acellular pertussis vaccine) is the preferred vaccine for all doses in the vaccination series, including completion of the series in children who have received 1 or more doses of whole cell DTP vaccine. Whole-cell DTP is an acceptable alternative to DTaP. The 4th dose (DTP or DTaP) may be administered as early as 12 mos of age, provided 6 mos have elapsed since the 3rd dose and if the child is unlikely to return at age 15–18 mos. Td (tetanus and diphtheria toxoids) is recommended at 11–12 years of age if at least 5 years have elapsed since the last dose of DTP, DTaP, or DT. Subsequent routine Td boosters are recommended every 10 years.

[5]Three H. influenzae type b (Hib) conjugate vaccines are licensed for infant use. If PRP-OMP (PedvaxHIB®[Merck]) is administered at 2 and 4 mos of age, a dose at 6 mos is not required.

[6]Two polio virus vaccines are currently licensed in the US: inactivated poliovirus vaccine (IPV) and oral poliovirus vaccine (OPV). The following schedules are all acceptable to the ACIP, the AAP, and the AAFP. Parents and providers may choose among these options.

1. 2 doses of IPV followed by 2 doses of OPV.

2. 4 doses of IPV.

3. 4 doses of OPV.

The ACIP recommends 2 doses of IPV at 2 and 4 mos of age followed by 2 doses of OPV at 12–18 mos and 4–6 years of age. IPV is the only polio virus vaccine recommended for immunocompromised persons and their household contacts.

[7]The 2nd dose of MMR is recommended routinely at 4–6 years of age but may be administered during any visit, provided at least 1 mo has elapsed since receipt of the 1st dose and that both doses are administered beginning at or after 12 mos of age. Those who have not previously received the 2nd dose should complete the schedule no later than the 11–12 year-old visit.

[8]Susceptible children may receive Varicella vaccine (Var) at any visit after the first birthday, and those who lack a reliable history of chickenpox should be immunized during the 11–12 year-old visit. Susceptible children 13 years of age or older should receive 2 doses, at least 1 month apart.

Immunization schedule for the Unites States, Centers for Disease Control and Prevention, 1998

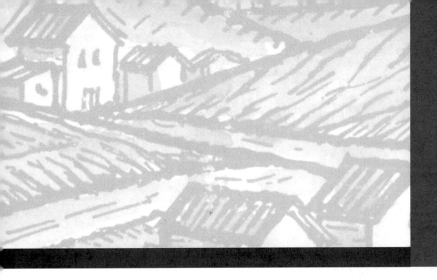

CHAPTER 1
Caring in Community Health Nursing

American Nurses Association. (1980). *A conceptual model of community health nursing* (ANA Pub. No. Ch-10). Kansas City, MO: Author.

American Public Health Association. (1981). *The definition and role of public health nursing practice in the delivery of health care: A statement of the public health nursing section*. Washington, DC: Author.

American Public Health Association, Public Health Nursing Section. (1996). *The definition and role of public health nursing—A statement of the Public Health Nursing Section*. Washington, DC: Author.

Association of Community Health Nursing Educators, Task Force on Basic Community Health Nursing Education. (1990). *Essentials of baccalaureate nursing education for entry level community health nursing practice*. Louisville, KY: Author.

Benner, P., & Wrubel, J. (1989). *The primacy of caring: Stress and coping in health and illness*. Menlo Park, CA: Addison-Wesley.

Breslow, L. (1990). A health promotion primer for the 1990s. *Health Affairs, 9*(2), 6–21.

Brown, L. (1986). The experience of care: Patient perspectives. *Topics in Clinical Nursing, 8,* 56–62.

Buhler-Wilkerson, K. (1993). Bringing care to the people: Lillian Wald's legacy to public health nursing. *American Journal of Public Health, 83*(12), 1778–1786.

Callahan, D. (1990). *What kind of life: Limits of medical progress*. Simon & Schuster.

Fawcett, J. (1995). *Analysis and evaluation of conceptual models of nursing*. (3rd ed.). Philadelphia: F. A. Davis.

Freeman, R. B. (1963). *Public health nursing practice* (3rd ed.). Philadelphia: W. B. Saunders.

Fry, S. T. (1991). A theory of caring: Pitfalls and promises. In D. A. Gaut & M. M. Leininger (Eds.), *Caring: The compassionate healer* (pp. 161–172). New York: National League for Nursing.

Fry, S. T. (1993). The ethic of care: Nursing's excellence for a troubled world. In D. A. Gaut (Ed.), *A global agenda for caring* (p. 30). New York: National League for Nursing.

Gadow, S. A. (1980). Existential advocacy: Philosophical foundation of nursing. In S. Spicker & S. Gadow (Eds.), *Nursing images and ideals: Opening dialogue with the humanities* (pp. 79–101). New York: Springer Publishing.

Gadow, S. A. (1985). Nurse and patient: The caring relationship. In A. Bishop & J. R. Scudder (Eds.), *Caring, curing, coping: Nurse, physician, patient relationships* (pp. 31–43). Birmingham: University of Alabama.

Gaut, D. A. (1981). Conceptual analysis of caring: Research method. In M. Leininger (Ed.), *Caring: An essential human need* (pp. 17–24). Thorofare, NJ: Charles B. Slack.

Gaut, D. A., (1989). A philosophic orientation to caring research. In M. M. Leininger (Ed.). *Care: The essence of nursing and Health* (pp. 17–25). Detroit, MI: Wayne State University Press.

Gaut, D. (1993a). A vision of wholeness for nursing. *Journal of Holistic Nursing, 11*(2), 164–171.

Gaut, D. (Ed.). (1993b). *A global agenda for caring*. New York: National League for Nursing.

Gaut, D. A., & Leininger, M. M. (Eds.). (1991). *Caring: The compassionate healer*. New York: National League for Nursing.

Gaylin, W. (1976). *Caring*. New York: Avon.

Gilligan, C. (1977). In a different voice: Women's conceptions of self and of morality. *Harvard Educational Review, 47,* 481–517.

Hanlon, J., & Pickett, G. (1984) *Public health: Administration and practice* (8th ed.). St. Louis, MO: Times Mirror/Mosby.

Henderson, V. (1993). Health is everybody's business. In M. Styles & P. Moccia (Eds.), *On nursing: A literary celebration, an anthology* (pp. 38–42). New York: National League for Nursing.

Institute of Medicine, Committee for the Study of the Future of Public Health. (1988). *The future of public health*. Washington, DC: National Academy Press.

Kickbusch, I. (1989). *The new public health orientation for the city*. In *WHO Healthy Cities Papers, No. 4.* (pp. 43–54). Copenhagen, Denmark: FADL Publishers.

Lakomy, J. M. (1993). The interdisciplinary meanings of human caring. In D. A. Gaut (Ed.), *A global agenda for caring* (pp. 181–189). New York: National League for Nursing.

Larson, P. L. (1986). Cancer nurses' perceptions of caring. *Cancer Nursing, 9*(2), 86–91.

Leavell, H. R., & Clark, E. G. (1958). *Preventive medicine for the doctor in his community*. New York: McGraw Hill.

Leininger, M. (1977). The phenomenon of caring: Caring—The essence and central focus of nursing. *Nursing Research Report, 12*(1), 2–14.

Leininger, M. M. (1991). *Culture care diversity and universality: A theory of nursing*. New York: National League for Nursing.

Leininger, M. M. (Ed.) (1984). *Care: The essence of nursing and health*. Thorofare, NJ: Charles B. Slack.

Mayeroff, M. (1971). *On caring*. New York: Harper & Row.

McKinlay, J. B. (1979). A case for refocusing upstream: The political economy of illness. In E. G. Jaco (Ed.), *Patients, physicians, and illness* (3rd ed., pp. 9–25). New York: The Free Press.

Milio, N. (1981). *Promoting health through public policy*. Philadelphia: F. A. Davis.

Morse, J. M., Solberg, S. M., Neander, W. (1990). Concepts of caring and caring as a concept. *Advances in Nursing Science, 13*(1), 1–14.

Muecke, M. A. (1984). Community health diagnosis in nursing. *Public Health Nursing, 1,* 23–35.

Nijuis, H. G. (1989). Contemporary municipal health departments in the Netherlands: A proposed potential for new public health. In World Health Organization, The new public health in an urban context: Paradoxes and solutions, *WHO Healthy Cities Papers No. 4* (pp. 17–39). Copenhagen, Denmark: FADL Publishers.

Noack, H. (1987). Concepts of health and health promotion. In T. Abelin, Z. J. Brzezinski, & V. D. L. Carstairs (Eds.), *Health promotion and protection* (WHO Regional Publications, European series 22). Copenhagen, Denmark: World Health Organization and the International Epidemiological Association.

Noddings, N. (1984). *Caring: A feminine approach to ethics and moral education*. Berkeley, CA: University of California Press.

Ottawa Charter for Health Promotion. (1987). *Health Promotion, 1*(4), iii.

Pellegrino, E. (1985). The caring ethic: The relation of physician to patient. In A. H. Bishop & J. R. Scudder (Eds.), *Caring, curing, coping: Nurse, physician, patient relationships* (pp. 8–30). Birmingham: University of Alabama Press.

Pender, N. (1996). *Health promotion in nursing practice* (3rd ed.). Stamford, CT: Appleton & Lange.

Pickett, G., & Hanlon, J. (1990). *Public health administration and practice*. St. Louis, MO: Times Mirror/Mosby College Publishing.

Ray, M. (1981). A philosophical analysis of caring within nursing. In M. Leininger (Ed.), *Caring: An essential human need* (pp. 25–36). Thorofare, NJ: Charles B. Slack.

Ray, M. (1987). Health care economics and human caring in nursing: Why the moral conflict must be resolved. *Family and Community Health, 10,* 35–43.

Roach, M. S. (1989). *The human act of caring: A blueprint for the health professions.* Ottawa, Canada: Canadian Hospital Association.

Roach, M. S. (1991). The call to consciousness: Compassion in today's health world. In D. A. Gaut & M. M. Leininger (Eds.), *Caring: The compassionate healer* (pp. 7–17). New York: National League for Nursing.

Salmon, M. E. (1993). Public health policy forum: Public health nursing—The opportunity of a century. *American Journal of Public Health, 12*(83), 1674–1675.

Shugars, D. A., O'Neil, E. H., & Bader, J. D. (Eds.). (1991). *Healthy America: Practitioners for 2005.* Durham, NC: The Pew Health Professionals Commission.

U.S. Department of Health and Human Services. (1991). *Healthy people 2000: National health promotion and disease prevention objectives.* Rockville, MD: Author.

Wald, L. D. (1971). *The house on Henry Street.* New York: Dover Publications.

Watson, J. (1985) *Nursing: Human science and human care: a theory of nursing.* Norwalk, CT: Appleton Century-Crofts.

Watson, J. M. (1988). New dimensions of human caring theory. *Nursing Science Quarterly, 1*(4), 175–181.

Williams, C. A. (1996). Community-based population-focused practice: The foundation of specialization in public health nursing. In M. Stanhope & J. Lancaster, *Community health nursing: Process and practice for promoting health* (4th ed.) (pp. 21–33). St. Louis, MO: Mosby-Yearbook.

World Health Organization. (1974). *Chronicle of WHO, 1,* 1–2.

World Health Organization. (1988a). A guide to assessing healthy cities. *WHO Healthy Cities Papers, No. 3.* Copenhagen, Denmark: FADL Publishers.

World Health Organization. (1988b). Promoting health in the urban context. *WHO Healthy Cities Papers, No. 1.* Copenhagen, Denmark: FADL Publishers.

World Health Organization. (1989). The new public health in an urban context: Paradoxes and solutions. *WHO Healthy Cities Papers, No. 4.* Copenhagen, Denmark: FADL Publishers.

World Health Organization, Health and Welfare Canada, Canadian Public Health Association. (1986). *Ottawa charter for health promotion.* Copenhagen, Denmark: FADL Publishers.

World Health Organization, Regional Office for Europe. (1984). *Health promotion: A discussion document on the concepts and principles.* Copenhagen, Denmark: WHO Europe, FADL Publishers.

Zerwekh, J. V. (1993). Commentary: Going to the people—Public health nursing today and tomorrow. *American Journal of Public Health, 83*(12), 1676–1678.

CHAPTER 2
Historical Development of Community Health Nursing

Allen, C. E. (1991). Holistic concepts and the professionalism of public health nursing. *Public Health Nursing. 8*(2), 74–80.

American Public Health Association. (1993). *A century of caring: A celebration of public health nursing in the United States, 1893–1993.* Washington, DC: USPHS Division of Nursing.

Anderson, C. L., Morton, R. F., & Green, L. W. (1978). *Community health* (3rd ed.). St. Louis, MO: Mosby.

Ashton, J. (1992). *Healthy cities.* Buckingham, England: Open University Press.

Basch, P. F. (1990). *Textbook of International Health.* New York: Oxford University Press.

Booth, R. (1989). Summary. *Journal of Professional Nursing, 5*(5), 271–272.

Brainard, A. M. (1985). *The evolution of public health nursing.* New York: Garland. [Reprinted from Brainard, A. M. (1922). *The evolution of public health nursing.* Philadelphia: W. B. Saunders.]

Browne, H. (1966). A tribute to Mary Breckinridge. *Nursing Outlook, 14,* 5.

Buhler-Wilkerson, K. (1985). Public health nursing: In sickness or health. *American Journal of Public Health, 75,* 1155–1161.

Cassedy, J. H. (1962). Hygeia: A midvictorian dream of a city of health. *Journal of the History of Medicine, 17*(2), 217–228.

Chadwick, H. D. (1937). The diseases of the inhabitants of the Commonwealth. *New England Journal of Medicine, 216,* 8.

Cohen, I. B. (1984). Florence Nightingale. *Scientific American, 250*(3), 128–137.

Deloughery, G. L. (1977). *History and trends of professional nursing* (8th ed.). St. Louis, MO: Mosby.

Dock, L. L., & Stewart, I. M. (1925). *A short history of nursing: From the earliest time to the present day.* New York: G. P. Putnam.

Dock, L. L. & Stewart, I. M. (1938). *A short history of nursing* (4th ed.). New York: Putnam.

Dolan, J. (1978). *History of nursing.* Philadelphia: Saunders.

Donahue, M. P. (1991). Why nursing history? *Journal of Professional Nursing, 7*(2), 77.

Duhl, L. (1992). Healthy cities: Myth or reality. In J. Ashton, *Healthy cities* (pp. 15–21). Buckingham, England: Open University Press.

Duhl, L., & Hancock, T. (1988). Community self-evaluation: A guide to assessing healthy cities. *Healthy Cities Papers,* Copenhagen: FADL.

Fagin, C. (1978). Primary care as an academic discipline. *Nursing Outlook, 26,* 750–753.

Fee, E. (1991). The origins and development of public health in the United States. In W. Holland, R. Detels, & G. Knox (Eds.), *Oxford textbook of public health* (2nd ed., pp. 3–22). Oxford, England: Oxford University Press.

Finer, S. E. (1952). *The life and times of Sir Edwin Chadwick.* London: Methuen.

Ford, L. C., & Silver, H. K. (1967). The expanded role of the nurse in child care. *Nursing Outlook, 15*(9), 43–45.

Freeman, R. (1964). *Public health nursing practice* (3rd ed.). Philadelphia: W. B. Saunders.

Friedman, E. (1990). Troubled past of an invisible profession. *Journal of American Medical Association, 264,* 2851–2855, 2958.

Gardner, M. S. (1919). *Public health nursing.* New York: Macmillan.

Gardner, M. S. (1952). *Public health nursing* (3rd ed.). New York: Macmillan.

Ginzberg, E. (1985). *American medicine: The power shifts.* Totowa, NJ: Rowman & Allanheld.

Goldwater, M., & Zusy, M. (1990). *Prescription for nurses effective political action.* Philadelphia: Mosby.

Goodnow, M. (1933). *Outlines of nursing history.* Philadelphia: W. B. Saunders.

Green, L. W. (1996). Commentary. In U.S. Department of Health and Human Services, Public Health Service, *Healthy People 2000: Midcourse review and 1995 revisions.* Sudbury, MA: Jones & Bartlett.

Grier, B., & Grier, M. (1978). Contributions of the passionate statistician. *Research in Nursing and Health, 1,* 103–109.

Hamilton, D. (1989). The cost of caring: The Metropolitan Life Insurance company's visiting nurse service, 1909–1953. *Bulletin of the History of Medicine, 63,* 414–434.

Hanlon, J. (1964). *Principles of public health administration.* St. Louis, MO: Mosby.

Hanlon, J., & Pickett, G. (1984). *Public health: administration and practice* (8th ed.). St. Louis, MO: Times Mirror/Mosby.

Harding, H. O. (1926). Health opportunities in Harlem. *Opportunity: Journal of Negro Life, 4,* 386–387.

Haupt, A. C. (1953). Forty years of teamwork in public health nursing. *American Journal of Nursing, 53,* 81–84.

Health Targets and Implementation Committee. (1988). *Health for all Australians: Report to the Australian Health Ministers' Advisory Council and the Australian Health Ministers' Conference.* Canberra, Australia: Australian Government Publishing Service.

Igoe, J. B. (1980). Changing patterns in school health nursing. *Nursing Outlook, 28,* 486–492.

Jensen, D. M. (1959). *History and trends of professional nursing.* (4th ed.). St. Louis, MO: Mosby.

Kalisch, P. L., & Kalisch, B. J. (1982). *Politics of nursing.* Philadelphia:

Kalisch, P. L., & Kalisch, B. J. (1995). *The advance of American nursing* (3rd ed.). Philadelphia: Lippincott.

Kaufman, M., Hawkins, J. W., Higgins, L. P., & Friedman, A. H. (1988). *Dictionary of American nursing bibliography.* Westport, CT: Greenwood Press.

Keeling, A., & Ramos, C. (1995). The role of nursing history in preparing nursing for the future. *N & HC: Perspectives on Community, 16*(1), 30–34.

Kelly, L. Y. (1971). *Dimensions of professional nursing* (4th ed.). New York: Macmillan.

Kelly, L. Y. (1981). *Dimensions of professional nursing* (5th ed.). New York: Macmillan.

Kelly, L. Y. (1991). *Dimensions of professional nursing* (6th ed.). New York: Pergaman Press.

Kiernan, F. (1952). *Citizens on the march: History of the New York Tuberculosis and Health Association.* New York: New York Tuberculosis and Health Association.

Lamont, L., & Lees, P. (1994). Practicing community health nursing in the context of primary health care. In C. Cooney (Ed.), *Primary health care: The way to the future* (pp. 313–329). Sydney, Australia: Prentice Hall.

Lancaster, J. (1996). History of community health and community health nursing. In M. Stanhope, & J. Lancaster, *Community health nursing: Process and practice for promoting health.* (4th ed.). (pp. 3–19). St. Louis, MO: Mosby.

Lee, P. R. (1996). Foreword. In U.S. Department of Health and Human Services, Public Health Service, *Healthy People 2000: Midcourse review and 1995 revisions.* Sudbury, MA: Jones & Bartlett.

Maynard, T. (1939). *The apostle of charity: The life of St. Vincent de Paul.* New York: Dial Press.

McKeown, T. (1976). *The role of medicine—Dream, mirage, or nemesis.* London: Nuffield Provincial Hospitals Trust.

McNeil, E. E. (1967). *Transition in public health nursing.* John Sundwall lecture. University of Michigan, February 27.

Mosley, M. O. (1995). Mabel K. Staupers: A pioneer in professional nursing. *N & HC: Perspectives on Community, 16*(1), 12–17.

National Organization of Public Health Nursing. (1944). Approval of Skidmore College of Nursing as preparing students for public health nursing. *Public Health Nursing, 36,* 371.

Nightingale, F.(1867). Letter to the editor, Macmillan magazine as cited in M. Styles & P. Moccial. (1993). *On nursing: A literary celebration.* New York: National League for Nursing.

Nightingale, F. (1969). *Notes on nursing: What it is and what it is not.* New York: Dover. (Original work published in 1859.)

Novak, J. C. (1988). The social mandate and historical bases for nursing's role in health promotion. *Journal of Professional Nursing, 4*(2), 80–87.

Olds, D. L., Eckenrode, J., Henderson, J. R., C. R., Kitzman, H., Powers, J., Cole, R., Sidora, K., Movis, P., Pettitt, L. M., Frackey, D. (1997). Long-term effects of home visitation on maternal life course and child abuse and neglect: Fifteen-year follow-up of a randomized trial. *Journal of American Medical Association, 278*(8), 637–643.

Osofsky, G. (1966). *Harlem tragedy: An emergency slum. Harlem: The making of a ghetto.* New York: Harper and Row.

Pickett, G., & Hanlon, J. (1990). *Public health administration and practice* (9th ed.). St. Louis, MO: Times Mirror/Mosby.

Public Health Service. (1958). *General organization, functions, procedures, and forms.* Washington, DC: U.S. Government Printing Office.

Roberts, D. E., & Heinrich, J. (1985). Public health nursing comes of age. *American Journal of Public Health, 75*(10), 1162–1172.

Roberts, M. M. (1954). *American nursing, history and interpretation.* New York: Macmillan.

Rodgers, B. L. (1989). Concepts, analysis and the development of nursing knowledge: The evolutionary cycle. *Journal of Advanced Nursing, 14.*

Rosen, G. (1958). *A history of public health.* New York: MD Publications.

Ruth, M. V., & Partridge, K. B. (1978). Differences in perceptions of education and practice. *Nursing Outlook, 26,* 622–628.

Smillie, W. G. (1952). *Preventive medicine and public health* (2nd ed.). New York: Macmillan.

Styles, M. (1992). Commentary: Nightingale: The enduring symbol. In *Nightingale, notes on nursing* (commemorative edition). Philadelphia: J. B. Lippincott.

Tinkham, C. W., & Voorhies, E. F. (1977). *Community health nursing: Evolution and practice.* New York: Appleton Century Croft.

U.S. Department of Health and Human Services. (1990). *Healthy people 2000: National health promotion and disease prevention objectives. Summary report.* Washington, DC: Author.

Wald, L. (1971). *The house on Henry Street.* New York: Dover. (Reprinted from 1915 edition, New York: Henry Holt & Co.)

Walker, L., & Avant, K. (1995). *Strategies for theory construction in nursing* (3rd ed.). Norwalk, CT: Appleton & Lange.

Waters, Y. (1912). *Visiting nursing in the United States.* New York: Charities Publication Committee, The Russell Sage Foundation.

Wilde, M. H. (1997). The caring connection in nursing: A concept analysis. *International Journal for Human Caring, 1*(1), 18–24.

Winslow, E. E. (1923). *The evolution and significance of the modern public health campaign.* New Haven, CT: Yale University Press.

World Health Organization, Regional Office for Europe. (1985). *Targets for health for all.* Copenhagen, Denmark: Author.

World Health Organization, Regional Office for Europe. (1991). *Targets for health for all.* Copenhagen, Denmark: Author.

CHAPTER 3
Health Care Delivery in the United States

American Nurses Association. (1993). Nursing's agenda for reform.

American Nursing Home Association (1970–71). *Nursing Home Fact Book 3.* Washington, DC: Author.

Association of State and Territorial Health Officials. (1994). Public health and prevention are essential to health care reform. Washington, DC: Author.

Aydellotte, M. K., Barger, S. E., Branstetter, E., Fehring, R. J., Lindgren, K., Lundeen, S., & Riesch, S. K. (1987). *The nursing center: Concept and design.* Kansas City: American Nurses Association.

Davis, K., Collins, K. S., & Morris, C. (1994). Managed care: Promise and concerns. *Health Affairs, 13*(4), 178–185.

DeLaw, N., Greenberg, G., & Kinchen, K. A. (1992). A layman's guide to the U.S. health care system. *Health Care Financing Review, 14*(1), 151–169.

Eisenberg, D. M., Kessler, R. C., Foster, C., Norlock, F. E., Calkins, D. R., & Delbanco, T. L. (1993). Unconventional medicine in the United States: Prevalence, costs, and patterns of use. *New England Journal of Medicine, 328,* 246–252.

Elazar, D. (1966). *American federalism: A view from the states.* New York: Crowell.

Ellencweig, A. Y., & Yoshpe, R. B. (1984). Definition of public health. *Public Health Review, 12,* 65–78.

Employee Benefit Research Institute. (1997). *Sources of health insurance and characteristics of the uninsured: Analysis of the March, 1997 Current Population Survey* (ERBI Issue Brief No. 192) December 1997, Washington, DC: Author.

Fogel, B. S., Brock, D., Goldscheider, F., & Royall, D. (1994). *Cognitive dysfunction and the need for long-term care: Implications for public policy.* Washington, DC: Public Policy Institute, American Association of Retired Persons.

Glass, L. (1989). The historic origin of nursing centers. In *Nursing centers: Meeting the demand for quality health care* (pp. 21–33). New York: National League for Nursing Press.

Holahan, J., Zuckerman, S., Evans, A., & Rangarajan, S. (1998). Medicaid managed care in thirteen states. *Health Affairs 17*(1), 43–63.

Institute of Medicine, Committee for the Study of the Future of Public Health. (1988). *The future of public health.* Washington, DC: National Academy Press.

Judy, R., & D'Amico, C. (1997) *Work force 2020.* Indianapolis, IN: Hudson Institute.

Koop, C. E. (1991). *Koop.* New York: Random House.

Kopf, E. W. (1991). Florence Nightingale as statistician. In B. W. Spradley (Ed.), *Readings in community health nursing* (4th ed., pp. 274–285). Philadelphia: J. B. Lippincott.

Kuhn, T. (1986). *The structure of scientific revolutions.* New York: New American Libraries.

Letsch, S. (1993). National health care spending in 1991. *Health Affairs, 12*(1), 94–110.

Lockhart, C. (1992). *Influences on the healthcare system.* Tempe, AZ: C. Lockhart Associates.

Lockhart, C. (1994). Community nursing centers: An analysis of status and needs. In B. Murphy (Ed.), *Nursing centers: The time is now* (pp. 2–18). New York: National League for Nursing Press.

Luft, H. S., & Trauner, J. B. (1981). *The operations and performance of health maintenance organizations.* National Center for Health Services Research, U.S. Department of Health and Human Services. Washington, DC: U.S. Government Printing Office.

Mackey, T., & Adams, J. (1994). The use of health risk appraisal in a nursing center: Costs and benefits. In B. Murphy (Ed.), *Nursing centers: The time is now* (pp. 254–265). New York: National League for Nursing Press.

Manning, M. (1984). *The hospice alternative: Living with dying.* London: Souvenir Press.

Morgan, P. A. (1986). Developing a freestanding ambulatory surgery center. *The College Review,* Fall.

Mundinger, M. O. (1983). *Home care controversy: Too little, too late, too costly.* Rockville, MD: Aspen Systems Corporation.

Priester, R. (1992). *Taking values seriously: A values framework for the U.S. health care system*. Minneapolis: Center for Biomedical Ethics, University of Minnesota.

Rakich, J. S., Longest, B. B., & Darr, K. (1992). *Managing health services organizations* (3rd ed.). Baltimore, MD: Health Professions Press.

Random House Webster's College Dictionary. (1992). New York: Random House.

Riesch, S. K. (1990). *A review of the state of the art of research on nursing centers. Differentiating nursing practice: Into the twenty-first century*. From proceedings of the 18th annual Conference of the American Academy of Nursing. NLN 41-2281, 91–104.

Safriet, B. J. (1992). Health care dollars and regulatory sense: The role of advanced practice nursing. *Yale Journal of Regulation, 9*(2), 417–488.

Sharp, N. (1992). Community nursing centers: Coming of age. *Nursing Management, 23*(8), 18–20.

Stryker, R. (1988). Historical obstacles to management of nursing homes. In G. K. Gordon & R. Stryker (Eds.), *Creative long-term care administration* (2nd ed., pp. 6–7). Springfield, IL: Charles C. Thomas.

Sullivan, C. B., & Rice, T. (1991). The Health insurance picture in 1990. *Health Affairs, 10*(2) 104–115.

U.S. Department of Health and Human Services, Public Health Service. (1994). *For a healthy nation—Returns on investment in public health*. Washington, DC: Author.

U.S. Department of Health and Human Services. (1991). *Healthy People 2000: National health promotion and disease prevention objectives* (DHHS Publication No. [PHS]91-50212). Washington, DC: Author.

Williams, S. J., & Torrens, P. R. (Eds.) (1999). *Introduction to health services* (5th ed.). Albany, NY: Delmar Publishers.

World Health Organization. (1978). *Primary health care*. Geneva, Switzerland: Author.

CHAPTER 4
Health Care Economics

Abel-Smith, B. (1992). Cost containment and new priorities in the European community. *The Milbank Quarterly, 70*(3), 393–415.

Agency for Health Care Policy and Research. (1997). *Access to health care in America, 1996*. Rockville, MD: MEPS Highlights No. 3. AHCPR pub. No. 98-0002.

Altman, S. H., & Cohen, A. B. (1993). The need for a national global budget. *Health Affairs, 12*, 194–203.

American Nurses' Association. (1995). *Agenda for health care reform*. Washington, DC: Author.

America's bubble economy. (1998b, April 18). *The Economist, 347*(8064), 4, 19–22.

Ashby, J. L., & Greene, T. F. (1993). Implications of a global budget for facility-based health spending. *Inquiry, 30*(4), 362–371.

Barker, J. A. (1992). *Paradigms: The business of discovering the future*. New York: Harper Press.

Berrand, N. L., & Schroeder, S. A. (1994). Lessons from the states. *Inquiry, 31*(1), 10–13.

Bodenheimer, T. S., & Grumbach, K. (1998). *Understanding health policy: A clinical approach*. Stamford: Appleton & Lange.

Congressional Budget Office. (1993, March). *Analysis of president's budgetary proposals*. Washington, DC: Author.

Congressional Budget Office. (1995, September). *Analysis of the administration health proposal*. Washington, DC: Author.

Congressional Budget Office. (1998, January). *The economic and budget outlook: Fiscal years 1999–2008*. Washington, DC: Author.

Davis, K. (1994). Availability of medical care and its financing. In P. Lee & C. Estes (Eds.), *The nation's health* (4th ed., pp. 296–302). Boston: Jones & Bartlett.

DeLaw, N., Greenberg, G., & Kinchen, K. A. (1992). A layman's guide to the U.S. health care system. *Health Care Financing Review, 14*(1), 151–169.

Duffy, J. (1993). *Economics*. Lincoln, NE: Cliff.

Enthoven, A. C. (1993). The history and principles of managed competition. *Health Affairs, 12*, 24–48.

Enthoven, A. C. (1994). Why not the Clinton health plan? *Inquiry, 31*(2), 129–136.

Enthoven, A. C. (1996, April). Driving down costs while maintaining quality. *Kaiser Permanente Teleconference*. Oakland, CA.

Enthoven, A. C., & Kronick R. (1994). Universal health insurance through incentive programs. In P. Lee & C. Estes (Eds.), *The nation's health* (4th ed., pp. 284–291). Boston: Jones & Bartlett.

Fry, S. T. (1994). *Ethics in nursing practice: A guide to ethical decision making*. International Council of Nurses. Geneva, Switzerland.

Health Care Finance Administration. (1996, March 11), [Online], HCFA.gov.

Health Care Finance Administration. (1997a, May 12), [Online], HCFA.gov.

Health Care Finance Administration. (1997b, January 27). *Medicare Bulletin*. Washington, DC: Author.

Health Care Finance Administration. (1997c, April 21). *Medical Expenditures Panel Survey*. Washington, DC: Author.

Health Care Finance Administration. (1998a, January). *Medicare Bulletin*. Washington, DC: Author.

Health Care Finance Administration. (1998b, April). *Medicaid Bulletin*. Washinton, DC: Author.

Health Care Finance Administration. (1998c, March 18). *Medical Expenditures Panel Survey*. Washington, DC: Author.

Himmelstein, D. U., Woolhandler, S., & Wolf, S. M. (1992). The vanishing health care safety net: New data on uninsured Americans. *International Journal of Health, 22*, 381.

How HMOs decide your fate. (1998, March 9). *U.S. News and World Report*.

Inglehart, J. K. (1994). The American health care system: Managed care. In P. Lee & C. Estes (Eds.), *The nation's health* (4th ed., pp. 231–233). Boston: Jones & Bartlett.

Kronick, R. (1993). Perspectives: Design issues in managed care. *Health Affairs*, (Suppl. 12), 87–98.

Lamm, R. D. (1994). The brave new world of health care. In P. Lee & C. Estes (Eds.), *The nation's health* (4th ed., p. 152). Boston: Jones & Bartlett.

Lee, P. R., & Estes, C. L. (1994). *The nation's health* (4th ed.). Boston: Jones & Bartlett.

Leininger, M. M. (Ed.). (1981). *Caring: An essential human need*. Thorofare, NJ: Charles B. Slack. (Reprinted in 1988 by Wayne State University Press, Detroit, MI).

Levit, K. R., Olin, G. L., & Letsch, S. W. (1992). American health insurance coverage, 1980–91. *Health Affairs, 14*(1), pp. 31–57.

Litman, T. J. (1994). Government and health: The political aspects of health care: A sociopolitical overview. In P. Lee & C. Estes (Eds.), *The nation's health* (4th ed., pp. 107–120). Boston: Jones & Bartlett.

Lundberg, G. D. (1994). National health care reform: The aura of inevitability intensifies. In P. Lee & C. Estes (Eds.), *The nation's health* (4th ed., pp. 238–244). Boston: Jones & Bartlett.

Mechanic, D. (1994). Managed care: Rhetoric and realities. *Inquiry, 31*(2), 124–128.

Patients or profits. (1998, March 7). *The Economist, 346*(8058), 6, 23–24.

Prospective Payment Assessment Commission. (1997). *Medicare and the American health care system. Report to the Congress. June 1997*. Washington, DC: Author.

Reinhardt, U. E. (1993). Reorganizing the financial flows in U.S. health care delivery. *Heath Affairs, 12*, 172–193.

Reinhardt, U. E. (1994). Providing access to health care and controlling costs: The universal dilemma. In P. Lee & C. Estes (Eds.), *The nation's health* (4th ed., pp. 263–278). Boston: Jones & Bartlett.

Schieber, G. J., & Poullier, J. P. (1991). International health spending: Issues and trends. *Health Affairs, 10*(1), 106–116.

Schieber, G. J., Poullier, J. P., & Greenwald, L. M. (1992). U.S. health expenditure performance: An international comparison and data update. *Health Care Financing Review, 13*(4), 1–15.

Staines, V. S. (1993). Impact of managed care on national health spending. *Health Affairs, 12* (Suppl. 3), 248–257.

U.S. Bureau of the Census. (1997, November 10). *Insured and uninsured U. S. Citizens*. Washington, DC: U.S. Government Printing Office.

U.S. Department of Labor. (1997). *The Employed and Insured and the Employed and Un-insured*. Washington, DC: U.S. Government Printing Office.

Walsey, T. P. (1992). *What has government done to our health care?* New York: CATO Institute.

Wessels, W. J. (1993). *Economics*. New York: Barron's Business Review Press.

White House Fact Sheet. (1998, April 6). The Health of America. Washington, DC: U.S. Government Printing Office.

Wilbur, K. (1996). *A brief history of everything*. Boston: Shambhala.

Wilson, E. O. (1998). *Consilience: The unity of knowledge*. New York: Knopf.

Woolhandler, S., & Himmelstein D. U. (1997). Costs of care and administration at for-profit and other hospitals in the United States. *New England Journal of Medicine, 336*(11), 769–774.

World Health Organization. (1996, March 13). *Health statistics*.

World Health Organization. (1997, May 12). *Health statistics.*
World Health Organization. (1998, October 1). *Health statistics.*

CHAPTER 5
Philosophical and Ethical Perspectives

Aiken, T. D., & Catalano, J. T. (1994). *Legal, ethical, and political issues in nursing.* Philadelphia: F. A. Davis.

American Health Consultants. (1994). The new face of bioethics: County ethics committee reviews health and social service decisions. *Medical Ethics Advisor, 10*(9), 114–115.

American Health Consultants. (1995). Changes in accreditation thrust ethics committees into new roles. *Medical Ethics Advisor, 11*(1), 1–4.

American Nurses Association. (1985). *Code for nurses, with interpretive statements.* Kansas City, MO: Author.

Annas, G. J. (1978). Patient's rights movement. In W. T. Reich (Ed.), *Encyclopedia of bioethics.* Vol. 3. New York: Free Press.

Beauchamp, T. L., & Childress, J. F. (1994). *Principles of biomedical ethics* (4th ed.). New York: Oxford University Press.

Beauchamp, T. L., & Walters, L. R. (1994). *Contemporary issues in bioethics* (4th ed.). Belmont, CA: Wadsworth.

Benjamin, M., & Curtis, J. (1992). *Ethics in nursing* (3rd ed.). New York: Oxford University Press.

Burkhardt, M. A., & Nathaniel, A. K. (1998). *Ethics and issues in contemporary nursing.* Albany, NY: Delmar Publishers.

Canadian Nurses Association. (1997). *Code for ethics for nursing.* Ottowa, Canada: Author.

Collopy, B., Dubler, N., & Zuckerman, C. (1990). The ethics of home care: Autonomy and accommodation. *The Hastings Center Report, 20*(2, Special Suppl.), 1–16.

Daniels, N. (1979). Rights to health care and distributive justice: programmed worries. *Journal of Medical Philosophy,* 4, 174–191.

DeLaune, S., & Ladner, P. (1998). *Fundamentals of nursing: Standards and practices.* Albany, NY: Delmar Publishers.

DuBose, E. R., Hamel, R., & O'Connell, L. J. (Eds.). (1994). *A matter of principles? Ferment in U.S. bioethics.* Valley Forge, PA: Trinity.

Ellis, J. R., & Hartley, C. L. (1997). *Nursing in today's world: Challenges, issues, and trends* (6th ed.). Philadelphia: J. B. Lippincott.

Gudorf, C. E. (1994). A feminist critique of biomedical principlism. In E. R. DuBose, R. Hamel, & L. J. O'Connell (Eds.), *A matter of principles? Ferment in U.S. bioethics* (pp. 164–181). Valley Forge, PA: Trinity.

Husted, G. L., & Husted, J. H. (1995). *Ethical decision making in nursing.* (2nd ed). St. Louis, MO: Mosby Yearbook.

International Council of Nurses. (1973). *ICN code for nurses: Ethical concepts applied to nursing.* Geneva, Switzerland: Imprimeries Populaires.

Joint Commission on Accreditation of Healthcare Organizations. (1990). *1991 Joint Commission accreditation manual for hospitals,* Vol. 1, Standards. Oakbrook Terrace: IL: Author.

Joint Commission on Accreditation of Healthcare Organizations. (1994). *Joint Commission 1995 accreditation manual for hospitals,* Vol. 1, Standards. Oakbrook Terrace, IL: Author.

Joint Commission on Accreditation of Healthcare Organizations. (1996). *Joint Commission 1996 accreditation manual for hospitals,* Vol. 1, Standards. Oakbrook Terrace, IL: Author

Kane, R. A., & Caplan, A. L. (Eds.) (1993). *Ethical conflicts in the management of home care.* New York: Springer.

Kane, R. A., Penrod, J. D., & Kivnick, H. Q. (1993). Ethics and case management: Preliminary results of an empirical study. In R. A. Kane & A. L. Caplan (Eds.), *Ethical conflicts in the management of home care* (pp. 7–25). New York: Springer.

Kuehl, K. S., Shapiro, S., & Sivasubramanian, K. N. (1992). Should a school honor a student's DNR order? Case history of S. A. *Kennedy Institute of Ethics Journal, 2*(1), 1–3.

Leddy, S., & Pepper, J. M. (1998). Conceptual bases of professional nursing (4th ed.). Philadelphia: J. B. Lippincott.

Leininger, M. M. (1990). *Ethical and moral dimensions of care.* Detroit, MI: Wayne State University.

Manning, R. C. (1992). *Speaking from the heart: A feminist perspective on ethics.* Lanham, MD: Rowman & Littlefield.

Mappes, T. A., & Zembaty, J. S. (1991). *Biomedical ethics* (3rd ed.) New York: McGraw-Hill.

Mason, L. (1995). The Denver community bioethics committee: Healthcare decisions in adult protection and long-term care settings. *Healthcare Ethics Committee Forum, 7*(5), 284–289.

Mitchell, C. (1990). Ethical dilemmas. *Critical Care Nursing Clinics of North America, 2*(3), 427–430.

Munson, R. (1996). *Intervention and reflection: Basic issues in medical ethics* (5th ed.). Belmont, CA: Wadsworth.

Pence, G. E. (1990). Classic cases in medical ethics. New York: McGraw Hill. (Chapter 7, The Baby Doe Case, p. 136–163).

President's Commission. (1983). *Deciding to forego life-sustaining treatment: Ethical, medical and legal issues in treatment decisions.* Washington, DC: U.S. Government Printing Office.

Reckling, JA. B. (1989). Abandonment of patients by home health nursing agencies: An ethical analysis of the dilemma. *Advances in Nursing Science, 11*(3), 70–81.

Ross, J. W., Glaser, J. W., Rasinski-Gregory, D., McIver, Gibson, J., & Bayley, C. (1993). Health care ethics committees: The next generation. Chicago, IL: American Hospital Association.

Runes, D. D. (Ed.). (1983). *Dictionary of philosophy.* Totowa, NJ: Rowman & Allanheld.

Scofield, G. R. (1992). A lawyer responds: A student's right to forgo CPR. *Kennedy Institute of Ethics Journal, 2*(1), 4–12.

Sherwin, S. (1992). *No longer patient: Feminist ethics and health care.* Philadelphia: Temple University.

Silva, M. C. (1990). *Ethical decision making in nursing administration.* Norwalk, CT: Appleton & Lange.

Smith, D. H., & Veatch, R. M. (Eds.). (1987). *Guidelines on the termination of life-sustaining treatment and the care of the dying: A report by the Hastings Center.* Bloomington, IN: Indiana University.

Strike, K. A. (1992). An educator responds: A school's interest in denying the request. *Kennedy Institute of Ethics Journal, 2*(1), 19–23.

Walker, N. U. (1993). Keeping moral space open: New images of ethics consulting. *Hastings Center Report, 23*(2), 33–40.

Younger, S. J. (1992). A physician/ethicist responds: A student's rights are not so simple. *Kennedy Institute of Ethics Journal, 2*(1), 13–18.

CHAPTER 6
Cultural and Spiritual Perspectives

Adair, M. (1984). *Working inside out: Tools for change.* Oakland, CA: Wingbow.

Andrews, M. (1995). Transcultural perspectives in the nursing care of children and adolescents. In M. Andrews & J. Boyle (Eds.). *Transcultural concepts in nursing care* (2nd ed., pp. 123–179). Philadelphia: J. B. Lippincott.

Arrien, A. (1993). *The four-fold way: Walking the paths of the warrior, teacher, healer and visionary.* San Francisco: Harper.

Azzam, A. (1964). *The eternal message of Muhammad.* New York: New American Library.

Barrington, R. (1997, November). *Stories from an urban Indian clinic: A case history for clinical application.* Paper presented at the Nurse Healers—Professional Associates meeting, Vancouver, BC.

Birnbaum, R. (1979). *The healing Buddha.* Boulder, CO: Shambhala.

Blofeld, J. (1970). *The Tantric mysticism of Tibet.* New York: Arkana.

Boyle, J. (1995). Alterations in lifestyle: Transcultural concepts in chronic illness. In M. Andrews & J. Boyle (Eds.). *Transcultural concepts in nursing care* (2nd ed., pp. 237–252). Philadelphia: J. B. Lippincott.

Burkhardt, M. (1991). Spirituality and children: Nursing considerations. *Journal of Holistic Nursing, 9*(2), 31–40.

Chapman, L. (1987). Developing a useful perspective on spiritual health: Love, joy, peace and fulfillment. *American Journal of Health Promotion,* 12–17.

Chinn, P., & Wheeler, C. (1991). *Peace and power: A handbook of feminist process* (3rd ed.). New York: National League for Nursing. #15-2404.

Dossey, L. (1993). A new era in healing? *NAPRA Trade Journal.* 17.

Duggan, R. (1996). Complementary medicine: Transforming influence or footnote to history? *Alternative Therapies in Health & Medicine, 1*(2). 28–33.

Eisenberg, D., Kessler, R., & Foster, C., Norlock, F., Calkins, D. & Delbanco, T. L. (1993). Unconventional medicine in the United States: Prevalence, costs, and patterns of use. *New England Journal of Medicine, 328*(4), 246–252.

Frankl, V. (1939). *Man's search for meaning.* New York: Pocket Books.

Frisch, N., & Kelley, J. (1996). *Healing life's crises: A guide for nurses.* Albany, NY: Delmar Publishers.

Giger, J. M., & Davidhizar, R. E. (1995). *Transcultural nursing.* (2nd ed.). St. Louis, MO: Mosby-Yearbook.

Griffiths, B. (1984). Science today and the new creation. In S. Grof, (Ed.).

Ancient wisdom in modern science. Albany, NY: State University of New York.

Grossman, D. (1994). Enhancing your "cultural competence." *American Journal of Nursing,* 58–62.

Heinberg, R. (1989). *Memories and visions of paradise: Exploring the universal myth of a golden age.* Los Angeles: Jeremy P. Tarcher.

Hover-Kramer, D. (1993). *Healing touch: A resource for health care professionals.* Albany, NY: Delmar Publishers.

Illich, I. (1977). *Limits to medicine.* London: Marion Boyars.

Jonas, W. (1996). Issues of concern for the Office of Alternative Medicine. *Bridges, 7*(2), 1–14.

Keegan, L. (1994). *The nurse as healer.* Albany, NY: Delmar Publlishers.

Kleinman, A. (1980). *Patients and healers in the context of culture.* Berkeley, CA: University of California.

Krieger, D. (1979). *The Therapeutic Touch: How to use your hands to help or to heal.* New York: Prentice Hall.

Krieger, D. (1993). *Accepting your power to heal: The personal practice of Therapeutic Touch.* Santa Fe, NM: Bear.

Kunz, D. (1991). *The personal aura.* Wheaton, IL: Theosophical Publishing House.

Kunz, D. (1992). In J. Quinn (Producer), Video II: The method. *Therapeutic Touch: Healing through human energy fields* [videotape series]. New York: National League for Nursing.

Lad, V. (1984). *Ayurveda, the science of self-healing.* Santa Fe, NM: Lotus.

Lauderdale, J., & Greener, D. (1995). Transcultural nursing care of the childbearing family. In M. Andrews & J. Boyle (Eds.), *Transcultural concepts in nursing care* (2nd ed., pp. 99–122). Philadelphia: J. B. Lippincott.

Leininger, M. (1978). *Transcultural nursing: Concepts, theories, and practices.* New York: John Wiley.

Leininger, M. (1984). Care: The essence of nursing and health. In M. Leininger (Ed.), *Care: The essence of nursing and health.* (pp. 3–15). Thorofare, NJ: Slack.

Leininger, M. (1991). The theory of culture care diversity and universality. In M. Leininger (Ed.). *Culture care diversity and universality: A theory of nursing.* (pp. 5–68). New York: National League for Nursing.

Lionberger, H. (1986). An interpretive study of nurses' practice of Therapeutic Touch (Doctoral dissertation, University of California, San Francisco, 1985). *Dissertation Abstracts International, 46,* 2624B.

Macrae, J. (1987). *Therapeutic Touch: A practical guide.* New York: Alfred A. Knopf.

McDowell, B. (1994). The National Institutes of Health Office of Alternative Medicine: Evaluating research outcomes. *Alternative & Complementary Therapies, 1*(1), 17–25.

Mitchell, S. (1991). *The Gospel according to Jesus.* New York: Harper Collins.

Nagai-Jacobson, M. G., & Burkhardt, M. A. (1989). Spirituality: Cornerstone of holistic nursing practice. *Holistic Nursing Practice, 3*(3), 18–26.

Nasr, S. (1971). *Islam and the plight of modern man.* London: Longman.

Newman, M. (1994). *Health as expanding consciousness* (2nd ed.). New York: National League for Nursing.

North American Nursing Diagnosis Association. (1999). *Nursing diagnosis: Definitions and classification 1999–2000.* Philadelphia, PA: North American Nursing Diagnosis Association.

Nurse Healers—Professional Associates, Inc. (1992). *Therapeutic Touch teaching guidelines: Beginner's level Krieger/Kunz method.* New York: Author.

Nurse Healers—Professional Associates, Inc. (1994). *Therapeutic Touch: Teaching guidelines: Intermediate level Krieger/Kunz method.* New York: Author.

Office of Alternative Medicine. (1995, December). OAM funds eight research centers to evaluate alternative treatments. *Newsletter.*

Office of Alternative Medicine. (1997). Classification of alternative medicine practices. Available Internet: http://altmed.od.nih.gov/oam/what-is-cam/classify.shtml

Orque, M. S., Bloch, B., & Monroy L. S. A. (1984). *Ethnic nursing care.* St. Louis: C. V. Mosby.

Pender, N. J. (1996). *Health promotion in nursing practice* (3rd ed.). Stamford, CT: Appleton & Lange.

Quinn, J. (1992, Producer). Video I: Theory and research. *Therapeutic Touch: Healing through human energy fields* [videotape series]. New York: National League for Nursing.

Quinn, J., & Strelkauskas, A. (1993). Psychoimmunologic effects of Therapeutic Touch on practitioners and recently bereaved recipients: A pilot study. *Advances in Nursing Science, 15*(4), 13–26.

Rogers, M. E. (1990). Nursing: Science of unitary, irreducible, human beings: Update 1990. In E. A. M. Barrett (Ed.), *Visions of Rogers' science-based nursing.* (Pub. No. 15-2285). New York: National League for Nursing.

Ross, N. W. (1966). *Three ways of Asian wisdom.* New York: Simon & Schuster.

Ross, N. W. (1980). *Buddhism: A way of life and thought.* New York: Vintage.

Schubert, P. (1989). Mutual connectedness: Holistic nursing practice under varying conditions of intimacy (Doctoral dissertation, University of California, San Francisco, 1989). *Dissertation Abstracts International, 50,* 4987B.

Schubert, P., & Lionberger, H. (1995). Mutual connectedness: A study of client–nurse interaction using the Grounded Theory method. *Journal of Holistic Nursing, 13*(2), 102–116.

Smith, C. (1995). The lived experience of staying healthy in rural African American families. *Nursing Science Quarterly, 8*(1), 17–21.

Spector, R. (1996). *Cultural diversity in health and illness* (4th ed.). Stamford, CT: Appleton & Lange.

Steinberg, M. (1974). *Basic Judaism.* New York: Harcourt, Brace & World.

Stoll, R. (1989). The essence of spirituality. In V. B. Carson, *Spiritual dimensions of nursing practice* (pp. 4–23). Philadelphia: W. B. Saunders.

Stuart, E., Deckro, J., & Mandle, C. (1989). Spirituality in health and healing: A clinical program. *Holistic Nursing Practice, 3*(3), 35–44.

Touba, N. (1995). *Female genital mutilation: A call for global action.* New York: Women, Ink.

Travelbee, J. (1971). *Interpersonal aspects of nursing* (2nd ed.). Philadelphia: Davis.

Tripp-Reimer, T., Brink, P. J., & Saunders, J. M. (1984). Cultural assessment: Content and process. *Nursing Outlook, 32*(2) 78–82.

Viswananda (1938/1992). Unity of religions. In Ramakrishna Mission Institute of Culture (1992), *The Religions of the world. Proceedings of the Sri Ramakrishna Centenary Parliament of Religions, 1 March–8 March, 1937,* 235–237. Calcutta, India: The Ramakrishna Mission Institute of Culture.

Wirth, D. (1990). The effect of non-contact Therapeutic Touch on the healing rate of full thickness dermal wounds. *Subtle Energies, 1*(1), 1–20.

Wolf, F. A. (1996). *The spiritual universe: How quantum physics proves the existence of the soul.* New York: Simon & Schuster.

CHAPTER 7
Environmental Perspective

American Nurses Association (1995). *Nursing: A social policy statement.* Washington, DC: Author.

Bohm, D. (1980). *Wholeness and the implicate order.* London: Rutledge & Kegan Paul.

Bureau of Labor Statistics (1995a, April 26). Work injuries and illnesses by selected characteristics, 1993. *Department of Labor News.* Washington, DC: Department of Labor.

Bureau of Labor Statistics (1995b, May 15). National census of fatal occupational injuries, 1993. *Department of Labor News.* Washington, DC: Department of Labor.

California Public Health Foundation. (1992). *Kids and the environment: Toxic hazards: A course on pediatric environmental health.* Berkeley, CA: Author.

Center for Biomedical Ethics. (1992). *Taking values seriously: A values framework for the U.S. health care system.* Minneapolis: University of Minnesota.

Chivian, E., McCally, M., Hu, H., & Haines, A. (1993). *Critical condition: Human health and the environment.* Cambridge, MA: Massachusetts Institute of Technology.

Colodzin, B. (1993). Respect and "real work." *Noetic Sciences Review, 25,* 30–31.

Dass, R. (1993). Compassion: The delicate balance. In R. Walsh, & F. Vaughan (Eds.), *Paths beyond ego: The transpersonal vision* (pp. 234–236). Los Angeles: Jeremy P. Tarcher/Perigee.

Ehrlich, P., & Ehrlich, A. (1990). *The population explosion.* New York: Simon & Schuster.

Harrison, P. (1992). *The third revolution: Environment, population and a sustainable world.* London/New York: I. B. Taurus, distributed by St. Martin's Press, New York.

Herbert, N. (1987). *Quantum reality: Beyond the new physics.* Garden City, NY: Anchor.

Institute of Medicine. (1995). *Nursing, health, and the environment.* Washington, DC: National Academy Press.

Josten, L., Clarke, P., Ostwald, S., Stoskopf, C., & Shannon, M. (1995). Public health nursing education: Back to the future for public health sciences. *Family & Community Health, 18*(1), 36–48.

Kennedy, P. (1993). *Preparing for the twenty-first century.* New York: Random House.

Kim, H. S. (1983). *The nature of theoretical thinking.* East Norwalk, CT: Appleton-Century-Crofts.

Lum, M. (1995). Environmental public health: Future direction, future skills. *Family & Community Health, 18*(1), 24–35.

Maslow, A. (1962). Health as transcendence of the environment. *Journal of Humanistic Psychology, 9*(1), 12–20.

Miringoff, M. (1995). *1995 index of social health: Monitoring the social well-being of the nation.* Tarrytown, NY: Institute for Innovation in Social Policy, Fordham Graduate Center.

Moos, R. (1979). Social-ecological perspectives on health. In G. Stone, F. Cohen, & N. Adler, (Eds.), *Health psychology: A handbook.* (pp. 523–547) San Francisco: Jossey-Bass.

National Research Council. (1993). *Pesticides in the diets of infants and children.* Washington, DC: National Academy Press.

Neufeld, A., & Harrison, M. (1990). The development of nursing diagnoses for aggregates and groups. *Public Health Nursing, 7*(4), 251–252.

Neufer, L. (1994). The role of the community health nurse in environmental health. *Public Health Nursing, 11*(3), 155–162.

Newman, M. (1994). *Health as expanding consciousness* (2nd ed.). St. Louis, MO: C. V. Mosby.

Nightingale, F. (1860/1969). *Notes on nursing.* New York: Dover.

Phillips, L. (1995). Chattanooga Creek: Case study of the public health nursing role in environmental health. *Public Health Nursing, 12*(5), 335–340.

Powers, A. (1988). Social networks, social support, and elderly institutionalized people. *Advances in Nursing Science, 10*(2), 40–58.

Public Health Service. (1994). *Public health in America.* Washington DC: Author.

Puntillo, K. (1992). *A model of environment.* Unpublished paper for class syllabus. Rohnert Park, CA: Sonoma State University.

Rogers, M. (1990). Nursing: Science of Unitary, Irreducible, Human Beings: Update 1990. In Barrett, E. A. M. (Ed.), *Visions of Rogers' science-based nursing.* (pp. 5–11). New York: National League for Nursing.

Salmon, M. (1995). Public health policy: Creating a healthy future for the American public. *Family & Community Health, 18*(1), 1–11.

Schmoll, H., Tewes, U., & Plotnikoff, N. (1992). *Psychoneuroimmunology: Interactions between the brain, nervous system, behavior, endocrine & immune systems.* Lewiston, NY: Hogrefe & Huber.

Schubert, P. (1989). Mutual connectedness: Holistic nursing practice under various conditions of intimacy. (Doctoral dissertation, University of California, San Francisco, 1989). *Dissertation Abstracts International, 50,* 4987B.

Schubert, P., & Lionberger, H. (1995). Mutual connectedness: A study of client–nurse interaction using the Grounded Theory method. *Journal of Holistic Nursing, 13*(2), 102–116.

Social Health. (1996, October 31). *Rachel's Environment & Health Weekly.* Annapolis, MD: Environmental Research Foundation.

Sorrell, J. M. (1994). Remembrance of things past through writing: Esthetic patterns of knowing in nursing. *Advances in Nursing Science, 17*(1), 60–70.

Tiedje, L., & Wood, J. (1995). Sensitizing nurses for a changing environmental health role. *Public Health Nursing, 12*(6), 359–365.

U.S. Department of Health and Human Services. (1992a). Environmental health: Resource list. In *Healthy People 2000: National health promotion and disease prevention objectives.* Washington, DC: Author.

U.S. Department of Health and Human Services. (1992b). *Healthy People 2000: Public Health Service Action.* Washington, DC: Author.

U.S. Department of Health and Human Services. (1996). *Healthy People 2000: Midcourse review and 1995 revisions.* Sudbury, MA: Jones & Bartlett.

von Bertalanffy, L. (1968). *General Systems Theory.* New York: George Braziller.

Welp, E., Kogevinas, M., Andersen, A., Bellander, T., Biocca, M., Coggon, D., Esteve, J., Gennaro, V., Kolstad, H., Lundberg, I., Lynge, E., Partanen, T., Spence, A., Boffetta, P., Ferro, G. & Saracci, R. (1996). Exposure to styrene and mortality from nervous system diseases and mental disorders, *American Journal of Epidemiology, 144*(7), 623–633.

Whitehead, A. (1969). *Process and reality: An essay in cosmology.* New York: The Free Press.

Williams, C. (1995). Beyond the Institute of Medicine report: A critical analysis and public health forecast. *Family & Community Health, 18*(1), 12–23.

CHAPTER 8
Caring Communication and Client Teaching/Learning

American Nurses Association. (1990). *Survival skills in the workplace: What every nurse should know.* Kansas City, MO: Author.

Andrews, M. M. (19950. Transcultural nursing. In M. M. Andrews & J. A. Boyle. *Transcultural concepts in nursing care* (2nd ed., pp. 49–96). Philadelphia: J. B. Lippincott.

Arnold, E., & Boggs, K. (1995). *Interpersonal relationships* (2nd ed.). Philadelphia: W. B. Saunders.

Babcock, D., & Miller, M. (1994). *Client education: Theory and practice.* St. Louis, MO: Mosby.

Balzer-Riley, J. (1996). *Communications in nursing: Communicating assertively and responsibly in nursing: A guidebook* (3rd ed.). St. Louis, MO: Mosby.

Boyd, M. D. (1992). Strategies for effective health teaching. In N. I. Whitman, B. A. Graham, C. J. Gleit, & N. I. Whitman, *Teaching in nursing practice: A professional model* (3rd ed., pp. 201–228). Stamford, CT: Appleton & Lange.

Brown, S. J. (1995). An interviewing style for nursing assessment. *Journal of Advanced Nursing, 21,* 340–343.

Carol, E. M. (1989). *Guidelines for intercultural communication.* Unpublished manuscript.

Cushnie, P. (1988). Conflict: Developing resolution skills. *American Operating Room Nurses Journal, 47*(3), 732–742.

Davis, T. C., Crouch, M. A., Wills, G., Miller, S., & Abdehou, D. M. (1990). The gap between patient reading comprehension and the readability of patient education materials. *Journal of Family Practice, 31,* 533–538.

Dixon, E., & Park, R. (1990). Do patients understand written health information? *Nursing Outlook, 36,* 278–281.

Freire, P. (1983). *Education for critical consciousness* (2nd ed.). New York: Continuum Press.

Gordon, T. (1970). *Parent effectiveness training: The "no-lose" program for raising responsible children.* New York: Peter H. Wyden.

Graham, B. A., & Gleit, C. J. (1998). Teaching in selected settings. M. D. Boyd, B. A. Graham, C. J. Gleit, & N. I. Whitman. *Teaching in nursing practice: A professional model* (3rd ed., pp. 41–63). Stamford, CT: Appleton & Lange.

Hartmann, R. A., & Kochar, M. S. (1994). The provision of patient and family education. *Patient Education and Counseling, 24,* 101–108.

Hatton, D. C., & Webb, T. (1993). Information transmission in bilingual, bicultural contexts: A field study of community health nurses and interpreters. *Journal of Community Health Nursing, 10*(3), 137–147.

King, I. (1981). *A theory for nursing: Systems, concepts, process.* New York: John Wiley & Sons.

Knowles, M. (1990). *The adult learner* (4th ed.). Houston, TX: Gulf.

Krieger, D. (1993). *Accepting your power to heal: The personal practice of Therapeutic Touch.* Sante Fe, NM: Bear.

Loomis, M. (1979). *Group process for nurses.* St. Louis, MO: C. V. Mosby.

McMaster, P. L., & Connell, C. M. (1994). Health education interventions among Native Americans: A review and analysis. *Health Education Quarterly, 21,* 521–538.

Murphy, P. W., Davis, T. C., Long, S. W., Jackson, R. H., & Decker, B. C. (1993). Rapid estimate of adult literacy in medicine (REALM): A quick reading test for patients. *Journal of Reading, 37,* 124–130.

Northouse, P. G., & Northouse, L. L. (1997). *Health communication: Strategies for health professionals* (3rd ed.). Norwalk, CT: Appleton & Lange.

Nurss, J. R., Baker, D. W., Davis, T. C., Parker, R. M., & Williams, M. V. (1995). Difficulties in functional health literacy screening in Spanish-speaking adults. *Journal of Reading, 38,* 632–637.

Orlando, I. (1961). *The dynamic nurse–patient relationship.* New York: G. P. Putnams & Sons.

Orlando, I. (1972). *The discipline and teaching of nursing process.* New York: G. P. Putnams & Sons.

Peplau, H. E. (1952). *Interpersonal relations in nursing.* New York: G. P. Putnam & Sons.

Peplau, H. E. (1960). Talking with patients. *American Journal of Nursing, 60,* 964.

Rankin, S. H., & Stallings, K. D. (1996). *Patient education: Issues, principles, and guidelines* (3rd ed.). Philadelphia: J. B. Lippincott.

Rogers, C. R. (1951). *Client-centered therapy.* Boston: Houghton.

Rogers, M. E. (1990). Nursing: Science of Unitary, Irreducible Human Beings: Update 1990. In E. A. Manhart Barrett (Ed.), *Visions of Rogers' science-based nursing.* New York: National League for Nursing.

Schubert, P. E. (1989). Mutual connectedness: Holistic

under varying conditions of intimacy (Doctoral dissertation, University of California, San Francisco, 1989). *Dissertation Abstracts International, 50,* 4987B.

Schubert, P. E., & Lionberger, H. J. (1995). Mutual connectedness: A study of client–nurse interaction using the Grounded Theory method. *Journal of Holistic Nursing, 13*(2), 102–116.

Smith, S. (1992). *Communications in nursing: Communicating assertively and responsibly in nursing: A guidebook* (2nd ed.). St. Louis, MO: Mosby.

Snyder, M. (1993). Critical thinking: A foundation for consumer-focused care. *The Journal of Consumer Education in Nursing, 24,* 206–210.

Stuart, G. W., & Sundeen, S. J. (1991). *Principles and practice of psychiatric nursing* (4th ed.). St. Louis, MO: Mosby-Yearbook.

Tones, K., Tilford, S., & Robinson, Y. (1990). *Health education: Effectiveness and efficiency.* New York: Chapman and Hall.

Travelbee, J. (1963). What do we mean by rapport? *American Journal of Nursing, 63,* 70–72.

Travelbee, J. (1964). What is wrong with sympathy? *American Journal of Nursing, 64,* 68–71.

Travelbee, J. (1971). *Interpersonal aspects of nursing* (2nd ed.). Philadelphia: F. A. Davis.

Tripp-Reimer, T. (1989). Cross-cultural perspectives on patient teaching. *Nursing Clinics of North America, 24,* 613–614.

Truax, C., & Carkhuff, R. (1967). *Toward effective counseling and psychotherapy: Training and practice.* Chicago: Aldine.

Tuckman, B. (1965). Developmental sequences in small groups. *Psychological Bulletin, 63*(6), 384–399.

U.S. Department of Health and Human Services. (1996). *Healthy People: 2000: Midcourse review and 1995 revisions.* Sudbury, MA: Jones & Bartlett.

Wallerstein, N., & Bernstein, E. (1988). Empowerment education: Freire's ideas adapted to health education. *Health Education Quarterly, 15,* 379–394.

Wallerstein, N., & Bernstein, E. (1994). Introduction to community empowerment, participatory education, and health. *Health Education Quarterly, 21,* 141–148.

Weaver, S. K., & Wilson, J. E. (1994). Moving toward patient empowerment. *Nursing & Health Care, 15,* 480–483.

Whitman, N. I. (1998). Assessment of the learner. In M. D. Boyd, B. A. Graham, C. J. Gleit, & N. I. Whitman. *Teaching in nursing practice: A professional model* (3rd ed., pp. 157–180). Stamford, CT: Appleton & Lange.

Witte, K., & Morrison, K. (1995). Intercultural and cross-cultural health communication. In R. L. Wiseman (Ed.), *Intercultural communication theory.* Thousand Oaks, CA: Sage.

Yalom, I. (1975). *The theory and practice of group psychotherapy* (2nd ed.). New York: Basic Books.

Yalom, I. (1983). *Inpatient group psychotherapy.* New York: Basic Books.

CHAPTER 9
Health-Promotion and Disease-Prevention Perspectives

Barger, S., & Rosenfeld, P. (1993). Models in community health care. *Nursing and Health Care, 14*(8), 426–431.

Becker, M. H. (1974). *The Health Belief Model and personal health behavior.* Thorofare, NJ: Charles B. Slack.

Benson, H. (1975). *The relaxation response.* New York: William Morrow.

Bresler, D. (1991). Health promotion and chronic pain: Challenges and choices. In A. Kaplan, (Ed.), *Health promotion and chronic illnesses: Discovering a new quality of health* (pp. 139–151). World Health Organization. Cologne: The Federal Centre.

Burmeister, M. (1994a). *Jin Shin Jyutsu is: Book I* (6th ed.). Scottsdale, [AZ]: Jin Shin Jyutsu.

[...] (undated). *Jin Shin Jyutsu Is: Book I Project summary sheet.* [Jin Shin] Jyutsu, Inc. 8719 E. San Alberto, Scottsdale, AZ

[...] 95). *Living well: Health in your hands* [...] ollins.

[...] *g herbs: The ultimate guide to the cu-* [...] *cines.* Emmaus, PA: Rodale.

[...] Dead tired. San Francisco: *San Francisco*

[...] d Prevention. (1994). *Ten leading causes* [...] *es.* Atlanta, GA: Author.

[...] /December). Your health depends on sleep.

Donatelle, R. J., & Davis, L. G. (1998). *Access to health* (2nd ed.). Englewood Cliffs, NJ: Prentice Hall.

Edlin, G., & Golanty, E. (1992). *Health and wellness: A holistic approach* (4th ed.). Boston: Jones & Bartlett.

Friedman, H., Thomas, W., Klein, A., & Friedman, L. (1996). *Psychoneuroimmunology.* Boca Raton, FL: CRC Press.

Hardman, J., Limbrid, L., Molinoff, P., Rudden, R., & Goodman-Gilman, A. (1996). *Goodman & Gilman's pharmacological basis of therapeutics* (9th ed.). New York: McGraw-Hill.

Health and Welfare Canada: Minister of Supply and Services Canada. (1992). *Canada's food guide to healthy eating.*

Keegan, L. (1996). *Healing nutrition.* Albany, NY: Delmar Publishers.

McCuen, G. (1993). *Health care and human values.* Hudson, WI: Gem.

Memmler, R., Cohen B., & Wood, D. (1996). *The human body in health and disease* (8th ed.). New York: J. P. Lippincott.

Messina, M., & Barnes, S. (1991). The role of soy products in reducing the risk of cancer. *Journal of the National Cancer Institute, 83,* 541–546.

National Research Council. (1989). Recommended dietary allowances (10th ed.). Washington, DC: National Academy Press.

National Wellness Institute, Inc. (1997). *Lifestyle Assessment Questionnaire.* Stevens Point, WI: Authors.

Neuman, B. (1990). Health as a continuum based on the Neuman Systems Model. *Nursing Science Quarterly, 3*(3), 129–135.

Newman, M. (1994). *Health as expanding consciousness* (2nd ed.). New York: National League for Nursing.

Niknian, M, Lefebvre, C., & Carleton, R. (1991). Are people more health conscious? A longitudinal study of the community. *American Journal of Public Health, 81*(2), 205–207.

Pender, N. J. (1996). *Health promotion in nursing practice* (3rd ed.). Stanford, CT: Appleton & Lange.

Plotnikoff, N., Faith, R., & Murgo, A. (1991). *Stress and immunity.* Boca Raton, FL: CRC Press.

Rew, L. (1996). *Nurse as healer: Awareness in healing.* Albany, NY: Delmar Publishers.

Rogers, M. (1990). Nursing: Science of Unitary, Irreducible Human Beings: Update 1990. In E. A. M. Barrett, (Ed.), *Visions of Rogers' science-based nursing* (pp. 5–11). New York: National League for Nursing.

Rosenstock, I. (1966). Why people use health services. *Millbank Memorial Fund Quarterly, 44* 99–127.

Rossman, M. (1993). *Mind/body medicine: How to use your mind for better health.* New York: Consumer Reports Books.

Rossman, M., & Bresler, D. (1994). *Interactive guided imagery: Clinical techniques for brief therapy and health psychology: A training workbook* (5th ed.). Mill Valley, CA: Academy for Guided Imagery.

Schubert, P. (1989). *Mutual connectedness: Holistic nursing practice under varying conditions of intimacy* (Doctoral dissertation, University of California, San Francisco, 1989). *Dissertation Abstracts International, 50,* 1987B.

Schubert P., & Lionberger, H. (1995). Mutual connectedness: A study of client–nurse interaction using the Grounded Theory method. *Journal of Holistic Nursing, 13*(2), 102–116.

Shames, K. (1996). *Nurse as healer: Creative imagery in nursing.* Albany, NY: Delmar Publishers.

Smith, C. (1981). The idea of health: A philosophical inquiry. *Advances in Nursing Science, 3,* 43–50.

Swinford, P. C., & Webster, J. A. (1989). *Promoting wellness: A nurse's handbook.* Rockville, MD: Aspen.

Takaki, R. (1993). *A different mirror: A history of multicultural America.* Boston: Little, Brown & Co.

Thibodeaux, G. & Patton, L. (1997). *The human body in health and disease.* (2nd ed.). St. Louis, MO: Mosby.

Travis, J. W. (1977). *Wellness workbook for health professionals.* Berkeley, CA: Ten Speed Press.

U.S. Department of Agriculture, Human Nutrition Information Service. (1992). *Food Guide Pyramid: A guide to daily food choices.* Washington, DC: Author.

U.S. Department of Agriculture & U.S. Department of Health and Human Services. (1995). *Nutrition and your health: Dietary guidelines for Americans* (4th ed.). Washington DC: Author.

U.S. Department of Agriculture & U.S. Department of Health and Human Services. (1995, December). Third report on nutrition monitoring in the United States: Executive summary. Washington, DC: Author.

U.S. Department of Health and Human Services. (1979). *Healthy people: The Surgeon General's report on health promotion and disease prevention.* Washington DC: Author.

U.S. Department of Health and Human Services. *Promoting health/pre-*

venting disease: Objectives for the nation. (1980). Washington, DC: Author.

U.S. Department of Health and Human Services. (1990). *Healthy people 2000: National health promotion and disease prevention objectives.* Washington, DC: Author.

U.S. Department of Health and Human Services. (1992). *Healthy People 2000: Public health service action.* Washington DC: Author.

U.S. Department of Health and Human Services. (1996). *Healthy People 2000: Midcourse review and 1995 revisions.* Sudbury, MA: Jones & Bartlett.

World Health Organization. (1974). *Chronicle of WHO, 1,* 1–2.

World Health Organization. (1981). *Global strategy for Health for All by the Year 2000.* Geneva, Switzerland: Author.

World Health Organization. (1986). Ottawa Charter for Health Promotion. *Health Promotion, 1*(4), iii.

Zahourek, R. (1988). *Relaxation and imagery: Tools for therapeutic communication and intervention.* Philadelphia: W. B. Saunders.

CHAPTER 10
Population-Focused Practice

American Public Health Association, Public Health Nursing Section. (1996). *The definition and role of public health nursing—A statement of the APHA Public Health Nursing Section* (pp. 1–4). Washington, DC: American Public Health Association.

Anderson, I. (1996). Aboriginal well-being. In C. Grbich (Ed.), *Health in Australia: Sociological concepts and issues.* Australia: Prentice Hall.

Ashton, J., & Seymour, H. (1988). *The new public health.* Philadelphia: Open University Press, Milton Keynes.

Bastian, H. (1989). A guide to WHO and "WHO speak," *Consumer Health Forum,* 9, 15.

Baum, F., Fry, D., & Lennie, I. (Eds.). (1992). *Community health policy and practice in Australia.* Sydney: Pluto Press.

Beck, U. (1989). On the way to the industrial risk-society: Outline of an argument. *Thesis Eleven,* 23, 86–105.

Black, D., Townsend, P., & Davidson, N. (1982). Great Britain: Working group on inequalities in health. *Inequalities in Health: The Black Report,* Harmondsworth: Penguin.

Blane, D. (1987). The value of labour-power and health. In Graham Scambler (Ed.), *Sociological theory and medical sociology.* London: Tavistock Publications.

Bracht, N., & Tsouros, A. (1990). Principles and strategies of effective community participation. *Health Promotion International, 5*(3), 99–208.

Brown, L., Donovan, J., & Islip, R. (1988). A guidebook for leaders of new parents' groups, *AECA 18th National Conference,* Canberra, Australia.

Cheek, J., & Willis, E. (1998). Health risk analysis and sociomedical technologies of the self—Private health insurance gets into health promotion. *Australian Journal of Social Issues, 33*(12), 119–132.

Commonwealth Department of Health, Housing and Community Services. (1993). *Towards health for all and health promotion: The evaluation of the national better health program.* Canberra, Australia: AGPS.

Foucault, M. (1980). Power/Knowledge: Selected interviews and other writings, 1972–1977. (C. Gordon, trans.). Brighton: Harvester Press.

Gardner, H. (1992). Health policy: Development, implementation, and evaluation in Australia. Melbourne: Churchill Livingstone.

Hawe, P., Degeling, D., Hall, J., & Brierley, A. (1990). *Evaluating health promotion.* New South Wales: MacLennan & Petty.

Health Targets and Implementation (Health for All) Committee. (1988). *Health for all Australians: Report to the Australian Health Ministers' Advisory Council and the Australian Health Ministers Conference,* Canberra: Australian Government Printing Service.

Institute of Medicine, Committee for the Study of the Future of Public Health. (1988). *The future of public health.* Washington, DC: National Academy Press.

Jackson, T., Mitchel, S., & Wright, M. (1989). The community development continuum. *Community Health Studies, 13*(1).

Keck, C. W. & Scutchfield, E. D. (1997). The future of public health. In F. D. Scutchfield & C. W. Keck, *Principles of public health practice.* Albany, New York: Delmar Publishers.

Labonte, R. (1990). Heart health inequalities in Canada: Models, theory and planning, *Health Promotion International, 7*(2), 119–128.

Lord, J., & McKillop, F. (1990, Fall). A study of personal empowerment: Implications for health promotion. *Health Promotion.*

Lundberg O. (1991). Causal explanations for class inequalities in health—An empirical analysis. *Social Science and Medicine, 32*(4), 385–393.

McKeown, T. (1962). Reasons for the decline of mortality in England and Wales during the nineteenth century. *Population Studies, 16*(2), 94–122.

McKnight, J. (1986). *The need for oldness.* Paper presented at the Center on Aging, McGraw Medical Center. Northwestern University, Evanston, Illinois.

McPherson, P. (1992). Health for all Australians. In Heather Gardner (Ed.), *Health policy: Development, implementation and evaluation in Australia* (p. 120). Melbourne: Churchill Livingstone.

Mosely, H. (1988). Is there a middle way? Categorical programmes for primary health care. *Social Science and Medicine, 26*(9), 907–908.

National Association for County Health Officials. (1994). *Blueprint for a healthy community: A guide for local health departments.* Washington, DC: Author.

National Centre for Epidemiology and Population Health. (1991). *The role of primary health care in health promotion in Australia.* Commonwealth Department of Health, Housing and Community Services and National Better Health Program, Canberra, Australia: Author.

Newell, K. (1988). Selective primary health care: The counter revolution. *Social Science and Medicine, 26*(9), 903–906.

Nutbeam, D. (1986). Health promotion glossary. *Health Promotion, 1*(1), 113–127.

Peterson, A. (1994 June) Community development and health promotion: Empowerment or regulation? *Australian Journal of Public Health, 18*(2), 213–217.

Power, T., & Parke, R. (1984). Social network factors and the transition to parenthood. *Sex Roles, 10*(11/12), 949–972.

Powles, J., & Salzberg, M. (1989). Work, class or life-style? Explaining inequalities in health. In G. Lupton and J. Najman (Eds.), *Sociology of health and illness: Australian readings* (pp. 135–168). South Melbourne: MacMillan.

Scheyner, S., Landefeld, J. S., & Sandifer, F. H. (1981). Biomedical research and illness: 1900–1979. *Millbank Memorial Fund Quarterly/Health and Society, 59*(1).

Sorlie, P. D., Backlund, E., and Keller, J. B. (1995). U.S. mortality by economic, demographic, and social characteristics: The national longitudinal mortality study. *American Journal of Public Health, 85*(7), 949–956.

Stacey, M. (1988). Strengthening communities. *Health Promotion, 2*(4), 321.

Telleen, S., Herzog A., & Kilbane, T. (1989, July). Impact of a family support program on mothers' social support and parenting stress. *American Journal of Orthopsychiatry, 59*(3) 410–419.

U.S. Department of Health and Human Services. (1991). *Healthy people 2000: National health promotion and disease prevention objectives.* Washington, DC: Author.

Vagero, D. (1991). Inequalities in health: Some theoretical and empirical problems. *Social Science and Medicine, 32*(4), 367–371.

Walsh, J. (1988). Selectivity within primary health care. *Social Science and Medicine, 26*(9), 899–902.

Washington State Department of Health. (1994). *Public health improvement plan.* Olympia, WA: Author.

Warren, K. S. (1988). The evolution of selective primary health care. *Social Science and Medicine, 26*(9), 891–898.

Williams, C. A. (1996). Community-based population-focused practice: The foundation of specialization in public health nursing. In M. Stanhope & J. Lancaster, *Community health nursing: Promoting health of aggregates, families, and individuals* (pp. 21–13). St. Louis, MO: Mosby.

Willis, E. (1990). *Advanced nursing studies 3.* Adelaide, Australia: The Flinders University of South Australia, Master of Nursing, School of Nursing.

Wisner, B. (1988). GOBI versus PHC? Some dangers of selective primary health care. *Social Science and Medicine, 26*(9), 963–969.

World Health Organization. (1978a). *Declaration of Alma Ata.* Geneva: Author.

World Health Organization. (1978b). *Primary health care: Report of the international conference on primary health care.* Geneva: Author.

World Health Organization. (1986). *Ottawa Charter for Health Promotion.* Ottawa, Canada: Author.

World Health Organization. (1988, June). *Summary report—European conference on nursing.* Vienna, Austria: Author.

World Health Organization. (1991). Supportive environments for health: The Sundsvall statement. *The Sundsvall Conference on Health Promotion.* Sundsvall, Sweden.

World Health Organization. (1993). *Implementation of the global strat-*

egy for health for all: Second evaluation. Eighth report on the world health situation, Vol. 1, Global Review, Geneva: Author.

World Health Organization & Commonwealth Department of Community Services and Health. (1988). *Proceedings of the Second International Conference of Health Promotion*, April 5–9. Adelaide, Australia: World Health Organization, p. 2.

World Health Organization Regional Office for Europe. (1985). *Primary health care in industrialised countries.* Report of 1983 Conference in Bordeaux on Primary Health Care in Industrialised Countries, Euro Reports and Studies #95. Copenhagen, Denmark: Author.

CHAPTER 11
Epidemiology

Freeman, R. (1963). *Public health nursing practice* (3rd ed.). Philadelphia: W. B. Saunders.

Friedman, G. (1987). *Primer of epidemiology.* New York: McGraw-Hill.

Green, L. (1990). *Community health.* St. Louis, MO: Times-Mirror/Mosby.

Green, L., & Kreuter, M. (1991). *Health promotion planning: An educational and environmental approach.* Mountain View: Mayfield Publishing.

Greenberg, R., Daniels, S. R., Flanders, W. D., Eley, J. W., & Boring III, J. R. (1996). (1993). *Medical epidemiology.* (2nd ed.). Stamford, CT: Appleton & Lange.

Hennekens, C., & Buring, J. (1987). *Epidemiology in medicine.* Boston: Little, Brown, and Company.

Last, J. (1995). *Dictionary of epidemiology.* New York: Oxford University Press.

Lilienfeld, D., & Stolley, P. (1994). *Foundations of epidemiology.* New York: Oxford University Press.

Morton, R., Hebel, J. & McCarter, R. (1996). *A study guide to epidemiology and biostatistics.* Gaithersburg, MD: Aspen Publishers.

National Center for Health Services. (1990). *Healthy people 2000.* Washington DC: U.S. Government Printing Office.

Staff. (1996, June). Major findings from the Nurses' Health Study, 1998 through 1994. *Nurses Health Study Newsletter*, 6.

Teutsch, S., Churchill, R., & Elliott, R. (1994). *Principles and practice of public health surveillance.* New York: Oxford University Press.

U.S. Department of Health and Human Services. (1990). *Healthy people 2000.* Washington, DC: Author.

U.S. Department of Health and Human Services. (1996). *Healthy people 2000.* Midcourse review and 1995 revisions. Sudbury, MA: Jones & Bartlett.

CHAPTER 12
Assessing the Community

American Public Health Association. (1991). *Healthy communities 2000 model standards: Guidelines for community attainment of the year 2000 national health objectives.* Washington, DC: Author.

Anderson, E., & McFarlane, J. (1988). *Community as client: Application of the nursing process.* Philadelphia: J. B. Lippincott.

Arnstein, S. (1971). Eight rungs on the ladder of citizen participation. In E. S. Cahn, & B. A. Passett (Eds.), *Citizen participation: Effecting community change* (pp. 69–91). New York: Praeger Publishers.

Auer, J. (1988). *Exploring legislative arrangements for promoting primary health care in Australia.* Adelaide, Australia: Social Health Branch, South Australian Health Commission.

Barton, J. A., Smith, M. C., Brown, N. J., & Supples, J. M. (1993). Methodological issues in a team approach to community health needs assessment. *Nursing Outlook, 41*(6).

Baum, F. (1992). Researching community health: Evaluation and needs assessment that makes an impact. In F. Baum, D. Fry, & I. Lennie (Eds.), *Community health: Policy and practice in Australia.* Sydney, Australia: Pluto Press in association with Australian Community Health Association.

Baum, F. E. (1995). Researching public health: Behind the qualitative–quantitative debate. *Social Science and Medicine, 40*(4), 459–468.

Baum, F. E., & Cooke, R. D. (1988). Community-health needs assessment: Use of the Nottingham health profile in an Australian study. *Medical Journal of Australia, 150*, 581–590.

Becker, M. H. (1986). The tyranny of health promotion. *Public Health Review, 14*, 15–25.

Billings, J. R., & Cowley, S. (1995). Approaches to community needs assessment: A literature review. *Journal of Advanced Nursing, 22*, 721–730.

Bowling, A. (1992). *"Local voices" in purchasing health care: An exploratory exercise in public consultation in priority setting.* London: Needs Assessment Unit, St Bartholomew's Hospital Medical College.

Bradshaw, J. (1972, March 30). The concept of social need. *New Society*, 640–643.

Brennan, A. (1992). The Altona Clean Air Project. *Health Issues, 32*, 18–20.

Brown, V. (1985). Towards an epidemiology of health: A basis for planning community health programs. *Health Policy, 4*, 331–340.

Bryson, L., & Mowbray, M. (1981). "Community": The spray-on solution. *Australian Journal of Social Issues, 16*(4), 255–267.

Chalmers, K., & Kristajanson, L. (1989). The theoretical basis for nursing at the community level: A comparison of three models. *Journal of Advanced Nursing, 14*, 569–574.

Chu, C. (1994). Assessing community needs and integrated environmental impact assessment. In C. Chu, & R. Simpson (Eds.), *Ecological public health: From vision to practice.* Nathan, Queensland: Institute of Applied Environmental Research, Griffith University and Ontario, Centre for Health Promotion, University of Toronto.

Clark, D. B. (1973). The concept of community: A re-examination. *Sociological Review, 21*(3), 397–415.

Cooney, C. (1994). Community assessment: A vital component of Primary Health Care Objectives. In C. Cooney (Ed.), *Primary health care: The way to the future.* Sydney, Australia: Prentice Hall.

Courtney, R., Ballard, E., Fauver, S., Gariota, M., & Holland, L. (1996). The partnership model: Working with individuals, families and communities toward a new vision of health. *Public Health Nursing, 13*(3), 177–186.

Daly, H. E., & Cobb, J. B. (1989). *For the common good: Redirecting the economy toward community, the environment and a sustainable future.* Boston: Beacon Press.

De Bella, S., Martin, L., & Siddall, S. (1986). *Nurses' role in health care planning.* Norwalk, CT: Appleton-Century-Crofts.

Dewar, T. (1990, July). *Community partnerships seminar three.* Paper presented at Durham, NH: Sponsor W. K. Kellogg Foundation.

Eng, E., Salmon, M. E., & Mullan, F. (1992). Community empowerment: The critical base for primary health care. *Family and Community Health, 15*(1), 1–12.

Epp, J. (1986). *Achieving health for all: A Framework for health promotion.* Ottawa, Canada: National Health and Welfare.

Ewles, L., & Simnett, I. (1992). *Promoting health: A practical guide.* London: Scutari Press.

Flynn, B. C., Ray, D. W., & Rider, M. S. (1994). Empowering communities: Action research through Healthy Cities. *Health Education Quarterly, 21*(3), 395–405.

Gilmore, G. D., Campbell, M. D., & Becker, B. (1989). *Needs assessment strategies for health education and health promotion.* Indianapolis: Benchmark Press.

Goeppinger, J., & Baglioni, A. J. (1985). Community competence: A positive approach to needs assessment. *American Journal of Community Psychology, 13*(5), 507–523.

Green, L. W., & Kreuter, M. W. (1991). *Health promotion planning: An educational and environmental approach.* Mountain View: Mayfield.

Hancock, T., & Duhl, L. (1985). World Health Organization Healthy Cities Project: Promoting health in the urban context. Copenhagen, Denmark: The WHO Healthy Cities Project Office, FADL Publishers.

Hawe, P. (1994). Capturing the meaning of "community" in community intervention evaluation: Some contributions from community psychology. *Health Promotion International, 9*(3), 199–210.

Hawe, P., Degeling, D., & Hall, J. (1990). *Evaluating health promotion: A health worker's guide.* Sydney, Australia: MacLennan and Petty.

Hawtin, Hughes, & Percy-Smith. (1994). *Community profiling: Auditing social needs.* Buckingham, U.K.: Open University Press.

Hayes, M. V., & Willms, S. (1990). Healthy community indicators: The perils of the search and the paucity of the find. *Health Promotion International, 5*(2), 161–166.

Health Targets and Implementation Committee. (1988). *Health for All Australians.* Canberra, Australia: Australian Government Publishing Service.

Henderson, P., & Thomas, D. N. (1987). *Skills in neighbourhood work.* Sydney, Australia: Allen and Unwin.

Institute of Medicine. (1988). *The future of public health.* Washington, DC: National Academy Press.

Kang, R. (1995). Building community capacity for health promotion: A challenge for public health nurses. *Public Health Nursing, 12*(5), 312–318.

Katz, M. F., & Kreuter, M. W. (1997). Community assessment and empowerment. In F. D. Scutchfield & C. W. Keck. *Principles of public health practice* (pp. 147–1570). Albany, New York: Delmar Publishers.

Kelly, J. G. (1988). *A guide to conducting prevention research in the community: First steps.* New York: Haworth.

Kreuter, M. W. (1984). Health promotion: The role of public health in the community for free exchange. *Health Promotions Monographs, 4.* New York: Columbia University, Center for Health Promotion.

Kuehnert, P. L. (1995). The interactive and organizational model of community as client: A model for public health nursing practice. *Public Health Nursing, 12*(1), 9–17.

Labonte, R. (1989). Community empowerment: The need for political analysis. *Canadian Journal of Public Health, 80,* 87–88.

Labonte, R. (1994). Health promotion and empowerment: Reflections on professional practice. *Health Education Quarterly, 21*(2), 253–268.

Matrice, D., & Brown, V. (1990). *Widening the research focus: Consumer roles in public health research.* Curtin, Australian Capital Territory: Consumers' Health Forum.

McBride, T. (1988). Poverty action in a community health center. *Health Issues,* September, (15), 24–27.

McKenzie, J. F., & Jurs, J. L. (1993). *Planning, implementing, and evaluating health programs: A primer.* New York: Macmillan.

McKnight, J. (1986, Fall). *The need for oldness.* Paper presented at the Center for Aging, McGraw Medical Center, Northwestern University, Evanston, IL.

McTaggart, R. (1991). Principles for participatory action research. *Adult Education Quarterly, 41*(3), 168–187.

Minkler, M. (1994). Ten commitments for community health education. *Health Education Research, 9*(4), 527–534.

Murphy, B., Cockburn, J., & Murphy, M. (1992). Focus groups in health research. *Health Promotion Journal of Australia, 2*(2), 37–40.

Murray, C. J., & Lopez, A. D. (1996). *Summary: The Global Burden of Disease and Inquiry Series.* Cambridge, MA: The Harvard School of Public Health on behalf of the World Health Organization and the World Bank. Harvard University Press.

Oakley, P. (1989). *Community involvement in health development.* Geneva, Switzerland: World Health Organization.

Ong, B. N., Humphris, G., Annett, H., & Rifkin, S. (1991). Rapid appraisal in an urban setting, An example from the developed world. *Social Science and Medicine, 32*(8), 909–915.

Patrick, D. L. (1986). Measurement of health and quality of life. In D. L. Patrick, & G. Scambler (Eds.), *Sociology as applied to medicine.* London: Bailliere Tindall.

Peckham, S., & Spanton, J. (1994). Community development approaches to health needs assessment. *Health Visitor, 67*(4), 124–125.

Rains, J. W., & Ray, D. W. (1995). Participatory action research for community health promotion. *Public Health Nursing, 12*(4), 256–261.

Rissel, C. (1991). The tyranny of needs assessment in health. *Evaluation Journal of Australia, 3*(1), 26–31.

Rissel, C. (1996). A communitarian correction for health outcomes in New South Wales? *Australian Journal of Primary Health—Interchange, 2*(2), 36–45.

Robertson, A., & Minkler, M. (1994). New health promotion movement: A critical examination. *Health Education Quarterly, 21*(3), 295–312.

Rorden, J. W., & McLennan, J. (1992). *Community health nursing: Theory and practice.* Sydney, Australia: Harcourt Brace.

Ruffing-Rahal, M. A. (1987). Resident/provider contrasts in community health priorities. *Public Health Nursing, 4*(4), 242–246.

Russell, C. K., Gregory, D. M., Wotton, D., Mordoch, E., & Counts, M. M. (1996). ACTION: Application and extension of the GENESIS community analysis model. *Public Health Nursing, 13*(3), 187–194.

Ryan, W. (1976). *Blaming the victim.* New York: Vintage Books.

Shuster, G. F., & Goeppinger, J. (1996). Community as client: Using the nursing process to promote health. In M. Stanhope, & J. Lancaster, *Community health nursing: Process and practice for promoting health.* (4th ed.). pp. 289–314. St. Louis, MO: C. V. Mosby.

Southern Community Health Research Unit. (1991). *Planning healthy communities: A guide to community needs assessment.* Bedford Park, South Australia: Southern Community Health Research Unit.

Stalker, K. (1993). The best laid plans . . . gang aft agley? Assessing population needs in Scotland. *Health and Social Care, 2,* 1–9.

Stevens, P. E. 1996. Focus groups: Collecting aggregate-level data to understand community health phenomena. *Public Health Nursing, 13* 3, 170–176.

Stoner, M. H., Magilvy, J. K. and Schultz, P. R. 1992. Community analysis in community health nursing practice: The GENESIS model, *Public Health Nursing, 9* 4, 223–227.

Twelvetrees, A. 1987. *Community work.* London: Macmillan.

U.S. Department of Health and Human Services. 1991. *Healthy people 2000: National health promotion and disease prevention objectives.* Washington, DC: Author.

Van de Ven, A. H. and Delbecq, A. L. 1972. The nominal group process as a research instrument for exploratory health studies. *American Journal of Public Health, 62,* 337–342.

Wadsworth, Y. 1988. *Participatory research and development in primary health care by community groups: Report to the National Health and Medical Research Council Public Health Research and Development Committee.* Deakin, ACT: Consumers' Health Forum.

Wallerstein, N. (1992, January/February). Powerlessness, empowerment, and health: Implications for health promotion programs. *American Journal of Health Promotion, 6*(3), 197–205.

Wass, A. 1994. *Promoting health: The primary health care approach.* Sydney: Harcourt Brace and Company.

Wass, A. 1995. Health workers and communities working together—Challenges for a meaningful partnership. In *Primary health care: Working together, proceedings of the sixth annual Primary Health Care Conference,* 23–24 November. Sydney, Australia: Faculty of Nursing, Cumberland, University of Sydney.

World Health Organization. (1978). The Declaration of Alma-Ata. Reproduced in *World Health,* 1988, August/September, 16–17.

World Health Organization, Health and Welfare Canada, Canadian Public Health Association. (1986). *Ottawa Charter for Health Promotion.* Copenhagen, Denmark: FADL Publishers.

CHAPTER 13
Program Planning, Implementation, and Evaluation

American Nurses Association. (1991). *Nursing's agenda for health care reform.* Kansas City, MO: Author.

American Public Health Association. (1991). *Healthy communities 2000: Model standards for community attainment of the year 2000 national health objectives* (3rd ed.). Washington DC: Author.

Attridge, C., Budgen, C., Hilton, A., McDavid, J., Molzahn, A., & Purlis, M. E. (1997). The Comox Valley nursing centre demonstration project: How did it work? *Canadian Nurse, 93*(2), 34–38.

Bassett-Smith, J. (1997). *Toward critical scholarship for research in nursing.* (Unpublished doctoral candidacy paper, University of Victoria), British Columbia, Canada.

Bateson, M. C. (1990). *Composing a life.* New York: Penguin Books.

Baum, F. (1993). Healthy Cities and change: Social movement or bureaucratic tool? *Health Promotion International, 8*(1), 31–40.

Baum, F., & Sanders, D. (1995). Can health promotion and primary health care achieve Health for All without a return to their more radical agenda? *Health Promotion International, 10*(2), 149–160.

Bent, K. N. (1993). Perspectives on critical and feminist theory in developing nursing praxis. *Journal of Professional Nursing, 9*(5), 296–303.

Bless, C., Murphy, D., & Vinson, N. (1995). Nurses' role in primary health care. *National Health and Welfare: Perspectives on Community, 16*(2), 70–76.

Borich, G. D., & Jemelka, R. P. (1982). *Programs and systems: An evaluation perspective.* New York: Academic Press.

Bracht, N. (Ed.) (1990). *Health promotion at the community level.* Newbury Park, CA: Sage.

Bracht, N., Finnigan, J., Rissel, C., Weisbrod, R., Gleason, J., Corbett, J., & Veblen-Mortensen, S. (1994). Community ownership and program continuation following a health demonstration project. Health Education Research 9(2) 243–255.

Bracht, N., & Kingsbury, L. (1990) Community organization principles in health promotion: A five stage model. In N. Bracht (Ed.), *Health promotion at the community level* (pp. 66–89). Newbury Park, CA: Sage.

British Columbia Ministry of Health. (1989). *Healthy communities: The process.* Victoria, British Columbia, Canada: Author.

Budgen, C. M. (1987). Modeling: A method for program development. *Journal of Nursing Administration, 17*(12), 19–25.

Budgen, C., & Bates, M. (1996). Campus Health Services project evaluation report. Kelowna, B.C., Canada: Okanagan University College, Department of Nursing.

Butterfield, P. G. (1990). Thinking upstream: Nurturing a conceptual understanding of the societal context of health behavior. *Advances in Nursing Science, 12*(2), 1–8.

Canadian Nurses Association. (1997). *Code of ethics.* Ottawa, Canada: Author.

Chalmers, K., & Bramadat, I. (1996). Community development: theoretical and practical issues for community health nursing in Canada. *Journal of Advanced Nursing, 24*, 719–726.

Chinn, P. (1995). *Peace and power: Building communities for the future* (4th ed.). New York: National League for Nursing.

Clarke, H. F., Beddome, G., & Whyte, N. B. (1993). Public health nurses' vision of the future reflects changing paradigms. *Image, 25* (4), 305–310.

Covey, S., Merrill, A., & Merrill, R. (1997). *First things first every day: Because where you're headed is more important than how fast you're going.* New York: Simon & Schuster.

Creese, A. (1994). Global trends in health care reform. *World Health Forum, 15*, 317–322.

Daniel, M. (1997). *Effectiveness of community directed diabetes prevention and control in a rural aboriginal population.* (Unpublished doctoral dissertation, University of British Columbia), Vancouver, B.C., Canada.

Daniel, M., Gamble, D., (1996). *Aboriginal community-directed diabetes prevention and control: The Okanagen Diabetes Project.* (National Health and Research Development Program Project No. 6610-2022ND). Ottawa, Canada: Health Canada.

Dignan, M. B., & Carr, P. A. (1992). *Program planning for health education and promotion* (2nd ed.). Philadelphia, PA: Lea & Febiger.

Dignan, M., Tillgren, P., & Michielutte, R. (1994). Developing process evaluation for community-based health education, research and practice: A role for the diffusion model. *Health Values, 18*(5), 56–59.

Drevdahl, D. (1995). Coming to voice: The power of emancipatory community interventions. *Advances in Nursing Science, 18*(2), 13–24.

Eng, E., Salmon, M. E., & Mullan, F. (1992). Community empowerment: The critical base for primary health care. *Family Community Health, 15*(1), 1–12.

English, J. (1995). Community development. In M. Stewart (Ed.), *Community nursing: Promoting Canadians' health* (pp. 513–531). Toronto, Canada: W. B. Saunders.

Epp, J. (1986). *Achieving Health for All: A framework for health promotion.* Ottawa, Canada: National Health and Welfare.

Evans, R., & Stoddart, G. (1990). Producing health, consuming health care. *Social Science & Medicine, 31*(12), 1347–1363.

Flick, L., Reese, C., Rogers, G., Fletcher, P., & Sonn, J. (1994). Building community for health: Lessons from a seven year old neighborhood/university partnership. *Health Education Quarterly, 21*(3), 369–380.

Flynn, B., Ray, D., & Rider, M. (1994). Empowering communities: Action research through healthy cities. *Health Education Quarterly, 21*(3), 395–405.

Frank, J. W. (1995). Why "population health"? *Canadian Journal of Public Health, 86*(3), 162–164.

Freire, P. (1970/1993). *Pedagogy of the oppressed* (20th ed.). New York: Continuum.

Goodman, R., Steckler, A., Hoover, S., & Schwartz, R. (1993). A critique of contemporary community health promotion approaches based on a qualitative review of six programs in Maine. *American Journal of Health Promotion, 7*(3), 208–220.

Grace, V. M. (1991). The marketing of empowerment and the construction of the health consumer: A critique of health promotion. *International Journal of Health Services, 21*(2), 329–343.

Green, L., & Kreuter, M. (1991). *Health promotion planning: An educational and environmental approach.* Mountain View, CA: Mayfield.

Green, L., & Kreuter, M. (1993). Are community organization and health promotion one process or two? Commentary. *American Journal of Health Promotion, 7*(3) 221.

Green, L., & Raeburn, J. (1990). Contemporary developments in health promotion: Definitions and challenges. In N. Bracht (Ed.), *Health promotion at the community level* (pp. 29–42). Newbury Park, CA: Sage.

Hagedorn, S. (1995). The politics of caring: The role of activism in primary care. *Advances in Nursing Science, 17*(4), 1–11.

Hale, C., Arnold, F., & Travis, M. (1994). *Planning and evaluating health programs,* Albany, NY: Delmar Publishers.

Hamilton, N., & Bhatti, T. (1996). *Population health promotion: An integrated model of population health and health promotion* (Rep.). Ottawa, Canada: Health Promotion Development Division.

Hammer, M., & Champy, J. (1994). *Reengineering the corporation: A manifesto for business revolution.* New York: Harper Business/Collins.

Hancock, T. (1993). Health, human development and the community ecosystem: Three ecological models. *Health Promotion International, 8*(1), 41–47.

Health and Community Services Agency. (1998). *Circle of health.* Charlottetown, Prince Edward Island, Canada: Author.

Higgins, J., & Green, L. (1994). The APHA criteria for development of health promotion programs applied to four Healthy Community projects in British Columbia. *Health Promotion International, 9*(4), 311–319.

Hills, M., Lindsey, E., Chisamore, M., Bassett-Smith, J., Abbott, K., & Fournier-Chalmers, J. (1994). University–college collaboration: Rethinking curriculum development in nursing education. *Journal of Nursing Education, 33*, 220–225.

Hutchison, R. R., & Quartaro, E. G. (1995). High-risk vulnerable population and volunteers: A model of education and service collaboration. *Journal of Community Health Nursing, 12*(2), 111–119.

Kendall, J. (1992) Fighting back: Promoting emancipatory nursing actions. *Advances in Nursing Science, 15*(2), 1–15.

Labonte, R. (1993). Health promotion & empowerment frameworks: Practice frameworks. *Issues in health promotion series, No. 3.* Toronto, Canada: University of Toronto.

Labonte, R. (1994). Death of program, birth of metaphor: The development of health promotion in Canada. In A. Pederson, M. O'Neill, & I. Rootman (Eds.), *Health promotion in Canada* (pp. 72–90). Toronto, Canada: W. B. Saunders.

Lalonde, M. (1974). *A new perspective on the health of Canadians: A working document.* Ottawa, Canada: Government of Canada.

Leonard, V. W. (1991). A Heideggerian phenomenologic perspective on the concept of the person. *Advances in Nursing Science, 11*(4), 40–55.

Lindsey, E., & Hartrick, G. (1996). Health-promoting nursing practice: The demise of the nursing process? *Journal of Advanced Nursing, 23*, 106–112.

Maglacas, A. M. (1988). Health for All: Nursing's role. *Nursing Outlook, 36*(2), 66–72.

Mahler, H. (1985, June). Nurses lead the way. *World Health Organization Features, 97.*

Manson-Singer, S. (1994). The Canadian Healthy Communities project: Creating a social movement. In A. Pederson, M. O'Neill, & I. Rootman (Eds.), *Health promotion in Canada* (pp. 72–90). Toronto, Canada: W. B. Saunders.

Marlatt, G., & Gordon, J. (Eds.). (1985). *Relapse prevention.* New York: Guilford Press.

McKenzie, J. F., & Smeltzer, J. (1997). *Planning, implementing, and evaluating health promotion programs: A primer* (2nd ed.). Boston: Allyn & Bacon.

McKnight, J., & Kretzmann, J. (1992, Winter). Mapping community capacity. *New Designs,* 9–15.

Minkler, M. (1990). Improving health through community organization. In K. Glanz, F. M. Lewis, & B. K. Rimer (Eds.), *Health behavior and health education* (pp. 257–285). San Francisco: Jossey Bass.

Moccia, P. (1990). Re-claiming our communities. *Nursing Outlook, 38*(2), 73–76.

Mullett, J. (1995). *Program performance evaluation framework for Regional Health Boards and Community Health Councils.* Unpublished paper. Victoria, British Columbia, Canada: Ministry of Health.

Oullet, F., Durand, D., & Forget, G. (1994). Preliminary results of an evaluation of three Healthy Cities initiatives in the Montreal area. *Health Promotion International, 9*(3), 153–159.

Parcel, G., Perry, C., & Taylor, W. (1990). Beyond demonstration: Diffusion of health promotion innovations. In N. Bracht (Ed.), *Health promotion at the community level* (pp. 229–251). Newbury Park, CA: Sage.

Pederson, A., O'Neill, M., & Rootman, I. (1994). *Health promotion in Canada: Provincial, national and international perspectives.* Toronto, Canada: W. B. Saunders.

Pirie, P. (1990). Evaluating health promotion programs: Basic questions and approaches. In N. Bracht (Ed.), *Health promotion at the community level* (pp. 201–208). Newbury Park. CA: Sage.

Porter-O'Grady, T. (1994). Building partnerships in health care: Creating whole system change. *Nursing & Health Care, 15*(1), 34–38.

Pratt, L. (1997, September). RN with a cause. *Chatelaine,* 76–81, Toronto, Canada: Maclean-Hunter.

Prochaska, J., Redding, C., Harlow, L., Rossi, J., & Velicer, W. (1994). The transtheoretical model of change and HIV prevention: A review. *Health Education Quarterly, 21*(4), 471–486.

Province of British Columbia. (1989). *Healthy Communities: The process.* Victoria, British Columbia, Canada: Province of British Columbia Ministry of Health and Ministry of Responsibility for Seniors.

Provincial Health Officer. (1996). *A report on the health of British Columbians: Annual report 1995.* Victoria, British Columbia, Canada: Ministry of Health.

Registered Nurses Association of British Columbia. (1994). *Creating the new health care: A nursing perspective.* Vancouver, Canada: Author.

Rissel, C. (1994). Empowerment: The holy grail of health promotion? *Health Promotion International, 9*(1), 39–47.

Ritchie, J. (1997). Happenings: The national forum on health. *Canadian Journal of Nursing Research, 29*(2), 119–128.

Roberts, S. J. (1983). Oppressed group behavior: Implications for nursing. *Advances in Nursing Science, 5*(4), 21–30.

Robertson, A., & Minkler, M. (1994). New health promotion movement: A critical examination. *Health Education Quarterly, 21*(3), 295–312.

Skelton, R. (1994). Nursing and empowerment: Concepts and strategies. *Journal of Advanced Nursing, 19*, 415–423.

Smith, G. (1997). *Shaping the future health system through community based approaches.* Keynote presentation at the 21st Quadrennial International Congress of Nurses, Vancouver, British Columbia, Canada.

Stachtchenko, S., & Jecinek, M. (1990, January/February). Conceptual differences between prevention and health promotion: Research implications for community health programs. *Canadian Journal of Public Health, 81*, 53–59.

Steckler, A., Orville, K., Eng, E., & Dawson, L. (1992). Summary of a formative evaluation of PATCH. *Journal of Health Education, 23*(3), 174–178.

Steingraber, S. (1997). *Living downstream: An ecologist's look at cancer & the environment.* Menlo Park, CA: Addison-Wesley.

Steuart, G. W. (1959/1993). The importance of programme planning. *Health Education Quarterly* (Suppl.), (470) 6–22, S21–27.

Stevens, P. (1989). A critical reconceptualization of the environment in nursing. *Advances in Nursing Science, 11*(4), 56–68.

Stewart, M. J. (Ed.). (1995). *Community nursing: Promoting Canadians' health.* Toronto, Canada: W. B. Saunders.

Stokols, D. (1992). Establishing and maintaining healthy environments: Toward a social ecology of health promotion. *American Psychologist, 47*(1), 6–22.

Stoto, M. A., Behrens, R., & Rosemont, C. (Eds.). (1990). *Healthy people 2000: Citizens chart the course.* Washington, DC: National Academy.

U.S. Department of Health and Human Services. (1992). *Healthy people 2000: Summary report.* Sudbury, MA: Jones & Bartlett.

U.S. Department of Health and Human Services. (1996). *Healthy people 2000: Midcourse review and 1995 revisions.* Sudbury, MA: Jones & Bartlett.

Vail, S. (1995, December). Making tough decisions. *Canadian Nurse, 91*(12), 59–60.

Vail, S. (1997). A question of values. *Canadian Nurse, 93*(10), 59–60.

Vail, S., & Shetowsky, B. (1997). Keeping up with health care technologies. *Canadian Nurse, 93*(7), 59–60.

Van Norstrand, C. H. (1993). *Gender responsible leadership: Detecting bias implementing interventions.* Newbury Park, CA: Sage.

Verhey, M. (1997). *Partners in power: Client education for the 21st century.* Paper presented at the 21st Quadrennial International Congress of Nurses, Vancouver, British Columbia, Canada.

Wallerstein, N. (1992). Powerlessness, empowerment, and health: Implications for health promotion. *American Journal of Health Promotion, 6*(3), 197–205.

Wallerstein, N., & Bernstein, E. (1988). Empowerment education: Friere's ideas adapted to health education. *Health Education Quarterly, 15*(4), 379–394.

Waring, M. (1996). *Three masquerades: Essays on equality work and human rights.* Auckland, New Zealand: Auckland University Press.

Watson, J. (1988). *Nursing: Human science and human care: A theory of nursing.* New York: National League for Nursing.

White, J. (1995). Patterns of knowing: Review, critique, and update. *Advances in Nursing Science, 17*(4), 73–86.

Wolton, K., Amit, H., Kalma, S., Hillman, L., Hillman, D., & Cosway, N. (1995, January). *Basic concepts of international health.* Module. Ottawa, Canada: Canadian University Consortium for Health in Development.

Wong-Rieger, D., & David, L. (1995). Using program logic models to plan and evaluate education and prevention programs. In A. Love (Ed.), *Evaluation methods sourcebook II* (pp. 120–135). Ottawa, Canada: Canadian Evaluation Society.

World Health Organization. (1978). *Alma-Alta 1978: Report of the International Conference on Primary Health Care.* Geneva, Switzerland: Author.

World Health Organization. (1981). *Global strategy for Health for All by the year 2000.* Geneva, Switzerland: Author.

World Health Organization. (1986). *Ottawa charter for health promotion.* Ottawa, Canada: Canadian Public Health Association.

Zerwekh, J. (1992). The practice of empowerment and coercion by expert public health nurses. *Image, 24*(2), 101–105.

CHAPTER 14
The Varied Roles of Community Health Nursing

American Association of Occupational Health Nurses. (1994). *Standards of occupational health nursing practice.* AAOHN: Atlanta, GA: Author.

American Association of Occupational Health Nurses. (1994). *Standards of occupational health nursing practice.* AAOHN: Atlanta, GA: Author.

American Nurses Association. (1985). *Standards of nursing practice in correctional facilities.* Kansas City, MO: Author.

American Nurses Association. (1986a). *Standards of community health nursing practice.* Kansas City, MO: Author.

American Nurses Association. (1986b). *Standards of home health nursing practice.* Kansas City, MO: Author.

American Nurses' Association. (1987). *Standards and scope of hospice nursing practice.* Kansas City, MO: Author.

American Nurses Association. (1991). *Nursing's agenda for health care reform.* Kansas City, MO: Author.

American Nurses Association. (1995). *Scope and standards of nursing practice in correctional facilities.* Washington, DC: American Nurses Publishing.

American Public Health Association, Public Health Nursing Section. (1996). *The definition and role of public health nursing—A statement of the Public Health Nursing Section.* Washington, DC: Author.

Association of Community Health Nursing Educators. (1993). *Differentiated nursing practice in community health.* Lexington, KY: Author.

Atherton, R. A., & LeGendre, S. T. (1985). A description of nurse practitioners' practice in occupational health settings. *Occupational Health Nursing, 33*, 18–20.

Babcock, D. E., & Miller, M. A. (1994). *Client education: Theory and practice.* St. Louis, MO: C. V. Mosby.

Balzar-Riley, J. W. (1996). *Communication in nursing* (3rd ed.). St. Louis: Mosby Year-book.

Bandman, E. L., & Bandman, B. (1995). *Nursing ethics through the life span* (3rd ed.). Norwalk, CT: Appleton & Lange.

Barlow, R. (1992). Role of the occupational health nurse in the year 2000: Perspective view. *American Association of Occupational Health Nurses Journal, 40*, 463–467.

Boss, J., & Corbett, J. (1990). The developing practice of the parish nurse: An inner city experience. In P. Solari-Twadell, A. Djupe, & M. McDermott (Eds.), *Parish nursing: The developing practice* (pp. 77–103). Park Ridge, IL: National Parish Nurse Resource Center.

Bramlett, M. H., Gueldner, S. H., & Sowell, R. L. (1990). Consumer-centric advocacy: Its connection to nursing frameworks. *Nursing Science Quarterly, 3*, 156–161.

Bridges, M. J. (1981). Prison: A learning experience. *American Journal of Nursing, 81*, 744–745.

Brunk, Q. A. (1992). The clinical nurse specialist as an external consultant: A framework for practice. *Clinical Nurse Specialist, 6*, 2–4.

Burbach, C. A., & Brown, B. E. (1988). Community health and home health nursing: Keeping the concepts clear. *Nursing and Health Care, 9*, 97–100.

Butler, M. (1986). Forging a dual role: Administrator/consultant. *Nursing Administration Quarterly, 10*(4), 50–57.

Cary, A. H. (1996). Promoting continuity of care: Case management. In M. Stanhope & J. Lancaster, *Community health nursing: Process and practice for promoting health* (4th ed., pp. 357–374). St. Louis, MO: C. V. Mosby.

Chaisson, G. M. (1981). Correctional health care: Beyond the barriers. *American Journal of Nursing, 81*, 737–738.

Clark, M. J. (1996). Community health nursing. In M. J. Clark, *Nursing in the community* (pp. 55–73). Norwalk, CT: Appleton & Lange.

Clark, M. J. (1996). Community health nursing. In M. J. Clark (ed.). *Nursing in the community* (2nd ed.). Stamford, CT: Appleton & Lange, 55–73.

Clarke, B. A., & Strauss, S. S. (1992). Nursing role supplementation for adolescent parents: Prescriptive nursing practice. *Journal of Pediatric Nursing, 7*, 312–318.

Cookfair, J. M. (1996). *Nursing care in the community* (2nd ed.). St. Louis: Mosby Year-book.

Dalle Molle, C., & Allan, J. (1989). The need for a more holistic health care system. *American Association of Occupational Health Nurses Journal, 37*, 518–525.

DeBella, S. (1993). Health education. In J. M. Swanson & M. Albrecht, *Community health nursing: Promoting the health of aggregates* (pp. 163–185). Philadelphia: W. B. Saunders.

Downs, M. (1984). The hospice team. In S. Schraff (Ed.), *Hospice, the nursing perspective* (pp. 47–59). New York: National League for Nursing.

Elder, R. G., & Bullough, B. (1990). Nurse practitioners and clinical nurse specialists: Are the roles merging? *Clinical Nurse Specialist, 4,* 78–84.

Epstein, M. H., Nelson, C. M., Polsgrove L., Coutinho, M., Cumblad, C., & Quinn, K. (1993). A comprehensive community-based approach to serving students with emotional and behavioral disorders. *Journal of Emotional and Behavioral Disorders, 1,* 127–133.

Faris, J. (1995). Consumer relationships. In P. Wise, *Leading and managing in nursing* (pp. 392–409). St. Louis, MO: Mosby.

Farnsworth, B., & Gutterres, C. (1989). The role of school nurses in health promotion and prevention of illness. *Georgia Nursing, 49*(4), 4.

Feroli, K. L., Hobson, S. K., Miola, E. S, Scott, P. N., & Waterfield, G. D. (1992). School-based clinics: The Baltimore experience. *Journal of Pediatric Health Care, 6,* 127–131.

Gillespie, M., & Gartland, K. (1984). Organization and administration. In S. Schraff (Ed.), *Hospice, the nursing perspective* (pp. 17–34). New York: National League for Nursing.

Gurfolino, V. & Dumas, V. (1994). Hospice nursing. *Nursing Clinics of North America, 29*(3), 533–548.

Haag, A. B., & Glazner, L. K. (1992). A remembrance of the past, an investment for the future. *American Association of Occupational Health Nurses Journal, 40,* 56–60.

Hardy, M. E., & Conway, M. E. (1978). *Role theory: Perspectives for health professionals.* Norwalk, CT: Appleton-Century-Crofts.

Hart, B. G., & Moore, P. V. (1992). The aging work force: Challenge for the occupational health nurse. *American Association of Occupational Health Nurses Journal, 40,* 36–40.

Hazelton, J. H., Boyum, C. M., & Frost, M. H. (1993). Clinical nurse specialist subroles: Foundations for entrepreneurship. *Clinical Nurse Specialist, 7,* 40–45.

Heider, J. (1985). The ripple effect. In J. Heider, *The tao of leadership* (p. 107). Atlanta, GA: Humanics New Age.

Holst, L. (1987). The parish nurse. *Chronicle of Pastoral Care, 7,* 13–17.

Hospice Nurses Association. (1995). *Standards of hospice nursing practice and professional performance.* Pittsburgh, PA: Author.

Igoe, J. (1984). Current issues and future directions. In S. Schraff (Ed.), *Hospice, the nursing perspective* (pp. 153–168). New York: National League for Nursing.

Igoe, J. B., & Giordano, B. P. (1992). *Expanding school health services to serve families in the 21st century.* Washington, DC: American Nurses Publishing.

Igoe, J. B., & Speer, S. (1996). The community health nurse in the schools. In M. Stanhope & J. Lancaster, *Community health nursing: Process and practice for promoting health* (4th ed., pp. 879–906). St. Louis, MO: C. V. Mosby.

Jones, M. E., & Clark, D. W. (1990). Nurse practitioners develop leadership in community problem-solving. *Journal of the American Academy of Nurse Practitioners, 2,* 160–163.

Kane, R. A. (1990). What is case management anyway? In R. A. Kane, K. Urv-Wong, & C. King (Eds.), *Case management: What is it anyway?* (pp. 1–17). Minneapolis, MN: University of Minnesota Long-Term Care DECISIONS Resource Center.

Keegan, L. (1994). The nurse as healer. Albany, NY: Delmar Publishers.

Kenyon, V., Smith, E., Hefty, L. V., Bell, M. L., McNeil, J., & Martaus, T. (1990). Clinical competencies for community health nursing. *Public Health Nursing, 7*(1), 33–39.

Klainberg, M., Holzemer, S., Leonard, M., & Arnold, J. (1998). *Community health nursing: An alliance for health.* New York: McGraw–Hill.

Kohnke, M. F. (1980). The nurse as advocate. *American Journal of Nursing, 80,* 2038–2040.

Kosik, S. H. (1972). Patient advocacy or fighting the system? *American Journal of Nursing, 72,* 695–698.

Kuehnert, P. L. (1991). The public health policy advocate: Fostering the health of communities. *Clinical Nurse Specialist, 5,* 5–10.

Laffrey, S. C., & Page, G. (1989). Primary health care in public health nursing. *Journal of Advanced Nursing, 14,* 1044–1050.

Lange, F. C. (1987). *The nurse as an individual, group, or community consultant.* Norwalk, CT: Appleton-Century-Crofts.

Lee, R. K. (1992). The community health nurse manager. In M. Stanhope & J. Lancaster, *Community health nursing: Process and practice for promoting health* (3rd ed., pp. 648–661). St. Louis, MO: C. V. Mosby.

Little, L., (1981). A change process for prison health nursing. *American Journal of Nursing, 81,* 739–742.

LoBiondo-Wood, G., & Haber, J. (1994). *Nursing research: Methods, critical appraisal, and utilization.* St. Louis, MO: C. V. Mosby.

Lyon, J. C., & Stephany, T. M. (1993). Home health care. In J. M. Swanson & M. Albrecht, *Community health nursing: Promoting the health of aggregates* (pp. 626–639). Philadelphia: W. B. Saunders.

Maciag, M. E. (1993). Occupational health nursing in the 1990s: A dif-

ferent model of practice. *American Association of Occupational Health Nurses Journal, 41,* 39–45.

Marquis, B. L., & Huston, C. J. (1992). *Leadership roles and management functions in nursing: Theory and application.* Philadelphia: J. B. Lippincott.

Mason, D. J., Knight, K., Toughil, E., DeMaio, D., Beck, T. L., & Christopher, M. A. (1992). Promoting the community health clinical nurse specialist. *Clinical Nurse Specialist, 6,* 6–13.

Mayeroff, M. (1971). *On caring.* New York: Harper & Row.

Miller, M. A. (1989). Social, economic, and political forces affecting the future of occupational health nursing. *American Association of Occupational Health Nurses Journal, 37,* 361–366.

Miskelly, S. (1995). A parish nursing model: Applying the community health nursing process in a church community. *Journal of Community Health Nursing, 12,* 1–14.

Molloy, S. P. (1994). Defining case management. *Home Health Care Nurse 12*(3), 51–54.

Moritz, P. (1982). Health care in correctional facilities: A nursing challenge. *Nursing Outlook, 30,* 253–259.

Murphy, N. J. (1998). Nursing leadership in health policy decision making. In B. W. Spradley & J. Allender (eds.). *Readings in community health nursing.* Philadelphia: J. B. Lippincott, 555–561.

Murray, R. B., & Zentner, J. P. (1989). *Nursing assessment and health promotion through the life span.* Englewood Cliffs, NJ: Prentice-Hall.

Murray, R. B., & Zentner, J. P. (1997). *Nursing assessment and promotion strategies* (6th ed.). Stamford, CT: Appleton & Lange.

National Institute of Nursing Research. (1993). *National nursing research agenda: Setting nursing research priorities.* Bethesda, MD: Author.

National League for Nursing. (1993). *A vision for nursing education.* New York: Author.

Niskala, H. (1986) Competencies and skills required by nurses working in forensic areas. *Western Journal of Nursing Research, 8,* 400–413.

Ogle, B. (1990). What is forensic/correctional nursing. *The Florida Nurse, 38*(6), 12.

Ossler, C. C. (1992). The community health nurse in occupational health. In M. Stanhope & J. Lancaster, *Community health nursing: Process and practice for promoting health* (3rd ed., pp. 731–746). St. Louis, MO: C. V. Mosby.

Peternely-Taylor, C. A., & Hufft, A. G. (1997). Forensic psychiatric nursing. In B. S. Johnson, *Adaptation and growth: Psychiatric nursing* (4th ed.). Philadelphia: Lippincott-Raven.

Petrosino, B. (1984). Staffing and stress management. In S. Schraff (Ed.), *Hospice, the nursing perspective* (pp. 73–91). New York: National League for Nursing.

Proctor, S. T., Lordi, S. L., & Zaiger, D. S. (1993). *School nursing practice: Roles and standards.* Scarborough, ME: National Association of School Nurses.

Rankin, S. H., & Stallings, K. D. (1996). *Patient education: Issues, principles, practices* (3rd ed.). Philadelphia: J. B. Lippincott.

Rector, C. (1997). Innovative practice models in community health nursing. In B. W. Spradley & J. Allender (ed.). *Readings in community health nursing* (5th ed.). Philadelphia: J. B. Lippincott, 163–172.

Redford, L. (1992). Case management: The wave of the future. *Journal of Case Management, 1,* 5–8.

Reutter, L. G., & Ford, J. (1996). Perceptions of public health nursing: Views from the field. *Journal of Advanced Nursing, 24,* 7–15.

Rheaume, A., Frisch, S., Smith, A., & Kennedy, C. (1994). Case management and nursing practice. *Journal of Nursing Administration, 24,* 30–36.

Riner, M. B. (1989). Expanding services: The role of the community health nurse and the advanced practitioner. *Journal of Community Health Nursing, 6,* 223–230.

Riportella-Muller, R., Selby, M. L., Salmon, M. E., Quade, D., & Legault, C. (1991). Specialty roles in community health nursing: A national survey of educational needs. *Public Health Nursing, 8,* 81–89.

Robinson, M. B. (1985). Patient advocacy and the nurse: Is there a conflict of interest? *Nursing Forum, 22*(2), 58–63.

Rogers, B. (1989). Establishing research priorities in occupational health nursing. *American Association of Occupational Health Nurses Journal, 37,* 493–500.

Rogers, M., Riordan, J., & Swindle, D. (1991). Community-based nursing case management pays off. *Nursing Management, 22*(3), 30–34.

Rubin, S. (1988). Expanded role nurse: Part 1, role theory concepts. *Canadian Journal of Nursing Administration, 1*(2), 23–26.

Ryan, J. (1990). Society, the parish and the parish nurse. In P. Solari-Twadell, A. Djupe, & M. McDermott (Eds.), *Parish nursing: The developing practice* (pp. 41–53). Park Ridge, IL: National Parish Nurse Resource Center.

Samarel, N. (1989). Caring for the living and dying: A study of role transition. *International Journal of Nursing Studies, 26,* 313–326.

Schank, M., Weis, S., & Matheus, R. (1996). Parish nursing: Ministry of healing. *Geriatric Nursing, 17,* 11–13.

Schneider, B. (1989). Care planning in the aging network. In R. A. Kane, K. Urv-Wong, & C. King (Eds.), *Concepts in case management* (pp. 3–27). Minneapolis, MN: University of Minnesota Long-Term Care DECISIONS Resource Center.

Schneider, J. K. (1992). Clinical nurse specialist: Role definition as discharge planning coordinator. *Clinical Nurse Specialist, 6,* 36–39.

Schultz, S. J. (1984). Reimbursement issues. In S. Schraff (Ed.), *Hospice, the nursing perspective* (pp. 35–46). New York: National League for Nursing

Sellek, C. S., Sirles, A. T., & Sloan, R. H. (1992). The community health nurse clinician and family nurse practitioner in primary and ambulatory care. In M. Stanhope & J. Lancaster, *Community health nursing: Process and practice for promoting health* (3rd ed., pp. 635–645). St. Louis, MO: C. V. Mosby.

Shelov, S. P. (1994). Editorial: The children's agenda for the 1990s and beyond. *American Journal of Public Health, 84,* 1066–1067.

Snow, T., Giduz, E. H., McConnell, E. S., Sanchez & Wildman, D. S. (1988). *Handbook of geriatric practice essentials.* Rockville, MD: Aspen.

Solari-Twadell, A., & Westberg, G. (1991, September). Body, mind, and soul: The parish nurse offers physical, emotional, and spiritual care. *Health Progress,* 24–28.

Solari-Twadell, P. (1990). Models of parish nursing: A challenge in design. In P. Solari-Twadell, A. Djupe, & M. McDermott (Eds.), *Parish nursing: The developing practice* (pp. 57–76). Park Ridge, IL: National Parish Nurse Resource Center.

Spector, R. (1984). What makes hospice unique? In S. Schraff (Ed.), *Hospice, the nursing perspective* (pp. 1–15). New York: National League for Nursing.

Spradley, B. W. (1990). Roles and settings for community health nursing practice. In B. W. Spradley, *Community health nursing: Concepts and practice* (3rd ed., pp. 191–209). Glenview, IL: Scott, Foresman/Little, Brown Higher Education.

Spradley, B. W., & Allender, J. A. (1996). *Community health nursing: Concepts and practice.* (4th ed.). Philadelphia: J. B. Lippincott.

Spradley, B. W., & Dorsey, B. (1992). Health of the home care population. In M. Stanhope & J. Lancaster, *Community health nursing: Process and practice for promoting health* (3rd ed., pp. 625–644). St. Louis, MO: C. V. Mosby.

Stanhope, M. (1992). The community health nurse in home health and hospice care. In M. Stanhope & J. Lancaster. *Community health nursing: Process and practice for promoting health* (4th ed., pp. 805–834). St. Louis, MO: C. V. Mosby.

Strong, A. G. (1992). Case management and the CNS. *Clinical Nurse Specialist, 6,* 64.

Thompson, L. (1989). The occupational health nurse as an employee assistance program provider. *American Association of Occupational Health Nurses Journal, 37,* 501–507.

Thurber, F., Berry, B., & Cameron, M. E. (1991). The role of school nursing in the United States. *Journal of Pediatric Health Care, 5,* 135–140.

Travers, P. H., & McDougall, C. E. (1997). The occupational health nurse: Roles and responsibilities, current and future trends. In J. M. Swanson & M. Nies, *Community health nursing: Promoting the health of aggregates* (pp. 767–795). Philadelphia: W. B. Saunders.

Urbano, M. T., vonWindeguth, B., Siderits, P., Parker, J., & Studenic-Lewis, C. (1991). Developing case managers for chronically ill children: Florida's registered nurse specialist program. *Journal of Continuing Education in Nursing, 22*(2), 62–66.

Van Hoozer, H. L., Bratton, B. D., Ostmoe, P. M., Weinholtz, D., Craft, M. J., Gjerde, C. L., & Albanese, M. A. (1987). *The teaching process: Theory and practice in nursing.* Norwalk, CT: Appleton-Century-Croft.

Wagner, J. D., & Menke, M. E. (1992). Case management of homeless families. *Clinical Nurse Specialist, 6,* 65–71.

Westberg, G. (1990). A historical perspective: Wholistic health and the parish nurse. In P. Solari-Twadell, A. Djupe, & M. McDermott (Eds.), *Parish nursing: The developing practice* (pp. 27–39). Park Ridge, IL: National Parish Nurse Resource Center.

White, M. S. (1982). Construct for public health nursing. *Nursing Outlook, 30,* 527–530.

Williams, C. A. (1996). Community-based population focused practice: The foundation of specialization in public health nursing. In M. Stanhope & J. Lancaster. *Community heatlh nursing: Promoting health of aggregates, families, and individuals* (4th ed.). St. Louis: Mosby, 21–33.

Wright, S., Johnson, M., & Purdy, E. (1991). The nurse as consultant. *Nursing Standard, 6*(5), 31–34.

Zanga, J. R., & Oda, D. S. (1987). School health services. *Journal of School Health, 57,* 413–416.

Zerwekh, J. (1993). Commentary: Going to the people—Public health nursing today and tomorrow. *American Journal of Public Health, 83*(12), 1676–1678.

CHAPTER 15
The Home Visit

Balzer-Riley, J. W. (1996). *Communications in nursing* (3rd ed.). St. Louis, MO: Mosby-Year Book.

Byrd, M. E. (1995a). A concept analysis of home visiting. *Public Health Nursing, 12,* 83–89.

Byrd, M. E. (1995b). The home visiting process in the contexts of the voluntary vs. required visit: Examples from fieldwork. *Public Health Nursing, 12,* 196–202.

D'Avanzo, C. E., Frye, B., & Froman, R. (1994). Stress in Cambodian refugee families. *Image: Journal of Nursing Scholarship, 26,* 100–105.

Davis, L. L., & Grant, J. S. (1994). Constructing the reality of recovery: Family home care management strategies. *Advances in Nursing Science, 17*(2), 66–76.

Deal, L. W. (1993). The effectiveness of community health nursing interventions: A literature review. *Public Health Nursing, 5,* 315–323.

Humphrey, C. J., & Milone-Nuzzo, P. (1991). *Home care nursing: An orientation to practice.* Norwalk, CT: Appleton & Lange.

Janosik, E. H. (1994). *Crisis counseling: A contemporary approach* (2nd ed.). Boston: Jones & Bartlett.

Klass, C. S. (1996). *Home visiting: Promoting healthy parent and child development.* Baltimore: Paul H. Brookes.

Kozier, B., Erb, G., Blais, K., & Wilkinson, J. M. (1995). *Fundamentals of nursing: Concepts, process and practice* (5th ed.). Redwood City, CA: Addison-Wesley.

Kristjanson, L. J., & Chalmers, K. I. (1991). Preventive work with families: Issues facing public health nurses. *Journal of Advanced Nursing, 16,* 147–153.

Murray, R. B., & Zentner, J. P. (1997). Nursing assessment and health promotion (6th ed.). Englewood Cliffs, NJ: Appleton & Lange.

Rice, R. (1993). Principles of universal precautions/body substance isolation. *Home Healthcare Nurse, 11*(4), 55–59.

Rice, R. (1994). Procedures in home care: Safety in the community. *Home Healthcare Nurse, 12*(3), 70.

Ruskin, J. (1865). Sesame and lilies, of king's treasures: of Queen's gardens. Section 68. As quoted in J. Bartlett, *Bartlett's familiar quotations* (13th + centennial ed.). Boston: Little Brown & Co.

Sloan, M. R., & Schommer, B. T. (1991). The process of contracting in community health nursing. In B. W. Spradley (Ed.), *Readings in community health nursing* (4th ed., pp. 304–312). Philadelphia: J. B. Lippincott.

Thomas, R. B., Barnard, K. E., & Sumner, G. A. (1993). Family nursing diagnosis as a framework for family assessment. In S. L. Feetham, S. B. Meister, J. M. Bell, & C. L. Gilliss (Eds.), *The nursing of families* (pp. 127–136). Newbury Park, CA: Sage.

Wright, L. M., & Leahey, M. W. (1994). *Nurses and families: A guide to family assessment and intervention* (2nd ed.). Philadelphia: F. A. Davis.

Zerwekh, J. V. (1991). A family caregiving model for public health nursing. *Nursing Outlook, 39,* 213–217.

Zerwekh, J. V. (1992a). Laying the groundwork for family self-help: Locating families, building trust, and building strength. *Public Health Nursing, 9*(1), 15–21.

Zerwekh, J. V. (1992b). Public health nursing legacy: Historical practical wisdom. *Nursing and Health Care, 13,* 84–91.

Zerwekh, J. V. (1997). Making the connection during home visits: Narratives of expert nurses. *International Journal for Human Caring, 1*(1), 25–29.

CHAPTER 16
Care of Infants, Children, and Adolescents

Alan Guttmacher Institute. (1994). *Sex and America's teenagers.* New York: Author.

Center on Budget and Policy Priorities. (1994). *Despite economic recov-*

ery, poverty and income trends are disappointing in 1993. Washington, DC: Author.

Centers for Disease Control and Prevention. (1990). Selected behaviors that increase risk for HIV infection among high school students—U.S. 1990. *Morbidity and Mortality Weekly Reports (MMWR) 41,* 33–35.

Centers for Disease Control and Prevention. (1993). *HIV/AIDS Surveillance Reports, 5*(2).

Centers for Disease Control and Prevention. (1994b). *Summary of 1991 report: Preventing lead poisoning in young children.* Washington DC: Author.

Centers for Disease Control and Prevention. (1996a). Exposure to second-hand smoke widespread. *HHS NEWS.* Washington DC: U. S. Department of Health and Human Services.

Centers for Disease Control and Prevention. (1996b). Youth risk behavior surveillance—United States, 1995. *Morbidity and Mortality Weekly Reports (MMWR), 45*(SS-4).

Centers for Disease Control and Prevention. (1996c). Youth risk behavior surveillance—United States, 1995. *Morbidity and Mortality Weekly Reports (MMWR), 45*(SS-r), 1–86.

Centers for Disease Control and Prevention. (1998). *Recommended Childhood Immunization schedule for the United States, January–December 1998.* Atlanta: National Immunization Program.

Child Welfare League of America. (1997). *Comprehensive sexuality education: Adolescents and abstinence* [on-line]. HN3898@handsnet.org

Children's Defense Fund. (1996a). *Healthy start: Frequently asked questions. Head Start FAQs.* Washington, DC: Author.

Children's Defense Fund. (1996b, November 22). *Summary of legislation affecting children in 1996* [On-line].

Children's Defense Fund. (1997). *The state of America's children yearbook 1998.* Washington, DC: Author.

Children's Defense Fund. (1998a). Moments in America for Children. *CDF Report 190.* Washington, DC: Author.

Children's Defense Fund. (1998b). *Poverty matters: The cost of child poverty in America.* Washington, DC: Author.

Cunningham, F. G., MacDonald, P. C., Gant, N. F., Leveno, K. J., Gilstrap, L. C. Hankins, G. D. V., & Clark, S. L. (1997). *Williams obstetrics* (20th ed.). Norwalk, CT: Appleton & Lange.

Dacey, J., & Travers, J. (1996). *Human development across the lifespan* (3rd ed.). Madison, WI: Brown & Benchmark.

Duvall, E., & Miller, B. (1984). *Marriage and family development* (6th ed.). New York: Harper & Row.

Earls, F. (1994). Violence and today's youth. *Future of Children, 4*(3).

Edelman, M. (1997). New CDF report on state of America's children finds child well-being lagging despite economic recovery. In Children's Defense Fund, *The state of America's children yearbook 1997.* Washington DC: Children's Defense Fund.

Eggert, L. L. (1994). Prevention research program: Reconnecting at-risk youth. *Issues in Mental Health Nursing, 15,* 107–135.

Flaskerud, J. H., & Ungvarski, P. J. (1995). *HIV/AIDS: A guide to nursing care* (2nd ed.). Philadelphia: W. B. Saunders.

Futterman, D., & Hein, K. (1992). Medical care and HIV infected adolescents. *AIDS Clinical Care, 4,* 95–93.

Gill, C. (1995). Protecting our children: Where have we gone and where should we go from here? *Journal of Psychosocial Nursing, 33*(3), 31–35.

Gilliss, C. L. (1993). Family nursing research, theory and practice. In G. D. Wegner & R. J. Alexander (Eds.), *Readings in family nursing* (pp. 34–42). Philadelphia: J. B. Lippincott.

Hatcher, R. A. (1994). *Contraceptive technology* (16 ed.). New York: Irvington.

Hatton, D. (1997). Managing health problems among homeless women with children in a transitional shelter. *Image: Journal of Nursing Scholarship, 29*(1).

Institute of Medicine. (1995). *Nursing, health, and the environment.* Washington, DC: National Academy Press.

Jahiel, R. J. (1992). Empirical studies of homeless populations in the 1970s and 1980s. In R. I. Jahiel (Ed.), *Homelessness: A prevention-oriented approach* (pp. 40–56). Baltimore: Johns Hopkins University.

Joffe, G. M., Symmas, R., Alverson, D., & Chilton, L. (1995). The effect of a comprehensive prematurity prevention program on the number of admissions to the neonatal intensive care unit. *Journal of Perinatology, 15*(4), 305–309.

Johnston, L., O'Malley, P., & Bachman, J. (1994). *National survey results on drug use from the monitoring the future study, 1975–1993.* Rockville, MD: National Institute on Drug Abuse.

Johnston, L., O'Malley, P., & Bachman, J. (1995). *National survey results on drug use from the monitoring the future study, 1975–1994.* Rockville, MD: National Institute on Drug Abuse.

Koop, C. E. (1992). Violence in America: A public health emergency. *Journal of the American Medical Association, 267,* 3075–3076.

Kunins, H., Hein, K., Futterman, D., Tapley, E., & Elliot, A. S. (1993). Guide to adolescent HIV/AIDS program development. *Journal of Adolescent Health, 14,* 1S-140S.

Lankford, T. (1994). *Foundations of normal and therapeutic nutrition* (2nd ed.). Albany, NY: Delmar Publishers.

Lemone, P., & Burke, K. R. (1996). *Medical–surgical nursing: Critical thinking in client care.* Menlo Park, CA: Addison-Wesley.

Lewis, C., Battisich, V., & Schaps, E. (1990). School-based primary prevention: What is an effective program? *New Directions for Child Development, 50,* 35–39.

Lewit, E., Baker, L., Corman, H., & Shiono, P. (1995). The direct cost of low birth weight. *The Future of Children, 5*(1), 1–23.

McCormick, M., & Richardson, D. (1995). Access to neonatal intensive care: Low birthweight. *The Future of Children 5*(1), 1–16.

Mendoza, F. (1994). The health of Latino children in the U.S. *The Future of Children, 14* (3), .

Moon, M. W. (1995). Nursing care of the adolescent. In J. H. Flaskerud & P. J. Ungvarski, *HIV/AIDS: A guide to nursing care* (2nd ed.). Philadelphia: W. B. Saunders.

Murray, R., & Zentner, J. (1997). *Health assessment and promotion strategies through the life span.* Stamford, CT: Appleton & Lange.

National Center for Health Statistics, Division of Vital Statistics. (1994). Rates of teen deaths by accident, homicide or suicide, 1994 [On-line].

National Center for Injury Prevention and Control. (1997). *Fact sheet: Childhood injury.* Atlanta, GA: Division of Unintentional Injury Prevention.

National SAFE KIDS Campaign. (1996). *Trends in unintentional childhood injury prevention since the launch of the National SAFE KIDS Campaign.* Washington, DC: Author.

Nelsen, J. (1997). *Positive discipline.* New York: Ballantine.

Petersen, E. (1995). 14 tips for teens. The National Parenting Center, Woodland Hills, CA. *ParenTalk Newsletter.*

Schubert, P., & Lionberger, H. (1995). Mutual connectedness: A study of client–nurse interaction using the Grounded Theory method. *Journal of Holistic Nursing, 13*(2), 102–116.

Sells, C. W., & Blum, R. (1996). Morbidity and mortality among U.S. adolescents: An overview of data and trends. *American Journal of Public Health, 86*(4), 513–519.

Sherman, A. (1994). *Wasting America's future: The Children's Defense Fund report on the costs of child poverty.* Boston: Beacon.

Sidel, R. (1996). *Keeping women and children last: America's war on the poor.* New York: Penguin Books.

Singh, G., & Yu, S. (1996). U.S. childhood mortality, 1950 through 1993: Trends and socioeconomic differentials. *American Journal of Public Health, 86*(4), 505–512.

Strauss, A., & Corbin, J. (1994). Grounded theory methodology. In N. K. Denzin & Y. S. Lincoln (Eds.), *Handbook of qualitative research* (pp. 273–285). Thousand Oaks, CA: Sage.

U.S. Advisory Board on Child Abuse and Neglect. (1995). *A nation's shame: Fatal child abuse and neglect.* Washington, DC: Author.

U.S. Census Bureau. (1996). *Statistical abstract of the U.S.* Washington, DC: U.S. Government Printing Office.

U.S. Conference of Mayors. (1997). *Status report on hunger and homelessness in America's cities.* Washington, DC: Author.

U.S. Department of Commerce. (1993). *U.S. statistical abstracts* (11th ed.). Washington, DC: Author.

U.S. Department of Health and Human Services. (1996b). *Trends in the well-being of America's children and youth: 1996.* Washington, DC: Author.

U.S. Department of Health and Human Services. (1996c). Vital statistics report shows broad gains in the nation's health. *Births and Deaths: United States, 1995, 45*(3, Suppl. 2). Washington DC: Public Health Service.

U.S. Department of Health and Human Services. (1996d). *Healthy people 2000: Midcourse review and 1995 revisions.* Sudbury, MA: Jones & Bartlett.

U.S. Department of Health and Human Services. (1997, September). *Sexually transmitted disease surveillance, 1996.* Atlanta: Centers for Disease Control and Prevention. Available online at http://wonder.cdc.gov/wonder/STD/STDD016.PCW.html

Wehr, E., & Jameson, E. (1994). Beyond benefits: The importance of a pediatric standard in private insurance contracts to ensure health care access for children. *The Future of Children, 4*(3).

Weiss, R. A. (1993). How does HIV cause AIDS? *Science, 260,* 1273–1279.

Wheeler, S. (1993). Substance abuse during pregnancy. *Primary Care, 20*(1), 191–203.

Whitney, E. N., & Rolfes, S. R. (1996). *Understanding nutrition* (7th ed.). St. Paul, MN: West.

Wong, D. (1997). *Essentials of pediatric nursing*. St. Louis, MO: Mosby-Yearbook.

Worthington-Roberts, B. S., & Williams, S. R. (1996). *Nutrition throughout the life cycle* (3rd ed.). St. Louis, MO: Mosby-Yearbook.

CHAPTER 17
Care of Young, Middle, and Older Adults

Alford, D. M. (1995). Nurses' role with the elderly in a nurse-managed clinic. In M. Stanley & P. G. Beare (Eds.), *Gerontological nursing* (pp. 115–121). Philadelphia: F. A. Davis.

Andrews, M. M., & Boyle, J. S. (1995). *Transcultural concepts in nursing care* (2nd ed.). Philadelphia: Lippincott.

Angelucci, D., & Lawrence, M. (1995). Death and dying. In M. Stanley & P. G. Beare (Eds.), *Gerontological nursing* (pp. 400–414). Philadelphia: F. A. Davis.

Anglin, L. T. (1994). Historical perspectives: Influences of the past. In J. Zerwekh & J. C. Claborn (Eds.), *Nursing today* (pp. 29–49). Philadelphia: W. B. Saunders.

Banani, S. (1987). Life's rainbow. In S. Martz (Ed.), *When I am an old woman I shall wear purple* (p. 181). Manhattan Beach, CA: Papier-Mache Press.

Blazer, D. (1991). Suicide risk factors in the elderly: An epidemiological study. *Journal of Geriatric Psychiatry, 24*(2), 175–190.

Brewster, K. L., Billy, J. O., & Grady, W. R. (1993, March). Social context and adolescent behavior: The impact of community on the transition to sexual activity. *Social Forces, 71*, 713–740.

Burlew, L. D., Jones, J., & Emerson, P. (1991), Exercise and the elderly: A group counseling approach. *Journal for Specialists in Group Work, 16*, 152–158.

Centers for Disease Control and Prevention. (1997). *CDC Surveillance Summaries*. Morbidity and Mortality Weekly Reports (MMWR), 34.

Centers for Disease Control and Prevention (Division of HIV/AIDS Prevention). (1998). *Update: Cricitcal need to pay attention to HIV prevention for women: Minority and young women bear greatest burden.* Available online: www.cdc.gov/nchstp/hiv_aids.

Cole, P. M., & Putnam, F. W. (1992). Effect of incest on self and social functioning: A developmental psychopathology perspective. *Journal of Consulting and Clinical Psychology, 60*, 174–184.

Dacey, J. S., & Travers, J. F. (1996). *Human development across the lifespan* (3rd ed.). Madison, WI: Brown & Benchmark.

Dawson, C., & Whitfield, H. (1996). Subfertility and male sexual dysfunction. *British Medical Journal, 312*, 902–904.

DeBuono, B. A. (1996). *Communities working together for a healthier New York*. Report to the Commissioner of Health from New York State Public Health Council, September, 1996.

Doenges, M. E., Moorhouse, M. F., & Burley, J. T. (1995). *Application of nursing process and nursing diagnosis* (2nd ed.). Philadelphia: F. A. Davis.

Dorgan, C. A. (Ed.). (1995). *Statistical record of health and medicine*. New York: International Thompson Publishing.

Ebersole, P., & Hess, P. (1994). *Toward healthy aging: Human needs and nursing response* (4th ed.). St. Louis, MO: Mosby.

Edelman, C. L., & Mandle, C. L. (1994). *Health promotion throughout the lifespan* (3rd ed.). St. Louis, MO: Mosby.

Erikson, E. H. (1963). *Childhood and society* (2nd ed.). New York: W. W. Norton.

Ferraro, K. F. (1992). Cohort changes in images of older adults, 1974–1981. *The Gerontologist, 32*, 296–304.

Gallman, R. L. (1995). The sensory system and its problems in the elderly. In M. Stanley & P. G. Beare (Eds.), *Gerontological nursing* (pp. 135–147). Philadelphia: F. A. Davis.

Haight, B. K., & Leech, K. (1995). Family dynamics. In M. Stanley & P. G. Beare (Eds.), *Gerontological nursing* (p. 365). Philadelphia: F. A. Davis.

Harvey, C. D. H., Bond, J. B., Jr., & Greenwood, L. J. (1991). Satisfaction, happiness, and self-esteem of older rural parents. *Canadian Journal of Community Mental Health, 10*(2), 31–46.

Jarvis, C. (1992). *Physical examination and health assessment*. Philadelphia: W. B. Saunders.

Jecker, N. S. (1995). Ethical issues in gerontological nursing. In M. Stanley & P. G. Beare (Eds.), *Gerontological nursing* (pp. 51–62). Philadelphia: F. A. Davis.

Johnson, B. S. (1993). *Psychiatric–mental health nursing* (3rd ed.). Philadelphia: J. B. Lippincott.

Johnson, L. H., & Johnson, M. A. (1995). Dementia in the elderly. In M. Stanley & P. G. Beare (Eds.), *Gerontological nursing* (pp. 493–504). Philadelphia: F. A. Davis.

Jung, C. (1933). *Modern man in search of a soul*. New York: Harcourt, Brace & World.

Kennedy, G. E. (1992). Shared activities of grandparents and grandchildren. *Psychological Reports, 70*, 211–227.

Lefrancois, G. R. (1996). *The lifespan* (5th ed.). Belmont, CA: Wadsworth.

Leitenberg, H., Greenwald, E., & Cado, S. (1992). A retrospective study of long-term methods of coping with having been sexually abused during childhood. *Child Abuse and Neglect, 16*, 399–407.

Levinson, D. J. (1978). *The seasons of a man's life*. New York: Alfred A. Knopf.

Levinson, D. J. (1986). A conception of adult development. *American Psychologist, 41*, 3–13.

McFall, S., & Miller, B. H. (1992). Caregiver burden and nursing home admission of frail elderly persons. *Journal of Gerontology: SOCIAL SCIENCES, 47*, 573–579.

Mellins, C. A., Blum, M. J., Boyd-Davis, S. L., & Gatz, M. (1993). Family network perspectives on caregiving. *Generations, 17*(1), 21–24.

Milgram, G. G. (1993). Adolescents, alcohol and aggression. *Journal of the Study of Alcohol* (Suppl. 11), 53–61.

Moyer, M. S. (1992). Sibling relationships among older adults. *Generations, 16*(3), 55–58.

Murray, R. B., & Zentner, J. P. (1997). *Nursing assessment and health promotion strategies through the lifespan* (6th ed.). Englewood Cliffs, NJ: Prentice-Hall.

Panayotoff, K. G. (1993). The impact of continuing education on the health of older adults. *Educational Gerontology, 19*(1), 9–20.

Pattillo, M. M. (1995). The musculoskeletal system and its problems in the elderly. In M. Stanley & P. G. Beare (Eds.), *Gerontological nursing* (pp. 161–173). Philadelphia: F. A. Davis.

Rosenberg, H. M., Ventura, S. J., Maurer, J. D., et al. (1996). Births and deaths: United States, 1995. *Monthly Vital Statistics Report, 45*(3) supp. 2., p. 31. Hyattsville, MD: National Center for Health Statistics.

Roussel, L. A. (1995). The neurological system and its problems in the elderly. In M. Stanley & P. G. Beare (Eds.), *Gerontological nursing* (pp. 174–188). Philadelphia: F. A. Davis.

Sarna, L. (1995). Cancer in the elderly. In M. Stanley & P. G. Beare (Eds.), *Gerontological nursing* (pp. 323–337). Philadelphia: F. A. Davis.

Schulman, B. H., & Sperry, L. (1992). Consultation with adult children of aging parents. *Individual Psychology, 48*, 427–431.

Sheehy, G. (1995). *New passages*. New York: Random House.

Silverstein, M., & Bengtson, V. L. (1991). Do close parent–child relations reduce the mortality risk of older parents? *Journal of Health and Social Behavior, 32*, 382–395.

Sims, L. K., D'Amico, D., Stiesmeyer, J. K., & Webster, J. A. (1995). *Health assessment in nursing*. Redwood City, CA: Addison-Wesley.

Smith, S. F., & Smith, C. M. (1990). *Personal health choices*. Boston: Jones & Bartlett.

Speare, A., Jr., & Avery, R. (1993). Who helps whom in older parent–child families. *Journal of Gerontology: SOCIAL SCIENCES, 48*, 564–573.

Staab, A. S., & Hodges, L. C. (1996). *Essentials of gerontological nursing*. Philadelphia: Lippincott.

Stanley, M., & Beare, P. G. (1995). Theories of aging. In M. Stanley & P. G. Beare (Eds.), *Gerontological nursing* (pp. 13–16). Philadelphia: F. A. Davis.

Stein, L. M., & Bienenfeld, D. (1992). Hearing impairment and its impact on elderly patients with cognitive, behavioral, or psychiatric disorders: A literature review. *Journal of Geriatric Psychiatry, 25*, 145–156.

Tyler, T. R., & Schuller, R. A. (1991). Aging and attitude change. *Journal of Personality and Social Psychology, 61*, 689–697.

U.S. Bureau of the Census. (1995). *Statistical abstract of the United States: 1995* (115th ed.). Washington, DC: Author.

U.S. Centers for Disease Control. (1992). *HIV/AIDS surveillance report*. Atlanta, GA: Author.

U.S. Department of Health and Human Services. (1990). *Healthy people 2000: National health promotion and disease prevention objectives* (DHHS Publication No. [PHS] 91-50212). Washington, DC: U.S. Government Printing Office.

Ward, R. A., & Spitze, G. (1992). Consequences of parent–adult child coresidence. *Journal of Family Issues, 13*, 553–572.

Wasaha, S., & Angelopoulos, F. M. (1996). What every woman should know about menopause. *American Journal of Nursing, 96*(1), 24–33.

Wendell, D. A., Onorato, I. M., McCray, E., Allen, D. M., & Sweeney, P.

A. (1992). Youth at risk: Sex, drugs, and human immunodeficiency virus. *American Journal of Disabled Children, 146,* 76–81.

Wiersema, L. A. (1995). The integumentary system and its problems in the elderly. In M. Stanley & P. G. Beare (Eds.), *Gerontological nursing* (pp. 148–160). Philadelphia: F. A. Davis.

Wold, G. (1993). *Basic geriatric nursing.* St. Louis, MO: Mosby.

CHAPTER 18
Frameworks for Assessing Families

Ackermann, M. L., Brink, S. A., Clanton, J. A., Jones, C. G., Marriner-Tomey, A., Moody, S. L., Perlich, G. L., Price, D. L. & Prusinski, B. B. (1994). Imogene King: Theory of goal attainment. In A. Marriner-Tomey (Ed.), *Nursing theorists and their work* (3rd ed., pp. 305–322). St. Louis, MO: Mosby-Yearbook.

Aerts, E. (1993). Bringing the institution back in. In P. A. Cowan, D. Field, D. A. Hansen, A. Skolnick, & G. E. Swanson (Eds.), *Family, self, and society: Toward a new agenda for family research* (pp. 3–41). Hillsdale, NJ: Lawrence Erlbaum Associates.

Allgeier, A. R., & Allgeier, E. R. (1995). *Sexual interactions* (4th ed.). Lexington, MA: D. C. Health.

Andrews, M. M. (1995). Transcultural nursing care. In M. M. Andrews & J. S. Boyle (Eds.), *Transcultural concepts in nursing care* (2nd ed., pp. 49–96). Philadelphia: J. B. Lippincott.

Associated Press. (1994, February 15). Welfare cases rise as debate over reform heats up. *Marin Independent Journal,* A7.

Baker, D. (1996). *King's Theory and case management of high-risk senior citizens within a health maintenance organization.* Unpublished paper.

Becvar, D. S., & Becvar, R. J. (1996). *Family therapy: A systematic integration* (3rd ed.). Needham Heights, MA: Allyn & Bacon.

Blue, C. L., Brubaker, K. M., Fine, J. M., Kirsch, M. J., Papazian, K. R., Riester, C. M., & Sobiech, M. A. (1994). Sister Callista Roy: Adaptation model. In A. Marriner-Tomey (Ed.), *Nursing theorists and their work* (3rd ed., pp. 246–268). St. Louis, MO: Mosby-Yearbook.

Bronfenbrenner, U. (1977). Toward an experimental ecology of human development. *American Psychologist, 7,* 513–531.

Carter, B., & McGoldrick, M. (1989). Overview: The changing family life cycle—A framework for family therapy. In B. Carter, & M. McGoldrick (Eds.), *The changing family life cycle* (pp. 3–28). Boston: Allyn & Bacon.

Combrinck-Graham, L. (1985). A developmental model for family systems. *Family Process, 24,* 139–150.

Craft, M. J., & Willadsen, J. A. (1992). Interventions related to family. *Nursing Clinics of North America, 27,* 517–529.

Cuellar, I., & Glazer, M. (1996). The impact of culture on the family. In M. Harway (Ed.), *Treating the changing family: Handling normative and unusual events.* American Counseling Association. New York: John Wiley & Sons.

Danielson, C. B., Hamel-Bissell, B., & Winstead-Fry, P. (1993). *Families in health and illness: Perspectives on coping and intervention.* St. Louis, MO: Mosby.

David, L. L. (1996). Dementia caregiving studies: A typology for family interventions. *Journal of Family Nursing, 2*(3), 30–55.

Dawson, D. A. (1991). Family structure and children's health and well-being: Data from the 1988 national health interview survey on child health. *Journal of Marriage and the Family, 53,* 573–584.

Donnelly, E. (1993). Health promotion, families, and the diagnostic process. In G. D. Wegner & R. J. Alexander (Eds.), *Readings in family nursing* (pp. 271–279). Philadelphia: J. B. Lippincott.

Duvall, E. M. (1977). *Marriage and family development.* Philadelphia: J. B. Lippincott.

Duvall, E. M., & Miller, B. C. (1985). *Marriage and family development* (6th ed.). New York: Harper and Row.

Falco, S. M., & Lobo, M. L. (1995). Martha E. Rogers. In J. B. George (Ed.), *Nursing theories* (4th ed., pp. 229–248). Norwalk, CT: Appleton & Lange.

Friedman, M. M. (1998). *Family nursing: Theory and practice* (4th ed.). Stamford, CT: Appleton & Lange.

Geissler, E. M. (1991). Transcultural nursing and nursing diagnoses. *Nursing and Health Care, 12,* 190–203.

Gilliss, C. L. (1993). Family nursing research, theory and practice. In G. D. Wegner & R. J. Alexander (Eds.), *Reading in family nursing* (pp. 34–42). Philadelphia: J. B. Lippincott.

Givens, C. & Fortier, L. D. (1992). *Practicing eternity.* San Diego: Paradigm.

Hanson, S. M. H. & Boyd, S. T. (1996). *Family health care nursing: Theory, practice, and research.* Philadelphia: F. A. Davis.

Hare, J., & Richards, L. (1993). Children raised by lesbian couples: Does context of birth affect father and partner involvement? *Family Relations, 42,* 249–255.

Harway, M., & Wexler, K. (1996). Setting the stage for understanding and treating the changing family. In M. Harway (Ed.). *Treating the changing family: Handling normative and unusual events.* New York: John Wiley & Sons.

Holman, A. M. (1983). *Family assessment: Tools for understanding and intervention.* Newbury Park, CA: Sage.

King, I. M. (1981). *A theory for nursing: Systems, concepts, process.* New York: John Wiley.

King, I. M. (1986). *Curriculum and instruction in nursing.* Norwalk, CT: Appleton-Century-Crofts.

King, I. M. (1994). Quality of life and goal attainment. *Nursing Science Quality, 7,* 29–32.

Lapp, C. A., Diemert, C. A., & Enestvedt, R. (1993). Family-based practice: Discussion of a tool merging assessment with intervention. In G. D. Wegner & R. J. Alexander (Eds.), *Reading in family nursing* (pp. 280–287). Philadelphia: J. B. Lippincott.

Lindgren, C. L. (1993). The caregiver career. *Image, 25,* 214–219.

Macklin, E. D. (1987). Nontraditional family forms. In M. B. Sussman & S. K. Stienmetz (Eds.), *Handbook of marriage and the family.* New York: Plenum.

Magilvy, J. K., Congdon, J. G., & Martinez, R. (1994). Circles of care: Home care and community support for rural older adults. *Advances in Nursing Science 16*(3), 22–23.

Marciano, T. (1991). A postscript on wider families: Traditional family assumptions and cautionary notes. *Marriage and Family Review, 17,* 159–163.

Marciano, T., & Sussman, M. B. (1991). Wider families: An overview. *Marriage and Family Review, 17,* 1–7.

Martin, K. S., & Scheet, N. J. (1992). *The Omaha system: Applications for community health nursing.* Philadelphia: W. B. Saunders.

Neuman, B. (1983). Family intervention using the Betty Neuman health care systems model. In I. W. Clements & F. B. Roberts (Eds.), *Family health: A theoretical approach to nursing care* (pp. 161–175). New York: John Wiley & Sons.

North American Nursing Diagnosis Association. (1999). Nursing diagnosis: Definitions and Classification, 1999–2000. Philadelphia, PA: North American Nursing Diagnosis Association.

Otto, H. A. (1963). Criteria for assessing family strength. *Family Process, 2,* 329338.

Pepin, J. I. (1992). Family caring and caring in nursing. *Image, 24,* 127–131.

Petze, C. F. (1991). Health promotion for the well family. In B. W. Spradley (Ed.), *Readings in community health nursing* (4th ed., pp. 355–364). New York: J. B. Lippincott.

Pinderhughes, E. B. (1983). Empowerment for our clients and for ourselves. *Social Casework: The Journal of Contemporary Social Work, 6,* 331–338.

Reutter, L. (1991). Family health assessment—An integrated approach. In B. W. Spradley (Ed.), *Readings in community health nursing* (4th ed., pp. 341–354). New York: J. B. Lippincott.

Richards, W. R., Burgess, D. E., Petersen. F. R., & McCarthy, D. L. (1993). Genograms: A psychosocial assessment tool for hospice. *Hospice Journal, 9*(1), 1–12.

Rogers, M. (1990). Nursing: Science of Unitary, Irreducible, Human Beings: Update 1990. In E. A. M. Barrett (Ed.), *Visions of Rogers' science-based nursing* (pp. 5–11). New York: National League of Nursing.

Rogers, M. E. (1992). Nursing science and the space age. *Nursing Science Quarterly, 5,* 27–34.

Rosenberg, E. B. (1992). *The adoption life cycle: The children and their families through the years.* New York: The Free Press.

Roy, Sr. C. (1983). Roy adaptation model. In I. W. Clements & F. B. Roberts (Eds.), *Family health: A theoretical approach to nursing care* (pp. 255–278). New York: John Wiley & Sons.

Rubin, R. M., & Riney, B. J. (1994). *Working wives and dual-earner families.* Wesport, CT: Praeger.

Solomon, C. M. (1992). Work/family ideas that break boundaries. *Personnel Journal, 71*(10), 112–117.

Spector, R. E. (1996). *Cultural diversity in health and illness* (4th ed.). Stamford, CT: Appleton & Lange.

Spiegel, J. (1982). An ecological model of ethnic families. In M. McGoldrick, J. K. Pearce, & J. Giordano (Eds.), *Ethnicity and family therapy* (pp. 31–51). New York: Guilford.

Staples, R. (1989). Family life in the 21st century: An analysis of old forms, current trends, and future scenarios. In C. L. Gilliss, B. L. Highley, B. M. Roberts, & I. M. Martinson (Eds.), *Toward a science of family nursing* (pp. 156–170). Menlo Park, CA: Addison-Wesley.

Szapoeznik, J. B. Kurtines, W. M. (1993). Family psychology and cultural diversity. *American Psychologist 18,* 400–407.

Talento, B. (1995). Jean Watson. In J. B. George (Ed.), *Nursing theories* (4th ed., pp. 317–333). Norwalk, CT: Appleton & Lange.

Thomas, R. B., Barnard, K. E., & Sumner, G. A. (1993). Family nursing diagnosis as a framework for family assessment. In S. L. Feetham, S. B. Meister, J. M. Bell, & C. L. Gilliss (Eds.), *The nursing of families* (pp. 127–136). New York: Sage.

Tomlinson, P. S., & Anderson, K. H. (1995). Family health and the Neuman systems model. In B. Neuman (Ed.), *The Neuman systems model* (3rd ed., pp. 133–144). Norwalk, CT: Appleton & Lange.

U.S. Bureau of the Census. (1992). *Statistical abstracts of the United States* (112th ed.). Washington, DC: Government Printing Office.

U.S. Bureau of the Census. (1995). *Statisical abstracts of the United States: 1995* (115th ed). Washington, DC: U.S. Government Printing Office.

U.S. Department of Health and Human Services. (1995). *Healthy people 2000: Summary report.* Boston: Jones & Bartlett.

von Bertalanffy, L. (1950). The theory of open systems in physics and biology. *Science, 111,* 25–29.

Wallerstein, J. S. (1995). The early psychological tasks of marriage: Part 1. *American Journal of Orthopsychiatry, 65,* 640–650.

Wallerstein, J. S. (1996). The psychological tasks of marriage: Part 2. *American Journal of Orthopsychiatry, 66,* 217–227.

Wallerstein, J. S., & Blakeslee, S. (1995). *The good marriage: How and why love lasts.* New York: Houghton Mifflin.

Walsh, W. M. (1992). Twenty major issues in remarriage families. *Journal of Counseling and Development, 70,* 709–715.

Whall, A. L. (1991). Family system theory: Relationship to nursing conceptual models. In A. L. Whall & J. Fawcett (Eds.), *Family theory development in nursing: State of the science and art* (pp. 317–341). Philadelphia: F. A. Davis.

Wright, L. M., & Leahey, M. (1994). *Nurses and families: A guide to family assessment and intervention* (2nd ed.). Philadelphia: F. A. Davis.

CHAPTER 19
Family Functions and Processes

Acock, A. C., & Demo, D. H. (1994). *Family diversity and well-being.* Thousand Oaks, CA: Sage.

Antai-Otong, D. (Ed.) (1995). *Psychiatric nursing: Biological and behavioral concepts.* Philadelphia: W. B. Saunders.

Arnold, E., & Boggs, K. U. (1995). *Interpersonal relationships: Professional communication skills for nursing* (2nd ed.). Philadelphia: W. B. Saunders.

Babcock, D. E., & Miller, M. A. (1994). *Client education: Theory and practice.* St. Louis, MO: Mosby-Yearbook.

Ball, F. L. J., Cowan, P., & Cowan, C. P. (1995). Who's got the power? Gender differences in partners' perceptions of influence during marital problem-solving discussions. *Family Process, Inc. 34,* 303–321.

Beavers, W. R., & Hampson, R. B. (1993). Measuring family competence: The Beavers Systems Model. In F. Walsh (Ed.), *Normal family processes.* (2nd ed., pp. 73–103). New York: Guilford.

Becvar, D. S., & Becvar, R. J. (1996). *Family therapy: A systematic integration* (3rd ed.). Needham Heights, MA: Allyn & Bacon.

Bisagni, G. M., & Eckenrode, J. (1995). The role of work identity in women's adjustment to divorce. *American Journal of Orthopsychiatry, 65,* 574–583.

Carey, R. (1989). How values affect the mutual goal setting process with multiproblem families. *Journal of Community Health Nursing, 6*(1), 7–14.

Carson, V. B., & Arnold, E. N. (1996). *Mental health nursing: The nurse–patient journey.* Philadelphia: W. B. Saunders.

Charmaz, K. (1991) *Good days and bad days.* New Brunswick, NJ: Rutgers University.

Crosbie-Burnett, M., & Helmbrecht, L. (1993). A descriptive empirical study of gay male stepfamilies. *Family Relations, 42,* 256–262.

Curran, D. (1983). *Traits of a healthy family.* Minneapolis, MN: Winston.

D'Avanzo, C. E., Frye, B., & Froman, R. (1994). Stress in Cambodian refugee families. *Image: Journal of Nursing Scholarship, 26,* 100–105.

Doornbos, M. M. (1996). The strengths of families coping with serious mental illness. *Archives of Psychiatric Nursing, 10,* 214–219.

Epstein, N. B., Bishop, D., Ryan, C., Miller, I., & Keitner, G. (1993) The McMaster Model: View of healthy family functioning. In F. Walsh

(Ed.). *Normal family processes* (2nd ed., pp. 138–160). New York: Guilford.

Friedman, M. M. (1998). *Family nursing theory and practice: Research* (4th ed.). Stamford, CT: Appleton & Lange.

Galvin, K. M., & Brommel, B. J. (1986). *Family communication, cohesion, and change.* Glenview, IL: Scott, Foresman.

Garbarino, J. (1993). Reinventing fatherhood. *Families in Society: The Journal of Contemporary Human Services, 74,* 51–54.

Gelles, R. J. (1995). *Contemporary families: A sociological view.* Thousand Oaks, CA: Sage.

Hanson, S. M. H., & Boyd, S. T. (1996). *Family health care nursing: Theory, practice, and research.* Philadelphia: F. A. Davis.

Heiney, S. P. (1993). Assessing and intervening with dysfunctional families. In G. D. Wegner & R. J. Alexander (Eds.), *Readings in family nursing* (pp. 357–367). Philadelphia: J. P. Lippincott.

Ide, B. A., Tobias, C., Kay, M., Monk, J., & de Zapien, J. G. (1990). A comparison of coping strategies used effectively by older Anglo and Mexican-American widows: A longitudinal study. *Health Care for Women International, 11,* 237–249.

Janosik, E. H. (1994). *Crisis counseling* (2nd ed.). Boston: Jones & Bartlett.

Janosik, E. H. & Green, E. (1992). *Family life: Process and practice.* Boston: Jones & Bartlett.

McCubbin, M. A. (1989). Family stress and family strengths: A comparison of single- and two-parent families with handicapped children. *Research in Nursing and Health, 12,* 101–110.

McCubbin, M. A. (1993). Family stress theory and the development of nursing knowledge about family adaptation. In S. L. Feetham, S. B. Meister, J. M. Bell, & C. L. Gilliss (Eds.), *The nursing of families* (pp. 46–58). Newbury Park, CA: Sage.

McCubbin, M. A., & McCubbin, H. I. (1989). Theoretical orientation to family stress and coping. In C. R. Figley (Ed.), *Treating stress in families* (pp. 3–43). New York: Brunner/Mazel.

McCubbin, M. A., & McCubbin, H. I. (1993). Families coping with illness: The resiliency model of family stress, adjustment, and adaptation. In C. B. Danielson, B. Hamel-Bissell, & P. Winstead-Frye, *Families, health, and illness* (pp. 21–63). St. Louis, MO: Mosby-Yearbook.

McCubbin, H. I., Olson, D. H., & Larsen, A. S. (1987). F-COPES: Family crisis oriented personal scales. In H. McCubbin & A. Thompson (Eds.), *Family assessment inventories for research and practice* (pp. 197–207). Madison, WI: University of Wisconsin, Madison.

McCubbin, H. L., Patterson, J. M., & Wilson, I. (1987). FILE: Family inventory of life events and changes. In H. McCubbin & A. Thompson (Eds.), (pp. 197–207). *Family assessment inventories for research and practice.* Madison, WI: University of Wisconsin, Madison.

McGoldrick, M., Heiman, M, & Carter, B. (1993). The changing family life cycle: A perspective on normalcy. In F. Walsh (Ed.), *Normal family processes* (2nd ed., pp. 405–443). New York: Guilford.

Mercer, R. T., & Ferketich, S. L. (1990). Predictors of family functioning eight months following birth. *Nursing Research, 39,* 70–75.

Moorehouse, M. J. (1993). Work and family dynamics. In P. A. Cowan, D. Field, D. A. Hansen, A. Skolnick, & G. E. Swanson (Eds.), *Family, self, and society: Toward a new agenda for family research* (pp. 265–386). Hillsdale, NJ: Laurence Erlbaum Associates.

Moos, R. H., & Moos, B. S. (1981). *Family environment scale manual.* Palo Alto, CA: Consulting Psychologists.

Moriarty, H. J. (1990). Key issues in the family research process: Strategies for nurse researchers. *Advances in Nursing Science, 12*(3), 1–14.

Olson, D. H. (1993). Circumplex model of marital and family systems: Assessing family functioning. In F. Walsh (Ed.), *Normal family processes* (2nd ed., pp. 104–137). New York: Guilford.

Olson, D. H., Portner, J., & Lavee, Y. (1985). *FACES III.* St. Paul, MN: University of Minnesota.

Pratt, L. (1976). *Family structure and effective health behavior. The energized family.* Boston: Houghton-Mifflin.

Smilkstein, G., Ashworth, C., & Montano, D. (1982). Validity and reliability of the family APGAR as a test of family function. *Journal of Family Practice, 15,* 303–311.

Stevenson-Hinde, J., & Akister, J. (1996). The McMaster model of family functioning: Observer and parental ratings in a nonclinical sample. *Family Process, 34,* 337–347.

Strober, M. H. (1988). Two earner families. In M. H. Strober & S. F. Dornbusch (Eds.), *Feminism, children and the new family* (pp. 161–190). New York: Guilford.

Tomlinson, P. S. (1996). Marital relationship change in the transition to parenthood: A reexamination as interpreted through transition theory. *Journal of Family Nursing, 2,* 286–305.

U.S. Bureau of the Census. (1995). *Statistical abstracts of the United States* (115th ed.). Washington, DC: U.S. Government Printing Office.

U.S. Bureau of the Census, Current Population Reports. (1992). *Studies in household and family formation* (Series P23-179). Washington, DC: U.S. Government Printing Office.

U.S. Department of Health and Human Services. (1990). *Identifying successful families: An overview of constructs and selected measures.* Washington, DC: U.S. Government Printing Office.

Voydanoff, P. (1993). Work and family relationships. In T. H. Brubaker, *Family relations: Challenges for the future* (pp. 98–111). Newbury Park, CA: Sage.

Walsh, F. (1993). Conceptualization of normal family processes. In F. Walsh (Ed.), *Normal family processes* (2nd ed., pp. 3–69). New York: Guilford.

Wright, L. M., & Leahey, M. W. (1994). *Nurses and families: A guide to family assessment and intervention* (2nd ed.). Philadelphia: F. A. Davis.

Zacks, E., Green, R. J., & Marrow, J. (1988). Comparing lesbian and heterosexual couples on the curcumplex model: An initial investigation. *Family Process, 27,* 471–484.

CHAPTER 20
Communicable Diseases

Ackers, M. L., Herwaldt, B. L. (1997). An outbreak in 1996 of cyclosporiasis associated with imported raspberries. *The New England Journal of Medicine, 336*(22), 1548–1557.

AIDS fear brings syphilis decline. (1994, November 7). *AIDS Weekly,* 10.

Anderson, L. (1994). AIDS/STDs-Overview magnitude, Cost to society. Paper presented at the "Women's Health Care: Developing Public Policy" Conference, Colorado Springs, Colorado.

Anderson, R. N., Kochanek, K. D., & Murphy S. L. (1997). Report of final mortality statistics 1995. *Monthly Vital Statistics Report, 45*(11) (Suppl. 2), Hyattsville, MD: National Center for Health Statistics.

Benenson, A. S. ed. (1995). *Control of communicable diseases in man* (16th ed.). Washington DC: American Public Health Association.

Bloom, A. S., Curran, J. W., Elsner, L. G., Gwinn, M., Mofenson, L. M., Moore, J. S., Moseley, R. R., Peterson, H. B., Rogers, M. F., Simonds, R. J. (1995). U.S. Public Health Service recommendations for human immunodeficiency virus counseling and voluntary testing for pregnant women, Part 1. *Morbidity and Mortality Weekly Report, 44*(RR-7), i–7.

Boutotte, J. (1993, May). T.B. The second time around. *Nursing '93,* 42–49.

Bowie, W. R. (1994). STDs in '94: The new CDC guidelines. *Patient Care, 28*(7), 29–53.

Cardo, D. M., Culver, D. H., Cresielski, L. A., Srirzstavz, P. U., Marcus, I. Z., Abitebonl, D., Heptonstall, J., Ippolito, G., Lot, F., McKiblen, P. S., & Bell, D. M. (1997). A cell-control study of HIV seroconversion in health care workers after percutaneous exposure. *New England Journal of Medicine, 337,* 1485–1490.

Carpenter, C. C. J., Fischl, M. A., Hammer, S. M., Hirsch, M. S., Jacobsen, D. M., Katzenstein, D. A., Montaner, J. S. G., Richman, D. D., Saag, M. S., Schooley, R. T., Thompson, M. A., Vella, S., Yeni, P. G., & Volberding, P. A. (1997). Antiretroviral therapy for HIV infection in 1997: Updated recommendations of the International AIDS Society USA Panel. *Journal of the American Medical Association, 277*(24),1962–1969.

Cassel G. H. (1994). New and emerging infections in the face of a funding crisis. *ASM News, 60*(5), 251–254.

Centers for Disease Control and Prevention. (1987). Revision of the CDC surveillance case description for acquired immunodeficiency syndrome. *Morbidity and Mortality Weekly Report, 36* (Suppl. 73), 1–155.

Centers for Disease Control and Prevention. (1988a). Update: Universal precautions for prevention of transmission of HIV, hepatitis B virus and other bloodborne pathogens in health care settings. *Morbidity and Mortality Weekly Report, 37,* 377–388.

Centers for Disease Control. (1988b). Use of BCG vaccines in the control of tuberculosis: A joint statement by the ACIP and the Advisory Committee for Elimination of Tuberculosis. *Morbidity and Mortality Weekly Report, 37,* 663–675.

Centers for Disease Control and Prevention. (1990). Health objectives for the nation: Healthy people 2000: National health promotion and disease prevention objectives for the year 2000. *Morbidity and Mortality Weekly Report, 39,* 689–697.

Centers for Disease Control and Prevention. (1991). Rabies prevention—United States. Recommendations of the Immunization Practices Advisory Committee (ACIP). *Morbidity and Mortality Weekly Report, 40,* 1–19.

Centers for Disease Control and Prevention. (1992). *Division of STD/HIV Prevention, 1991. Annual Report.* Atlanta, GA: Author.

Centers for Disease Control and Prevention. (1993a). Special focus: Surveillance for sexually transmitted diseases. *Morbidity and Mortality Weekly Report, 42*(RR-5), 1–25.

Centers for Disease Control and Prevention. (1993b). Standards for pediatric immunization practices. *Morbidity and Mortality Weekly Report, 42*(RR-5), 1–14.

Centers for Disease Control and Prevention. (1994). Addressing emerging infectious disease threats: A prevention strategy for the United States. Atlanta, GA: Public Health Service, U.S. Department of Health and Human Services.

Centers for Disease Control and Prevention. (1995). *Sexually transmitted disease surveillance, 1994.* Atlanta, GA: Author.

Centers for Disease Control and Prevention. (1996a). Human rabies—Connecticut, 1995. *Morbidity and Mortality Weekly Report, 45,* 207–209

Centers for Disease Control and Prevention. (1996b). Infectious diseases designated as notifiable at the national level—United States. *Morbidity and Mortality Weekly Report, 25*(3), 32.

Centers for Disease Control and Prevention. (1996c). The manual for the surveillance of vaccine-preventable diseases. Atlanta, GA: Author.

Centers for Disease Control and Prevention. (1996d). Surveillance for foodborne disease outbreaks, United States, 1988–1992. *Morbidity and Mortality Weekly Report, 45,* 1–66.

Centers for Disease Control and Prevention. (1997a). *AIDS information: Statistical projections and trends.* [Online].

Centers for Disease Control and Prevention. (1997b). *AIDS information: Transfusions and HIV infection* [Online].

Centers for Disease Control and Prevention. (1997c). *AIDS information: Transmission* [Online].

Centers for Disease Control and Prevention. (1997d). Case definitions for infectious conditions under public health surveillance. *Morbidity and Mortality Weekly Report, 46*(RR-10), 19.

Centers for Disease Control and Prevention. (1997e). *The concept of emergence.* Atlanta, GA: Author.

Centers for Disease Control and Prevention. (1997f). Female/adult/adolescent AIDS cases by exposure and ethnicity. *HIV/AIDS Surveillance Report 1997, 9*(1), 10.

Centers for Disease Control and Prevention. (1997g). Hantavirus pulmonary syndrome—Chile, 1997. *Morbidity and Mortality Weekly Report, 46*(40), 949.

Centers for Disease Control and Prevention. (1997h). Hepatitis A associated with consumption of frozen strawberries—Michigan, March, 1997. *Morbidity and Mortality Weekly Report, 46*(13), 288.

Centers for Disease Control and Prevention. (1997i). Provisional cases of selected notifiable diseases, United States, *Morbidity and Mortality Weekly Report, 46*(51, Dec. 26), 1236–1239.

Centers for Disease Control and Prevention. (1997j). Risk factors for acute hepatitis, 1972–1993. Centers for Disease Control and Prevention. Atlanta, GA: Author.

Centers for Disease Control and Prevention. (1997k). Summary of notifiable diseases, United States, 1996. *Morbidity and Mortality Weekly Report, 45*(53), 3.

Centers for Disease Control and Prevention. (1997l). An unusual hantavirus outbreak in southern Argentina: Person to person transmission? *Emerging Infectious Diseases, 3*(2), 171–174.

Centers for Disease Control and Prevention. (1997m). Update: Trends in AIDS incidence—United States, 1996. *Morbidity and Mortality Weekly Report, 46*(37), 165–173.

Centers for Disease Control and Prevention. (1998a). Information on Lyme Disease: perspectives.

Centers for Disease Control and Prevention. (1998b). 1998 Diseases, *Morbidity and Mortality Weekly Report, 47*(RR-1), 99–105.

Centers for Disease Control and Prevention. (1998c). Tuberculosis Morbidity—United States, 1997. *Morbidity and Mortality Weekly Report, 47*(13), 253–257.

Childs, J. E., Kaufman, A. F., Peters, C. T. & Ehrenburg, R. L. (1993). Hantavirus infection—Southwestern United States: Interim recommendations for risk reduction. *Morbidity and Mortality Weekly Report, 42*(RR-11), 1–13.

Coburn, T., & Pelosi, N. (1997). Should HIV be treated like other infectious disease? *Insight on the News, 13*(32), 24.

Deasy, J. (1996). The bite of rabies: Prevention and control strategies for rabies zoonosis. *Physician Assistant, 20*(10), 49–57.

De Vincent-Hayes, N. (1995). Hepatitis. *Current Health, 22*(4), 20–22.

Donovan, P. (1993). Testing positive: Sexually transmitted disease and the public health response. New York: Alan Guttmacher Institute.

Edmunds W. J., Medley, G. F., Nokes, D. J., Hall, A. J., & Whittle, H. C. (1993). The influence of age on the development of the hepatitis B carrier state. *Proceedings of the Royal Society of London, series B: Biological Sciences, 253,* 197–201.

Eng T. R., & Butler W. T. (Eds.). (1996). *The hidden epidemic: Confronting sexually transmitted diseases.* Committee on Prevention and Control of Sexually Transmitted Diseases. Institute of Medicine. Washington DC: National Academy Press.

Enria, D., Padula, P., Segura, E. L., Pini, N., Edelstein, A., Posse, C. R., Weissenbacher, M. C. (1995). Hantavirus pulmonary syndrome in Argentina. Possibility of person-to-person transmission. *Medicina (Buenos Aires), 58,* 709–711.

Flores, J. L. (1995). Syphilis: A tale of twisted treponemes. *Western Journal of Medicine, 163*(6), 552.

Gerchufsky, M. (1996). Human papilloma virus. *Advance for Nurse Practitioners 4*(5), pp. 21–26.

Getty, V. (1997, April 25). Hepatitis A in Michigan. *USDA News Release, April 25.*

Gordis, L. (1996). *Epidemiology.* Philadelphia: W. B. Saunders.

Hanlon, J. J., & Pickett, G. E. (1979). *Public health administration and practice.* St. Louis, MO: C. V. Mosby Company.

Healy, B. (1995). *A new prescription for women's health: Getting the best medical care in a man's world.* New York, NY: Penquin Books.

Hemming, V. G., Palmer, A. L., Sinnot, J. T., & Glaser, V. (1997). Bracing for the cold and flu season. *Patient Care, 31*(15), 47–54.

Henderson, C. (1997, February 10). The link between HIV and other STDs. *AIDS Weekly Plus,* 16.

Hook, E., & Hansfield, H. (1990). Gonococcal infections in the adult. In K. K. Holmes, P. Mardh, P. F. Sparling, P. J. Wiesner (Eds.), *Sexually transmitted diseases.* New York: McGraw-Hill.

Hutchinson, C. M., Hook, E. W., Shepherd, M., Verley, J., & Rompalo, A. M. (1994). Altered clinical presentation of early syphilis in patients with human immunodeficiency virus infection. *Annals of Internal Medicine, 121*(2), 94–100.

Jones, R. B., & Wasserheit, J. N. (1991). Introduction to the biology and natural history of sexually transmitted diseases. In J. N. Wasserheit, S. O. Aral, K. K. Holmes (Eds.), *Research issues in human behavior and sexually transmitted diseases in the AIDS era* (pp. 11–37). Washington, DC: American Society for Microbiology.

Kuss, T., Proulx-Girouard, L., Lovitt, S., Katz, C. B. Y., Kennelly, P. (1997). A public health nursing model. *Public Health Nursing, 14*(2), 81–91.

LaPook, J. (1995). Hepatitis. In *The Columbia University College of Physicians and Surgeons Complete Home Medical Guide* (3rd ed., pp. 596–597). New York, NY: Crown Publishing Group.

Leccese, C. (1997). The best news yet: AIDS in 1997. *Advance for Nurse Practitioners, 5*(12), 25–30.

Lederberg, J., & Shope R. E. (1992). *Emerging infections: Microbial threats to health in the United States.* Washington, DC: National Academy Press.

Mandell, G. L., Bennett, J. E., & Dolin, R. (Eds.). (1995). *Principles and practices of infectious diseases* (4th ed.). New York: Churchill-Livinston.

Morse, S. (1993). *Emerging viruses.* New York, NY: Oxford University Press.

NJMC National Tuberculosis Center. (1997). Epidemiology of TB.

O'Casey, S. (1949). *Inishfallen: Fare thee well.* Vol 1. New York: Macmillan.

Peters, S. (1997a). The state of pediatric immunizations today. *ADVANCE for Nurse Practitioners, 5*(2), 43–49.

Peters, S. (1997b). Influenza update: An overview of the 1996–97 flu season. *ADVANCE for Nurse Practitioners, 5*(1), 33–38.

Plotkin, S. A. (1996). Varicella vaccine (commentary). *Pediatrics, 97*(2), 251–253.

Rodier, G. (1997). WHO response to epidemics. *World Health, 50*(1), 7–9.

Rupprecht, C. E., & Smith, J. S. (1994). Raccoon rabies—The re-emergence of an epizootic in a densely populated area. *Seminars in Virology, 5,* 155–164.

Satchell, M., & Hedges, S. J. (1997). The next bad beef scandal: Cattle feed now contain things like chicken manure and dead cats. *U.S. News & World Report, 123*(8), 22–25.

Shafer, R. W., Winters, M. A., Pelrer, S., and Merigan, T. C. (1998). Multiple concurrent reverse transcriptase and protease mutations and multi-drug resistance of HIV-1 isolated from heavily treated patients. *Annals of Internal Medicine, 128,* 906–911.

Sjogren, M. H. (1994). Serologic diagnosis of viral hepatitis. *Gastroenterology Clinics of North America, 23,* 457–477.

SmithKline Beecham. (1997, February 3). PR Newswire.

Stein, R. (1993). The ABC's of hepatitis. *American Health, 12*(5), 65–70.

Strausbaugh, L. J. (1997). Emerging infectious diseases: A challenge to all. *American Family Physician, 55*(1), 111–118.

Tauxe, R. (1997). Emerging foodborne diseases: An evolving public health challenge. *Emerging Infectious Diseases, 3,* 425–434.

Uhaa, I. J., Dato, V. M., Sorhage, F. E., Beckly, J. W., Roscoe, D. E., Gorsky, R. D., & Fishbein, D. B. (1992). Benefits and costs of using an orally absorbed vaccine to control rabies in raccoons. *Journal of the American Veterinary Medical Association, 201,* 1873–1882.

Walker, D. H., Barbour, A. G., Oliver, J. H., Lane, R. S., Dumler, J. S., Dennis, D. T., Persing, D. H., Azad, A. F., & McSweegan, E. (1996). Emerging bacterial zoonotic and vector-borne diseases: Ecological and epidemiological factors. *Journal of the American Medical Association, 275*(6), 463–470.

Wang, J. F. (1997). Attitudes, concerns, and fear of acquired immunodeficiency syndrome among registered nurses in the United States. *Holistic Nursing Practice, 11*(2), 36–50.

Wilson, M. E. (1994). Disease in evolution: Introduction. In M. E. Wilson, R. Levins, & A. Spielman (Eds.), *Disease in evolution: Global changes and emergence of infectious disease* (pp. 1–12). New York: New York Academy of Sciences.

World Health Organization. (1997a, March 26). Pap cytology screening: Most of the benefits reaped? *WHO and EUROGIN report on cervical cancer control.* Geneva, Switzerland: Author.

World Health Organization. (1997b). *Global causes of death, 1996* [Online]. Available: http://www.who.ch/whr/1997/fig2e.gif

CHAPTER 21
Chronic Illness

Airhihenbuwa, C., & Harrison, I. (1993). Traditional medicine in Africa: Past, present, and future. In P. Conrad & E. Gallagher (Eds.), *Health and health care in developing countries.* Philadelphia: Temple University Press.

American Cancer Society. (1997). *Cancer facts & figures—1997.* Atlanta: Author.

American Nurses Association. Community Health Nurse Division. (1986). *Standards of community health nursing practice.* (Publication. No CH-10). Kansas City, MO: Author.

American Public Health Association. Public Health Nursing Section. (1981). *The definition and role of public health nursing in the delivery of health care.* Washington, DC: Author.

Americans with Disability Act of 1990. Pub. L. No. 101-336, 104 Stat. 328 (1991).

Anderson, J. M. (1991). Immigrant women speak of chronic illness: The social construction of the devalued self. *Journal of Advanced Nursing, 16,* 710–717.

Baker, N. (1996). Psychosocial adaptation of the child, adolescent, and family with physical illness. In P. D. Barry, *Psychosocial nursing: Care of physically ill patients and their families* (3rd ed., pp. 505–524). Philadelphia: Lippincott-Raven.

Bauer, T., & Barron, C. (1995). Nursing interventions for spiritual care: Preferences of the community based elderly. *Journal of Holistic Nursing, 13*(3), 268–279.

Benner, P., & Wrubel, J. (1989). *The primacy of caring.* Menlo Park, CA: Addison-Wesley.

Boland, D., & Sims, S. L. (1996). Family care giving at home as a solitary journey. *IMAGE: Journal of Nursing Scholarship, 28*(1), 55–58.

Callaghan, D. (1992). *Living with diabetes: A qualitative study.* (Unpublished master's thesis, University of Manchester), Manchester, England.

Callaghan, D., & Williams, A. (1994). Living with diabetes: Issues for nursing practice. *Journal of Advanced Nursing, 20,* 132–139.

Canadian Charter of Rights and Freedom. (1982). Government of Canada: Ottawa.

Canadian Public Health Association. (1990). *Community health—public health nursing in Canada.* Ottawa: Author.

Centers for Disease Control and Prevention. (1993). Burden of chronic illness. *Morbidity and Mortality Weekly Report, 42,* 926–930.

Centers for Disease Control and Prevention. (1995). Advance report of final mortality statistics, 1992. *Monthly Vital Statistics Report, 43*(6), 3–15.

Central Statistical Office. (1990). *Social Trends* 20. London: Her Majesty's Stationary Office.

Charmaz, K. (1983). Loss of self: A fundamental form of suffering in the chronically ill. *Sociology of Health and Illness, 5*(2), 168–195.

Charmaz, K. (1991). *Good days, bad days: The self in chronic illness and time.* New Brunswick, NJ: Rutgers University Press.

Coates, V., & Boore, J. (1995). Self-management of chronic illness: Implications for nursing. *International Journal of Nursing Studies, 32*(6), 628–640.

Cohen, C. A., Pushkar Gold, D., Shulman, K. I., & Zucchero, C. A. (1994). Positive aspects of caregiving: An overlooked variable in research. *Canadian Journal of Aging, 13*(3), 378–391.

Collins, J. G. (1997). Prevalence of selected chronic conditions: United States, 1990–92. *National Center for Health Statistics, Vital Health Statistics, 10*(1994).

Conrad, P. (1987). The experience of chronic illness: Recent and new directions. In J. A. Roth & P. Conrad (Eds.), *Research in the sociology of health care: The experiences and management of chronic illness.* Greenwich, CT: JAI Press.

Conrad, P. (1990). Qualitative research on chronic illness: A commentary on method and conceptual development. *Social Science and Medicine, 30*(11), 1257–1263.

Conrad, P., & Gallagher, E. (1993). Introduction. In P. Conrad & E. Gallagher (Eds.), *Health and health care in developing countries.* Philadelphia: Temple University Press.

Corbin, J., & Strauss, A. L. (1987). Accompaniments of chronic illness: Changes in body, self, biography, and biographical time. *Sociology of Health Care, 6,* 249–281.

Corbin, J., & Strauss, A. L. (1988). *Unending work and care: Managing chronic illness at home.* San Francisco: Jossey-Bass.

Day, J. C. (1996). *Population projections of the United States by age, sex, race, and Hispanic origin: 1995–2050.* (U.S. Bureau of the Census, Current Population Reports, P25–1130). Washington, DC: U.S. Government Printing Office.

Epp, J. (1986). *Achieving health for all: A framework for health promotion.* Ottawa: National Health and Welfare.

Fahlberg, L. L., Poulin, A. L., Girdano, D. A., & Dusek, D. E. (1991). Empowerment as an emerging approach in health education. *Journal of Health Education, 22*(3), 185–193.

Ficke, H. (1995). Being a caregiver and a bread winner, too. *BC Caregiver News, 1*(3), 1.

Funnel, M., Anderson, M. R., Arnold, M. A., Barr, P. A., Donnelly, M., Johnson, P. D., Taylor-Moon, D., & White, N. H. (1991). Empowerment: An idea whose time has come in diabetes education. *Diabetes Education, 17*(1), 37–41.

Gerhardt, U. (1990). Qualitative research on illness: The issue and the story. *Social Science and Medicine, 30*(11), 1161–1172.

Harkness, G. A. (1995). *Epidemiology in nursing practice.* St. Louis: C. V. Mosby.

Hartrick, G., Lindsey, A. E., & Hills, M. (1994). Family nursing assessment: Meeting the challenge of health promotion. *Journal of Advanced Nursing, 20,* 85–91.

Health and Welfare Canada. (1987). *Active health report: Perspective on Canada's health promotion survey: 1985.* Ottawa: Ministry of Supply and Services.

Hymovich, D. P., & Hagopian, G. A. (1992). *Chronic illness in children and adults: A psychosocial approach.* Philadelphia: Saunders.

Kozier, B., Erb, G., & Blais, K. (1992). *Concepts and issues in nursing practice.* (2nd ed.). Redwood City, CA: Addison-Wesley.

Kozier, B., Erb, G., Blias, K., & Wilkinson, J. M. (1995). *Fundamentals of nursing: Concepts, process, and practice.* Redwood City, CA: Addison-Wesley.

Labonte, R. (1990). Empowerment: Notes on community and professional dimensions. *Canadian Research on Social Policy, 26,* 64–75.

Lamb, R. M. (1988). *Health promotion: Holistic guidelines for nurses in Canada.* Vancouver, Canada: Kiernan & Associates.

Lazarus, R., & Folkman, S. (1984). *Stress, appraisal and coping.* New York: Springer.

Lindsey, L. (1993). *Health within illness: Experiences of the chronically ill/disabled.* (Unpublished doctoral dissertation, University of Victoria), Victoria, British Columbia, Canada.

Lindsey, L. (1995). The gift of healing in chronic illness/disability. *Journal of Holistic Nursing, 13*(4), 287–305.

Lindsey, L. (1996). Health within illness: Experiences of chronically disabled people. *Journal of Advanced Nursing, 24,* 465–472.

Lubkin, I. M. (1995). *Chronic illness: Impact and interventions.* Boston: Jones & Bartlett.

McKie, C. (1993). Population aging: Baby boomers into the 21st century. *Canadian Social Trends, 29,* 2–6.

Meeberg, G. A. (1993). Quality of life: A concept analysis. *Journal of Advanced Nursing, 18,* 32–38.

Michael, S. R. (1996). Integrating chronic illness into one's life: A phenomenological inquiry. *Journal of Holistic Nursing, 14*(3), 251–267.

Miller, J. F. (1992a). Analysis of coping with illness. In J. F. Miller, (1992).

Coping with chronic illness. (2nd ed.). Philadelphia: F. A. Davis, pp. 19–49.

Miller, J. F. (1992b). Concept development of powerlessness: A nursing diagnosis. In J. F. Miller *Coping with chronic illness.* (2nd ed., pp. 50–81). Philadelphia: F. A. Davis.

Miller, J. F. (1992c). Patient power resources. In J. F. Miller *Coping with chronic illness* (2nd ed, pp. 3–18). Philadelphia: F. A. Davis.

Mishel, M. H., & Braden, C. J. (1988). Finding meaning: Antecedents of uncertainty in illness. *Nursing Research, 37*(2), 98–103, 127.

Mumma, C. M. (1992). Nursing role in management: Stroke client. In S. Lewis & L. C. Collier (Eds.), *Medical-surgical nursing assessment and management of clinical problems.* (3rd ed., pp. 1557–1578). St. Louis: C. V. Mosby.

National Center for Health Statistics. (1994). *Health, United States, 1993.* Hyattsville, MD: Public Health Service.

National Center for Health Statistics. (1996). DHHS release latest progress report on prevention. *1996 Fact Sheet.* Hyattsville, MD: Public Health Service.

Nyhlin, T. K. (1990). Diabetes patients facing long-term complications: Coping with uncertainty. *Journal of Advanced Nursing, 15,* 1021–1029.

Roberson, M. H. B. (1992). The meaning of compliance: Patient perspectives. *Qualitative Health Research, 2*(1), 7–26.

Rutman, D. (1995). *Caregiving as women's work: Women's experiences of powerfulness and powerlessness.* Victoria, Canada: University of Victoria.

Stapleton, S. (1992). Decreasing powerlessness in the chronically ill: A prototypical plan. In J. Miller (Ed.), *Coping with chronic illness* (2nd ed.). Philadelphia: F. A. Davis.

Statistics Canada. (1994). *Health status of Canadians: Report of the 1991 general social survey.* (Publication number 11-612E 8). Ottawa: Author.

Strauss, A. L. (1975). *Chronic illness and quality of life.* St. Louis: C. V. Mosby.

Subedi, J., & Subedi, S. (1993). The contribution of modern medicine in a traditional system: The case of Nepal. In P. Conrad & E. Gallagher (Eds.), *Health and health care in developing countries.* Philadelphia: Temple University Press.

Thorne, S. E. (1993). *Negotiating health care: The social context of chronic illness.* Newbury Park, CA: Sage.

Tomm, K. (1988). Interventive interviewing: Part III. Intending to ask linear, circular, strategic, or reflexive questions? *Family Process, 27*(1), 1–15.

U.S. Department of Health and Human Services. (1991). *Vital and health statistics: Current estimates from the national health interview survey, 1990.* Hyattsville, MD: Author.

U.S. Department of Health and Human Services. (1992). *Healthy people 2000: National health promotion and disease prevention objectives. Summary report.* Boston: Jones & Bartlett.

U.S. Department of Health and Human Services. (1996). *Healthy people 2000: Midcourse review and 1995 revisions.* Boston: Jones & Bartlett.

Wallace, R. B., & Rohrer, J. E. (1990). Aging, quantitative health status assessment and the effectiveness of medical care. In R. L. Kane, J. G. Evans, & D. MacFadyen (Eds.), *Improving the health of older people: A world view.* Oxford: Oxford University Press.

Walton, J. (1996). Spiritual relationships: A concept analysis. *Journal of Holistic Nursing, 14*(3), 237–250.

Watson, J. (1988). *Nursing: Human science and human care: A theory of nursing.* New York: National League for Nurses.

Washington Department of Health. (1993). *A progress report from the Washington state core government public health functions task force. Core public health functions.* Olympia, WA: Author.

World Bank. (1993). *World development report: 1993 investing in health.* Executive summary. Washington, DC: Oxford University Press.

World Health Organization. (1974). *Community health nursing.* (WHO Expert Committee Report No. 558). Geneva: Author.

World Health Organization. (1978). *Alma-Ata 1978: Primary health care. Report of the international conference on primary health care.* Geneva: Author.

World Health Organization. (1985). *Report of a WHO study group.* Technical Report Series 727. Geneva: Author.

World Health Organization. (1986). *Ottawa charter for health promotion.* Ottawa, Ontario, Canada: World Health Organization, Health and Welfare Canada, and Canadian Public Health Association.

Wright, L. M., & Leahey, M. (1994). *Nurses and families: A guide to family assessment and intervention* (2nd ed.). Philadelphia: F. A. Davis.

Wuest, J. (1993). Removing the shackles: A feminist critique of noncompliance. *Nursing Outlook, 41*(5), 217–224.

Zarate, A. O. (1994). *International mortality chartbook: Levels and trends, 1955–91.* Hyattsville, MD: Public Health Service.

CHAPTER 22
Developmental Disabilities

Adams, M. J., & Hollowell, J. G. (1992). Community-based projects for the prevention of developmental disabilities: Community involvement and evaluation of interventions. *Mental Retardation, 30,* 331–336.

American Academy of Pediatrics, Committee on Genetics. (1996a). Health supervision for children with fragile X syndrome. *Pediatrics, 98,* 297–300.

American Academy of Pediatrics, Committee on Genetics. (1996b). Newborn screening fact sheet. *Pediatrics, 98,* 473–501.

American Association on Mental Retardation. (1992). *Mental retardation: definition, classification, and systems of support* (9th ed.). Washington, DC: author.

American Psychiatric Association. (1994). *Diagnostic and statistical manual of mental disorders* (4th ed.). Washington, DC: Author.

Americans with Disabilities Act of 1990, PL 101-336. (July 26, 1990). Title 42, U.S.C. 12101 et seq.: *U.S. Statutes at Large,* 104, 327–378.

Batshaw, M. L., & Perret, Y. M. (1992). *Children with disabilities: a medical primer* (3rd ed.). Baltimore, MD: Paul H. Brookes Publishing Co.

Bennett, F. (1994, May). *A pediatric overview of early developmental intervention.* Paper presented at workshop, Best practices in early intervention. Far Northern Regional Center, Redding, CA.

Blondis, T. (1996). Attention deficit disorders and hyperactivity. In A. J. Capute & P. J. Accardo (Eds.), *Developmental disabilities in infancy and childhood,* Vol. 2, (2nd ed., pp. 417–436). Baltimore: Paul H. Brookes Publishing.

Blondis, T., & Roizen, N. (1996). Management of attention deficit disorders and hyperactivity. In A. J. Capute, & P. J. Accardo (Eds.), *Developmental disabilities in infancy and childhood,* Vol. 2 (2nd ed., pp. 437–449). Baltimore: Paul H. Brookes Publishing.

Booth, T., & Booth, W. (1994). Working with parents with mental retardation: Lessons from research. *Journal of Developmental and Physical Disabilities, 6,* 23–41.

Boyle, C., Decoufle, P., & Holmgreen, P. (1994). Contribution of developmental disabilities to childhood mortality in the United States: A multiple-cause-of-death analysis. *Pediatrics and Perinatal Epidemiology, 8* (4), 411–422.

Capute, A. J., & Accardo, P. J. (1996a). Cerebral palsy. In A. J. Capute & P. J. Accardo (Eds.), *Developmental disabilities in infancy and childhood,* Vol. 2, (2nd ed., pp. 81–94). Baltimore: Paul H. Brookes Publishing Co.

Capute, A. J., & Accardo, P. J. (1996b). A neurodevelopmental perspective on the continuum of developmental disabilities. In A. J. Capute & P. J. Accardo (Eds.), *Developmental disabilities in infancy and childhood,* Vol 1, (2nd ed., pp. 1–22). Baltimore: Paul H. Brookes Publishing Co.

Cefalo, R., & Moos, M-K. (1995). *Preconceptional health care: A practical guide* (2nd ed.). St. Louis: C. V. Mosby.

Centers for Disease Control and Prevention. (1995). Disabilities among children aged 17 and under, U. S. 1991–1992. *Morbidity and Mortality Weekly Report,* 44(33), 609–613.

Centers for Disease Control and Prevention, Division of Birth Defects and Developmental Disabilities (January, 1997). *Mission statement* [Online].

Criscione, T., Walsh, K., & Kastner, T. (1995). An evaluation of care coordination in controlling inpatient hospital utilization of people with developmental disabilities. *Mental Retardation, 33,* 364–373.

Curry, D. M., & Duby, J. C. (1994). Developmental surveillance by pediatric nurses. *Pediatric Nursing, 20,* 40–44.

Deal, L. (1994). The effectiveness of community health nursing interventions: a literature review. *Public Health Nursing, 11,* 315–323.

DeRogatis, M. (1993). A different reflection. *Nursing Outlook, 41,* 235–237.

Developmental Disabilities Assistance and Bill of Rights Act (1990). PL 101-496, Title 42, U.S.C. 6000 et seq.: *U. S. Statutes at Large,* 43 CFR 1385-1388.

Dzienkowski, R., Smith, K., Dillow, K, & Yucha, C. (1996). Cerebral palsy: A comprehensive review. *Nurse Practitioner, 21,* 45–59.

Edgerton, R. (1991). Preface. In R. Edgerton and M. Gaston (Eds.), *"I've seen it all": Lives of older persons with mental retardation in the community* (pp. viii–x). Baltimore: Paul H. Brookes Publishing.

Edgerton, R., Gaston, M., Kelly, H., & Ward, T. (1994). Health care for

aging people with mental retardation. *Mental Retardation, 32,* 146–150.

Education for All Handicapped Children Act of 1975, PL 94–142. (August 23, 1977). Title 20, U.S.C. 6000 et seq.: *U.S. Statutes at Large,* 89, 773–796.

Farrell, S., & Pimental, A. (1996). Interdisciplinary team process in developmental disabilities. In A. J. Capute & P. J. Accardo (Eds.), *Developmental disabilities in infancy and childhood,* Vol. 1 (2nd ed., pp. 431–441). Baltimore: Paul H. Brookes Publishing.

Feeg, V. (1994). Forward. In S. P. Roth & J. S. Morse (Eds.), *A life-span approach to nursing care for individuals with developmental disabilities* (pp. ix–x). Baltimore: Paul H. Brookes Publishing.

Fletcher, R., & Poindexter, A. (1996). Current trends in mental health care for persons with mental retardation. *Journal of Rehabilitation, 62*(1), pp. 23–26.

Frank, J. (1994). The role of the nurse in seizure management. In S. P. Roth & J. S. Morse (Eds.), *A life-span approach to nursing care for individuals with developmental disabilities* (pp. 219–248). Baltimore: Paul H. Brookes Publishing.

Gabriel, S. R. (1994). The developmentally disabled, psychiatrically impaired client: Proper treatment of dual diagnosis. *Journal of Psychosocial Nursing and Mental Health Services, 32,* 35–39.

Groce, N. E., & Zola, I. K. (1993). Multiculturalism, chronic illness and disability. *Pediatrics, 91,* (Suppl.), 1048–1055.

Harper, D. (1996). Emerging rehabilitation needs of adults with developmental disabilities. *Journal of Rehabilitation, 62*(1), pp. 7–10.

Hayden, M., Lukin, C., Braddock, D., & Smith, G. (1995). Growth in self-advocacy organizations. *Mental Retardation, 33,* 342.

Howell, L. (1994). The unborn surgical patient: A nursing frontier. *Nursing Clinics of North America, 29,* 681–694.

Hunt, N. (1967). *The world of Nigel Hunt: The diary of a mongoloid youth.* New York: Garrett Publications.

Individuals with Disabilities Education Act of 1990 PL 101–476. (October 30, 1990). Title 20, U.S.C., 1400 et. seq.: *U. S. Statutes at Large,* 104, 1103–1151.

Jenkins, J., Covington, C., & Plotnick, J. (1994). Early childhood intervention: The law. *American Journal of Maternal Child Nursing, 19,* pp. 135–143.

Johnson, C. (1996). Transition in adolescents with disabilities. In A. J. Capute & P. J. Accardo (Eds.), *Developmental disabilities in infancy and childhood* Vol. 1,(2nd ed., pp. 549–570). Baltimore: Paul H. Brookes Publishing.

Kaatz, J. (1992). Enhancing the parenting skills of developmentally disabled parents: A nursing perspective. *Journal of Community Health Nursing, 9,* 209–219.

Keltner, B. (1994). Home environments of mothers with mental retardation. *Mental Retardation, 32,* 123–127.

Kersbergen, A. (1996). Case management: A rich history of coordinating care to control costs. *Nursing Outlook, 44,* pp. 169–172.

Kramer, R. A., Allen, P., & Gergen, P. J. (1995). Health and social characteristics and children's cognitive functioning: Results from a national cohort. *American Journal of Public Health, 85,* 312–318.

Levy, S. (1996). Nonpharmacologic management of disorders of behavior and attention. In A. J. Capute & P. J. Accardo (Eds.), *Developmental disabilities in infancy and childhood,* Vol. 2, (2nd ed., pp. 451–457). Baltimore: Paul H. Brookes Publishing.

Lipkin, P. (1996). The epidemiology of the developmental disabilities. In A. J. Capute & P. J. Accardo (Eds.), *Developmental disabilities in infancy and childhood* Vol. 1, (2nd ed., pp. 137–156). Baltimore: Paul H. Brookes Publishing.

Madiros, M. (1989). Conception of childhood disability among Mexican-American parents. *Medical Anthropologist, 12,* 55–68.

Meyers, B. (1996). Psychiatric problems in people with developmental disabilities. In A. J. Capute & P. J. Accardo (Eds.), *Developmental disabilities in infancy and childhood* Vol. 2, (2nd ed., pp. 289–316). Baltimore: Paul H. Brookes Publishing.

Minihan, P., Dean, P., & Lyon, C. (1993). Managing the care of patients with mental retardation: A survey of physicians. *Mental Retardation, 31,* 239–246.

Morse, J. & Colatarci, S. (1994). The impact of technology. In S. P. Roth & J. S. Morse (Eds.), *A life-span approach to nursing care for individuals with developmental disabilities* (pp. 351–383). Baltimore: Paul H. Brookes Publishing.

Morse, J. & Roth, S. (1994). Sexuality: The nurse's role. In S. P. Roth & J. S. Morse (Eds.), *A life-span approach to nursing care for individuals with developmental disabilities* (pp. 281–304). Baltimore: Paul H. Brookes Publishing.

Murphy, K., Molnar, G., & Lankasky, K. (1995). Medical and functional status of adults with cerebral palsy. *Developmental Medicine and Child Neurology, 37,* 1075–1084.

National Information Center for Children and Youth with Disabilities. (1993). *General information about epilepsy.* Washington, DC: Author.

National Information Center for Children and Youth with Disabilities. (1994). *Children with disabilities: Understanding sibling issues.* Washington, DC: Author.

Natvig, D. A. (1994). The role of the nurse as a case manager/qualified mental retardation professional. In S. P. Roth & J. S. Morse (Eds.), *A life-span approach to nursing care for individuals with developmental disabilities* (pp. 385–400). Baltimore: Paul H. Brookes Publishing.

Nehring, W. M. (1994). The nurse whose specialty is developmental disabilities. *Pediatric Nursing, 20,* 78–81.

Nelson, K. B. (1996). The epidemiology and etiology of cerebral palsy. In A. J. Capute & P. J. Accardo (Eds.), *Developmental disabilities in infancy and childhood,* Vol. 2, (2nd ed., pp. 73–79). Baltimore: Paul H. Brookes Publishing.

Niebuhr, V. N., & Smith, L. R. (1993). The school nurse's role in attention deficit hyperactivity disorder. *Journal of School Health, 63*(2), 112–115.

Nutt, L., & Malone, M. (1992). Gerontology services. In P. McGaughlin & P. Wehman (Eds.), *Developmental disabilities: A handbook for best practices* (pp. 277–297). Boston: Andover Medical Publishers.

O'Brien, D. R. (1994). Health maintenance and promotion in adults. In S. P. Roth & J. S. Morse (Eds.), *A life-span approach to nursing care for individuals with developmental disabilities* (pp. 171–192). Baltimore: Paul H. Brookes Publishing.

The President's Panel on Mental Retardation. (1962). *A proposed program for national action to combat mental retardation.* Washington, DC: U.S. Government Printing Office.

Prouty, R., & Lakin, C. (1996). Residential services for persons with developmental disabilities: Status and trends through 1995. Executive summary. *Research and Training Center on Community Living, Institute on Community Integration.* (Report No. 48). Minneapolis: University of Minnesota, Research and Training Center on Community Living.

Rice, B. R. (1994). Self-care deficit nursing theory and the care of persons with developmental disabilities. In S. P. Roth & J. S. Morse (Eds.), *A life-span approach to nursing care for individuals with developmental disabilities* (pp. 105–118). Baltimore: Paul H. Brookes Publishing.

Rogers, P., Roizen, N., & Capone, G. (1996). Down Syndrome. In A. J. Capute & P. J. Accardo (Eds.), *Developmental disabilities in infancy and childhood,* Vol. 2, (2nd ed., pp. 221–244). Baltimore: Paul H. Brookes Publishing.

Roizen, N., Blondis, T., Irwin, M., Rubinoff, A., Kieffer, J., & Stein, M. (1996). Psychiatric and developmental disorders in families with children with attention deficit hyperactivity disorder. *Archives of Pediatrics and Adolescent Medicine, 150*(2), 203–206.

Scheerenberger, R. C. (1987). *A history of mental retardation: A quarter century of progress.* Baltimore: Paul H. Brookes Publishing.

Seltzer, G. B. & Luchterhand, C. (1994). Health and well-being of older persons with developmental disabilities. In M. M. Seltzer, M. W. Krause, & M. P. Janicki (Eds.), *Life course perspectives in adulthood and old age* (pp. 109–142). Washington, DC: American Association on Mental Retardation.

Smith R. (Ed.) (1993). *Children with mental retardation: A parent's guide.* Rockville, MD: Woodbine House.

Sobsey, D. (1994). *Violence and abuse in the lives of people with disabilities: The end of silent acceptance?* Baltimore: Paul H. Brookes Publishing.

Spencer, E. (1960). *The light in the piazza.* New York: McGraw-Hill.

Steadham, C. I. (1994). Health maintenance and promotion: Infancy through adolescence. In S. P. Roth & J. S. Morse (Eds.), *A life-span approach to nursing care for individuals with developmental disabilities* (pp. 147–170). Baltimore: Paul H. Brookes Publishing.

Strauss, D., & Kastner, T. (1996). Comparative mortality of people with mental retardation in institutions and in the community. *American Journal on Mental Retardation, 101,* 26–40.

Szymanski, E. M., & Maxwell, C. H. (1996). Career development of people with developmental disabilities: An ecological model. *Journal of Rehabilitation, 62,* 48–55.

Toleman, B. C., Brown, M. C., & Roth, S. P. (1994). Supporting positive behaviors. In S. P. Roth & J. S. Morse (Eds.), *A life-span approach to nursing care for individuals with developmental disabilities* (pp. 249–280). Baltimore: Paul H. Brookes Publishing.

Trent, J. W., Jr. (1994). *Inventing the feeble mind: A history of mental retardation in the United States.* Berkeley: University of California Press.

U.S. Department of Health and Human Services. (1996). *Healthy people 2000: Midcourse review and 1995 revision.* Sudbury, MA: Jones & Bartlett.

Whiteman, T. & Novotni, M., with Peterson, R. (1995). *Adult ADD.* Colorado Springs, CO: Pinon Press.

Wolfensberger, W. (1972). *Normalization: The principle of normalization in human services.* Toronto: The National Institute on Mental Retardation.

Zigman, W. B., Seltzer, G. B., & Silverman, W. P. (1994). Behavioral and mental health changes associated with aging. In M. Seltzer, M. Krause, & M. Janacki (Eds.), *Life course perspectives on adulthood and old age* (pp. 67–92). Washington, DC: American Association on Mental Retardation.

CHAPTER 23
Mental Health and Illness

American Nurses Association, American Psychiatric Nursing Association, Association of Child and Adolescent Psychiatric Nurses & Society for Education and Research in Psychiatric-Mental Health Nursing. (1994). *Statement on psychiatric-mental health clinical nursing practice and standards of psychiatric-mental health clinical nursing practice.* Washington, DC: American Nurses Publishing.

American Psychiatric Association. (1993). *Idea and information exchange for disaster response.* Washington, DC: Author

American Psychiatric Association. (1994). *Diagnostic and statistical manual of mental disorders* (4th ed.). Washington, DC: Author.

Bisbee, C. (1991). *Educating patients and families about mental illness: A practical guide.* Rockville, MD: Aspen Publications.

Bonger, B., Berman, A. L., Maris, R. W., Silverman, M. M., Harris, E. A., & Packman, W. L. (1998). *Risk management with suicidal patients.* New York: Guilford.

Bradshaw, T., Everitt J. (1995). Providing support to families. *Nursing Times 91*(32) 28–30.

Brooker, C., Falloon, I., Butterworth, A., Goldberg, D., Graham-Hole, V., Hillier, V. (1994). The outcome of training community psychiatric nurses to deliver psychosocial intervention. *British Journal of Psychiatry, 165*(2), 222–230.

Brown, D., Leary, J., Carson, J., Bartlett, J., and Fagin, L. (1995). Stress and the community mental health nurse: The development of a measure. *Journal of Psychiatric and Mental Health Nursing, 2*(1), 9–12.

Carson, L., Leary, J., de Villiers, N., Fagin, L., and Radmall, J. (1995). Stress in mental health nurses: Comparison of ward and community staff. *British Journal of Nursing, 4*(10), 579–582.

Centers for Disease Control. (1990). *Vital statistics.* Washington, DC: National Center for Health Statistics, U.S. Public Health Service.

Centers for Disease Control and Prevention. (1997, August 29). *CDC Surveillance Summaries. Morbidity and Mortality Weekly Report, 34.*

Centers for Disease Control and Prevention. (1997, November 14). *CDC Surveillance Summaries. Morbidity and Mortality Weekly Report, 46* (No.SS-6).

Firestone, R. W. (1997). *Suicide and the inner voice: Risk assessment, treatment, and case management.* Thousand Oaks, CA: Sage.

Foderaaro, L. (1995, April 24). Albany Plans House Calls to Monitor the Mentally Ill. *New York Times* pp. 35, 39.

Ford, J. and Rigby, P. (1996). Aftercare under supervision: Implications for CMHNs. *British Journal of Nursing, 5*(21), 1312–1316.

Freud, S. (1938). In Brill A. A. (Ed. and Trans.), *The basic writings of Sigmund Freud.* New York: The Modern Library.

Frisch, N. C., & Frisch, L. E. (1998). The client who is suicidal. In N. C. Frisch & L. E. Frisch. *Psychiatric mental health nursing* (pp. 293–317). Albany, NY: Delmar Publishers.

Golden, B. (1994). *Mental health screening.* Unpublished.

Gournay, K. (1995). Mental health nurses working purposefully with people with serious and enduring mental illness—an international perspective. *International Journal of Nursing Studies, Aug: 32*(4): 341–352.

Hanily, F. (1995). Mental health teams in the community. *Nursing Standard, 10*(10), 35–37.

Hellwig, K. (1993). Psychiatric home care nursing: Managing patients in the community setting. *Journal of Psychosocial Nursing, 31*(12), 21–24.

Kaplan, H. I., Sadock, B. J., Grebb, J. A. (1998). *Synopsis of psychiatry: Behavioral sciences, clinical psychiatry.* Baltimore: Williams & Wilkins.

Kessler, R. C., McGonagle, K. A., Zhao, S., Nelson, C., Hughes, M., Eshleman, S., Wittchen, H. U., & Kendler, K. S. (1994). Lifetime and 12-

month prevalence of DSM-III-R psychiatric disorders in the United States. *Archives of General Psychiatry, 51*(8), 8–19.

Kuchur, S. P., Potter, L. B., James, S. P., & Powell, K. E. (1995). *Suicide in the United States, 1980–1992. (Violence Surveillance Summary Series Summary No. 1.)* Atlanta, GA: National Center for Injury Prevention and Control, Center for Disease Control.

Kwakwa J. (1995). Alternative to hospital-based mental health care. *Nursing Times, 91*(23), 38–9.

Maslow, A. H. (1962). *Toward a psychology of living.* Princeton, NJ: Van Nostrand.

Martin, K. S., & Scheet, N. J. (1992). *The Omaha system: Applications for community health nursing.* Philadelphia: W. B. Saunders.

Meleis, A. L. (1997). *Theoretical nursing: Development and progress* (3rd ed.). Philadelphia: Lippincott-Raven.

Murray R. B., Baier M. (1993). Use of therapeutic milieu in a community setting. *Journal of Psychosocial Nursing, 31*(10), 11–16.

National Advisory Mental Health Council. (1993). Health care reform for Americans with severe mental illness: Report of the National Advisory Mental Health Council. *American Journal of Psychiatry* 150, 1447–1465.

National Alliance for the Mentally Ill. (1993). *History of NAMI.* Arlington, VA: Author.

National Institute of Mental Health (1998a). *WWW.nimh.nih.gov/research/suichart.htm*

National Institute of Mental Health (1998b). *WWW.nimh.nih.gov/research/suifact.htm*

North American Nursing Diagnosis Association. (1999). *NANDA nursing diagnoses: Definitions and classification 1999–2000.* Philadelphia: Author.

Orem, D. E. (1991). *Nursing concepts of practice* (4th ed.) St. Louis: Mosby-Yearbook.

Peplau, H. E. (1952). *Interpersonal relations in nursing.* New York: G. P. Putnam's Sons.

Porter, R. (1989). *A social history of madness: The world through the eyes of the insane.* New York: E. P. Dutton.

Pritchard, C. (1995). Suicide—the ultimate rejection? Bristol, PA: Open University.

Skinner, B. F. (1953). *Science and human behavior.* New York: Macmillan.

Slay, J. (1993). Medicare syndrome: Chained and bound. *Journal of Psychosocial Nursing, 31*(9), 48.

Sullivan, H. S. (1953). In H. S. Perry, and M. L. Gawel, (Eds.), *The interpersonal theory of psychiatry.* New York: W. W. Norton & Co.

Thobaben, M., & Kozlac J. (1990). Home health care's unique role in serving the elderly mentally ill. *Home Healthcare Nurse, 8*(4), 37–9.

U.S. Department of Health and Human Services. (1991). *Healthy people 2000: National health promotion and disease prevention objectives.* (DHS Publication No. (PHS) 91-50212.) Washington DC: U.S. Government Printing Office.

U.S. Department of Health and Human Services. (1996). *Healthy people 2000: Midcourse review and 1995 revisions.* Sudbury, MA: Jones & Bartlett.

Uys, L. R., Subedar, H., & Lewis, W. (1995). Educating nurses for primary psychiatric care: A South African perspective. *Archives of Psychiatric Nursing, Dec 9*(6): 348–353.

Valente, S. M. (1993). Evaluating suicide risk in the medically ill patient. *Nurse Practitioner, 18*(9), 41–50.

Vellenga, B. A., Christenson, J. (1994). Persistent and severely mentally ill clients' perceptions of their mental illness. *Issues in Mental Health Nursing 15,* 359–371.

Weiden, P., & Havens, L. (1994). Psychotherapeutic management techniques in the treatment of out-patients with schizophrenia. *Hospital and Community Psychiatry, 45*(6), 549–555.

World Health Organization. (1992). *Psychosocial consequences of disasters: Prevention and management.* Geneva: Author.

Youngkin, E. Q., & Davis M. S. (1998). *Women's health: A primary care clinical guide.* Stamford, CT: Appleton & Lange.

CHAPTER 24
Family and Community Violence

American Psychiatric Association. (1994). *Diagnostic and statistical manual of mental disorders* (4th ed.). Washington, DC: Author.

Bandura, A. (1973). *Aggression: A social learning analysis.* Englewood Cliffs, NJ: Prentice-Hall.

Barnett, O. W., Miller-Perrin, C. L., & Perrin, R. D. (1997). *Family violence across the lifespan.* Thousand Oaks, CA: Sage.

Baron, R. A. (1977). *Human aggression.* New York: Plenum.

Benton, D., & Marshall, C. (1991). Elder abuse. *Clinics in Geriatric Medicine, 7*(4), 831–845.

Black, C. A., & DeBlassie, R. R. (1993). Sexual abuse in male children and adolescents: Indicators, effects, and treatments. *Adolescence, 28*(109), 122–133.

Blau, G. M., Whewell, M. C., Gullotta, T. P., & Bloom, M. (1994). The prevention and treatment of child abuse in households of substance abusers: A research demonstration progress report. *Child Welfare League of America, LXXIII*(1), 83–90.

Bogard, M. (1992). Values in conflict: Challenges to family therapists' thinking. *Journal of Marital and Family Therapy, 18*(3), 245–256.

Bourg, S., & Stock, H. V. (1994). A review of domestic violence arrest statistics in a police department using a pro-arrest police: Are pro-arrest policies enough? *Journal of Family Violence, 9,* 177–192.

Bourne, R., Chadwick, D. L., Kanda, M. B., & Ricci, L. R. (1993). When you suspect child abuse. *Patient Care, 27*(3), 22–54.

Brody, A. L., & Green, R. (1994). Review of recent literature on the treatment of sexual offenders. *Bulletin of the American Academy of Psychiatry and the Law, 22*(3), 343–356.

Buntain-Ricklefs, J. J., Kemper, K. J., Bell, M., & Babonis, T. (1993). Punishments: What predicts adult approval. *Child Abuse and Neglect, 18*(11), 945–955.

Burgess, A. W., Burgess, A. G., & Douglas, J. E. (1994). Examining violence in the workplace. *Journal of Psychosocial Nursing, 32*(7), 11–18; 53.

Burgess, A. W., & Holmstrom, L. L. (1974). Adaptive strategies and recovery from rape. *American Journal of Psychiatry, 136,* 1278–1282.

Butler, M. J. (1995). Domestic violence—A nursing imperative. *Journal of Holistic Nursing, 13*(1), 54–69.

Butler, R. N., Finkel, S. I., Lewis, M. I., Sherman, F. T., & Sutherland, T. (1992). Aging and mental health: Prevention of caregiver overload, abuse and neglect. *Geriatrics, 47*(7), 53–58.

Campbell, J., & Humphreys, J. (1984). *Nursing care of victims of violence.* Reston, VA: Reston Publishing.

Campell, J. C. (1992). Violence against women. *Nursing and Health Care, 13,* 467–470.

Carden, A. D. (1994). Wife abuse and the wife abuser—Review and recommendations. *The Counseling Psychologist, 22*(4), 539–582.

Centers for Disease Control and Prevention. (1992). Prevention of violence and injuries due to violence. *Morbidity and Mortality Weekly Report, 41*(RR-6), 5–7.

Centers for Disease Control and Prevention. (1997). Rates of homicide, suicide, and firearm–related death among children–26 industrialized countries. *Morbidity and Mortality Weekly Report, 46* (pp. 101–145).

Centerwall, B. S. (1992). Television and violence. *Journal of the American Medical Association, 267,* 3059–3063.

Centerwall, B. S. (1995). Race, socioeconomic status, and domestic homicide. *Journal of the American Medical Association, 273,* 1755–1758.

Clarke, P. N., Pendry, N. C., & Kim, Y. S. (1997). Patterns of violence in homeless women. *Western Journal of Nursing Research, 19,* 490–500.

Community United Against Violence (1998) [On-line]. Available at www.xq.com/cuav.truths.

Council on Ethical and Judicial Affairs, American Medical Association. (1992). Physicians and domestic violence: Ethical considerations. *Journal of the American Medical Association, 267,* 3190–3193.

Crowell, N. A., & Burgess, A. W. (eds.). (1996). Understanding violence against women. Washington, DC: National Academy Press.

Cummings, P., Koepsell, T. D., Grossman, D. C., Savarino, J., & Thompson, R. S. (1997). The association between the purchase of a handgun and homicide or suicide. *American Journal of Public Health, 87,* 974–978.

D'Antonio, I. J., Darwish, A. M., & McLean, M. (1993). Child maltreatment: International perspectives. *Maternal Child Nursing Journal, 21*(2), 39–52.

Davidson, L. D. (1992). Violence to children and youths in urban communities. In D. F. Schwarz (Ed.), *Children and violence, Report of the Twenty-Third Ross Roundtable on Critical Approaches to Common Pediatric Problems* (pp. 21–29). Columbus, Ohio: Ross Laboratories.

Delong, M. F. (1995, February). Caring for the elderly. *Nurseweek,* 10–11.

Devlin, B. K., & Reynolds, E. (1994). Child abuse: How to recognize it, how to intervene. *American Journal of Nursing, 94*(3), 28–32.

Dobash, R. E., & Dobash, R. P. (1992). *Women, violence, and social change.* New York: Routledge.

Dunn, K. (1995). Domestic violence. *Nursing News, 45*(4), 6–7.

Erhart, J. K., and Sandler, B. R. (1985). *Myths and realities about rape.* Washington, DC: Project on the Status and Education of Women.

Else, L., Wonderlich, S. A., Beatty, W. W., Christie, D. W., and Stanton,

R. D. (1993). Personality characteristics of men who physically abuse women. *Hospital and Community Psychiatry, 44*(1), 54–58.

Fingerhut, L. A., Ingram, D. D., & Feldman, J. J. (1992). Firearm and non-firearm homicide among persons 15 through 19 years of age: Differences by level of urbanization, United States, 1979–1989. *Journal of the American Medical Association, 267,* 3048–3058.

Fingerhut, L. A., Ingram, D. D., & Feldman, J. J. Homicide rates among U.S. teenagers and young adults: Differences by mechanism, level of urbanization, race, and sex, 1987–1995. *JAMA, 280,*(5), pp. 423–427.

Flannery, Jr., R. B. (1997). *Violence in America: Coping with drugs, distressed families, inadequate schooling, and acts of hate.* New York: Continuum.

Freedberg, L. (April 3, 1997). Boston's big turnaround on crime among teens. *San Francisco Chronicle,* 1, 5.

Frenken, J. (1994). Treatment of incest perpetrators: A five-phase model. *Child Abuse and Neglect, 18*(4), 357–365.

Fromme, E. (1977). *The anatomy of human destructiveness.* Harmondsworth, England: Penguin.

Gage, R. B. (1990). Consequences of children's exposure to spouse abuse. *Pediatric Nursing, 16*(3), 258–260.

Garrett, D. (1995). Violent behaviors among African-American adolescents. *Adolescence, 30* (117), 207–216.

Gelles, R. J., & Loseke, D. R. (Eds.). (1993). *Current controversies on family violence.* Newberry Park: Sage.

Hart, P. D. (1994, February 9). *The January 1994 Wall Street Journal/NBC Poll* (No. 4045). Washington, DC: Hart-Teeter.

Hegar, R. L., Zuravin, S. J., & Orme, J. G. (1993). Can we predict severe child abuse? *Violence Update, 4* (1), 2–4.

Heide, K. M. (ed.). (1995). *Why kids kill parents.* Thousand Oaks, CA: Sage.

Hennes, H. (1998). Review of violence statistics among children and adolescents in the U.S. *Pediatric Clinics of North America, 45*(2), 269–280.

Herek, G. M., & Berrill, K. T. (1992). *Hate crimes: Confronting violence against lesbians and gay men.* Newbury Park: Sage.

Herman, J. L. (1992). *Trauma and recovery.* New York: Basic Books.

Hyman, A., Schillinger, D., & Bernard, L. (1995). Laws mandating reporting of domestic violence: Do they promote patient well-being? *Journal of the American Medical Association, 273,* 1781–1787.

Island, D. & Letellier, P. (1991). *Men who beat the men who love them: Battered gay men and domestic violence.* Binghamton, NY: Harrington Park.

Jenny, C., Roesler, T. A., & Poyer, K. L. (1994). Are children at risk for sexual abuse by homosexuals? *Pediatrics, 94*(1), 41–46.

Johnson, B. S. (1997). *Psychiatric-mental health nursing: Adaptation and growth* (4th ed.). Philadelphia: Lippincott.

Kaplan, H. B. (1975). *Self-attitudes of deviant behavior.* Pacific Palisades, CA: Goodyear.

Kellerman, A. L. (1994). Annotation: Firearm-related violence—What we don't know is killing us. *American Journal of Public Health, 84*(4), 541–542.

Kellerman, A. L., & Mercy, J. A. (1992). Men, women and murder: Gender-specific differences in rates of fatal violence and victimization. *Journal of Trauma, 33*(1), 3–4.

Kelly, T. H., & Cherek, D. R. (1993). Effects of alcohol on free operant aggressive behavior. *Journal of Studies on Alcohol, 11* (September Suppl.), 40–51.

Kershner, R. (1996). Adolescents' attitudes toward rape. *Adolescence, 31*(121), 9–33.

Kilpatrick, D. G., Edmunds, C. N., & Seymour, A. (1992). *Rape in America: A report to the nation.* Fort Worth, TX: National Victim Center and Crime Victims Research and Treatment Center.

King, M. C. & Ryan, J. R. (1989). Abused women: Dispelling myths and encouraging intervention. *Nurse Practitioner, 14*(5), 47–57.

Klaus, P., and Rand, M. (1992). Special report: Family violence. Bureau of Justice.

Klinger, R. L. (1995). Gay violence. *Journal of Gay and Lesbian Psychotherapy, 2*(3), 119–134.

Koop, E. C., & Lundberg, G. D. (1992). Violence in America: A public health emergency. *Journal of the American Medical Association, 267,* 3075–3076.

Lacayo, R. (1996, January 29). Law and order. *Time,* pp. 29–33.

Lewis, B. G. (1987). Psychosocial factors related to wife abuse. *Journal of Family Violence, 2*(1) 1–10.

Lie, G., Schlitt, R., Bush, J., Montagne, M. & Reyes, L. (1991). Lesbians in currently aggressive relationships: How frequently do they report aggressive past relationships? *Violence and Victims,* 6, 121–135.

Limandri, B. J. & Tilden, V. P. (1996). Nurses' reasoning in the assessment of family violence. *IMAGE: Journal of Nursing Scholarship, 28,* 247–252.

Loulan, J. (1987). *Lesbian passion: Loving ourselves and each other.* San Francisco: Spinsters/Aunt Lute.

Marques, J., Nelson, C., West, M. A., & Day, D. M. (1994). The relationship between treatment goals and recidivism among child molesters. *Behavioral Research Therapy, 32*(5), 577–588.

Marshall, W. L., & Pithers, W. D. (1994). A reconstruction of treatment outcomes with sex offenders. *Criminal Justice and Behavior, 21*(1), 10–27.

Martin, S. E. (1995). A cross burning is not just an arson: Police social construction of hate crimes in Baltimore County. *Criminology, 33*(3), 303–326.

Mason, J. (1992). Reducing youth violence: The physician's role. *Journal of the American Medical Association, 267,* 3003.

McKay, M. M. (1994). The link between domestic violence and child abuse: Assessment and treatment considerations. *Child Welfare League of America, 73*(1), 29–38.

Meehan, P. J., & O'Carroll, P. W. (1992). Gangs, drugs and homicide in Los Angeles. *AJDC, 146,* 683–687.

Milgram, G. G. (1993). Adolescents, alcohol and aggression. *Journal of Studies on Alcohol, 11* (September Suppl.).

Murman, D. (1992). Child sexual abuse. *Psychiatric and adolescent gynecology, 19,* 193–207.

Newberger, E. H., & Newberger, C. M. (1992). Treating children who witness violence. In D. F. Schwarz (Ed.), *Children and violence, Report of the Twenty-Third Ross Roundtable on Critical Approaches to Common Pediatric Problems* (pp. 118–125). Columbus, OH: Ross Laboratories.

Noel, N. L., & Yam, M. (1992). The pregnant battered woman. *Nursing Clinics of North America, 27*(4), 871–883.

Novello, A. (1992). A medical response to domestic violence. *Journal of the American Medical Association, 267,* 3132.

O'Donohue, W., & Letourneau, E. (1993). A brief group treatment for the modification of denial in child-sexual abusers: Outcome and follow-up. *Child Abuse and Neglect, 17,* 299–304.

Quina, K., and Carlson, N. I. (1989). *Rape, incest, and sexual harassment.* New York: Praeger Press.

Randall, T. (1992). Adolescents may experience home, school abuse; their future draws researchers' concerns. *Journal of the American Medical Association 267,* 3127–3131.

Rathus, S. A., Nevid, J. S., & Fichner-Rathus, L. (1997). *Human sexuality in a world of diversity* (3rd ed.). Boston: Allyn & Bacon.

Roane, T. H. (1992). Male victims of sexual abuse: A case review within a child protective team. *Child Welfare, 71*(3), 231–239.

Roberts, C., & Quillian, J. (1992). Preventing violence through primary care intervention. *Nurse Practitioner, 17*(8), 62–70.

Rosenberg, M. L., O'Carroll, P. W., & Powell, K. E. (1992). Let's be clear violence is a public health problem. *Journal of the American Medical Association, 267,* 3071–3072.

Saltzman, L. E., Mercy, J. A., O'Carroll, P. W., Rosenberg, M. L., & Rhodes, P. H. (1992). Weapon involvement and injury outcomes in family and intimate assaults. *Journal of the American Medical Association, 267,* 3043–3047.

Sheridan, D. J. (1993). The role of the battered woman specialist. *Journal of Psychosocial Nursing, 31*(11), 31–36.

Siann, G. (1985). *Accounting for aggression and violence.* London: Allen & Urwin.

Stanton, B., Baldwin, R. M., & Rachuba, L. A. (1997). A quarter century of violence in the United States: An epidemiological assessment. *Psychiatric Clinics in North America, 20*(2), 269–282.

Starling, S. P., Holden, J. R., & Jenny, C. (1995). Abusive head trauma: The relationship of perpetrators to their victims. *Pediatrics, 95*(2), 259–262.

Storr, A. (1968). *Human aggression.* Harmondsworth, England: Penguin.

Straus, M. A. (1992). Children as witnesses to marital violence: A risk factor for lifelong problems among a nationally representative sample of American men and women. In D. F. Schwartz (Eds.), *Children and violence, Report of the Twenty-Third Ross Roundtable on Critical Approaches to Common Pediatric Problems.* (pp. 98–104). Columbus, OH: Ross Laboratories.

Sutherland, S., & Scherl, D. J. (1970). Patterns of response among victims of rape. *American Journal of Orthopsychiatry, 40,* 503–511.

Taylor, S. P., & Chermack, S. T. (1993). Alcohol, drugs and human physical aggression. *Journal of Studies on Alcohol, 11* (September), 78–87.

Thobaben, M. (1998). Survivors of violence or abuse. In N. C. Frisch & L. F. Frisch. *Psychiatric Mental Health Nursing.* (pp. 559–605). Albany, NY: Delmar Publishers.

Toch, H. (1995). Foreword. In K. M. Heide, (ed.). *Why Kids Kill Parents.* (pp. ix–xii). Thousand Oaks, CA: Sage.

U.S. Department of Health and Human Services. (1990). *Healthy people 2000: National health promotion and disease prevention objectives.* DHHS Publication (Public Health Service No. 91–50212). Washington, DC: Public Health Service.

U.S. Department of Health and Human Services. (1996). *Healthy people 2000: Summary report.* Boston: Jones & Bartlett.

Van Horst, J. (1990). Preventing child abuse. *California Nursing Review, 12*(3), 42–45.

Virk, K. M., & Linnoila, M. (1993). Brain serotonin, type II alcoholism and impulsive violence. *Journal of Studies on Alcohol,* (Suppl. 11), 163–169.

Walker, L. E. (1979). *The battered woman.* New York: Harper & Row.

Wallach, L. B. (1993). Helping children cope with violence. *National Association for the Education of Young Children, 48*(4), 4–11.

Williams, A. (1993). Community health learning experiences and political activism: A model for baccalaureate curriculum revolution content. *Journal of Nursing Education, 32*(8), 352–355.

Yegidis, B. L. (1992). Family violence: Contemporary research findings and practice issues. *Community Mental Health Journal, 28*(6), 519–527.

CHAPTER 25
Substance Abuse

Abel, E. & Sokol, R. (1991). A revised conservative estimate of the incidence of FAS and its economic impact. *Alcoholism Clinical and Experimental Research, 15*(3), 514–524.

Agency for Health Care Policy and Research. (1996). Smoking cessation clinical practice guideline (consensus statement). *Journal of the American Medical Association, 275*(16), 1270–1281.

Ambrosone, C. B., Freudenheim, J. L., Graham, S., Marshall, J. R., Vena, J. E., Brasure, J. R., Michalek, A. M., Laughlin, R., Nemoto, T., Gillenwater, K. A., Harrington, A. M., & Shields, P. G. (1996). Cigarette smoking, N-acetyltransferase 2 genetic polymorphisms, and breast cancer risk. *Journal of the American Medical Association, 276*(18), 1494–1502.

American Psychiatric Association. (1994). *Diagnostic and statistical manual of mental disorders* (4th ed.), Washington, DC: Author.

Amodeo, M. (1995). The therapist's role in the drinking stage. In S., Brown, (Ed.), *Treating alcoholism* (pp. 95–132). San Francisco: Jossey-Bass.

Annas, G. J. (1996). Cowboys, camels and the first amendment. *New England Journal of Medicine, 335*(23), 1779–1784.

Atkinson, R. M., Ganzini, L., & Bernstein M. J. (1992). Alcohol and substance-use disorders in the elderly. In J. E. Birren, R. B. Sloane, & G. D. Cohen, (Eds.), *Handbook of mental health and aging* (2nd ed., pp. 515–555). Orlando, FL: Academic Press.

Bai, M. (1997). White storm warning. (Methamphetamine in the Midwest). *Newsweek, 129*(13), 66(2).

Baum, A. S., & Burnes, D. W. (1993). *A nation in denial: The truth about homelessness.* San Francisco: Westview Press.

Bean, M. (1984). Clinical implications of models for recovery from alcoholism. *Advances in Alcohol and Substance Abuse, 3,* 91–104.

Beary, K., Mudri, J. P., & Dorsch, L. (1996). Countering prescription fraud. *The Police Chief, 63*(3), 33–36.

Beebe, D. K., & Walley, E. (1995). Smokable methamphetamine ("ice"): An old drug in a different form. *American Family Physician, 51*(2), 449–454.

Beim, A. (1995). Quitting for good. *American Health, 14*(7), 88–90.

Blum, K., Cull, J. G., Braverman, E. R., & Comings, D. E. (1996). Reward deficiency syndrome. *American Scientist, 84*(2), 132–146.

Blumenstein, A. (1995). Youth violence, guns and the illicit-drug industry. *Journal of Criminal Law and Criminology, 86*(1), 10–36.

Broder, J. M. (1997). Cigarette maker concedes that smoking can cause cancer. *New York Times,* March 21, p. 1.

Brower, K. J., Eliopulos, G. A., Blow, F. C., Catlin, D. H., & Beresford, T. P. (1990). Evidence for physical and psychological dependence on anabolic androgenic steroids in eight weight lifters. *American Journal of Psychiatry, 147*(4), 510–512.

Brown, L. P. (1995). International drug trafficking. (Transcript of a speech delivered by the director of the Office of National Health Control Policy before the House Committee on the Judiciary Subcommittee on Crime and Criminal Justice, September 29, 1996). *Vital Speeches, 61*(6), 175–181.

Brown, S. (1995). Introduction: Treatment models. In S. Brown, (Ed.), *Treating alcoholism* (p. 17). San Francisco: Jossey-Bass.

Buckley, W. F. (1996). The California marijuana vote. *National Review, 48*(24), 62–64.

Calhoun, G. (1996). Prenatal substance afflicted children: An overview and review of the literature. *Education, 117*(1), 30–39.

Centers for Disease Control and Prevention. (1995a). Increasing morbidity and mortality associated with abuse of methamphetamine. *Morbidity and Mortality Weekly Report, 44*(47), 882–887.

Centers for Disease Control and Prevention. (1995b). Symptoms of substance abuse dependence associated with use of cigarettes, alcohol, and illicit drugs—United States, 1991–1992. *Morbidity and Mortality Weekly Report, 44*(44), 830–835.

Centers for Disease Control and Prevention. (1995c). Syringe exchange programs—United States, 1994–1995. *Journal of the American Medical Association, 274*(16), 1260–1262.

Centers for Disease Control and Prevention. (1996a). *HIV/AIDS surveillance report,* Washington DC: Author.

Centers for Disease Control and Prevention. (1996b). Scopolamine poisoning among heroin users. *Morbidity and Mortality Weekly Report, 45*(22), 457–461.

Chaisson, R. E., Baccheti, P., Osmond, D., Bradie, B. Sande, M. A., & Moss, A. R. (1989). Cocaine use and HIV infection in intravenous drug users in San Francisco. *Journal of the American Medical Association, 261,* 561–565.

Chapman, S. (1997). The lie of the needle: Clinton shoots down needle exchange. *New Republic, 216*(13), 11–13.

Coutinho, R. A. (1995). Needle exchange programs—Do they work? *American Journal of Public Health, 85*(11), 490–492.

Curtis, J. R., Geller, G., Stokes, E. J., Levin, D. M., & Moore, R. D. (1989). Characteristics, diagnosis and treatment of alcoholism in elderly patients. *Journal of the American Geriatric Society, 37,* 310–316.

Davenport, J. (1996) Macrocytic anemia. *American Family Physician, 53*(1), 155–163.

Delbanco, T. L. (1996). Patients who drink alcohol: Pain, pleasure and paradox (editorial). *Journal of the American Medical Association, 275*(10), 803–805.

Des Jarlais, D. C., Paone, D., Friedman, S. R., Peyser, N. Newman, R. G. (1995). Regulating controversial programs for unpopular people: Methadone maintenance and syringe exchange programs. *American Journal of Public Health, 85*(11), 1577(8).

Dority, B. (1997). The rights of Joe Camel and the Marlboro man. *The Humanist, 57*(1), 34–37.

Drake, R. E., & Mueser, K. T. (1996). Alcohol-use disorder and severe mental illness. *Alcohol Health and Research World, 20*(2), 86–94.

Dumas, L. (1991). Cocaine addicted women in home care. *Home Health Care Nurse, 10*(1), 12–17.

Dumas, L. (1992a). Addicted women: Profiles from the inner city, *Nursing Clinics of North America, 27*(4), 901–915.

Dumas, L. (1992b). Lung cancer in women: Rising epidemic, preventable disease. *Nursing Clinics of North America, 27*(4), 859–869.

Dumont, M. P. (1992). *Treating the poor.* Belmont, MA: Dympha Press.

Easley-Allen, C. (1992). Families in poverty. *Nursing Clinics of North America, 27,* 337–408.

Faltz, B. G. (1998). Substance abuse disorders. In A. Boyd & M. A. Nihart. *Psychiatric nursing: Contemporary practice.* Philadelphia: J. B. Lippincott Company.

Finkelstein, N. (1994). Treatment issues for alcohol-and-drug-dependent pregnant and parenting women. *Health and Social Work, 19*(1), 7–16.

Fishbein, D. H., & Pease, S. E. (1996). *The dynamics of drug abuse.* Boston: Allyn and Bacon.

Flexnor, S. B., & Hauck, L. C. (Eds.). (1993). *Random House unabridged dictionary* (2nd ed.). New York: Random House.

Flynn, J. C. (1991). *Cocaine: An in-depth look at the facts, science, history and future of the world's most addictive drug.* Secaucus, NJ: Carol Publishing.

Gold, M. (1991).*The good news about drugs and alcohol.* New York: Villard Press.

Goldberg, M. E. (1995). Substance-abusing women: False stereotypes and real needs. *Social Work, 40*(6), 789–799.

Gomberg, E. S. (1995). Older women and alcohol: Use and abuse. *Recent Developments in Alcoholism, 12,* 61–79.

Groark, C. M. (1992). Steroids. *Prevention Pipeline, 5*(1), 83–85.

Grube, J. W., & Wallack, L. (1994). Television beer advertising and drinking knowledge, beliefs and intentions among school children. *American Journal of Public Health, 84*(2), 254–260.

Hennessey, M. B. (1992). Identifying the woman with alcohol problems:

The nurse's role as gatekeeper. *Nursing Clinics of North America, 27*(4), 917–924.

Herbert, J. T., Hunt, B., & Dell, G. (1994). Counseling gay men and lesbians with alcohol problems. *Journal of Rehabilitation, 60*(2), 52–58.

Hewitt, B. G. (1995). The creation of the National Institute on Alcohol Abuse and Alcoholism: Responding to America's alcohol problem. *Alcohol Health and Research World, 19*(1), 12–17.

Hughes, T. L., & Smith, L. L. (1994). Is your colleague chemically dependent? *American Journal of Nursing, 94*(9), 30–35.

Igoe, J. (1994). School nursing. *Nursing Clinics of North America, 29*(3), pp. 443–457.

Julien, R. M. (1985). *A Primer of Drug Action* (4th ed.). New York: W. H. Freeman and Company.

Kinney, J. (1991). *Clinical manual of substance abuse*. St. Louis: Mosby-Yearbook.

Klatsky, A., Friedman, G., & Armstrong, M. (1990). Coffee use prior to myocardial infarction restudied: Heavier intake may increase the risk. *American Journal of Epidemiology, 132*, 479–488.

Lamarine, R. J. (1994). Selected health and behavioral effects related to the use of caffeine. *Journal of Community Health, 19*(6), 449–477.

Landry, M. & Smith, D. E. (1987). Crack: Anatomy of an addiction. *California Nursing Review, 9*(3), 28–31, 39–46.

Lehne, R. A. (1995). Pharmacology for nursing care (2nd ed.). Philadelphia: W. B. Saunders.

Leo, J. (1996). The voters go to pot. *U.S. News & World Report, 121*(17), 23.

Levine, H. G. (1978). The discovery of addiction: Changing conceptions of habitual drunkenness in America. *Journal of Studies on Alcohol, 39*(1), 143–169.

Liftik, J. (1995). Assessment. In S. Brown, (Ed.), *Treating alcoholism* (pp. 57–94). San Francisco: Jossey-Bass.

Ling, W. & Wesson, D. R. (1990). Drugs of abuse—Opiates. *Addiction medicine* (Special issue). *Western Journal of Medicine, 152*, 565–572.

Liu, S., Siegel, P. Z., Brewer, R. D., Mokdad, A. H., Sleet, D. A., & Serdula, M. (1997). Prevalence of alcohol impaired driving: Results from a national self-reported survey of health behaviors. *Journal of the American Medical Association, 277*(2), 122–126.

Lurie, P. & Drucker, E. (1997). An opportunity lost: HIV infections associated with lack of a national needle-exchange programme in the USA. *The Lancet, 349*(9052), 604–609.

Maher, L. (1992). Punishment and welfare: Crack cocaine and the regulation of mothering. *Women and Criminal Justice, 3*(2), 35–70.

Martin, S. E. (1997). Alcohol and homicide: A deadly combination of two American traditions. *Journal of Studies on Alcohol, 58*(1), 107.

Marzuk, A., Tardiff, K., Leon, A. C., Hirsch, C. S., Stajic, M., Portera, L., Hartwell, N., & Igbal, I. (1995). Fatal injuries after cocaine use as a leading cause of death among young adults in New York City. *New England Journal of Medicine, 332*(26), 1753–1758.

McCusker, J., Stoddard, A. M., Zapka, J. G., Morrison, C. S., Zorn, M., & Lewis, B. F. (1992). AIDS education for drug abusers: Evaluation of short-term effectiveness. *American Journal of Public Health, 82*(4), 533–540.

McKim, W. A. (1986). *Drugs and behavior: An introduction to behavioral pharmacology*. Upper Saddle River, NJ: Prentice Hall.

McKinlay, J. B. (1974). The case for refocussing upstream: The political economy of illness, applying behavioral science to cardiovascular risk. In *Proceedings of the American Heart Association Conference*, Seattle, WA.

McKinlay, J. B. (1993). Health promotion through healthy public policy: The contribution of complementary research methods. *Canadian Journal of Public Health, 4*(19), 109–117.

Meyer, R. E. (1996). The disease called addiction: Emerging evidence in a 200-year debate. *The Lancet, 347*(8995), 162–167.

Miller, N. S., & Gold, M. S. (1989). The diagnosis of marijuana (cannabis) dependence. *Journal of Substance Abuse Treatment, 6*, 183–192.

Miller, N. S., Gold, M. S., Cocores, J. A., & Pottash, A. C. (1988). Alcohol dependence and its medical consequences. *New York State Journal of Medicine*, (September), 476–481.

Monroe, J. (1996). A deadly narcotic: Heroin. *Current Health 2, 23*(2), 13–16.

Morganthau, T. (1997). The war over weed. *Newsweek, 129*(5), 20–23.

Mosher, J. F. (1994). Alcohol advertising and public health: An urgent call for action. *American Journal of Public Health, 84*(2), 180–182.

Myers, M. (1988). Effects of caffeine on blood pressure. *Archives of Internal Medicine, 148*, 1189–1193.

Myers, M. (1991). Caffeine and cardiac arrhythmias. *Annals of Internal Medicine, 114*, 147–150.

Nace, E. P. (1995). The dual diagnosis patient. In S. Brown, (Ed.), *Treating alcoholism* (pp. 163–193). San Francisco: Jossey-Bass.

National Center for Health Statistics. (1994). *Health United States*. Hyattsville, MD: Public Health Services.

National Center for Health Statistics. (1995). *Health United States*. Hyattsville, MD: Public Health Services.

Nelson, D. E., Giovino, G. A., Emont, S. L., Brackbill, R., Cameron, L. L., Peddicord, J., & Mowery, P. D. (1994). Trends in cigarette smoking among US physicians and nurses. *Journal of the American Medical Association, 271*(16), 1273–1276.

Nichols, W. D. (1995). Violence on campus: The intruded sanctuary. *FBI Law Enforcement Bulletin, 64*(6), 1–6.

O'Brien, C. P. & McLellan, A. T. (1996). Myths about the treatment of addiction. *The Lancet, 347*(8996), 237–241.

Olsen-Noll, C. G. & Bosworth, M. F. (1989). Alcohol abuse in the elderly. *American Family Physician, 39*, 173–179.

Oppenheimer, E. (1991). Alcohol and drug abuse among women—An overview. *British Journal of Psychiatry, 158* (Suppl. 10), 36–44.

Palmer, C. F. (1896). *Inebriety: Its source, prevention and cure* (3rd ed.). New York: Fleming H. Revell.

Pietinen, P., Geboers, J., & Kesteloot, H. (1988). Coffee consumption and serum cholesterol: An epidemiological study in Belgium. *International Journal of Epidemiology, 17*, 98–104.

Population Reference Bureau. (1989a). *America in the 21st Century: A demographic overview*, (pp. 1–8).

Population Reference Bureau. (1989b). *America in the 21st Century: Human resource development*, (pp. 8–11).

Portnoy, F. & Dumas, L. (1994). Nursing for the public good. *Nursing Clinics of North America, 29*(3), 371–376.

Prothrow-Stith, D. (1990). The epidemic of violence and its impact on the health care system. *Henry Ford Hospital Medical Journal, 38*(2, 3), 175–177.

Prothrow-Stith, D. (1996). *Violence prevention curriculum for Massachusetts*. Teen Age Health Teaching Modules. Newton, MA: Education Development Center.

Ray, O. (1983). *Drugs, society, and human behavior*. St. Louis: C. V. Mosby.

Reichman, M. E. (1994). Alcohol and breast cancer. *Alcohol, Health and Research World, 18*(3), 182–185.

Rodriguez, M. A. & Brindis, C. D. (1995). Violence and Latino youth: Prevention and methodological issues. *Public Health Reports, 110*(3), 260–268.

Rogers, A. (1997). Seeing through the haze: Can marijuana ever be good medicine? *Newsweek, 129*(2), 60.

Rosenberg, L. (1990). Coffee and tea consumption in relation to the risk of large bowel cancer: A review of epidemiological studies. *Cancer Letters, 52*, 163–171.

Rosenberg, L., Metzger, L. S., & Palmer, J. R. (1993). Alcohol consumption and risk of breast cancer: A review of the epidemiologic evidence. *Epidemiological Review, 15*, 133–144.

Schuckit, M. A. (1983). Alcoholism and other psychiatric disorders. *Hospital and Community Psychiatry, 34*(11), 1022–1027.

Schuckit, M. A., & Monteiro, M. G. (1988). Alcoholism, anxiety and depression. *British Journal of Addictions 83*(12), 1373–1380.

Shannon, I. R. (1990). Urban health challenges and opportunities. *Henry Ford Hospital Medical Journal: Urban Health Care Solutions for the 1990s, 38*(2, 3), 134–137.

Sluder, L. C., Kinnison, L. R. & Cates, D. (1996). Prenatal drug exposure: Meeting the challenge. *Childhood Education, 73*(2), 66–70.

Strain, E. C., Mumford, G. K., Silverman, K., & Griffiths, R. R. (1994). Caffeine dependence syndrome: Evidence from case histories and experimental examinations. *Journal of the American Medical Association, 272*(13), 1043–1049.

Streissguth, A. (1997). *Fetal alcohol syndrome: A guide for families and communities*. Baltimore: Brooks.

Sullivan, E. J., Handley, S. M., & Connors, H. (1994). The role of nurses in primary care: Managing alcohol abusing patients. *Alcohol, Health and Research World, 18*(2), 158–162.

Talashek, M. L., Laina, C. S., Gerace, M., & Starr, K. L. (1994). The substance abuse pandemic: Determinants to guide interventions. *Public Health Nursing 11*(2), 131–139.

Taylor, W. A. & Gold, M. S. (1990). Pharmacologic approaches to the treatment of cocaine dependence. In *Addiction medicine* (Special issue), *Western Journal of Medicine, 152*, 573–577.

Teinowitz, I. (1997). Justice Department backs FDA, sees cig ad/kids linkage. *Advertising Age, 68*(3) 39.

Tweed, S. H. (1989). Identifying the alcoholic client. *Nursing Clinics of North America, 24*(1), 13–32.

University of California. (1994, April). *Berkeley Wellness Letter, 10*(4), 7.

U.S. Department of Health and Human Services. (1990a). *Alcohol and Health*. DHHS Publication No. (ADM) 90–1656. Washington, DC: U.S. Government Printing Office.

U.S. Department of Health and Human Services. (1990b). *Healthy people 2000: National health promotion and disease prevention objectives.* DHHS Publication No. PHS 91–50212. Washington, DC: U.S. Government Printing Office.

U.S. Department of Health and Human Services. (1992). Alcohol related injuries and violence. *Prevention Pipeline 5*(3), 3–10.

U.S. Department of Health and Human Services. (1994a). *National household survey on drug abuse: Population estimates 1993.* DHHS Publication No. (SMA) 94–3017. Washington, DC: U.S. Government Printing Office.

U.S. Department of Health and Human Services. (1994b). *National survey results on drug use from the monitoring the future study, 1975–1993.* Vol. I: *Secondary school students.* NIH Publication No. 94–3809. Washington, DC: U.S. Government Printing Office.

U.S. Department of Health and Human Services. (1994c). *National survey results on drug use from the monitoring the future study, 1975–1993.* Vol. II: *College students and young adults.* NIH Publication No. 94–3810. Washington, DC: U.S. Government Printing Office.

U.S. Department of Health and Human Services. (1996). *Healthy People 2000: Midcourse review and 1995 revisions.* Sudbury, MA: Jones & Bartlett.

Valdiviesco, R., & Davis, C. (1988). U.S. Hispanics: Challenging Issues for the 1990s. *Population Trends and Public Policy*, No. 17, 1–16.

van Ameijden, E. J. C., van den Hoek, A. J. A. R., & Coutinho, R. A. (1994). Injecting risk behavior among drug users in Amsterdam, 1986–1992, and its relationship to AIDS prevention programs. *American Journal of Public Health, 84*(2), 275–282.

Wallace, J. (1977). Alcoholism from the inside out: A phenomenological analysis. In N. J. Estes, & M. E. Heinemann, (Eds.), *Alcoholism* (pp. 3–14). St. Louis: C. V. Mosby.

Waller, J. B. (1991). Epidemiology for identifying community Problems. *Henry Ford Hospital Medical Journal: Urban Health Care Solutions for the 1990s, 38*(2, 3).

Watters, J. K., Estilo, M. J., Clark, G. L., & Lorvick, J. (1994). Syringe and needle exchange as HIV/AIDS prevention for injection drug users. *Journal of the American Medical Association, 271*(2), 115–121.

Weiner, L. & Larsson, G. (1987, Summer). Clinical prevention of fetal alcohol effects, a reality: Evidence for the effectiveness of intervention. *Alcohol Health and Research World*, 60–65.

Weiner, L., Morse, B. & Garrido, P. (1989). FAS/FAE focusing prevention on women at risk. *International Journal of the Addictions, 24*(5), 385–395.

Weiner, L., Rosett, H. L., & Mason, E. A. (1985). Training professionals to identify and treat pregnant women who drink heavily. *Alcohol, Health and Research World, 1*, pp. 32–36.

Wheby, M. (1996). A rational approach to the anemia workup. *Patient Care, 30*(7)158(12).

Wilford, B. B. (1990) Abuse of prescription drugs. *Western Journal of Medicine, 152*(5), 609–612.

Wilsnack, S. & Wilsnack, R. (1991). Prevalence and magnitude of perinatal substance abuse exposures in California. *New England Journal of Medicine, 325*, 775–782.

Witters, W. L. & Venturelli, P. J. (1988). *Drugs and society* (2nd ed.). Boston: Jones & Bartlett.

Woody, G. (1996) The challenge of dual diagnosis (alcoholism and psychiatric disorder). *Alcohol, Health and Research World, 20*(2), 76–81.

Yost, D. A. (1996). Alcohol withdrawal syndrome. *American Family Physician, 54*(2), 657–666.

CHAPTER 26
Nutrition

Aday, L. A., Lee, E. S., Spears, B., Chung, C. W., Youssef, A., and Bloom, B. (1993). Health insurance and utilization of medical care for children with special health care needs. *Medical Care 31*(11), 1013–1026.

Addison, K. (1990). Cocaine: Effects on nutrient levels. *Journal of the American Dietetic Association*, September A–65 (Suppl., poster session).

American Dietetic Association. (1993). Nutrition, aging, and the continuum of health care. *Journal of the American Dietetic Association 93*(1), 80–82.

Banning, M. R. C. (1998). Risk factors for hypertension and cardiovascular disease. *Nursing Standard, 12*(22), 39–42.

Benjamin, R. (1996). Feeling poorly: The troubling verdict on poverty and health care in America. *National Forum 76*(3), 39–42.

Blot, W. J., Li, J. Y., Taylor, P. R., Guo, W., Dawsey, S. M., & Li, B. (1995). The Linxian trials: Mortality rates by vitamin-mineral intervention group. *American Journal of Clinical Nutrition, 62* (Suppl.), 1424S–1426S.

Bronner, Y. L. (1996). Nutritional status outcomes for children: Ethnic, cultural and environmental contexts. *Journal of the American Dietetic Association, 96*(9) 891–900, 903.

Cappuccio, F. P., Cook, D. G., Atkinson, R. W., & Strazzullo, P. (1997). Prevalence, detection, and management of cardiovascular risk factors in different ethnic groups in south London *Heart, 78*(6) 555–563.

Castro, F. G., Newcomb, M. D., & Kadish, K. (1987). Lifestyle differences between young adult cocaine users and their nonuser peers. *Journal of Drug Education, 17*(2), 89–111.

Centers for Disease Control and Prevention. (1992). Pediatric nutrition surveillance system, US, 1980–1991. *Morbidity and Mortality Weekly Report 41*(SS-7), 1–24.

Centers for Disease Control and Prevention. (1995a, November 24). First 500,000 AIDS cases—United States, 1995. *Morbidity and Mortality Weekly Report 44*, 849–853.

Centers for Disease Control and Prevention. (1995b, December). *HIV/AIDS Surveillance Report, 7*(2), 5–39.

Centers for Disease Control and Prevention. (1996). Update: Mortality attributable to HIV infection. *Morbidity and Mortality Weekly Report, 16*(45), 10–125.

Centers for Disease Control and Prevention. (1997). AIDS statistics. *Morbidity and Mortality Weekly Report. 46,* (8)168.

Chubon, S. J., Schulz, R. M., Lingle, E. W., and Coster-Schulz, M. A. (1994). Too many medications, too little money: How do patients cope? *Public Health Nursing, 11*(6), 412–415.

Cohn, L., & Deckelbaum, R. J. (1993). Early childhood nutrition: Eating today for tomorrow's health. *Pediatric Basics*, 66, 3.

Cookfair, J. M. (1996). *Nursing care in the community* (2nd ed.). St. Louis: Mosby.

Cornman, J. M. (1997). Questions for societies with "Third Age" populations. The extension-of-life working group, The Gerontological Society of America. *Academic Medicine, 72*(10), 856–862.

Crockett, E. G., Clancy, K. L., & Bowering, (1998). Comparing the cost of a thrifty food plan market basket in three areas of New York State. *Journal of Nutrition Education* (Suppl.), 725–795.

Davis, J., & Sherer, K. (1994). *Applied nutrition and diet therapy for nurses* (2nd ed., pp. 520–539, 545–559). Philadelphia: Saunders.

Dietitians teach chemically dependent patients the importance of nutrition in recovery. (1991, October 30). *American Dietetic Courier*, (10), 3–4.

Doweiko, H. E. (1999). *Concepts of chemical dependency.* Pacific Grove, CA: Brooks/Cole.

Edelstein, C. K. (1989). Early clues to anorexia and bulimia. *Patient Care, 23*(13), 155–175.

Fink, a., Hays, R. D., Moore, A. A., & Beck, J. C. (1996). Alcohol-related problems in older persons. Determinants, consequences, and screening. *Archives of Internal Medicine, 156*(11), 1150–1156.

Food Research and Action Center. (1998). *Fact sheet on hunger in the United States.* Washington, DC: Author.

Foulke, J. E. (1994, January/February). How to outsmart dangerous *E. coli* strain. *FDA Consumer, 28*(1), 7–11.

Friedman, M. M. (1992). *Family nursing: Theory and practice* (3rd ed.). Norwalk, CT: Appleton and Lange.

Frischknecht, R. (1998). Effect of training on muscle strength and motor function in the elderly. *Reproduction Nutritional Development, 38*(2), 167–174.

Giovannuci, E., Ascherio, A., Rimm, E. B., Meir, J. S., Colditz, G., & Willet, W. (1995). Intake of carotenoids and retinol in relation to risk of prostate cancer. *Journal of National Cancer Institute, 87*, 1767–1776.

Gloth, F. M., Gundberg, C. M., Hollis, B. W., Hadad, J. D., Tobin, J. D. (1995). Vitamin D deficiency in homebound elderly persons. *Journal of the American Medical Association, 274*(21), 1683–1686.

Goldstein, A. (1994, August 10). As patients differ so do ways of coping. *Washington Post*, pp. A1, A8.

Gram, L. (1988). Illness gendered poverty among the elderly. *Women's Health 12*(3/4), 103.

Green, L. W., & Kreuter, M. W. (1991). *Health promotion planning: An educational and environmental approach* (2nd ed.). Mountain View, CA: Mayfield.

Green, M. L., & H. J. (1987). *Nutrition in contemporary nursing practice* (2nd ed.). New York: John Wiley & Sons.

Grodner, M., Anderson, S. L., & DeYoung, S. (1996). *Foundations and clinical applications of nutrition: A nursing approach.* St. Louis, MO: Mosby-Yearbook.

Hommerson, S. (Ed.). (1992). *Practical guide to nutritional care.* Birmingham, AL: University of Alabama.

House, M. A. (1992, January 6). Cardiovascular effects of cocaine. *Journal of Cardiovascular Nursing* (2), 1–11.

Hsu, L. K. G. (1993). The outcome of eating disorder, part 1. Anorexia nervosa. *Eating Disorder Review* 4(6), 1–10.

Hughes, D. and Simpson, L. (1995). The role of social change in preventing low birth weight. *Future of Children* 5(2), 87–102.

Jaffe, M. S. and Skidmore-Roth, L. (1993). Home health: Nursing care plans (2nd ed.) St. Louis: Mosby.

Johnston, L., O'Malley, P., & Bachman, J. (1996). *News release, the rise in drug use among American teens continues in 1996.* Ann Arbor, MI: University of Michigan, Institute for Social Research.

Kohn, J. N. (1998). Preventing congestive heart failure. *American Family Physician, 57*(8), 1901–1904.

Kuczmarski, R. J. (1992, February). Relevance of overweight and weight gain in the United States. *American Journal of Clinical Nutrition 5* (Suppl. 2), 495S–502S.

Lieber, C. (1995). Medical disorders of alcoholism. *New England Journal of Medicine, 333*(16) 1058–1065.

Long, P. (1996). Winning at the losing game. *Health,* 62–68.

Mahan, L. K., & Escott-Stump, S. (1996). *Krause's food, nutrition and diet therapy* (9th ed.). Philadelphia: Saunders.

Maternal and Child Health Bureau. (1995). *Child Health USA '95.* Washington, DC: U.S. Government Printing Office.

Naeye, R. L. (1990). Maternal body weight and pregnancy outcome. *American Journal of Clinical Nutrition, 52*(2), 273–279.

Najman, J. M. (1993). Health and poverty: Past, present and prospects for the future. *Social Science Medicine, 36*(2), 157–166.

National Academy of Sciences/Institute of Medicine. (1990). *Nutrition during pregnancy.* Subcommittee on Nutritional Status and Weight Gain During Pregnancy. Washington, DC: National Academy Press.

Newcomb, M. D. (1992). Multiple proactive and risk factors for drug use and abuse: Cross-sectional and prospective findings. *Journal of Perspectives of Social Psychology, 63,* 280–296.

Nutrition Grand Rounds. (1994). New recommendations and principles for diabetes management. *Nutrition Reviews, 52*(7), 238–241.

Oakland, M. J. and Thomsen, P. A. (1990). Beliefs about the usage of vitamin/mineral supplements by elderly participants of rural congregate meal programs in central Iowa. *Journal of the American Dietetic Association 90*(5), 715–716.

Pappas, G. (1994). Elucidating the relationship between race, socioeconomic status and health. *American Journal of Public Health, 84*(6), 892–893.

Popkin, B. M. & Doak, C. M. (1998). *The obesity epidemic is a worldwide phenomenon.* Nutrition Review, 56(4), 106–114.

Popkin, B. M., Guilkey, D. K., Akin, J. S., Adair, L. S., Udry, J. R., Flieger, W. (1993). Nutrition, lactation, and birth spacing in Filipino women. *Demography 30*(3), 333–52.

Pories, W. J., Swanson, M. S., et al. (1995). Who would have thought it? An operation proves to be the most effective therapy for adult-onset diabetes mellitus. *American Surgery, 222,* 339–350.

Posner, B. M., Jette, A. M., Smith, K. W. and Miller, D. R. (1993, July). Nutrition and health risks in the elderly: The nutrition screening initiative. *American Journal of Public Health* (8), 972–978.

Prince, R., Devine, A., Dick I., et al. (1995). *Journal of Bone Mineral Research, 10,* 1068.

Rasco, C. (1992). Discouraging smoking: Interventions for pediatric nurse practitioners. *Journal of Pediatric Health Care* 6, 4.

Rees, J. M., Engelbert-Fenton, K. A., Gong, E. J., & Bach, C. M. (1992). Weight gain in adolescents during pregnancy: Rate related to birthweight outcome. *American Journal of Clinical Nutrition, 56*(5), 868–873.

Reid, I. R. (1996). Therapy of osteoporosis: Calcium, vitamin D, and exercise. *American Journal of Medical Science, 312,* 278–286.

Rice, A. E., & Ritchie, C. (1995). Relationships between international nongovernmental organizations and the United Nations. *Transnational Associations, 47*(5), 254–265.

Ryan, A. S., Treuth, M. S., Hunter, G. S., & Elahi, D. (1998). Resistive training maintains bone mineral density in postmenopausal women. *Calcified Tissue International, 62*(4), 295–299.

Saffel-Shriver, S., & Athas, B. (1993). Effective provisions of comprehensive nutrition case management for the elderly. *Journal of the American Dietetic Association, 93*(4), 439.

Sands, S. H. (1990). Bulimia, dissociation, and empathy: A self-psycho-

logical view. In C. L. Johnson (Ed.), *Psychodynamic treatment of anorexia nervosa and bulimia* (pp. 35–50). New York: Guilford Press.

Smith, M. M., & Lifschitz, F. (1990). Failure to thrive. *Contemporary Nutrition, 15*(5).

Streissguth, A. P., Aase, J. M., Sterling K. C., Randel, S. R., Ladue, R. K., Smith, D. F. (1991). Fetal alcohol syndrome in adolescents and adults. *Journal of the American Medical Association, 265*(15), 1961–1967.

Sugarman, H. J. (1996). Weight reduction after gastric bypass and hospital gastoplasty for morbid obesity. *European Journal of Surgery, 182*(2), 157–158.

Sugarman, H. J., Kellum, J. M., DeMaria, E. J., & Reines, H. D. (1996). Conversion of failed or complicated vertical bonded gastroplasty to gastric bypass in morbid obesity. *American Journal of Surgery, 171,* 263–269.

Townsend, C. (1994). *Nutrition and diet therapy* (6th ed.). Albany, NY: Delmar Publishers.

Treatment of Mild Hypertension Research Group. (1991). The treatment of mild hypertension study: A randomized, placebo-controlled trial of a nutritional hygienic regimen along with various drug nontherapies. *Archives of Internal Medicine 151*(7), 1413–1420.

U.S. Bureau of the Census. (1993). Population profile of the U.S. Current Population Report, Series P23–185. Washington, DC: U.S. Government Printing Office.

U.S. Bureau of the Census. (1995). *Income, poverty and valuation of non-cash benefits: Current population.* P–60, 188, Washington, DC: U.S. Department of Commerce.

U.S. Bureau of the Census. (1998, February 24). 1998 poverty guidelines for the 48 contiguous states and the District of Columbia. *Federal Register, 63*(36).

U.S. Department of Agriculture & Health and Human Services. (1995). *Third report on nutrition monitoring in the United States.* Washington, DC: U.S. Government Printing Office.

U.S. Department of Health and Human Services. (1990a). *Eating hints: Recipes for better nutrition during cancer treatment.* (NIH Publication No. 92-2079). Washington, DC: National Institutes of Health— National Cancer Institute.

U.S. Department of Health and Human Services. (1990). *Healthy people 2000: Citizens chart the course.* Washington, DC: Author.

U.S. Department of Health and Human Services. (1996). *Healthy people 2000: Midcourse review and 1995 revisions.* Sudbury, MA: Jones & Bartlett.

Waite, L. J. (1996). The demographic face of America's elderly. *Inquiry, 33,* 220–224.

Wallenstein, S. M. (1992). Geriatric mental health: A portrait of homelessness. *Journal of Psychosocial Nursing 30*(9), 20–24.

Waller, G. (1998). Perceived control in eating disorders: Relationship with reported sexual abuse. *International Journal of Eating Disorders, 23*(2), 213–216.

Weigle, D. S. (1990). Human obesity. Exploding the myths. *Western Journal of Medicine, 153,* 421–428.

Weisburger, J. H. (1991). Nutritional approach to cancer prevention with emphasis on vitamins, antioxidants, and carotenoids. *American Journal of Clinical Nutrition, 53* (Suppl.), 2265–2375.

Wheeler, M., & Mazur, M. L. (1997). Sugars and diabetes. *Diabetes Forecast, 50*(2), 38.

White, J. V. (1992). Nutrition Screening Initiative: Development and implementation of the public awareness checklist and screening tools. *Journal of the American Dietetic Association 92,* 163.

Wolf, N. (1991). *The beauty myth.* New York: Doubleday.

World Bank. (1993). *World development report 1993: Investing in health.* New York: Oxford University Press.

Yale, C. E. (1989). Gastric surgery for morbid obesity. Complications and long-term weight control. *Archives of Surgery, 124,* 941–946.

CHAPTER 27
Homelessness

Alperstein, G., Rappaport, C., & Flanigan, J. M. (1988). Health problems of homeless children in New York City. *American Journal of Public Health, 78*(9), 1232–1233.

Altman, J., Buckley, J., Taylor, M., & Doherty, S. (1984, January 2). Fighting back: Arizona and Massachusetts represent the extremes. *Newsweek,* p. 26.

Bassuk, E. L. (1983, Nov. 6). Addressing the needs of the homeless. *Boston Globe Magazine.*

Bassuk, E. L. (1993). Social and economic hardships of homeless and other poor women. *American Journal of Orthopsychiatry, 63*(3), 340–347.

Bassuk, E. (1995). Dilemmas in counting the homeless: An introduction. *American Journal of Orthopsychiatry, 65*(3), 318–319.

Bassuk, E. L., Buckner, J. C., Weinreb, L. F., Browne, A., Bassuk, S. S., Dawson, R., & Perloff, J. N. (1997). Homelessness in female-headed families: Childhood and adult risk and protective factors. *American Journal of Public Health, 87,* 241–248.

Bassuk, E., & Gerson, S. (1978) Deinstitutionalization and mental health services. *Scientific American, 238*(2), 46–53.

Bassuk, E. L., Rubin, L., & Lauriat, A. S. (1986). Characteristics of sheltered homeless families. *American Journal of Public Health, 76*(4),1097–1100.

Bassuk, E. L., Weinreb, L. F., Buckner, J. C., Browne, A., Salomon, A., & Bassuk, S. S. (1996). The characteristics and needs of sheltered homeless and low-income housed mothers. *Journal of the American Medical Association, 276*(8), 640–646.

Baum, A. S., & Burnes, D. W. (1993). *A nation in denial: The truth about homelessness.* San Francisco: Westview Press.

Baumohl, J. (ed.). (1996). *Homelessness in America.* Phoenix, AZ: Oryx.

Bogue, D. J. (1963). *Skid row on American cities.* University of Chicago: Community and Family Study Center.

Bond, L. S., Mazin, R., & Jiminez, M. V. (1992, Fall). Street youth and AIDS. *AIDS Education and Prevention,* (Suppl.), 14–23.

Breakey, W. R. (1997). Editorial: It's time for the public health community to declare war on homelessness. *American Journal of Public Health, 87,* 153–155.

Buckner, J. C., Bassuk, E. L., & Zima, B. T. (1993). Mental health issues affecting homeless women: Implications for interventions. *American Journal of Orthopsychiatry, 63*(3), 385–399.

Burt, M. R. (1992). *Over the edge: The growth of homelessness in the 1980s.* New York: Russell Sage Foundation (The Urban Institute Press, Washington, DC).

Centers for Disease Control and Prevention. (1992). Prevention and control of tuberculosis among homeless persons. *Morbidity and Mortality Weekly Report, 41*(RR-5), 13–23.

Centers for Disease Control and Prevention. (1993). *TB-HIV: The connection: what health care workers should know.* Washington, DC: U.S. Government Printing Office.

Centers for Disease Control and Prevention. (1994). *Core curriculum on tuberculosis: What the clinician should know* (3rd ed.). Washington, DC: U.S. Government Printing Office.

Cohen, C. I. (1994). Down and out in New York and London: A cross national comparison of homelessness. *Hospital and Community Psychiatry, 45*(8), 769–776.

Cohen, C. I., & Thompson, K. S. (1992). Homeless mentally ill or mentally ill homeless? *American Journal of Psychiatry, 149*(6), 816–23.

Cohen, E. L. & Cesta, T. G. (1997). *Nursing case management: From concept to evaluation* (2nd ed.). St. Louis: Mosby-Yearbook.

Dennis, D. L., Buckner, J. C., Lipton, F. R., & Levine, I. S. (1991). A decade of research and services for homeless mentally ill persons: Where do we stand? *American Psychologist, 46*(11), 1129–1138.

DiBlasio, F. A., & Belcher, J. R. (1993). Social work outreach to homeless people and the need to address self esteem. *Health and Social Work, 8*(4), 201.

Eighner, L. (1993). *Travels with Lisbeth.* New York: St. Martin's Press.

Federal Task Force on Homelessness and Severe Mental Illness. (1992). *Outcasts on Main Street: Report of the federal task force on homelessness and severe mental illness.* Rockville, MD: National Institute of Mental Health.

Ferguson. M. A. (1989). Psych nursing in a shelter for the homeless. *American Journal of Nursing, 89*(8), 1060–1062.

Fischer, P. J. & Breakey, W. R. (1991). The epidemiology of alcohol, drug, and mental disorders among homeless persons. *American Psychologist, 46*(11), 1115–28.

Fisher, B., Hovell, M., Hofstetter, C. R., & Hough, R. (1995). Risks associated with long-term homelessness among women: Battery, rape and HIV infection. *International Journal of Health Services, 25*(2), 351–69.

Gelberg, L., Gallagher, T. C., Andersen, R. M., & Koegel, P. (1987). Competing priorities as a barrier to medical care among homeless adults in Los Angeles. *American Journal of Public Health, 87,* 217–220.

Goldsmith, J. (1995). Breaking the barrier of not caring: Urban nursing. *Reflections, 21*(2), 8–10.

Goodman. L., Saxe, L., & Harvey, M. (1991). Homelessness as psychological trauma. *American Psychologist, 46*(11), 1219–1225.

Green, R. W. (1985). Infestations: Scabies and lice. In P. W. Brickner, L. K. Scharer, B. Conanan, A. Elvy, & M. Savarese, (Eds.), *Health care of homeless people* (pp. 35–55). New York: Springer Publishing.

Greene, J. M., Ennett, S. T., & Ringwalt, C. L. (1997). Substance use among runaway and homeless youth in three national samples. *American Journal of Public Health, 87,* 229–235.

Harrington, M. (1962). *The other America: Poverty in the United States.* Baltimore: Penguin Books.

Hector, M. G. (1992). Treatment of accidental hypothermia. *American Family Physician, 45*(2), 785–792.

Henderson, V. (1966). *The nature of nursing.* New York: MacMillan.

Herlihy-Starr, C. (Spring, 1982). They are their brother's keepers. *Boston College Magazine, XLV*(2), 16–19.

Jameson, S. (1995). Harsh Russian winter takes an early toll. *British Medical Journal, 311*(7017), 1385.

Jones, R. E. (1983). Street people and psychiatry: An introduction. *Hospital and Community Psychiatry, 34*(9), 807–811.

Kakuchi, S. (1996). Japan's painful changes. *MacLean's, 109*(2), 18–21.

Katz, J. L. (1996). Welfare overhaul law (provisions of the Personal Responsibility and Work Opportunity Reconciliation Act of 1996). *Congressional Quarterly Weekly Report, 54*(38), 2696–2706.

Kennedy, M., & Reed, B. (1996, January-February). Homeless in Massachusetts. *Dollars and Sense,* p. 27.

Kozol, J. (1988). *Rachel and her children: Homeless families in America.* New York: Crown Publishers.

Lebow, J. M., O'Connell, J. J., Oddleifson, S., Gallagher, K. M., Seage, G. R., & Freedberg, K. A. (1995). AIDS among the homeless of Boston: A cohort study. *Journal of Acquired Immune Deficiency Syndromes and Human Retrovirology, 8*(3), 292–296.

Lenehan, G., McInnis, B. N., O'Donnell, D., & Hennessey, M. (1985). A nurses' clinic for the homeless. *American Journal of Nursing, 85*(11), 1237–1240.

MacDonald, N. E., Fisher, W. A., Wells, G. A., Doherty, J. A., & Bowie, W. R. (1994). Canadian street youth: Correlates of sexual risk-taking activity. *Pediatric Infectious Disease Journal, 13*(8), 690–7.

Marin, M. V., & Vacha, E. F. (1994). Self-help strategies and resources among people at risk of homelessness: Empirical findings and social service policy. *Social Work, 39*(6), 649–657.

Mauch, D., & Mulkern, V. (1992). The McKinney Act. In P. O'Malley (Ed.), *Homelessness: New England and beyond* (pp. 419–430). Boston: University of Massachusetts Press.

McBride, K., & Mulcare, R. J. (1985). Peripheral vascular disease in the homeless. In P. W. Brickner, L. K. Scharer, B. Conanan, A. Elvy, & M. Savarese, (Eds.), *Health care of homeless people* (pp. 121–129). New York: Springer.

McGinnis, B. (1995). Tuberculosis among the homeless: The Pine Street Inn experience. In F. L. Cohen, & J. Durham, (Eds.), *Tuberculosis: A source book for nursing practice* (pp. 229–240). New York: Springer.

McInnis, B. (1988). A place for the homeless to call home. *National Commission on Nursing Implementation Project: Models for the future of nursing.* New York: National League for Nursing.

McMurray, D. (1990). Family breakdown causes homelessness. In L. Orr (Ed.), *The homeless: Opposing viewpoints* (pp. 71–74). San Diego, California: Greenhaven Press.

Murata, J., Mace, J. P., Strehlow, A. & Shuler, P. (1992). Disease patterns in homeless children: A comparison with national data. *Journal of Pediatric Nursing, 7*(3), 196–204.

National Coalition for the Homeless. (1997). Fact sheet #8: *Health care and homelessness.* Washington, DC: Author. Available from *http://nch.ari.net/*

National Coalition for the Homeless. (1997). *How many people experience homelessness?* NCH Fact sheet #2 Washington, DC: Author. Available on *http://nch.ari.net/numbers.html*

National Coalition for the Homeless. (1998). *Who is homeless?* Washington, DC: Author. Available on *http://nch.ari.net/numbers.html*

National Coalition for the Homeless (NCH). (1998). *Why are people homeless?* Washington, DC: Author. Available on *http://nch.ari.net/causes.html*

Peterson, K. (1997). The homeless mentally ill. In B. S. Johnson *Adaptation and growth: Psychiatric-mental health nursing* (4th ed.). Philadelphia: Lippincott. 727–742.

Redburn, F. S., & Buss T. F. (1986). *Responding to America's homeless: Public policy alternatives.* New York: Praeger.

Riesdorph-Ostrow, W. (1989). Deinstitutionalization: A public policy perspective. *Journal of Psychosocial Nursing, 27*(6), 4–8.

Ringwalt, C. L., Greene, J. M., Robertson, M., & McPheeters, M. M. (1998). The prevalence of homelessness among adolescents in the United States. *American Journal of Public Health, 88,* 1325–1329.

Rossi, P. H. (1994). Troubling families: Family homelessness in America. *American Behavioral Scientist, 37*(3), 342–395.

St. Lawrence, J. S., & Brasfield, T. L. (1995). HIV risk behavior among homeless adults. *AIDS Intervention and Prevention, 7*(1), 22–31.

Scanlan, B. C., & Brickner, P. W. (1990). Clinical concerns in the care of homeless persons. In P. W. Brickner, L. K. Scharer, B. A. Conanan, M. Savarese, & B. C. Scanlon, (Eds.), *Under the safety net* (pp. 69–81). New York: W. W. Norton.

Scharfman, S., Anderson, J. K. & Maus, W. (1989). Homeless veterans. *Veterans of Foreign Wars of the United States Magazine, 76*(6), 25(8).

Schmidt, W. E. (1992, January 5). Across Europe, faces of homeless become more visible and vexing, *New York Times*, pp. 1, 8.

Shinn, M., & Weitzman, B. C. (1996). Homeless families are different. In J. Baumohl (Ed.), *Homelessness in America*. Phoenix, AZ: Oryx.

Snyder, M. & Hombs, M. E. (1986, November-December). Sheltering the homeless: An American imperative. *State Government: The Journal of State Affairs*.

Somers, S. A., Rimel, R. W., Shmavonian, N., Waxman, L. D., Reyes, L. M. Wobido, S. L., & Brickner, P. W. (1990). Creation and evolution of a national health care for the homeless program. In P. W. Brickner, L. K. Scharer, B. Conanan, M. Savarese, & Scanlan, B. C. (Eds.), *Under the safety net*, (pp. 56–66). New York: W. W. Norton.

Strasser, J. A., Damrosch, S., & Gaines, J. (1991). Nutrition and the homeless person. *Journal of Community Health Nursing, 8*(2), 65–73.

Stricoff, R. L., Kennedy, J. T., Nattell, T. C., Weisfuse, I. B., & Novick, L. F. (1991). HIV seroprevalence in a facility for runaway and homeless adolescents. *American Journal of Public Health, 81* (Suppl.), 50–53.

Sugerman, S. T., Hergenroeder, A. C., Chacko, M. R., & Parcel, G. S. (1991). Acquired immunodeficiency syndrome and adolescents: Knowledge, attitudes and behaviors of runaway and homeless youths. *American Journal of Diseases of Children, 145*(4), 431–436.

Toro, P., & Rojansky, A. (1990). Homelessness: Some thoughts from an international perspective. *Community Psychologist, 24*(4), 8–11.

Tynes, L. L., Sautter, F. J., McDermott, B. E., & Winstead, D. K. (1993). Risk of HIV infection in the homeless and chronically mentally ill. *Southern Medical Journal, 86*(3), 276–81.

U.S. Conference of Mayors. (1990). *A status report on hunger and homelessness in America's cities*. Washington, DC: Author.

U.S. Conference of Mayors. (1995). *A status report on hunger and homelessness in America's cities*. Washington, DC: Author.

U.S. Conference of Mayors. (1996). A status report on hunger and homelessness in America's cities. Washington, DC: Author.

U.S. Department of Health and Human Services. (1990). *Healthy people 2000: National health promotion and disease prevention objectives.* (DHHS Publication No. PHS 91–50212). Washington, DC: U.S. Government Printing Office.

U.S. Department of Health and Human Services. (1996). *Healthy people 2000: Midcourse review and 1995 revisions*. Sudbury, MA: Jones & Bartlett.

U.S. Department of Housing and Urban Development. (1984). *A report to the secretary on homeless and emergency shelter*. Washington, DC: U.S. Government Printing Office.

Wagner, J., & Menke, E. M. (1991). Stressors and coping behaviors of homeless, poor, and low-income mothers. *Journal of Community Health Nursing, 8*(2), 75–84.

Watson, J. (1985). *Nursing: Human science and human care*. Norwalk, CT: Appleton-Century-Crofts.

Winick, M. (1985). Nutritional and vitamin deficiency states. In P. W. Brickner, L. K. Scharer, B. Conanan, A. Elvy, & M. Savarese, (Eds.), *Health care of homeless people* (pp. 103–108). New York: Springer.

Worsnop, R. L. (1996). Helping the homeless: The issues. *CQ Researcher, 26*, 75–91.

Wright, J. D. (1990). The health of homeless people: Evidence from the National Health Care for the Homeless Program. In P. W. Brickner, L. K. Scharer, B. Conanan, M. Savarese, & Scanlan, B. C. (Eds.). *Under the safety net* (pp. 15–31). New York: W. W. Norton.

Zima, B. T., Bussing, R., Forness, S. R., & Benjamin, B. (1997). Sheltered homeless children: Their eligibility and unmet need for special education evaluations. *American Journal of Public Health, 87*, 236–240.

Zima, B. T., Wells, K. B., & Freeman, H. E. (1994). Emotional and behavioral problems and severe academic delays among sheltered homeless children in Los Angeles County. *American Journal of Public Health, 84*(2), 260–264.

CHAPTER 28
Rural Health

Alcott, L. M. (1863). *Hospital sketches*. New York: Hurst & Company.

American Nurses Association, Rural/Frontier Health Care Task Force. (1996). *Rural/frontier nursing: The challenge to grow*. Washington, DC: Author.

Bigbee, J. L. (March 1993). The uniqueness of rural nursing. *Nursing Clinics of North America, 28*(1), 131–144.

Bushy, A. (1991). *Rural nursing*, Vol. 1. Newbury Park, CA: Sage.

Bushy, A. (1992). Rural nursing research priorities. *Journal of Nursing Administration, 22*(1), 50–56.

Bushy, A. (1993). Forward. *Family and Community Health, 16*(1), viii–ix.

Center for Health Policy. (1997a). *Factors affecting children's health: A rural profile, 1*(2). [Online]. Available: www.gmu.edu/departments/chp/rhr/brief2

Center for Health Policy. (1997b). *The current status of health care in rural America, 1*(1). [Online]. Available: www.gmu.edu/departments/chp/rhr/brief1

Centers for Disease Control and Prevention. (1992). Prevention and control of tuberculosis in migrant farm workers: Recommendations of the advisory council for the elimination of tuberculosis. *Morbidity and Mortality Weekly Report*, June 6.

Ciarlo, J. A. (1997). *States with frontier populations*. Available from: http:www.du.edu/frontier-hg/fronsta7.html

Ciarlo, J. A., Wachwitz, J. H., Wagenfield, M. O., Mohatt, D. F. (1996). *Focusing on "frontier": Isolated rural America, letter to the field No. 2*. Denver, CO: Frontier Mental Health Services Resources Network.

Colorado Migrant Health Program. (1998). Internet Page.

Cook, P. J., & Mizer, K. L. (1995). *The revised ERS county typology: An overview. Rural development research report 89*. Washington, DC: Rural Research Service, Economic Research Service, U.S. Department of Agriculture.

Frenzen, P. D. (1997, March). *Issues in rural health: How will measures to control medicare spending affect rural communities?* USDA Publication No. 734. Washington, DC: Department of Agriculture.

Goeppinger, J. (1993). Health promotion for rural populations: Partnership interventions. *Family Community Health, 16*(1), 1–10.

Gorman, C. (1997). The wired prairie. *Time* Special Issue, Heroes of Medicine, *150*(19), 61–63.

Grun, B. (1991). *The timetables of history* (3rd ed.). New York: Simon & Schuster.

Health Resources and Services Administration. (1998, February 11). *The migrant health program*. [Online].

Hornblower, M. (1996, November 25). Picking a new fight. *Time, 148*, 64–65.

Johnson-Webb, K. D., Baer, L. D., Gesler, W. M. (1997). What is rural? Issues and considerations. *Journal of Rural Health, 13*(3), 253–256.

Klassen, R. (1996, August). *Farming safety on-line*. Davis, CA: UC Agricultural Health & Safety Center at Davis, University of California, Davis.

Kurtz, J. (1997a). *Farm employers of migrant workers must follow specific safety rules*. http://www.mes.umn.edu/Documents/news.html

Kurtz, J. (1997b). *Good news—and bad: Is farming really getting safer*. http://www.mes.umn.edu/Documents/news.html

Lee, B. C., Jenkins, L. S., Westaby, J. D. (1997). Factors influencing exposure of children to major hazards on family farms. *Journal of Rural Health, 13*(3), 206–215.

Lee, H. J. (1993). Health perceptions of middle, "new middle," and older rural adults. *Family Community Health, 16*(1), 19–27.

Migrant Clinicians Network. (1997). *Redefining migration patterns in the migrant farmworker populations*. [Online].

Mohatt, D. F. (1997, November). *Access to mental health services in frontier America. Letter to the field no. 4*. http://www.du.edu/frontier_mh/letter4.html

Mulder, P. L., & Chang, A. F. (1997). Domestic violence in rural communities: A literature review and discussion. *The Journal of Rural Community Psychology*. [Online]: Available: www.marshall.edu/jrep/VolE1-/Mulder-Chang

National Center for Farmworker Health. (1997). *Who are America's farmworkers*. [Online].

National Rural Health Association. (1997, May). *Rural and frontier emergency medical services toward the year 2000*. Available: www.nrharural.org/pagefile/issuepaper/paper9.html. March 12, 1998.

National Rural Health Association. (1998, February). *Rural health services, rural communities and reform: A vision for health reform models for America's rural communities*. [Online].

National Rural Recruitment and Retention Network. (1997). *What is the Rural Recruitment and Retention Network (Triple R Net or 3R Net)?* [Online].

Pooley, E. (1997). The great escape. *Time, 150*(24), 52–63.

Rowley, T. D. (1996). The value of rural America. *Rural Development Perspectives, 12*(1), 2–4.

Rural Health Futures. (1997). *Telemedicine and distance learning*. [Online].

Sharpe, W. D. (1980). Introduction. In A. Novotny & C. Smith (Eds.), *Images of healing* (pp. 8–11). New York: Macmillan.

Turner, T., & Gunn, I. (1991). Issues in rural health nursing. In A. Bushy (Ed.), *Rural nursing*, Vol. 2 (pp. 105–110). Newbury Park, CA: Sage.

U.S. Census Bureau. (1992). *Census of population and housing, 1990.* [Online].

U.S. Census Bureau. (1995, October). *Urban and rural definitions.* [Online].

U.S. Census Bureau. (1997, September 24). *Selected historical census data: Urban and rural definitions and data.* [Online].

U.S. Department of Agriculture. (1997a). *Rural-urban continuum codes.* [Online].

U.S. Department of Agriculture. (1997b). *What is Rural?* [Online].

U.S. Department of Agriculture, Economic Research Service. (1997a). Births to unmarried mothers are rising faster in rural areas. *Rural Conditions and Trends, 8*(2), 66–69.

U.S. Department of Agriculture, Economic Research Service. (1997b). Nonmetro elders better off than metro elders on some measures, not on others. *Rural Conditions and Trends, 8*(2), 52–59.

U.S. Department of Agriculture, Economic Research Service. (1997c, April). *Racial/ethnic minorities in rural areas: Progress and stagnation.*

U.S. Department of Agriculture, Economic Research Service. (1997d). Rural poverty rate stabilizes. *Rural Conditions and Trends. 7*(3), 37–39.

U.S. Department of Agriculture, Economic Research Service. (1997e, February 10). *Understanding rural America.* [Online].

U.S. Department of Health and Human Services, Agency for Health Care Policy and Research. (1995). *Research in action: Improving health care for rural populations.* [Online].

U.S. Department of Health and Human Services, Center on Budget and Priorities. (1991). *Health care for the rural poor.* Washington, DC: Author.

U.S. Department of Health and Human Services, Indian Health Service. (1997). *Comprehensive health care program for American Indians and Alaska Natives.* Available from: http://www.hqe.ihs.gov

U.S. Department of Health and Human Services, National Institute for Occupational Safety and Health. (1996, April) *National occupational research agenda.* Document No. 705011. Washington, DC: Author.

U.S. Department of Health and Human Services, National Institute for Occupational Safety and Health. (1996, July). *Agriculture safety and health.* Document No. 705030. Washington, DC: Author.

U.S. Department of Health and Human Services, National Institute for Occupational Safety and Health. (1997, April) *National occupational safety and health.* Document No. 705010. Washington, DC: Author.

U.S. Department of Health and Human Services, Office of Evaluation and Inspections. (1994). *Hospital closure: 1994.* [Online].

U.S. Executive Office of the President. (1998). *Budget of the United States government fiscal year 1999.* [Online].

U.S. Office of Management & Budget. (1997). *Welcome to the Office of Management and Budget.* [Online].

University of California, San Francisco. The Center for Health Professions, Pew Health Profession Commission. (1995). *Critical challenges: Revitalizing the health professions for the twenty-first century.* [Online]. Available: www/futurehealth.ucsf.edu/summaries/challenges

Wagenfeld, M. O. (1994, July). *Mental health and substance abuse in underserved areas: Models of effective service delivery.* Helsinki, Finland: Federation for International Cooperation of Health Systems and Services Research Centers.

CHAPTER 29
Health Status: National and International Perspectives

Australian Bureau of Statistics. (1982). *Handicapped persons, Australia 1981* (No. 4343.0). Canberra, Australia: Australian Government Printing Office.

Australian Bureau of Statistics. (1990). *Disability and handicap, Australia 1988* (No. 4120.0). Canberra, Australia: Australian Government Printing Office.

Australian Bureau of Statistics. (1991). *1889–90, National health survey: Summary of results, Australia* (No. 4363.0). Canberra, Australia: Australian Government Printing Office.

Blane, D. (1995). Editorial: Social determinants of health-socioeconomic status, social class and ethnicity. *American Journal of Public Health, 85*(7), 903–904.

Brodney, K., & Dobkin, J. (1991). Resurgent tuberculosis in New York City: Human immunodeficiency virus, homelessness, and the decline of tuberculosis control programs. *American Review of Respiratory Disease, 144,* 745–749.

Brownson, R., Taylor, J., Bright, F., et al. (1991). Chronic disease prevention and control activities: United States, 1989. *Morbidity and Mortality Weekly Report, 40,* 459–463.

Canadian Public Health Association. (1992). *Human and ecosystem health.* Ottawa: Author.

Centers for Disease Control and Prevention. (1988). Tuberculosis, final data—United States, 1986. *Morbidity and Mortality Weekly Report, 36,* 817–820.

Centers for Disease Control and Prevention. (1993a). *AIDS: An expanding tragedy. The final report of the National Commission on AIDS.* Rockville, MD: Centers for Disease Control and Prevention National AIDS Clearing House.

Centers for Disease Control and Prevention. (1993b). Tuberculosis—Western Europe, 1974–1991. *Morbidity and Mortality Weekly Report, 42,* 628–631.

Centers for Disease Control and Prevention. (1994). Expanded tuberculosis surveillance and tuberculosis morbidity—United States, 1993. *Morbidity and Mortality Weekly Report, 43,* 361–366.

Centers for Disease Control and Prevention. (1995). Tuberculosis morbidity—United States, 1994. *Morbidity and Mortality Weekly Report, 44,* 387–389.

Centers for Disease Control and Prevention. (1996a). Tuberculosis morbidity—United States, 1995. *Morbidity and Mortality Weekly Report, 45,* 365–370.

Centers for Disease Control and Prevention. (1996b). Update: Mortality attributable to HIV infection among persons aged 25–44 years—United States. *Morbidity and Mortality Weekly Report, 45,* 121–125.

Dreher, M. (1996). Nursing: A cultural phenomenon. *Reflections: Sigma Theta Tau, International, 22*(4), 4.

Dubos, R., & Dubos, J. (1952). *The white plague: Tuberculosis, man, and society.* Boston, MA: Little, Brown, & Co.

Duhl, L., & Drake, J. (1995). Healthy cities: A systemic view of health. *Current Issues in Public Health, 1,* 105–109.

Elling, R. H. (1994). Theory and method for the cross-national study of health systems. *International Journal of Health Sciences, 24,* 285–309.

Fee, F. (1987). *Disease and discovery: A history of the Johns Hopkins School of Hygiene and Public Health, 1916–1939.* Baltimore, MD: Johns Hopkins University Press.

Foege, W. H., Rosenberg, M. L., & Mercy, J. A. (1995). Public health and violence prevention. *Current Issues in Public Health, 1*(1), 2–9.

Friedan, T. R. (1994). Tuberculosis control and social changes. *American Journal of Public Health, 84*(11), 1721–1723.

Hamburg, M. A. (1995). Tuberculosis and its control in the 1990s. *Current Issues in Public Health, 1*(2), 49–54.

Hancock, T., & Garrett, M. (1995). Beyond medicine: Health challenges and strategies in the 21st century. *Futures, 27*(9/10), 935–951.

Heggenhougen, H. K. (1995). The world mental health report. *Current Issues in Public Health, 1*(6), 267–271.

Hogue, C. J., & Hargraves, M. A. (1993). Class, race, and infant mortality in the United States. *American Journal of Public Health, 83*(1), 9–12.

Horiuchi, S. (1992). Global trends of age distribution, 1950–1990. In United Nations, *Changing population age structures, 1990–2105.* Geneva, Switzerland: Author.

Hunter, S. S. (1990). Levels of health development: A new tool for comparative research and policy formation. *Social Science Medicine, 31,* 433–444.

Jereb, J. A., Kelly, G. D., Dooley, S. W., et al (1991). Tuberculosis morbidity in the United States. Centers for Disease Control and Prevention, Surveillance Summary. *Morbidity and Mortality Weekly Report, 40,* 23–27.

Kickbusch, I. (1989). The new public health orientation for the city. In WHO Healthy Cities Papers, *The new public health in an urban context: Paradoxes and solutions* (pp. 43–54). Copenhagen, Denmark: FADL Publishers.

Lee, P. R., & Estes, C. L. (1994). *The nation's health* (4th ed.). Boston: Jones & Bartlett.

MacDorman, M. F., & Rosenberg, H. M. (1993). Trends in infant mortality by cause of death and other characteristics. *Vital Health Statistics* (pp. 93–185). Washington, DC: U.S. Public Health Service.

McKeown, T. (1978). Determinants of health. In P. R. Lee, & C. L. Estes, (Eds.). (1994). *The nation's health* (4th ed., pp. 6–13). Boston: Jones & Bartlett.

Murray, C. J., & Lopez, A. D. (1996). *Summary: The global burden of disease, global burden of disease and injury series.* Cambridge, MA: Harvard School of Public Health on behalf of the World Health Organization and the World Bank, Harvard University Press.

National Center for Health Statistics. (1992). *Health, United States 1981–1991, and Prevention Profile*, Publication No. PHS 92–1232. Hyattsville, MD: U.S. Department of Health and Human Services.

Nijhuis, H. G. (1989). Contemporary municipal health departments in the Netherlands: A proposed potential for new public health. In WHO Healthy Cities Paper, *The new public health in an urban context: Paradoxes and solutions* (pp. 17–39). Copenhagen, Denmark: FADL Publishers.

Ramos, M. (1997). Caring for patients, profession, and world: The social activism of Lavinia Lloyd Dock. *International Journal for Human Caring, 1*(1), 12–17.

Rice, D. (1994). Health status and national priority. In P. R. Lee, & C. L. Estes, (Eds.), *The nation's health* (4th ed.). Boston, MA: Jones & Bartlett.

Rosenberg, C. E. (1962). *The cholera years.* Chicago, IL: University of Chicago Press.

Rosenberg, M. L., & Fenley, M. A. (1990). *Violence in America: A public health approach.* New York: Oxford University Press.

Sepulveda, J., Lopez-Cervantes, M., Frenk, J., deLeon, J., Lezana-Fernandez, M., & Santos-Burgoa, C. (1992). Key issues in public health surveillance for the 1990s. In Centers for Disease Control and Prevention, U.S. Public Health and Human Services. Proceedings of the 1991 international symposium on public health surveillance. *Morbidity and Mortality Weekly Report*, 61–76.

Singh, G. P., & Yu, W. (1995). Infant mortality in the United States: Trends, differentials and projections, 1950 through 2010. *American Journal of Public Health, 85*(7), 957–964.

United Nations. (1992a). *Changing population age structures, 1990–2015: Demographic and economic consequences and implications.* Geneva: Switzerland: Author.

United Nations, Department of International Economic and Social Affairs. (1992b). *Long-range world population projections, two centuries of population growth, 1950–2150.* New York: Author.

U.S. Department of Health and Human Services. (1993). *Healthy People 2000 Review, 1992.* Hyattsville, MD: Author.

U.S. Department of Health and Human Services. (1996). *Healthy people 2000: Midcourse review and 1995 revisions.* Sudbury, MA: Jones & Bartlett.

Wilson, M. E. (1995). Anticipating new diseases. *Current Issues in Public Health, 1*(2), 90–95.

World Bank. (1993). *World development report 1993: Investing in health.* New York: Oxford University Press.

World Health Organization. (1991). *Statistics annuals 1990–1991.* Geneva, Switzerland: Author.

World Health Organization. (1992). *Global health situation and projections.* Geneva, Switzerland: Author.

World Health Organization. (1998). *Fifty facts from the World Health Report 1998: Global health situations and trends 1955–2025.* Geneva, Switzerland: Author.

Duckett, S. (1995). The council of Australian government's agenda—A Commonwealth perspective. In Health and Community Services Conference Proceedings. *Planning for Change.* Melbourne, Victoria, Australia: Department of Health and Community Services.

Katz, M. F., & Kreuter, M. W. (1997). Community assessment and empowerment. In E. D. Schutchfield & W. C. Keck (Eds.), *Principles of public health practice.* Albany, NY: Delmar Publishers.

Lasker, R. D., & the Committee on Medicine and Public Health. (1997). *Medicine and public health: The power of collaboration.* New York: New York Academy of Medicine.

Miotto Wright, M., Godue, C., Manfredi, M., & Korniewicz, D. M. (1998). Nursing education and international health in the United States, Latin America, and the Caribbean. *Image: Journal of Nursing Scholarship, 30*(1), 31–36.

Ohlson, V. M., & Styles, M. (1997). International nursing: The role of the International Council of Nurses and the World Health Organization. In J. C. McCloskey & H. Grace (Eds.), *Current issues in nursing* (5th ed.). St Louis, MO: C. V. Mosby.

Perfiljeva, G. (1997). Progress in Russia: Working together for change. *Reflections 23*(2), 8–9.

Picard, C., & DiVitto, S. (1997, Second quarter). Think and act both locally and globally. *Reflections*, 6–9.

Pike, S. (1995). Health promotion now: The development of policy. In S. Pike & D. Forster (Eds.), *Health promotion for all* (27–38). Edinburgh: Churchill Livingstone.

Pike, S., & Forster, D. (1995). *Health promotion for all.* Edinburgh: Churchill Livingstone.

Quinn, S. (1981). *What about me? Caring for the carers.* Geneva: International Council of Nurses.

Roach, M. S. (1995). The dominant paradigm of the modern world. In A. Boykin (Ed.), *Power, politics, and public policy: A matter of caring* (pp. 3–10). New York: National League for Nursing.

Ross Kerr, J. C. (1997). The Canadian health care system: Overview and issues. In J. C. McCloskey & H. Grace (Eds.), *Current issues in nursing* (5th ed., pp. 460–466). St. Louis, MO: C. V. Mosby.

Salmon, M. E. (1998). Guest Editorial—The future of public health nursing: A state of mind. Washington, DC: American Public Health Association, Public Health Nursing Section Newsletter, 3.

Smith, L. S. (1997). Nursing in Russia: Impact of recent political changes. In J. C. McCloskey & H. Grace (Eds.), *Current issues in nursing* (5th ed., pp. 686–694). St. Louis, MO: C. V. Mosby.

Splane, V. H., & Splane, R. B. (1994). International nursing leaders. In J. C. McCloskey & H. Grace (Eds.), *Current issues in nursing* (4th ed., pp. 49–56). St. Louis, MO: C. V. Mosby.

World Health Organization. (1978). *Alma Ata 1978: Primary health care.* Geneva, Switzerland: Author.

World Health Organization. (1986). *The Ottawa charter for health promotion.* Geneva, Switzerland: Author.

World Health Organization. (1993). *Health for all targets: The health policy for Europe* (updated ed.). Copenhagen: WHO, Regional Office for Europe.

Zamurs, A. (1995). Service development in the new environment. In Health and Community Services Conference Proceedings. *Planning for change* (pp. 21–24). Melbourne: Australia: Health and Community Services.

CHAPTER 30
Health Care Delivery Systems around the World

American Public Health Association. (1997). *The nation's health* (6), 24.

Ashton, J., & Seymour, H. (1988). *The new public health.* Philadelphia: Open University.

Basch, P. F. (1990). *Textbook of international health.* New York: Oxford University Press.

Berman, P. (1996). Health sector reform: A worldwide perspective. *Current Issues in Public Health, 2*(1), 34–38.

Bridges, D. (1965). *A history of the International Council of Nurses, 1899–1964.* Philadelphia: Lippincott.

Commonwealth Department of Health, Housing, and Community Services. (1992). *Annual report 91–92: Statistical supplement.* Canberra: Australian Government Printing Office.

Commonwealth Department of Human Services and Health. (1995). *Department of Human Services and Health: Statistical overview 1993–1994.* Canberra: Australian Government Printing Service.

Curtis, S., Petukhova, N., & Taket, A. (1995). Health care reforms in Russia: The example of St. Petersburg. *Social Science and Medicine, 40*(6), 755–765.

Dreher, M. C. (1997). Creating a multitude of opportunities for nurses to interact: Global sharing among nurses. *Reflections, 23*(2), 5.

CHAPTER 31
Power, Politics, and Public Policy

American Nurses Association. (1996). *Successes and challenges in the federal legislative arena.* ANA Policy Series. Washington, DC: Author.

Association of Community Health Nurse Educators. (1990). *Essentials of baccalaureate nursing education for entry level community health nursing practice.* Louisville, KY: Author.

Backer, B. A. (1993). Lillian Wald: Connecting caring with activism. *Nursing and Health Care, 14*(3), 128.

Bavier, A. (1995). Where research and practice meet—Opportunities at the Agency for Health Care Policy and Research. *Nursing Policy Forum, 1*(4), 21.

Brown, S. (1996). Incorporating political socialization theory into baccalaureate nursing education. *Nursing Outlook, 44*(3), 3.

Caterinicchio, M. J. (1995). AACN Perspective, Redefining nursing in the midst of health care reform. *Nursing Policy Forum, 1*(1), 9.

Chaffee, M. (1996). The nurse in Washington internship (NIWI). *Nursing Policy Forum, 2*(1), 24.

Cohen, S. S., Mason, D. J., Korner, C., Leavitt, J. K., Pulcini, J., & Sochalski, J. (1996). Stages of nursing's political development: Where we've been and where we ought to go. *Nursing Outlook, 44*(6), 259–266.

Flynn, B. C. (1995). Healthy Cities: Building partnerships for healthy public policy. *Nursing Policy Forum, 1*(6), 7.

Freed, L. (1996). *Political action handbook for nurses.* Santa Rosa, CA: Professor Publishing.

Hall-Long, B. A. (1995). Nursing's past, present, and future political experiences. *Nursing and Health Care: Perspectives on Community, 16*(1). p. 27.

Jennings, C. (1995). The time is now. *Nursing Policy Forum, 1*(1), 5.

Livsey, K. (1995). AAOHN Perspective—Leaders in workplace health and safety. *Nursing Policy Forum, 1*(1), p. 14.

MacPherson, K. I. (1987). Health care policy, values, and nursing. *Advances in Nursing Science, 9*(3), 1–11.

Mason, D. J., Talbott, S. W., and Leavitt, J. K., (Eds.). (1993). *Policy and politics for nurses: Action and change in the workplace, government, organization and community* (2nd ed.). Philadelphia: W. B. Saunders.

Milio, N. (1981). *Promoting health through public policy.* Philadelphia: F. A. Davis.

National League for Nursing. (1988). *Curriculum revolution: Mandate for change.* New York: Author.

Olds, D. L., Eckenrode, J., Henderson, C., Kitzman, H., Powers, J., Cole, R., Sidora, K., Morris, P., Pettit, L., Luckey, D. (1997). Long-term effects of home visitation on maternal life course and child abuse and neglect: Fifteen-year follow-up of a randomized trial. *Journal of the American Medical Association, 278,* 637–643.

Porter-O'Grady, T. (1994). Building partnerships in health care: Creating whole systems change. *Nursing and Health Care, 15*(1), 38.

Stanhope, M., & Lancaster, J. (1996). *Community health nursing: Promoting health of aggregates, families and individuals* (4th ed.). St. Louis: Mosby.

Swan, S. (1995). Anderson, R. AONE Perspective-meeting the needs of the future. *Nursing Policy Forum, 1*(1), 11.

Towers, J. (1995). AANP Perspectives—Nurse practitioners and health policy. *Nursing Policy Forum, 1*(1), 13.

Tri-Council for Nursing. (1991). *Nursing's agenda for health care reform.* Washington, DC: American Nurses Association.

U.S. Department of Health and Human Services. (1995). *Healthy people 2000: Midcourse review and 1995 revision.* Sudbury, MA: Jones & Bartlett.

Weis, D. (1995). Challenging our values—Directing health care reform. *Nursing Policy Forum, 1*(1), 26.

Williams, A. (1993). Community health learning experiences and political activism: A model for baccalaureate curriculum revolution content. *Journal of Nursing Education, 32*(8), 353.

CHAPTER 32
Visions for the Future

Anderson, E., & McFarlane, J. (1996). *Community as partner: theory and practice in nursing.* Philadelphia: Lippincott.

Ashton, J. (1991). The healthy cities project: A challenge for health education. *Health Education Quarterly, 18*(1), 39–48.

Barrett, E. A. M. (1990). Health patterning with clients in a private practice environment. In E. A. M. Barrett (Ed.), *Visions of Rogers' Science-Based Nursing* (pp. 105–115). New York: National League for Nursing.

Barrett, E. A. M. (1994). On the threshold of tomorrow. In V. M. Malinski, & E. A. M. Barrett, (Eds.), *Martha E. Rogers: Her life and her work* (pp. 271–275). Philadelphia: F. A. Davis.

Barrington, R. (1995). *Repatterning an urban Indian clinic through Rogerian Nursing Science and caring framework.* Paper presented at the regional meeting of the Society of Rogerian Scholars, San Diego, CA.

Belmont Vision Project. (1995). *Health care innovation: A vision for the 21st century: Creating the vision.* Alexandria, VA: Institute for Alternative Futures.

Bezold, C., & Hancock, T. (1994). Possible futures, preferable futures. *Health Care Forum Journal,* p.25.

Biester, D. J. (1994). Schools and health: A partnership for a healthier future. *Journal of Pediatric Nursing, 9,* 414–416.

Bryant, J. H., Zuberi, R. W., & Thaver, I. H. (1991). Alma Ata and health for all by the year 2000. *Infectious Disease Clinics of North America, 5,* 403–415.

Buhler-Wilkerson, K. (1993). Public health then and now. Bringing care to the people: Lillian Wald's legacy to public health nursing. *American Journal of Public Health, 83*(12), 1778–1786.

Bulechek, G., & McCloskey, J. (1992). Future directions. In G. M. Bulechek & J. C. McCloskey (Eds.), *Nursing interventions classification* (pp. 401–408). St. Louis, MO: Mosby Year-book.

Clarke, P., & Cody, W. (1994). Nursing theory-based practice in the home and community: The crux of professional nursing education. *Advances in Nursing Science, 17*(2), 41–53.

Congress, E., & Lyons, B. (1992). Cultural differences in health beliefs: Implications for social work practice in health care settings. *Social Work in Health Care, 17*(3), 81–96.

Fawcett, J. (1984). *Analysis and evaluation of conceptual models of nursing.* Philadelphia: F. A. Davis.

Fawcett, J. (1993). From a plethora of paradigms to parsimony in worldviews. *Nursing Science Quarterly, 6*(2), 56–58.

Flynn, B. (1992). Developing community leadership in healthy cities: The Indiana Model. *Nursing Outlook, 40*(3), 121–126.

Grace, H. K. (1995). Nurses make "Health for All" a reality. *Nursing and Health Care: Perspectives on Community, 16*(4), 172.

Gray, B. B. (1994). 21st century hospital will embody new concept. *Nurseweek, 7*(1), 22–23.

Hancock, T. (1993a, August). Towards a primary health services system for the 21st century: A personal reflection. Kleinburg, Ontario, Canada: Author.

Hancock, T. (1993b). The evolution, impact and significance of the healthy cities/healthy communities movement. *Journal of Public Health Policy, 14,* 5–18.

Hancock, T., & Bezold, C. (1994, March/April). Possible futures, preferable futures. *Healthcare Forum Journal,* 23–29.

Hancock, T., & Garrett, M. (1995). Beyond medicine: Health challenges and strategies in the 21st century. *Futures, 27*(9/10), 935–951.

Healthcare Forum. (1992). Bridging the leadership gap in healthcare. San Francisco: Author.

Healthcare Forum Leadership Center. (1992). *Bridging the leadership gap in healthcare.* San Francisco: Author.

Hudson-Rodd, N. (1994). Public health: People participating in the creation of healthy places. *Public Health Nursing, 11,* 119–126.

Jenkins, M. L., & Sullivan-Marx, E. M. (1994). Nurse practitioners and community health nurses. *Nursing Clinics of North America, 29,* 459–466.

King, I. (1981). *A theory for nursing.* New York: Wiley.

Knollmueller, R. (1994). Thinking about tomorrow for nursing: Changes and challenges. *Journal of Continuing Education in Nursing, 25*(5), 196–201.

Leininger, M. (1988). Leininger's theory of nursing: Cultural care diversity and universality. *Nursing Science Quarterly, 1,* 152–160.

Leininger, M. (Ed.). (1991). *Culture care diversity and universality: A theory of nursing.* Publication No. 15–2402. New York: National League for Nursing.

Lewis, J. M., & Farrell, M. (1995). Distance education: A strategy for leadership development. *Nursing and Health Care: Perspectives on Community, 16*(4), 184–187.

Madrid, M., & Barrett, E. A. M. (Eds.). (1994). *Rogers' scientific art of nursing practice.* New York: National League for Nursing.

Mason, D., Talbott, S., & Leavitt, J. (1993). *Policy and politics for nurses.* Philadelphia: W. B. Saunders.

Meservey, P. M. (1995). Fostering collaboration in a boundaryless organization. *Nursing and Health Care: Perspectives on Community, 16*(4), 234–236.

National League for Nursing. (1993). *A vision for nursing education.* New York: NLN Press.

Neuman, B. (1982). *The Neuman Systems Model: Application to nursing education and practice.* Norwalk, CT: Appleton-Century-Crofts.

Newman, M. (1990). Theory for nursing practice. *Nursing Science Quarterly, 7*(4), 153–157.

Newman, M. (1994). Health as expanding consciousness (2nd ed.). New York: National League for Nursing.

Nightingale, F. (1860/1969). *Notes on nursing: What it is and what it is not.* New York: Dover.

Orem. D. (1985). *Nursing: Concepts of practice* (3rd ed.). New York: Mc-Graw-Hill.

Parse, R. (1987). Man-living-health. In R. Parse, (Ed.), *Nursing science: Major paradigms, theories, and critiques* (pp. 159–179). Philadelphia: W. B. Saunders.

Passarelli, C. (1994). School nursing: Trends for the future. *Journal of School Health, 64,* 141–146.

Peacock, L. (1996, Summer). Editorial. *Bahm News,* p. 1. San Francisco: Bay Area Health Ministries.

Pew Health Professions Commission. (1995). Critical challenges: Revitalizing the health professions for the twenty-first century. http://-futurehealth.ucsf.edu/pubs.html

Phillips, J. R. (1994). A vision of nursing research priorities. *Nursing Science Quarterly, 7*(2), 52.

Quinn, J. F., & Strelkauskas, A. J. (1993). Psychoimmunologic effects of Therapeutic Touch on practitioners and recently bereaved recipients: A pilot study. *Advances in Nursing Science, 15*(4), 13–26.

Rathwell, T. (1992). Realities of health for all by the year 2000. *Social Science in Medicine, 35,* 541–547.

Reverby, S. M. (1993). From Lillian Wald to Hillary Rodham Clinton: What will happen to public health nursing? *American Journal of Public Health, 83*(12), 1662–1663.

Roach, M. S. (1991). The call to consciousness: Compassion in today's health world. In D. A. Gout & M. M. Leininger (Eds.), *Caring: The compassionate healer* (pp. 7–17). New York: National League for Nursing.

Rogers, M. E. (1988). Nursing science and art: A prospective. *Nursing Science Quarterly, 1,* 99–102.

Rogers, M. (1994). Nursing science evolves. In M. Madrid & E. A. M. Barrett (Eds.), *Rogers Scientific Art of Nursing Practice* (pp. 3–9). New York: National League for Nursing.

Roy, C. (1982). *Adaptation nursing: The Roy Conceptual Model applied.* St. Louis, MO: C. V. Mosby.

Salmon, M. E. (1993). Public health nursing—The opportunity of a century. *American Journal of Public Health, 83*(12), 1674–1675.

Salmon, M. E. (1994). School (health) nursing in the era of health care reform: What is the outlook? *Journal of School Health, 64,* 137–140.

Schoenhofer, S. O. (1993). What constitutes nursing research? *Nursing Science Quarterly, 6*(2), 59–60.

Schubert, P., & Lionberger, H. (1995). Mutual connectedness: A study of client-nurse interaction using the Grounded Theory method. *Journal of Holistic Nursing, 13*(2), 102–116.

Shalala, D. E. (1993). Nursing and society: The unfinished agenda for the 21st century. *Nursing and Health Care, 14,* 289–291.

Sims, T. W. (1994). Health care reform and nursing as window of opportunity: An interview with Connie Curran. *American Nephrology Nurses' Association Journal, 2,* 250–255.

Smith, G. R. (1995). Lessons learned: Challenges for the future. *Nursing and Health Care: Perspectives on Community, 16*(4), 188–191.

Styles, M. (1994). Nursing in the years to come. *World Health, 5,* 26–27.

Tietebaum, M., & Bieg, K. (1994). *Evaluation of the community-based health project, final report.* Bethesda, MD: Abt Associates.

Watson, J. (1985). *Nursing: Human science and human care, a theory of nursing.* Norwalk, CT: Appleton-Century-Crofts.

Wilber, K. (1996). *A brief history of everything.* Boston: Shambala.

World Health Organization. (1978). *Report on the international conference on primary health care, Alma Ata, 6–12 September.* Geneva: Author.

World Health Organization. (1981). *Global strategy for health for all by the year 2000.* Geneva: Author.

World Health Organization. (1986). *Promoting health in the urban context.* Copenhagen: The WHO Healthy Cities Project Office.

Zerwekh, J. (1993). Going to the people—Public health nursing today and tomorrow. *American Journal of Public Health, 83*(12), 1676–1618.50.

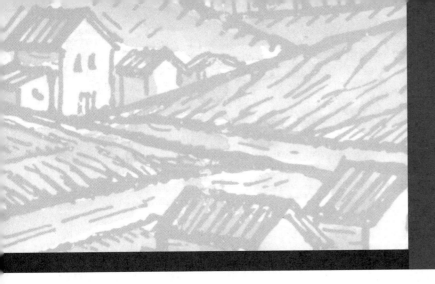

GLOSSARY

A

acculturation The process by which new members of a culture learn its ways and become part of that culture.

achieved role Role activities that are not ordinarily assigned but are earned.

acquaintance rape Rape by an individual known to the victim.

acquired immunity Immunity conferred by the transfer of antibodies from mother to child via the placenta or breastfeeding.

active immunity Immunity developed by introducing an infectious agent or vaccine into the host.

active listening Carefully listening to another and reflecting back content and meaning to check for accuracy and to facilitate further exploration.

activity center A place where persons needing extensive or pervasive supports can be taught self-care, social skills, homemaking, and leisure activities skills.

acupressure A system of applying pressure with the thumbs to acupoints along the meridians rather than inserting needles as in acupuncture.

adaptive skills Physical, emotional, and social abilities that permit an individual to function at an appropriate level in society.

advocacy Acting on behalf of an individual client or family by communicating needs to relevant persons or agencies or by serving as activist or policy planner for groups or populations by speaking, writing, or any other supportive action.

advocacy role Nursing role involving acting or speaking for someone who may be unable to act or speak for him- or herself.

advocate A person who speaks or acts for an individual or group of individuals who may be unable to speak for themselves.

aerobic conditioning Use of an exercise program planned to improve cardiorespiratory fitness; such a program requires a consistent supply of oxygen to the tissues over a sustained period of time. Conditioning requires steady, continuous movement, producing an increased, sustained heart rate equal to 60% to 85% of the person's maximum possible heart rate. Examples are vigorous walking, running, swimming, cycling, rowing, and cross-country skiing.

affective function A family function that provides affirmation, support, and respect for one another.

affirming Asserting or supporting the declarations of self or others.

ageism Any attitude or action constituting discrimination against an individual because of age.

agent A causative factor, such as a biological or chemical agent that must be present (or absent) in the environment for disease occurrence in a susceptible host.

aggregates Individuals, families, or other groupings who are associated because of similar social, personal, or health care needs; a defined group or population.

airborne transmission Microorganisms suspended in the air spread to a suitable port of entry.

alternative health care Therapies used in place of standard medical interventions (termed complementary health care when used in addition to standard medical interventions); considered to have insufficient documentation in the United States with regard to safety and effectiveness, are not generally taught in schools of medicine in the United States, and are not generally reimbursable for third-party payment (Office of Alternative Medicine, 1995)

amended Referring to a parliamentary or constitutional document (e.g., a bill), that is different from the original.

analytic epidemiologic studies Study designs that examine groups of individuals in order to make comparisons and associations and to determine causal relationships; also known as *cohort, cross-sectional,* and *case-control studies.*

andragogy Learning wherein the learner is actively involved in the learning process rather than a passive recipient of teaching.

anorexia nervosa A psychophysiological disorder, usually occurring in teenage women, characterized by an abnormal fear of becoming obese, a distorted self-image, a persistent aversion to food, and severe weight loss.

approach strategy Strategy used by an individual that signifies an effort to confront the challenges of a chronic illness.

assault A violent attack, either physical or verbal; an unlawful threat or unsuccessful attempt to do physical harm to another, causing a present fear of immediate harm.

assessment The systematic collection of data to assist in identifying the health status, assets, health needs and problems, and available resources of the community.

assets assessment Part of the planning process whereby health care professionals identify the resources and strengths of the client or community.

assimilated family style   A family acculturative style where there is full assimilation to the host culture.

association   The relationship between two or more events or variables.

assurance   The role of a public agency in ensuring that high-priority personal and community wide health services are available.

attack rate   The number of cases of disease in a specific population divided by the total population at risk for a limited time period, usually expressed as a percentage.

attention deficit/hyperactivity disorder   A neurobiologically based disability characterized by hyperactivity, impulsiveness, and inattentiveness.

attributable risk percentage (AR%)   A statistical measure that estimates the number of cases of a disease attributable to the exposure of interest.

author   The legislator who submits a bill in the legislative process.

autism   A behaviorally defined syndrome of neurological impairment of unknown etiology, characterized by severe impairment in development of reciprocal social interaction and communication and restricted interests and activities, with onset before age 3; a form of pervasive developmental disorder, also known as infantile autism, autistic disorder, or Kanner's syndrome.

autonomy   The principle of respect for persons that is based on the recognition of humans as unconditionally worthy agents, regardless of any special characteristics, conditions, or circumstances. Involves self-determination and the right to make choices for oneself.

B

basic research   Research designed to extend the base of knowledge in a discipline for the sake of knowledge production or theory construction, rather than for solving an immediate problem.

battered women   Women who are in physically and/or emotionally abusive relationships with their spouses or partners in which battering is ongoing.

batterer   One who beats or strikes another person.

beauty   The quality of being aesthetically pleasing to the senses; the harmonious experience of color, sound, form, order, fragrance, taste, and texture.

behavior modification   The changing of behavior by manipulating environmental stimuli.

beliefs   Ideas assumed and accepted as true on the basis of one's personal judgement.

beneficence   The ethical principle of doing or promoting good that requires abstention from injuring others and promotion of the legitimate interests of others primarily by preventing or avoiding possible harm.

best interest judgment   A proxy decision made on behalf of another based on what is thought to be in the best interest of the other in the circumstances and on what a reasonable person would decide in the given situation.

bias   An error in the study design caused by the tendency of researchers to expect certain conclusions on the basis of their own personal beliefs that results in incorrect conclusions regarding the association between potential risk factors and disease occurrence.

bioaccumulative   Accumulation over time of certain materials in the environment, due to inability to go through the natural process of decay; applies to products such as plastics.

biodiversity   The variety of life that now exists; vital to maintaining ecological balance.

biographical disruption   The change in people's self-image, relationships, and life plans that can accompany chronic illness.

biographical work   The work that a chronically ill person does to adjust to living with the impact of chronic illness on identity, body, and sense of time.

biological mother   A woman who gives birth to and raises her own children.

biometrics   The application of statistical methods to biological facts.

biopersistent   The quality of not decaying and continuing to exist for many years; usually applies to synthetic materials.

blended (or binuclear) family   The combination of two divorced families via remarriage.

blocker   Covert, informal family role used to meet the emotional needs of the individual whereby a member tends toward the negative regarding all ideas.

bonadaptation   Successful adaptation whereby the family is able to stabilize itself in a growth-producing way.

boundary   An abstract demarcation line composed of family rules that separates the focal system from its environment; may be more or less open.

bulimia nervosa   An eating disorder in which one alternates between abnormal craving for and aversion to food; characterized by episodes of excessive food intake followed by periods of fasting and self-induced vomiting or diarrhea.

C

cachexia   Weight loss, wasting of muscle, loss of appetite, general debility that can occur during a chronic disease.

capitation   A health insurance payment mechanism wherein a fixed amount is paid per person to cover health care services received or needed for a specific period of time.

caregiver   A person, usually a family member, who has the primary responsibility to care for at least one dependent member of the family.

caretaker   Covert informal family role used to meet the emotional needs of the individual and/or to maintain the family equilibrium whereby a member nurtures and cares for other members in need. May or may not have family permission to be a caretaker.

caring   Those assistive, enabling, supportive, or facilitative behaviors toward or for another individual or group to promote health, prevent disease, and facilitate healing.

carrier   A host that harbors an infectious agent without noticeable signs of disease or infection. The carrier state can exist while the host is healthy or during a specific time period in the natural history of the disease, when infection is not apparent. The carrier state can be of long or short duration.

case fatality rate   Deaths from a specific disease calculated by dividing the number of deaths from a specific disease in a given time period by the number of persons diagnosed with the disease.

case management   Coordinating and allocating services for clients to enhance continuity and appropriateness of care developed in response to client needs and problems.

case managers   Health care providers who serve as advocates for clients within the health care delivery system and coordinate their case.

case reports   Client (case) history studies used in epidemiologic descriptive studies.

case series   A compilation of case reports.

case-control study   An analytic epidemiologic study design that assembles study groups after a disease has occurred; also called a *retrospective study*.

cause-specific death rate   Number of deaths from a specific cause; expressed as a number per 100,000 population.

centering   Finding within one's self a sense of inner being that is quiet and at peace, a place where one feels integrated and focused.

Centers for Disease Control and Prevention (CDC)   An agency of the U.S. Department of Health and Human Services, whose mission is to promote health and quality of life by preventing and controlling disease, injury, and disability.

cerebral palsy   A group of disorders characterized by abnormal control of movement and posture, secondary to a static encephalopathy occurring prenatally, perinatally, or in early childhood.

chakras   Energy centers within the energy fields.

chaotic family   Crisis-prone family whose members rebound from one crisis to another.

chemical agents   Includes poisons and allergens.

child abuse   Physical or mental injury, sexual abuse or exploitation, negligent treatment, or maltreatment of a child by a person who is responsible for the child's welfare.

child neglect   The failure of a family to provide a child with basic needs of food, clothing, shelter, supervision, education, emotional affection, stimulation, or health care.

chronic disease   A long term physiological or psychological disorder.

chronic illness   A social phenomenon that accompanies a disease that cannot be cured and extends over a period of time.

circular questioning   Questions that are neutral, accepting, and exploratory and are used to expose patterns that connect persons, objects, actions, perceptions, ideas, feelings, events, beliefs, and context.

Circumplex Model of Marital and Family Systems   A map of types of marriages and family system attributes that mediate or buffer stressors and demands; illustrates the types of balanced and unbalanced relationships.

clarity   When verbal and nonverbal communication are congruent so that the message is clear to the receiver.

client cost sharing   Requirement that the client pay for a portion of the health care received.

client-centered   Client-focused; pertinent to all communication in helping relationships given the goal of client well-being.

clinical nurse specialist   An expert practitioner with graduate preparation in a nursing specialty.

closed questions   Questions that limit or restrict the client to provide only specific information; can usually be answered with one word or a short phrase; used to gather very specific information.

coalition   A collective that is characterized as a temporary alliance of diverse members who come together for joint action in support of a shared goal.

cognitive organization   The teacher's intellectual grasp of the material.

cohort study   An analytic epidemiologic study design that assembles study groups before disease occurrence to observe and compare the rates of a health outcome over time; also called a *prospective study*.

collaborate   To work with others to achieve common goals in a collegial manner.

collaborator   In interpreting, the interaction style wherein the interpreter and nurse function as colleagues and engage in interaction with the client as appropriate to the situation; one who works with others toward a common goal.

collective   A group that is brought together to pursue an agreed-upon goal, action, or set of actions.

communicable disease   A disease in a susceptible host that is caused by a potentially harmful infectious organism or its toxic products; spread by direct or indirect contact with an infectious agent (human, animal, or inanimate reservoir).

communication   The process of exchanging information through a common system of symbols, signs, and behaviors.

community   A group of people sharing common interests, needs, resources, and environment; an interrelating and interacting group of people with shared needs and interests.

community assessment   The process of critically examining the characteristics, resources, and needs of a community in collaboration with that community, in order to develop strategies to improve the health and quality of life of the community.

community capacity   The strengths, resources, and problem-solving abilities of a community.

community competence   The ability of a community to collaborate in identifying its problems and in effectively planning responses to those problems.

community health   Meeting collective needs by identifying problems and supporting community participation in the process within the community and society.

community health nurse generalist   The community health nurse prepared at the baccalaureate level. The focus of practice is individuals and families within a community context, with the primary responsibility being the population as a whole.

community health nurse specialist   The community health nurse prepared at the master's or doctoral level. Focus of practice for the master's-prepared nurse is the health of populations; the doctoral-prepared nurse focuses on population health, health policy, and research.

community health nursing   Synthesis of nursing and public health practice applied to promoting, protecting, and preserving the health of populations.

community of interest   A group of people who share values, beliefs, or interests on a particular issue.

community nursing centers   Nurse-managed settings established in underserved areas, where clients can receive monitoring, screening, treatment, and a variety of nursing services.

community organization   A multifaceted theoretical approach intended to create change at the community level; models include community development, social action, and social planning.

community participation   The active involvement of community members in assessing, planning, implementing, and evaluating health programs.

community partnership   The working relationship between the community health nurse or other health care professionals that involves participants from the community in the process of assessment, program planning, implementation, and evaluation. This process is opposed to one in which professionals carry out the process without input from the community at large.

comparative need   Need determined on the basis of comparison with another similar area, group, or person.

compassion   A quality of presence with another; an entering into the experience of the other; a sensitivity to pain and suffering of others.

complementary care therapies   Nonmedical interventions that people use in addition to standard medical care to promote health and healing.

compliance   A disposition or tendency to yield to others; submissiveness.

concept   An abstract version of the real world or of a concrete idea.

conflict   A difference between two or more persons when they hold seemingly incompatible ideas, interests, or values; can be spoken or unspoken.

conflict management   Efforts to work together while at the same time recognizing and accepting the conflicts inherent in the relationships involved.

conflict resolution   Methods to resolve conflicts by expressing concerns and differences of opinion until clarity and resolution are achieved.

consciousness   In the person–environment relationship, the organizing factor commonly experienced as awareness, thoughts, emotions, beliefs, and perceptions; the totality of thoughts, feelings, images, and impressions that shape our reality of person–environment processes.

consultant   One who provides clients with professional advice, services, or information to assist them in making informed decisions.

contact   A person who because of exposure to an infectious agent or environment has the potential for developing an infectious disease.

contacting phase   First phase of the home visit that includes the referral of the client (antecedent event), the preparation for the home visit, and the journey to the home; may be required or a request for service.

content-oriented groups   Those groups whose focus is to meet certain goals or to perform specific tasks.

contexts   The places or settings where community health nursing services are provided.

contextual family structure   The dimension of the family that includes ethnicity, race, social class, religion, and the environment.

contextual stimuli   In Roy's theory, all factors other than focal stimuli that contribute to adaptive behavior.

contextualism   Understanding the individual in the context of the family and the family in the context of the culture.

continuity   Connectedness of thought and coherence in the flow of language so that thought is easy to follow and understand; in community health nursing, the client's concerns are addressed through consistent interaction with the nurse.

continuum of care   Refers to the succession of services needed by the individual as he or she moves from one life stage to another.

contract   In the health care setting, a working agreement that is not legally binding between two or more parties; promotes self-care and facilitates a family focus on health needs.

conversational interview   Interview wherein clients tell their stories without interruption rather than answering questions from the nurse.

coordination   The efficient management and delivery of services without gaps and overlaps.

coordinator   Covert, informal family role, used to meet the emotional needs of the individual and/or to maintain the family equilibrium whereby a member organizes and plans family activities. May or may not have family permission to be coordinator.

co-payment   Cost-sharing arrangement whereby the person who is insured pays a specified charge.

coping   A strategy developed by people to enable them to live with chronic illness.

correctional health nursing   A branch of professional nursing that provides nursing services to clients in correctional facilities.

correlational study   A descriptive epidemiologic study design used to compare aggregate populations for potential exposures of disease.

cost analysis of health programs   An evaluation of the costs of a program in relation to health outcomes; requires consideration of the values and needs that gave rise to the program, the short- and long-term outcomes, and the human and material dimensions.

cost-plus reimbursement   Reimbursement based on what a service costs plus the addition of some percentage of profit.

counseling   Assisting clients in the use of problem-solving processes to decide on the course of action most appropriate for them.

crack   A freebase form of cocaine formed by mixing cocaine with baking soda and water and separating it from its hydrochloride base, making it usable for smoking.

crack babies   A term used to describe babies with physical problems and developmental delays secondary to the mother's prenatal use of cocaine.

created-environment   In the Neuman systems model, a protective, unconsciously derived environment that exists for all clients and acts as an intrapersonal protective shield against the reality of the environment.

creativity   The artistic and intellectual ability to produce new and original forms by bringing together in new ways elements already in existence.

critical thinking   Use of logic and analytical, intuitive and creative approaches to problem solving; involves looking at a situation from multiple perspectives; thoughtful and careful examination of beliefs, values, and action within the context of the whole picture of life; the educational process of the young adult learning to examine truth within the context of a breadth of knowledge.

cross-sectional survey   A descriptive epidemiologic study design that uses a representative sample of the population to collect information on current health status, personal characteristics, and potential risk factors or exposures at one point in time.

crystallized intelligence   Mental operation including skills acquired through education and acculturation.

cultural assessment   The collection, verification, and organization of data about the beliefs, values, and health care practices that clients share or have shared with others of the same culture.

cultural competence   The ability to communicate with people of various cultures, beliefs, and values to promote a positive outcome.

cultural diversity The great variety of cultural values, beliefs, and behavior; a term used to reflect appreciation for the richness of human experience in these areas.

cultural sensitivity Having the awareness and appreciation of cultural influences in health care and being respectful of differences in cultural belief systems and values.

cultural values Values that are desirable or preferred ways of acting or knowing something that over time are reinforced and sustained by the culture and ultimately govern one's action or decisions.

culture The values, beliefs, norms, and practices of a particular group that are learned and shared and that guide thought, decisions, and actions in a patterned way.

culture bound Being limited to one's own view of reality and, therefore, unable to accept or even consider the views of another culture.

cutting agents Substances added to street drugs to increase bulk (e.g., mannitol and starch), to mimic or enhance pharmacological effects (e.g., caffeine and lidocaine), or to combat side effects (e.g., vitamin C and dilantin).

D

date rape Rape by an individual the victim is dating.

decision making The process of "gaining the assent and commitment of family members to carry out a course of action or to maintain the status quo" (Friedman, 1992).

deep relaxation A state of relaxation wherein internal processes of mind and body are in balance and harmony, rendering the person's inner healing processes at their peak; usually intentionally induced and requiring practice.

degenerative disease Disease characterized by a breaking down of body tissues and organ systems, causing impeded performance and functioning.

deinstitutionalization The phenomenon of shifting the population experiencing major psychiatric disorders from large inpatient institutions into community-based care.

demand Buyers' willingness to purchase a particular product or service.

demography The statistical science or study of populations, related to age-specific categories, birth and death rates, marital status, and ethnicity.

deontology The ethical theory according to which actions are inherently right or wrong independent of the consequences; based on the morality of the action itself.

depressants An agent that depresses a body function or nerve activity.

descriptive epidemiologic studies Epidemiologic study designs that contribute to the description of a disease or condition by examining the essential features of person, place, and time.

designer drugs Analogues of known drugs created for their psychoactive properties.

determinants of health Factors that influence the risk for health outcomes.

detoxification The process of removing toxins from the body.

developmental approach to care A method of encouraging development and skill acquisition based on present developmental level rather than chronological age.

developmental assessment Observation and assessment of a child's skills in physical, social, and mental domains compared with established age-related norms.

developmental assessment tools Tools used by nurses and other care providers to assess developmental progress of children; observation and interviewing are used and the results recorded; the resulting record provides a measure of how the child is developing in different areas and serves as a tool that can be used in teaching parents how to determine potential readiness.

developmental disability A severe, chronic condition attributable to mental or physical impairment, or both, manifested before age 22 and likely to continue indefinitely, resulting in substantial limitations in three or more areas, including self-care, receptive and expressive language, and learning, and requiring a combination and sequence of special, interdisciplinary, or generic care, treatment, or other services, individually planned and coordinated, required for an extended period or throughout life.

developmental model of services Programs of care and instruction designed to promote skill acquisition to the highest level possible, regardless of age or severity of handicap.

developmental tasks The work that each family must complete at each stage of development before movement to the next stage is possible.

developmental theory Theory that families evolve through typical developmental stages during the life cycle; each stage is characterized by specific issues and tasks; also called the *life cycle approach*.

diagnosis-related group (DRG) System of classification for cost of inpatient services based on diagnosis, age, sex, and presence of complications.

differentiation A living system's capability to advance to a higher order of complexity and organization.

dimensions of environment The nature of and relationship among the various aspects of environment within the whole.

direct transmission Immediate transfer of disease from infected host to susceptible host.

directive approach The nurse defines the nature of the client's problem, prescribes appropriate solutions, and provides specific, concrete information needed for problem solving.

disability-adjusted life year (DALY) An internationally standardized measure that expresses years of life lost to premature death and years lived with a disability of specified severity and duration.

disease frequency Occurrence of disease as measured by various rates such as morbidity rate.

disease prevention Those activities or actions that seek to protect clients from potential or actual health threats and related harmful consequences.

disengaged family Family that is distanced or totally cut off from family relationships.

domestic violence A broad term encompassing a spectrum of violence within a family. It may (and usually does) refer to a husband battering his wife but more broadly addresses any intrafamilial violence such as elder or child abuse.

dominator Covert, informal family role, used to meet the emotional needs of the individual whereby a member tries to assert authority or superiority by manipulating the family or certain members of the family.

Down syndrome Condition of extra chromosome material on chromosome 21 or 22 with associated mental retardation and other conditions such as dysmorphic features and heart disease.

downstream thinking A microscopic focus that by nature is characterized primarily by short-term individual-based interventions.

dyscalculia Poor ability to learn or use mathematics.

dyslexia Poor ability to learn or work with visual symbols.

E

early intervention Services to infants and young children and their families designed to promote health, development, and family functioning. Services are interdisciplinary and individually designed.

ecological approach Incorporation of developmental, systems, and situational perspectives to understand the family within the multiperson environmental system within which the family is enmeshed; encompasses the following subsystems, the totality of which makes up the ecosystem: microsystem, mesosystem, exosystem, and macrosystem.

ecological balance The complex relationships among living things and between a specific organism and its environment.

ecological system The interrelationship between living things and their environment.

ecology The study of relations and interactions among all organisms within the total environment; in community health, the individual's interaction with his or her social, cultural, and physical environments.

ecomap A visual overview of the complex ecological system of the family, showing the family's organizational patterns and relationships.

economic function Maintenance of economic survival in society.

economic policy Course of action intended to influence or control the behavior of an economy.

economics Social science concerned with the ways that society allocates scarce resources (commonly known as goods and services) in the most cost-efficient way.

ecosystem The relationships and interactions among all subsystems including microsystem, mesosystem, exosystem, and macrosystem.

ecotoxicity Contamination of the planet with toxic chemicals that poison and have genetic, hormonal, immunological, and psychological consequences.

educator role Nursing roles that involve assisting others to gain knowledge, skills, or characteristics needed for living a healthy life.

ego One of Freud's three main theoretical elements (with id and superego) of the mental mechanism; its function is to mediate between the demands of the other two, serving as compromiser, adapter, and executor.

ego integrity versus despair Erikson's final conflict of development wherein the adult must accept his life as inevitable or, in failing this task, feel futility and hopelessness.

elder abuse A form of violence against older adults; may include physical abuse, neglect, intimidation, cruel punishment, financial abuse, abandonment, isolation, or other treatment resulting in physical harm or mental suffering; the deprivation by a custodian of goods or services necessary to avoid physical harm or mental suffering.

emerging diseases New, reemerging, or drug-resistant infections whose incidence in humans has increased within the past two decades or whose incidence threatens to increase in the near future (National Center for Infectious Diseases, 1996).

emotional abuse Verbal or behavioral actions that diminish another's self-worth and self-esteem so that he or she feels uncared for, inept, and worthless.

empathy The ability to understand the subjective world of another and then to communicate that understanding.

employee assistance programs (EAPs) Company-provided programs such as counseling, chemical rehabilitation, or stress management that are helpful in supporting workers' attempts at maintaining or restoring productivity.

empowerment The process whereby individuals feel increasingly in control of their own affairs.

empowerment education A particular approach to community education that is based on Freire's ideas and makes use of active learning methods to engage clients in determining their own needs and priorities.

empty nest syndrome Parents' response to children's leaving home, leaving the parents as a couple again.

enculturation The process of acquiring knowledge and internalizing values and attitudes about a culture.

endemic The constant presence of an infectious agent or disease within a defined geographic area.

energy In the Neuman Systems Model, an innately or genetically acquired primary and basic power resource for the client as a system; a resource for system empowerment toward achievement of the highest level of wellness; the force needed to meet the demands for system integrity.

energy field The whole of a person's being as reflected in one's presence via observation, sensation, or intuition.

enmeshed family Family in which individual needs are sacrificed for the group.

enthusiasm Teaching behavior characterized by interest in and excitement about the subject being taught.

entropy Tending toward maximum disorder and disintegration; occurs when a system is either too open or too closed, causing family dysfunction.

entry phase The second phase of the home visit; the nurse enters the home, begins to develop a plan with the client or family, and performs other activities as needed.

environment Internal and external factors that constitute the context for agent-host interactions; the aspect of existence perceived outside the self; this perception changes with alterations in awareness and expansion of consciousness; one of the concepts of nursing metaparadigm.

environmental hazards Those aspects of the environment that present real or potential danger to the human being, usually categorized as chemical, physical, mechanical, or psychosocial.

environmental health The study and prevention of environmental problems, especially those created by pollution; problems that may influence health and well-being of people.

epidemic A number of cases of an infectious agent or disease (outbreak) clearly in excess of the normally expected frequency of that disease in that population.

epidemiology An applied science that studies the distribution and determinants of health-related states or events in populations.

epilepsy A condition characterized by repeated abnormal electrical discharges from neurons in the cortex of the brain resulting in loss of consciousness, behavior changes, involuntary movements, altered muscle tone, or abnormal sensory phenomena.

epistemologic Pertaining to the nature and foundations of knowledge.

equifinality The quality of there being a characteristic final state regardless of initial state. For instance, people tend to develop habitual ways of behaving and communicating so that whatever the topic, their way of dealing with it will be the same.

equilibrium Self-regulation, or adaptation that results from a dynamic balance or steady state.

equipotentiality The quality of different end states being possible from the same initial conditions.

equity in health care The goal of equal access to medical or illness care, but may also refer to equal access to health and wellness care, education, a clean and caring environment, and the opportunity to fulfill one's life potential.

era A period or stage of development in Levinson's theory of development, which is divided into early adulthood, middle adulthood, and late adulthood.

eradication Via the extermination of infectious agents, irreversible termination of the ability to transmit infection after the successful global eradication of infection.

ergonomics The study of the relationship between individuals and their work or working environment, especially with regard to fitting jobs to the needs and abilities of workers.

ethics The study of the nature and justification of principles that guide human behaviors and are applied to special areas in which moral problems arise.

ethnicity A group whose members share a common social and cultural heritage passed on to successive generations, such that members feel a bond or sense of identity with one another.

ethnocentrism The belief that one's own lifeway is the "right" way or is at least better than another.

ethnomedicine Study of traditional healing systems within the field of medical anthropology.

ethno-nursing research A qualitative method of research developed by Madeleine Leininger for the collection and study of descriptive data regarding people, their worldview, ideas, and cultural practices related to the nursing phenomena of caring, health, and well-being within the environmental contexts of experience.

eudaemonistic A philosophy of health whereby the goal is full realization and actualization of one's intrinsic potential as a human being.

excluder In interpreting, the interaction style wherein the interpreter takes over the provider–client interaction, excluding the nurse from the conversation; explanations given to the nurse regarding those things that transpired during the interaction after the completion of the interaction.

existentialism A philosophical movement that proposes that humans are totally free and responsible for their acts and that this responsibility in itself constitutes the source of suffering in human existence.

exosystem The major institutions of the society.

expressed need Demand for services demonstrated by action: for example, putting a name on a waiting list.

expressive function The affective dimension of the family.

extended family Traditionally, those members of the nuclear family and other blood-related persons, usually the family of origin (grandparents, aunts, uncles, cousins), called "kin"; more recently, people who identify themselves as "family" but are not necessarily related by blood or through adoption.

external family structure The dimension of the family structure that includes extended family and the larger systems of the community.

F

failure to thrive (FTT) Lack of adequate growth in the absence of an organic defect during the first year of life; those infants falling below the 3rd percentile on growth charts are evaluated for either insufficient contact with the mother or lack of stimulation.

false-negative test A screening test result that is negative when the individual actually has the disease of interest.

false-positive test A screening test result that is positive when the individual does not have the disease of interest.

family A social context of two or more people characterized by mutual attachment, caring, long-term commitment, and responsibility to provide individual growth, supportive relationships, health of members and of the unit, and maintenance of the organization and system during constant individual, family, and societal change (Craft & Willadsen, 1992, p. 519).

family acculturative styles Ways in which the family can be understood as a cultural system; include the integrated bicultural, marginalized, traditional-oriented, nonresistive, assimilated, and separatist family styles.

family assessment The systematic collection and analysis of family data for the purpose of identifying the family's health-related strengths or problems.

family-centered nursing practice Set of principles that helps the nurse address the important health issues of families and individual family members; views the family as the basic unit of care.

family as client The family considered as a set of interacting parts; assessment of the dynamics among these parts renders the whole family the client.

family cohesion Emotional bonding among family members.

family communication Transactional process whereby meanings are created and shared with others; in the Circumplex Model, considered a facilitating dimension.

family as context The family considered as the context within which individuals are assessed; emphasis is placed primarily on the individual, keeping in mind that she or he is part of a larger system.

family flexibility Amount of change in the family's leadership, role relationships, and relationship rules.

family functions The ways that families meet the needs of individuals and purposes of the broader society.

family health tree A genogram that includes the family health history.

family interactional theories Those theories that focus on the ways that family members relate to the family and on internal family dynamics.

family myths Longstanding family beliefs that shape family members' interactions with one another and with the outside world; unchallenged by family members, who distort their perceptions if necessary to keep the myths secure.

family networks   Patterns of communication that families develop in order to deal with the needs of family living, specifically needs of regulating time and space, sharing resources, and organizing activities.

family of origin (or orientation)   The family unit into which a person is born.

family process function   Interactions between family members whereby they accomplish their instrumental and expressive tasks.

family of procreation   The family created for the purpose of raising children.

family roles   Repetitive patterns of behavior by which family members fulfill family functions.

family strengths   Characteristics that contribute to family unity and solidarity in order to manage the family's life successfully and to foster health and healing.

family structure   Refers to the role structure, value systems, communication processes, and power structure.

family systems theories   Those theories that emerge from sociology and psychology and are related to general systems theory, structural-functional approaches, and developmental theory but tend to focus on ways to change "dysfunctional" families.

family values   Principles, standards, or qualities that family members believe to be worthwhile and hold dear.

fecal/oral transmission   Transmission of an infectious agent directly via the hands or other objects that are contaminated with an infectious organism from human or animal feces and then placed in the mouth.

feedback   The process of providing a circular information loop so that the system can receive and respond to its own output. A self-corrective process whereby the system adjusts both internally and externally. Feedback can be negative or positive. Positive feedback refers to input that is returned to the system as information that moves the system toward change. Negative feedback promotes equilibrium and stability, not change.

fee-for-service   Method of paying health care providers for service or treatment, wherein a provider bills for each client encounter or service rendered and identified by a claim for payment.

feelings reflection   A statement on the part of the listener that reflects feelings expressed by the speaker as heard by the listener.

felt need   Those needs which people say they need.

fetal alcohol syndrome   A pattern of anomalies occurring in infants born to mothers who abused alcohol during pregnancy.

fidelity   The principle of promise keeping; the duty to keep one's promise or word.

finance controls   Cost-control strategy that attempts to limit the flow of funds into public or private health care insurance plans.

financing   Amount of dollars that flow from payors to an insurance plan, either private or governmental.

first-order change   Change in the degree of family functioning but not in the family system.

flow and transformation   The process whereby input travels through the system in its original state or transformed so that the system can use it.

fluid intelligence   Mental functioning that reflects relational thinking and the capability of thinking independently of culturally based content.

focal stimuli   In Roy's theory, factors that precipitate an adaptive response.

focal system   The particular system under study.

folk health system   The cultural health care practices used by people in addition to or in place of those used in the professional health care system.

food-borne illness   An illness resulting from food contaminated with infectious microorganisms.

formal roles   Roles explicitly assigned to family members as needed to keep the family functioning.

formal teaching   Prearranged, planned teaching.

formative program evaluation   An ongoing evaluation that provides information regarding program performance "along the way"; permits improvements while programming is happening.

fragile X syndrome   A condition of mutation of the X chromosome with associated mental retardation; expression of the condition differs in males and females.

freebase   A homemade refining process by which cocaine hydrochloride (HCl) is chemically "freed" from its HCl base to form a less stable but more potent drug.

frontier area   An area that has fewer than 6 or 7 persons per square mile.

G

general systems theory   The theory that the whole of any system is more than the sum of its parts, such that the whole can be understood only by study of the entire system in all its aspects; theory that describes the ways that units interact with larger and smaller units; used to explain the way that the family interacts with its members and with society.

generation gap   conflict between parents and adolescents.

generativity versus stagnation   Erikson's middle adult conflict wherein one seeks productivity as opposed to self-indulgence that leads to personal impoverishment.

genogram   A graph outlining a family's history over a period of time, usually over three generations.

geophagia   Also known as pica; a craving for nonfood substances such as clay or earth.

global budgeting   A strategy aimed at controlling health care spending by controlling the product of price and value.

global burden of disease (GBD)   A method of measurement of health status in a population that quantifies not only the number of deaths but also the impact of premature death and disability on a population.

go-between   Covert, informal family role, used to meet the emotional needs of the individual whereby a member transmits and monitors communication throughout the family.

gross domestic product (GDP)   All the goods and services produced for domestic use by a nation in one year.

growth   Increase in body size or changes in structure, function, and complexity of body cell content and metabolic and biochemical processes up to the point of maturity.

guest   A homeless person being housed temporarily in a hotel, shelter, boarding house, or the like.

guided imagery   An imaging process wherein the guide tells the person or group of persons what to imagine and how to progress through the exercise, leaving the individuals to respond silently in their own ways; used to facilitate inner healing processes.

H

harmonizer Covert, informal role used to meet the emotional needs of the individual member by mediating the differences that exist between other members.

hate crimes Acts of violence perpetrated against another because of that person's race, religion, culture, or sexual preference.

healing The natural and inner process of moving toward realization of one's full potential as a human being by letting go, accepting oneself, and experiencing transformation; the restoration of health, harmony, and well-being to the body, mind, spirit, and environment.

healing environment An environmental state that supports natural healing processes of the person and is characterized by caring, safety, nurturance, order, and beauty.

healing practices Practices intended to facilitate integration of one's whole self and relationships.

health Within the person–environment process, a state of well-being that is dependent on the nature of relationships within the system; one of the concepts of nursing's metaparadigm.

Health for All A movement initiated by the World Health Organization to improve health worldwide by reducing inequities that negatively affect health; strategies include primary health care and health promotion.

health balance The state of well-being resulting from the harmonious interaction of body, mind, spirit, and environment.

health behavior Those behaviors exhibited by persons that affect their health either constructively or destructively; may be consciously selected, although unconscious needs may thwart the person's ability to carry out conscious intentions.

health care function The provision of physical necessities to keep the family healthy; health care and health practices that influence the family's health status.

health care networks Systems of health care within communities that provide comprehensive care, including activities for disease prevention and health promotion as well as care for sickness.

health care policy Those public policies related to health and health services; actions taken by a government concerning health.

health communication Communication that centers on health-related issues of individuals and groups, encompassing feelings and attitudes as well as information.

health determinant A factor that helps to either create or diminish health.

health education Learning experiences designed to facilitate self-awareness, provide information, and support change through the teaching process for the purpose of promoting health.

health maintenance organization (HMO) A health care organization formed within certain areas that emphasize prevention, wellness, and coordination of primary care in an effort to decrease utilization of high-cost, high-tech, acute care services; an organization or set of related entities organized for the purpose of providing health benefits to an enrolled population for a predetermined fixed periodic amount to be paid by the purchaser (e.g., government, employer, individual). There are four general models of HMOs: staff, medical groups, independent practice associations, and networks.

health ministries Health care settings in which the clients or consumers, clergy, and health care professionals work together to preserve and promote the health of people within faith communities.

health potential The ability to cope with environmental changes.

health promotion Activities or interventions that identify the risk factors related to disease; the lifestyle changes related to disease prevention; the process of enabling individuals and communities to increase their control over and improve their health; these activities or strategies are directed toward developing the resources of clients to maintain or enhance their physical, social, emotional and spiritual well-being.

health-promotion model A model that depicts the multidimensional nature of people interacting with their environments in their pursuit of health.

health protection Those activities designed to maintain the current level of health, actively prevent disease, detect disease early, thwart disease processes, or maintain functioning within the constraints of disease.

health risk A precursor whose presence is associated with morbidity and/or mortality.

health risk communication Informing people about environmental health hazards and health risks.

helicy In Rogerian theory of the person–environment relationship the unpredictablity, diversity, and innovation of human and environmental field patterns.

hierarchy of systems The level of influence of one system with respect to another. The closer the supra- or subsystem to the focal system, the greater the influence.

holism The belief that living beings are interacting wholes who are more than the mere sum of their parts.

holistic healing therapies Based on the belief in the unity of body, mind, and soul and on ethnomedicine.

holistic health Integration of the whole being and implies feelings of well-being, positive attitudes, a sense of purpose, and spiritual development.

holistic medicine Views illness as an opportunity for learning, personal growth, and transformation.

holistic worldview The perception that everything in the universe is interconnected and that everything affects everything else.

home health nursing Skilled nursing and other related services provided to individuals and families in their places of residence for the purpose of promoting, maintaining, or restoring health.

homelessness Residing with relatives, living on the streets, or living in shelters during difficult times.

homeopathy A system of medical treatment based on the theory of treating certain diseases with very small doses of drugs that, in a healthy person in large doses, would produce symptoms like those of the disease.

homogeneity A situation in which all persons from a particular ethnic group or culture share the same beliefs, values, and behaviors.

homogenize The process of viewing members of any aggregate as similar and having no diversity of capability, personal style, economic status, or lifestyle preference.

horizontal transmission Transfer of disease or antibodies from person to person.

hospice A coordinated program of supportive, palliative services for terminally ill clients and their families.

host A person or living species capable of being infected.

house of origin The part of the legislature (Senate, House, Assembly) to which a bill is first introduced by its author; the author's house.

human aggregate dimension That aspect of environment comprising the set of characteristics that apply to the group of persons within the environment.

human development The patterned, orderly, lifelong changes in structure, thought, and behavior that evolve as a result of physical and mental capacity, experiences, and learning; the result of an integration of environmental, cultural, and psychological forces within the human being.

human diversity The myriad differences reflected in and among human beings and the human experience.

human field patterns In Roger's theory, irreducible, indivisible, multidimensional energy field patterns manifested by characteristics of the whole.

human responses The various ways human beings respond to environment; a significant aspect for assessment in the person–environment interrelationship.

I

id One of Freud's three main theoretical elements (with ego and superego) of the mental mechanism; the part of personality design that contains the unconscious and instinct.

idiopathic failure to thrive Lack of adequate growth wherein the infant falls below the 3rd percentile of growth, in the face of adequate parenting skills, good maternal-child attachment, and no apparent organic cause for the lack of growth.

imagery A quasi-perceptual event of which we are self-consciously aware and that exists in the absence of stimuli that produce genuine sensory or perceptual counterparts; a mental representation of reality, or fantasy; encompasses all five modes of perception (visual, auditory, kinesthetic, olfactory, and gustatory).

immunity An acquired resistance to specific diseases.

impact evaluation The determination of the immediate effects of a program and whether these effects are those that were intended; a form of outcome evaluation.

incest The crime of sexual relations between persons related by blood, especially between parents and children or brother and sister.

incidence The frequency of new cases of a health outcome in a specified population during a given time period.

incidence rate The rate of new cases of a condition or disease in a population in a specified time period; provides an estimate of the condition/disease risk in that population.

inclusion Requiring children with disabilities to have the most contact possible with children who do not have disabilities.

indemnity insurance Insurance benefits provided in cash that utilizes a payment method to the beneficiary rather than in services (service benefits); fee-for-service.

independent practice association model HMO Physicians providing care are organized into professional corporations or other legal entities that contract with the HMO; physicians maintain their own practices in their own offices.

indirect transmission Transfer of a disease by way of human host having contact with vehicles that support and transport the infectious agent.

indirectedness Teaching behavior whereby the teacher guides students to find their own way.

industrial hygiene That science and art devoted to the anticipation, recognition, evaluation, and control of those environmental factors or stresses in or from the workplace that may cause sickness, impaired health and well-being, or significant discomfort and inefficiency among workers or among citizens of the community.

infant mortality rate The number of deaths of infants under 1 year of age in a year divided by the number of live births in the same year per 1,000 live births; a measure of community and national health status.

infectious agents Bacteria, fungi, viruses, metazoa, and protozoa.

infectious disease A disease of human or animal caused by the entry and development of an infectious agent in the body.

inflation Rise in the general level of prices; an increase in the amount of money in circulation, resulting in a sudden fall in the value of money and an increase in prices.

informal roles Covert roles that meet the emotional needs of the individual and/or maintain the family equilibrium.

informal teaching Spontaneous teaching that takes advantage of a teachable moment without prior planning.

information gathering Using communication skills to obtain the information necessary to carry out the nursing process on behalf of the client.

information-sharing interviews Discussions centering on the request for and provision of information, with the focus being on content rather than on relationship or feelings.

inhalant substance A volatile substance purposely inhaled to produce intoxication.

inner aspect of aging One's relationship to oneself and contentment with aging.

input Energy, matter, and information that the system must receive and process in order to survive.

insider's perspective A person's lived experience.

instrumental function The activities that assist individuals in the management of their lives, such as cooking, housekeeping, paying bills, shopping, and doing laundry (activities of daily living).

integrality A principle of homeodynamics in the Rogerian Science of Unitary Human Beings; the continuous, mutual human field and environmental field process inherent in nature.

integrated bicultural family style A family acculturative style in which the elements of both cultures are integrated, resulting in a balanced acceptance of two or more cultures.

integrated health care system A network and linkages of services that enhance continuity of care.

integrative models of health Those models that address a broad range of biological, emotional, mental, social, and spiritual factors.

intentional injuries Injuries occurring secondary to intentional acts of violence.

interactive guided imagery A process wherein the nurse or health professional serves as a guide for the imagery process but stays in dialogue with the client while the client describes the inner experience and wherein the suggestions made by the guide depend on the client's responses.

interdisciplinary services Diagnostic, developmental, educational, or other services provided by members of different disciplines functioning as a team.

intergovernmental organizations Those organizations that deal with health concerns on an ongoing basis and collaborate with national governments, private foundations, and other efforts to improve health: e.g., the World Health Organization.

intermediate care facility Nursing home providing 24-hour care and supervision with restorative, supportive and preventive services. The degree of care is less than provided by a hospital or a skilled nursing facility but more than that provided in a small-group residence.

internal dimension That aspect of environment commonly referred to as aspects of the person; physical body composition, biochemistry, genetics, attitudes, beliefs, and life experience.

internal family structure The dimension of family structure that includes family composition, gender, rank order, subsystems, and boundaries.

International Council of Nurses (ICN) An international organization that represents 112 national nursing organizations as members, with as many as 1 million nurses; it is the primary organization to promote the advancement of nurses.

interpenetrating processes The theory that nothing is whole in itself and that everything exists throughout the whole of everything else.

interpersonal systems Those systems or patterns that involve more than one person in an exchange of energy, such as in communication.

intersectoral collaboration Coordinated action by sectors of a community from governmental officials to grassroots community organizations to plan and implement health care strategies.

intersectoral partnerships Working relationships between different sectors of the community or of society, such as education, business, and government.

intervention study Epidemiologic study design that is experimental in nature and used to test a hypothesis about a cause-and-effect relationship.

intimacy versus isolation Erikson's task of young adults whereby the individual develops close relationships with others or suffers loneliness and isolation.

intrafamilial violence Violence occurring within the family, between family members.

intrapersonal systems Those aspects of ourselves that we experience within ourselves, such as thoughts, beliefs, feelings, and attitudes; significant for both the nurse and client because they influence the nature of our relationships as well as our behavior.

investigator role The investigative role of the nurse involved in assessment of the environment and in data gathering; formulating a nursing diagnosis related to the community environment is inherent in the role.

ionizing radiation Radiation resulting from energy transferred through electromagnetic waves or subatomic particles; causes a variety of health effects as it passes through human tissue.

J

Jin Shin Jyutsu (JSJ) Developed and taught by Burmeister, a touch therapy similar in nature to acupressure wherein the nurse or provider holds "safety energy locks" along flows of energy to balance and harmonize the human energy field.

justice The principle of fairness that is served when an individual is given that which he or she is due, owed, deserves, or can legitimately claim.

K

killed A slang expression referring to a bill's defeat.

L

lacto-ovovegan diet A vegetarian diet that includes both dairy products and eggs.

lactovegan diet A vegetarian diet that includes dairy products but no eggs.

learned helplessness Decreasing motivation to respond to abusive treatment secondary to chronic feelings of helplessness and inability to control certain outcomes.

learning The process of gaining knowledge, skills, or understanding.

learning disability A generic term referring to a heterogeneous group of disorders characterized by significant difficulties in acquisition and use of listening, speaking, reading, writing, reasoning, or mathematical abilities.

learning need The gap between the information an individual knows and the information the individual needs in order to perform a function or to care for oneself.

learning process A process involving the whole person and reflected in a change of behavior; involves cognitive, affective, and psychomotor components.

legitimate power The shared agreement among family members to designate a person to be the leader and to make the decisions.

levels of prevention A three-level model of intervention (primary, secondary, tertiary) used in the epidemiologic approach, designed to prevent or to halt or reverse the process of pathological change as early as possible in order to prevent damage.

lobby The act of influencing legislators to take certain positions on prospective bills or issues.

locus of control The perception regarding source of control in one's life; internal locus of control is the perception that the person is in control, whereas external locus of control is the perception that outside influences are in control.

lose–win approach A destructive approach to conflict resolution whereby, regardless of his or her own needs, one person gives in to another person by being nonassertive and nonresponsible.

low birth weight (LBW) Neonate weight of less than 2,500 grams resulting from prematurity or being small for gestational age.

M

macroeconomics Subscience focusing on the aggregate performance of all markets in a market system and on the choices made by that large market system.

macrosystem The institutional patterns of the culture.

mainstreaming The philosophy and activities associated with providing services to persons with disabilities in community settings, especially in school programs, to promote their fullest participation with those who have no disabilities.

maladaptation Unsuccessful adaptation wherein the results are a more chaotic state, sacrificed family growth and development, and markedly lowered overall sense of well-being, trust, and sense of order and coherence in the family.

male climacteric A feeling of anxiety over signs of aging in late-middle-aged men.

managed care   A health service payment or delivery arrangement wherein the health plan attempts to control or coordinate use of services by its enrolled members in order to contain expenditures, improve quality, or both; arrangements usually involve a defined delivery system with providers who have some form of contractual arrangement with the plan.

managed care organization   An entity that integrates financing and management and the delivery of health care services to an enrolled population.

managed competition   An approach to health system reform wherein health plans compete to provide health insurance coverage for enrollees; relies on market incentives (namely more subscribers and revenue) to encourage health care plans to keep down the cost of care; typically, enrollees sign up with a purchasing entity that purchases the services of competing health plans, offering enrollees a choice of the contracting health plans; purchasing strategy aimed at obtaining maximum value for employers and consumers; rewards suppliers who do the most efficient job of providing health care services that improve quality, cut costs, and satisfy customers.

marginalized family style   A family acculturative style in which there is loss of identity with both the traditional culture and the majority culture.

market system   Mechanism whereby society allocates scarce resources.

martyr   Covert, informal family role used to meet the emotional needs of the individual whereby a member sacrifices his or her own needs for the sake of the other family members.

maternal mortality rate   Deaths of mothers at time of birth, expressed as a number per 100,000 live births.

maturation   The emergence of genetic potential for changes in form, structure, complexity, integration, organization, and function, both physically and mentally.

maturity   A state of complete growth or development that promotes physical and psychological well-being.

McMaster Model of Family Functioning   Describes a set of positive characteristics of a healthy family; focuses on the following six dimensions: problem solving, communication, role function, affective responsiveness, affective involvement, and behavior control.

meal site   A place where meals are offered to a specific population such as the elderly or women, or usually at a greatly reduced cost.

meanings reflection   A statement by the listener that reflects meanings and facts apparent in something expressed by the speaker, allowing for further exploration and clarification.

measures of association   Statistical analysis methods used to investigate the relationship between two or more variables or events.

mechanistic view   The perspective that the universe is made up of separate parts and together these parts create the whole.

Medicaid   A health program that is funded by federal and state taxes and pays for the health care of low-income persons.

medical assistive device   An appliance that replaces or augments inadequate body functions necessary to sustain life.

medical group model HMO   Physicians providing care in large multispecialty or primary care medical groups, who contract with the HMO and usually draw the majority of their income from the HMO subscribers; the HMO typically contracts with hospitals as needed but can own hospitals.

Medicare Part A   Government-run hospital insurance plan that helps pay for hospital, home health, skilled nursing facility, and hospice care for elderly and some disabled persons; financed primarily by payroll taxes paid by workers and employers.

Medicare Part B   Government-run insurance plan that pays for physician, outpatient hospital, and other services for the aged and disabled; financed primarily by transfers from the general fund (tax revenues) of the U.S. Treasury and by monthly premiums paid by beneficiaries.

menopause   Cessation of menstruation, or female climacteric.

Mental Hygiene Movement   Founded in 1909, later renamed the Mental Health Association, it is the leading voluntary citizens organization in mental health. It emphasizes education and public awareness techniques to promote prevention and effective treatment.

mental retardation   Significantly subaverage intellectual functioning existing with related limitations in adaptive skills such as communication, self-direction, self-care, social skills, health, academics, or work, with onset before age 18.

mesosystem   The interrelationships of the major settings of a person's life.

metropolitan area (MA)   An area containing core counties with one or more central cities of at least 50,000 residents or with a Census Bureau–defined urban area (a total metro area population of 100,000 or more).

microeconomics   Subscience focusing on the individual markets that make up the market systems and on the choices made by small economic units such as individual consumers and individual firms.

microsystem   The immediate setting within which a person fulfills his or her roles.

midlife crisis   The period of middle adulthood when the individual confronts his or her aging process.

midrange groups   Those groups that focus on both content or tasks and process.

migrant farm worker   A person employed in agricultural work of a seasonal or other temporary nature who is required to be absent overnight from his or her permanent place of residence.

minority   The label applied to race, ethnicity, religion, occupation, gender, or sexual orientation; implies less in number than the general population or having characteristics perceived as undesirable by those in power.

mode of transmission   The mechanism by which an infectious agent is transferred from an infected host to an uninfected host.

model   A representation of reality.

moral agency   The ability to act according to moral standards.

moral obligation   Duty to act in a particular way in response to ethical and moral norms.

morbidity rate   A disease rate, specifically prevalence and incidence rates of diseases in a population in a specified time period.

morphogenesis   A natural tendency of a normal social organization to grow.

morphostasis   A balance between stability and a tendency to grow.

mortality rate   The number of deaths from all causes divided by the total population at a particular time and place.

multicultural   A population made up of people from many and diverse cultures.

multidisciplinary   The combination or working together of many different professional disciplines or branches of learning.

multidisciplinary team   A group of health care professionals from diverse fields who work in a coordinated fashion toward a common goal.

mutation   An anomaly in the genetic makeup of an organism; responsible for antibiotic resistance.

N

natural history of a disease   The course that a disease would take from onset to resolution without intervention by humans.

natural immunity   Immunity conferred when the host acquires an infection and develops antibodies that protect against subsequent infection.

needle and syringe exchange programs   Programs in which intravenous drug users can exchange used needles and syringes for new ones; developed to help prevent the spread of HIV/AIDS.

needs assessment   The systematic appraisal of the type, depth, and nature of health needs and problems as perceived by clients, health providers, or both, in a given community.

negentropy   Tending toward maximum order; appropriate balance between openness and closedness is maintained.

network model HMO   Large, multispecialty physician group practices that serve clients from a number of sources and that contract with an HMO.

network therapy   An approach directed toward changing a family network that is reinforcing a dysfunctional stalemate.

neurotransmitter   Nervous system chemicals that facilitate the transmission of impulses across the synapses between neurons.

newborn screening   State programs providing blood tests on newborns to detect treatable conditions such as phenylketonuria, hypothyroidism, and galactosemia.

noncompliance   Failure to yield or obey. A term often used in a negative way to describe a client's failure to follow the treatment regimen prescribed by health care professionals.

nondirective approach   By asking open questions, the nurse encourages the client to seek solutions to his or her own problems and to express thoughts and feelings.

nonlegitimate power   Characterized by domination or exploitation that suggests power against another's will.

nonmaleficence   The principle of doing no harm.

nonmetropolitan areas   Areas outside the boundaries of metropolitan areas that do not have a city of at least 50,000 residents.

non-organic failure to thrive (NFTT)   Lack of adequate growth wherein the infant falls below the 3rd percentile on the growth charts and there is no physical cause for the lack of growth; usually accompanies inadequate parenting skills or lack of parental attachment to the child.

nonverbal behaviors   Those behaviors that communicate attitudes, meaning, or content to another, either intentionally or unintentionally, through gestures or other body language.

normalization   A principle of service to people with disabilities, particularly mental retardation, that requires culturally appropriate methods and services to be provided in culturally appropriate settings so the individual may participate in community life as fully as possible.

normalizing   A coping strategy used by people to control the impact of chronic illness on their lives.

normative need   Need identified as such by professional opinion.

nosocomial infection   An infection that develops in a health care setting and that was not present in the client at the time of admission.

nuclear family   Husband, wife, and their children (natural, adopted, or both).

nurse practitioner   An advanced practice nurse prepared to provide a full range of primary health care services.

nursing research   Development of nursing scientific knowledge by conducting research studies to test theory used in nursing practice.

nurturance   Things the environment provides that support health and healing, such as nutritious food, shelter, supplies, and respectful touch; also, the act of providing these things.

nutritive elements   Substances such as vitamins or proteins that, if excessive or deficient, act as an agent of disease.

O

obesity   The condition of being 20% above one's ideal weight.

observational studies   Nonexperimental studies that describe, compare, and explain disease occurrence.

occupational health nursing   Specialty nursing practice that provides health care services to workers and worker populations.

odds ratio   A statistical measure of association reflecting the ratio of two odds reflecting the relative risk (RR) when the specific risk of disease of both the exposed and the unexposed groups is low. Calculated when incidence rates are unavailable.

official international health organizations   Agencies throughout the world that participate in collaborative arrangements via official governmental structure.

open questions   Questions that do not restrict the client's responses but are instead intended to solicit the client's views, opinions, thoughts, and feelings; a means of getting clients to freely disclose information pertinent to their health.

open systems   Those systems, such as human beings, that exist in interrelationship with their environment, taking in and assimilating energy and eliminating waste.

openness/closedness   Extent to which a system permits or screens out input, or new information.

operant conditioning   The concept of seeking to discover what elicits a particular behavior and what subsequently reinforces it.

order   That element of the environment constituting methodical and harmonious arrangement of things.

organic failure to thrive (OFTT)   Lack of adequate growth wherein the infant falls below the 3rd percentile on the growth charts and the cause is a physical condition.

organizational dimension   That aspect of environment related to how time, space, and things are structured.

outcome evaluation   An assessment of change in a client's health status resulting from program implementation and whether this change was the intended result; requires selection of indicators sensitive to the program activities.

outer (or social) aspect of aging   One's relationship with society as one ages.

out-of-pocket expenses   Expenses not covered by a health care plan and, therefore, borne by the person.

output   The result of the system's processing of input.

ovovegan diet   A vegetarian diet that includes eggs but no dairy products.

P

palliative   Serving to alleviate without curing; nursing actions that reduce or lessen pain or other symptoms for terminally ill clients.

Pan American Health Organization (PAHO)   A health organization that focuses its efforts on the Americas; its major functions are to identify public health factors that are related to health and to distribute public health data that include epidemiologic information, information about the health systems within the countries, and various environmental issues.

pandemic   A worldwide outbreak of an epidemic disease.

panhandling   Begging, especially on the streets.

paradigm   A shared worldview, or a way of looking at the nature of things that leads to shared understandings of the way things work.

paradigm shift   Changing perceptions or worldviews by an individual, or perhaps by an entire society, about the nature of reality.

paraphrasing   Putting something that was said in different words to convey that which was heard or understood.

parish nursing   A community health nursing role in which a church or religious group provides services that promote health and facilitate healing to its members; a subspecialty of community health nursing that provides noninvasive health care services to the members of faith congregations.

partner abuse   Physical, emotional, or sexual abuse perpetrated by one partner in an intimate relationship against the other. This term is inclusive of same-sex partners, unmarried heterosexual partners, and unmarried heterosexual men who are abused by female partners.

partnership   The shared participation and agreement between a client and the nurse regarding the mutual identification of needs and resources, development of a plan, decisions regarding division of responsibilities, setting time limits, evaluation, and renegotiation; a relationship between individuals, groups, or organizations wherein the different participants in the relationship work together to achieve shared goals.

pathogenicity   The ability or power of an infectious agent to produce disease.

patriarchy   A male-dominated system in which males hold the majority of power; government rule, or domination, by men.

pattern appraisal   The term used in Rogerian nursing theory to address what is generally called *health assessment*, because organizational patterns of the human–environment interrelationship determine health in this philosophy or conceptual model for nursing practice.

patterns   Family behaviors, beliefs, and values that together make up the uniqueness that is the family; ways of behaving, feeling, believing, choosing, valuing, and perceiving that form a picture of the person–environment interrelationship.

pedagogy   Teacher-directed education.

peer education   Using peers of the target group to provide education in either a one-on-one or a group situation; frequently used with adolescents.

person   One of the concepts of nursing's metaparadigm reflecting wholeness in all dimensions of the human being as well as the inseparable and indivisible nature of the person–environment process.

person–environment interrelationship   The whole of the interpenetrating, inseparable process that makes up the person and environment.

pervasive developmental disorder   A group of conditions characterized by qualitative impairment in the development of reciprocal social interaction and verbal and nonverbal communication skills and in imaginative activity.

philanthropic foundations   Organizations that use funds from private endowments to support health-related projects.

physical agents   Agents of disease that must be present or absent for a problem to occur. Examples include radiation, excessive sun exposure, mechanical agents.

physical dimension   That aspect of environmental structures constituting the physical things we need for survival and safety, such as architecture, cleanliness, air, soil, water, food, and clothing.

physical environment of the family   The dwelling and the conditions both inside and outside.

pica   A craving for nonfood substances.

plumbism   A neurological condition caused by lead poisoning in children and that may be reversed in the early stages of the condition.

point of prevalence   The total number of persons with a disease at a specific point of time.

point-of-service plan   A managed care plan that combines features of both prepaid and fee-for-service insurance; enrollees decide whether to use the providers in the managed care network or nonnetwork providers at the time that care is sought; a sizable co-payment is usually charged for selecting the latter.

Policy   Governmental practice that guides and directs action in all spheres of social interaction such as national defense policy, environmental policy, economic policy, and health care policy.

policy development   Provision of leadership in developing comprehensive public health policies, including the use of scientific knowledge in decision making about policy.

policy framework   The policies in place that determine how the organizational framework is structured to meet the needs of society and individuals within that society.

political action/political activism   Activities and/or strategies involved in influencing the political process.

politics   A process by which one influences the decisions of others and exerts control over situations and events.

population   A statistical aggregate of separate individuals with similar or the same characteristics.

population approach (population-focused care)   An element of health promotion whereby focus is on communities or aggregates.

population density   The number of persons per square kilometers or square miles of land area; computed by dividing the total population of a geographic unit (e.g., a county) by its land area.

population-focused practice   Health care approach based on the notion that understanding the population's health is critical; focus is on diagnosing the population's health needs and assets and formulating interventions at the population level.

power Actual or potential ability of individual family members to change the behavior of other family members; also called *influence* and *dominance*; control or command over others; the ability to do or act; achievement of the desired result.

power bases Sources from which a family's power is derived.

power outcomes The final decision made, including who ultimately has control of the situation.

power processes Processes used in arriving at family decisions; also called *decision-making processes*.

power resources A person's physical, psychological, and social strengths.

powerlessness A sense of lack of control over the outcomes of one's life.

PRECEDE-PROCEED model A health–promotion planning framework useful in applying the epidemiologic approach to community health planning.

pre-existing condition A health problem that was diagnosed or treated before an insurance policy was issued.

preferred provider organization (PPO) A managed care health plan that contracts with networks or panels of providers to furnish services; providers are paid on a negotiated fee schedule. Unlike HMOs, PPOs do not provide the services themselves. Enrollees are offered a financial incentive to use providers on the preferred list, but they may use nonnetwork providers as well.

pregnancy-induced hypertension (PIH) Formerly known as toxemia; a condition of pregnancy that may cause physical harm to the mother and the fetus; characterized by hypertension, proteinuria, and edema; common among adolescents.

pregnancy outcome Health status of mother and infant at birth.

prenatal diagnosis Examination of the fetus by fetoscopy, amniocentesis, chorionic villus biopsy, ultrasound, or x-ray to detect abnormality.

prenatal risk assessment An assessment of a pregnant female for factors that may affect pregnancy outcome.

presbycusis Loss of hearing associated with aging.

presbyopia Farsightedness resulting from age-related changes in the elasticity of the lens of the eye.

prevalence The number of existing cases of a health outcome in a specified population at a designated place and time.

prevalence rate A proportion or percentage of a disease or condition in a population at any given time.

prevention Activities designed to intervene in the course of a disease or health-related conditions before pathology occurs (primary prevention); to detect and treat a disease early (secondary prevention); and to limit a disability or associated conditions (tertiary prevention).

prevention trials An epidemiologic intervention study design used to compare measures or interventions aimed at the prevention of disease.

primary care The term used in the United States to address entry into the health care delivery system, such as the physician who serves as the primary care provider.

primary health care A model for health care that emphasizes equity, accessibility (close to home), full participation by communities, acceptable and affordable technology, intersectoral collaboration, and care that is health promotive and disease preventive; based on practical, scientifically sound and socially acceptable methods and technology made universally accessible to individuals and families in the community and at a level the country can afford to maintain at every stage of development in the spirit of self-reliance and self-determination (World Health Organization, 1978, p. 3). The activities deemed necessary to meet the Health for All 2000 objectives.

primary prevention Activities designed to promote health and prevent disease processes or injuries.

principlism System of theory and practice whereby ethical decisions in health care are made exclusively via the formal application of ethical principles.

private organizations Privately owned organizations that provide financial and technical assistance for health care, employment, and access.

private voluntary organizations Organizations that provide different health care assistance programs; may be either religious or secular groups.

process-oriented groups Those groups that focus on relating and getting along with people.

process program evaluation An assessment of how well program activities are carried out; an account of that which actually happened or is happening in the program; involves interpretation of program outcomes in relation to process evaluation.

program A service designed to produce particular results.

program evaluation The process of inquiry to assess the performance of a program, to determine whether a service is needed, likely to be used, and actually assists clients.

program implementation The process of putting into action the program plan.

program planning The process of identifying the situation, deciding on a more desirable situation, and designing actions to create the desirable situation.

programming Processes that when carried out together produce a program and the desired results; involves assessment, planning, implementation, evaluation, and sequential and iterative work.

programming models Representations of approaches to programming that offer explanations of the processes involved and, therefore, guide the programmer.

project team Group of people who conduct a community assessment; responsible for development of a research plan and time frame and for collection and analysis of information already available.

prospective cost reimbursement A method of paying all health care providers in which rates are established in advance.

prospective study An epidemiologic study design that assembles study groups before disease occurrence.

pseudomutuality Long-term dysfunctional adaptive strategy that maintains family homeostasis at the expense of meeting the family's affective function.

psychoanalysis A treatment technique that uses free association and the interpretation of dreams to trace emotions and behaviors to repressed drives and instincts. By being made aware of the existence, origins, and inappropriate expression of these unconscious processes, the client's can eliminate or diminish the undesirable effects; a theory of psychology and a system of psychotherapy, developed by Freud.

psychological environment Developmental stages, family dynamics, and emotional strengths.

psychoneuroimmunology Study of the communication and interactions among the psyche, the nervous system, the immune system, the endocrine system, and other body systems via informational substances such as neuropeptides, hormones, and neurotransmitters.

psychotherapy The process of addressing symptom relief, resolution of problems, or personal growth through interacting in a prescribed way with a therapist.

public health Organized community efforts designed to protect health, promote health, and prevent disease.

public health nursing The field of nursing that synthesizes the public health, social, and nursing sciences to promote and protect the health of individuals, families, and communities.

public policy The decisions made by the government about how things should be done in order to best serve the people.

public speaking Using spoken words to communicate with many individuals at a time; community nurses often use this tool to teach or to exert influence in policy making.

Q

qualitative Data that consist of words and/or observations.

quantitative Data that is based on numbers.

quantum mechanics That branch of physics concerned with the energetic characteristics of matter at the subatomic level.

R

race Term applying to biological characteristics, such as skin color and bone structure, that are genetically transmitted from one generation to another.

rape Sexual contact occurring without the victim's consent, involving the use or threat of force, and involving sexual penetration of the victim's vagina, mouth, or rectum.

rapport A close, harmonious relationship between or among human beings.

rationing Limits placed on health care; including implicit rationing, which limits the capacity of the system and uses consumer triaging as a method of determining who will be served, and explicit rationing, whereby price and ability to pay are used to control costs.

reference group A group of others undergoing role transition.

regulatory finance controls Cost controls restricting the amount of state and federal tax revenues deposited into programs that fund health care programs such as Medicare and Medicaid.

rehabilitation A restoration to a former state of functioning or a limiting of impairment and disability to the lowest possible level.

reimbursement Flow of dollars from the insurance company to providers or hospitals.

reimbursement controls Cost-control strategies including price and utilization controls and patient cost sharing.

relationships In community nursing care, the connections among the client, significant others, and professionals that affect client health.

relative risk An epidemiologic measure of association that indicates the likelihood that an exposed group will develop a disease or condition relative to those not exposed.

religions A specific belief system regarding divine and superhuman power and involving a code of ethics and philosophical

assumptions that lead to certain rituals, worship, and conduct by believers.

repetitive motion injuries Injuries that occur over time (and usually on the job) as a result of repetitively performing the same motion.

reproductive function Ensures the continuity of both the family and society.

reservoir Any host or environment where an infectious agent normally lives and multiplies.

residual stimuli In Roy's theory, factors that may affect behavior but for which the effects are not validated.

Resiliency Model of Family Stress, Adjustment, and Adaptation Emphasizes family adaptation and includes family types and levels of vulnerability.

resonancy In the Rogerian theory of person–environment relationship, a continuous change of human and environmental energy wave patterns from lower to higher frequency; continuous evolution.

respect Trust that a person is capable of and has potential for learning and healing and can benefit from a caring environment.

retrospective cost reimbursement A reimbursement system that has no preestablished reimbursement rates; commonly referred to as the fee-for-service system.

retrospective study An epidemiologic study design that assembles study groups after disease occurrence.

risk The probability that an event, outcome, disease, or condition will develop in a specified time period.

risk factors Precursors to disease that increase one's risk of the disease (e.g., demographic variables, certain health practices, family history of disease, and certain physiological changes).

role A position in a social structure; a set of expectations associated with a position in a social structure; a set of behaviors associated with a position.

role accountability Pertaining to the procedures for ensuring that functions are fulfilled in the family.

role allocation Family's pattern in assigning roles.

role ambiguity Vague, ill-defined, or unclear role demands.

role clarification Mastering and incorporating new knowledge and role expectations.

role complementarity Mutual agreement about a role or modification of a role.

role conflict Result of contradictory or incompatible role expectations regarding one's role.

role enactment That which a person actually does in a particular role position.

role flexibility Openness of family to shifts in role behavior to maintain family equilibrium.

role incompetence Subjective feelings that may result when one's resources are inadequate to meet the demands of a role.

role incongruity Result of role expectations' not being in agreement with self-perception, disposition, attitudes, and values.

role modeling The process of enacting a role that others can observe and emulate.

role overload Having insufficient time to carry out all expected role functions.

role overqualification Situation resulting when one's resources are in excess of those necessary for the job.

role performance Achievement in a particular role position in response to role expectations.

role rehearsal The internal preparation and overt practice of new role behaviors.

role socialization The process by which persons acquire knowledge, skills, and dispositions that enable them to fulfill assigned roles.

role strain Result of role stress and reflected in feelings of frustration and tension.

role stress Result of difficult, conflicting, or impossible demands being placed on a family member.

role taking Change in overt behavior and inner definition of self resulting in new roles' being both internally and externally validated.

role transition A process of learning new role behaviors, reviewing previously learned material, and mediating conflicts between different role expectations.

rules Characteristic relationship patterns within which a system operates; express the values of the system and the roles appropriate to behavior within the system; distinguish the system from other systems and, therefore, from the system boundaries; explicit or implicit regulations regarding what is acceptable or unacceptable to which the family is expected to adhere.

rural area An area with fewer than 2,500 residents and open territories.

rural health clinics Clinics that are certified under federal law to provide care in underserved areas within sparsely populated areas.

rural nursing The practice of professional nursing within the physical and sociocultural context of sparsely populated communities that involves continual interaction of the rural environment, the nurse, and the nurse's practice.

S

safety That component of environment that protects and keeps a person secure, unharmed, and free from danger.

safety energy locks In Jin Shin Jyutsu, those points along the energy pathways that are held by the practitioner to open up and balance the energy flow.

sandwich generation Middle adults on whom demands are placed by adolescent and young adult offspring as well as aging parents.

scapegoating Avoidance of threatening issues by blaming a family member rather than dealing with the issues. One member of the family is "chosen" to be negatively labeled and stigmatized while the rest of the family achieves unity and cohesiveness.

school nursing A branch of community health nursing that seeks to identify or prevent school health problems and intervene to remedy or reduce these problems.

scope of practice The customary practice of a profession, taking into account the ways whereby legislation defines the practice of the profession within a particular area (local, state, or national).

seamless care The term used to describe an integrated health care delivery system in which a client may move or be moved from one part of the system to another in a way that is most effective and efficient for health and healing.

seasonal farm worker A person employed in agricultural work of a seasonal or temporary nature who is not required to be absent overnight from his or her permanent place of residence.

secondary prevention Actions taken for the purpose of detecting disease in the early stages before there are clinically evident signs and symptoms present; early diagnosis and treatment.

secondhand smoke Tobacco smoke inhaled indirectly, from the environment; exposure determined by cotinine (the chemical metabolized by the body from nicotine) blood levels.

second-order change Change that occurs in times of stress or crisis and involves an adjustment in established family patterns.

sedative A depressant drug that produces soothing or relaxing effects at lower doses and induces sleep at higher doses.

self-care An individual's acts and decisions to sustain life, health, well-being, and safety in the environment; personal health care performed by the client, often in collaboration with health care providers.

self-determination The right and responsibility of one to decide and direct one's choices.

self-efficacy The power to produce effects and intended results on one's own health and in one's own life.

self-esteem Feelings about oneself and how one measures up to that which one expects. People with high self-esteem see themselves as measuring up to their expectations for themselves; conversely, people with low self-esteem recognize a great disparity between who they actually are and their expectations of who they should be.

sensitivity The probability that an individual who has the disease of interest will have a positive screening test result.

separatist family style A family acculturative style in which the family does not feel comfortable assimilating and actively opposes doing so.

sheltered employment A work center where supports are available and individual productivity may be set at noncompetitive levels.

shelters Facilities established to assist homeless people. Services offered vary from those that simply provide a place to get in out of the weather to those that offer a wide range of services. Some are specialized to deal with specific populations such as runaway youth and battered women.

Sigma Theta Tau International International honor society of nursing whose purpose is to promote excellence in nursing education, practice, and research.

small-group communication The verbal and nonverbal communication that occurs among a small number of persons who are somewhat independent of one another.

small-group residence A facility licensed to provide housing, food, and programs to no more than 15 clients.

social dimension The aspect or dimension of environment provided by that aspect comprising social relationships, connection, and support.

social environment Religion, race, culture, social class, economic status, and external resources such as school, church, and health resources.

social justice The entitlement of all persons to basic necessities, such as adequate income and health protection, and the acceptance of collective action and obligation to make such possible.

social support   A perceived sense of support from a complex network of interpersonal ties and from backup support systems for nurturance.

social systems   Those systems that involve groups of different sizes and populations and their organizational processes and patterns of energy. Communication within and among these systems is a significant aspect of community nursing, and the nurse with communication skills applicable to a variety of social systems can be influential in the community.

socialization   Lifelong process of assuming the norms and values for the many family roles that are required of family members.

soup kitchen   A place where food is offered either free or at greatly reduced price to individuals in need.

specificity   The probability that an individual who does not have the disease of interest will have a negative screening test result.

spirit   The spark of the divine within each person that gives meaning and direction to life.

spiritual assessment   The collection, verification, and organization of data regarding the client's beliefs and feelings about such things as the meaning of life, love, hope, forgiveness, and life after death, as well as the client's degree of connectedness to self, others, and a larger purpose in life. Spirituality refers to a sense of oneness with all of creation and of humanity and to the search for and discovery of life meaning and purpose.

spirituality   The human belief system pertaining to humankind's innermost concerns and values, ultimatley affecting behavior, relationship to the world, and relationship to God. (Stuart, Deckro, & Mandle, 1989)

sponsor   An individual or group who conceives of and may draft a bill to be presented in the legislature by a legislator.

spousal abuse   Physical, emotional, or sexual abuse perpetrated by either a husband or a wife against the marriage partner; marital rape.

staff model HMO   Physicians providing care are generally salaried by the HMO and usually limit their practices to subscribers of the HMO; typically, the hospitals are also owned or otherwise affiliated with the HMO, but some services may be contracted to selected hospitals and providers.

steering committee   Group of people from outside the project team who oversee the project, providing outside advice and ensuring that the project achieves its goals.

stigma   The disgrace or reproach experienced by mentally ill people and their families. In general it can be assigned to anyone who is perceived by others to be in a discredited position.

story telling   The sharing of stories between people, sometimes from one's life and sometimes in the form of parables, myths, and metaphors. Life meanings change as stories are shared in different life contexts.

stress   Both a response and a stimulus as well as the interaction of person and environment; the response to stress is a critical determinant in health and illness.

stress response   The nonspecific response of the body to any demand, which Selye called the general adaptation response.

stressors   Environmental pressures that trigger the stress response.

structural-functional framework   Framework focusing on interaction of the family and its internal-external environment; deemphasizes the importance of growth, change, and disequilibrium of a family over time.

structure building   The period of development in young adulthood when the person fashions a lifestyle.

subenvironments   An idea similar to dimensions of environment; used for the sake of analysis and assessment of environments.

substance substitution   Non-nutritious foods such as sugar, caffeine, and nicotine or excessive food taken to replace alcohol.

substituted judgment   A proxy decision for another based on an understanding of what the other would decide were that person able to decide on his or her own behalf.

subsystems   The smaller units or systems of which a larger unit or system consists.

summative program evaluation   The retrospective assessment of how well a program performed up to the point of evaluation; a method used to assess program outcomes.

summative reflection   A statement on the part of the nurse that sums up a conversation so that both nurse and client understand those things that have been accomplished so far and those things that remain to be done, clarifying and bringing closure to an interaction.

superego   One of Freud's three main theoretical elements (with id and ego) of the mental mechanism; the part of the personality structure associated with ethics, standards, and self-criticism, formed by identification with important persons, especially parents, early in life.

Superfund site   A hazardous waste site designated by the U. S. Environmental Protection Agency as being a threat to human health.

supply   A seller's willingness to supply a particular product or service at a cost.

supported employment   A job coach or other support ensures success at a competitive job.

suprasystem   The larger system of which smaller systems are a part.

surrogate mother   A woman who, for someone other than herself, carries a child conceived from an egg not necessarily her own.

surveillance   The systematic collection and evaluation of all aspects of disease occurrence and spread, resulting in information that may be useful in the control of the disease.

system   A goal-directed unit made up of interdependent, interacting parts that endure over a period of time. According to Rogers, the parts are interpenetrating processes within the larger system throughout the whole.

T

teaching   Helping another gain knowledge, understanding, and/or skills by instructing, demonstrating, or guiding the learning process in some way.

teaching/learning process   The teacher–learner interaction wherein each participant communicates information, emotions, perceptions, and attitudes to the other.

teaching strategies   Specific actions taken by the teacher to strengthen teaching, provide focus, and encourage client involvement.

technology-assisted   Dependent upon a device that substitutes for a body function.

telemedicine   The practice of health care delivery, diagnosis, consultation, treatment, transfer of data, and education through interactive audio, video, or data communications technology.

teleology   The ethical theory that determines rightness or wrongness solely on the basis of an estimate of the probable outcome; a theory of purpose, ends, goals, or final causes.

teratogenic effects   The disruption of normal fetal development by an agent such as a drug or substance, affecting the genetic structure of the fetus and causing malformations.

termination phase   The third phase of the home visit; the nurse summarizes accomplishments, discusses plans for the next visit, discusses referrals, and prepares documentation for the visit as prescribed by the agency for which the nurse is working.

tertiary prevention   The treatment, care, and rehabilitation of people who have acquired acute or chronic disease, with the goal of limiting disability and minimizing the extent and severity of health problems.

testimony   Communicating to a committee or the legislature evidence in support of a fact, statement, or bill.

theory-based nursing practice   Nursing practice using the conceptual models and theories of the nurse theorists that define nursing in terms of the nursing metaparadigm: health, person, environment, and nursing.

therapeutic communication   Communication that helps the client cope with stress, get along with other people, adapt to situations that cannot be changed, and overcome emotional and mental blocks that prevent evolution of one's potential as a human being.

therapeutic interview   Discussion with one skilled in listening that focuses on exploring relationship and feeling issues, relieving emotional tension, and gaining insight.

Therapeutic Touch (TT)   A holistic therapy whereby there is a consciously directed manipulation of energy; the practitioner uses the hands to facilitate the healing process.

therapeutic trials   An epidemiologic intervention study design used to compare measures or interventions aimed at therapeutic benefits.

third-party payor   Entity other than the provider or consumer that is responsible for total or partial payment of health care costs.

touch therapy   One of multiple energy-releasing and balancing modalities that use the hands to promote health and facilitate healing in the receiver or client.

toxicology   The science or study of poisons.

traditional family   Usually children, a legal marriage, blood kinship bonds, and a lifestyle that has its genesis in the family.

traditional-oriented nonresistive style   A family acculturative style that is composed of first-generation parents and children who are traditionally oriented and have had little exposure to the host country.

transactional field theory   Theory that views the individual in the context of his or her transactional field, which is composed of all aspects of that individual's life.

transactions   Interactions between the client and persons in relationship with the client that affect health in some way.

transcultural   A situation in which there is more than one cultural belief system at work; in nursing, there is often a difference in belief systems between the nurse and the client.

transcultural nursing   A client–nurse relationship wherein the parties are from different cultures; the nurse works within the cultural framework of the client as well as within the health care system of which the nurse is a part.

transition   A period of approximately five years within the developmental era designed by Levinson to explain developmental stages.

triangling   Reduction of tension in a dyadic relationship by introducing a third member who absorbs and diffuses the ongoing tension in the relationship.

U

uncertainty   The inability to make meaning of or predict life events.

unemployment rate   The number of people not working as a percentage of the civilian labor force age 16 years or older.

unicultural   A situation in which all parties share the same cultural beliefs, values, and health care practices.

unintentional injury   Accidental injury, a major health problem for children and the leading cause of death and disability in children under the age of 14.

United Nations Children's Fund (UNICEF)   International organization that was originally formed to assist the children who lived in European war countries but currently has a worldwide focus.

universality   The commonalities of all human beings; the aspects we recognize that unite the species.

upstream thinking   Identifying and modifying those economic, political, and environmental variables that are contributing factors to poor health worldwide.

urban   An area that includes all territory, population, and housing units in an urban area and in places of 2,500 or more persons outside urban areas.

urban area (UA)   An area that includes a central city and a surrounding densely settled territory that together have a minimum population of 50,000 persons.

usual and customary reimbursement   Arrangement whereby the provider agrees to accept a predetermined level of reimbursement for service.

utilitarianism   The ethical theory used to determine whether actions are wrong or right depending on their outcomes, the utility of an action being based on whether that action brings about a greater number of good consequences as opposed to evil consequences and, by extension, greater good than evil in the world as a whole; one type of teleology.

utilization controls   Cost-control strategy aimed at the supply side of the health care market, whereby a provider is evaluated against other providers who supply similar services so as to determine cost of care in relation to quality and outcomes.

utilization review (UR)   The review of services delivered by a health care provider or supplier to determine whether the services are medically necessary; may be performed on a concurrent or retrospective basis.

V

validation   An aspect of mutual problem solving; asking for input from the client regarding thoughts and feelings at each step and phase of the nursing process.

values   Beliefs held by a person.

vector   An agent that actively carries a germ to a susceptible host.

vegans Vegetarians who eat no meat, eggs, or dairy products.

vegetarian diet A diet composed of only grains, fruits, and vegetables and no meat; variations may include or not include eating fish, dairy products, and/or eggs.

veracity The principle of truth telling; the duty to tell the truth.

vertical transmission Disease or antibody transfer from mother to child.

very low birth weight Neonate weight of 1,500 grams or less.

veto Power of a chief executive to reject bills passed by the legislature.

violence against women A broad term encompassing physical violence, rape, homicide, genital mutilation, denial of rights because of gender, and female infanticide.

virulence An agent's degree of pathogenicity, or ability to invade and harm the host.

visualization In the imagery process, the use of visual pictures in the mind as opposed to hearing, smell, touch, taste, and movement.

vital statistics Systematically tabulated data on vital events such as births, deaths, marriages, divorces, adoptions, annulments, separations, and health events that are based on registration of these events.

voice box In interpreting, the interaction style wherein the interpreter attempts to translate word for word.

vulnerable families Families in which physical and emotional resources are so insufficient that critical tasks and family functions are threatened.

W

warmth Conveying to others that you like to be with them and that you accept them as they are; extending warmth enhances closeness and makes the nurse more approachable from the perspective of both clients and colleagues.

wellness Moving toward the fulfillment of one's potential as a human being; physically, emotionally, mentally, and spiritually; a dynamic state of health wherein individuals, families, and population groups progress to a higher level of functioning.

wider family Relationships that emerge from lifestyle and are voluntary and independent of necessary biological or kin connections; participants may or may not share a common dwelling.

wife abuse Physical, emotional, or sexual abuse perpetrated by a husband against his wife.

windshield survey Observation of a community while driving a car or riding public transportation in order to collect data for a community assessment.

win–lose approach A destructive form of conflict resolution whereby without regard for the concerns and wishes of the other person, one person gets what he or she wants by "bulldozing" the other person; an aggressive and nonresponsible approach.

win–win approach A constructive form of conflict resolution whereby, via assertiveness and responsibility, both parties gain something and are happy with the outcome.

Z

zoonosis An infection that can be transmitted from animals to humans.

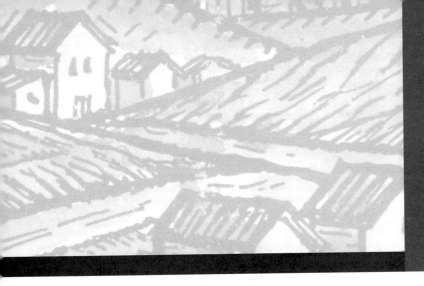

INDEX

Note: Page numbers in *italics* indicate illustrations; page numbers followed by "t" indicate tables; page numbers followed by "b" indicate boxed material.